IMMUNOLOGY

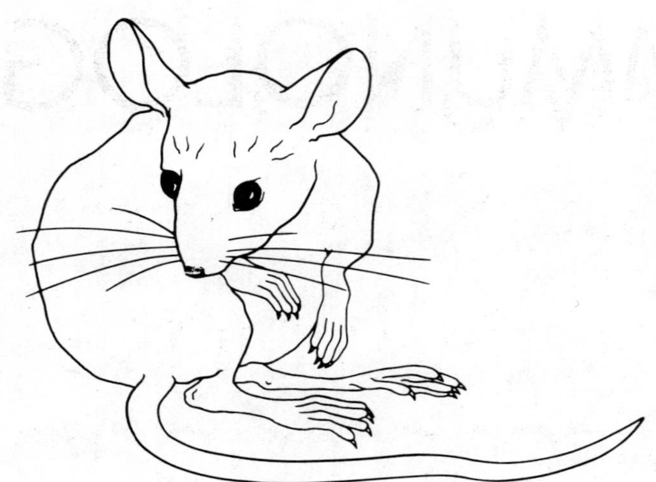

IMMUNOLOGY
The Science of Self–Nonself Discrimination

Jan Klein
Abteilung Immungenetik
Max-Planck-Institut für Biologie
Tübingen, Federal Republic of Germany

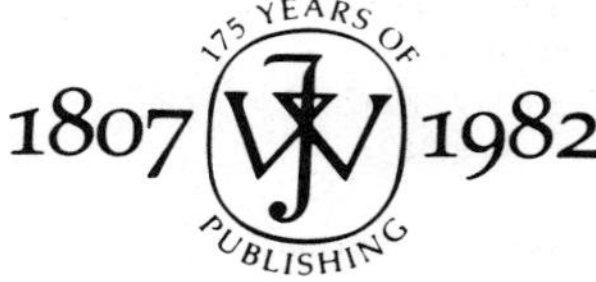

A Wiley-Interscience Publication
JOHN WILEY & SONS
New York · Chichester · Brisbane · Toronto · Singapore

Library of Congress Cataloging in Publication Data:

Klein, Jan, 1936–
Immunology: the science of self-nonself discrimination.
"A Wiley-Interscience publication."
Includes index.
1. Immunology. I. Title. [DNLM: 1. Allergy and immunology. QW 504 K54i]
QR181.K53 591.2'9 82-2632
ISBN 0-471-05124-1 AACR2

Printed in the United States of America

10 9 8 7 6 5 4 3 2 1

To

DAGMAR

NORMAN

DANIEL

and

PAVEL

PREFACE

Before you begin—a few answers to questions you might not have thought to ask.

Why did I write this book?

I have a confession to make: when I started to work on the book, I knew little immunology. I knew something about one branch—the one I am actively involved in—but next to nothing about the rest. Every time the new issue of the *Journal of Immunology* arrived, I paged through it and immediately became depressed at how little I understood. At conferences I was greatly impressed by the speakers because I could not comprehend most of what they were talking about. When teaching a course on my specialty, I was constantly afraid that students would ask questions outside my area of expertise and I would not be able to answer them. Finally, I decided to do something about my appalling lack of knowledge: I decided to write a textbook of immunology. So, in contrast to most authors—who undoubtedly write textbooks for the very noble goal of educating their students, I wrote this book for the very egotistical reason of educating myself.

For whom did I write the book?

Having answered the question of *why* I wrote it, I need not answer for *whom* the book is intended: why, obviously, for me—and for anyone who is in a situation similar to the one I was in three years ago when I started. It is for students of any specialty who, for some reason or other, know nothing and are required to learn everything about immunology; for biologists who have just discovered immunology and find it fascinating, but do not know where to begin to learn more about this discipline; for physicians who are interested in the body's defense not just because it bears on this or that disease, but because it is a remarkable biological phenomenon. And it is perhaps even for fellow immunologists who, from time to time, feel they need an overview of their field.

How is the book organized?

Before starting to write my own version of immunology, I looked up the textbooks already available (there are, in fact, quite a few) to get an idea of how others have treated the subject. But with the characteristic arrogance of the beginner, I decided to do it differently. I thought that immunology was more than a pastiche science, a collage of drawings and photos clipped from different sources. I came to the conclusion that, if immunology were to be considered an independent scientific discipline, it should have its own internal structure and its own logic. So I decided to abandon the traditional division of the textbook, with sections on immunochemistry, immunobiology, immunopathology, immunogenetics, and so on, and I tried instead to find a more natural organization.

I thought that a more logical approach would be to first define the subject of study, then describe the physical scaffolding on which immunological reactions take place, then describe these reactions themselves, and finally discuss how the reactions fulfill their functions on the battlefields of the body. So I divided the book into four parts, as a composer divides a symphony into four movements.

Part One serves as an introduction to the subject—explaining what immunology encompasses, giving a view of why and how immunological processes might have originated and evolved, and ending with a brief history of immunology. The historical sketch is written to serve as an introduction to the individual topics covered in the text.

Part Two is the slow movement of the symphony. It is organized like a series of Chinese boxes—the largest box containing a smaller box, which contains a still smaller box, and so on. I start with the organism, move to the immunologically important organs and tissues, then to cells, and finally to molecules. Each "box" is viewed in a broad biological perspective: I not only describe the organ, cell, or molecule, but also discuss its possible evolutionary origin, its ontogenic origin, and its pathology.

Part Three, the symphony's *scherzo*, describes what the major triad of immunology—macrophages, T lymphocytes, and B lymphocytes—does: what kinds of reaction the cells are involved in, how an immunologist learns about these reactions, how the cells interact, and what the natural function of the cells involved in immunological processes could be.

Part Four is the synthetic movement of the symphony. It uses all the knowledge accumulated in the first three parts to describe how the body—in particular, the mammalian body—may defend itself from various external and internal insults. The book ends with my own evaluation of the current situation in immunological sciences.

What is the best way to use this book?

I realize that not everyone will want to read this textbook from cover to cover, although, if one wants an overview of what is known about bodily defense, one should do just that. For those who will read only parts of the book, I have tried to make the individual chapters as self-contained as possible; this has led, in spots, to a certain repetitiousness of the text, which I hope will not bother the reader of the entire book. Frequent cross-references should help the reader select those sections that interest him or her or that contain detailed information about matters that he does not fully understand in the context of a particular chapter. Cross-references are also given for terms that had to be used before they could be explained in detail (for instance, I had to use the term "antibody" before I could devote a whole chapter to it). Many of the basic terms are introduced and explained in the chapter that deals with the history of immunology. A beginner should not skip this chapter.

I know that students—and sometimes their teachers too—often use words the precise meanings of which have never been explained to them. I have therefore included brief definitions and etymological derivations of terms when they are used for the first time, because knowing the origin of a word often helps one remember what the word actually means.

To understand immunology, one must know the basics of biology, medicine, histology, cytology, genetics, virology, pathology, cell biology, and biochemistry. A reader who knows all these disciplines should read only the chapters and ignore the appendices. But anyone who has forgotten most of what was learned in biochemistry class, or who could use a refresher in the principles of genetics should first read the appropriate appendix, and *then* the chapter. The appendices summarize the most fundamental knowledge necessary for understanding the corresponding chapters. They should save the reader the trouble of consulting many other books to understand this one.

Modern scientific texts often look like Swiss cheese, they are so riddled with references. Authors often feel they must fortify every statement they make by referring to a work from which the statement follows. Such texts are difficult to read because the constant mention of names, dates, and numbers disrupts the train of thought. I have eliminated reference citations from the text altogether and moved them to the ends of the chapters, where they are grouped under two headings. *General* references are books or reviews that cover a given topic in greater detail than my chapter does and that also contain many additional references to original works. *Original Articles* refers to the work of the authors who are mentioned by name in the text. These represent the "classics" of immunology, from its scientific beginnings to the present day. Anyone who intends to make immunology his or her profession should take the time to read these works, even those published in the nineteenth century. It is a worthwhile investment; one gets a completely different perspective on the discipline by systematically sifting through its milestone works.

Why so many references to works of art?

The percolation of arts into this science textbook is not an affected pose. It is an expression of a belief—which I share with Aldous Huxley—that "art and literature and science are one."

It is also a gentle reminder to those who confront immunology all too intensely that there are things to enjoy beyond the laboratory. And it is an expression of the view that even so specialized a discipline as immunology has its connections to even the most seemingly unrelated parts of the overall system of human endeavor.

To whom is credit due?

To many—only some of whom can be mentioned here. To Drs. Max D. Cooper, William C. Davis, Thomas J. Gill III, Berenice Kinddred, Zoltan Nagy, Heinz Schwarz, Günther Vogel, Edward K. Wakeland, and Paul Singer, who read portions of this manuscript and made invaluable suggestions. To Drs. Peter Andrews, N. Michael Green, David E. Harrison, Catherine Neauport-Sautes, John J. Owen, Fred S. Rosen, and S. John Singer, who supplied some of the photographs reproduced here. To Dr. Marika Pla for helping me to find many of the references. To Rosemary Franklin, who, with dedication and patience, transcribed hundreds of yards of tape and typed, edited, and otherwise helped out whenever asked. To Elizabeth Davis and Korina Bartels, who typed page after page of what must have looked to them like a Sanskrit text. To Pamela Erbe, who, with a skill I admire, put the final touches on the manuscript. To the illustrators, Ladina Ribi, Klaus Lamberty, and Erich Freiberg; it was a continual joy for me to see my primitive sketches transformed into beautiful drawings. To Eva Illgen, who prepared most of the photographic material used in this book. To Lynne Yakes, who kept the *Abteilung* running smoothly and so freed me from many worries. To all who have permitted me to reproduce published or unpublished material. To Josef Haydn for his 104 symphonies, which made drafting of illustrations an enjoyable task. And finally, to my wife and children, who resigned themselves to seeing their husband and father only occasionally.

How does it feel to live with a book for three years?

There were long moments during the writing when I thought I knew how Lindbergh must have felt halfway across the Atlantic Ocean: masses of water behind him and masses of water before him. And the doubt: will I last? will the engine last? The "loneliness of the long-distance runner." Writing a book about it is a good way to learn immunology, but I cannot recommend it to anyone as a pleasant way to pass the afternoons.

JAN KLEIN

Tübingen, Federal Republic of Germany
July 1982

CONTENTS

THE FIRST MOVEMENT
Initiation

CHAPTER 1

IMMUNOLOGY: WHAT IS IT ALL ABOUT?

1.1 FOUR THREATS TO INDIVIDUALITY

An organism is a miracle of harmony. Its individual parts—organs, tissues, cells, and subcellular organelles—have divided among themselves the functions necessary for the sustenance of life and interact with one another in a complex but precisely defined manner. However, this delicate system of interactions can easily be disturbed by any agent that endangers the body's integrity. The four main threats to an organism's integrity are these.

Fusion of Individuals. In a jungle or at the bottom of the sea, organisms—especially plants, but also all kinds of sessile animals—are often in such close proximity that they are in constant danger of losing their individuality by fusion. Ridiculous? Not at all, since we know, for example, that two mice, when joined surgically side-to-side, unite their bodies into a single *parabiont* that can live for many months. And even in the human, partial fusion of embryos sometimes occurs naturally, resulting in Siamese twins that can often lead paranormal lives. At the cellular level, experimental fusion has been accomplished between cells of widely different species, such as mouse and human, and many monstrous, interspecific hybrid cell lines grow in laboratories all over the world. So the *potential* for fusion of individuals exists in all phyla of the animal and plant kingdoms. But only in the imagination of an artist (Fig. 1.1) does an all-out fusion occur; in reality, organisms keep pretty much separate, no matter how near to one another they live and grow.

Organ and Tissue Damage. A thorn stuck in the body (Fig. 1.2), an extremity lost during a fight, an abrasion after a fall, a tissue succumbing to an attack by bacteria—any of these can be a source of harmful substances that may endanger the integrity and welfare of an individual.

Parasitism. A parasite is an organism that lives on another organism and depends on it for nourishment. Parasitism exists in all phyla, and every species is host to numerous parasites. The harm they cause ranges from hardly noticeable effects to partial or complete destruction of the host. Disease-causing parasites, particularly those of microscopic size (*microorganisms*), are referred to as *pathogenic organisms* or *pathogens* (Gr. *pathos*, disease, *-gen*, to produce), and the ability of a parasite to cause disease is termed *pathogenicity*. Invasion of host tissues by pathogens is known as *infection* and diseases communicable from host to host as

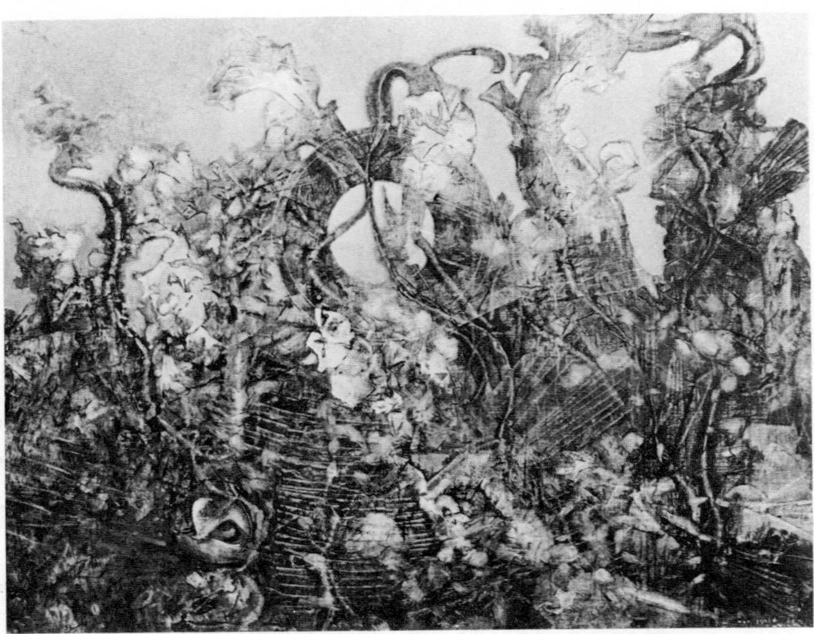

Figure 1.1. The first threat to the body's integrity. In Max Ernst's vision of *The Last Forest*, living matter is a fused continuum. In the real world as well, organisms are in constant danger of losing their individuality through fusion of their bodies.

infectious diseases. Frequently, infectious diseases affect many individuals, causing an *epidemic* (Gr. *epi-*, upon, *demos*, the people), which may wipe out populations and sometimes even endanger an entire species' existence. Luckily, our generation knows about the horrors of past epidemics primarily from such safely distant sources as the paintings of Pieter Breughel the Elder and Hieronymus Bosch (Fig. 1.3), and from such vivid verbal descriptions as those of Alessandro Manzoni and Albert Camus.

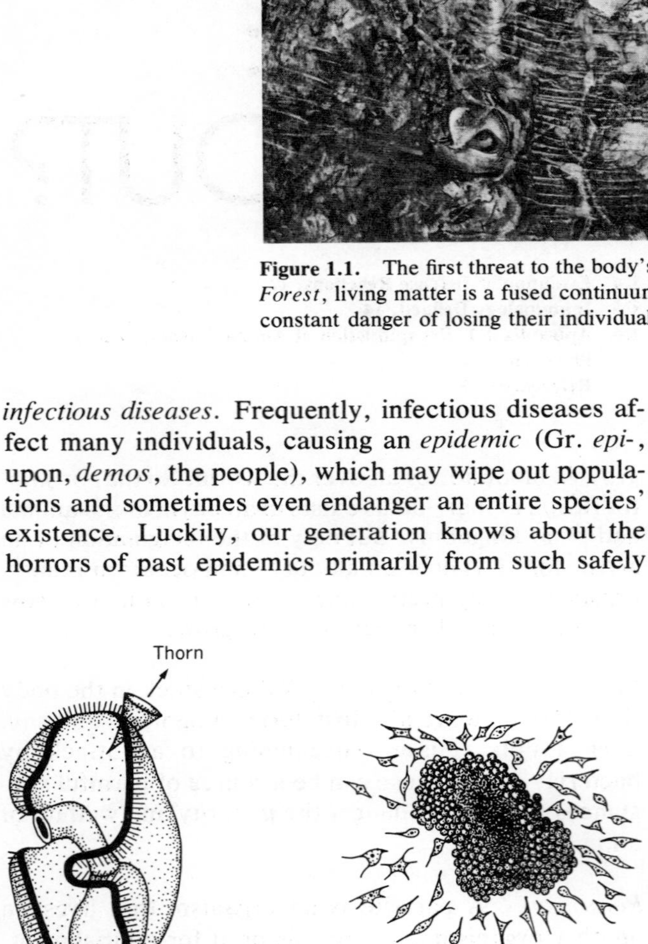

Thorn

(a) (b)

Figure 1.2. The second threat to the body's integrity. A rose thorn in a bipinnaria. In a famous experiment, the Russian immunologist Elie Metchnikoff stuck a splinter into a starfish larva (*a*). The next day the foreign body was surrounded by macrophages (*b*). Metchnikoff concluded that the body defends itself against foreign particles that threaten its integrity by mobilizing cells of a special type, which attempt to eliminate the foreign matter. (Note: none of the figures in this text has been drawn to proportion.)

Neoplasia. A multicellular organism results from a number of cell divisions, each division being preceded by a duplication of genetic material. During this duplication, copying errors may occur and a variant (mutant) cell may be produced. Sometimes the appearance of such cells may be stimulated by factors such as viruses or certain chemical substances. Some of the mutant cells may escape the normal regulatory mechanisms and begin to divide in an uncontrolled manner, developing into *neoplasms* (Gr. *neos*, new, *plasma*, thing formed) or *tumors* (Fig. 1.4), which may cripple or kill the host.

1.2 DEFENSE OF INDIVIDUALITY

To protect themselves against these threats to their individuality, organisms have developed a large variety of *defense reactions*. Some of these are easily noticeable: animals run from danger, fight it physically, or hide and disguise themselves. Others are more subtle and less conspicuous, for they take place largely within the animal's body. It is these *intraor-*

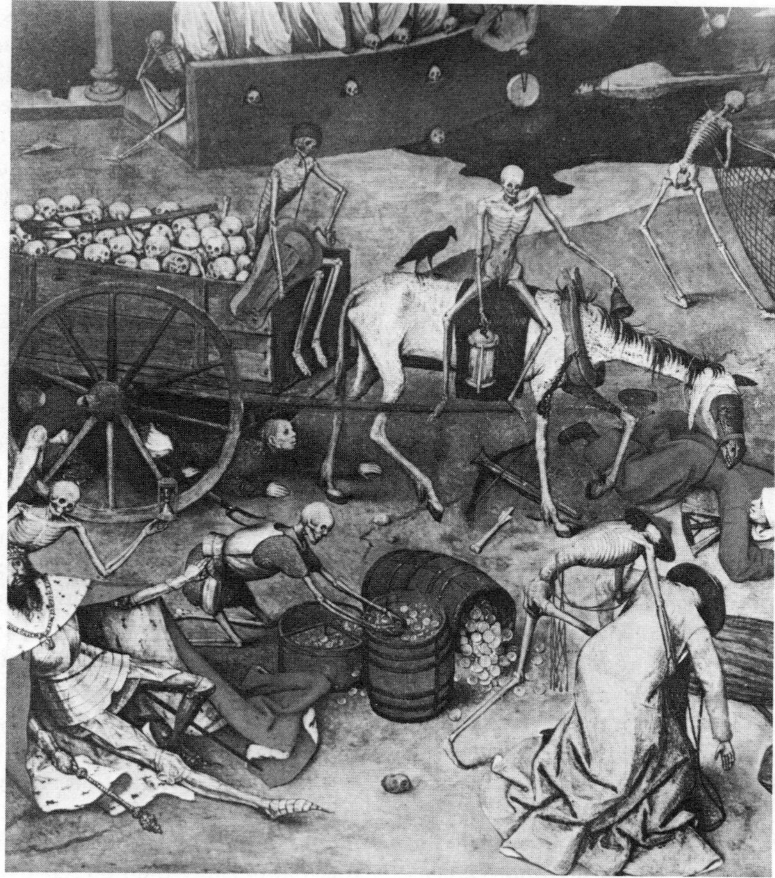

Figure 1.3. The third threat to the body's integrity. Before they were checked by modern medicine, epidemics of infectious disease ravaged humanity like the Fourth Horseman of the Apocalypse, turning the Medieval landscape into one large graveyard. This representation is from a painting by Pieter Breughel.

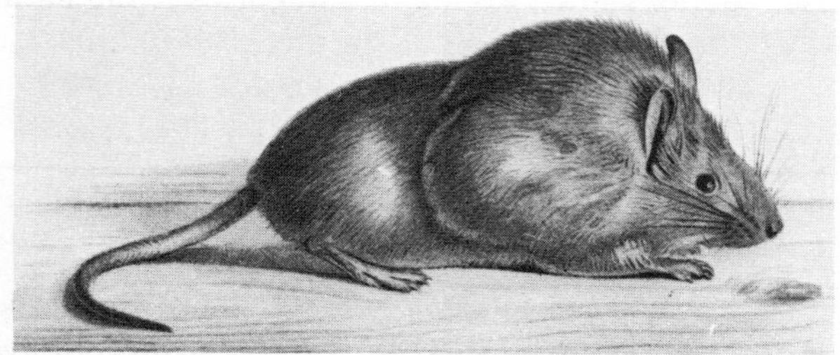

Figure 1.4. The fourth threat to the body's integrity. Looking like a monstrous hunchback, this mouse carries a tumor that arose from uncontrolled growth of a single cell of the mouse's own body—a growth that was not arrested because of a failure of the protective mechanisms. This drawing is from a work by Carl O. Jensen, who, in 1903, was among the first to transplant a tumor successfully from one mouse to another. (See C. O. Jensen: *Centralbl. Bakteriol. Parasitenk. Infektionskrankh.* **34:**28–34, 122–143, 1903.)

ganismic defense reactions with which we shall concern ourselves in this book.

There are three phases to each intraorganismic defense reaction: *recognition*, *processing*, and *response*. *Recognition* is a noncovalent interaction between two molecules, one carrying certain information, and another capable of receiving this information. The former is a *signal molecule*, the latter a *receptor*. Recognition allows organisms to discriminate between *self*—that is, everything constituting an integral part of a given individual—and *nonself*, or all the rest. The smallest unit of the nonself world capable of eliciting a defense reaction is an *antigen*. Theoretically, recognition can be either positive or negative. In *positive recognition*, an organism recognizes nonself actively and reacts to it; in *negative recognition*, an organism actively recognizes self and the reaction to nonself is merely the consequence of a failure to recognize it as self.

Processing, the second step in a defense reaction, is the transmission of the received signal from the receptor to other molecules and the analysis of the signal's information by these molecules. A decision, the nature of which depends upon the result of this analysis, is made about the action to be taken against the stimulus.

In the third, *response* (or *effector*), phase of a defense reaction, the individual acts (effects a response, often via effector molecules) to eliminate a threat from the nonself world.

Defense reactions can display various degrees of specificity, where *specificity* is defined as the ability to discriminate among the various nonself stimuli. This discrimination occurs in the recognition phase, when the signal molecule reacts with the receptor. The receptor would be absolutely specific if it reacted with only one particular molecule and not with any other molecule. However, such a situation never occurs: a receptor is always able to recognize several molecules while failing to react with others. The number of molecules recognized by a receptor determines its *degree of specificity*. A receptor capable of recognizing only a few different molecules is said to be *highly specific*; on the other end of the scale, a receptor that recognizes a large number of molecules relatively indiscriminately is said to be *nonspecific*. The fact that certain receptors recognize only certain molecules is explained by the assumption that spatial arrangements of atoms in the recognizing and recognized molecules are *complementary*. In other words, where one molecule has a protruding group of atoms, the other has a matching depression, and where one is charged positively, the other is charged negatively. This *stereospecificity* allows the surfaces of interacting molecules to come so close to one another that weak binding forces can occur between them.

In some defense reactions, the response to a given stimulus always proceeds at the same speed, no matter how often the reaction is evoked. In other reactions, the second response comes faster and is often more vigorous than the first, as if the system has remembered that it has done the same thing before. The secondary reaction is therefore called *anamnestic* (Gr. *anamnesis*, a recalling to mind, a remembering) and defense reactions displaying this ability are said to have a *memory*.

1.3 TYPES OF DEFENSE REACTION

There is hardly a living thing on earth that does not possess some form of defense reaction. Even seemingly inert plants can defend themselves against pathogens, are well-protected against injury, and have a low incidence of neoplasms. They produce fungitoxic substances, reject genetically incompatible grafts, and can heal their wounds. They also possess highly sophisticated systems governing fusion of their gametes. However, since by far the most developed defense reactions are found in the animal kingdom, we shall focus our attention on the animal phyla.

Considering the great diversity of the animal world, it is not surprising to find not one, but many different forms of defense reaction. They differ in their degree of specificity, speed of response, presence or absence of memory, mode of processing stimulating signals, and the manner in which effector functions are carried out. To orient ourselves in this maze of reactions, we shall classify them according to their most conspicuous features (Table 1.1). However, we should be aware that this classification is a gross oversimplification of a complex situation, and that it is artificial since, in many cases, we know virtually nothing about the mechanism of these reactions.

The main dividing line that groups the various defense reactions into two major categories is the nature

Table 1.1 Classification of Defense Reactions

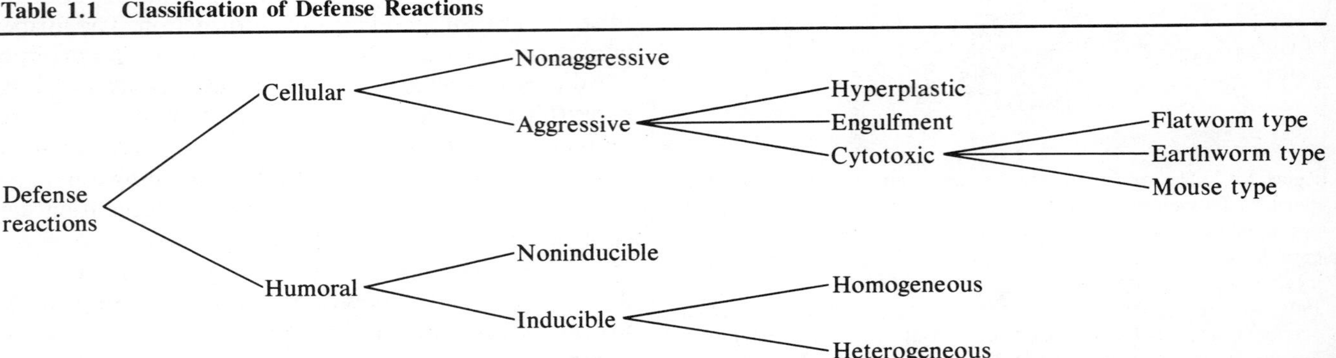

of the effector mechanism. Reactions mediated by soluble products in body fluids are referred to as *humoral* (L. *humor*, liquid), and those mediated directly by cells are referred to as *cellular*. Humoral reactions can be studied experimentally by obtaining body fluids, mixing them with an antigen, and observing the antigen's alteration. Cellular reactions can be studied by exposing cells, tissues, or the whole body to an antigen and following the antigen's fate, the response of the cells, or both. When the antigen itself is carried by cells, contact between the antigen-carrying cells and the cells reacting with them can be established simply by mixing the two cell types together, by grafting (transplanting) tissue or organs of one individual (donor) onto another (recipient, host), or by joining two bodies surgically (*parabiosis*). When no adverse reaction occurs during this contact, the cells, tissues, or bodies are said to be *histocompatible* (Gr. *histos*, tissue); when a reaction does occur, they are *histoincompatible*.

Depending on the outcome of the interaction between the antigen and the responding cells, cellular reactions can be further divided into *nonaggressive*, in which no cell death or tissue damage occurs, and *aggressive* reactions, in which destruction occurs because of hostile action by the host, the donor tissue, or both. This hostile action can consist of *hyperplasia* (an abnormal increase in the rate of cell division), *engulfment* (swallowing up of the foreign material), or *rejection* (destruction of tissue by specialized effector cells).

Humoral reactions can be divided roughly into *inducible* and *noninducible*, depending on whether the level of the humoral factor is increased by the exposure of an organism to an antigen. Examples of the above-described reactions follow.

1.3.1 Nonaggressive Cellular Reactions

The only expression of incompatibility in nonaggressive reactions is a failure to establish contact among interacting cells. We shall give three examples of this type of reaction, one each from three animal phyla: *Protozoa* (*Difflugia*), *Porifera* (sponges), and *Cnidaria* (corals).

Difflugia (Fig. 1.5) is a one-celled protozoan that abounds on the muddy bottoms of stagnant ponds. It hides in a pear-shaped shell composed of foreign particles cemented together. The shell has a single aperture, through which the cell sends out slender projections referred to as *pseudopodia* (Gr. *pseudēs*, false, *podus*, foot). In 1923 William A. Kepner and D. Reynold described an experiment in which they cut off these projections from the main body. They observed that both the body and the projections moved toward each other and eventually fused. A projection amputated from one individual fused with the body of another, provided the two protozoans belonged to the same species and had been grown in the same medium. A pseudopod of one species, however, would not fuse with the body of another species, nor would a pseudopod of an individual grown in one type of medium fuse with a body grown in another medium. The cells were, in such instances, incompatible.

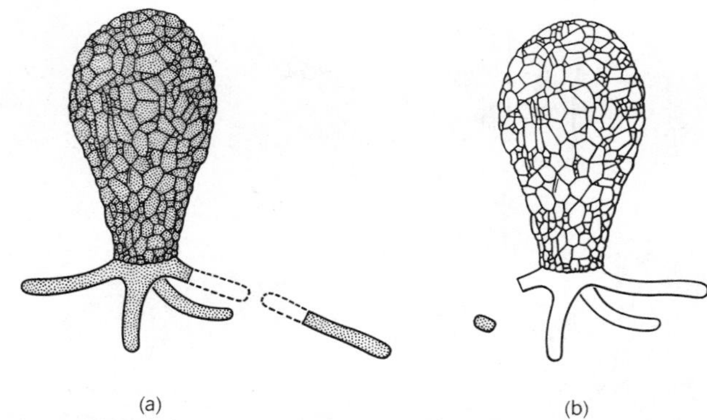

Figure 1.5. Nonaggressive incompatibility reaction in *Difflugia*. (*a*) (*a*) A pseudopod severed from a cell fuses with a cell of the same species, grown in the same medium. (*b*) A pseudopod from one species does not fuse with a cell of another species or a cell grown in a different medium.

Sponges (Fig. 1.6) are aquatic, mostly marine animals whose bodies are essentially double-walled, porous bags attached at one end to various objects in the water. H. V. Wilson demonstrated in 1907 that one can cut a sponge into small pieces and prepare a suspension of single cells by straining the pieces through finely meshed cloth. If one then lets the suspension settle into a dish of water, one observes that, as soon as the cells attach to the substrate, they begin to move around actively, adhering to one another upon contact. They form minute balls in which canals soon appear. Cells in the balls begin to differentiate, and after a few days, functional sponges develop. The whole body reconstitutes itself from dissociated cells! One can then prepare two cell suspensions, each from a different species of sponge, mix them together, and ask the question: will the cells be able to tell that they come from two different parents? The answer is yes—in most cases they will. In the mixed suspension, the two cell types sort themselves out and reconstitute the two parental species. Apparently, the cells somehow recognize one another, and only cells from the same species adhere.

Corals (Fig. 1.7) are warm-water colonial animals (polyps) enclosed in stony, often exquisitely colored protective cups. The individual polyps resemble small

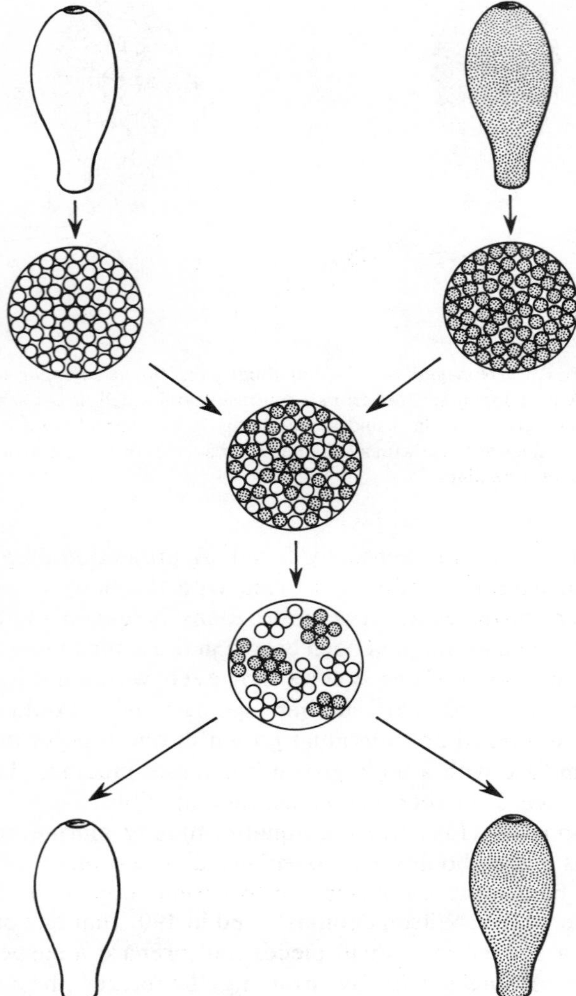

Figure 1.6. Nonaggressive incompatibility reaction in sponges. A mixture of dissociated cells obtained from two different species of sponge sorts itself out, and the cells aggregate to form parental body types. (Simplified and highly schematic)

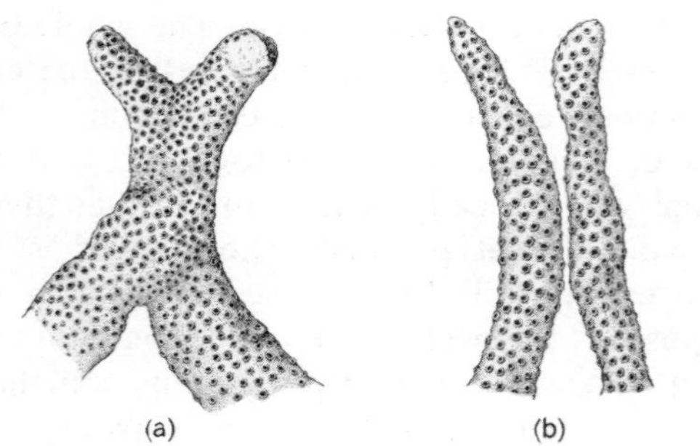

Figure 1.7. Nonaggressive incompatibility reaction in corals. (*a*) Fusion of two corals belonging to the same species. (*b*) Contact avoidance reaction between corals belonging to two different species. (*a*) is based on a photograph in W. H. Hildemann, D. S. Lithicum, and D. C. Vann, *Immunogenetics* **2**:269–284, 1975.)

sea anemones with their tentacles spread out from openings in the cup. William H. Hildemann and his co-workers demonstrated that when two branches of living corals are tied together with a nylon filament, their soft tissues unite and the branches are cemented together, provided they belong to the same species. Corals belonging to different species usually do not fuse and their branches remain separated by a narrow gap, as if trying to avoid contact with each other.

In all three instances incompatible cells simply ignore one another so that grafts fail to fuse, cells do not aggregate, and bodies do not unite. Whether the mechanism of these three nonaggressive reactions is the same is not known.

1.3.2 Aggressive Cellular Reactions

Hyperplastic Reactions

Corals also provide an example of a hyperplastic reaction, in which the death of one individual ensues because of abnormal growth of another individual. The example is taken from a work by Frances B. Ivker, published in 1972 (Fig. 1.8). When stemlike parts (sto-

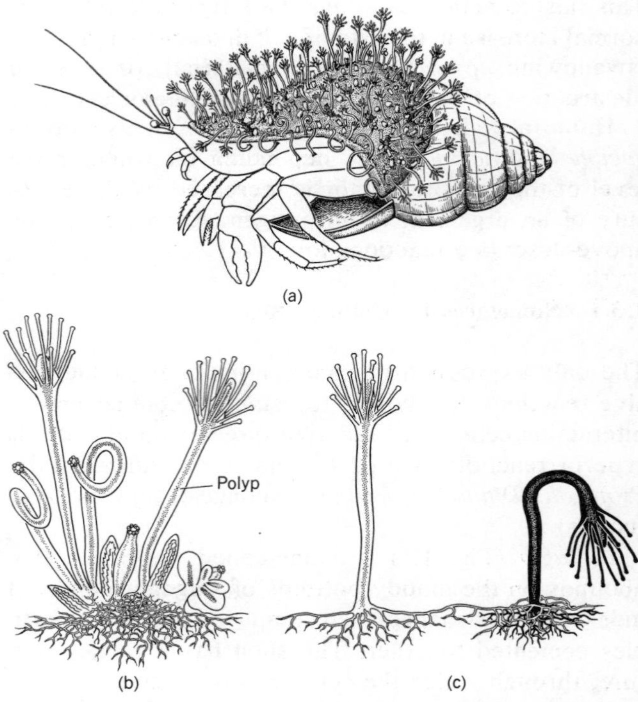

Figure 1.8. Aggressive incompatibility (hyperplastic) reaction in corals. (*a*) Colonies of *Hydractinia* corals growing on a snail shell inhabited by a hermit crab. (*b*) Detail of *Hydractinia* colony. (*c*) One colony of *Hydractinia* (left) strangling another colony (right). (*a*) is redrawn from C. Hauenschild, *Roux Arch. Entwicklungsmechanik* **147**:1–41, 1954.)

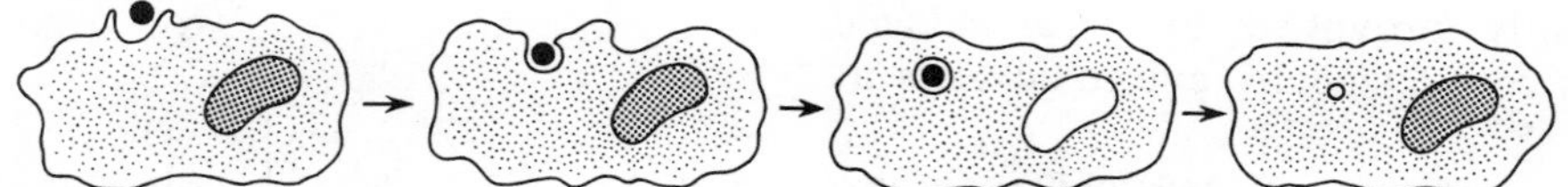

Figure 1.9. Pinocytosis of foreign material by a cell. If the engulfed particle were large, this drawing could also represent phagocytosis.

lons) of the coral *Hydractinia echinata* are placed into a dish containing sea water, they attach to the bottom and grow into new coral colonies. Colonies derived from the same stock fuse upon contact; colonies derived from different stocks display a hyperplastic reaction. In the latter case, one of the two colonies starts to produce abnormal stolons that lift off the ground, lose contact with the substrate, and form hyperplastic, tangled masses. The hyperplastic stolons eventually cut off the feeding polyps from the rest of the normal colony, preventing normal food supply, and thus eventually causing death by "strangulation." Once the hyperplastic stolons completely cover the underlying colony and reach the substrate, they return to a normal growth pattern.

A certain genetically controlled hierarchy of overgrowth seems to exist among colonies of different origin. Thus, for example, if colony A is able to overgrow colony B, and colony B is able to overgrow C, then A is usually able to overgrow C.

Engulfment Reactions

Three types of engulfment reaction, depending on the size of the foreign material, can be distinguished (Fig. 1.9). When the engulfed material is a fluid droplet, the process is termed *pinocytosis* (Gr. *pineo*, to drink, *kytos*, cell); when it is a small particle, such as a bacterium, one uses the term *phagocytosis* (Gr. *phagein*, to eat, *kytos*, cell); and when it is a large multicellular parasite, one refers to the process as *encapsulation*. In pinocytosis and phagocytosis, a droplet or particle is engulfed by a single cell, while encapsulation of a single parasite is accomplished by a multitude of cells.

Pinocytosis and *phagocytosis* (Fig. 1.9) were discovered by Ernst Haeckel in *Tethys fimbria,* a small mollusc found in the Mediterranean Sea and the Atlantic Ocean. When one injects blood vessels of this animal with indigo dye, one finds that within a few hours many of the blood cells (hemocytes) are packed with fine indigo particles. A closer study revealed that upon contacting a particle, the cytoplasm of the hemocyte sends out projections that envelop and swallow up the foreign matter, just as an amoeba swallows a food particle. The engulfed substance remains in a small, fluid-filled space (vacuole) into which enzymes are then released from the cytoplasm, destroying it. After digestion of the particle, the vacuole decreases in size until it completely disappears.

Encapsulation (Fig. 1.10) was first observed in the larvae of the oriental cockroach *Blatta orientalis* (reviewed by George Salt, 1963). When invaded with *Spirura rytipleuritis*, a tiny nematode worm, the larvae defend themselves by imprisoning the parasite in a small capsule. Encapsulation starts with the host's hemocytes congregating on the worm's body surface, flattening, and organizing themselves into multiple layers around the parasite. Later, the cells begin to secrete a nonliving connective tissue substance, first in the inner and then also in the outer layers of the capsule. Still later, the cells degenerate and the capsule becomes totally acellular. In some cases, the parasite is covered by a layer of dark pigment (melanin), which is produced by the host in a process called *melanization* (Gr. *melas*, black). Deprived of nutrients, the prisoner dies in the capsule.

Cellular Cytotoxic Reactions

These reactions are primarily against intracellular parasites—in particular, against viruses. When a virus invades a cell, the best defense strategy for the host is to destroy the cell before the virus has a chance to multiply in it. This destruction is accomplished by specialized, *cytotoxic* (*killer*, *cytolytic*, *effector*) *cells* that bind to the infected *target cell*, cause changes in the permeability of its membrane, and thus bring about cell lysis (disintegration of inner cell structure). The

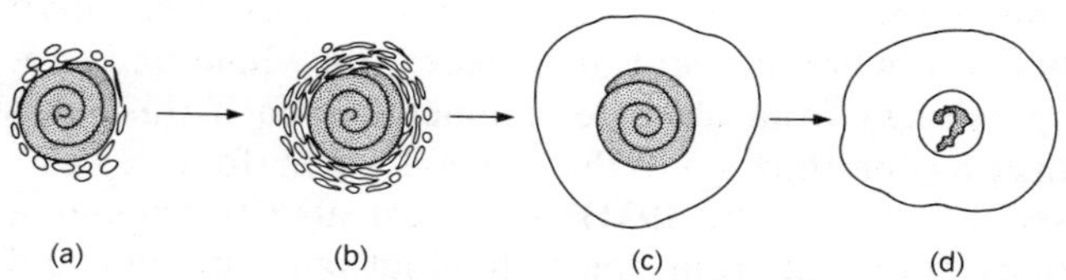

Figure 1.10. Encapsulation of a parasite (a nematode worm—stippled area). (*a*) Host's hematocytes surround the worm. (*b*) The surrounding cells flatten and arrange themselves in multiple layers. (*c*) Cells of the capsule secrete connective tissue substance and then degenerate. (*d*) Parasite shrinks and dies.

binding is apparently provoked by virus-induced membrane changes recognized by cytotoxic cells as nonself.

The same cytotoxic (Gr. *kytos*, cell) cells can also attack normal, noninfected cells of another individual if these are artificially introduced (transplanted) into a host and if they differ from the host cells in their membrane structure. The cytotoxic defense reaction can therefore be studied conveniently by *transplantation* (grafting) of cells, tissues, or organs from one individual to another. In this principally experimental situation, the reaction of the host to the *transplant* (graft) depends to a large degree on the genetic relationship between host and donor. If the donor and the host carry the same genes, their cell membranes have the same structure, and the cytotoxic cells of the host are unable to distinguish the transplant from the host's own tissues. The host *accepts* such a transplant as if it were part of its own body. This relationship between two genetically identical individuals is referred to as *syngeneic* (Gr. *syngenes*, congenital).

If, on the other hand, the donor and host differ in genes coding for cell membrane molecules, the transplanted cells are recognized as nonself and *rejected*—that is, destroyed by the host's cytotoxic cells. The relationship between two genetically dissimilar individuals is referred to as *allogeneic* (Gr. *allos*, other, *genos*, kin) when the individuals belong to the same species, and as *xenogeneic* (Gr. *xenos*, stranger) when they are members of two different species. We shall distinguish three types of cytotoxic reaction, based on the properties of the killer cells. Once again, examples from different animal phyla will help us describe them. These three types vary in sophistication, from the most primitive type, found in flatworms, through the more complex earthworm type, to the most evolved type, found in mice. Although one might surmise that these three types of reaction represent three different stages in the evolution of the cytotoxic response, there is no direct evidence to support this notion.

Flatworm-Type Cytotoxic Reaction. The flatworm (*Platyhelminthes*) has long been a favorite experimental animal for the study of regeneration and differentiation because when it is cut into pieces, its whole body reconstitutes from a single fragment, even if this is as little as one-thirtieth of the original worm (for a review, see E. Korschelt, 1931). One can also transplant a body fragment from one individual onto another and create monstrous worms with two heads, two bodies, or two tails. When transplantation is between individuals of the same species, the grafts are almost always accepted and retained for as long as the worm lives (Fig. 1.11). By contrast, grafts between two different species at first heal in, but are later rejected. The mechanism of this rejection is unknown, but some zoologists suspect that the destruction is effected by so-called type I cells, which are characterized by a large nucleus and scanty cytoplasm, and thus resemble the lymphocytes of more advanced animal forms.

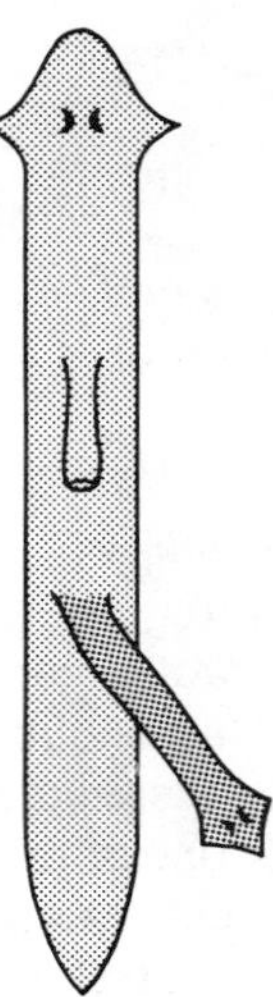

Figure 1.11. A successful transplant of one flatworm (dark stippling) onto another (light stippling).

Earthworm-Type Cytotoxic Reaction. Like flatworms, earthworms too have an eminently good regeneration capacity and are thus highly suitable animals for transplantation studies. Work by Ernst Joest, O. Rabes, Pierre Valembois, P. Duprat, Edwin L. Cooper and others has demonstrated that transplantation between individuals of the same species sometimes succeeds, at other times fails, depending to a large degree on the worms' origin. Transplants between individuals collected at the same locality are usually retained by the host permanently, whereas grafts between individuals from different localities are usually rejected. Because of interbreeding, two worms from the same locality are apparently more similar to each other than worms from different localities. Grafts exchanged between individuals belonging to different species are almost always rejected, despite the fact that they originally heal in (Fig. 1.12). Rejection usually does not start before day 30, and sometimes starts as late as 150 days after transplantation. Graft destruction is probably carried out by coelomocytes, cells present in the fluid that bathes the body cavity, or *coelom*. This destruction is slow, sometimes requiring several weeks for completion.

Worms that have rejected one graft often reject a

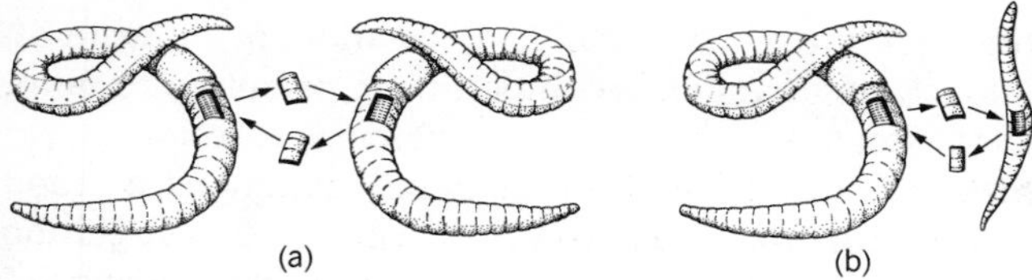

Figure 1.12. Transplantation of tissues in earthworms. (*a*) Grafts exchanged between individuals of the same species survive, especially if the two worms come from the same geographical area. (*b*) Grafts between different species of earthworm are rejected.

second graft from the same donor more rapidly than the first one, while rejecting a graft from an unrelated donor with normal (unaccelerated) speed. The cytotoxic reaction in earthworms thus shows both memory (the cells learn from their exposure to the first graft and attack a second graft in an accelerated manner) and specificity (learned behavior pertains only to the second graft carrying the same antigens as the first one). However, both memory and specificity are relatively poorly expressed: they are present only sometimes and are not very potent since even the secondary graft rejection is still relatively slow and the worm fails to recognize some allogeneic transplants altogether.

Mouse-Type Cytotoxic Reaction. We shall deal with this reaction in great detail later; here we shall point out only three of its features. First, this reaction is very vigorous and has a well-developed memory component. First grafts are usually rejected within a few weeks, and second grafts from the same donor within a few days. Second, this reaction is exquisitely specific. Mouse X that has rejected graft Y rejects a second graft Y in an accelerated manner, and rejects graft Z with normal speed. Third, this vigorous rejection is elicited by one major system of cell membrane-bound molecules that are encoded by a set of closely linked genes referred to as the *major histocompatibility complex* (MHC). The MHC molecules act as both stimulators and targets of the cytotoxic reaction.

In summary, the three types of cytotoxic reaction differ in these main features.

Flatworm-type. Only xenogeneic grafts are rejected; there is no evidence of memory; specificity of the reaction is low.

Earthworm-type. Both allogeneic and xenogeneic grafts are rejected; rejection is slow; memory is present, but weak; specificity of the reaction is higher than in the flatworm-type.

Mouse-type. All nonsyngeneic grafts are rejected; rejection is vigorous; memory is strongly expressed; specificity is high; stimulatory and target antigens are controlled by a single genetic complex.

Humoral Reactions

The tissues of multicellular organisms are bathed in bodily fluids. In primitive forms, these fluids percolate freely through the intercellular spaces, whereas in more advanced forms, networks of transport vessels, constituting the *circulatory* or *vasculatory system*, appear. One of the many functions of the bodily fluids is to disseminate elements of bodily defense, be they cellular or humoral.

There is a bewildering variety of humoral defense factors in plant and animal bodies, but only a few of these factors have been characterized to any appreciable degree of precision. Regarding most of the others, we know only that they exist and somehow participate in defense reactions; their specific function, origin, structure, and interrelationship are all unknown. For this reason, we shall not deal with all factors here; instead we shall limit ourselves to a few selected examples. We shall divide the factors into two classes—noninducible and inducible.

Noninducible Humoral Factors. These are secreted into the bodily fluid at a steady rate that is independent of the presence or absence of antigens. Of the many noninducible factors that probably exist in nature, we shall give only two examples.

Snail Agglutinin. J. Cantuzène discovered in 1916 that bacteria injected into the vascular system of the land snail *Helix pomatia* are rapidly cleared from the circulation: within two hours after injection, 90 percent of the bacteria are eliminated. Although most of the invaders are disposed of by phagocytosis, other defense reactions are also in operation. One of these is agglutination (gluing) of individual bacteria into clumps, which are then removed from the circulation. The *agglutinin*, the substance gluing bacteria together, is secreted by the digestive gland, a paired organ disgorging into the snail's stomach and considered by zoologists to be the primitive liver. Snail agglutinin is a glycoprotein with a molecular weight of some 100,000 daltons and with a specificity for certain carbohydrate molecules. Since these molecules are also present on certain types of human erythrocytes, snail agglutinin can be used for the study of human blood groups. The snail uses agglutinin not only against bacteria, but also against larvae of various parasites. Substances resembling snail agglutinin have been found in many other molluscs and in other invertebrates.

Human Complement. Human serum contains a complex system of proteins which, under certain circumstances, can assemble into a supermolecular structure capable of punching holes in the cell membrane. In addition, certain components of this *complement system*, which is present not only in the human but also in most other vertebrates, are involved in a variety of other defense reactions. (More about complement in Chapter 9.)

Inducible Humoral Factors. These factors are either completely absent prior to antigenic stimulation, or present in only a low amount. Exposure of an organism to an antigen causes a rapid increase in factor production; cessation of antigenic stimulation results in gradual disappearance of the factor from the circulation.

Our two examples of inducible factors—lobster bactericidin and mammalian antibodies—differ in their degree of heterogeneity and specificity. *Bactericidin* is a homogeneous substance with a highly restricted range of reactivity; *antibodies* are heterogeneous mixtures of molecules, with each molecule highly specific for only a few antigens, but with the entire antibody population covering virtually all existing antigens.

Lobster Bactericidin. E. Edward Evans and his colleagues reported in 1968 that an invasion of bacteria into the circulation of the spiny lobster *Panulirus* results in the appearance of a substance that kills the invaders. There is very little, if any, of this substance present in an uninfected lobster, but within one or two days after infection, there is a tremendous increase in bactericidin production and the level remains elevated for as long as the infection lasts. A second infection often results in an even more vigorous response, but this enhanced response can be induced even with bacteria unrelated to those that caused the first infection. The response thus has a certain degree of memory but a low degree of specificity. The bactericidin is a high-molecular weight substance, the chemical nature of which is unknown.

Vertebrate Antibodies. Antibodies (immunoglobulins) are proteins of a characteristic structure (tetramers consisting of two longer and two shorter polypeptide chains). They bind to antigens with exquisite specificity and neutralize their potentially harmful effects. (More about antibodies in Chapter 6.)

1.4 EVOLUTION OF DEFENSE REACTIONS

Since defense reactions are one of the principal attributes of living matter, they very likely appeared when life first arose on earth and, as did life in general, underwent a gradual evolution from primitive to more sophisticated forms. At first, defense reactions were probably tied to such other bodily functions as food processing, waste disposal, or cell-to-cell recognition during embryonal differentiation. Later, when the need for defense increased, cells specialized to this function emerged. These cells wandered through tissues, searching for nonself matter, and, when they found it, disposed of it in one of two ways: by swallowing up the material just as their predecessors swallowed food particles, or by secreting soluble substances to neutralize the material's harmful effects. When organisms developed circulatory systems, defense cells tied in with them and thus became much more effective at patrolling tissues and reaching sites where they were needed.

The original defense cells had some sort of recognition system that allowed them to distinguish self from nonself. But this recognition was relatively unsophisticated and inefficient: the cells distinguished self from nonself, but could not differentiate between and respond specifically to the various forms of nonself. Later, when the demands on the defense system increased even more and the primitive cells could no longer meet them, natural selection began to work in favor of more specialized and efficient defense mechanisms. The specialization of defense cells occurred in two ways. First, the cells developed a division of labor, so that each cell type specialized in one phase of the defense reaction (i.e., recognition, transfer of signals, and effector functions). Several cell types that were related in their origin and function thus emerged. This diversification in turn required a mechanism assuring a coordinated action of these cells, a requirement fulfilled with the emergence of special *regulatory* cells that could either enhance (*helper cells*) or suppress (*suppressor cells*) the response of other cells. Second, cells involved in recognition progressively increased the specificity of their receptors and their memory capacity. No longer did one cell recognize a broad spectrum of nonself agents; rather, each cell became specialized in the recognition of a small segment of the spectrum, so that the defense cell population became progressively more heterogeneous. The speed with which defense cells—in particular, lymphocytes—were able to recall previous experience with the same antigen and the duration of this memory also increased gradually, progressively shortening the dangerous period between recognition of a pathogen and activation of effector mechanisms.

The original, less sophisticated defense cell mechanisms were not discarded by the evolving organisms;

instead they were kept to handle cruder defense assignments. More advanced life forms thus possess two basic types of defense cell—the less sophisticated *macrophages* (Gr. *makros*, large, *phagein*, eat) and the highly sophisticated *lymphocytes* (L. *lympha*, water, Gr. *kytos*, cell). Macrophages continue to dispose of nonself matter in the way they learned from their amoeba-like ancestors, by engulfment and digestion.

Phagocytosis is probably the most widely distributed defense reaction, occurring in virtually all phyla of the animal world. Macrophages, however, also possess several other functions that they probably inherited from their ancestors—for example, the secretion of relatively nonspecific humoral factors facilitating phagocytosis and other defense reactions. Among the variety of factors produced by macrophages, one group has gained particular prominence. These factors, called *complement components*, have the ability to assemble on a cell membrane to form a multimolecular structure, open up holes in the membrane, and thus to kill target cells.

While macrophages can attack virtually any nonself entity, be it a bacterial cell, a multicellular parasite, or a particle of nonliving matter, lymphocytes seem to have specialized in attacking only one kind of cell—self cells (i.e., cells of the animal's own body) that have been altered by an infectious agent (e.g., a virus) or by the neoplastic process. To carry out the attack, they first need to identify the attacked cell via two markers, one signaling that the cell was originally part of the animal's self world, and another indicating that the cell is no longer of the self type. The latter marker could be any one of the several types of membrane alteration appearing in the aberrant cell; for the former, evolutionarily more advanced animals developed a particular set of molecules, all controlled by a single gene cluster, the *major histocompatibility complex* (MHC). In addition to serving as self markers, MHC molecules probably also play other roles in the animal's defense mechanisms, perhaps by participating in the effector stage of defense.

Like macrophages, lymphocytes too have maintained a double role in defense reactions: they have learned not only to attack other cells directly, but also to make soluble factors that either regulate (enhance or suppress) the response of other cells in the defense machinery or combat threats from the nonself world. Among the latter factors, the highest degree of specificity and heterogeneity has been achieved by the *immunoglobulins*.

The defense system's progressively increasing sophistication gradually changed the overall defense strategy. While the system was relatively nonspecific, it operated on the "survival of the fittest" principle. There was a set of genes coding for receptors able to recognize certain pathogenic parasites and to trigger defense reactions against them. When a new pathogen or a new variant of an existing pathogen appeared in the environment, most individuals of a given population became defenseless, because they did not possess the appropriate receptor to recognize the new threat. These individuals died. But in each population, there were a few individuals with receptor molecules that had been changed by mutation in the corresponding genes so that they could recognize the new pathogen. These individuals survived and became the stock from which a new, resistant population derived.

The "survival of the fittest" strategy can operate only in species that produce large numbers of relatively short-lived progeny. Species with fewer progeny and longer generation time have a low probability of developing genetic variants that can adapt rapidly to a new threat. Such species have developed a new defense strategy that can cope more efficiently with dangerous situations. In this strategy, the process of selection of the fittest has been transposed from the population level to the level of cells within an individual. Each individual possesses a group of cells (lymphocytes) that can divide rapidly and can, in each division, generate changes in the genes coding for defense receptors. In this fashion, an individual produces a heterogeneous lymphocyte population consisting of variant receptors that cover a wide spectrum of antigens and are thus prepared for all occasions. When such an individual encounters a pathogen with a variant antigen, it will very likely have in its body a lymphocyte or group of lymphocytes capable of recognizing it. The antigen will stimulate these cells, which will expand into a population that can liquidate the pathogen efficiently. An essential component of this new defense strategy is a *generator of diversity* (GOD), or a genetic mechanism that rapidly produces many variants from a limited number of genes in a limited number of somatic cell generations.

The evolution of the new defense strategy was probably tied to the emergence of vertebrates, which generally have few progeny, are relatively long-lived, and have small populations. Moreover, they usually have more complex bodies than invertebrates, which makes them more vulnerable to threats from the nonself world. They simply cannot afford the "survival of the fittest" strategy.

The new strategy called for a considerably higher number of defense cells than the old one had. The defense cells, because of this requirement and because of the increasing interactions among them, were no longer distributed diffusely throughout the body. Instead they aggregated in nodules, where they could communicate with one another. These nodules were mostly on the gut wall, the inner surface of which is exposed to elements from the nonself world and so is very vulnerable to this world's assaults. Apparently, the nodules were present in the most primitive vertebrates, and then, during vertebrate evolution, they became organizationally more complex, acquired an architecture of their own, and turned into discrete bodily parts—the *lymphoid organs*.

One of the most important functions of the newly arisen lymphoid organs was to provide conditions for lymphocyte differentiation. This differentiation evolved along two main lines—one leading to a cell capable of interacting with other cells through its cell-bound receptors and either regulating their activity (helper or suppressor lymphocyte) or killing them (cytotoxic lymphocyte), and another line leading to a cell capable of secreting specific receptor molecules (immunoglobulins). Since the conditions necessary for differentiation along these two lines were not the same, two different lymphoid organs evolved to separate the lines—the *thymus* for the differentiation of regulatory and cytotoxic lymphocytes, and the *bursa of Fabricius* (or a homologous organ) for differentiation of immunoglobulin-producing lymphocytes. Lymphocytes differentiating under the influence of the thymus are, therefore, referred to as *thymus-derived* or *T lymphocytes*, and those differentiating in the bursa as *bursa-derived* or *B lymphocytes*. When exactly during evolution the major steps in this highly speculative scheme occurred is not known and might never be known with certainty. What kind of defense reactions extinct species possessed we can only guess, for defense reactions leave no fossils. Nor do we know much about the defense reactions of animals living today, except for those of birds and mammals. How do the various types of reaction relate to one another? Are they all offshoots of one major evolutionary line, or do they represent independent attempts at solving the defense problems? The answers to these questions are unknown. The phylogeny of defense reactions is a fascinating and wide-open area of investigation for students interested in solving difficult biological puzzles.

1.5 IMMUNOLOGY DEFINED

The branch of biology concerned with the study of defense reactions is *immunology*, a term understood differently by different investigators. Some, including the author, use the word in its broadest sense, that is, to denote the study of *all* types of defense reaction, including those found in all animal and plant phyla, and encompassing even the most primitive reactions, which have a low degree of specificity and no memory. Other scientists, particularly those working in medically oriented disciplines, use the word in a narrower sense, and understand immunology to be the study of only the most advanced types of defense reaction, those with a high degree of specificity and memory. Immunology in this narrow sense deals almost exclusively with vertebrates, and among vertebrates, with mammals in particular. The word "immunology" derives from the Latin *immunis*, meaning "free of burden," where the burden might be a tax imposed by Caesar, a law affecting an individual, or a disease. Persons resistant to certain diseases are therefore said to be *immune* to them, and the status of a specific resistance to a disease is referred to as *immunity*. Used in this sense, immunology has an even more restricted meaning, referring to defense reactions that confer resistance to those pathogens that cause infectious diseases.

In this book we use the word "immunology" in its broader sense whenever possible. However, our knowledge of prevertebrate immunology is so limited that we have already covered most of its important aspects in this chapter. The rest of the book, therefore, is devoted primarily to vertebrate immunology.

1.6 APPENDIX 1.1: RECAPITULATION OF ANIMAL TAXONOMY AND PHYLOGENY

To summarize the evolution of life on earth, biologists draw a tree with its branches arranged to show the purported origin of groups of organisms, or *phyla*. (The complete evolutionary history of a group of organisms is then referred to as *phylogeny*.) Because our knowledge of evolution is still quite incomplete and subject to different interpretations, there are many ways of drawing a *phyletic tree*. One such drawing, depicted in Figure 1.13, shows five main stems, representing five kingdoms of life: bacteria, blue-green algae, fungi, plants, and animals.

The animal kingdom, which is our primary concern here, derives from one-celled organisms with complex structures, the *Protozoa* (Gr. *protos*, first, *zoon*, animal). Most protozoans live as single, free cells, but some organize themselves into colonies in which individual cells, although joined together, still function as units that carry out all life-associated activities. One group of colonial protozoans—perhaps that from

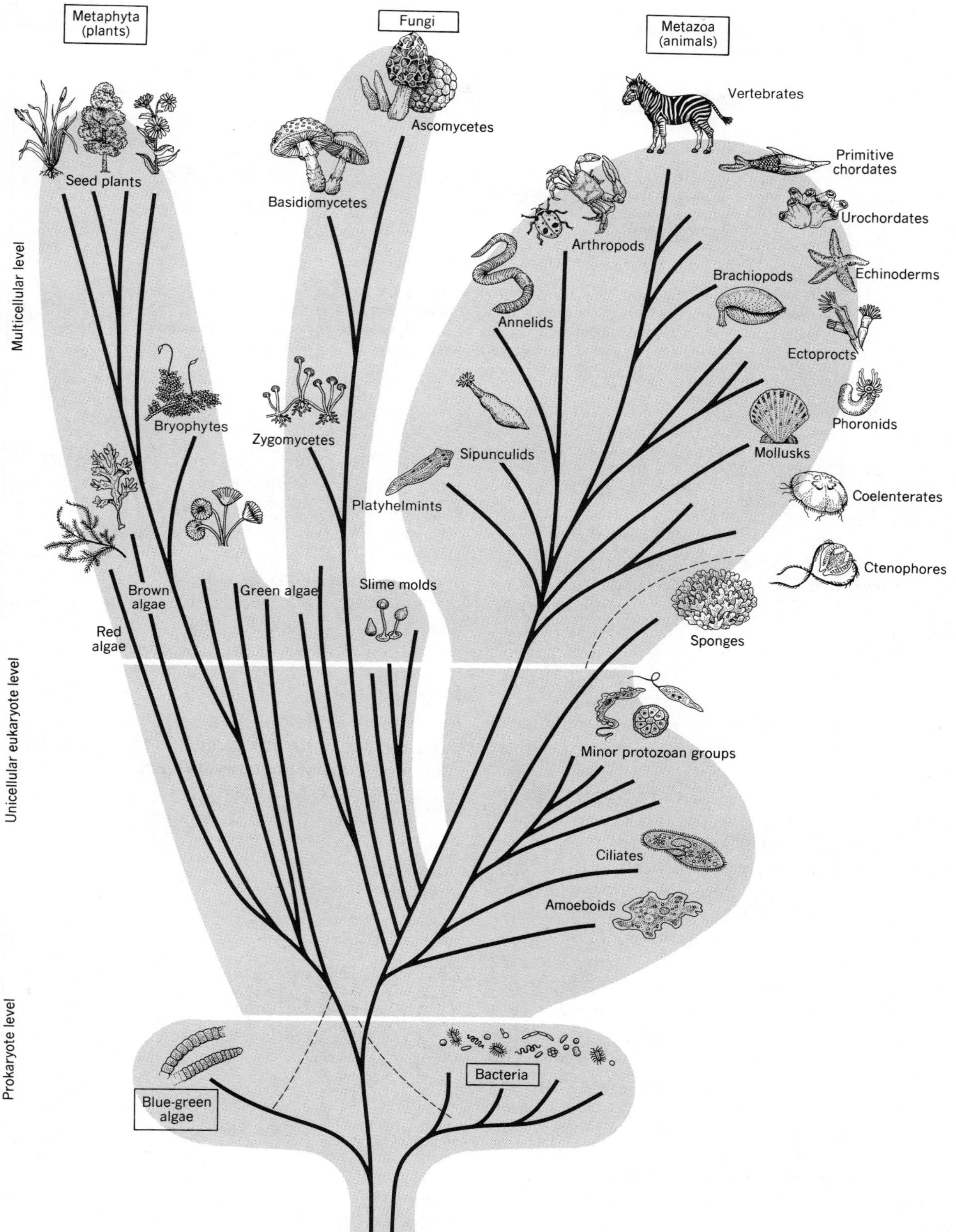

Figure 1.13. Kingdoms of the living world. [Redrawn from J. W. Valentine, *Sci. Am.* **239** (Sept.):104–117, 1978.]

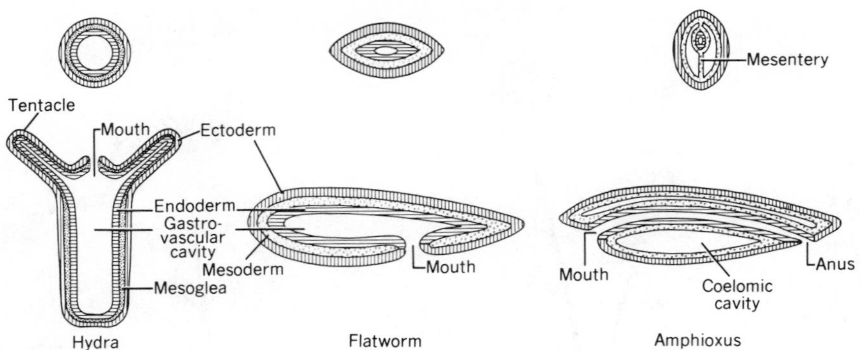

Figure 1.14. Three basic body plans in transverse (upper part) and sagittal (lower part) sections. The hydra is a representative of acoelomate animals with radial symmetry; the flatworm is an acoelomate with bilateral symmetry; and the amphioxus is a coelomate animal with bilateral symmetry. Acoelomate animals have no bodily cavity. In coelomate animals, a bodily cavity (coelom) exists, bounded by the mesoderm.

which the present-day *Choanoflagellida* [organisms with a conical collar (choana; Gr. *choane*, funnel) about their flagellate cells] derived—gave rise to the most primitive *Metazoa* (many-celled organisms), represented today by *Porifera* (L. *porus*, pore, *fero*, to bear), or sponges. Another group evolved into *Coelenterata* (Gr. *koilos*, hollow, *enteron*, intestine), represented by jellyfishes, sea anemones, and hydras, and all other *Metazoa*. Certain marine *Coelenterata* have a complicated life cycle, in which, at one stage, they change into a ball-like ciliated larva—a *planula*. Zoologists believe that this larva resembles the ancestral form from which all *Metazoa* except *Porifera* evolved.

The evolution of more advanced *Metazoa* led to three important changes in body organization. First, body symmetry changed from the radial type of the *Coelenterata* (Fig. 1.14), in which parts of the body radiate from a central axis like spokes of a wheel, to the bilateral type of the *Platyhelminthes* (flatworms; Fig. 1.14), in which the body is divisible into two equal halves along a central plane. Second, to the two cell layers of the *Porifera* and *Coelenterata* (the outer *ectoderm* and the inner *endoderm*), *Platyhelminthes*, for the first time, added the *mesoderm* (Fig. 1.14), a third layer inserted between the ecto- and endoderm. [In *Porifera* and *Coelenterata* the space between ecto- and endoderm is filled with the *mesoglea*—a gelatinous matrix with a few scattered cells (Gr. *mesos*, middle, *glia*, glue).] Third, cavities developed in the body. In *Platyhelminthes*, the mesoderm is a solid sheet of cells, but in some other phyla—for example, in the *Aschelminthes* ("cavity worms")—a *pseudocoelom*, a cavity between the endoderm and mesoderm, appears. In still more advanced *Metazoa*, the mesoderm itself splits into two sheets, one attached to the ectoderm and the other to the endoderm. The cavity between the two mesodermal sheets is the *coelom*. The mesodermal sheet attached to the ectoderm forms the muscles of the body wall, which are involved primarily in locomotion, whereas the endoderm-associated mesoderm gives rise to the muscles of the digestive tract. The development of the coelom changed the body from the double-walled sack of the *Porifera*, *Coelenterata*, and *Platyhelminthes* into the "tube within a tube" organization of the more advanced *Metazoa*, with the outer tube representing the body wall and the inner tube the wall of the digestive tract.

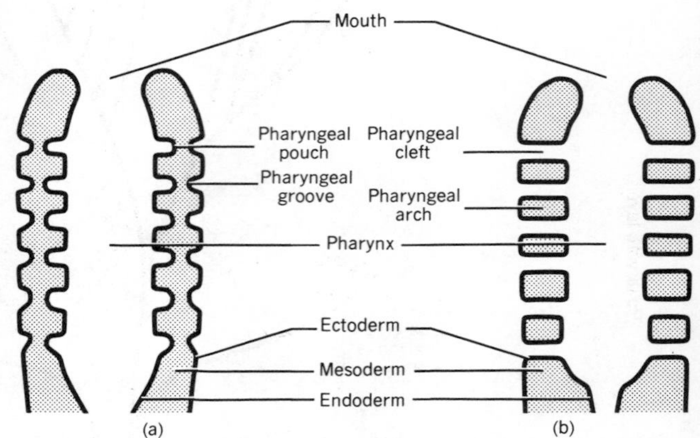

Figure 1.15. Diagram depicting the pharyngeal clefts in chordate embryos before (*a*) and after (*b*) connection with the outside world has been established.

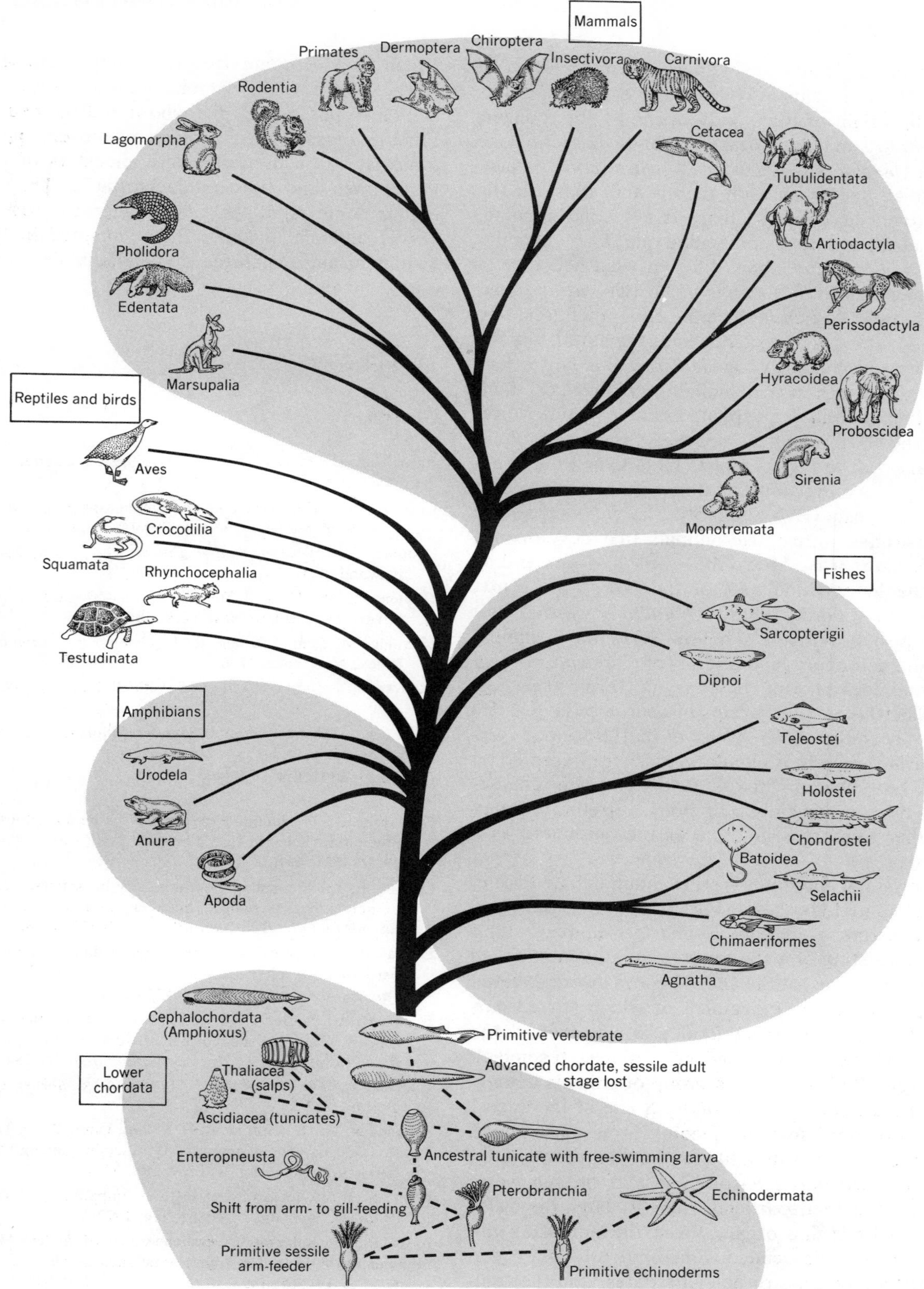

Figure 1.16. Phyletic tree of *Chordata*, showing the postulated origin of vertebrates. [Redrawn and modified from J. W. Valentine, *Sci. Am.* **239** (Sept.):104–117, 1978.]

After the development of the coelom, the stem of the phyletic tree splits into two major branches, differing in the origin of their body openings. In sponges, *Coelenterata*, and flatworms, the body has only one opening (*blastopore*; Gr. *blastos*, germ, *poros*, opening), which serves as both mouth and anus. In the more advanced *Metazoa*, there is a second opening, usually at the end opposite the first one. The two major branches of *Metazoa*, then, differ in what becomes of the blastopore. In *protostome phyla* (Gr. *protos*, first, *stoma*, mouth), which include annelids, molluscs, and arthropods, the blastopore becomes the mouth and the anus forms secondarily; in *deuterostome phyla* (Gr. *deuteros*, second), which include echinoderms, tunicates, hemichordates, cephalochordates, and vertebrates, the blastopore becomes the anus and the mouth forms anew. The two branches have gone their separate ways since Precambrian times, that is, for at least 500 million years. Evolutionarily, the most successful deuterostomes were those animals that developed a flexible, supportive rod—the *notochord*—extending along the longitudinal axis of the body (Gr. *notos*, back, *chorde*, cord). These *Chordata* ("corded animals") also developed a hollow *nerve tube* running above the notochord, and a series of paired *pharyngeal slits* along each side of the pharynx (throat; see Fig. 1.15). The three major groups of chordates (Fig. 1.16) are the sea squirts or *Urochordata* (barrel-shaped, sessile, marine animals), *Cephalochordata* (represented by a single type, the amphioxus), and *Vertebrata* (characterized by a cartilaginous or bony vertebral column that either reinforces or replaces the notochord as a supportive rod).

The origin of chordates is still a much-debated issue. The prevailing hypothesis (Fig. 1.16) is that the chordate ancestors were sessile marine animals, their bodies consisting of a stalk with a mouth, surrounded by outspread arms, at the end. The arms were covered with small cilia, the movement of which stirred currents of water containing food particles toward the mouth. These "arm feeders" much resembled present-day *Pterobranchia*, a group of animals belonging to the division *Hemichordata*. Some of the ancestral pterobranchs lost the feeding arms and instead developed a set of slits (gills) in the wall of the stalk, which widened into a barrel. The slits filtered water and collected food particles from it; later they also became a breathing organ. From the ancestral gill-feeding forms descended *Enteropneusta* or acorn worms, another class of hemichordates, and the tunicates. The latter are sessile, like their ancestors, but some of them pass through a developmental stage in which they become free-swimming, tadpole-shaped larvae. The larvae are among the most primitive forms known to possess the notochord and the neural tube. For this reason, most zoologists consider the ancient tunicates to be the immediate ancestors of primitive vertebrates and of cephalochordates. They believe that at some point the larvae failed to grow up into sessile animals; instead, they remained in the free-swimming state, matured sexually, and developed into a new species.

REFERENCES

General

Barnes, R. D.: *Invertebrate Zoology*, 3rd ed. Saunders, Philadelphia, 1974.

Cooper, E. L. (Ed.): *Invertebrate Immunology. Contemporary Topics in Immunobiology* Vol. 4. Plenum, New York, 1974.

Cooper, E. L.: *Comparative Immunology*. Prentice-Hall, Englewood Cliffs, New Jersey, 1976.

Hildemann, W. H. and Benedict, A. A. (Eds.): *Immunologic Phylogeny*. Plenum, New York, 1975.

Manning, M. J. and Turner, R. J.: *Comparative Immunobiology*. Wiley, New York, 1976.

Romer, A. S.: *The Vertebrate Body*, 4th ed. Saunders, Philadelphia, 1970.

Villee, C. A.: *Biology*, 7th ed. Saunders, Philadelphia, 1972.

Original Articles

Cantuzène, J.: Production expérimentale d'hemoagglutinines et de précipitines chez helix pomatia. *C. R. Soc. Biol.* (*Paris*) **79**:528–531, 1916.

Cooper, E. L.: Transplantation immunity in Annelids. I. Rejection of xenografts exchanged between *Lumbricus terrestris* and *Eisenia foetida*. *Transplantation* **6**:322–337, 1968.

Duprat, P.: Mise en évidence immunitaires dans les homogreffes de paroi du corps chez le Lombricien *Eisenia foetida typica*. *C.R. Soc. Acad. Sci.* (*Paris*) **259**:4177–4180, 1964.

Evans, E. E., Painter, B., Evans, M. L., Weinheimer, P., and Acton, R. T.: An induced bactericidin in the spiny lobster, *Panulirus argus*. *Proc. Soc. Exp. Biol. Med.* **128**:394–398, 1968.

Haeckel, E.: *Die Radiolarien*. (*Rhizopoda Radiaria*). G. Reimer, Berlin, 1862.

Hildemann, W. H., Linthicum, D. S., and Vann, D. C.: Transplantation and immunoincompatibility reactions among reef-building corals. *Immunogenetics* **2**:269–284, 1975.

Ivker, F. B.: A hierarchy of histo-incompatibility in *Hydractinia echinata*. *Biol. Bull.* **143**:162–174, 1972.

Joest, E.: Transplantationsversuche an *Lumbriciden*. Morphologie und Physiologie der Transplantationen. *Arch. f. Entw. Mech. Org.* **5**:419–569, 1897.

Kepner, W. A. and Reynold, D.: Reactions of cell bodies and pseudopodial fragments of *Difflugia*. *Biol. Bull.* **44**:22–46, 1923.

Korschelt, E.: *Regeneration und Transplantation*. II. Band: *Transplantation*. Borntraeger, Berlin, 1931.

Rabes, O.: Transplantationsversuche an *Lumbriciden*. Histologie und Physiologie der Transplantationen. *Arch. f. Entw. Mech. Org.* **13**:239–352, 1902.

Salt, G.: The defence reactions of insects to metazoan parasites. *Parasitology* **53**:527–642, 1963.

Valembois, P.: Recherches sur la nature de la réaction antigreffe chez le Lombricien *Eisenia foetida Sav. C. R. Acad. Sci. (Paris)* **257**:3489–3490, 1963.

Wilson, H. V.: On some phenomena of coalescence and regeneration in sponges. *J. Exp. Zool.* **5**:245–258, 1907.

CHAPTER 2

HISTORY OF IMMUNOLOGY

2.1 AN IMMUNOLOGIST'S *HÖLLENFAHRT*

"*Tief ist der Brunnen der Vergangenheit*," ("deep is the well of the past") writes Thomas Mann in *Joseph und seine Brüder*.

Where did immunology begin? Was it in the seventeenth century, when parents intentionally infected their children with mild forms of smallpox[1] to protect them from a more severe infection?[2] Or in first-century B.C. Pontus, where King Mithridates VI is said to have taken to drinking a little poison every day in the hope that it would protect him from a fatal dose served to him by a murderer?[3] Or did immunology begin in fifth-century B.C. Athens, of which Thucydides, the great historian of the Peloponnesian War, writes:

> Yet it was with those who had recovered from the disease that the sick and the dying found most com-

[1] Smallpox is a disease caused by a virus which, when inhaled, enters cells lining the throat and trachea, multiplies in them, and is then disseminated by the bloodstream throughout the body. When it reaches the skin, it multiplies in the epidermal cells and causes characteristic lesions, primarily on the face, chest, and arms. The lesions start as small bumps, which then enlarge, fill with fluid, inflame, swell, and break out into pustules. Next, a soft crust forms over the pustules, which later falls off, revealing characteristic pocks, or depressed scars, which gave the disease its name. (The original name was "small pokkes," distinguishing the disease from "great pokkes," or syphilis.) Great smallpox epidemics of the past left two of five victims dead and the rest disfigured (and often blind) for life. In modern times, except for a few remaining pockets in certain underdeveloped countries, smallpox has been eradicated from the earth.

[2] The western world learned of this practice mainly from Mary Pierrepont, an English beauty, who, against her father's wishes, eloped in 1712 with Edward Wortley Montagu, a grandson of the first Earl of Sandwich. When Montague was appointed ambassador to Turkey, Lady Mary, who by then had lost her beauty because of smallpox, accompanied him on his mission. After she had learned about the Turkish method of smallpox protection, she not only had her own children variolated, but after her return to England, passionately agitated in favor of variolation. (Latin *varus* means pimple; the scholarly name of smallpox is *variola*, and the technique of artificial exposure to smallpox is referred to as *variolation*.)

[3] The treatment must have been effective, since it is said that when, in old age, Mithridates tried to kill himself, the poison he took failed to work.

passion. These knew what it was from experience, and had now no fear for themselves; for the same man was never attacked twice—never at least fatally. And such persons not only received the congratulations of others, but themselves also, in the elation of the moment, half entertained the vain hope that they were for the future safe from any disease whatsoever?[4]

No, Athens cannot have been the birthplace of immunology, because, long before that time, the ancient Chinese made children inhale a powder from the crusts shed by a patient recovering from smallpox. And before the Chinese. . . .

Thomas Mann is right: history—including the history of immunology—is like a trip into a bottomless pit. Nevertheless, we can more or less arbitrarily divide immunological history into two periods, one in which it resembled Mann's *Höllenfahrt*, and one more familiar to us, in which the signposts of recorded experiments guide us on our journey. The dividing line between these two periods—a sort of B.C. and A.D. division—is 1798, the year in which Edward Jenner published *An Inquiry into the Causes and Effects of the Variolae Vaccinae*.

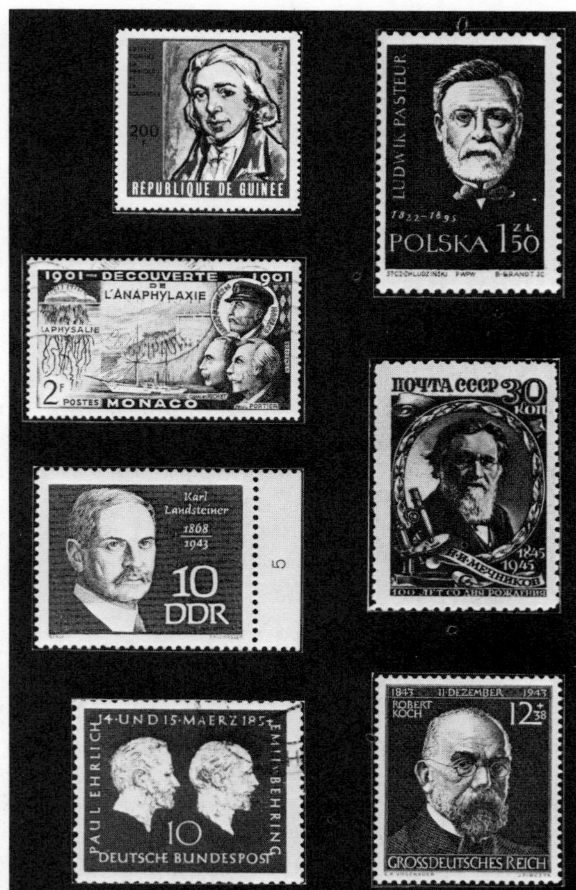

Figure 2.1. The immunological hall of fame: immunologists on postage stamps. Left column from top to bottom: Edward Jenner, Charles Richet and Paul Portier, Karl Landsteiner, Paul Ehrlich and Emil von Behring. Right column from top to bottom: Louis Pasteur, Elie Metchnikoff, Robert Koch. (Stamps from the collection of Dr. Eugene D. Rosenblum.)

2.2 JENNER AND SMALLPOX VACCINE

Edward Jenner (Fig. 2.1) was an English country physician, a contemporary of the painter Thomas Gainsborough. There are stories about Jenner which, like Gainsborough's paintings, embody an element of rococo, so that it becomes difficult to separate *Dichtung* and *Wahrheit*, or the fanciful additions of later storytellers from the truth of what really happened.

One story goes like this. One day, Jenner examined a milkmaid who complained of fever, backache, and vomiting. He thought that she might be coming down with smallpox, but she had a ready answer: "I cannot take that disease, for I have had the cowpox." Jenner was, of course, familiar with cowpox, a disease that produces sores on cows' udders, and, when passed on to the people who milk the cows, causes pustules like those seen in smallpox. He also knew that, unlike smallpox, cowpox is almost never fatal. He realized that the girl was suggesting that cowpox protects against smallpox.

Her simple statement aroused his curiosity, and when he checked out her claim, he found that it seemed to be true: he could not find a single person who had contracted smallpox after having had cowpox. So Jenner decided to do an experiment. He found another milkmaid, named Sarah Nelmes, who was sick with cowpox, took some material from a pustule on her hand, and injected it into the arm of eight-year-old James Phipps. Six weeks later, after the boy's reaction to the cowpox injection had subsided, Jenner inoculated Phipps with smallpox. Shocking? Unethical? Yes, but let us not forget that eighteenth-century ethical standards were different from those of today. And after all, it worked out well for James Phipps: he became immune to smallpox. (Jenner inoculated him with smallpox 20 times to prove his point!)

[4] Thucydides: *The Complete Writings of Thucydides: The Peloponnesian War*. transl. J. H. Finley, Jr., The Modern Library, New York, 1951, p. 112.

In 1798 Jenner published a 70-page pamphlet describing his experience, the now famous *Inquiry*, in which he called his technique *vaccination*, from the Latin word *vacca*, meaning cow. After a period of initial resistance by a few physicians, the practice of smallpox vaccination spread quickly, the disease began to disappear, Jenner became a hero, and this rococo little melodrama was retold in every immunology textbook. It is a nice story, so why not tell it here, too, as long as we take it as *Dichtung*, and not as factual truth? The cold reality was probably somewhat different and not half so interesting. In fact, we are not even sure that Jenner vaccinated with cowpox. Some historians suggest that his vaccine was contaminated by an attenuated form of human smallpox virus. The truth may never be known.

2.3 PASTEUR AND CHICKEN CHOLERA

Another legendary figure in the history of immunology is Louis Pasteur (Fig. 2.1), the discoverer of molecular asymmetry, the mechanism of fermentation, and anaerobic life, and one of the founders of bacteriology. Like Jenner, Pasteur is the subject of many stories that season the facts liberally with fancy; one of these stories is important to an understanding of the history of immunology.

In 1878, Pasteur was much interested in chicken cholera, a disease unrelated to human cholera, but as devastating to fowl populations as human cholera once was to humanity. Afflicted birds stop eating, their feathers stand grotesquely on end, they weaken, and most of them die. Pasteur was working to find out all about the organism causing this disease, and soon succeeded in growing pure cultures of the causative agent, a bacterium later called *Pasteurella multocida*. But then—so the story goes—his work was interrupted by summer vacation, for in Europe then as today, all work stopped in summer, even in the laboratory. When he returned from his holiday, Pasteur resumed his studies. He injected some chickens with a culture of bacteria that had been lying around for several weeks. The chickens got sick, but recovered within a few days: apparently, the bacteria had been so weakened that they were no longer fatal.

Pasteur then wanted to inject fresh chickens with fresh bacteria, but his assistant told him—at least according to the script written by Paul de Kruif—that they were low on chickens. So Pasteur injected the remaining fresh chickens and those that had recovered from the mild infection. When the fresh ones died and the recovered ones again recovered, Pasteur realized that he had just accomplished with chicken cholera what Jenner had accomplished with smallpox 100 years earlier. He called the culture containing weakened (attenuated) bacteria *vaccine* and began a largely successful search for similar vaccines against other infectious diseases. Vaccines against swine erysipelas, sheep anthrax, and rabies followed, and with them came the realization that the body, when conditioned in the right way, can defend itself against infectious diseases.

2.4 THE HUMORAL THEORY OF IMMUNITY

Pasteur was too busy chasing germs and producing vaccines to worry about the mechanisms by which those vaccines prevent disease. This area of inquiry he left to his pupils and followers. The first clue to the mechanism of disease prevention came from the studies of Emile Roux and Alexandre J. E. Yersin on diphtheria, a disease that causes the formation of a membrane in the patient's throat (Gr. *diphthera*, skin or leather). *Corynebacterium diphtheriae*, the bacterium causing this disease, always localizes in the diphtheritic membrane and almost never disseminates to other organs. Yet, diphtheric lesions are found in almost all organs, including those in which no *C. diphtheriae* occur. To explain this paradox, Roux and Yersin postulated that bacteria in the throat release a powerful poison, or *toxin*, which spreads throughout the body via the bloodstream, causing the diphtheric lesions. And indeed, when they filtered cultures of *C. diphtheriae* through porcelain filters, which retain bacteria but allow soluble substances to pass through, they observed that animals injected with the filtrate died, although no diphtherial microorganisms could be found in their bodies. Similar toxins were later demonstrated in association with other infectious diseases.

This line of investigation was taken a step further by Emil von Behring and Shibasaburo Kitasato, who injected serum from animals resistant to diphtheria into normal animals and demonstrated that the normal animals became resistant to the disease. Behring and Kitasato concluded, therefore, that the blood (serum) of resistant animals contains a substance, *antitoxin*, that can neutralize the toxic effects of bacteria. This antitoxin is highly specific in that it neutralizes the diphtheria toxin, but not toxins produced by other bacteria.

In 1897 Rudolf Kraus obtained visual proof of the reaction between toxin and antitoxin by demonstrating that a bacterial filtrate became clouded with a precipitate when mixed with serum from immune animals (*immune serum,* or *antiserum*). The antiserum thus contained *precipitins,* substances separating toxins out from a solution. At about the same time, Richard Pfeiffer, Max von Gruber, and Herbert E. Durham discovered that an antiserum reacted not only with bacterial products, but also with the bacteria themselves. Pfeiffer observed that certain antisera dissolve (*lyse*) bacterial cells, and he attributed this reaction to *bacteriolysins*. Gruber and Durham reported that certain other antisera glue (agglutinate) bacteria together, and they attributed this activity to *agglutinins*. A long debate then ensued as to whether antitoxins, precipitins, bacteriolysins, agglutinins, and several other factors discovered later (e.g., opsonins, reagins, and conglutinins) were different forms of the same substance or different substances. This debate was not resolved until 1930, when finally the *unitarian concept* of a single group of substances prevailed. To emphasize the unity of these substances, a single term, *antibodies*, was applied to their various forms. This term was a translation of the German *Antikörper,* first used in 1900 by Karl Landsteiner. Substances stimulating the appearance of antibodies were then designated *antigens* (Gr. *anti*, against, *genès*, born, become).

In 1893 Hans Büchner discovered yet another serum factor—one involved in immune reactions, yet distinct from antibodies. Büchner reported that certain antisera, when fresh, killed (lysed) bacteria, but when heated to 56°C, lost their activity. Two years later, Jules Bordet definitely established the presence of this heat-labile factor by demonstrating that heating of a goat antiserum to *Vibrio cholerae* for one hour at 58°C resulted in the loss of the antiserum's lytic effect. But when Bordet added fresh (normal) serum from nonimmunized guinea pigs to the heated antiserum, he found that the lytic power of the mixture reappeared. He therefore concluded that the goat antiserum contained two kinds of substance: specific, thermostable antibodies and nonspecific (shared by goats and guinea pigs), thermolabile *alexin* (from the Greek "to defend"). The term "alexin" was later replaced by *complement*.

At first, microbiologists believed that antibodies could be generated only against microorganisms, as a part of the host's defense reaction. But toward the end of the nineteenth century, evidence indicating that this concept was incorrect gradually accumulated. At that time several investigators, almost simultaneously, found evidence of antibodies produced against nonmicrobial, totally innocuous substances. In 1898, Jules Bordet obtained antibodies that agglutinated or lysed erythrocytes. Other investigators made antibodies to milk, eggwhite, and many other substances of nonbacterial origin. These results suggested that almost any substance, when introduced in a proper form into the body, could act as an antigen and initiate antibody production. Even more striking was the observation that all of these antibodies seemed to be incredibly specific: antigen X produced an antibody, anti-X, that reacted with X, but not with Y; anti-Y reacted with Y, but not with X or Z, and so forth. Scientists immediately found many ways of using this antibody specificity and thus founded an entirely new science—*serology*, the study of the reaction of serum antibody with antigens. Contemporary immunologists still rely heavily on serology and on reactions mediated by antibodies (*serological reactions*).

2.5 CHEMISTRY OF ANTIBODIES AND ANTIGENS

Once the unitarian hypothesis had been accepted, the main question remaining to be answered was that of the chemical nature of antibodies. Several experiments suggested indirectly that antibodies are proteins, but proof of this thesis required isolation of pure antibodies, which was no easy task. Among the first to succeed were Lloyd D. Felton and G. H. Bailey in 1926. These investigators isolated a substance from pneumococcal bacteria that was a pure polysaccharide without a trace of protein. They then injected this preparation into a horse and obtained antiserum specifically reactive with the polysaccharide. When they added the purified polysaccharide to the antiserum, a precipitate—presumably representing the antigen-antibody complex—fell out from the mixture. When Felton and Bailey isolated the precipitate and analyzed it chemically, they discovered that, in addition to polysaccharide (the antigen), the precipitate contained a large amount of protein inseparable from the antigen. They therefore concluded that the protein was antibody bound to the antigen.

Having established the proteinaceous nature of antibodies, chemistry-oriented immunologists asked another question: what kind of proteins are antibodies? They knew that serum could be separated into two fractions by the addition of neutral salts such as ammonium sulfate. The fraction that precipitated ("salted out'') with addition of ammonium sulfate was termed *globulin* (because it was thought to be related to hemoglobin); the soluble fraction was designated *albumin*, because when heated, it coagulated and hardened into stuff resembling eggwhite, or *album ovi*.

Further fractionation of serum became possible in 1937, when Arne W. Tiselius developed an apparatus in which electric current separated proteins according to their charge. When Tiselius applied this technique of *electrophoresis* to a serum, he not only could separate albumin from globulin, but also split globulin into three fractions, which he designated alpha, beta, and gamma. To determine which of the newly resolved serum fractions contained antibodies, Tiselius joined forces with Elvin A. Kabat. When these two scientists immunized rabbits with ovalbumin, a protein of eggwhite, and subjected the antiserum to electrophoresis, they observed that the antiserum's gamma globulin peak was higher than that of a serum from normal, unimmunized rabbits (see Fig. 6.2). They then added ovalbumin to the antiserum, removed the resultant antigen-antibody precipitate by centrifugation, and put the remaining antiserum into the electrophoretic apparatus. The gamma globulin level was now indistinguishable from that of normal rabbit serum. This experiment proved that antibodies are *gamma globulins*. Later, some investigators found antibody activity in other globulin fractions, but all attempts to find an antibody that is not a globulin have failed. Globulins with antibody activity were designated by J. F. Heremans as *immunoglobulins*.

The most puzzling thing about antibodies is how they manage to distinguish so many antigens with such great specificity. One of the first hypotheses of antibody specificity, which proved to be correct in principle, was advanced in 1900 by Paul Ehrlich. According to Ehrlich, the basis for the specific interaction between antigens and antibodies is the stereoscopic complementarity of the two kinds of molecule. He theorized that the antibody molecule is shaped to fit a particular antigen and only that antigen, like a key that fits only one lock.

Concurrently with the studies on antibodies, progress had also been made in elucidating the nature of antigens. At first, immunologists thought that antigens, like antibodies, could only be proteins. But then, in 1923, Michael Heidelberger and Oswald T. Avery isolated an antigen from the capsules of pneumococci and established that the antigen was a polysaccharide with a high molecular weight. Apparently, antigens could be either proteins or carbohydrates.

The question of what makes a molecule antigenic was investigated by Karl Landsteiner and his collaborators. From 1917 onward, Landsteiner had been attaching small organic molecules, similar to those shown in Figure 10.5, to proteins such as egg albumin and studying the immune response to such conjugates. He demonstrated that the small molecule induced antibodies only when attached to the large one, but once antibodies had been formed, the small molecule, without the assistance of the large one, reacted with them. Landsteiner named the substance that can bind antibodies but cannot induce them *hapten*, and termed the molecule to which the hapten must be attached to stimulate antibody production the *carrier*. By replacing one hapten with another, Landsteiner and his colleagues demonstrated that even a slight change in the molecule could dramatically change its reactivity with specific antibodies.

How do antibodies react with antigens? The most striking visible result of the antigen-antibody reaction is the precipitate formed when an antiserum is mixed with a soluble antigen. Several explanations of how precipitation occurs were offered, but the correct one was suggested by John R. Marrack in 1934. According to Marrack's *lattice theory*, both the antigen and antibody have more than one binding site, so that one antibody molecule can connect itself to more than one antigen molecule and vice versa. A lattice of interlocking aggregate, the precipitate, is thus formed.

As early as 1907, Svante Arrhenius had become so impressed by what chemistry offered to immunology that he suggested a name, *immunochemistry*, denoting a new science combining the two. Thirty years later, when the boom in chemical immunology began, the name was remembered and accepted.

2.6 CELLULAR THEORY OF IMMUNITY

While some microbiologists at the end of the nineteenth century had been collecting evidence that immunity is mediated by soluble substances (antibodies) present in body fluids (*humor*; hence the designation *humoral theory of immunity*), others had been trying to demonstrate that immunity is mediated primarily by cells. The founder of the *cellular theory of immunity* was the Russian zoologist Elie Metchnikoff. According to Metchnikoff, the idea that cells, rather than fluids, protect animal bodies from invaders occurred to him as a sudden inspiration one day when he was observing large, amoeboid, mobile cells—*macrophages*, as he called them—as they moved about in transparent starfish larvae (see Fig. 1.2). Metchnikoff speculated that the macrophages might be ingesting intruders and, to test this idea, he stuck a rose thorn under the skin of a starfish larva. When, the next day, he found the thorn surrounded by macrophages, he considered his theory proved.

The proponents of the cellular theory could not deny the existence of humoral factors, but they argued that the function of antibodies is merely to prepare "food" (the invading microorganisms) for ingestion by macrophages. Their argument was strongly supported by an observation made in 1903 by Almroth E. Wright and Stewart R. Douglas, who developed a simple method for quantitation of phagocytosis. The method consisted of preparing leukocytes from peripheral blood, removing all traces of serum by repeated washing, and mixing the leukocytes with a known number of bacteria. After incubation of the mixture for 30 minutes at 37°C, Wright and Douglas smeared the suspension on a microscope slide, stained the cells, and counted the number of bacteria ingested by individual cells. They noticed that the *phagocytic index*—that is, the average number of bacteria per leukocyte—was always higher when they incubated the suspension in normal serum rather than in physiological salt solution, and still higher when they replaced normal serum with an antiserum. Apparently, normal serum contained a substance enhancing phagocytosis, and the level of this substance increased after immunization. They named this hypothetical substance *opsonin* (from the Greek "to prepare food for") and referred to the enhancement of leukocyte activity as *opsonization*.

The followers of the cellular theory quickly extended the findings of Wright and Douglas by claiming that all antibodies act on a similar principle. In this, however, they were wrong, since opsonins were later found to be a special class of antibody. Nevertheless, the cellular theory was an important contribution to immunology that pointed out the existence of alternatives to humoral immunity. Macrophages indeed carry out immunological functions, but alas, nonspecific ones. However, as was later discovered, other cells, primarily lymphocytes, are involved in defense reactions in quite specific ways.

The idea of lymphocyte involvement in immunity can be traced back to Robert Koch (Fig. 2.1) and his work on tuberculosis (consumption, phthisis). This disease is caused by *Mycobacterium tuberculosis*, a slender, slightly bent or curved bacillus isolated by Koch in 1882. When inhaled, the bacillus settles in the lungs and causes the formation of small nodules, or tubercles, which eventually become necrotic and often calcify. Koch was able to transfer the disease from humans to guinea pigs and, in the process, observed an interesting phenomenon that was later to bear his name. Specifically, when he took guinea pigs that, four to six weeks earlier, had been inoculated with *M. tuberculosis* and reinjected them with the bacillus, he observed that the inoculation site underwent characteristic changes. On the first or second day after inoculation, the area darkened and hardened; on succeeding days, it became necrotic and eventually sloughed off, leaving a shallow ulcer. This *tuberculin reaction* (*Koch phenomenon*) can also be elicited by injecting dead bacilli, concentrated filtrate of the medium in which the bacilli have been grown (the *old tuberculin*, or OT), or a protein precipitated by trichloracetic acid from the medium (*purified protein derivative*, or PPD). Later, when other investigators gathered evidence that a tuberculin-like reaction could also develop in the absence of tuberculosis or any other bacterial disease, a broader term for these reactions was needed. The one eventually adopted was *delayed-type hypersensitivity*, or *DTH*. This term emphasizes the two most conspicuous aspects of the reaction: first, its resemblance to other types of hypersensitivity—a resemblance that later turned out to be spurious, and second, the late onset of the reaction compared to other hypersensitivities (see below). A clue to the nature of DTH came from the study of a different type of hypersensitivity reaction.

Around the turn of the century, several physicians noticed that some patients using drugs such as Salvarsan or Novocain had a reaction characterized by redness of the skin and itching, oozing vesicular lesions that later became scaly or encrusted. Since a similar reaction developed in some patients who had come into contact with a variety of substances—including mercury, poison ivy, cosmetics, or many simple compounds such as picric acid—this condition was termed *contact sensitivity* or *contact dermatitis*. Among those interested in contact sensitivity was Karl Landsteiner, who systematically investigated the reaction, attempting to determine whether antibodies play a role in it. He and Merrill W. Chase sensitized an animal to a particular compound, injected serum from this animal into an untreated one, and tested the new host for contact sensitivity. But they discovered that the reaction could not be transferred in this fashion, and hence that antibodies circulating in the blood did not seem to cause this reaction. However, when they isolated lymphocytes from the sensitive donor animal, the new recipient of the cell suspension became as sensitive as the donor, indicating that contact sensitivity is transferable by cells (lymphocytes).

Landsteiner and Chase published a description of their experiment in 1942. Three years later, they reported that they had been able to transfer the tuberculin reaction in the same way, proving that both delayed hypersensitivity and contact sensitivity are mediated by cells, rather than by circulating antibodies. Cells were also implicated in other types of immune phenomena, particularly in the *allograft reaction*, which we shall discuss later. The study of the cellular mechanisms of immunity became the subject of *cellular immunology*.

2.7 CELLS AND ANTIBODIES

Immunologists knew that antibodies, like all other serum proteins, must be produced by cells, but for a long time the identity of these cells remained unknown. The most likely candidates were macrophages, lymphocytes, and plasma cells, and each of these three cell types was, at one time or another, considered as the source of antibodies. Macrophages were soon excluded, since no *direct* evidence that they produced antibodies could be found. The choice was then between lymphocytes and plasma cells, and there seemed to be evidence supporting the role of both cell types. The issue was resolved in 1948 by Astrid E. Fagraeus, who studied tissue fragments from spleens of immunized rabbits at various intervals during antibody response and found that lymphocytes transform progressively into plasma cells, which then secrete antibodies.

The identification of the antibody-producing cells immediately raised another question: how did plasma cells manage to make antibodies against virtually every conceivable antigen? Many ingenious solutions to this riddle were proposed, but as experimental data accumulated against them each was discounted. Finally, in 1957, F. Macfarlane Burnet proposed a hypothesis that seemed to fit all the new data. A similar hypothesis was proposed independently by David W. Talmage, and Burnet and Talmage had both drawn on ideas developed in 1955 by Niels K. Jerne. Burnet's hypothesis states that an unimmunized individual is a mosaic of lymphocyte clones, with each clone being derived from a single parent cell. Lymphocytes comprising one clone can produce only one kind of antibody (reactive with only one antigen) and they display this type on their surfaces as an antigen receptor. When an antigen enters the body, it is bound by a clone of cells, each cell carrying an antibody specific for this antigen. This binding stimulates the clone, which then expands and begins to secrete the one antibody type. An antigen thus *selects* from a vast variety of lymphocytes a *clone* capable of producing antibodies to this antigen. According to this *clonal selection hypothesis*, clonal diversification occurs during the latter part of fetal development, through somatic mutation of immunoglobulin genes. Clones expressing antibodies to antigens present in the fetus (self molecules) are arrested in their development and eliminated, so that an individual normally does not develop immunity against its own tissues. Foreign antigens introduced artificially into the fetus at the time of clonal diversification trick the immune system into recognizing them as self molecules and make the individual *tolerant* of them.

The clonal selection hypothesis made two main predictions, both of which were confirmed experimentally. The first prediction—that antibodies would be found on the surface of normal lymphocytes—was confirmed by the *immunofluorescence technique*, developed in 1941 by Albert H. Coons. This confirmation consisted of producing antibodies to immunoglobulins isolated from the serum (in other words, obtaining antibodies against antibodies), tagging them with fluorescein isocyanate (a compound emitting fluorescent light when irradiated with ultraviolet rays), and then demonstrating that the labeled antibodies bind to the surface of certain lymphocytes.

The second prediction of the clonal selection hypothesis was that an individual would be tolerant of nonself molecules to which it had been exposed as a fetus. In fact, evidence for this thesis existed *before* the clonal selection hypothesis had been formulated. In 1945, Ray D. Owen reported that many nonidentical cattle twins are chimeras—that is, each twin has a small number of blood cells from its sibling in its bloodstream. The explanation for this finding was provided by the discovery that nonidentical cattle twins, unlike human twins, share a common placenta, by way of which blood cells from the two fetuses often mix (Fig. 2.2). Using Owen's findings, Burnet then argued that adult twins are able to tolerate each other's blood cells because of their having been mixed during the fetal stage.

An artificial induction of immunological tolerance was first accomplished in 1953 by Peter B. Medawar and his colleagues, and by Milan Hašek. Medawar, Rupert E. Billingham, and Leslie Brent injected spleen cells of mouse strain X into newborn mice of strain Y and then demonstrated that the adult Y-strain mice tolerated X-strain skin grafts, while untreated Y mice re-

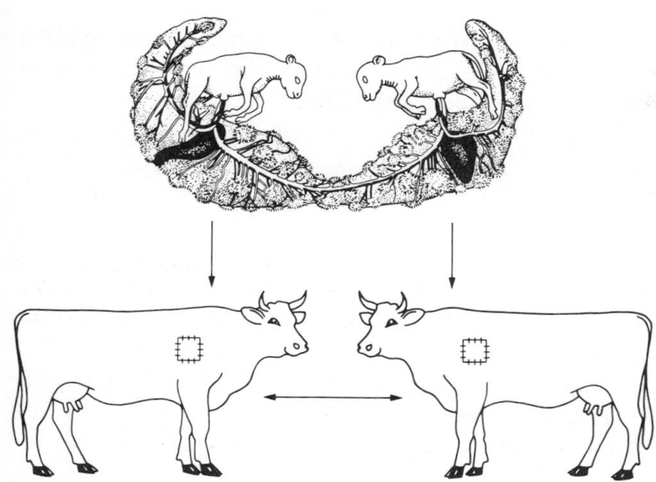

Figure 2.2. Nonidentical cattle embryos sharing a common placenta (top). Skin grafts exchanged between the adults are mutually accepted (bottom), indicating that the animals are chimeras as a result of blood mixing in embryonic life.

jected them. Hašek joined the circulatory systems of two chicken embryos in their corresponding eggs, and proved that the hatched birds were chimeras—similar to Owen's cattle chimeras—that tolerated each other's tissues. In both instances, exposure of a newborn animal or an embryo to foreign tissue elicited immunological tolerance to this tissue, as predicted by Burnet's hypothesis.

2.8 THE TWO ARMS OF IMMUNITY

By the 1950s, immunologists generally accepted the idea that there are two types of immune reaction in mammals: humoral reactions mediated by antibodies, and cellular reactions mediated primarily by macrophages and lymphocytes. But since antibodies are also produced by lymphocytes (or, more precisely, by their progeny, the plasma cells), an important question remained: what is the relationship between the lymphocytes involved in the two types of immune response? Are the lymphocytes responsible for cellular immunity different from those involved in humoral response—or is there only one type of lymphocyte that responds differently, depending upon the nature of the stimulus? The answers to these questions emerged only after immunologists had assimilated and comprehended several seemingly unrelated observations.

The first observation concerned a tiny pouch, the *bursa of Fabricius*, that opens into the posterior (cloacal) portion of the digestive tract of birds. Since the discovery of this gland by the sixteenth-century Paduan anatomist Hieronymus Fabricius Aquapendente, zoologists had tried to discover its function, but it was not until 1956 that one of them, Bruce Glick, finally succeeded. Glick sought a clue to the bursa's function by removing it surgically and observing the effect of this *bursectomy* upon birds, but as far as he could ascertain, the birds remained normal. But then the Three Princes of Serendip intervened. Unaware that the birds had been bursectomized, Glick's colleague, Timothy S. Chang, used some of them in a class demonstration of antibody formation. To Chang's great embarrassment, the demonstration failed, for the chickens did not respond to the inoculated antigen. When Glick heard about this incident and realized that these were the birds that had been bursectomized, he suspected that the bursa might be involved in antibody synthesis. Later research proved him right: the avian bursa *is* essential to antibody production.

Six years after the publication of Glick's and Chang's finding, Noel L. Warner, Aleksander Szenberg, and F. Macfarlane Burnet discovered that bursectomized chickens reject skin grafts as rapidly as do sham-operated birds. (The term refers to the practice of operating on an animal to produce a surgical trauma comparable to that in the experimental—in this case, bursectomized—animals, thereby providing further control over variables.) It thus became clear that whatever effect the bursa had on immunity, it concerned the humoral and not the cellular reaction. (Although mammals have no bursa of Fabricius, they presumably possess an organ that acts as a bursa equivalent.)

The second important observation pertaining to the relationship between humoral and cellular immunity was made on mammalian thymus, an organ that—like the bursa—had puzzled zoologists since its discovery in 1522 by Jacopo Berengario da Carpi. At first, many zoologists thought that the thymus was an endocrine (hormone-secreting) gland; but when the organ was found to contain lymphocytes, immunologists claimed it as their province. Increasingly, it was suspected that the thymus might be involved in antibody synthesis, but when it was removed surgically, ambiguous results were obtained: sometimes this thymectomy depressed antibody response; at other times it seemed to have no effect. It was not until 1961 that two investigators, Jacques F. A. P. Miller and Robert A. Good, thought of thymectomizing animals at birth and testing their immunological capacity by grafting foreign skin to them.

This time the results were quite unambiguous: the grafts survived much longer on thymectomized animals than on sham-operated controls. Miller, Good, and their colleagues concluded that the mammalian thymus is somehow involved in cellular immunity.

When combined, these two sets of experiments pointed to a dichotomy in the immune system wherein the bursa influences antibody response and the thymus influences cellular reactions. This dichotomy was further indicated by a third set of observations made on human patients by Ogden C. Bruton, Robert A. Good, Angelo M. DiGeorge, and others. These investigators described a whole spectrum of diseases affecting the immune system of the human. The interesting point is that some of these *immunodeficiency diseases* affected only humoral immunity, leaving cellular immunity intact, whereas others impaired primarily cellular immunity, affecting humoral immunity only moderately. Moreover, impairment of cellular immunity usually occurred together with a defect in the development of the thymus.

The realization that cellular and humoral immunity are governed by different organs led some immunologists to speculate that there are two different kinds of lymphocyte—one processed by the bursa and involved primarily in humoral immunity, and the other processed by the thymus and involved primarily in cellular immunity. Experimental evidence supporting this concept of lymphocyte duality was provided by William A. Ford, James E. Till, Ernest A. McCulloch, James L. Gowans, Malcolm A. S. Moore, and John J. T. Owen, who devised ingenious ways of tagging lymphocytes with visible markers and using these markers to follow the lymphocytes as they traveled through the body. These investigators observed that there are indeed two pathways of lymphocyte development: one passes through the thymus and leads to *thymus-derived lymphocytes,* or *T cells,* and the other passes through the bursa, leading to *bursa-derived lymphocytes,* or *B cells*.

There remained but one observation that did not fit into this division-of-labor scheme of the immune system: neonatal thymectomies *did* suppress antibody response to certain antigens. But this odd bit of information was finally fit into the jigsaw puzzle when Henry N. Claman, Anthony J. S. Davies, Graham F. Mitchell, and Jacques F. A. P. Miller demonstrated that certain T cells assist in the transformation of B lymphocytes into plasma cells, thereby enhancing antibody response. Thus, removal of the thymus not only inhibits cellular immunity, but depresses antibody response by preventing helper T cells from maturing.

This revised two-arm concept of the immune system has been widely accepted, and has become the cornerstone of cellular immunology.

2.9 THE DISCOVERY OF INJURIOUS ANTIBODIES

Until the end of the nineteenth century, most immunologists were convinced that antibodies always protect and never injure the body that produces them. The first indication that this concept might be fallacious came from the studies of Paul J. Portier and Charles R. Richet on the reaction of dogs to certain animal venoms. We will let Richet tell his own story.

> In tropical waters, *Coelenterata* are to be found floating on the surface, also known as *Physalia* (Portuguese galleys). The basic structure of these creatures is a pocket filled with air so that they can float like a bladder. A bucco-anal cavity is subjoined to this pocket, with very long tentacles which hang in the water. These feelers sometimes run to two or three meters long and are equipped with small devices which adhere like sucking cups to objects encountered. Within each of these innumerable suction-cups is a pin-point which drives into the foreign body that is being touched. At the same time, this pin-point causes penetration of a subtle but strong poison, which is contained in the tentacles, so that contact with a feeler of the *Physalia* is tantamount to a multiple injection of poison. On touching a *Physalia* an acute sensation of pain is felt immediately, due to the penetration of this liquid venom. This is similar in relative intensity to a swimmer's mishap when he bumps into a jelly-fish in the water.
>
> During a cruise on the yacht of Prince Albert of Monaco, the Prince advised me to study *Physalia* poison, together with our friends Georges Richard and Paul Portier. We found that it is easily dissolved in glycerol and that by injecting this glycerol solution, the symptoms of *Physalia* poisoning are reproduced.
>
> When I came back to France and had no more *Physalia* to study, I hit upon the idea of making a comparative study of the tentacles of the *Actinia* (*Actinia equina, Anemone sulcata*) which can be obtained in large quantities, for *Actinia* abound on all the rocky shores of Europe.
>
> Now *Actinia* tentacles, treated with glycerol, give off their poison into the glycerol and the extract is toxic. I therefore set about finding how toxic it was, with Portier. This was quite difficult to do, as it is a slowly acting poison and three or four days must elapse before it can be known if the dose be fatal or not. I was using a solution of one kilo of glycerol to one

> kilo of tentacles. The lethal dose was of the order of 0.1 liquid per kilo live weight of subject.
>
> But certain of the dogs survived, either because the dose was not strong enough or for some other reason. At the end of two, three, or four weeks, as they seemed normal, I made use of them for a new experiment.
>
> An unexpected phenomenon arose, which we thought extraordinary. A dog when injected previously even with the smallest dose, say of 0.005 liquid per kilo, immediately showed serious symptoms: vomiting, blood diarrhoea, syncope, unconsciousness, asphyxia, and death. This basic experiment was repeated at various times and by 1902 we were able to state three main factors: (1) a subject that had a previous injection is far more sensitive than a new subject; (2) that the symptoms characteristic of the second injection, namely swift and total depression of the nervous system, do not in any way resemble the symptoms characterizing the first injection; (3) a three or four week period must elapse before the anaphylactic state results. This is the period of incubation.[5]

Richet and Portier called the new phenomenon *anaphylaxis*, meaning a state in which an organism is rendered hypersensitive, instead of being protected (Gr. *phylaxis*, protection; anaphylaxis is therefore the opposite of protection).

In 1907, five years after the discovery of anaphylaxis, Richet established that the anaphylactic state could be transferred to untreated dogs with serum from anaphylactic animals, indicating that the reaction is mediated by humoral factors. Evidence that these factors are probably antibodies was provided by William H. Schultz and Henry H. Dale. In an attempt to demonstrate anaphylaxis in vitro, these investigators isolated strips of the small intestine, uterus, and heart from anaphylactic animals, and after removing all the blood, suspended these strips in an isotonic solution. When they added the sensitizing antigen to the solution, the smooth muscle in these organs contracted, a phenomenon now referred to as the *Schultz-Dale reaction.* Schultz and Dale drew two conclusions from their experiment: first, since anaphylaxis depends on the presence of an antigen and since it is specific (antigens unrelated to the sensitizing antigen do not elicit contraction), it must be triggered by an antigen-antibody interaction; and second, since washing of the organs by forcing fluids through them (perfusion) does not remove the antibodies, the latter must be bound to the tissues.

[5] Nobel Lecture, December 11, 1913.

In 1911, Dale and Patrick P. Laidlaw obtained an important clue concerning the mechanism of anaphylaxis by demonstrating that histamine—an amine that Dale had isolated previously from ergot (a fungus growth on cereal grains)—causes contraction of smooth muscles when used in vitro and symptoms resembling anaphylactic shock when administered intravenously to an animal. Dale and Laidlaw therefore suggested that histamine or a histamine-like substance might be involved in the anaphylactic reaction. Later, histamine was indeed isolated from animal tissues, and in 1953 it was shown by James F. Riley to be stored predominantly in mast cells.

Mast cells were described in 1877 by Paul Ehrlich, who, while testing new aniline dyes for use in histological techniques, discovered that certain connective tissue cells contain large granules that have a tendency to alter the shade of the dyes (an effect called metachromasia). Since such cells are more numerous in the connective tissue of well-fed animals, Ehrlich called them *Mastzellen* (well-fed cells). The function of mast cells remained unknown, but Riley's discovery suggested that they might be involved in anaphylaxis.

On another front, gradual progress in characterizing the mysterious anaphylactic antibodies, referred to as *reagins*, had been made. Several investigators had established that reagins indeed differ from other antibodies in that they can bind firmly to tissues, specifically to mast cells. At last the pieces of the puzzle began to fall into place and an understanding of the anaphylactic mechanism emerged.

During the sensitization period, specific reaginic antibodies are produced, which attach themselves firmly to mast cells. Upon restimulation, the antigen binds to the fixed antibodies, initiating reactions leading to degranulation (loss of granules) of mast cells and release of pharmacologically active substances such as histamine. These substances then cause capillary dilation, an increase in capillary permeability, contraction of smooth muscle, an increase in gastric secretion, and a generalized *anaphylactic shock*.

In 1921, Carl W. Prausnitz and Heinz Küstner described a new type of anaphylactic reaction referred to as *cutaneous anaphylaxis*. The discovery came about as follows. One day Küstner, a prominent German gynecologist, complained to Prausnitz about an affliction he had been suffering since the age of six. Every time he ate the merest trace of fish, he began to sneeze, cough, and vomit, his whole body started to itch, and his skin became covered with small wheals. After about ten or 12 hours, the symptoms disappeared and he felt good again. Prausnitz thought that his colleague's sufferings resembled the symptoms of an anaphylactic reaction, and decided to test this diagnosis by injecting Küstner's serum and a fish extract into his own skin. Within a few seconds, the test area had become hot, red, and softly swollen. The reaction reached a maximum after about 15 minutes, and then began to fade away. In this uncomplicated experiment, Prausnitz established two things: first, he found conditions in which anaphylaxis can occur locally in the skin (hence the name cutaneous anaphylaxis), and second, he developed a simple procedure that can be used for detecting food hypersensitivities. The procedure later became known as the *Prausnitz-Küstner*, or *P-K*, *test*.

Between 1903 and 1905, N. Maurice Arthus, Clemens P. von Pirquet, and Bela Schick discovered another category of reactions they believed to be anaphylactic. Arthus injected normal horse serum, 5 ml every six days, under the skin of a rabbit and observed that after the first three injections, the inoculum formed a bleb, which spread so rapidly that after one or two hours the injection site looked almost like normal skin. But after a fourth injection, rather than fading, the bleb rapidly became more conspicuous, developing within from 10 to 30 minutes into a pronounced swelling (edema), that reached its maximum within two to four hours. The swelling later reddened and became hemorrhagic and necrotic. Still later, the black crust covering the wound fell off and the wound healed. This phenomenon was named, after its discoverer, the *Arthus reaction*.

Pirquet and Schick observed a peculiar illness in some patients who had been treated with antibacterial serum made in another species (for example, horse antidiphtheria serum). This illness, which they called *serum sickness*, appears after an eight- to 12-day latent period, and is characterized by transient skin eruptions (urticaria), fever, swelling, and frequently, lymph node enlargement. In a few days, these symptoms vanish and patients recover completely. Pirquet and Schick thought serum sickness to be related to anaphylaxis, but we now know that both the Arthus reaction and serum sickness develop through a different mechanism. However, anaphylaxis, the Arthus reaction, and serum sickness have one common characteristic—an increased sensitivity (instead of resistance) to the inducing agent. For this reason these illnesses are classified as *hypersensitivities*, and since they develop shortly after injection of a challenging antigen, are referred to as *immediate hypersensitivities* (as opposed to delayed hypersensitivities). Pirquet believed that immunity and hypersensitivity are opposite forms of the same phenomenon and in 1906 suggested that this phenomenon be designated *allergy* (from the Greek *allos*, other, and *ergon*, action). The word "allergy" gradually became synonymous with hypersensitivity.

Investigations into the mechanism of hypersensitivity opened up a new field of study, *immunopathology*, a science dealing with the tissue-damaging effects of immune reactions.

2.10 ANTIBODIES AND GENES

The last chapter in the history of modern immunology starts at the beginning of this century. At that time, immunologists had discovered that antibodies can be made not only to pathogenic microorganisms, but also to many innocuous particles—to erythrocytes, for example. Some immunologists even found antibodies to erythrocytes in the blood of normal, unimmunized individuals. The origin of such antibodies was a much-debated question, but most immunologists believed that the antibodies were relics of past encounters with infectious microorganisms. Among those who investigated hemagglutinating antibodies on this premise was Karl Landsteiner, who soon discovered that hemagglutinins present in human sera have nothing to do with disease, since they appear in the blood of perfectly normal individuals with no history of infectious diseases. At the same time, there seemed to be certain regularities in the way that sera of certain individuals agglutinated erythrocytes of other individuals. By testing a large number of blood samples, Landsteiner demonstrated in 1901 that humans can be divided into three groups: A, B, and C. Sera of individuals belonging to group A agglutinate erythrocytes of other group-A and of group-C individuals; group-B sera agglutinate group-A, but not other group-B and group-C erythrocytes; and group-C sera agglutinate both group-A and group-B erythrocytes, but not other group-C erythrocytes. (The designation of the third group, C, was later changed to O, to indicate that if an individual is not of group A or B, he is of no—zero—group.) Later, several investigators discovered a fourth group of individuals (AB), whose sera fail to agglutinate erythrocytes of the remaining three groups, but whose erythrocytes are agglutinated by sera of individuals possessing any of these groups.

Landsteiner's work produced several results. First, it confirmed an earlier observation that antibodies can be present in the serum of individuals who have not been intentionally immunized. Such antibodies are sometimes referred to as *natural*. Second, it confirmed the existence of antibodies distinguishing individuals of the same species. Bordet had previously referred to such antibodies as *isoantibodies* or *isohemagglutinins*; however, a more proper designation is *alloantibodies* and *allohemagglutinins*. The antigens with which alloantibodies react are referred to as *alloantigens*. Third, Landsteiner's definition of *blood groups* made possible a more rational and less risky blood exchange (transfusion) among humans. Until then, the consequences of blood transfusion had been totally unpredictable. Finally, the stability of human blood groups during an individual's life suggested that the groups might be inherited and, as such, useful for the resolution of paternity disputes. The mode of inheritance of the ABO blood groups was firmly established in 1910 by Emil von Dungern and Ludwik Hirszfeld.

The increasing importance of blood grouping in medicine led to a search for more blood groups in humans and animals. This search, in turn, made geneticists aware of the possibilities that immunological methods had to offer for the study of inheritance. The encroachment of immunology upon the territory of genetics eventually resulted in the creation of a new scientific discipline, designated by M. Robert Irwin in 1936 *immunogenetics*.

One of the investigators searching for blood groups in animals was Peter A. Gorer, who worked with mice. Gorer chose the mouse for two reasons. First, it was one of the few species in which inbred strains (that is, lines of genetically identical animals) were available. Such lines were developed by Clarence C. Little, Leonell C. Strong, Walter E. Heston, Jacob Furth, and others. Second, Gorer was interested in genes controlling tumor growth, and most of the work on such genes had been done with mice.

In the first quarter of this century, Carl O. Jensen, Leo Loeb, Ernest E. Tyzzer, and Clarence C. Little established that a tumor from one individual can be transplanted successfully to another individual, provided the two individuals have certain matching genes. The number of these susceptibility genes varies according to the tumor (and the host) used. In some instances, up to 15 susceptibility genes determine whether a given tumor will grow, while in other instances there are only two or three such genes. Little's work suggested that the same genes determine whether *any* transplant, not just a tumor, is accepted by a host; the genes thus appeared to control tissue compatibility in general.

Gorer thought that some of these genes might be related to blood-group genes, but to test his idea he first had to describe blood groups of the mouse. Eventually, he succeeded in identifying four such groups, which he designated I through IV. One of these, group II, proved to be identical to a gene controlling tumor growth and tissue compatibility in general. And so, when George D. Snell later designated the genes determining the outcome of tissue transplantation (normal and malignant) as *histocompatibility genes,* Gorer agreed to change the designation of this blood-group gene to *histocompatibility-2,* or *H-2*. Gorer's, and later Snell's, work established that histocompatibility genes control tissue compatibility by coding for antigens that differ among individuals of the same species. Thus, when a tissue (a tumor, piece of skin, or blood cells) is transplanted from one individual to another, the antigens of the allograft elicit an immune response in the host, leading to the rejection of the transplant.

The nature of this *allograft reaction* was elucidated by Peter B. Medawar and N. Avrion Mitchison. Medawar and his co-workers pointed out that the reaction resembles delayed-type hypersensitivity, and Mitchison proved that immunity to allografts can be transferred, as delayed-type hypersensitivity can, to another animal with lymphocytes, but not with serum. Because of this latter finding, allograft reaction to histocompatibility antigens was classified as a cellular immune reaction.

Gorer and Snell later demonstrated that *H-2* is unique among histocompatibility genes in that it is complex (consists of several closely linked genes) and has a major effect on graft rejection. When still later, Jean Dausset, Jon J. van Rood, and Rose Payne discovered a similar gene complex in the human, and other investigators described homologous genetic systems in other species, the term *major histocompatibility complex,* or *MHC,* was applied to these systems. Numerous discoveries have shown that the MHC is closely tied to immune response and that, in addition to its involvement in graft rejection, it plays a major role in the immune processes of various organisms. The investigation of the MHC's role in immunity has become one of the most exciting endeavors in modern immunology.

2.11 EPILOGUE

Reading this chapter, the reader has probably gotten the impression that the history of immunology is a succession of brilliant discoveries fitting together like pieces of a puzzle, the design of which was known in advance. Nothing could be further from the truth. In reality, the progress of the science has been slow and tortuous. There have been periods during which all the carefully accumulated data seemingly contradicted each other, all was confusion, and nobody seemed to know what to do next. There have been blind alleys, irreproducible results, erroneously interpreted data, and misleading experiments. There have been controversies, skirmishes—yes, even battles in which great salvos were fired by the opposing sides. Even breakthroughs, when they came, did not appear out of the clear blue sky; the groundwork had been laid by slight advances and numerous bits of seemingly unimportant information. Often, some investigators came close to the solution, only to lose to those more fortunate by a matter of months, or even weeks—the Scotts and Amundsens in their race to the South Pole.

In writing this chapter, I have truncated the history of immunology, choosing only the discoveries that lay along a straight line and ignoring the dead ends, controversies, false ideas, and scraps of preliminary information. Had I not done so, I would still be sitting in my study, writing.

2.12 APPENDIX 2.1: CHRONOLOGICAL LIST OF MAJOR EVENTS IN THE HISTORY OF IMMUNOLOGY (*WITH REFERENCE NUMBERS*)

Year	Investigator and Event	Reference Number
1798	Edward Jenner Smallpox vaccination	48
1862	Ernst Haeckel Phagocytosis	41
1877	Paul Ehrlich Mast cells	25
1879	Louis Pasteur Attenuation of chicken cholera bacteria	75
1883	Elie Metchnikoff Cellular theory of immunity	64
1885	Louis Pasteur Rabies vaccination	76
1888	Pierre P. E. Roux and Alexandre J. E. Yersin Bacterial toxins	87
1888	George H. F. Nuttall Bactericidal action of blood	68
1890	Emil von Behring and Shibasaburo Kitasato Antitoxins	7
1891	Robert Koch Delayed-type hypersensitivity	51
1893	Hans Büchner Inactivation of antisera by heating	12
1894	Richard Pfeiffer Bacteriolysis	78
1895	Jules Bordet Complement and antibody activities in bacteriolysis	9
1896	Max von Gruber and Herbert E. Durham Specific agglutination	40
1896	Georges F. I. Widal and Arthur Sicard Test for the diagnosis of typhoid (Widal test) on the basis of the Gruber-Durham reaction	96
1897	Rudolf Kraus Precipitation test	52
1900	Paul Ehrlich Theory of antibody formation	26
1901	Jules Bordet and Octave Gengou Complement-fixation reaction	10
1901	Karl Landsteiner A, B, and O blood groups	54
1901–1908	Carl O. Jensen and Leo Loeb Transplantable tumors	49, 60
1902	Paul J. Portier and Charles R. Richet Anaphylaxis	82
1903	N. Maurice Arthus Specific necrotic lesions; Arthus phenomenon	2
1903	Almroth E. Wright and Stewart R. Douglas Opsonization reactions	98
1904	F. Obermeyer and E. P. Pick Altered protein antigens	69
1905	Clemens P. von Pirquet and Bela Schick Serum sickness	80
1906	Clemens P. von Pirquet Introduction of the term *allergy*	79

Year	Investigator and Event	Reference Number
1907	Svante Arrhenius Introduction of the term *immunochemistry*	1
1910	William H. Schultz and Henry H. Dale Schultz-Dale test for anaphylaxis	88
1910	Emil von Dungern and Ludwik Hirszfeld Inheritance of ABO blood groups	23
1910	F. Peyton Rous Viral immunology	86
1911	Henry H. Dale and Patrick P. Laidlaw Allergic contraction of muscle by histamine	19
1914	Clarence C. Little Genetics theory of tumor transplantation	59
1915–1920	Leonell C. Strong, Clarence C. Little, and others Inbred mouse strains	91
1917	Karl Landsteiner Haptens	55
1921	Carl W. Prausnitz and Heinz Küstner Cutaneous reactions	83
1923	Michael Heidelberger and Oswald T. Avery Polysaccharides as antigens	43
1924	L. Aschoff Reticuloendothelial system	3
1926	Lloyd D. Felton and G. H. Bailey Isolation of pure antibody preparation	30
1929	Michael Heidelberger and Forrest E. Kendall Quantitative chemical serology	44
1934–1938	John R. Marrack Antigen-antibody reaction	61
1936	M. Robert Irwin and Leon J. Cole Introduction of the term *immunogenetics*	45
1936	Peter A. Gorer Identification of the H-2 antigen	36
1939	Arne W. Tiselius and Elvin A. Kabat Demonstration of antibodies as gamma globulins	93
1940	Karl Landsteiner and Alexander S. Wiener Discovery of Rh antigens	56
1941	Albert H. Coons and others Immunofluorescence	18
1942	Jules T. Freund and Katherine McDermott Adjuvants	32
1942	Karl Landsteiner and Merrill W. Chase Cellular transfer of sensitivity in guinea pigs	57
1942–1949	Lloyd D. Felton Immunological unresponsiveness	31, 29
1944	Peter B. Medawar Immunological theory of allograft reaction	63
1945	Ray D. Owen Vascular anastomoses between bovine twins	74
1945	Merrill W. Chase Cellular transfer of hypersensitivity to tuberculin	15
1945	Robin R. A. Coombs, A. E. Mourant, and R. R. Race Antiglobulin test	17
1946	Jacques Oudin Precipitin reaction in gels	71
1948–1949	Örjan Ouchterlony and Stephen D. Elek Double diffusion of antigens and antibodies in gels	70, 27
1948	Astrid E. Fagraeus Demonstration of antibody formation by plasma cells	28
1948	George D. Snell Congenic mouse lines	90
1949	F. Macfarlane Burnet and Frank Fenner Theory of acquired immunological tolerance	14

Appendix 2.1 (*Continued*)

Year	Investigator and Event	Reference Number
1950	Richard K. Gershon and K. Kondo Discovery suppressor T cells	33
1952	Ogden C. Bruton Agammaglobulinemia in humans	11
1953	Morten Simonsen and W. J. Dempster Graft-versus-host reaction	89, 22
1953	James F. Riley and Geoffrey B. West Histamine in mast cells	84
1953	Rupert E. Billingham, Leslie Brent, Peter B. Medawar, and Milan Hašek Immunological tolerance	8, 42
1955	Pierre Grabar and Curtis A. Williams, Jr. Immunoelectrophoresis	38
1955–1959	Niels K. Jerne, David W. Talmage, and F. Macfarlane Burnet Clonal selection theory	50, 13, 92
1956	Jacques Oudin and R. Grubb Allotypy	39, 72
1956	Bruce Glick, Timothy S. Chang, and R. G. Jaap Involvement of bursa of Fabricius in antibody response	34
1957	Ernest Witebsky and his colleagues Induction of autoimmunity in animals	97
1957	Alick Isaacs and Jean Lindenmann Interferon	46
1958–1962	Jean Dausset, Jon J. van Rood, and Rose Payne Human leukocyte antigens	20, 85, 77
1959–1962	Rodney R. Porter, Gerald M. Edelman, and others Structure of antibody molecules	81, 24
1959	James L. Gowans and others Lymphocyte circulation	37
1960	Rosalyn S. Yalow and Solomon A. Berson Radioimmunoassay	99
1961–1962	Jacques F. A. P. Miller, Robert A. Good, and others Involvement of thymus in cellular immunity	65, 35
	Noel L. Warner, Aleksander Szenberg, and F. Macfarlane Burnet Dissociation of cellular and humoral reactions	95
1963	Jacques Oudin, Henry G. Kunkel, and others Idiotypy	73, 53
1963	Baruj Benacerraf, Hugh O. McDevitt, and others Immune reponse genes	58, 62
1964	Barbara Bain and her co-workers, Fritz H. Bach, and Kurt Hirschhorn Mixed lymphocyte reaction	6, 4
1964–1968	Anthony J. S. Davies, Henry N. Claman, Jacques F. A. P. Miller, Graham F. Mitchell, and others T-B cell cooperation	21, 16, 66
1965	Thomas B. Tomasi and his colleagues Secretory immunoglobulins	94
1967	Kimishige Ishizaka and Teruko Ishizaka Identification of IgE as the reaginic antibody	47
1970	N. Avrion Mitchison, Klaus Rajewsky, and R. B. Taylor Carrier effect	67
1971	Donald W. Bailey Recombinant inbred strains	5
1974	Rolf M. Zinkernagel and Peter C. Doherty MHC restriction	100

2.13 APPENDIX 2.2: NOBEL PRIZES FOR IMMUNOLOGICAL RESEARCH

Year	Name	Country	Prize for
1901	Emil von Behring	Germany	Serum therapy
1905	Robert Koch	Germany	Tuberculosis research
1908	Paul Ehrlich	Germany	Work on immunity
	Elie Metchnikoff	Russia	Work on phagocytosis
1913	Charles R. Richet	France	Discovery of anaphylaxis
1919	Jules Bordet	Belgium	Discovery of complement
1930	Karl Landsteiner	U.S.A.	Discovery of human blood groups
1951	Max Theiler	South Africa	Yellow fever vaccine
1957	Daniel Bovet	Italy	Antihistamine research
1960	F. Macfarlane Burnet	Australia	Discovery of immunologic tolerance
	Peter B. Medawar	Great Britain	
1972	Gerald M. Edelman	U.S.A.	Research on immunoglobin
	Rodney R. Porter	Great Britain	
1977	Rosalyn S. Yalow	U.S.A.	Development of radioimmunoassay
1980	George D. Snell	U.S.A.	Work on the major
	Jean Dausset	France	histocompatibility complex
	Baruj Benacerraf	U.S.A.	

REFERENCES

General

Bulloch, W.: *The History of Bacteriology*. Oxford University Press, London, 1938.

Collard, P.: *The Development of Microbiology*. Cambridge University Press, Cambridge, 1976.

Kruif, P., de: *Microbe Hunters*. Harcourt, Brace, and World, New York, 1953.

Landsteiner, K.: *The Specificity of Serological Reactions*, rev. ed. Dover, New York, 1962.

Lechevalier, H. A. and Solotorovsky, M.: *Three Centuries of Microbiology*. Dover, New York, 1974.

Metchnikoff, E.: *L'Immunité dans les Maladies Infectieuses*. Masson, Paris, 1901.

Metchnikoff, E.: *Lectures on the Comparative Pathology of Inflammation*. Dover, New York, 1968.

Parish, H. F.: *A History of Immunization*. Livingstone, Edinburgh, 1965.

Original Articles[6]: The 100 Classical Papers

Arrhenius, S.: *Immunochemistry*. Macmillan, New York, 1907. (1)

Arthus, N. M.: Injections répétées de sérum de cheval chez le lapin. *C. R. Soc. Biol. (Paris)* **55**:817–820, 1903. (2)

Aschoff, L.: Das reticulo-endotheliale System. *Ergeb. Inn. Med. Kinderheilkd.* **26**:1–118, 1924. (3)

[6] Numbers in parentheses refer to Appendix 2.1.

Bach, F. and Hirschhorn, K.: Lymphocyte interaction: a potential histocompatibility test *in vitro*. *Science* **143**:813–814, 1964. (4)

Bailey, D. W.: Recombinant-inbred strains, an aid to finding identity, linkage, and function of histocompatibility and other genes. *Transplantation* **11**:325–327, 1971. (5)

Bain, B., Vaz, M. R., and Lowenstein, L.: The development of large immature mononuclear cells in mixed lymphocyte cultures. *Blood* **23**:108–116, 1964. (6)

Behring, E., von and Kitasato, S.: Über das Zustandekommen der Diphtherie-Immunität und der Tetanus-Immunität bei Thieren. *Dtsch. Med. Wochenschr.* **16**:1113–1114, 1890. (7)

Billingham, R. E., Brent, L., and Medawar, P. B.: Actively acquired tolerance of foreign cells. *Nature* **172**:603–606, 1953. (8)

Bordet, J.: Les leucocytes et les propriétés actives du sérum chez les vaccinés. *Ann. Inst. Pasteur* **9**:462–509, 1895. (9)

Bordet, J. and Gengou, O.: Sur l'existence des substances sensibilitrices dans la plupart des sérums antimicrobiens. *Ann. Inst. Pasteur* **15**:289–302, 1901. (10)

Bruton, O. C.: Agammaglobulinemia. *Pediatrics* **9**:722–728, 1952. (11)

Büchner, H.: Ueber Bakteriengifte und Gegengifte. *Münch. Med. Wochenschr.* **40**:449–452, 1893. (12)

Burnet, F. M.: *The Clonal Selection Theory of Acquired Immunity*. Cambridge University Press, London, 1959. (13)

Burnet, F. M. and Fenner, F.: *The Production of Antibodies*. Macmillan, London, 1949. (14)

Chase, M. W.: The cellular transfer of cutaneous hypersensitivity to tuberculin. *Proc. Soc. Biol. Med.* **59**:134–135, 1945. (15)

Claman, H. N., Chaperon, E. A., and Triplett, R. F.: Thymus-marrow cell combinations. Synergism in antibody production. *Proc. Soc. Exp. Biol. Med.* **122**:1167–1171, 1966. (16)

Coombs, R. R. A., Mourant, A. E., and Race, R. R.: A new test for the detection of weak and "incomplete" Rh agglutinins. *Br. J. Exp. Pathol.* **6**:255–266, 1945. (17)

Coons, A. H., Creech, H. J., and Jones, R. N.: Immunological properties of an antibody containing a fluorescent group. *Proc. Soc. Exp. Biol. Med.* **47**:200–202, 1941. (18)

Dale, H. H. and Laidlaw, P. P.: The physiological action of β-iminazolylethylamine. *J. Physiol.* **41**:318–344, 1911. (19)

Dausset, J.: Iso-leuco-anticorps. *Acta Haematol. (Basel)* **20**:156–166, 1958. (20)

Davies, A. J. S., Leuchars, E., Wallis, V., Marchant, R., and Elliott, E. V.: The failure of thymus-derived cells to produce antibody. *Transplantation* **5**:222–231, 1967. (21)

Dempster, W. J.: Kidney homotransplantation. *Br. J. Surg.* **40**:447–465, 1953. (22)

Dungern, E., von and Hirszfeld, L.: Über Vererbung gruppenspezifischer Strukturen des Blutes. *Z. Immunforsch.* **6**:284–292, 1910. (23)

Edelman, G. M.: Dissociation of γ-globulin. *J. Am. Chem. Soc.* **81**:3155–3156, 1959. (24)

Ehrlich, P.: Beitäge zur Kenntnis der Anilinfärbungen und ihrer Verwendung in der mikroskopischen Technik. *Arch. Mikr. Anat.* **13**:263–277, 1877. (25)

Ehrlich, P.: On immunity with special reference to cell life. *Proc. R. Soc. Lond. (Biol)* **66**:424–428, 1900. (26)

Elek, S. D.: The plate virulence test for diphtheria. *J. Clin. Pathol.* **2**:250–258, 1949. (27)

Fagraeus, A.: *Antibody Production in Relation to the Development of Plasma Cells.* Doctoral thesis. Esselte Co., Stockholm, 1948. (28)

Felton, L. D.: The significance of antigen in animal tissues. *J. Immunol.* **61**:107–117, 1949. (29)

Felton, L. D. and Bailey, G. H.: Biologic significance of the soluble specific substances of pneumococci. *J. Inf. Dis.* **38**:131–144, 1926. (30)

Felton, L. D. and Ottinger, B.: Pneumococcus polysaccharide as a paralyzing agent on the mechanism of immunity in white mice. *J. Bacteriol.* **43**:94–95, 1942 (Abstract). (31)

Freund, J. and McDermott, K.: Sensitization to horse serum by means of adjuvants. *Proc. Soc. Exp. Biol. Med.* **49**:548–553, 1942, (32)

Gershon, R. K. and Kondo, K.: Cell interactions in the induction of tolerance: the role of thymic lymphocytes. *Immunology* **18**:723–737, 1970. (33)

Glick, B., Chang, T. S., and Jaap, R. G.: The bursa of Fabricius and antibody production. *Poultry Sci.* **35**:224–225, 1956. (34)

Good, R. A., Dalmasso, A. O., Martinez, C., Archer, O. K., Pierce, J. C., and Papermaster, B. W.: The role of the thymus in development of immunologic capacity in rabbits and mice. *J. Exp. Med.* **116**:773–796, 1962. (35)

Gorer, P. A.: The detection of antigenic differences in mouse erythrocytes by the employment of immune sera. *Br. J. Exp. Pathol.* **17**:42–50, 1936. (36)

Gowans, J. L.: The life history of lymphocytes. *Br. Med. Bull.* **15**:50–53, 1959. (37)

Grabar, P. and Williams, C. A., Jr.: Method of immunoelectrophoretic analysis of mixtures of antigenic substances. *Biochim. Biophys. Acta* **17**:67–74, 1955. (38)

Grubb, R.: Agglutination of erythrocytes coated with "incomplete" anti-Rh by certain rheumatoid arthritis sera and some other sera. *Acta Pathol. Microbiol. Scand.* **39**:195–197, 1956. (39)

Gruber, M., von and Durham, H. E.: Eine neue Methode zur raschen Erkennung des Choleravibrio und des Typhusbacillus. *Münch. Med. Wochenschr.* **43**:285–286, 1896. (40)

Haeckel, E.: *Die Radiolarien. (Rhizopoda Radiaria).* G. Reimer, Berlin, 1862. (41)

Hašek, M.: Parabiosis of birds during embryonic development. *Česk. Biol.* **2**:265–270, 1953. (42)

Heidelberger, M. and Avery, O. T.: The soluble specific substance of Pneumococcus. *J. Exp. Med.* **38**:73–79, 1923. (43)

Heidelberger, M. and Kendall, F. E.: A quantitative study of the precipitin reaction between type III pneumococcus polysaccharide and purified homologous antibody. *J. Exp. Med.* **50**:809–823, 1929. (44)

Irwin, M. R. and Cole, L. J.: Immunogenetic studies of species hybrids in doves and the separation of species-specific substances in the backcross. *J. Exp. Zool.* **73**:85–108, 1936. (45)

Isaacs, A. and Lindenmann, J.: Virus interference. I. The interferon. *Proc. R. Soc. Lond. (Biol.)* **147**:258–267, 1957. (46)

Ishizaka, K. and Ishizaka, T.: Identification of γE antibodies as a carrier of reaginic activity. *J. Immunol.* **99**:1187–1198, 1967. (47)

Jenner, E.: *An Inquiry into the Causes and Effects of the Variolae Vaccinae, a Disease Discovered in Some of the Western Counties of England, Particularly Gloucestershire, and Known by the Name of the Cow Pox.* Sampson Low, Soho, London, 1798. (48)

Jensen, C. O.: Experimentelle Untersuchungen über Krebs bei Mäusen. *Zentralbl. Bakteriol. Parasitol. Infect.* **34**:28–34, 122–143, 1903. (49)

Jerne, N. K.: The natural-selection theory of antibody formation. *Proc. Natl. Acad. Sci. U.S.A.* **41**:849–857, 1955. (50)

Koch, R.: Fortsetzung der Mitteilungen über ein Heilmittel gegen Tuberkulose. *Dtsch. Med. Wochenschr.* **9**:101–102, 1891. (51)

Kraus, R.: Über spezifische Reaktionen in keimfreien Filtraten aus Cholera, Typhus and Pestbouillonculturen, erzeugt durch homologes Serum. *Wien. Klin. Wochenschr.* **10**:736–738, 1897. (52)

Kunkel, H. G., Mannik, M., and Williams, R. C.: Individual antigenic specificity of isolated antibodies. *Science* **140**:1218–1219, 1963. (53)

Landsteiner, K.: Über Agglutinationserscheinungen normalen menschlichen Blutes. *Wien. Klin. Wochenschr.* **14**:1132–1134, 1901. (54)

Landsteiner, K.: Über die Antigeneigenschaften von methyliertem Eiweiss. *Z. Immunforsch.* **26**:122–133, 1917. (55)

Landsteiner, K. and Wiener, A. S.: An agglutinable factor in human blood recognized by immune sera for rhesus blood. *Proc. Soc. Exp. Biol. Med.* **43**:223, 1940. (56)

Landsteiner, K. and Chase, M. W.: Experiments on transfer of cutaneous sensitivity to simple compounds. *Proc. Soc. Exp. Biol. Med.* **49**:688–690, 1942. (57)

Levine, B. B., Ojeda, A., and Benacerraf, B.: Studies on artificial antigens. III. The genetic control of the immune response to hapten poly-L-lysine conjugates in guinea pigs. *J. Exp. Med.* **118**:953–957, 1963. (58)

Little, C. C.: A possible Mendelian explanation for a type inheritance apparently non-Mendelian in nature. *Science* **40**:904–906, 1914. (59)

Loeb, L.: On transplantation of tumors. *J. Med. Res.* **6**:28–39, 1901. (60)

Marrack, J. R.: *The Chemistry of Antigens and Antibodies* MCR Special Report Series, No. 230 (1938) and No. 194 (1934). London: Medical Research Council, 1930. (61)

McDevitt, H. O. and Chinitz, A.: Genetic control of the antibody response: relationship between immune response and histocompatibility (H-2) type. *Science* **163**:1207–1208, 1969. (62)

Medawar, P. B.: The behavior and fate of skin autografts and skin homografts in rabbits. *J. Anat.* **78**:176–199, 1944. (63)

Metchnikoff, E.: Untersuchungen über die intracelluläre Verdauung bei wirbellosen Tieren. *Arb. Zool. Inst. Wien und Zool. Station Triest* **5**:141–168, 1883. (64)

Miller, J. F. A. P.: Immunological function of the thymus. *Lancet* **2**:748–749, 1961. (65)

Mitchell, G. F. and Miller, J. F. A. P.: Immunological activity of thymus and thoracic duct lymphocytes. *Proc. Natl. Acad. Sci. U.S.A.* **59**:296–303, 1968. (66)

Mitchison, N. A., Rajewsky, K., and Taylor, R. B.: Cooperation of antigenic determinants of cells in the induction of antibodies. *In* J. Šterzl and I. Řiha (Eds.): *Developmental Aspects of Antibody Formation and Structure,* Vol. 2, pp. 547–561, Academia, Prague, 1970. (67)

Nutall, G.: Experimente über die bakterienfeindlichen Einflüsse des tierischen Körpers. *Z. Hyg. Infekt. Krankh.* **4**:353–394, 1888. (68)

Obermeyer, F. and Pick, E. P.: Beiträge zur Kenntnisse der Präzipitinbildung. Über den Begriff der Art- und Zustandsspezifizität (originäle und konstitutive Gruppierung) und die Beeinflussung der chemischen Eigenart des Tierkörpers. *Wien. Klin. Wochenschr.* **17**:265–267, 1904. (69)

Ouchterlony, Ö.: In vitro method for testing the toxin-producing capacity of diphtheria bacteria. *Acta Pathol. Microbiol. Scand.* **25**:186–191, 1948. (70)

Oudin, J.: Méthode d'analyze immunochimique par précipitation spécifique en milieu gélifie. *C. R. Acad. Sci. (Paris)* **222**:115–116, 1946. (71)

Oudin, J.: Réaction de précipitation spécifique entre des sérums d'animaux de même espèce. *C. R. Acad. Sci. (Paris)* **242**:2489–2490, 1956. (72)

Oudin, J. and Michel, M.: Une nouvelle forme d'allotypie des globulines du sérum de lapin apparemment liée à la fonction et à la spécificité anticorps. *C. R. Acad. Sci. (Paris)* **257**:805–808, 1963. (73)

Owen, R. D.: Immunogenetic consequences of vascular anastomoses between bovine twins. *Science* **102**:400–401, 1945. (74)

Pasteur, L.: De l'atténuation du virus du choléra des poules. *C. R. Acad. Sci. (Paris)* **91**:673–680, 1880. (75)

Pasteur, L.: Méthode pour prevenir la rage après morsure. *C. R. Acad. Sci. (Paris)* **101**:765–773, 1885. (76)

Payne, R.: The development and persistence of leukoagglutinins in parous women. *Blood* **19**:411–424, 1962. (77)

Pfeiffer, R.: Weitere Untersuchungen über das Wesen der Choleraimmunität und über specifische baktericide Prozesse. *Z. Hyg. Infekt. Krankh.* **18**:1–16, 1894. (78)

Pirquet, C., von: Allergie. *Münch. Med. Wochenschr.* **53**:1457–1458, 1906. (79)

Pirquet, C., von and Schick, B.: *Serum Sickness.* Franz Denticke, Leipzig, 1905. (80)

Porter, R. R.: The hydrolysis of rabbit γ-globulin and antibodies with crystalline papain. *Biochem. J.* **73**:119–126, 1959. (81)

Portier, P. and Richet, C.: De l'action anaphylactique de certains venins. *C. R. Soc. Biol. (Paris)* **54**:170–172, 1902. (82)

Prausnitz, C. and Küstner, H.: Studien über Überempfindlichkeit. *Zentralbl. Bacteriol.* **86**:160–169, 1921. (83)

Riley, J. F. and West, G. B.: The presence of histamine in tissue mast cells. *J. Physiol.* **120**:528–537, 1953. (84)

Rood, J. J., van: *Leucocyte Grouping. A Method and Its Application.* Doctoral thesis. Drukkerij Pasmans, Den Haag, 1962. (85)

Rous, F. P.: A transmissible avian neoplasm (sarcoma of the common fowl). *J. Exp. Med.* **12**:696–704, 1910. (86)

Roux, P. P. E. and Yersin, A. J. E.: Contribution à l'étude de la diphthérie. *Ann. Inst. Pasteur* **2**:629–661, 1888. (87)

Schultz, W. H.: Physiological studies in anaphylaxis. II. 1. Reaction of smooth muscle from guinea pigs rendered tolerant to large doses of serum. *J. Pharmacol.* **2**:221–229, 1910. (88)

Simonsen, M.: Biological incompatibility in kidney transplantation in dogs. *Acta Pathol. Microbiol. Scand.* **32**:36–84, 1953. (89)

Snell, G. D.: Methods for the study of histocompatibility genes. *J. Genet.* **49**:87–108, 1948. (90)

Strong, L. C.: The origin of some inbred mice. *Cancer Res.* **2**:531–539, 1942. (91)

Talmage, D. W.: Immunological specificity. *Science* **129**:1643–1648, 1959. (92)

Tiselius, A. and Kabat, E. A.: An electrophoretic study of immune sera and purified antibody preparations. *J. Exp. Med.* **69**:119–131, 1939. (93)

Tomasi, T. B., Tan, E. M., Solomon, A., and Prendergast, R. A.: Characteristics of an immune system common to certain external secretions. *J. Exp. Med.* **121**:101–124, 1965. (94)

Warner, N. L., Szenberg, A., and Burnet, F. M.: The immunological role of different lymphoid organs in the chicken. I. Dissociation of immunological responsiveness. *Aust. J. Exp. Biol. Med. Sci.* **40**:373–388, 1962. (95)

Widal, G. F. I. and Sicard, A.: Recherches de la réaction agglutinante dans le sang et le sérum desséchés des typhiques et dans la sérosité des vésicatoires. *Bull. Mem. Soc. Med. Hop. Paris* **13**:681–682, 1896. (96)

Witebsky, E., Rose, N. R., Terplan, K., Paine, J. R., and Egan, R. W.: Chronic thyroiditis and autoimmunization. *J. Am. Med. Assoc.* **164**:1439–1447, 1957 (97)

Wright, A. E. and Douglas, S. R.: An experimental investigation of the role of the blood fluids in connection with phagocytosis. *Proc. R. Soc. Lond. (Biol.)* **72**:357–370, 1903. (98)

Yalow, R. S. and Berson, S. A.: Immunoassay of endogenous plasma insulin in man. *J. Clin. Invest.* **39**:1157–1175, 1960. (99)

Zinkernagel, R. M. and Doherty, P. C.: Restriction of *in vitro* T cell-mediated cytotoxicity in lymphocytic choriomeningitis within a syngeneic or semiallogeneic system. *Nature* **248**:701–702, 1974. (100)

THE SECOND MOVEMENT
Structure

CHAPTER 3

THE EXPERIMENTAL ANIMAL

3.1 STRAINS OF EXPERIMENTAL ANIMALS

William Blake's dictum that "the true method of knowledge is experiment" also applies to immunology: experiments and observation are this discipline's primary sources of information. In an experiment, a researcher deliberately sets up conditions that will lead to his obtaining an answer to a particular question. Every so often, however, situations occur naturally that answer a question without the researcher's direct intervention. In these "experiments of nature," the researcher assumes the role of mere observer.

The subject of an experiment or observation is an animal (Fig. 3.1). Some animals are better suited for immunological research than others, and the choice is dictated by the type of question asked. For example, if the question concerns some genetic aspect of immunology, the animal of choice will probably be the mouse, since it breeds rapidly, produces large numbers of progeny, and is genetically well-characterized. The mouse is not, of course, suitable for experiments in which large amounts of material (animal tissue) are needed. A larger animal—the rabbit, for instance—is more appropriate then.

Ideally, in an experiment, all conditions will be constant, excepting one variable related to the question asked. But the main cause of variability in animal experimentation is the animal itself; sex, age, health, genetic background—all of these factors may influence the outcome of an experiment dramatically. For this reason, immunologists prefer to work with animals of known ancestry—that is, with defined *strains* or *lines*. Depending upon their degree of genetic variability, a strain may be one of five kinds—random-bred, inbred, congenic, coisogenic, and recombinant inbred (Fig. 3.2; the last kind is shown in Fig. 3.8). The choice of a particular strain depends on the particular experiment and on the type of question posed. The different strains, their derivations, and examples of their use are described below; the genetic terminology used in this description is explained in the appendix to this chapter.

3.2 RANDOM-BRED STRAINS

A random-bred strain is a group (population) of animals in which an individual of one sex has an equal probability of mating with any individual of the opposite sex. As a result of this *random mating,* no two individuals in the population are genetically the same. This genetic variability usually concerns from 30 to 40 percent of loci; in other words, any two individuals have different alleles at from 30 to 40 percent of their

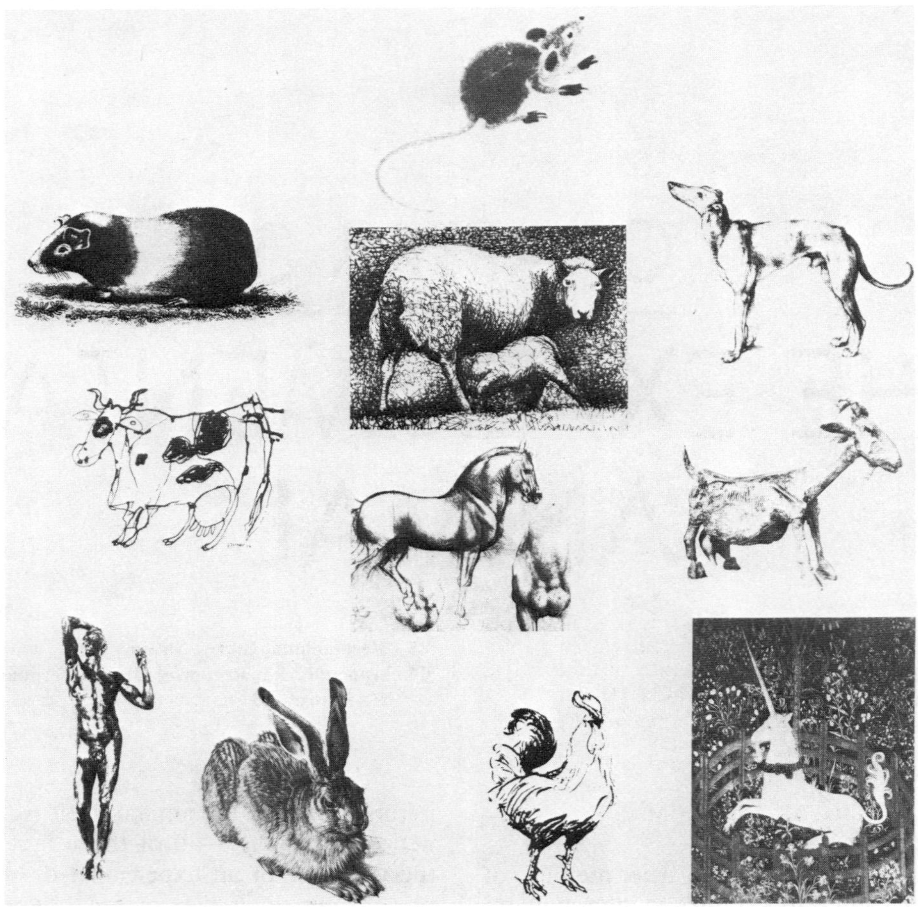

Figure 3.1. Top ten experimental animals in immunology, and an eleventh, the mythical ideal. Can you name the artists who drew these figures—or the animals, for that matter?

First row: mouse or rat (Chi Pai Shih). *Second row:* guinea pig (anonymous), sheep (Henry Moore), dog (Albrecht Dürer). *Third row:* cow (Jean Dubuffet), horse (Leonardo da Vinci), goat (Pablo Picasso). *Fourth row:* human (Auguste Rodin), rabbit or hare (Albrecht Dürer), cock or chicken (Henri de Toulouse-Lautrec), unicorn (anonymous: the captive unicorn from "The Lady and the Unicorn" tapestry series at the Cluny Museum, Paris).

loci and the same alleles at all the remaining loci. The loci at which only one allele exists are referred to as *monomorphic*, and those with two or more alleles as *polymorphic*. One can thus define *genetic polymorphism* as the presence in a population of two or more alleles at a single locus in frequencies that cannot be explained by recurrent mutations.

To maintain a random-bred strain in the laboratory, the immunologist must take special precautions to assure that mating is random. To avoid unintentional selection during the matings, the researcher numbers the animals and selects individuals for further mating from tables of random numbers. It is important to realize, however, that when an animal colony is small and closed (that is, no new animals are introduced into it), genetic dissimilarity among individuals is eventually lost, no matter how one varies the matings. The reasons for this drift of small populations toward genetic homogeneity will become apparent from the discussion of inbreeding in the next section. A true random-breeding population probably does not exist, but many natural populations approach random-bred status.

Random-bred animals are used mainly by those geneticists and immunogeneticists who are interested in the polymorphism of genetic loci and in the way polymorphisms are influenced by selection. Such animals are also rich sources of genetic variants—new alleles or new gene combinations—for the study of gene functions.

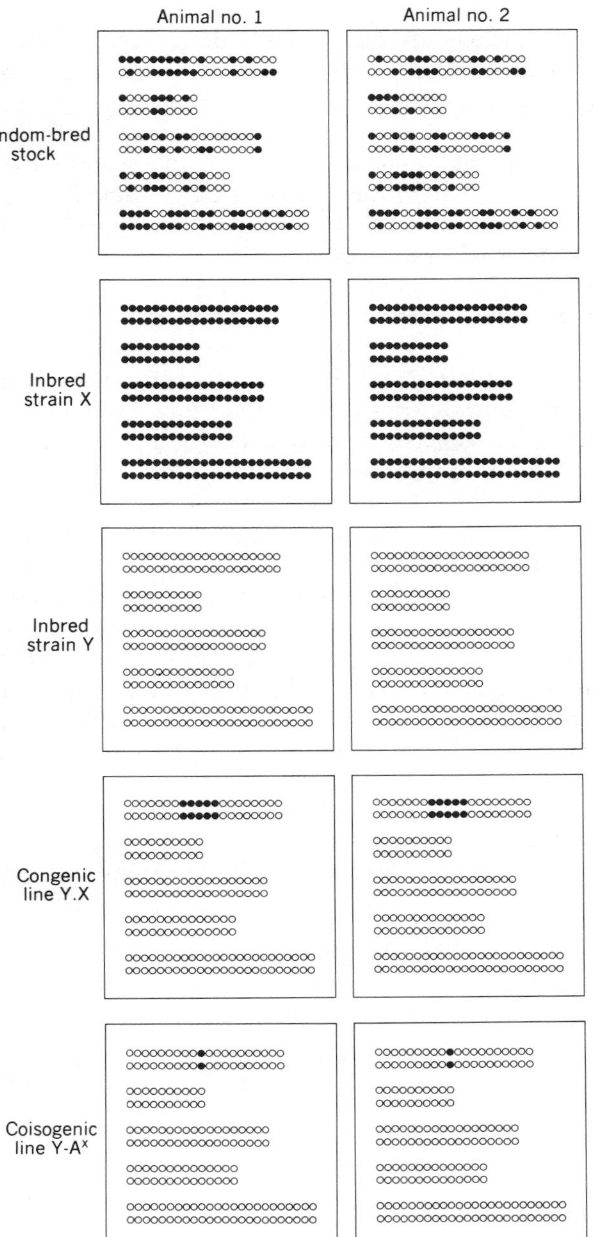

Figure 3.2. Genetic definitions of various animal stocks, strains, and lines. Each rectangle represents the genes of a single hypothetical animal, each circle corresponds to one gene, open and closed circles to alleles at a given locus, each string to one chromosome, paired strings to homologous chromosomes. *Outbred stock*: each animal is homozygous at some loci and heterozygous at others; two animals have the same alleles at some loci and different alleles at others. *Inbred strain*: each animal is homozygous at all loci; two animals have the same alleles at corresponding loci. Two inbred strains have different alleles at at least some of their loci; here, for simplicity, the two strains are depicted as carrying different alleles at all of their loci—a situation that never occurs. *Congenic line*: the line depicted is like inbred strain Y except that it has a few genes from strain X in the first pair of chromosomes. *Coisogenic line*: the line depicted is like inbred strain Y except that it has one pair of *A* genes from strain X.

Random breeding must be distinguished from *outbreeding*, which is the mating of individuals less closely related than individuals chosen at random from a population.

3.3 INBRED STRAINS

In contrast to outbreeding, *inbreeding* is the mating of individuals more closely related than mates chosen at random from a population. Ideally, an *inbred strain* is a population of genetically identical animals.

The speed with which inbred status is achieved depends upon the degree of relatedness between the mated individuals. The quickest way to produce an inbred strain is to mate brothers with sisters, but mating among any other relatives will also result in genetic homogeneity.

Why individuals become genetically homogeneous by matings with relatives can be explained by analogy (Fig. 3.3) or mathematically. Figure 3.3 depicts a game I played with two marbles—one black and one white—to illustrate how an inbred strain is produced. I started with two ''animals,'' each carrying nine ''loci'' (the twin circles shown in the figure; there are nine pairs because there are two alleles at each locus). I drew the animals from a random-bred population, which means that I determined the two alleles (O, or open, and C, or closed, circles) at each locus by drawing one of the two marbles from a bag. White represented open and black indicated closed. As you can see in the figure, for the first animal, I drew an OO combination at the first locus, a CO combination at the second locus, a CO combination at the third locus, and so on. All of these pairings were by chance. Also by chance, animals became heterozygous (OC or CO combinations) at 44 percent of the loci; they were homozygous (CC or OO) at the remaining 56 percent.

Then I produced ''gametes'' from the two animals (single rectangles). Gametes, of course, have only one of the two alleles at each locus; which one is, again, determined by chance. So I had to draw again, but only for the heterozygous loci (OC or CO), because a homozygous locus (CC or OO) has only one allelic type and so can provide only gametes carrying this type. The results of my drawing are shown in the second row of rectangles. In the first gamete I happened to draw a C allele at the second locus, a C allele at the third locus, and so on. Then I simulated fertilization by combining—at random—one gamete from one animal with another gamete from the second animal. I took care, of course, not to mix open or closed circles at different loci (circles from position 1 go again to posi-

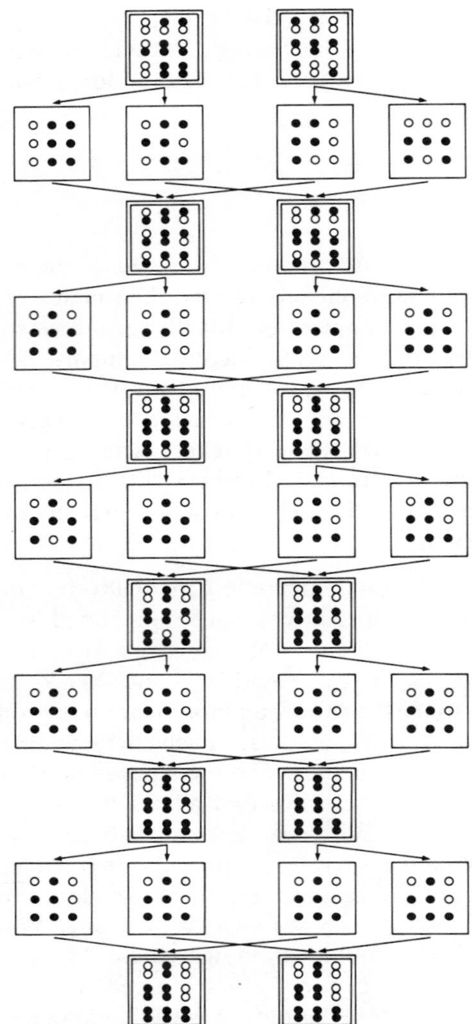

Figure 3.3. The marbles of the inbreeding game. The two double rectangles at the top represent two animals, each carrying nine "loci" (nine twin circles—twin because there are two alleles at each locus). Explanation in text.

tion 1, those from position 2 go again to position 2, and so on). I repeated the whole procedure again and again for several "generations," always generating gametes from the animals, fertilizing the gametes, and producing new animals.

The important point is that whenever a locus became homozygous, the allele carried by the gamete at that locus was "fixed" (it became invariable); whenever a locus became homozygous for the same allele in *both* animals, the allele was fixed for all the progeny of all the generations derived from those two animals. This fixation occurs because there is no external source of variability, barring mutations. And so, if, for instance, an O allele at locus 5 becomes homozygous in both animals, the progeny of the two animals will never again have a C allele at that locus. You can see that the longer I played the game, the more loci became homozygous for the same allele in both parental animals. And after five generations, *all* loci were homozygous, and the two animals became indistinguishable. I produced identical twins, whose progeny will be an inbred strain. When you play the game, you may have to play it for a few generations more or perhaps a few less, but the final result will be the same: you will end up with identical animals. If you don't believe it, try it yourself. Animals, of course, have not nine, but thousands of loci, so the achievement of genetic homogeneity by inbreeding takes somewhat longer than in this simplified analogy. But in the end, they do indeed achieve it.

We can also explain the achievement of genetic homogeneity mathematically.

Let us consider a single locus with two alleles, A and a. There can be three genotypes with respect to these alleles: AA, Aa, and aa. Let us assume that we start inbreeding with a population in which all three genotypes are present. Since any genotype can mate with any of the other two genotypes, there will be four mating combinations occurring with probabilities p_n, q_n, r_n, and v_n, where n is the mating generation, and where $p + q + r + v = 1$. The probabilities of the various mating combinations are as follows.

$$\begin{pmatrix} AA \times AA \\ aa \times aa \end{pmatrix} = p_n$$

$$(AA \times aa) = q_n$$

$$\begin{pmatrix} AA \times Aa \\ aa \times Aa \end{pmatrix} = r_n$$

$$(Aa \times Aa) = v_n$$

The animals become inbred (for the particular allelic pair) when $p = 1$, that is, when mating occurs only among homozygotes and all heterozygotes have been eliminated from the population. When does this situation occur? To answer this question, we must determine how the frequencies of the individual mating combinations change from one generation to another (from n to $n + 1$). Let us, therefore, consider the individual mating combinations one by one and see what kind of offspring they produce.

Matings $(AA \times AA)$ and $(aa \times aa)$ produce AA and aa progeny, respectively, which in turn produce $(AA \times AA)$ or $(aa \times aa)$ matings—that is, the same matings as those in the preceding generation.

Mating $(AA \times aa)$ produces only Aa offspring,

Table 3.1 Frequencies of Mating Types in Two Consecutive Generations of Brother-to-Sister Breeding (Explanation in Text)

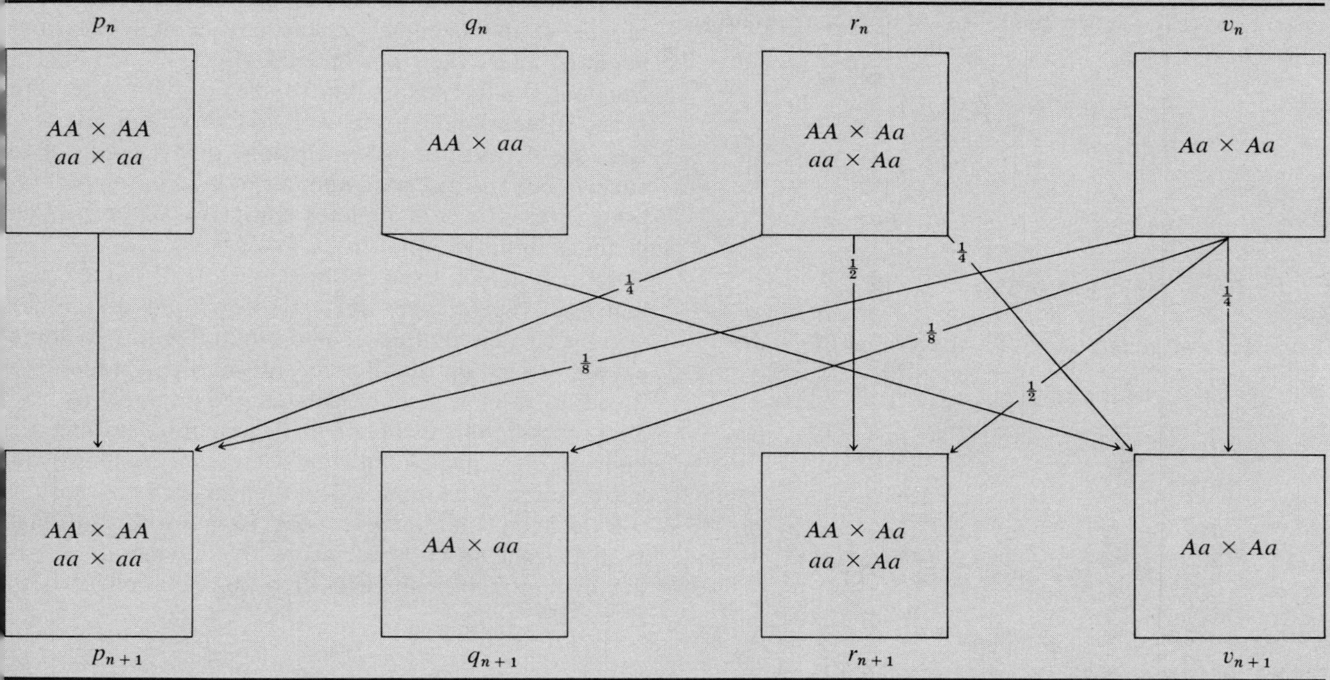

which yield only $(Aa \times Aa)$ matings in the next generation.

Mating $(AA \times Aa)$ produces half offspring with the AA genotype and half with the Aa genotype, which in turn yield the following matings in the next generation.

	$\frac{1}{2}AA$	$\frac{1}{2}Aa$
$\frac{1}{2}AA$	$\frac{1}{4}(AA \times AA)$	$\frac{1}{4}(AA \times Aa)$
$\frac{1}{2}Aa$	$\frac{1}{4}(AA \times Aa)$	$\frac{1}{4}(Aa \times Aa)$

The total is $\frac{1}{4}(AA \times AA)$, $\frac{1}{2}(AA \times Aa)$, and $\frac{1}{4}(Aa \times Aa)$. The $(aa \times Aa)$ mating produces a similar result, except that A and a are reversed.

Mating $(Aa \times Aa)$ produces:

	$\frac{1}{2}A$	$\frac{1}{2}a$
$\frac{1}{2}A$	$\frac{1}{4}AA$	$\frac{1}{4}Aa$
$\frac{1}{2}a$	$\frac{1}{4}Aa$	$\frac{1}{4}aa$

with the total of $\frac{1}{4}AA$, $\frac{1}{2}Aa$, and $\frac{1}{4}aa$ offspring. These offspring yield the following mating combinations in the next generation:

	$\frac{1}{4}AA$	$\frac{1}{2}Aa$	$\frac{1}{4}aa$
$\frac{1}{4}AA$	$\frac{1}{16}(AA \times AA)$	$\frac{1}{8}(AA \times Aa)$	$\frac{1}{16}(AA \times aa)$
$\frac{1}{2}Aa$	$\frac{1}{8}(AA \times Aa)$	$\frac{1}{4}(Aa \times Aa)$	$\frac{1}{8}(aa \times Aa)$
$\frac{1}{4}aa$	$\frac{1}{16}(AA \times aa)$	$\frac{1}{8}(aa \times Aa)$	$\frac{1}{16}(aa \times aa)$

The total is:

$$\begin{pmatrix} AA \times AA \\ aa \times aa \end{pmatrix} \quad \tfrac{1}{16} + \tfrac{1}{16} = \tfrac{1}{8}$$

$$(AA \times aa) \quad \tfrac{1}{16} + \tfrac{1}{16} = \tfrac{1}{8}$$

$$\begin{pmatrix} AA \times Aa \\ aa \times Aa \end{pmatrix} \quad \tfrac{1}{8} + \tfrac{1}{8} + \tfrac{1}{8} + \tfrac{1}{8} = \tfrac{4}{8} = \tfrac{1}{2}$$

$$(Aa \times Aa) \quad \tfrac{1}{4}$$

The relationships between two generations can then be summarized as in Table 3.1. From this table we can see that:

$$p_{n+1} = p_n + \tfrac{1}{4}r_n + \tfrac{1}{8}v_n$$

$$q_{n+1} = \tfrac{1}{8}v_n$$

$$r_{n+1} = \tfrac{1}{2}r_n + \tfrac{1}{2}v_n$$

$$v_{n+1} = q_n + \tfrac{1}{4}r_n + \tfrac{1}{4}v_n$$

Using these equations we can express the frequency of matings between homozygotes as:

$$p_{n+1} = p_n + \tfrac{1}{4}r_n + \tfrac{1}{8}v_n$$

and this formula is then used to calculate the progression of inbreeding in successive generations.

If the first mating is ($Aa \times Aa$), then in the first generation (F_1) the probabilities of the four mating combinations are:

$$p_1 = 0 + 0 + \tfrac{1}{8}, \text{ or } 0.125$$

$$q_1 = \tfrac{1}{8}, \text{ or } 0.125$$

$$r_1 = 0 + \tfrac{1}{2}, \text{ or } 0.500$$

$$v_1 = 0 + 0 + \tfrac{1}{4}, \text{ or } 0.250$$

In the second generation (F_2), the probabilities are:

$$p_2 = 0.125 + \tfrac{1}{4} + \tfrac{1}{8}, \text{ or } 0.281$$

$$q_2 = \tfrac{1}{8}, \text{ or } 0.031$$

$$r_2 = \tfrac{1}{2} + \tfrac{1}{2}, \text{ or } 0.375$$

$$v_2 = 0.125 + \tfrac{1}{4} + \tfrac{1}{4}, \text{ or } 0.312$$

and so on. When one calculates the p for the first 20 F generations, one sees that the probability of homozygosity increases, at first rapidly, and much more slowly in later generations (Fig. 3.4). After 20 generations of brother-to-sister mating, p reaches a value close to 1.0 (though theoretically, it can never reach 1.0), the animals are homozygous at most of the loci, and the line is inbred.

The production of an inbred strain is not as simple as it might seem. The major complication is the *inbreeding depression*, which sets in after a few generations of brother-to-sister mating, resulting in a decline in some or all components of biological fitness. This decline is caused mainly by deleterious genes harbored by each individual at a certain frequency. Since such genes are usually recessive, their effect in a heterozygous individual is masked by the dominant normal alleles. However, as inbreeding proceeds, the deleterious genes too become increasingly homozygous and begin to exert their detrimental effects. Components frequently affected are body size, growth rate, life span, susceptibility to disease, viability, and fertility. Because of inbreeding depression, many lines fail to survive beyond a certain number of inbreeding generations. Presently existing lines comprise only a fraction of those initiated in the past.

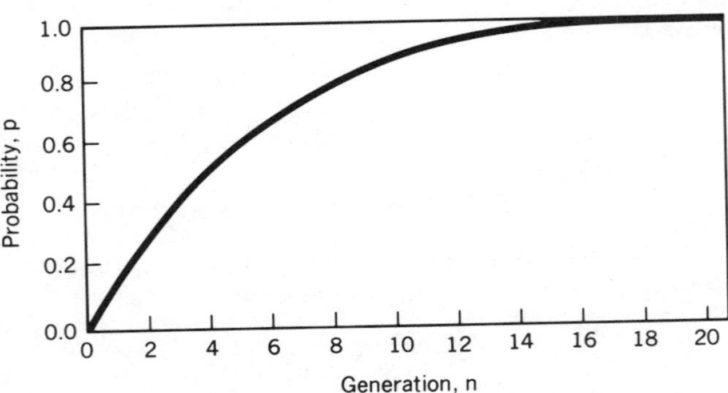

Figure 3.4. Probability of homozygosity at locus *A* during the first 20 generations of brother-sister mating (inbreeding).

Inbred strains exist in the mouse, rat, guinea pig, hamster, rabbit, and domestic fowl. Several other species live in conditions favoring inbreeding to some extent. Even in the human, primarily a randomly breeding animal, several isolated geographical or religious communities with a high degree of inbreeding are known. The species with most (several hundred) inbred strains is the mouse, and their major repository is the Jackson Laboratory, near Bar Harbor, Maine, U.S.A. Each strain is designated by a symbol consisting of letters or numbers, or a combination of both (Fig. 3.5).

3.4 COISOGENIC AND CONGENIC LINES

The need for coisogenic and congenic lines can best be explained using the following example. Immunologists have known for some time that acceptance or rejection of grafts exchanged between two mice is controlled by several genetic loci, which we shall refer to here as loci 1, 2, 3, 4, and so on. When the two mice differ at any one of these loci, they reject the grafts; when they are identical at all loci, they accept the grafts as their own tissue. This situation poses a serious problem for an immunologist who wants to study one of these loci—say, locus 12. Since the two mice differ not only at this locus but also, say, at loci 3, 7, 9, 17, and others, the investigator will be unable to tell what effect locus 12 alone has; whatever this effect might be, it will be masked by the combined effect of the other loci. To learn about the role of locus 12, the researcher would have to have mice differing at this locus but identical at all other loci. Only then would he know that the rejection was caused by a difference at locus 12, and not, for instance, by a difference at locus 3 or 7. Two animals (lines) that are genetically identical save for a difference at one locus are called *coisogenic* (L. *co*, together with, Gr. *iso*, alike, identical).

Two inbred mice become coisogenic when a mutation occurs in one of them. When the mutant is inbred and a line homozygous for the mutant allele is derived from it, this line becomes coisogenic with the original

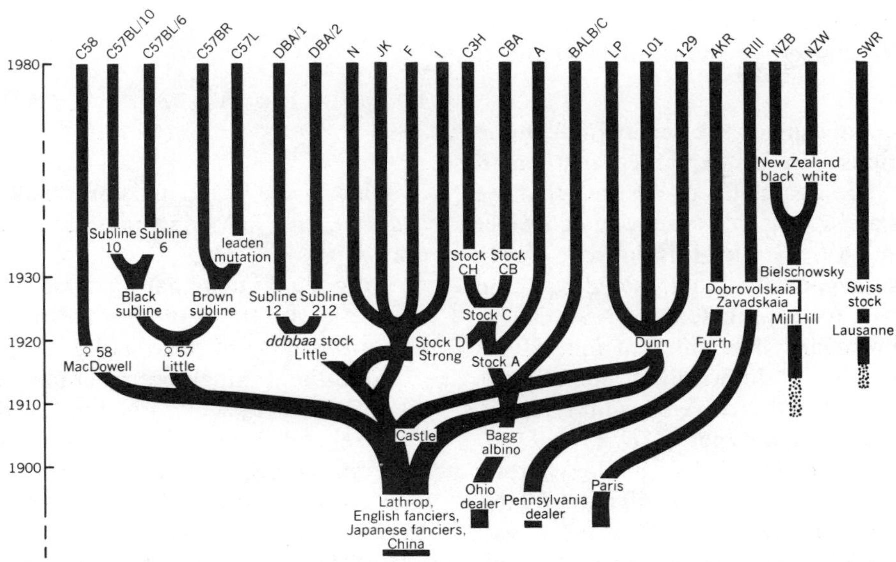

Figure 3.5. Pedigree of the more common inbred mouse strains and the time scale of their development.

inbred strain. However, mutations are random events and researchers wanting a coisogenic line with a difference at a particular locus (number 12, for example) cannot wait until a mutation occurs at this locus by chance. A compromise solution is to develop so-called *congenic lines*, which differ from their partner strains in a short chromosomal region. This region is likely to contain more than one locus, but with luck, the additional loci might not interfere with the study of the one locus in question.

In contrast to coisogenic lines, which can be produced only by mutation, congenic lines can be obtained by successive backcrossing to the same strain for a certain number of generations and by repeated selection in each generation for a particular gene.

The simplest mating design for the production of a congenic line is depicted in Figure 3.6. Here we start with two strains, 1 and 2, that differ at locus *D*. Strain 1, which must be inbred, is a *d*/*d* homozygote, and strain 2, which may or not be inbred, is a *D*/*D* homozygote. To study the effect of the *D* gene, we must produce a line that is genetically identical to strain 1, but carries the *D* allele. To this end, we cross the two strains and backcross the resulting F_1 hybrid to strain 1. In the backcross generation, the *D* gene has segregated so that half the progeny is *D*/*d* and the other half *d*/*d*. We type (or score) the animals, select one of the *D*/*d* individuals for further mating (backcrossing) to strain 1, and repeat this procedure for 12 generations. When we obtain the progeny of the twelfth backcross, we intercross two *D*/*d* individuals and obtain *D*/*D* animals. By brother-to-sister mating of the *D*/*D* animals

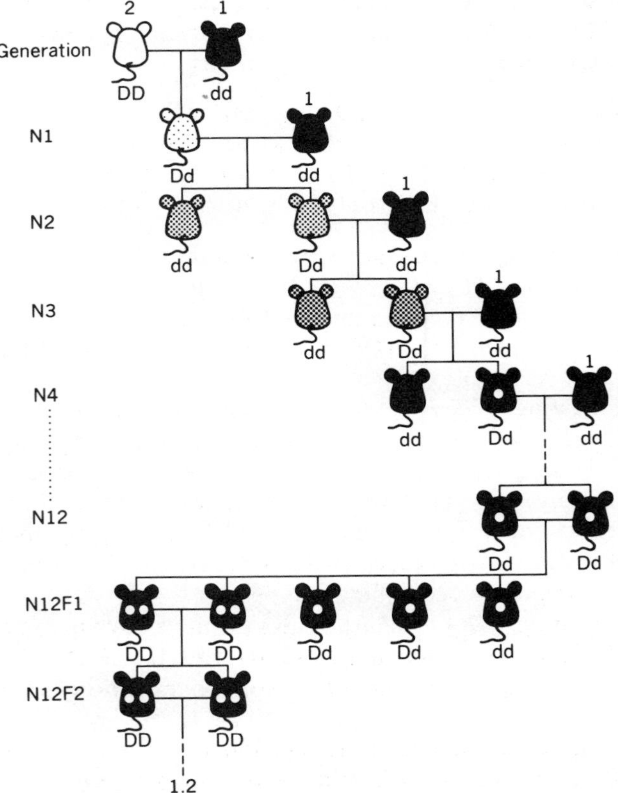

Figure 3.6. A scheme of congenic-line production by repeated backcrossing to strain 1 and selection in each segregating generation for the *D* allele donated by strain 2. The successive generations of matings of *Dd* individuals with strain H1 are designated N1, N2, N3, and so on. After 12 such generations, two *Dd* individuals are intercrossed and *dd* individuals are selected and mated *inter se*. The intercrossing generations are then designated F1, F2, F3, and so on.

we obtain a line 1.2 that is very similar to strain 1, but which carries the D instead of the d allele at the D locus.

The effect of backcrossing on the genetic makeup of successive generations can be explained mathematically as follows. Once again, let us assume that we have two strains, 1 and 2, but this time let us consider two loci, $A(a)$ and $D(d)$. Strain 1 is inbred, which means that it is homozygous at all loci, including A and D, its genotype being, for example, Ad/Ad. Strain 2 is random-bred, which means that different individuals may carry different alleles at different loci, including A and D. Let us assume that there are four individuals, each with one of four genotypes—AD/Ad, aD/ad, AD/ad, and aD/Ad (ignoring DD and dd homozygotes).

We wish to produce a third line that will carry all the genes of strain 1, except one: at the D locus it will carry the dominant allele. (The strain's genotype will be AD/AD.) To produce such a line, we mate the inbred strain with those individuals of the random-bred strain that carry the dominant D allele. Because these individuals are of four types, we get four mating combinations, each with a certain probability:

COMBINATION I $(AD/Ad \times Ad/Ad) = p_n$
COMBINATION II $(aD/ad \times Ad/Ad) = q_n$
COMBINATION III $(AD/ad \times Ad/Ad) = r_n$
COMBINATION IV $(aD/Ad \times Ad/Ad) = v_n.$

The result of these matings is as follows.

Mating $(AD/Ad \times Ad/Ad)$ produces two types of progeny (the recombinant and the parental types are indistinguishable), AD/Ad and Ad/Ad, with equal frequencies.

Mating $(aD/ad \times Ad/Ad)$ also produces two types of progeny, aD/Ad and ad/Ad, with equal frequencies.

Mating $(AD/ad \times Ad/Ad)$ produces four types of progeny, two parental (i.e., AD/Ad and ad/Ad) and two recombinant (i.e., aD/Ad and Ad/Ad). If the frequency of recombination between $A(a)$ and $D(d)$ is c, the ratio of parental to recombinant types is $(1 - c):c$.

Mating $(aD/Ad \times Ad/Ad)$ also produces two parental and two recombinant types: aD/Ad, Ad/Ad, AD/Ad, and ad/Ad, in a parental-to-recombinant ratio of $(1 - c):c$.

Because our goal is to introduce the dominant D allele into the inbred strain, we discard all the dd progeny from the four mating combinations, and for further mating use only individuals carrying the D allele, which are as follows.

FROM MATING I AD/Ad
FROM MATING II aD/Ad
FROM MATING III AD/Ad and aD/Ad in a ratio $(1 - c):c$
FROM MATING IV aD/Ad and AD/Ad in a ratio $(1 - c):c$

When these individuals are backcrossed to strain 1 (Ad/Ad), the following mating combinations are obtained.

From the original mating combination I, only mating $(AD/Ad \times Ad/Ad)$ is obtained, which is combination I. The probability of this mating is p_n.

From the original mating combination II, only mating $(aD/Ad \times Ad/Ad)$ is obtained, which is combination IV. The probability of this mating is v_n.

From the original mating combination III, two matings are obtained, $(AD/Ad \times Ad/Ad)$ and $(aD/Ad \times Ad/Ad)$, with probabilities $(1 - c)r_n$ and cr_n, respectively; these represent mating combinations I and IV, respectively.

From the original mating combination IV, two matings are obtained, $(aD/Ad \times Ad/Ad)$ and $(AD/Ad \times Ad/Ad)$, with probabilities $(1 - c)v_n$ and cv_n, respectively; these represent mating combinations IV and I, respectively.

So, in the first generation of backcross mating, combinations II and III are eliminated and only combinations I and IV remain. The overall relationship between two consecutive generations is summarized in Table 3.2. From this table, the frequencies of the individual matings in the $n + 1$ generation can be written as follows.

$$p_{n+1} = p_n + (1 - c)r_n + cv_n$$

$$q_{n+1} = 0$$

$$r_{n+1} = 0$$

$$v_{n+1} = q_n + cr_n + (1 - c)v_n$$

Since $q_{n+1} = 0$ and $r_{n+1} = 0$, we can write the equations for the next generation as follows.

$$p_{n+2} = p_n + cv_n$$

$$v_{n+2} = (1 - c)v_n$$

Thus

$$v_2 = (1 - c)v_1$$

$$v_3 = (1 - c)v_2 = (1 - c)(1 - c)v_1 = (1 - c)^2 v_1$$

Table 3.2 Frequencies of Mating Types in Two Consecutive Generations of Backcrossing (Explanation in Text)

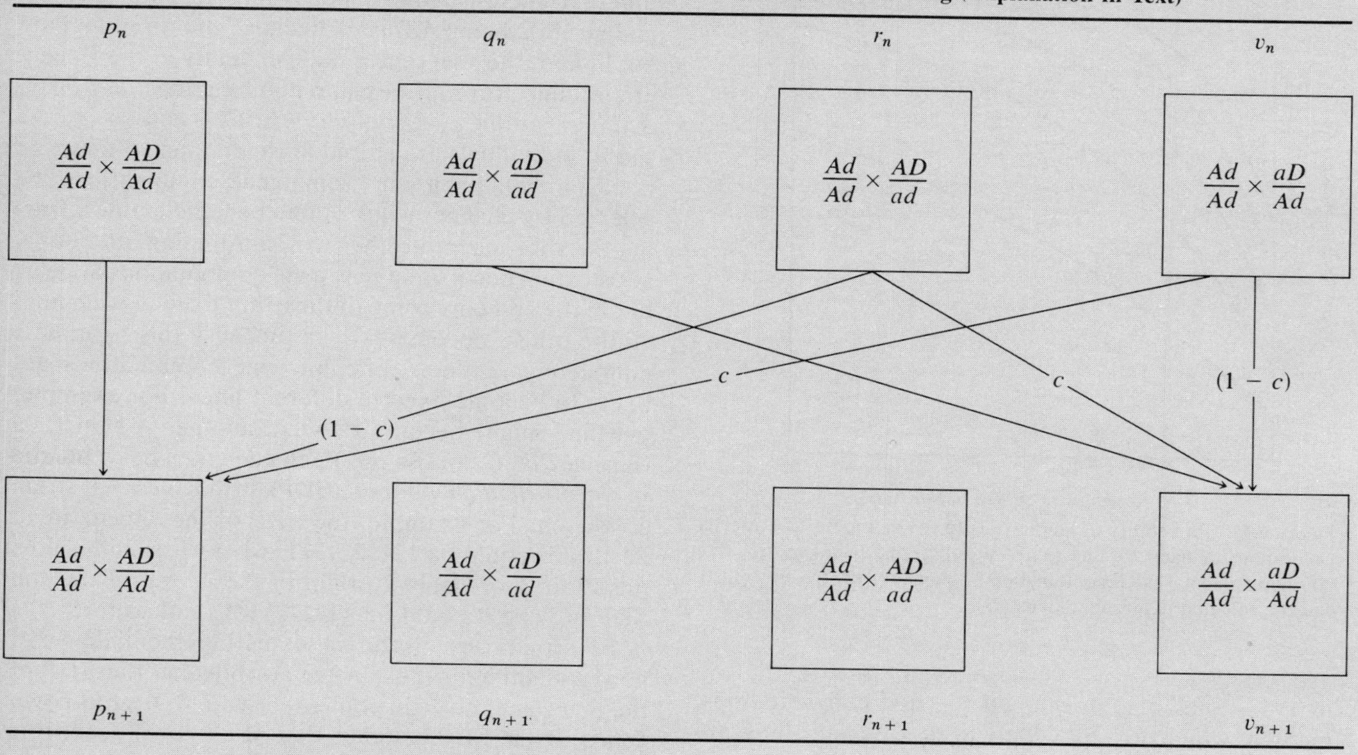

$$v_4 = (1 - c)v_3 = (1 - c)(1 - c)^2 v_1 = (1 - c)^3 v_1$$

$$\vdots$$

$$v_n = (1 - c)^{n-1} v_1.$$

If $v_1 = 1$, as is the case when the initial mating is of type I (that is, if $q_o = 1$), then

$$v_n = (1 - c)^{n-1}$$

Since $p_n + v_n = 1$, then

$$p_n = 1 - v_n$$

and

$$p_n = 1 - (1 - c)^{n-1}$$

This last equation gives the probability of homozygosity at a given locus in the nth generation. If $c = 0.5$ (no linkage between loci A and D), the value of p in successive generations (n = 1, 2, 3, etc.) is 1, $\frac{1}{2}$, $\frac{3}{4}$, $\frac{7}{8}$, $\frac{5}{16}$, $\frac{31}{32}$. . . .

Figure 3.7 depicts how values of p for different c values change in succeeding generations. We can see that after 12 backcross generations, most loci not linked to D are of strain 1 origin. However, chromosomal segments on both sides of D are still of strain 2 origin, and if strain 2 differed at any loci positioned in these segments, multiple differences would remain between the congenic line and strain 1. Although in most instances the additional differences do not interfere with an experiment, one must always keep in mind that a congenic line may differ from its inbred partner by more than one gene.

A congenic line is denominated in one of two ways, the more common of which is by a symbol derived from the designations of the two strains involved in its production. The inbred strain is listed first and the donor strain second; the two symbols are separated by a period. For example, B10.A is a congenic line carrying a gene (*H-2*^{a}) of the A strain on the C57BL/10 (abbreviated B10) strain background. A congenic line can also be designated by the locus at which if differs from the inbred strain, so the B10.A line can be also written as B10-*H-2*^{a}.

The idea of coisogenic and congenic lines was introduced into immunological research by George D. Snell

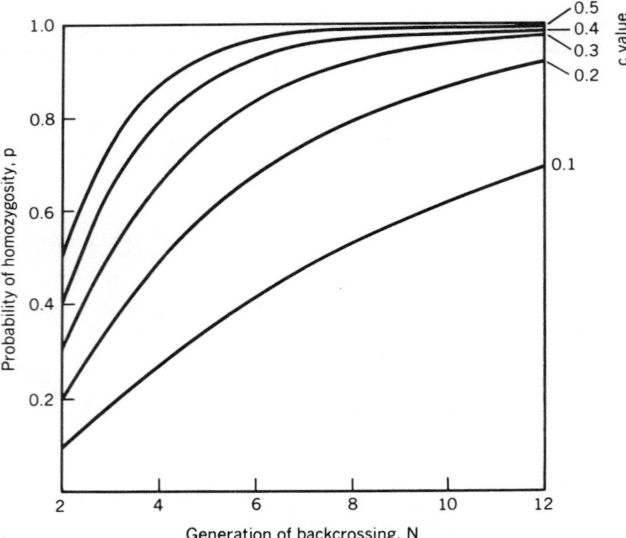

Figure 3.7. Probability of homozygosity (p) at a locus (D) after N generations of backcrossing to an inbred strain, calculated for five different values of the recombination frequency (c) between locus A and the selected differential locus (D).

in 1948. Snell also developed the first congenic lines, many of which are still widely used. Congenic lines are available in the mouse, rat, and domestic fowl.

3.5 RECOMBINANT INBRED STRAINS

Recombinant inbred (RI) strains are derived by a process that involves crossing two inbred strains (1 and 2), intercrossing the resulting F_1 hybrids, mating together several F_2 progeny, and producing an inbred line from each of the F_2 crosses by continuous brother-to-sister mating. Figure 3.8 diagrams what happens to the genes in such lines.

For simplicity, let us consider only three loci—*A*, *B*, and *C*—and let us assume that strains 1 and 2 carry different alleles at these loci, strain 1 being *aaBBCC* and strain 2 being *AAbbcc*. Because the three loci are not linked, they segregate independently in the F_2 generation and form all possible combinations: *aaBBCC*, *AAbbcc*, *AaBbCc*, *AAbbCC*, *aaBBCC*, and so on. As the F_2 individuals are paired at random and a new line is begun from each pair, some gene combinations are selected by chance, while others become extinct. During the subsequent brother-to-sister mating, additional segregation occurs and new gene combinations appear, but in the end only some of these are fixed in each line; all the others become extinct. Because this fixation is completely random, different gene combinations are likely to become fixed in different lines. For example, one line might become *aabbcc*, another *AAbbCC*, a third *aaBBCC*, and so on. Each gene then has a unique *strain distribution pattern* (SDP) in a given RI strain collection. For example, the SDP of the *A* gene in 10 RI strains could be 1211221211, where 1 or 2 indicates the strain 1 or strain 2 origin of the *A* or *a* allele; the SDP of gene *B* could be 1121221121, and so forth.

RI strains are useful in detecting the linkage of newly identified genes. After establishing the SDP of the new gene, one can compare it with SDPs of known genes. If the SDP matches that of a known gene, it is likely that the two genes are linked.

The idea of RI strains was conceived and the first set of these strains was produced by Donald W. Bailey in 1971. So far RI strains are available only in the mouse.

3.6 APPENDIX 3.1: REVIEW OF GENETIC TERMINOLOGY

Figure 3.9 is a diagram of a cell with a nucleus, cytoplasm, and cell membrane. In the nucleus are four

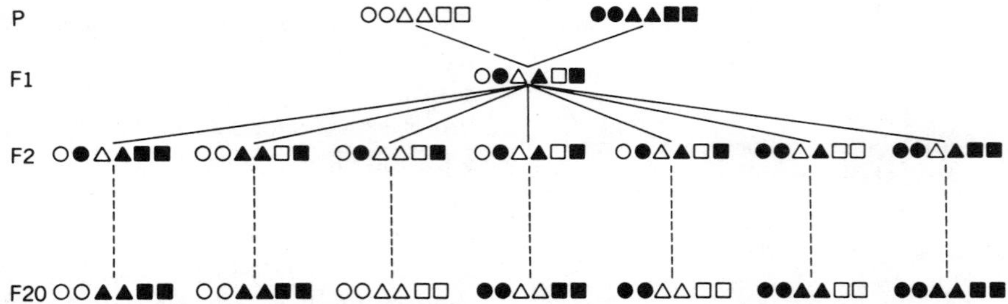

Figure 3.8. Diagrammatic representation of the principle involved in the production of recombinant inbred strains. Different symbols indicate different genes; open and closed symbols indicate alleles at the individual loci. Explanation in text. (From J. Klein: *Biology of the Mouse Histocompatibility-2 Complex*. Springer-Verlag, New York, 1975.)

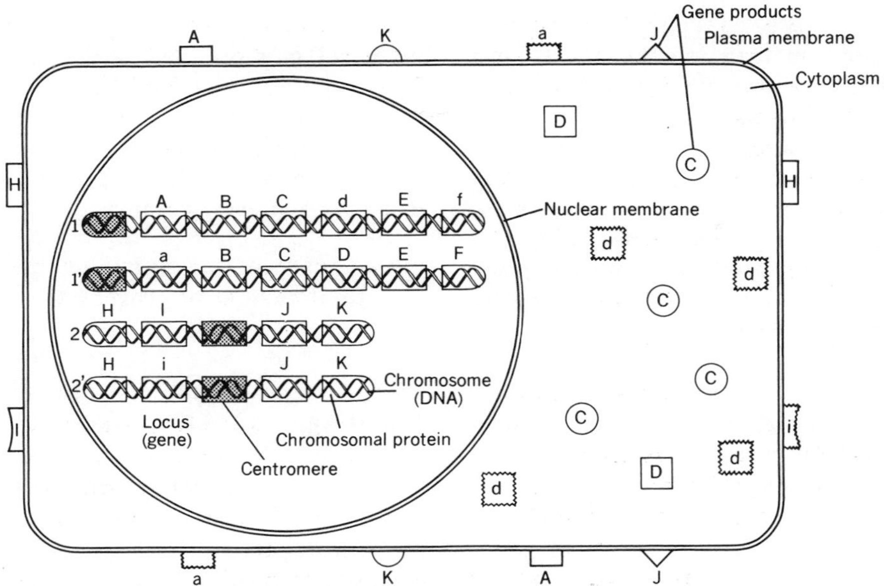

Figure 3.9. A geneticist's view of a cell. Everything in the figure is distorted—the length of the chromosome, the length of the gene, the size of the gene products, the number of chromosomes. *A* and *a* are alleles of gene *A* at locus *A*; *D* and *d* are alleles of gene *D* at locus *D*. *A*, *B*, *C*, *d*, *E*, and *f* are linked genes, all in one linkage group (linkage group I). *H*, *I*, *J*, and *K* are linked genes, all in another linkage group (linkage group II). Examples of unlinked genes (that are in different linkage groups and hence segregate independently) are *A* and *H*, *A* and *I*, and *B* and *H*. An example of closely linked genes is *C* and *d*. An example of loosely linked genes is *A* and *f*. 1 and 1′ are homologous chromosomes; 2 and 2′ are homologous chromosomes; 1 and 2 are nonhomologous chromosomes. 1 and 1′ are acrocentric (telocentric) chromosomes; 2 and 2′ are metacentric chromosomes. The cell is homozygous at *B*, *C*, *E*, *H*, *J*, and *K* loci; it is heterozygous at *A*, *D*, *F*, and *I* loci. Genes *A*(*a*), *C*, *D*(*d*), *H*, *I*(*i*), *J*, and *K* are expressed, but genes *B* and *F*(*f*) are not in this particular cell. *A*, *B*, *C*, *D*, *E*, *F*, *H*, *I*, *J*, and *K* are dominant alleles; *a*, *d*, *f*, and *i* are recessive alleles. The genotype of the cell is *A*/*a C*/*C D*/*d E*/*E G*/*G H*/*H I*/*i J*/*J K*/*K*. The phenotype is A C D E G H I J.

chromosomes, each consisting of chromosomal proteins and a single, continuous *DNA* double helix. Each chromosome also possesses a site, the *centromere*, to which fibers attach when the cell divides; these fibers pull the chromosome toward one of the two poles established during mitosis. The two chromosomes with centromeres situated along the length of the arm are referred to as *metacentric*; the two with centromeres at their ends are *telocentric* or *acrocentric*. The chromosomal end opposite the centromere is known as the *telomere*. Structurally similar chromosomes in each pair are referred to as *homologous*; chromosomes belonging to different pairs are *nonhomologous*.

The DNA double helix is divided into segments (*genes*) of a certain length, with each segment responsible for a single trait, represented in Figure 3.9 by individual molecules. Because the division into genes is exactly the same in two homologous chromosomes, there are pairs of genes (*alleles*) that always occupy the same position, or *locus*, in the chromosome. When one of the two alleles controls a demonstrable trait and the other does not, the former is called *dominant* and the latter *recessive*. Dominance and recessiveness are relative terms defined by the geneticist's ability or inability to detect a trait attributable to a given gene. In reality, most alleles are *codominant*—that is, both alleles at a given locus code for products, only one of which may manifest itself as a detectable trait.

A cell or animal carrying two identical genes (alleles) at the same locus is said to be *homozygous*; a cell or animal with different alleles at the same locus is *heterozygous*. Genes located on the same (or homologous) chromosome are said to be *linked*; genes on nonhomologous chromosomes segregate independently. Genes in a single chromosome form a *linkage group*, in which those adjacent or close to each other are said to be *closely linked*, while those some distance apart are *loosely linked*. Homologous chromosomes and linkage groups are assigned numbers—chromosomes according to their lengths (the longest being number 1) and other morphological features, and linkage groups according to their order of discovery (the first demonstrated linkage between two genes being linkage group I). Once linkage groups are identified with their corresponding chromosomes (which, in some species, can take a long time), only the chromosome numbers are used. A group of genes characterizing a cell or individual constitutes a *genotype*; a group of traits controlled by this genotype is the *phenotype*.

Genes are designated by symbols consisting of letters and numbers, which are italicized when used in publications; symbols of gene products are printed in roman type. When dominant and recessive genes are discussed generally, they are referred to by capital and small letters, respectively (e.g., *A*, *B*, *C*, or *a*, *b*, *c*). Mating (*cross*) of two individuals is indicated by an "×" between the gene symbols. The following types of cross are distinguished, based upon the genetic constitution (*zygosity*) of mating individuals.

INCROSS	$AA \times AA$ or $aa \times aa$
CROSS	$AA \times aa$
BACKCROSS	$AA \times Aa$ or $aa \times Aa$
INTERCROSS	$Aa \times Aa$

The two individuals that are crossbred are referred to as parents (symbols P_1 and P_2); the progeny of this first cross is known as the *first filial generation* (F_1), the progeny of an intercross between two F_1 hybrids as the *second filial generation* (F_2), and the progeny of a cross between F_1 and P_1 or P_2 as the *backcross* (*BC*) *generation*.

A cross involving a heterozygous individual leads to *segregation* of genes (and their corresponding traits) among the progeny. When a cross involves two alleles at a single locus, the ratio of segregants depends on the dominance-recessivity relationship between the two alleles. When two loci are involved, the segregant ratio depends, in addition, on the linkage relationship of the two loci. For example, an *AB*/*ab* individual that is heterozygous at two loci (*A* and *B*) produces four types of progeny—*AB*, *ab*, *Ab*, and *aB*—when mated to another individual. (For simplicity, the genetic contribution of the second parent is ignored here.) The *AB* and *ab* are the *parental types*; the *Ab* and *aB* are the *recombinant types*.

If *A* and *B* are not linked (they are on nonhomologous chromosomes), the expected proportion is 50 percent parental and 50 percent recombinant types. If the two genes *are* linked, the proportion of recombinant types will be more than zero and less than 50 percent. The proportion of recombinant types is used to express the strength of the linkage (and thus the relative distance) between two genes. The linkage is expressed in terms of *recombination frequency*, which is calculated using the following formula.

$$\frac{\text{number of recombinant individuals}}{\text{total number of progeny}} \quad \text{or}$$

$$\frac{Ab + aB}{AB + ab + Ab + aB}$$

The recombination frequency multiplied by 100 is the *percent of recombination*, with one percent taken as a unit of a distance on the *linkage* (*genetic*) *map*. The unit is designated as one *centimorgan*, or 1 cM. Therefore, if, for instance, 10 recombinant individuals are found among 200 progeny scored, the recombination frequency is 10/200 or 0.05, and the distance between the two loci is 5 map units (cM).

Recombinant types are obtained in crosses involving linked genes because genes in homologous chromosomes exchange places. This exchange is thought to occur via a mechanism called *crossingover*, in which homologous chromosomes break at corresponding positions and reunite in a reciprocal fashion. The frequency of crossingover between two loci is a function of their distance: the closer the two loci, the lower the probability that a break will occur between them.

To establish whether two loci, *A* (*a*) and *B* (*b*), are linked, a geneticist sets up an appropriate mating scheme, counts the individual phenotypes among the progeny, and determines how close the numbers are to those the linkage or nonlinkage hypothesis leads one to expect. If he uses a large enough sample, he can determine the linkage relationship of the two loci with certainty. However, this approach is not possible in the human, where mating is beyond the geneticist's control and where one mating usually produces only one offspring; in this case the researcher must be content to determine the odds for any set of data's being caused by linkage or by independent segregation. One method for doing so consists of the following steps.

Calculate the probability, P_y, that the observed data are the result of independent segregation.

Calculate the probability, P_x, that the same data result from linkage of two loci. (Calculate separately the probabilities for different degrees of linkage—say, 0.05, 0.1, 0.2, 0.3, and 0.4.)

Calculate the odds, P, for or against linkage from the formula $P = P_x/P_x$.

Calculate the *log of the odds* or the *lod score* z from the formula $z = \log_{10} P_x/P_y$. (The use of logarithms instead of probabilities is advantageous in that scores obtained from different families can be added and a combined score, $z = \Sigma i$, determined.) If the score for a particular recombination frequency is greater than one, the relationship is more likely to be linkage than independent segregation, and vice versa. The higher the numerator, the higher the probability of linkage. Thus, if the odds are, say, 1000 : 1, linkage of the A and B loci is likely; if the odds are 1 : 100, the loci are probably not linked.

Let us consider, as an example, a family of four in which the father is a double heterozygote, *AaBb*, the mother is a double homozygote, *aabb*, and both children are double heterozygotes, like the father. Such a mating is called a *double backcross* or *test cross*. The father can produce four types of gamete—*AB*, *Ab*, *aB*, and *ab*. If the A and B loci were not linked, all four types would be produced with equal probability, so that the probability that the children would receive the *AB* gene combination is one in four. If the A and B loci were linked, the probability that A and B would be transmitted simultaneously to the progeny would depend on the phase of the two genes in the father. If the A and B genes were carried by the same chromosomes (that is, in a *coupling phase* or *cis configuration*), and if there were no crossingover between the A and B loci, the probability that the children would receive *AB* genes would be one in two. If the A and B genes were carried by different chromosomes of a given homologous pair (where the genes would be in *repulsion phase* or *trans configuration*), the probability of their simultaneous transmission by a single gamete would be zero (assuming again that no crossingover were to occur between the two tightly linked loci). So the P_x/P_y ratio for the $AaBb \times aabb$ cross and the two *AaBb* children resulting from this cross is (1/2) (1/4) = 2, in favor of close linkage. Likelihood ratios for various degrees of linkage can be calculated in the same way, but for other mating types, the calculations are more complicated.

REFERENCES

General

Altman, P. L. and Katz, D. D. (Eds.): *Inbred and Genetically Defined Strains of Laboratory Animals*, Parts 1 and 2. Federation of American Societies for Experimental Biology, Bethesda, Maryland, 1979.

Bernischke, K., Garner, F. M., and Jones, T. C. (Eds.): *Pathology of Laboratory Animals*, Vols. 1 and 2. Springer-Verlag, New York, 1978.

Festing, M. F. W.: *Inbred Strains in Biomedical Research*. Macmillan, London, 1979.

Green, E. L. and Doolittle, D. P.: Systems of mating used in mammalian genetics. *In* W. J. Burdette (Ed.): *Methodology in Mammalian Genetics*, pp. 3–55, Holden-Day, San Francisco, 1963.

Green, E. L. (Ed.): *Biology of the Laboratory Mouse*, 2nd ed. McGraw-Hill, New York, 1966.

Green, M. C.: Methods for testing linkage. *In* W. J. Burdette (Ed.): *Methodology in Mammalian Genetics*, pp. 56–82, Holden-Day, San Francisco, 1963.

Lane-Petter, W. (Ed.): *Animals for Research. Principles of Breeding and Management*. Academic, London, 1963.

Li, C. C.: *Population Genetics*. University of Chicago Press, Chicago, 1955.

Strickberger, M. W.: *Genetics*, 2nd ed. Macmillan, New York, 1976.

Vogel, F. and Motulsky, A. G.: *Human Genetics. Problems and Approaches*. Springer-Verlag, Berlin, 1979.

CHAPTER 4

THE ORGANS OF IMMUNE RESPONSE

The two main cell types involved in vertebrate immunity are phagocytes and lymphocytes. The body's phagocytic cells are referred to collectively as the *reticuloendothelial system*; the assemblage of lymphocytes, their precursors, derivatives, and supportive cells will be referred to here as the *lymphoid system*. In this chapter we describe the tissues and organs forming the two systems, and in the next chapter we deal with the cells themselves. Both chapters require a certain knowledge of basic histology, the science concerned with tissue structure and organization, and the reader who is unfamiliar with this discipline should first read the appendix to this chapter, in which basic histological terms are reviewed.

4.1 RETICULOENDOTHELIAL SYSTEM

Early in the twentieth century, histologists discovered that dyes such as lithium carmine or trypan blue, when injected into the bloodstream, are taken up by certain cells and stored in their cytoplasm. Because the dyes stain live cells, histologists refer to them as *vital dyes*. The German pathologist K. A. Ludwig Aschoff made a thorough study of the cell types that store vital dyes and concluded that these cells belong to one of four categories (Fig. 4.1): macrophages in tissues (histiocytes) and blood (monocytes); microglia of the central nervous system; endothelial cells lining the dilated blood vessels (sinuses) in the liver (Kupffer cells), spleen, bone marrow, adrenal cortex, and anterior lobe of the pituitary; and reticular cells of lymphoid tissues. Aschoff believed that all these cells were part of a single system concerned primarily with phagocytic defense reactions, and because endothelial and reticular cells were important parts of it, he named it the *reticuloendothelial system* (RES).

However, more recent investigations have revealed that Aschoff was wrong in thinking that endothelial cells of the sinuses and the reticular cells of the connective tissue were involved in defense-related phagocytosis, and in including them on that basis in the

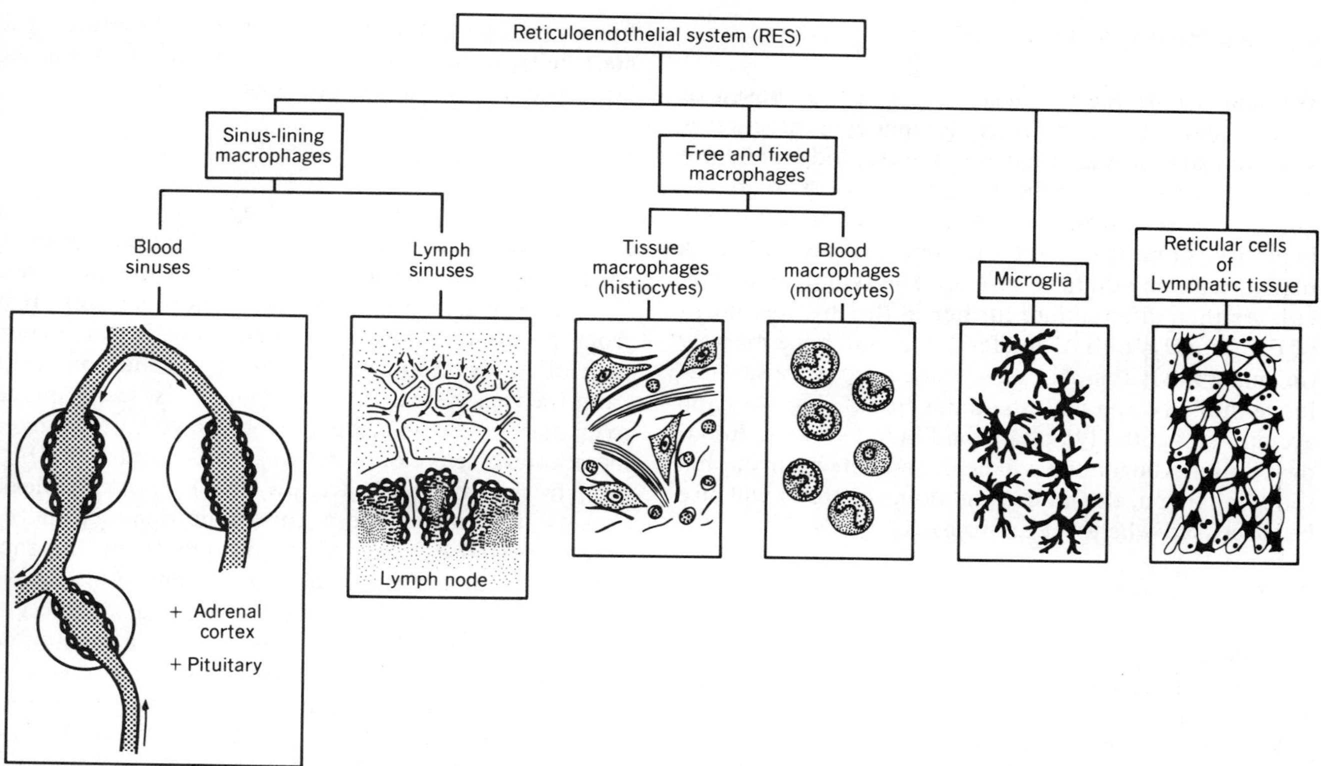

Figure 4.1. The original concept of the reticuloendothelial system (RES).

reticuloendothelial system. For although these cells can take up particles, this phagocytosis is different from that carried out by typical macrophages. Some immunologists have therefore suggested abandoning the term "reticuloendothelial system" altogether and replacing it with another, the *mononuclear phagocyte system* (MPS), which includes only cells involved in defense-related phagocytosis. Cells included in the MPS must meet four criteria: they must be derived from bone marrow precursor cells; they must have a characteristic morphology; they must be able to attach themselves firmly to glass; and they must show high phagocytic activity characterized by the involvement of immunoglobulins and serum complement. Cells meeting these criteria are monocytes and macrophages (free and fixed; Fig. 4.2), both of which are thought to be part of a common differentiation pathway that progresses as follows: stem cell → precursor cells → monocyte → macrophage. The organs in which most MPS cells are localized are the bone marrow, peripheral blood, connective tissue, liver, lungs, lymph nodes, spleen, and nervous system. Polymorphonuclear leukocytes are arbitrarily excluded from the MPS, even though they meet some of the criteria qualifying them for membership in the system.

The effort to replace the term RES with MPS, however, has not been completely successful. Many immunologists remain loyal to the RES designation, but those who do generally use the term in its modern connotation.

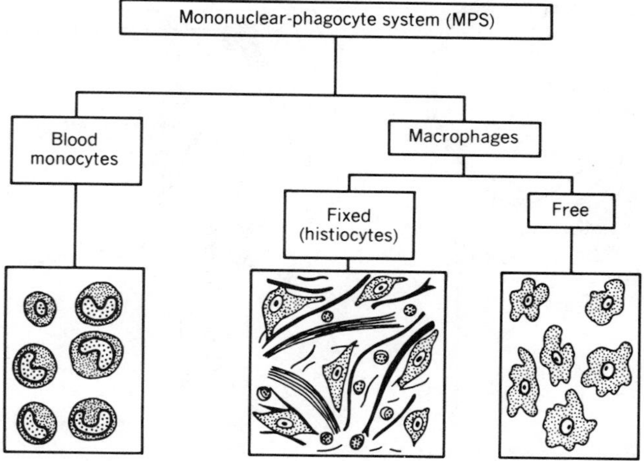

Figure 4.2. The new concept of the reticuloendothelial—or, more properly—mononuclear-phagocyte system (MPS).

4.2 LYMPHOID SYSTEM

We shall define the *lymphoid system* as composed of tissues and organs in which lymphocyte precursors and their derivatives originate, mature, lodge, and are moved. Organs of lymphocyte precursor origin are the yolk sac, liver, spleen, bursa of Fabricius, bone marrow in embryos or fetuses, and the bone marrow and bursa of Fabricius in adults (Fig. 4.3). The lymphocyte precursors then differentiate further in the thymus, bursa of Fabricius (in birds), and fetal liver and bone marrow (in mammals); lymphocytes seeded from these sites lodge in the lymph nodes and the spleen (Fig. 4.4) and are moved via the lymphatic and blood vessels. In our description, the human will be the model organism, but for comparison, the mouse and domestic fowl will also be discussed whenever appropriate.

4.2.1 Organs of Stem Cell Origin

Lymphocytes are derived from *hematopoietic stem cells,* which are also the precursors of all other blood cells, including erythrocytes (Gr. *haima*, blood, *poiēsis*, a making; see also next chapter). The stem cells themselves are derived from the mesenchymal tissue of the embryo. The location of hematopoietic stem cells—and thus the site of hematopoiesis (blood formation) and lymphopoiesis (lymphocyte formation)—changes with the organism's development (Fig. 4.5). The earliest blood-forming cells appear in the yolk sac; then, as the hematopoietic activity of the yolk sac fades away, it is gradually taken over by the fetal liver and spleen, and later by the bursa of Fabricius and the bone marrow. In an adult mammal, the bone marrow is the major source of hematopoietic stem cells; in an adult bird, stem cells are found in the bone marrow and in the bursa of Fabricius.

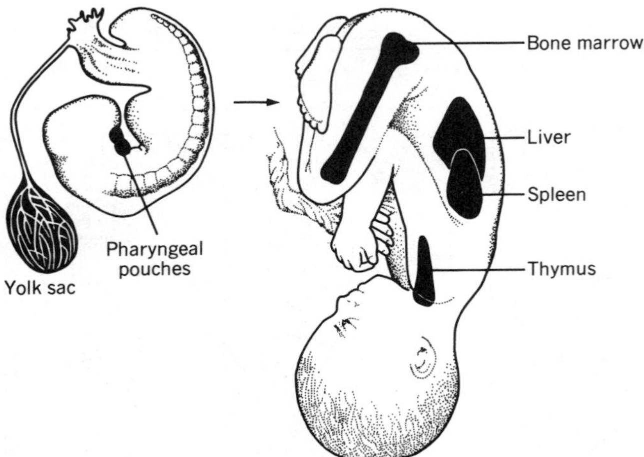

Figure 4.3. Organs of lymphocyte origin in the human fetus.

Yolk Sac

If one takes a newly laid bird egg, allows it to float freely in water until it comes to rest, and then opens it by cutting away the uppermost part of the shell, one finds a circular, whitish area lying atop the yolk. It is from this area that the embryo develops. At the beginning of its development, the embryo sends out cells from the region near the future gut; these cells spread over and nearly enclose the entire yolk, forming a membranous envelop—the *yolk sac*—around it (Fig. 4.6). In the yolk sac's wall, a rich network of blood vessels is formed. These collect nutrients from the yolk (digested by the activity of cells lining the sac' inner surface) and carry them to the embryo.

Although mammalian embryos develop from eggs containing little yolk, they, too, possess a membrane that corresponds to the yolk sac of bird embryos (Fig. 4.7). The wall of the mammalian embryo's yolk sac, like that of the bird embryo, is the site where the first blood cells appear. At the time of blood formation, the mammalian yolk sac wall consists of two layers: the inner endoderm and the outer mesoderm (Fig. 4.8). The mesoderm can be distinguished further into a more differentiated surface layer and an undifferentiated mesenchyme that forms the sac's middle layer. Some of the mesenchymal cells aggregate into nests, the *blood islands*, and the most superficial cells of these nests assemble into a wall—an endothelium—that encloses the island. The endothelial wall forms a primitive blood vessel, and the cells of the island become primitive hematopoietic cells. Elongation of blood vessels occurs by fusion of individual blood islands.

The mammalian yolk sac is a vestigial organ. Because the mammalian egg has such a small supply of nutrients, the embryo must connect its own circulatory system to that of its mother early in its development. This connection is established via the placenta, which develops primarily from another extraembryonic layer—the chorion (Fig. 4.7). As soon as the placenta becomes vascularized and begins to supply nutrients to the embryo, the yolk sac regresses and is reduced to a small remnant in the umbilical cord. The developing embryo, of course, needs a continuing source of blood-forming cells, and so as the yolk sac atrophies, another organ—the fetal liver—gradually takes over the hematopoietic function.

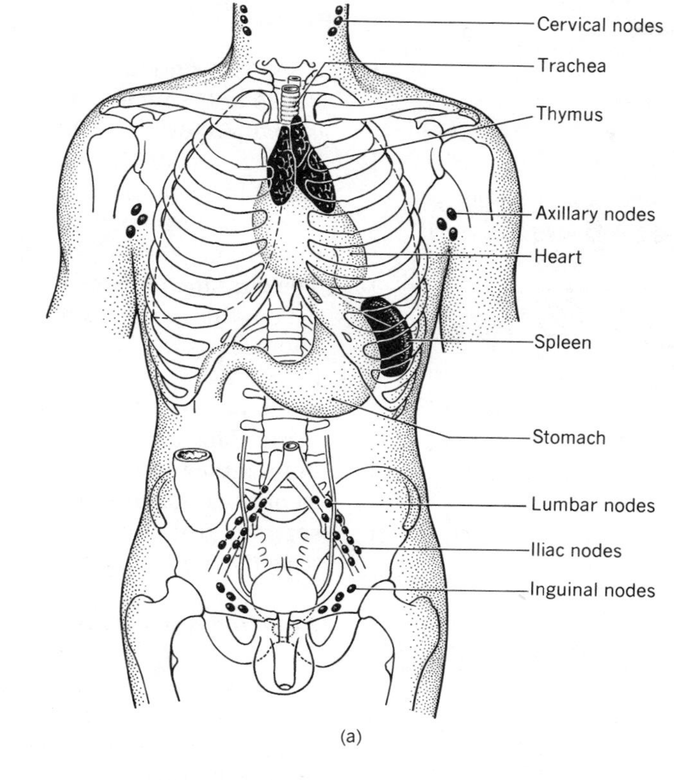

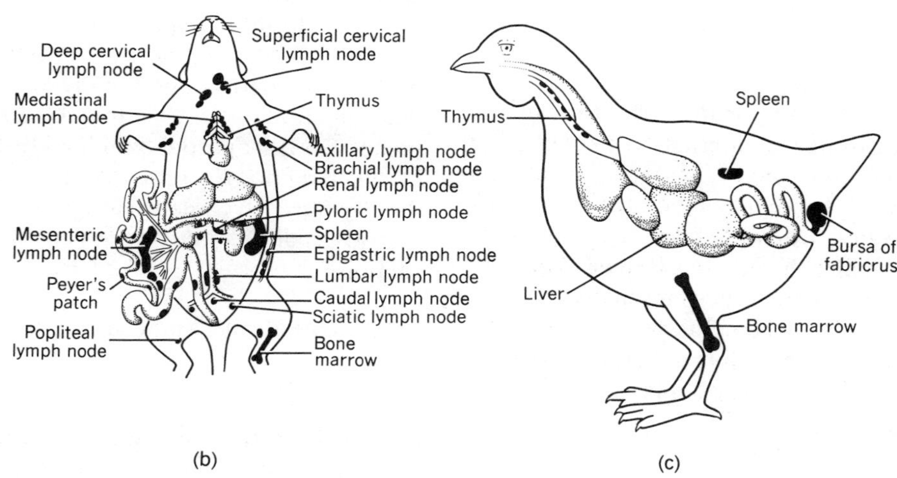

Figure 4.4. Organs of lymphocyte maturation and lodging in an adult human (*a*), mouse (*b*), and domestic fowl (*c*). [*b* is modified from T. B. Dunn, *J. Natl. Cancer Inst.* **14:**1281–1434, 1954; *c* modified from M. Burnet, *Sci. Am.* **207** (Nov.), 1962.]

Fetal Liver

The assumption of the hematopoietic function by the liver moves the site of blood formation from outside the embryo into the embryo proper. However, the new site of hematopoiesis is not far from the original one, since the liver develops from the gut near the gut's opening into the yolk sac (Fig. 4.9). At this site, the gut endoderm forms a pocket-like protrusion, from which the endodermal cells begin to migrate forward and form solid strands or cords. The strands then form a mesh that encloses the blood vessels in the region

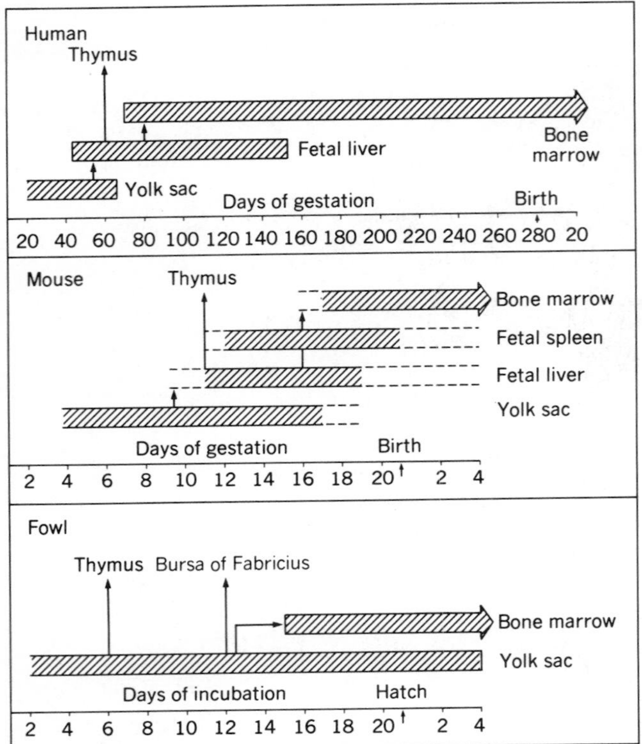

Figure 4.5. Timetable of hematopoietic stem-cell production in various organs of human, mouse, and fowl embryos.

close to the heart. The complicated structure of the adult liver emerges from the interaction between the liver cell cords and the blood vessels. During its growth, the liver mesh becomes embedded in the surrounding mesenchyme derived from the so-called *transverse septum*, which in turn is derived from the amnion. Either these or some other mesenchymal cells then become the source of hematopoietic stem cells. Blood formation in the fetal liver therefore occurs extravascularly—outside the blood vessels.

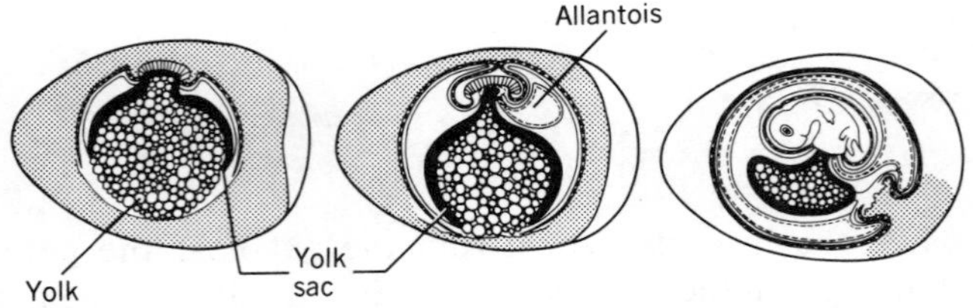

Figure 4.6. Three successive stages (from left to right) of fowl embryo development, showing how the yolk sac membrane envelops the yolk. The yolk sac is the earliest site wherein stem cells giving rise to lymphocytes are found. (From W. J. Hamilton and H. W. Mossman: *Human Embryology*. Williams and Wilkins, Baltimore, 1972.)

Fetal Spleen

As was mentioned earlier, the embryo's gut at first opens in the middle and connects to the yolk sac. The eventual closing of this opening is accomplished by a constriction of the mesoderm surrounding the gut, a stricture that closes the endoderm completely but leaves a curtain of mesodermal tissue on the dorsal (back) and ventral (belly) side of the gut (Fig. 4.10). The gut thus remains suspended on these two curtains, called the *dorsal* and *ventral mesentery* (Gr. *mesos*, middle, *enteron*, intestine). The spleen develops from the dorsal mesentery as a small thickening of mesodermal cells in the vicinity of the future stomach (Fig. 4.10). The mesenchymal cells of the thickened area differentiate in two directions: some remain connected to one another, forming a reticular mesh, while others separate from the rest, become free cells, and possibly transform into hematopoietic stem cells.

Fetal and Adult Bone Marrow

In birds, the final destinations of hematopoietic stem cell migration are the bone marrow and bursa of Fabricius. Both organs probably function not only as stem-cell reservoirs but also as sites of differentiation of stem cells into lymphocyte precursors. In mammals, virtually all hematopoietic stem cells eventually end up in the bone marrow, and in the adult animal this organ then functions both as a source of stem cells and as a place of at least partial lymphocyte differentiation; part of the lymphocyte precursors differentiate further in the thymus. All three organs—bone marrow, bursa of Fabricius, and thymus—are described in the following section.

4.2.2 Organs of Lymphocyte Generation

Bone Marrow

Development of Bone and Bone Marrow. The cellular content of bone cavities is referred to as *bone marrow*. In the human embryo, the first bone to develop marrow is the clavicle (collarbone), which, like all other bones, develops from the mesenchyme. At the site of bone formation, mesenchymal cells retract their cytoplasmic processes, round off, and multiply rapidly, forming a dense agglomerate shaped like the future bone (Fig. 4.11). The rounded cells, or *chondroblasts* (Gr. *chondros*, cartilage, *blastos*, germ), secrete an intercellular matrix consisting of collagenous fibers and an amorphous substance. This matrix separates individual cells, transforming them into *chondrocytes* (Gr.

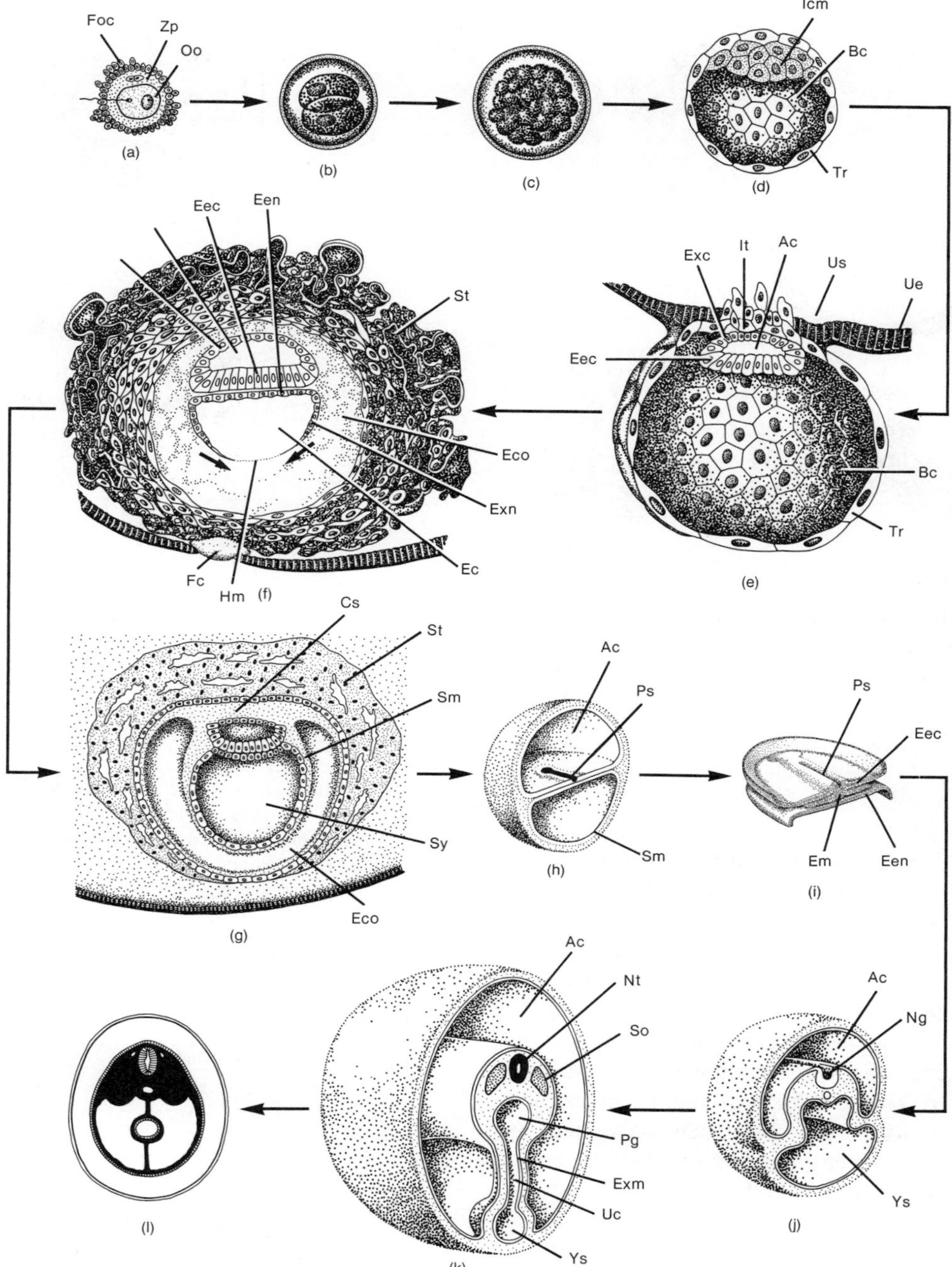

Figure 4.7. Early development of human embryo and yolk sac formation. (*a*) Fertilization. (*b*) First-cleavage stage. (*c*) Morula. (*d*) Blastocyst. (*e*) Implantation. (*f*) Formation of embryonic endoderm. (*g*) Formation of secondary yolk sac. (*h*) and (*i*) Formation of primitive streak. (*j*) Formation of neural groove. (*k*) Formation of neural tube, primitive gut, and yolk sac. (*l*) Formation of definitive gut. Ac, amniotic activity; Bc, blastocyst cavity; Cs, connective stalk; Ec, exocoelomic cavity (primitive yolk sac); Eco, extraembryonic coelom containing somatopleuric mesoderm; Eec, embryonic ectoderm; Een, embryonic endoderm; Em, embryonic mesoderm; Exc, extraembryonic ectoderm; Exm, extraembryonic mesoderm; Exn, extraembryonic endoderm; Fc, fibrin coagulum; Foc, follicular cells; Hm, Heuser's membrane; Icm, inner cell mass; It, invading trophoblast; Ng, neural groove; Nt, neural tube; Oo, oocyte; Pg, primitive gut; Ps, primitive streak; Sm, somatic mesoderm; So, somite; St, syncytial trophoblast; Sy, secondary yolk sac; Tr, trophoblast; Uc, umbilical cord; Ue, uterine epithelium; Us, uterine stroma; Ys, yolk sac; Zp, zona pellucida.

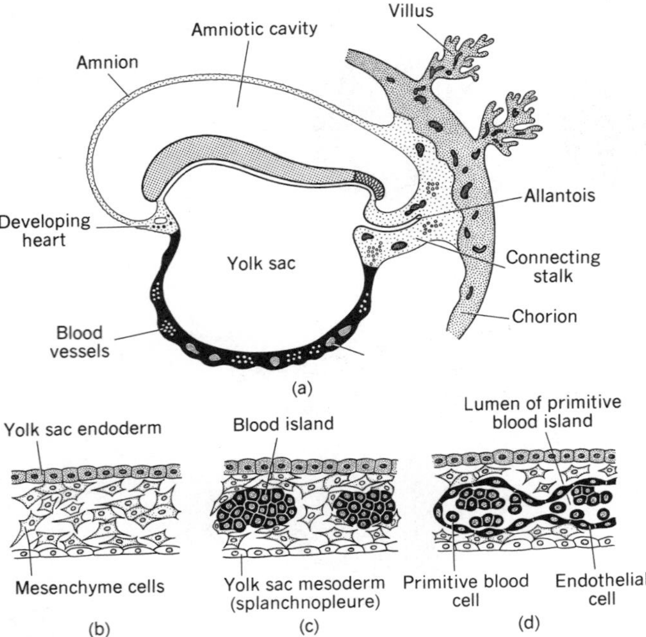

Figure 4.8. Blood and blood vessel formation in a 19-day-old human embryo. Hemopoiesis first occurs in the yolk sac wall (*a* and *b*) with the appearance of blood islands (*c*) and primitive blood vessels (*d*). In *b*, *c*, and *d*, the yolk sac wall is magnified to show three successive stages of blood vessel formation. (From J. Langman: *Medical Embryology*. Williams and Wilkins, Baltimore, 1975.)

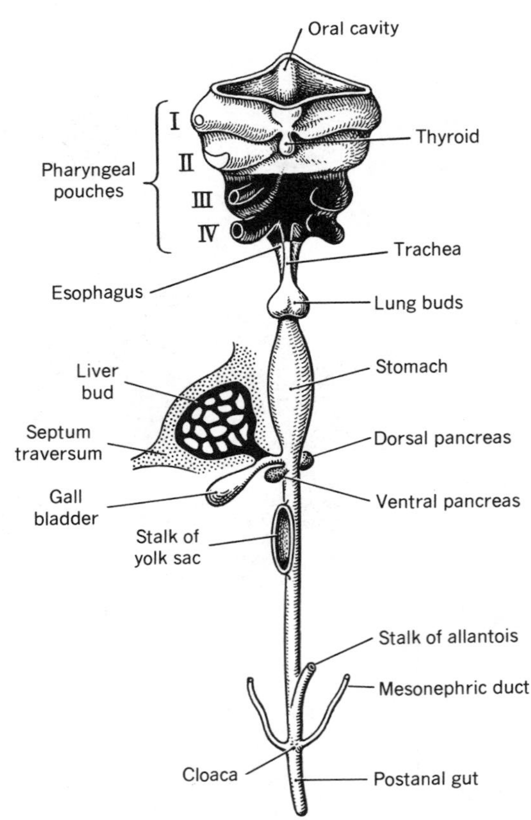

Figure 4.9. The digestive system of a five-week-old human embryo with pharyngeal pouches, some of which develop into the thymus, and with fetal liver. (Modified from H. Wang: *An Outline of Human Embryology*. Williams and Wilkins, Baltimore, 1972.)

kytos, a hollow or cell), and the entire tissue develops into a *cartilage*. Then, minute granules of calcium salts are deposited in the intercellular matrix, particularly in the vicinity of cells, and the cartilage calcifies. In the second month of intrauterine development, the cartilaginous clavicle is penetrated by blood and connective tissue cells that destroy the chondrocytes and dissolve the uncalcified cartilaginous matrix, leaving only the calcified matrix—in the form of septa, ridges, and canyons. The empty spaces are then colonized by capillaries and undifferentiated mesenchymal cells. Some of the undifferentiated cells develop into *osteoblasts* (Gr. *osteon*, bone, *blastos*, germ), which form a bony matrix on the remnants of the calcified cartilage matrix, while others develop into hematopoietic stem cells, filling the cavities that remain after destruction of the cartilage. Concurrently with the formation of new bone tissue, the bone formed in the central areas is destroyed and resorbed by specialized cells—the *osteoclasts* (Gr. *osteon*, bone, *klastos*, broken). This resorption creates a hollow space in the bone's center that also becomes filled with bone marrow cells. After the formation of the clavicular bone marrow, marrow forms in other embryonic bones—in the shoulder blades (scapulae), the innominate bones, and the bones of the skull, ribs, and vertebrae. At first, the marrow plays primarily a bone-forming role (which it retains throughout the individual's life); only later does it assume a hematopoietic function.

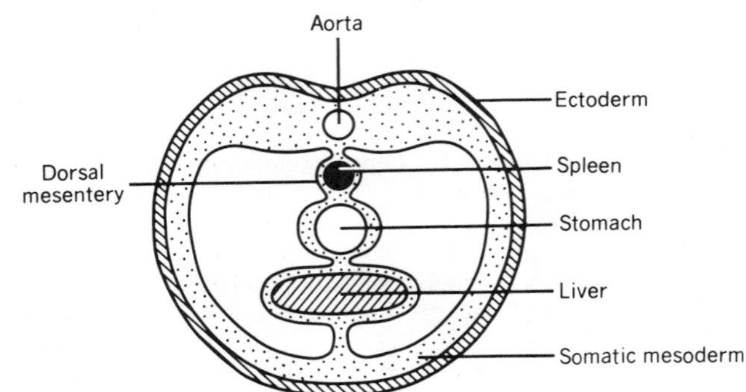

Figure 4.10. Diagrammatic transverse section through human embryo, showing spleen development from mesenchymal cells of the dorsal mesentery.

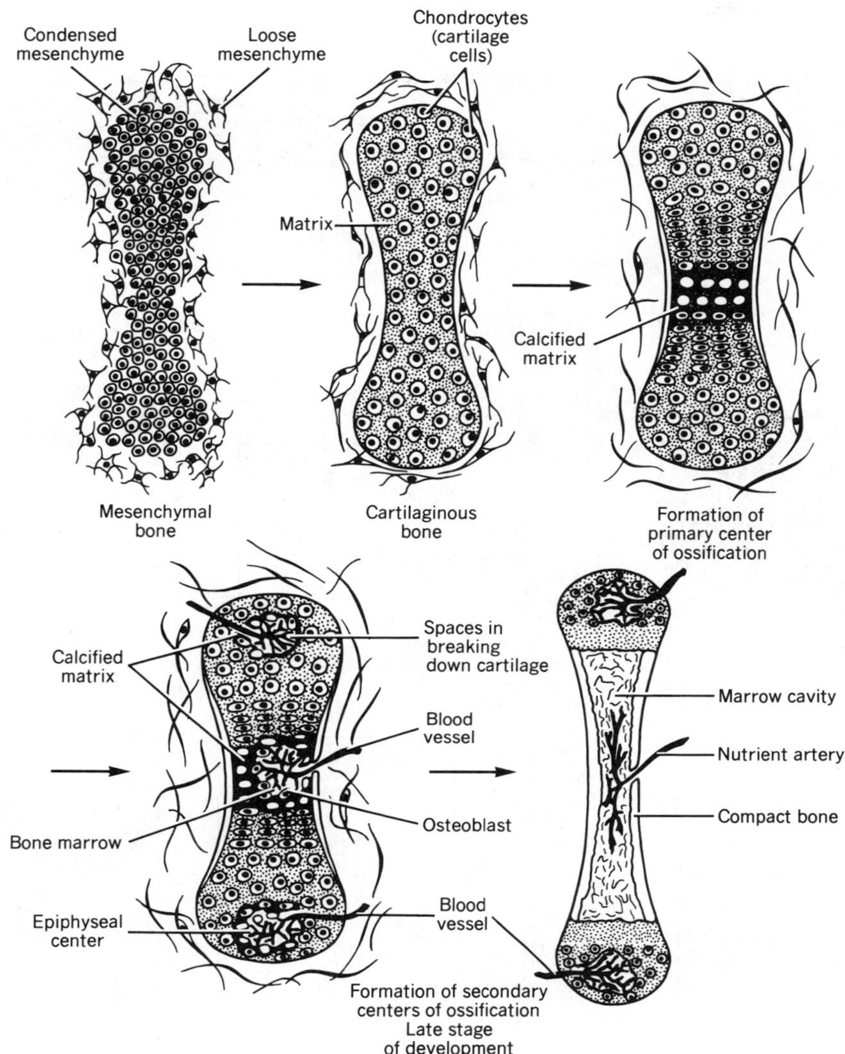

Figure 4.11. Stages in the development of a long bone from undifferentiated mesenchyme. (From R. S. Snell: *Clinical Embryology for Medical Students*. Little, Brown, Boston, 1975.)

The development of a bone from a cartilaginous template as described for the clavicle is characteristic of the short and long bones. Most of the flat bones develop directly from primitive mesenchymal cells, without going through the cartilaginous stage.

Organization of Adult Bone Marrow. There are two types of bone marrow, red and yellow, in an adult human being. The *red bone marrow* derives its color from the abundance of erythrocytes and their precursors, while *yellow bone marrow* owes its hue to the presence of numerous fat (adipose) cells. The red marrow produces blood cells, while the yellow marrow is normally hematopoietically inactive, although it can convert into a blood-forming tissue in stress situations. In a newborn, all the marrow is red; in an adult, red marrow remains only in the breast bone, vertebrae, ribs, clavicles, and bones of the pelvis and skull. The description below applies to the red marrow.

In long and short bones, the marrow occupies the central cavity (Fig. 4.11), the surface of which is often rugged, with many protruding ridges, shelves, and spikes (Fig. 4.12*b*). The protrusions (*trabeculae*, from

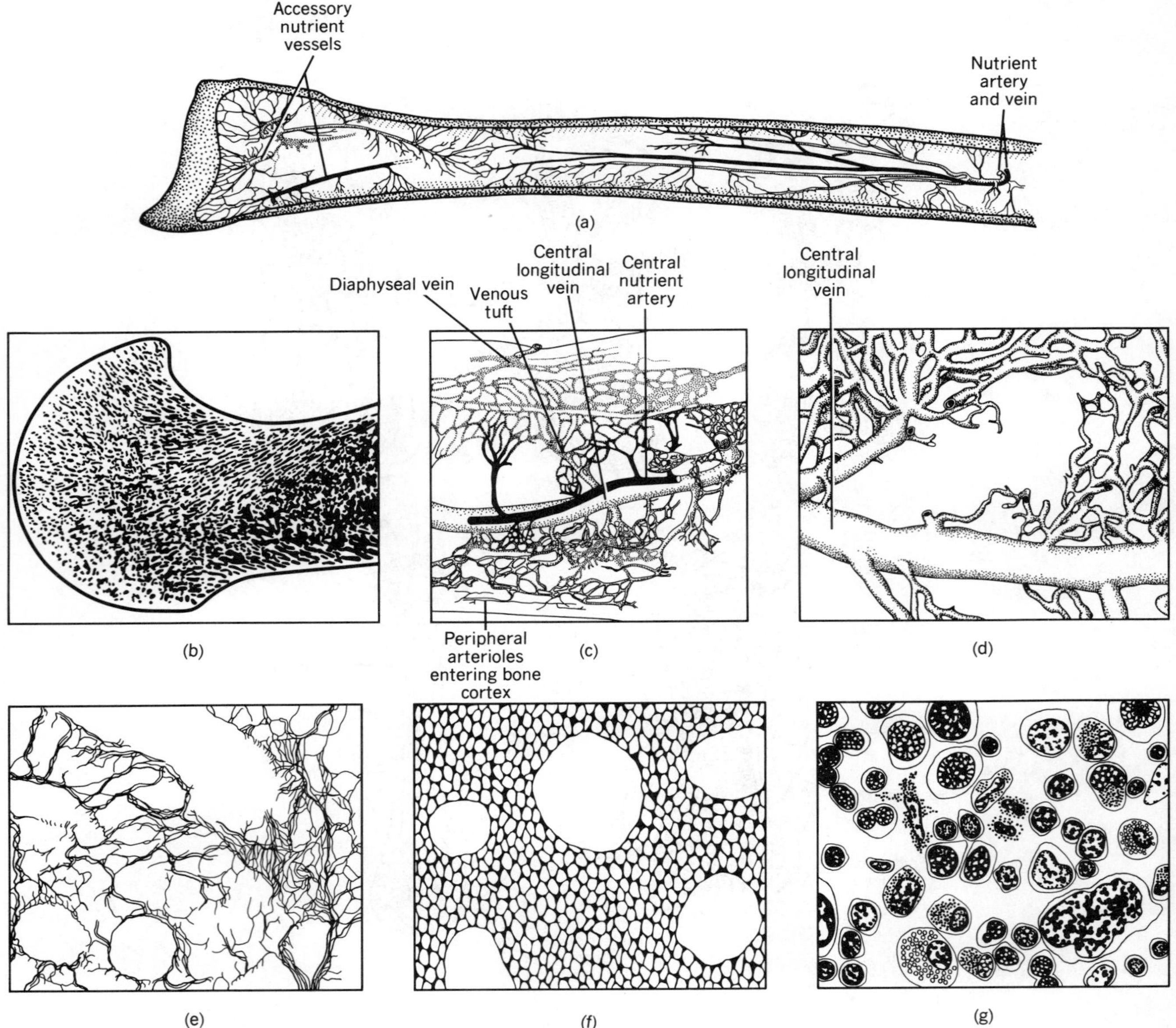

Figure 4.12. Organization of adult bone marrow. (*a*) Section through a long bone, showing the main blood vessels. (*b*) Section through head and neck of a long bone, showing spongelike trabeculae. The meshes of the sponge are occupied by bone marrow. (*c*) Section showing the relationship of main blood vessels. (*d*) The system of veins and sinuses. (*e*) Framework of reticular fibers. (*f*) Framework of reticular cells. (*g*) Hematopoietic cells filling the framework.

L. *trab*, a beam) may be interconnected, forming a labyrinth of chambers and passageways. The internal surface of some bones, however, may be relatively smooth. Lining the internal bone surface is the *endosteum* (Gr. *endon*, within, *osteon*, bone), consisting of a single layer of osteoblasts (bone-forming cells) and osteoclasts (bone-destroying cells).

In a long bone, the main blood supply is provided by the *nutrient artery*, which enters the marrow at about the midshaft and branches out into two (''left-hand'' and ''right-hand'') *central longitudinal arteries* (Fig. 4.12*a* and *c*). These run along the bone's longitudinal axis, sending out radial branches toward the marrow's periphery. The smaller arteries branch out further into arterial capillaries that are connected with a rich network of venous *sinuses* (L. *sinus*, cavity, channel; see Fig. 4.12*d*). The blood from these sinuses is collected by radial veins and then leaves the marrow via the *central longitudinal vein*, which runs parallel to the central longitudinal artery. The circulation system of the bone marrow is thus a closed one. (The venous sinuses are a specialty of hematopoietic organs, and we shall describe them in the section dealing with the spleen.)

The space between the blood vessels is occupied by the *reticular framework*, consisting of irregularly branching, interconnected reticular cells and fibers (Fig. 4.12*e* and *f*). The framework resembles a sponge, the pores of which are filled with hematopoietic cells; its function is to provide support for the free cells of the hematopoietic tissue. Originally some histologists thought that the framework was phagocytically active, but more recent work has demonstrated that the phagocytic activity of the reticular cells is negligible. An older hypothesis, that the reticular cells are stem cells, has also been disproved by recent studies.

The *hematopoietic tissue* (Fig. 4.12*g*) fills the pores of the reticular network. It contains, in addition to hematopoietic cells (lymphocytes compose about 10 percent of all bone marrow cells), fat cells, macrophages, and mast cells. The individual cell types have a tendency to localize in specific areas of the hematopoietic compartment; so megakaryocytes lie close to the reticular cells of the venous sinuses, erythrocytes are also found near the sinuses, granulocytes are produced in nests some distance from the sinuses, and lymphocytes are usually found in compact clusters surrounding small radial arteries.

In mammals, the initial stages of blood formation occur entirely in the hematopoietic tissue outside the blood vessels, but some of the later stages of blood-cell maturation occur intravascularly. To enter the circulatory system, newly formed cells must pass through the sinus wall. This passage is not a simple filtering through—the cells are too large for that—but is rather an active "burrowing." A passing cell must first push aside the reticular cells around the pore, make a hole in the basal membrane or in the cytoplasm of the endothelial cell (if present), and then squeeze through the tunnel thus formed into the sinus. Once there, blood cells, including lymphocyte precursors, become part of the circulatory system and are disseminated throughout the body.

Bursa of Fabricius

In birds, the digestive, urinary, and reproductive tracts open into a common chamber—the *cloaca* (L. sewer). In this chamber's ceiling is a small opening that leads through a short tunnel to a round or pear-shaped pocket referred to as the *bursa of Fabricius*, after the Italian anatomist and embryologist Hieronymus Fabricius Ab Aquapendente (1537–1619).

In the chicken embryo, the bursa of Fabricius (Fig. 4.13) develops from the endodermal epithelium of the primitive cloaca on the fourth or fifth day of embryogenesis. At that time, cells at one site of epithelium proliferate, forming a small protrusion that pushes forward along the cloaca. From the floor of this protrusion, fingerlike projections grow into the pocket, creating multiple folds or *plicae* (Fig. 4.13*a*, *b*). At 11 or 12 days of embryonic development, nodular foci called *follicles* begin to form from the epithelium lining the pocket's inner surface (Fig. 4.13*c*, *d*). The cells within these follicles differentiate into the peripheral *cortex* and the central *medulla*, separated by a layer of epithelial cells, including a basement membrane (Fig. 4.13*d*). The epithelium at the corticomedullary junction is a continuation of the epithelial layer lining the pocket. Later in development, epithelial cells of the medulla become stellate or reticular and are surrounded by a rich network of capillaries from the underlying connective tissue. During the seventh or eighth day of embryonic life, lymphocyte precursors begin to migrate from the yolk sac into the bursa. By the tenth day, they enter the epithelium by passing through the basement membrane, are induced to be-

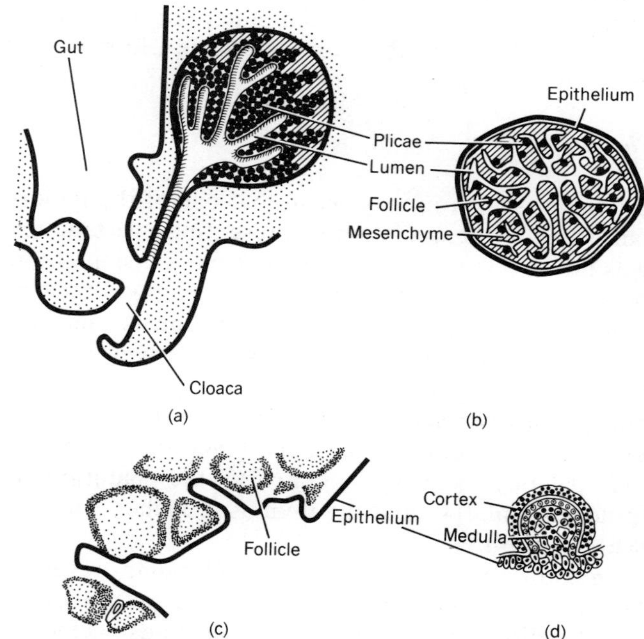

Figure 4.13. Bursa of Fabricius of a chicken embryo. (*a*) Sagittal section of the cloacal region. (*b*) Transverse section through the bursa. (*c*) Portion of plical epithelium with follicles. (*d*) Lymphoid follicle. (Based, in part, on J. Jolly: *Arch. Anat. Microsc.* **16**:363–547, 1915.)

come lymphocytes, which proliferate in the medulla of developing follicles, and then enter the cortex, again passing through the basement membrane. The immigration of lymphocyte precursors transforms the originally epithelial nodule into a *lymphoid follicle*. The number of lymphocytes in the follicles increases rapidly, partly because of immigration of new lymphocyte precursors, but mainly owing to repeated divisions of the lymphocytes already residing in the bursa. The mean generation time of follicular lymphocytes is seven to nine hours.

During their residence in the follicles, the precursors transform into mature cells that leave the bursa as *bursa-derived* or *B lymphocytes* (*B cells*). The maturation of B lymphocytes is driven by the follicular environment and proceeds in steps. (The individual maturation steps will be described in the next chapter.) The emigrating B lymphocytes are carried by the bloodstream to peripheral lymphoid organs, primarily the spleen. In adult mammals, which lack the bursa of Fabricius, this B-lymphocyte differentiation process takes place in the bone marrow. The bursa of Fabricius undergoes age-dependent *physiological involution*: in the domestic fowl, bursal activity begins to decline at about seven to 13 weeks after hatching, when the birds become sexually mature, and the organ gradually diminishes in size. Involution (L. *involvo*, to roll up) can also be induced artificially by injecting the birds with androgenic hormones. Injection of hormones into eggs early in embryonic life arrests bursal development almost completely.

Thymus

Development. You may recall that one of the important steps in the evolution of present-day vertebrates was the development of gill clefts from a fusion of the pharyngeal pouches and grooves (Fig. 1.14). To a certain extent, the mammalian embryo repeats this step by developing four pouches in the pharyngeal area (Figs. 4.9 and 4.14). But instead of developing into gills, these *pharyngeal pouches* become the primordia of several important organs: the inner ear (pouch 1), the palatine tonsils (pouch 2), the parathyroid (pouches 3 and 4), and the thymus (pouches 3 and 4; see Fig. 4.14).

In the sixth week of human embryonic development, the third pharyngeal pouch begins to grow rapidly, forming a saclike protrusion that bends backward toward the digestive tract and becomes the thymus rudiment (Fig. 4.14). Because the cells at the bottom of the sac divide more rapidly than those around its opening, the rudiment assumes a bulbous shape. The lumen

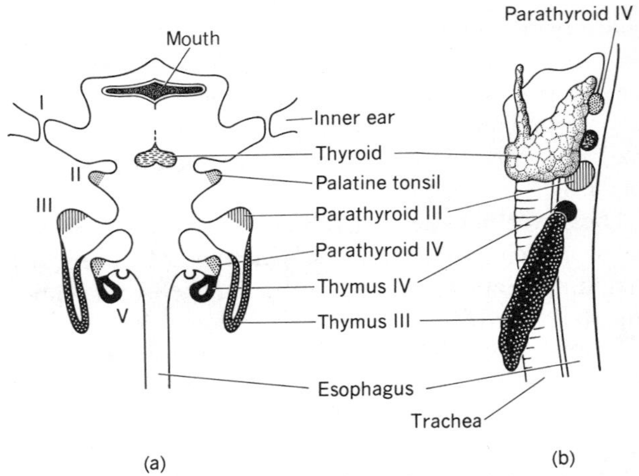

Figure 4.14. Development of the thymus from the third pharyngeal pouch. (*a*) Ventral view of embryonic pharynx, showing the downgrowth of the third pouch. (*b*) View of late embryonic pharynx, showing the disposition of the pouch derivatives. (Modified from H. Wang: *An Outline of Human Embryology*. Williams and Wilkins, Baltimore, 1972.)

of this sac is lost during this rapid growth, the tip of the bulb severs its connection with the pharynx, and the thymic rudiment slides down under the breastbone, where it establishes contact with a similar bulbous rudiment developing from the pouch on the opposite side of the pharynx. (The pouches are paired and the organ primordia develop symmetrically.) The two thymic primordia partially fuse at the surface, but the definitive organ never entirely loses its paired character. The thymic rudiment developing from the fourth pouch is believed to become embedded in the thyroid, and so not to contribute, at least in human embryos, to the organization of the definitive thymus. It is the epithelium (endoderm) of the third pharyngeal pouch that produces the thymic rudiment. As it grows, it pushes into the mesoderm that surrounds the primitive gut, and some of the mesenchymal tissue becomes trapped in the thymus. The mesenchymal tissue also provides the initial stimulus for the differentiation of the endoderm into the thymic rudiment. However, this differentiation proceeds only to a certain stage, where it stops, unless a second stimulus is provided by the arriving lymphocyte precursors. In human embryos, lymphocyte precursors first begin to arrive in the thymic rudiment in the third month of intrauterine life, while the rudiment is still connected to the pharynx. The precursors or stem cells come primarily from the hematopoietic organs that are active at the time—the yolk sac and fetal liver (Fig. 4.5). In the mouse, precursor cells first arrive in the thymic anlage at 12 days of gestation and the cell immigration proceeds in waves from then on. The lymphocyte precursors interact with the epithelial cells in a two-way fashion: the epithelial cells induce lymphoid differentiation, and they themselves are induced to develop further by the lymphoid cells. The first visible consequence of this differentiation is the regrouping of the originally uniformly distributed lymphocyte precursors into areas of dense and light concentration—the future cortex and medulla of the definitive thymus. Lymphocyte precursors migrate to the thymus via the bloodstream, and with the arrival of the first wave, the rudiment is invaded by blood vessels and becomes vascularized. At this time, the thymus epithelium also begins to produce thymic hormones (see Chapter 5).

An important method of studying the origin of cells in the thymus was developed by Nicole M. Le Douarin and her co-workers. The method is based on the observation that the interphase nuclei in embryonic cells of the Japanese quail contain a large amount of heterochromatin visible after staining for DNA. This feature distinguishes embryonic quail cells from those of other birds, including the domestic fowl, which contain very little heterochromatin in their nuclei. Le Douarin and her co-workers used this distinguishing feature to determine the origin of cells in chicken embryos grafted with pieces of quail tissue and to follow, for example, the seeding of the thymus anlage with cells from other organs.

Structure. At puberty, the human thymus consists of two elongated, pyramidal lobes, joined superficially, yet clearly separate, as if each individual had two thymuses rather than one (Fig. 4.15). The pyramid's base rests upon the pericardium (the heart-enclosing membrane), and its tip is at the upper end of the breastbone (Fig. 4.4*a*). A similar bilobate thymic structure exists in most mammals, but the thymus of guinea pigs and birds consists of strings of nodules located along the jugular veins of the neck (Fig. 4.15).

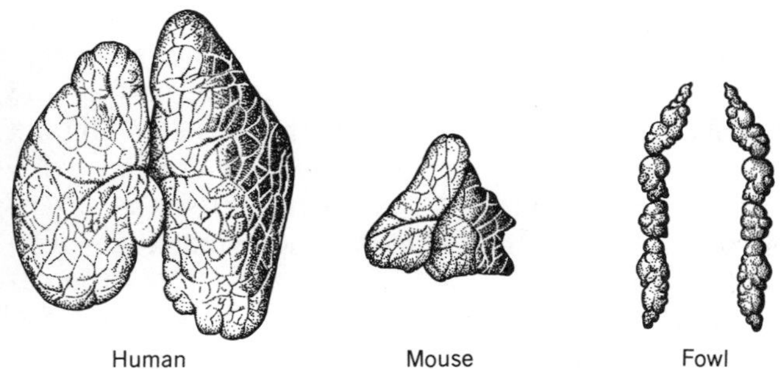

Figure 4.15. Thymuses of a young human, mouse, and domestic fowl.

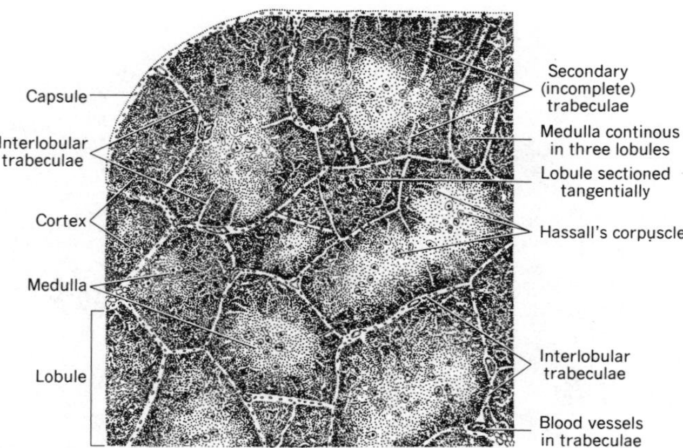

Figure 4.16. Structural components of the thymus. This is how a section looks when stained with hematoxylin and eosin. (Redrawn from M. S. H. DiFiore, R. E. Mancini, and E. D. P. De Robertis: *New Atlas of Histology*. Lea and Febiger, Philadelphia, 1977.)

If one takes one lobe of the human thymus, prepares a thin histological section from it, and stains the section with hematoxylin and eosin (a common histological stain), one sees something similar to what is pictured in Figure 4.16. The lobe is enclosed in a membranous *capsule,* which sends numerous partitions (*septa*) into the thymus, dividing the organ into small *lobules*. The cellular content of each lobule is differentiated into two regions—the darkly staining peripheral *cortex* and the lightly staining inner *medulla.* Closer examination reveals that the difference in staining is caused by the accumulation of darkly staining *lymphocytes* in the cortex and the prevalence of lightly staining *epithelial cells* in the medulla. Although epithelial cells do occur in the cortex, they are often obscured by the masses of lymphocytes. The medulla also contains groups of epithelial cells tightly wound about one another in a concentric pattern—the so-called thymic or *Hassall's corpuscles*, named after the nineteenth century English physician Arthur H. Hassall. Scattered throughout the thymic epithelium are numerous *blood vessels*.

Using this basic knowledge obtained from a two-dimensional section, we shall attempt to construct a three-dimensional view of the thymus (Fig. 4.17) by taking the individual structural elements one by one and considering each separately before putting them together again.

The first element to consider is the *capsule* and its *septa*, which may be visualized as a walnut shell from which the meat has been removed (Fig. 4.17*d*). The capsule and septa are made of dense connective tissue, rich in collagenous fibers and infiltrated with variable numbers of macrophages, plasma cells, mast cells,

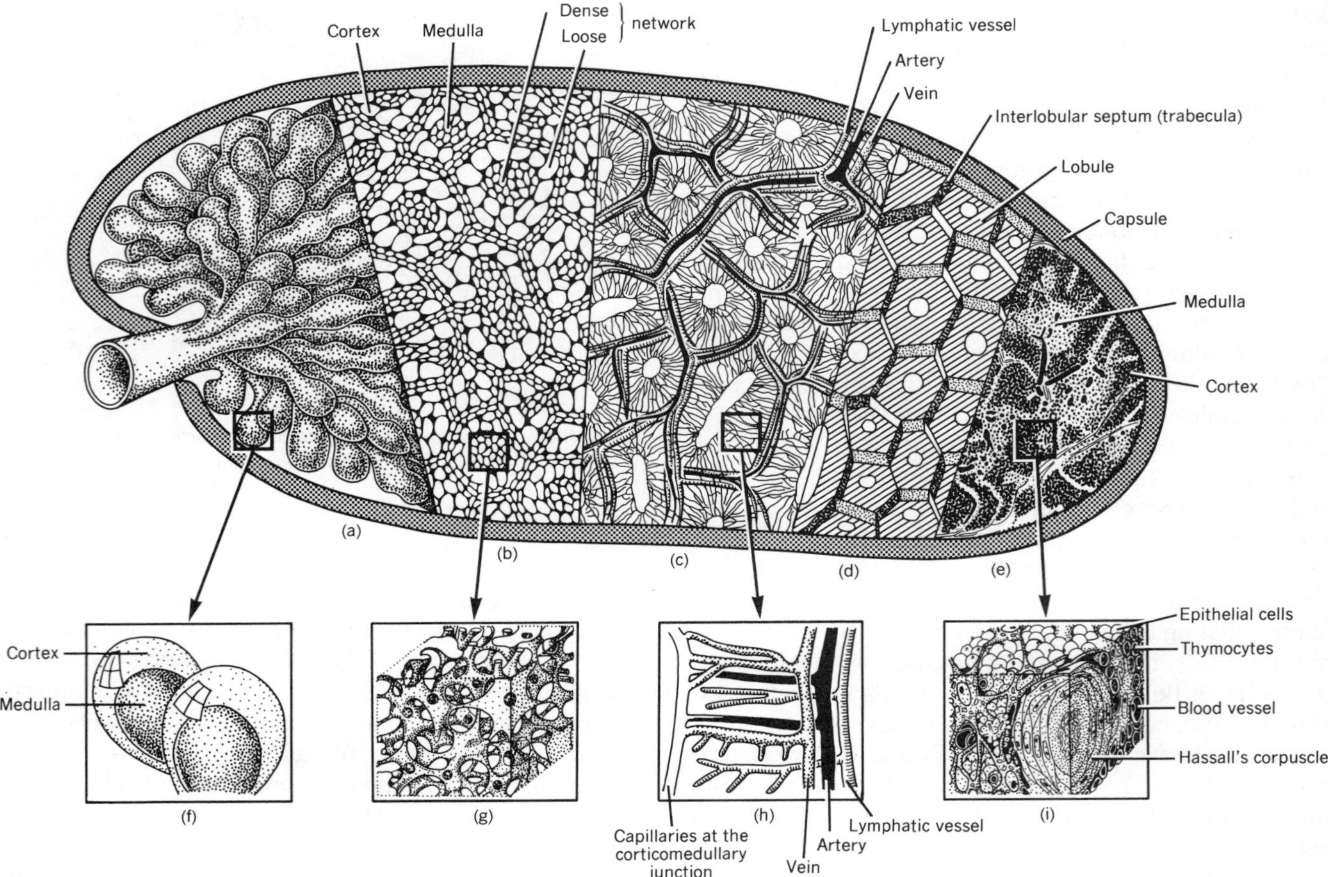

Figure 4.17. Structural organization of the thymus. (*a*) Strands of medulla in a three-dimensional view (cortex not shown). (*b*) Section showing only epithelial cells—densely packed in the medulla and on the surface of each lobule, and loosely organized in the cortex. (*c*) System of blood and lymphatic vessels running along the septae, ramifying in the cortex of each lobule but not entering the medulla. (*d*) The trabecular and septal system dividing the organ's interior into lobules. (*e*) The system of thymocytes filling the meshes of the epithelial framework. (*f*) Three-dimensional view of two lobules with cortex covering the medulla in a caplike fashion. (*g*) Three-dimensional view of epithelial framework from the medulla. (*h*) Diagram showing relation of arteries, veins, capillaries, and lymphatic vessels in a lobule. (*i*) A cube of cortical tissue with epithelial cells, thymocytes, and a Hassall's corpuscle. (*i*) is based on R. V. Krstić: *Die Gewebe des Menschen und der Säugetiere*. Springer-Verlag, Berlin, 1978.)

granulocytes, and other cells. Some of the septal walls are pierced by blood vessels that supply the thymus.

The vessels entering the thymus branch out from the subclavian artery, enter the medulla through the septa, and then branch into smaller arteries and arterioles running along the corticomedullary junction (Fig. 4.17*c* and *h*). The arterioles pass into arterial capillaries, which enter the cortex, run toward its periphery, and then return to the corticomedullary junction as venous capillaries. Blood from the venous capillaries collects in venules and then in veins running parallel to the arterioles of the corticomedullary junction. These veins drain into medullary veins, which in turn empty into the innominate vein.

The circulatory system of the thymus is not only closed, but also well insulated, forming what is sometimes referred to as the *blood-thymus barrier*. In the larger vessels, the blood is separated from thymic cells by four layers: the innermost layer of vascular endothelium, the endothelial basal membrane, a layer of perivascular connective tissue (which is part of the septal connective tissue), and another basal membrane derived from the outermost layer of epithelial cells. (The layer of perivascular connective tissue is absent in the capillaries.) So, to get into the bloodstream or to get from the blood to the thymic tissue, a cell or molecule must pass through four layers—a formidable task even for the very elastic blood cells. However, the blood-thymus barrier is not an absolute one, for experiments have shown that in the cortex, blood vessels are permeable only to soluble, low-molecular-weight substances, whereas in the medulla, even small particles and high-molecular-weight substances can pass through the vessels' four walls. Furthermore, in the medulla, cells have been seen passing through blood vessels; this is not surprising, since it is known that cells enter and leave the thymus, which could be accomplished only via the blood vessels. However, the blood–thymus barrier is much weaker in the medulla than in the cortex, and in the fetal and neonatal period, the thymic blood vessels appear to be more permeable to the passage of cells and molecules than in later life. Moreover, most lymphocyte precursors arrive in the thymus when it is not vascularized. At all stages of life, both the admittance of cells into and the departure of cells out of the thymus are highly selective processes that permit the immigration of only certain cells. How this selective admission and departure are accomplished is not known, but some kind of Maxwell's demon must surely be at work here. There are no afferent lymphatic vessels draining into the thymus, but there are efferent vessels that originate in the medulla and drain into the mediastinal lymph nodes (the mediastinum is the middle partition of the chest cavity).

Superimposed upon the mesh of septa and blood vessels is a mesh formed by *epithelial cells* (Fig. 4.17*b* and *g*). Unlike typical epithelium with closely aggregated cells and limited intercellular space, the thymic epithelium contains loosely connected cells with abundant space between them. Epithelial cells are more tightly aggregated in the medulla than in the cortex, where they are stellate in form and are connected only by their long cytoplasmic extensions. The spongelike appearance of the thymus epithelium led early histologists to believe that they were dealing with reticular connective tissue, and to this day, the epithelial thymic compartment is sometimes referred to as *reticular* or *epithelial reticular cells*. But the tissue is clearly epithelial in origin, and its other morphological characteristics—such as the lack of intercellular material and fibrils and the presence of desmosomes (tight junctions typical of epithelial cells)—support this contention. The loose arrangement of the thymic epithelium is secondary in that the originally aggregated cells are pushed apart by the masses of lymphocytes generated in the thymus.

In the medulla of the human or the guinea pig, some of the epithelial cells are arranged concentrically into nodules, or *Hassall's corpuscles* (Fig. 4.17*i*), the innermost cells of which often die and lyse, leaving a hollow space. Sometimes the cells on the periphery of these corpuscles fuse. The function of Hassall's corpuscles—if they have a special function—is unknown. They are sparse in some species—in healthy mice, for example—and abundant in others, especially following stress.

The interstices of the meshwork created by the septa, blood vessels, and epithelial cells are packed with *thymocytes* (Fig. 4.17*e*)—cells that represent a special class of lymphocyte. About 90 percent of thymocytes reside in the cortex; the remaining 10 percent occur in the medulla. Cortical and medullary thymocytes differ both biochemically and functionally, and these differences are believed to reflect different stages of thymocyte maturation. We shall return to this topic in the next chapter; here it suffices to mention that thymocyte precursors are believed to arrive in the thymic cortex, interact with the thymic epithelium, mature during this interaction, move into the medulla, and depart from both cortex and medulla via blood or lymphatic vessels. But this description applies only to a small minority of thymocytes; the majority apparently die without ever leaving the thymus. Immunologists estimate that more than 90 percent of thymocytes die in this "lymphocyte graveyard" and are replaced by new ones. New cells derive through the proliferation of precursor cells, supplied originally by the fetal hematopoietic organs and in postnatal life by the bone marrow. The proliferation rate of thymic lymphocytes must, therefore, be astounding! The cells that leave the thymus each day—and we know that these constitute a minority of thymocytes—can replace the lymphocyte population of the blood four times over.

Lymphocytes released from the thymus are referred to as *thymus-derived*, or *T lymphocytes* (*T cells*). It appears that there are two populations of such cells, one migrating to the spleen (*spleen-seeking lymphocytes*) and another to the lymph nodes (*lymph node-seeking lymphocytes*). The two populations differ in several characteristics, as will be discussed in the next chapter.

In this section we have dissected the thymus, isolated its various components, and described them. To imagine the thymus in a three-dimensional view, we must mentally reassemble its components by superimposing the different sectional views in Figure 4.17. This, then, is how the thymus looks in reality.

Involution. The thymus reaches its greatest relative weight (with respect to the body) at birth. Absolute thymic weight increases until puberty, after which it declines progressively to 50 percent or less of its peak value. This age-associated decrease in thymic weight, referred to as the *physiological involution*, is accompanied by changes in thymus structure: the rate of thymocyte proliferation, which reaches its peak value

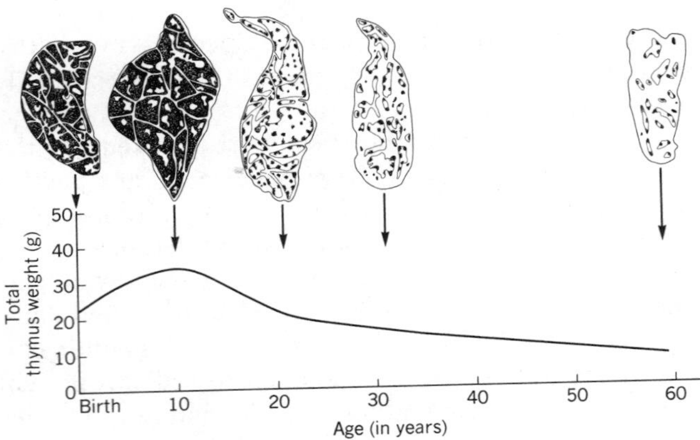

Figure 4.18. Changes in human thymus weight, size, and morphology with age.

during late fetal life and early infancy, declines by 50 percent or more, thymocytes begin to disappear from the cortex, the lobules diminish in size, and the septa broaden (Fig. 4.18). This involution, believed to reflect a general decline in thymus function, may be controlled hormonally since castration slows it down, while injection of corticosteroid hormones accelerates it. Occasionally, transient involution may also occur during childhood as a consequence of a stressful accident (e.g., severe burning), infection, or corticosteroid treatment (so-called *stress* or *acute involution*).

4.2.3 Organs of Lymphocyte Lodging

Upon maturation in the primary lymphoid organs, lymphocytes migrate to the *secondary (peripheral) lymphoid organs* and either lodge in them or continue to circulate through the body, always coming back to these organs as if to their home base. The secondary lymphoid organs are the spleen, lymph nodes, diffuse lymphoid tissues, and solitary and aggregated lymphoid follicles.

Spleen

Location and Appearance. To locate your own spleen, put your left hand on your left flank and touch the lower ribs. The spleen is just beneath them, behind the stomach (Fig. 4.4*a*). Normally it cannot be palpated, but if it enlarges, it extends below the ribs and can be felt.

In the past, when personality characteristics were attributed to the presence in greater or lesser degree of certain bodily fluids, or "humors," the spleen was thought to be the seat of the emotions controlled by black bile. This was the humor that produced, among other passions, bad temper, and so "spleen" became synonymous with melancholy and malice. Remember Baudelaire's "*Quand le ciel bas et lourd pese comme un courereté. . . .*"

When the low and heavy sky presses like a lid
On the groaning heart, a prey to slow cares,
And when from a horizon holding the whole orb
There is cast at us a dark sky more sad than
night. . . .

Appropriately enough, the stanza is from a poem called "Spleen" and defines what was felt to be the splenic temperament. Of course, the spleen has nothing to do with these or any other emotions. Its true function is a much more prosaic one, related to immunity and hematopoiesis.

The human spleen is an oblong, purplish, fist-sized organ (Fig. 4.19). Its surface is smooth except for an indented region—the *hilum*—where blood vessels enter and leave it.

Structure. In explaining the spleen's internal organization, we shall use the same approach as for the thymus, first describing the appearance of a histological section, and then composing a three-dimensional picture of its individual components.

A histological section of the spleen, stained with hematoxylin and eosin, looks like one of Georges Seurat's paintings, with lots of blue spots and pink smudges arranged in a revealing pattern (Fig. 4.20). As in the case of the thymus, this section reveals a

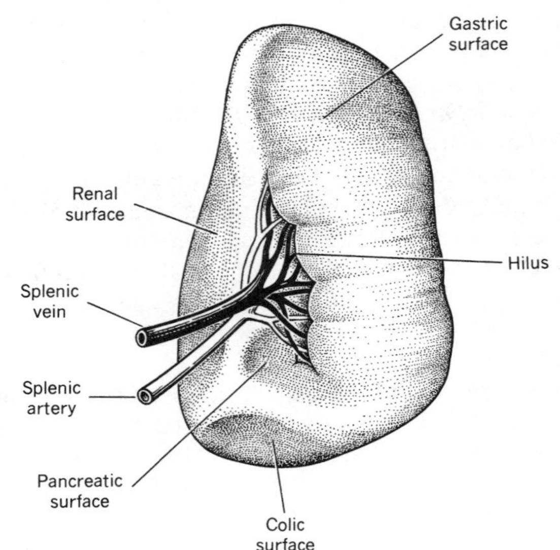

Figure 4.19. The human spleen.

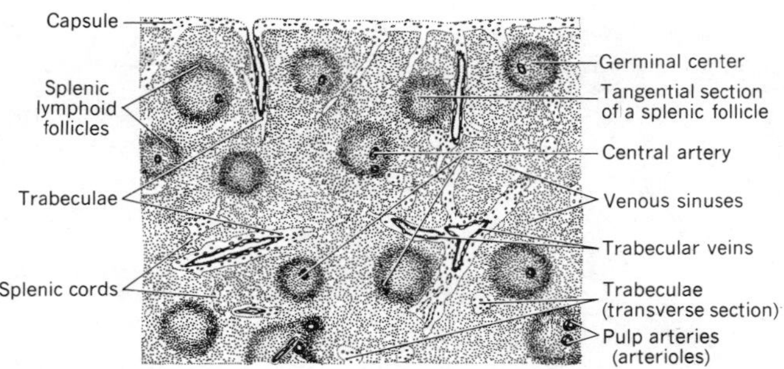

Figure 4.20. A histological section through the spleen. (Redrawn from M. S. H. Di Fiori, R. E. Mancini, and E. D. P. De Robertis: *New Atlas of Histology*. Lea and Febiger, Philadelphia, 1977.)

walnut-like organization, with the *capsule* and *trabeculae* corresponding to the shell and its septa, and the splenic *pulp* or *parenchyma* resembling the nut's meat. Histological staining allows two types of element to be distinguished: circles or rectangles of densely concentrated blue spots (lymphocytes), and a largely pink background. The circles, which often have a light center containing an eccentrically located blood vessel, are referred to as *white pulp*, and the background is called the *red pulp*. These names derive from the fact that white pulp consists mostly of white blood cells (lymphocytes) and red pulp mostly of red cells or their precursors. The area between the white and red pulp is referred to as the *marginal zone*.

Having examined a histological section, let us now try to construct a three-dimensional view of the spleen (Figs. 4.21 and 4.22). There are four main structural elements: the framework of reticular fibers, the framework of reticular cells, the components of the circulatory system, and the free cells.

The *framework of reticular fibers* (Fig. 4.21*a*) becomes visible when one macerates the spleen for weeks in water and then digests it with the enzyme pancreatin. On such preparations the collagenous fibrils are seen to be sprouting out of the capsule and trabeculae into the red pulp, where they form an intricate structure that somewhat resembles a leafless tree.

Superimposed on the fibrilar framework is the *framework of reticular cells* (Fig. 4.21*c*), an assembly of stellate, interconnected elements that resembles a sponge. The reticular cells are everywhere in the spleen, except in the sinuses and vessels. In the red pulp, the stellate cells are arranged in an irregular pat-

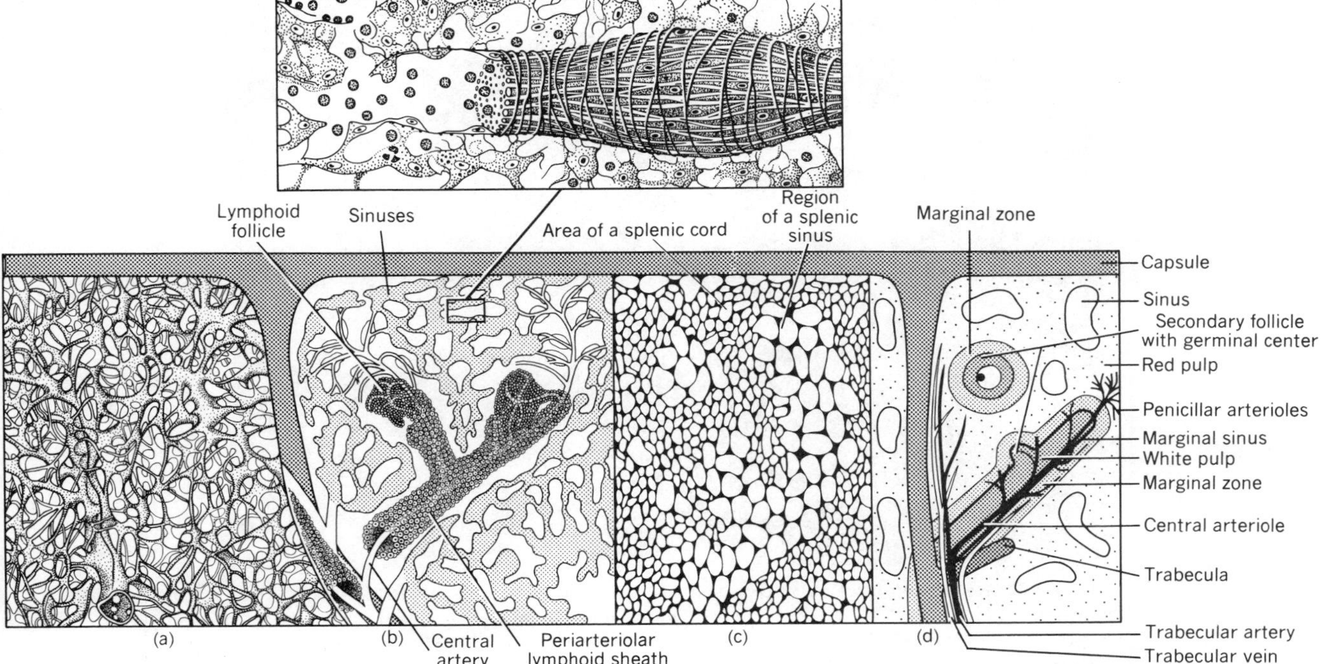

Figure 4.21. Histological organization of the spleen. The individual panels depict its different structural components. (*a*) Framework of reticular fibers; it remains when all cells are digested away. (*b*) Circulatory system of arteries, sinuses, and veins; the central artery is shown surrounded by the periarterial lymphoid sheath with lymphoid follicles. (*c*) Framework of reticular cells. (*d*) Diagrammatic representation of the spleen's main structural features. (*e*) An enlarged sinus containing red blood cells and surrounded by reticular cells of the framework. (The lymphocyte component of the spleen is shown in Figure 4.20.)

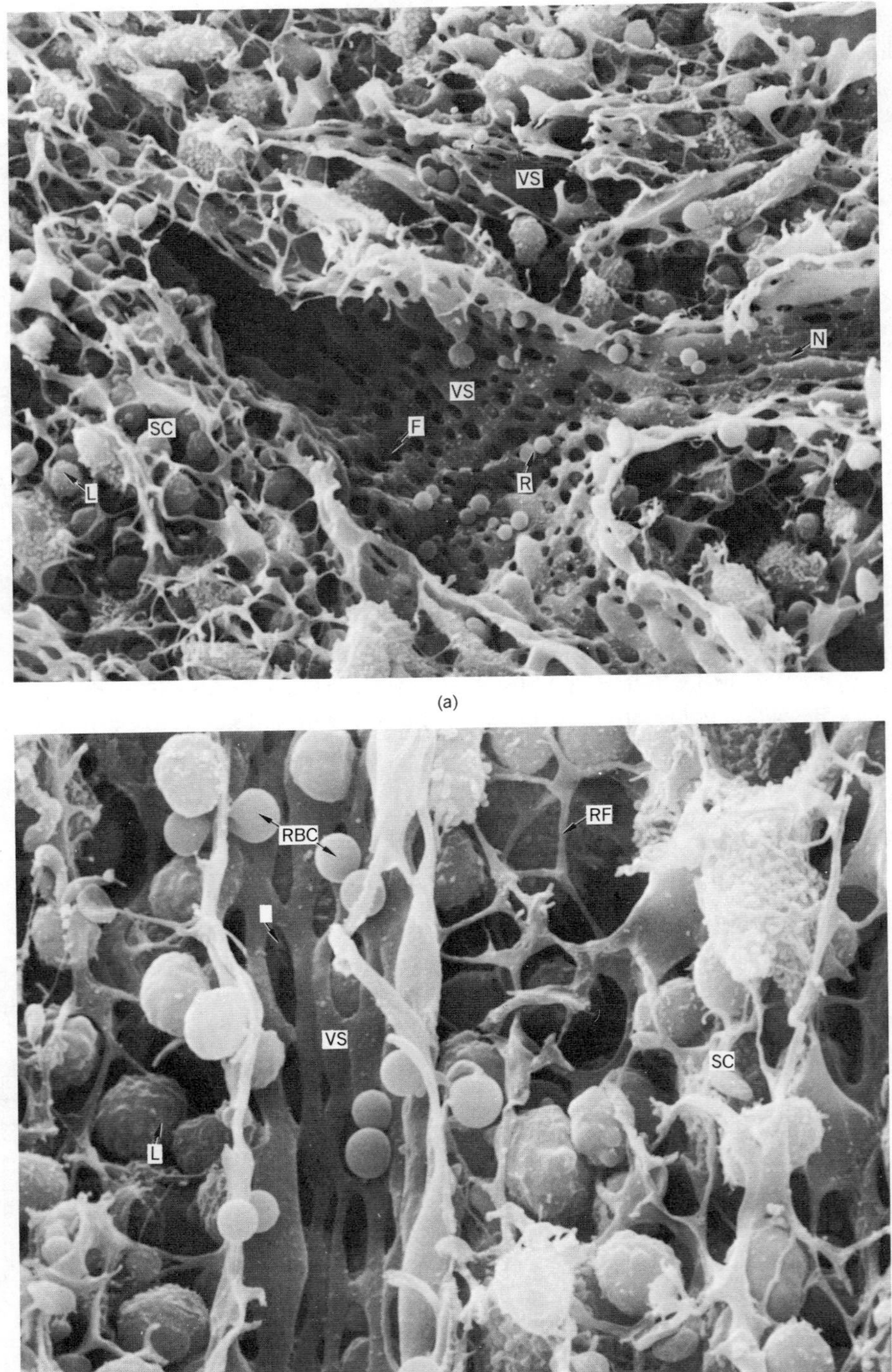

Figure 4.22. Scanning electron micrograph of a portion of rat spleen with a venous sinus, shown in (*a*) lower (x 1000) and (*b*) higher (x 2400) magnifications. In the upper part of the sinus in (*b*), a red blood cell is seen squeezing through the sinus wall, perforated by numerous fenestrations. F, fenestrations; L, lymphocyte; N, nucleus; SC, splenic cords; RBC, red blood cell; RF, reticular fiber; VS, venous sinus. (Micrograph: Dr. Peter Andrews.)

ern, whereas in the white pulp flattened cells are ar-ranged into layers that form the wall of a cylinder, with he inside of the cylinder interwoven with a loose, ir-regular, spongelike mass.

The third main structural component of the spleen, he *circulatory system*, consists of arteries, veins, capil-laries, sinuses, and lymphatic vessels (Fig. 4.21*b*). The nain arteries and veins are enclosed in the hollow passageways of the trabeculae, but the thinner vessels run independently of the trabecular system. The spleen's sole source of blood is the *splenic artery*, which divides into numerous branches before entering the organ at the hilus (Fig. 4.19). These branches, in turn, ramify into subdivisions, which diverge further and run through the trabeculae as *trabecular arteries*. Upon leaving the trabecular system, these enter the white pulp as *central arterioles*, which give off, almost at right angles, many branches of thinner arterioles that either end on the outer surface of the white pulp or extend all the way to the marginal zone. The main trunk of the central arterioles passes through the entire length of the white pulp cylinder, and when it leaves the cylin-der, it branches out, like a tuft of hair, into straight, thin *penicillar arterioles* (L. *penicillus*, a hair-pencil). These either end as such or become even thinner *arte-rial capillaries*, often enclosed in a spherical, eliptical, or cylindrical sheath of closely packed macrophages. The blood discharged into the pulp is collected in *ven-ous sinuses*, which are barrel-shaped vessels that ex-pand or contract, depending on the volume of blood passing through them. The sinus wall is perforated with small openings through which cells can pass, like particles through pores of a filter (Fig. 4.21*e*). Unlike regular blood vessels, sinuses are not always lined with endothelial cells, but if an inner endothelial sheet is present, it consists of a single layer of flat cells resting on a basement membrane. In most instances the sinus wall is formed by long, slim, rod-shaped *reticular* (*ad-ventitial*) *cells* arranged parallel to the long axis of the sinus. These cells are so slim that their nuclei often protrude into the sinus lumen. Wound around the sinus wall are circular, occasionally branching reticular fi-bers, which are fitted into grooves on the reticular cells' outer surface. The reticular cells and fibers connect with cells and fibers of the reticular framework.

Most of the sinuses are located in the red pulp but some—the so-called *marginal sinuses*—envelop the white pulp at the border between the periarteriolar lymphoid sheath and the marginal zone. The marginal sinuses are homologous to the postcapillary venules of the lymph node (see below), and as such, represent the sites where the lymphocytes leave the blood brought into each sinus by a branch of the central arteriole and enter the splenic parenchymal tissue. However, the sinus does not completely enclose the sheath; at a few sites it is interrupted by *bridging channels* that cross the marginal zone and connect the white pulp with the red pulp. The individual sinuses—in both the white and red pulp—drain into *veins of the pulp*, which then enter the trabecular system. The *trabecular veins*, in turn, drain into *splenic veins*, which carry blood to the *portal vein*.

Histologists have long argued among themselves whether splenic blood circulation is closed or open. Observations on live animals have shown that blood passes unobstructed through the spleen, as if through continuous channels. Yet histological sections provide no evidence for the existence of such channels; on the contrary, they reveal that most of the arteries open into the reticular mesh and have no direct connection to the sinuses. These findings can be reconciled by assuming that, depending on the physiological state, the interstices in the reticular mesh are either plugged or open, and that temporary channels connecting arte-rial endings with the sinus can be formed. To enter the sinus, however, cells must still squeeze through its wall.

The spleen contains only efferent *lymphatic vessels* that carry lymph out of the organ; there are no vessels bringing lymph in. The efferent vessels originate in the white pulp, where they lie in close association with the central artery near the trabeculae; from here they enter the trabecular system, and after leaving the spleen, drain into the thoracic duct.

In the meshes of the fibrilar and cellular networks are *free cells*, the fourth basic structural component of the spleen. In the white pulp, free cells consist predom-inantly of lymphocytes arranged concentrically in a cylindrical fashion around the central artery (Fig. 4.21*b*). The cylinder, also referred to as the *periarterio-lar lymphoid sheath* (PALS), contains nests of spheri-cally arranged lymphocytes—the so-called *lymphoid follicles* (*nodules*). In some follicles, lymphocyte con-centration is higher at the periphery than in the center, and such follicles are said to have *mantles* and *germinal centers*. The follicles often push the central artery to one side, placing it in an eccentric location. In histolog-ical sections, follicles, and often the lymphoid sheaths too (depending on how the sections are cut), appear as circles (Fig. 4.20). The follicles contain mostly B lym-phocytes, the sheaths mostly T lymphocytes. Scat-tered throughout the white pulp are the so-called *den-dritic cells* that will be described in the next chapter. The pulp immediately surrounding the periarteriolar lymphoid sheaths is referred to as the *marginal zone*. Here most of the arterioles end, spilling blood into the

Table 4.1 Main Structural Elements of Spleen Parenchyme

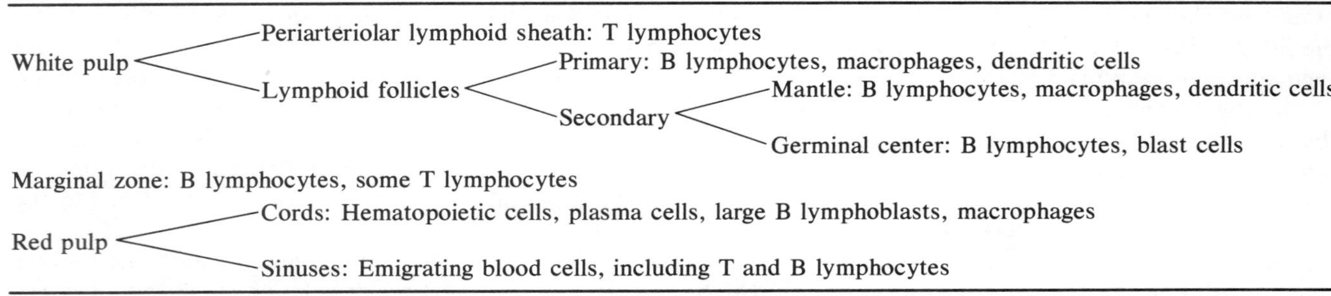

Region	Component	Subdivision	Part	Cells
White pulp	Periarteriolar lymphoid sheath			T lymphocytes
	Lymphoid follicles	Primary		B lymphocytes, macrophages, dendritic cells
		Secondary	Mantle	B lymphocytes, macrophages, dendritic cells
			Germinal center	B lymphocytes, blast cells
Marginal zone				B lymphocytes, some T lymphocytes
Red pulp	Cords			Hematopoietic cells, plasma cells, large B lymphoblasts, macrophages
	Sinuses			Emigrating blood cells, including T and B lymphocytes

reticular framework. In contrast to the red pulp, the marginal zone contains no sinuses (but see below). The predominant cells of the *red pulp* are macrophages, but the pulpal interstices also contain large numbers of red blood cells, platelets, B lymphocytes, and plasma cells. Scattered throughout the framework are the sinuses; the pulpal tissue lying between the sinuses is referred to as the *splenic cords*. The main structural elements of the spleen and their dominant cell types are summarized in Table 4.1.

The ratio of white pulp to red pulp varies, depending on the immune status of an individual. Normally, the white pulp constitutes about 20 percent of the spleen, but in highly immunized animals the pulp may comprise more than half the splenic volume. The histology of the white pulp changes upon stimulation with an antigen. These changes are similar to those occurring in the lymph node, as described in the next section. The main hallmarks of these alterations are the appearance of blast cells in the periarteriolar lymphoid sheath, cellular proliferation and the appearance of young plasma cells in the germinal centers of the lymphoid follicles, the appearance of intermediate and mature plasma cells in the marginal zone, and the passage of plasma cells into the red pulp.

Function. Although spleen is not essential for survival (an individual can lead a normal life without it), it nevertheless has an important function as a discriminatory filter for blood cells and fluids and as an organ of immunity. In its filtering role, the spleen sorts out blood cells, sends them to different compartments, examines them for imperfections, stores some of them, concentrates others, and separates blood from plasma. The sorting process begins after the arterioles have discharged their content into the marginal sinuses and these into the spongework of the marginal zone. As the blood filters through the mesh, *red blood cells* continue their movement toward the red pulp and pass through the splenic cords into the sinuses. But "pass" is the wrong word—in actuality they must *push through* the masses of macrophages filling the cords. And as the red cells squeeze through, the macrophages feel and examine each of them—like a blind Polyphemus feeling his sheep while searching for Odysseus. Cells showing any defect are stopped and devoured on the spot. *Lymphocytes* from the blood enter the spleen by traversing the walls of the marginal sinus and then migrate to their respective domains—B cells to the follicles and T cells to the periarterial lymphoid sheath. They leave the spleen by migrating across the white pulp to the marginal zone, crossing via so-called *bridging channels* to the red pulp, and then entering the veins in the red pulp; some lymphocytes may also leave via efferent lymphatics. *Monocytes* are removed from the circulation and set on a course that transforms them into macrophages. *Blood plasma* is taken up by the sinuses, only to be expelled again by their constriction and forced to move toward the lymphatic vessels, where it becomes part of the lymph. Any particulate *foreign matter* present in the blood is taken up by macrophages and processed.

The immune function of the spleen is to trap and process particles and substances capable of eliciting immune reactions, and to provide a "home" for lymphocytes and macrophages—a place where these cells can interact and go about the business of defense.

Lymph Nodes

Lymph nodes are spherical or bean-shaped bodies that may be as small as a pinhead or as large as a walnut. They are distributed all over the body, but particularly large lymph nodes are found in the armpits (axillary nodes), groin (inguinal nodes), neck, and mesentery (Fig. 4.4*a*).

The basic lymph node structure is similar to that of other lymphoid organs (Fig. 4.23). Each node is enveloped by a connective tissue *capsule* sending many *trabecular projections* into the node's interior. The intertrabecular spaces are occupied by a *reticular spongework* and by *free cells*, mostly lymphocytes,

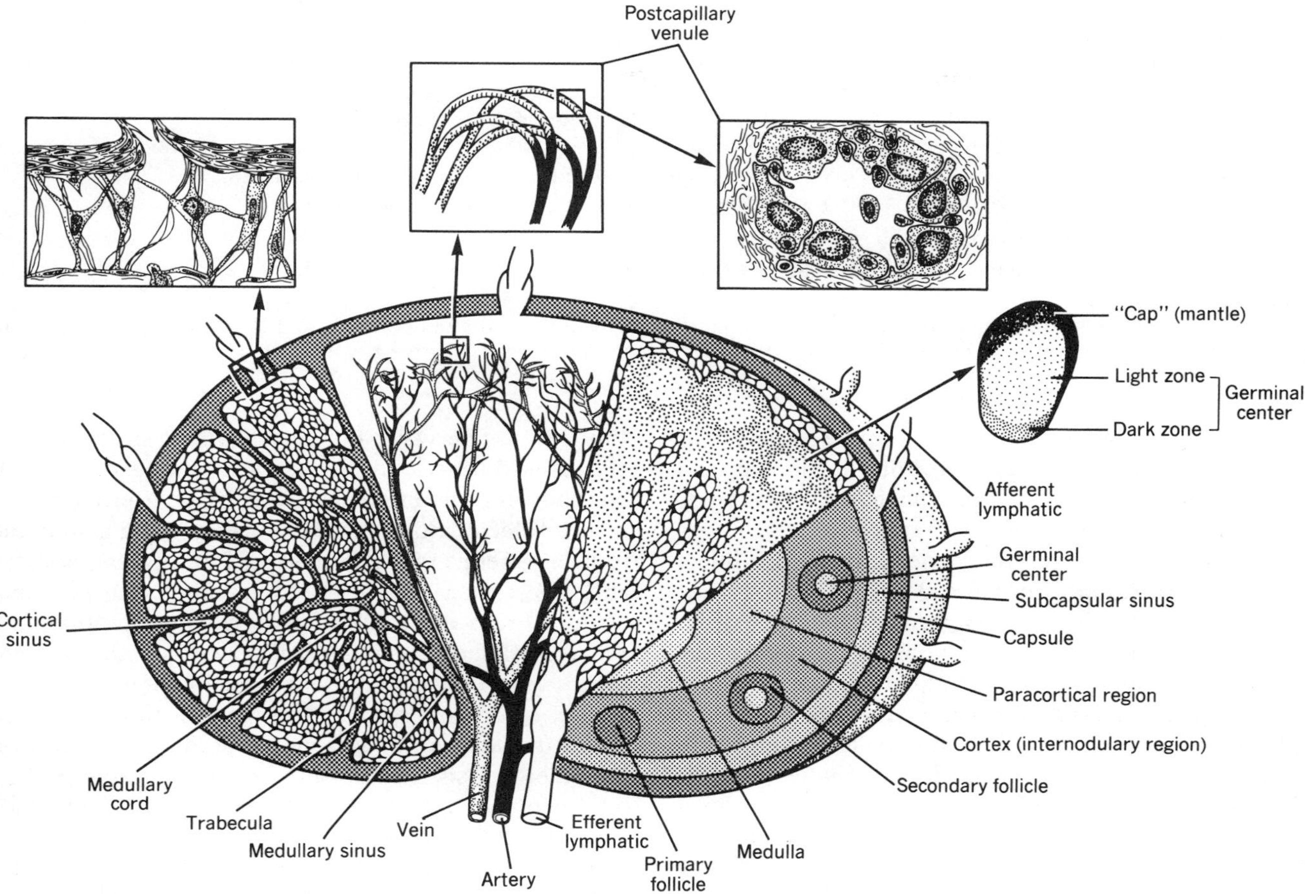

Figure 4.23. Histological organization of a lymph node. The four wedges of the node represent, from left to right, the reticular framework, the circulatory system, the cellular components, and the main structural features in diagram. The four drawings outside the node itself are magnified views of the indicated areas. The third from the left shows the passage of lymphocytes through the postcapillary venule.

lodged in the mesh. The node's periphery (*cortex*) contains more lymphocytes than its interior (*medulla*), many of them aggregated into nestlike *follicles* or *nodules*. Follicles that have a uniform density are referred to as *primary*, while those that have more lymphocytes on their periphery than in their interior are referred to as *secondary*. The central region of a secondary follicle is the *germinal center*; the peripheral region, often reduced to a cap or crescent, is the *mantle*. The lymphocytes in the follicles are primarily B cells and the germinal center is the site of B-cell proliferation and differentiation. Other elements found in germinal centers are blast cells, macrophages, dendritic cells, and a few T lymphocytes. The follicles are separated from one another by *interfollicular* or *internodular tissue* (*diffuse cortex*) and the cortex is separated from the medulla by a *paracortical region*. Most lymphocytes in the interfollicular and paracortical regions are T cells.

The nodal interior is penetrated by numerous channels, or *sinuses*, with walls formed by reticular cells; in contrast to splenic and marrow sinuses, nodal sinuses do not contain blood. The largest channel—perhaps one should say lake—is the *subcapsular sinus* located just beneath the capsule. It drains into numerous *cortical* (*trabecular*) *sinuses*, which often run along the trabecular projections; in the medulla, the cortical sinuses become *medullary* and these then converge into the same area—the nodal *hilus*—and connect to the *efferent lymphatic channels*. The sinuses are lined with phagocytic cells and contain emigrating T and B lymphocytes and blast cells. The mesh between the medullary sinuses, referred to as the *medullary cords*, is dominated by plasma cells and large lymphoblasts. A summary of lymphoid cell distribution in the different regions of a lymph node is given in Table 4.2.

Lymph nodes usually lie directly in the path of lymphatic vessels. The *afferent vessels* pierce the nodal capsule at many different points on the capsule's sur-

Table 4.2 Main Structural Elements of Lymph Node Parenchyma

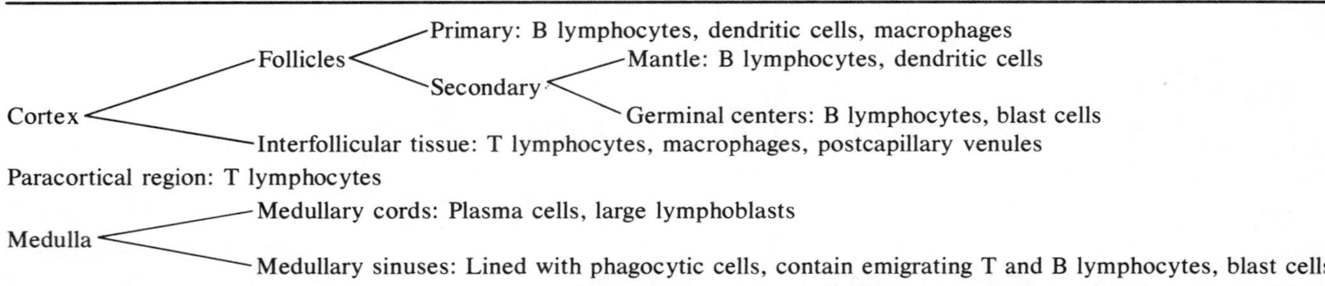

Cortex
- Follicles
  - Primary: B lymphocytes, dendritic cells, macrophages
  - Secondary
    - Mantle: B lymphocytes, dendritic cells
    - Germinal centers: B lymphocytes, blast cells
- Interfollicular tissue: T lymphocytes, macrophages, postcapillary venules

Paracortical region: T lymphocytes

Medulla
- Medullary cords: Plasma cells, large lymphoblasts
- Medullary sinuses: Lined with phagocytic cells, contain emigrating T and B lymphocytes, blast cells

face, and discharge their contents into the subcapsular sinus. This content then percolates through the cortical and medullary sinuses toward the hilus, where it is collected by *efferent lymphatic vessels*.

Several *arteries* enter the node through the hilus, branch out, run along the trabeculae, and, upon reaching the cortex, split into numerous *capillaries* (Fig. 4.23). A particularly dense network of capillaries surrounds the cortical follicles. Capillaries then pass into *venules*, which merge into veins that run along the trabecular system and leave the node through the hilus. The *postcapillary venules* (i.e., venules immediately following the capillaries in the cortex) have a characteristic lining of cuboidal endothelium. To leave the bloodstream, cells must pass through this epithelial layer (inset, Fig. 4.23); to accomplish this feat, they must make themselves as small as possible and even push out the membrane of the endothelial cells.

Two facts should be emphasized about the lymph node structure. First, it is a *dynamic* structure in which both the liquids and free cells are constantly on the move, entering the lymph node in the cortical region from afferent lymphatics and postcapillary venules, migrating via the wide channels through the medulla toward the hilus, and leaving the node by way of efferent lymphatic vessels; the only relatively stable structural element is the scaffolding of the reticular spongework. Second, the node structure changes, depending on the immune status of an organism. In a nonimmune animal, the node is relatively small and its cortical region contains mostly primary follicles. Lymphocytes from the blood enter the node by traversing the walls of the postcapillary venules; the T cells remain in the interfollicular cortex and the B cells enter the follicles. Both cell types then percolate "down" through the node toward the hilus and leave the node via the efferent lymphatics. Upon immunization, small T lymphocytes entering the node via postcapillary venules begin to transform into large blasts and to proliferate in the interfollicular region (see Chapter 13, Fig. 13.7). The wave of T-cell division in the diffuse cortex is followed by the transformation of small B lymphocytes into large blasts and by their proliferation in the follicle. Some of the T cells migrate into the follicle, where a focus of dividing T and B lymphocytes and macrophages forms the beginning of a germinal center. From this region of active proliferation, the progeny of these dividing cells push into the follicle, often compressing it into a crescent. Therefore, in an active secondary follicle one can distinguish three zones: the dense (dark) zone of proliferating cells on the pole opposite the capsule; the less densely packed (and hence lighter) central region of mostly nondividing cells; and a dense crescent of the compressed original follicular tissue on the pole close to the capsule. (The dark zone of proliferating cells and the light zone comprise the germinal center; see inset in Fig. 4.23.) The differentiated progeny of B cells in the germinal center (mostly plasma cells) then move out of the center toward the hilus; some of these cells settle between the sinuses of the medulla, forming the medullary cords; others percolate through the nodal tissue and leave the node via the efferent lymphatic vessels. The activated T and B lymphocytes secrete soluble factors, some of which cause local vessel dilatation, allowing leakage (transudation) of plasma from blood vessels into extravascular spaces; other factors attract macrophages and granulocytes into the node, and these then plug some of the medullary sinuses, causing a slowing down of lymph drainage into efferent lymphatics. The accumulation of fluids and cells leads to lymph node enlargement—the "swollen glands" characteristic of infection. As the antigenic stimulation of the node subsides, the node's histological appearance and size return to normal. Similar changes also occur in other lymphoid organs—for example, the spleen—containing structures homologous to the lymph node follicle.

Besides providing residence for lymphocytes and macrophages, lymph nodes perform three other funcions: they capture infectious agents and any other par- iculate matter present in the fluids brought into them ›y the lymphatic vessels, they process the foreign ma- erial (primarily through phagocytosis), and they pro- ride the cellular scaffolding necessary for interactions ›f immune cells.

During embryogenesis, lymph nodes originate from the mesenchyme in circumscribed areas between blood and lymphatic vessels (Fig. 4.24). In each such area, the mesenchyme condenses into a bulb-shaped anlage, which is infiltrated by blood-borne lymphocytes. The lymphatic vessel widens into a flat sac, indented by the outgrowth of the anlage. Cords of mesenchymal cells then invade the sac and divide it into a maze of

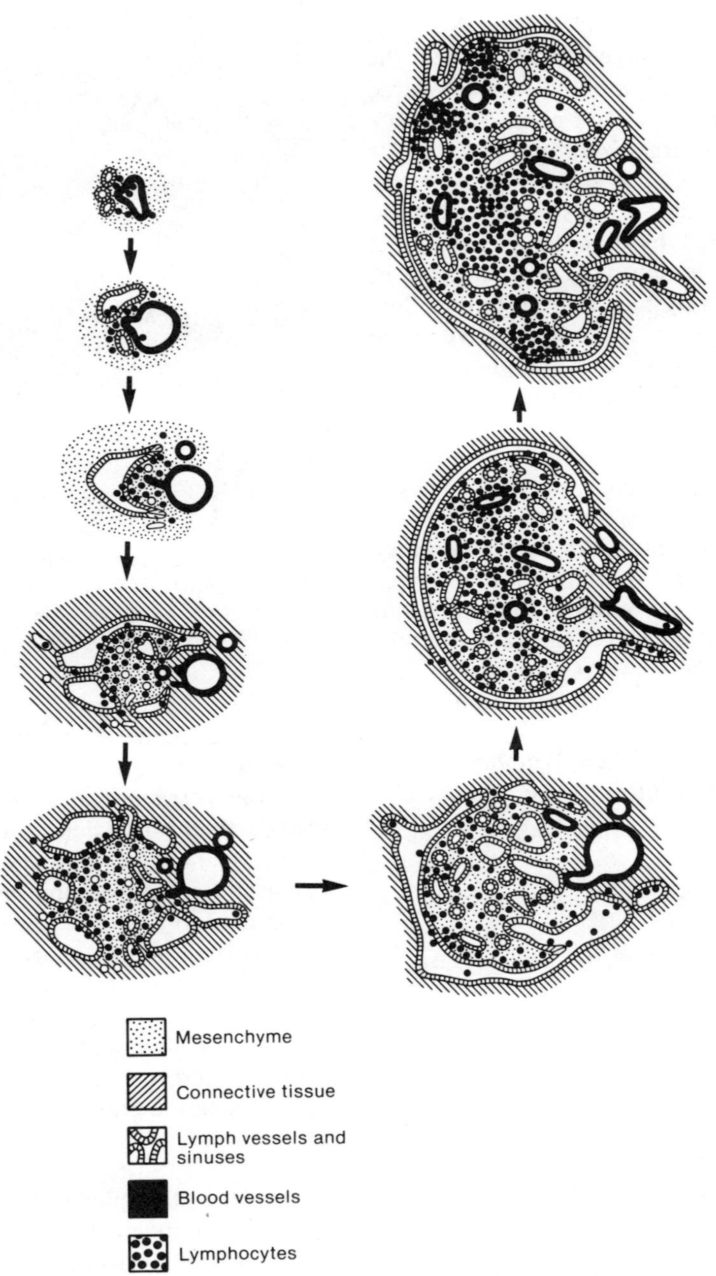

Figure 4.24. Ontogeny of a lymph node. Explanation in the text. (Modified from P. Eikelenboom, J. J. J. Nassy, J. Post, J. C. M. B. Versteeg, and H. C. Langevoort: *Anat. Rec.* **190**:201–216, 1978.)

channels and spaces—the future sinuses of the adult node. Some of the mesenchymal cells transform into connective tissue, which, on the anlage's surface, gives rise to the capsule, and inside, between the channels, condenses into trabeculae. Almost simultaneously, an ingrowth of blood vessels occurs along the developing trabeculae and into the anlage interior.

Other Types of Lymphoid Tissue

In addition to the highly organized lymph nodes, the body contains other types of lymphoid tissue, related to the nodes but usually not so complex. This tissue can either be diffuse or organized into solitary or aggregated follicles (nodules). It differs from lymph nodes in two main ways. First, it does not filter lymph; although often surrounded by lymphatic vessels, it does not intercept them, lymph does not perforate it, and the vessels serve merely to drain the tissue. Second, it does not possess sinuses and a connective tissue capsule. The main function of this lymphoid tissue is defense. A description of some of the major types follows.

Diffuse Lymphoid Tissue. Lamina propria (the layer of connective tissue immediately underlying the basement membrane of an epithelium) in the respiratory and digestive tracts contains scattered lymphocytes and mature plasma cells, sometimes clustered into nests, but never organized into a recognizable pattern (Fig. 4.25). The number of lymphocytes in this diffuse lymphoid tissue increases during infection.

Solitary Lymphoid Follicles. When lymphocytes in the connective tissue cluster into a dense, clearly circumscribed sphere, usually surrounded by a net of draining lymphatic capillaries, the aggregate is referred to as the *lymphoid follicle* (nodule) (Fig. 4.26). It corresponds to the follicles found in the cortex of lymph nodes. The location of these follicles is not fixed: they come and go, depending on the conditions in a given organ at a given time. Some of them develop *germinal centers*—light-staining areas of rapidly proliferating cells. Lymphatic follicles have an organ distribution similar to that of the diffuse lymphoid tissue, being particularly abundant in the connective tissues of the digestive and respiratory tracts. Histologists have estimated that the bowels of a healthy child contain some 15,000 follicles.

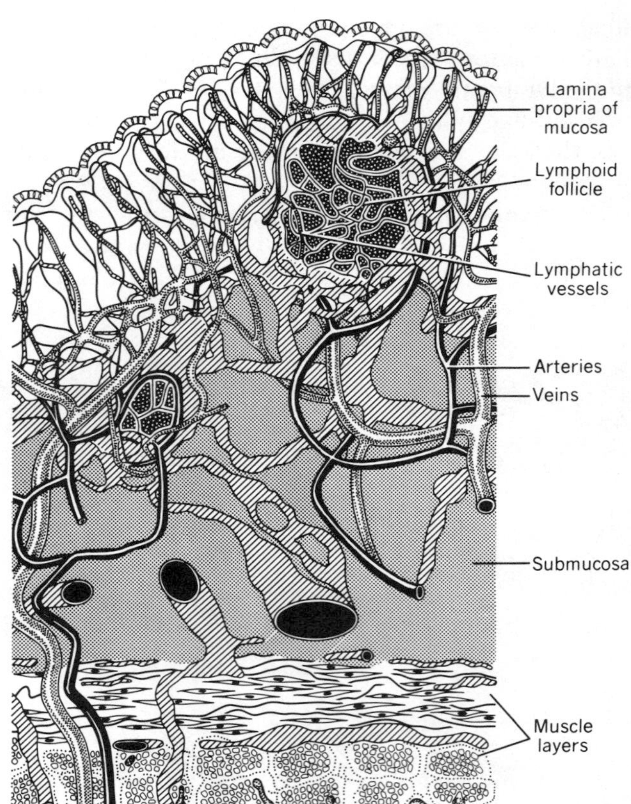

Figure 4.26. Lymphoid follicles in the colonic wall of a human infant. (From O. F. Kampmeier: *Evolution and Comparative Morphology of the Lymphatic System*. C. C. Thomas, Springfield, Illinois, 1969.)

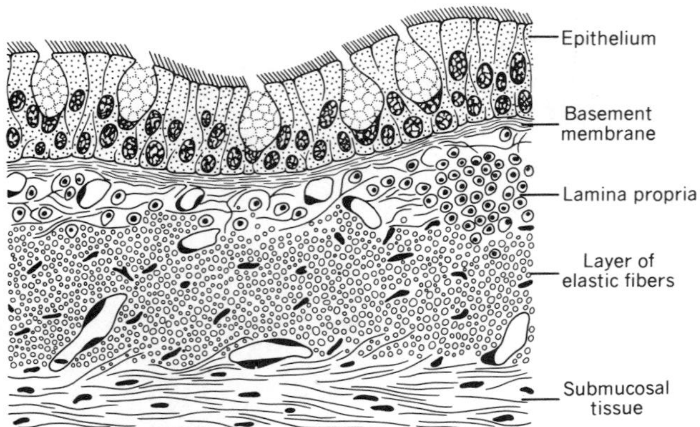

Figure 4.25. Diffuse lymphoid tissue in the lamina propria of the mucous membrane covering the inner surface of adult human trachea. (Modified from O. F. Kampmeier: *Evolution and Comparative Morphology of the Lymphatic System*. C. C. Thomas, Springfield, Illinois, 1969.)

Aggregated Lymphoid Follicles. This category of lymphoid tissue includes three types—the tonsils of the mouth, pharynx, and larynx; the Peyer's patches of the small intestine; and the vermiform appendix of the large bowel.

The four main *tonsils*—the palatine, lingual, pharyngeal, and tubal (Fig. 4.27)—form a ring (''chain

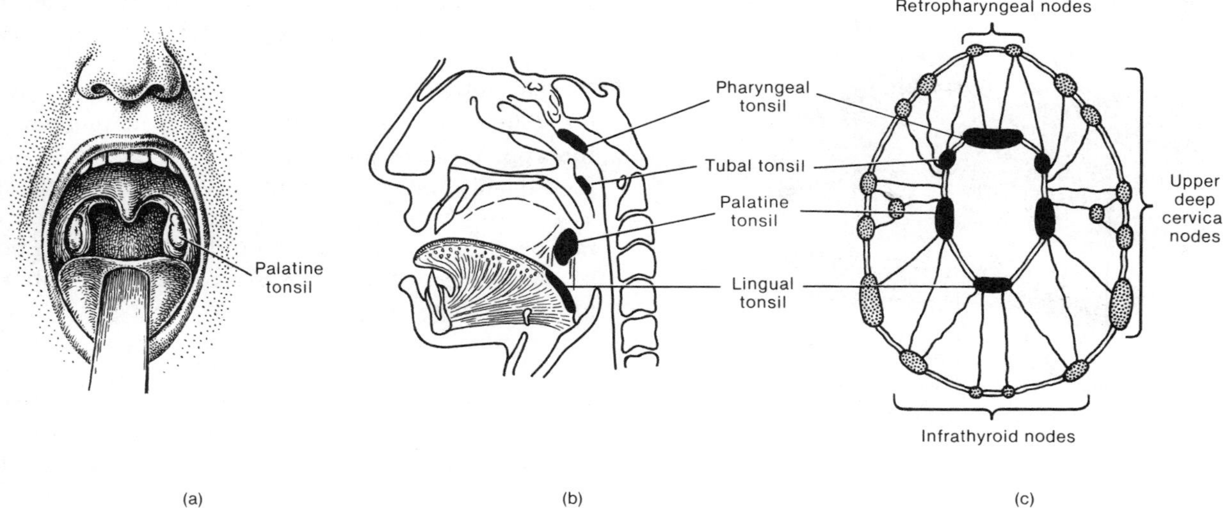

Figure 4.27. Human tonsils. (*a*) Palatine tonsils visible in an open mouth. (*b*) Section through the head showing location of tonsils. (*c*) Lymphatic drainage of tonsils.

of fortresses'') about the openings into the mouth and nose. The largest of these, the palatine tonsils, are located at each side of the entrance to the throat and are what the layperson means by ''tonsils.'' Each palatine tonsil is about the size and shape of an almond and consists of an outer layer of stratified squamous epithelium surrounding an inner layer of connective tissue. The epithelium contains so many lymphoid nodules that, in a histological section, it almost disappears under them (Fig. 4.28). The tonsil's surface is furrowed by many grooves and wrinkles (*crypts*) penetrating deep into the interior. Each tonsil is surrounded by a net of draining lymphatic capillaries which, without penetrating the organ, collect fluids and cells from the tonsil and carry them to the nearest lymph node. The organization of the other three tonsils is similar to that of the palatine tonsils. The paired *lingual tonsils* are located at the base of the tongue (L. *lingua*, tongue), directly in front of the epiglottis—a leaf-shaped plate of elastic cartilage at the root of the tongue. The unpaired *pharyngeal tonsils*, also known as the *adenoids* (Gr. *adēn*, gland, *eidos*, appearance), appear as a thickening and wrinkling of the mucosa at the rear of the nasopharynx, and the *tubal tonsils* consist of a small mass of lymphoid tissue lying just at the opening of the auditory (Eustachian) tube. Behind these four tonsils, in the wall of the larynx, diffuse lymphoid tissue sometimes condenses into nodules referred to as *laryngeal tonsils*.

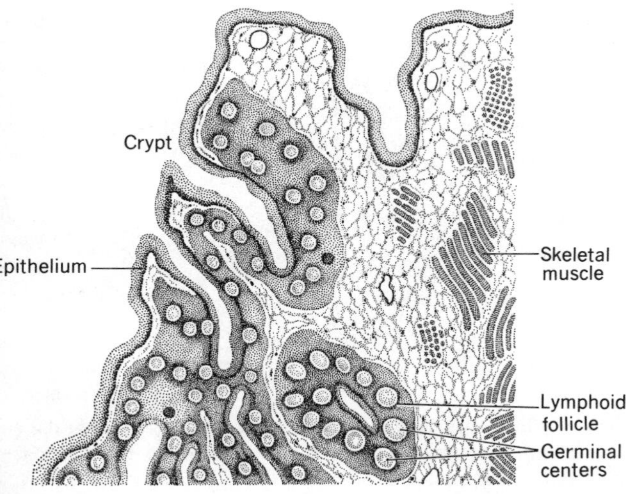

Figure 4.28. Cross section through a portion of a palatine tonsil. (Modified from L. C. Junqueira, J. Cameiro, and A. Contopoulos: *Basic Histology*. Lange, Los Altos, California, 1977.)

The inner surface of the ileum, the distal segment of the small intestine, is covered with a great number of minute, fingerlike projections—the intestinal villi; but scattered among the villi are groups of bare, dome-shaped structures that look somewhat like nests of puffballs in the grass (Fig. 4.29*a*). The groups are called *Peyer's patches* after the Swiss anatomist Johann K. Peyer (1653–1712), and under each dome is a single lymphoid follicle. In mammals, each intestine may contain as many as 200 patches (30 to 40 large ones and many smaller ones) and each patch may contain up to 70 lymphoid follicles; birds possess only one Peyer's patch. The epithelium of the dome overlying each follicle is comprised of specialized cells characterized by

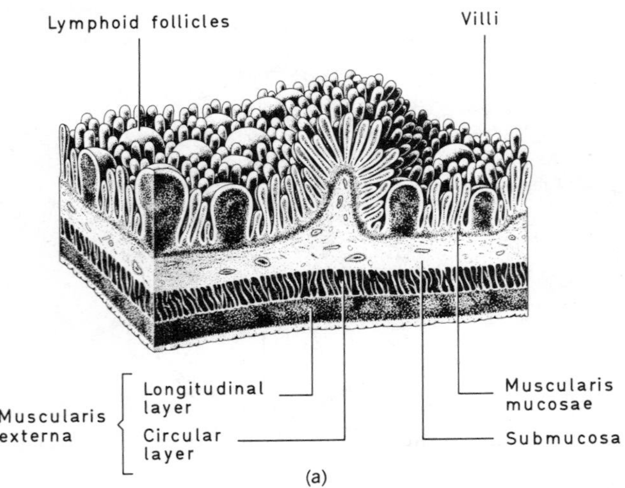

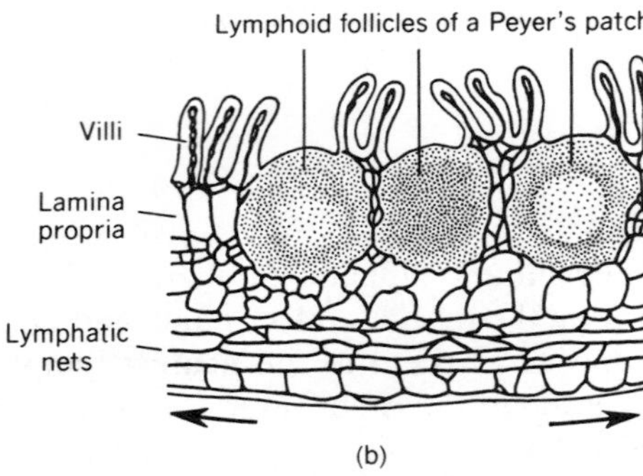

Figure 4.29. Peyer's patches. (*a*) Block of intestinal tissue with one Peyer's patch. (*b*) Diagram of the lymphatic vessels draining the area of a Peyer's patch. (*a* from W. M. Copenhaver, R. B. Bunge, and M. B. Bunge: *Bailey's Textbook of Histology*. Williams and Wilkins, Baltimore, 1971; *b* from O. F. Kampmeier: *Evolution and Comparative Morphology of the Lymphatic System*. C. C. Thomas, Springfield, Illinois, 1969.)

the presence of many microfolds and hence referred to as *M cells*. In contrast to the villous epithelium, the epithelium of the bare areas does not contain any mucus-secreting goblet cells and is not typically columnar. The M cells are thought to be involved in absorbing antigens and passing them on to the lymphoid cells in the nodule. The egg-shaped follicles are accumulations of B lymphocytes that are either uniformly distributed or differentiated into a mantle and a germinal center (Fig. 4.29*b*). T lymphocytes are found in the interfollicular regions.

A third site of lymphoid nodule aggregation is the *vermiform appendix* (L. *vermis*, worm; here worm-shaped). The inner surface of the appendix is marked by crypts similar to those in the tonsils, and underneath this surface is a band of tightly aggregated follicles (Fig. 4.30). Because its lymphoid tissue resembles that of the tonsils, the appendix is sometimes called the *abdominal tonsil*. The average number of nodules in the appendix is about 200.

The diffuse lymphoid tissue of the lamina propria, the solitary lymphoid follicles, Peyer's patches, and the appendix are all believed to belong to a single, functionally interconnected system called the *gut-associated lymphoid tissue*, or *GALT*. Some immunologists also include the tonsils and lymph nodes of the mesentery in this system. GALT is important in processing antigens entering the body from the gastrointestinal tract. A similar system—*bronchial-associated lymphoid tissue*, or *BALT*—may exist in association with the respiratory tract and may be primarily involved in handling inhaled antigens. We shall have more to say about GALT and BALT in Chapter 13.

4.2.4 Organs of Lymphocyte Migration

We have learned that lymphocyte precursors originate at one place in the body, are induced to begin lymphoid differentiation at other places, and settle down in still different places. But some lymphocytes never settle down; they continue migrating through the body until they wear out—which may take years—and are destroyed. Many macrophages, too, are constantly on the move, migrating from organ to organ throughout their entire life span. This migration of lymphocytes and macrophages takes place in the two vascular systems—the lymphatic and blood vessels.

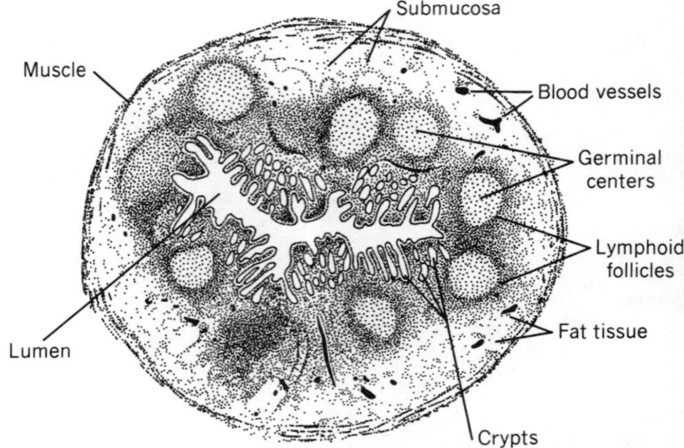

Figure 4.30. Cross section through the appendix, showing the accumulation of lymphoid follicles underneath the inner surface. (Based on J. Sobotta: *Atlas und Lehrbuch der Histologie und Mikroskopischen Anatomie des Menschen*. Lehmanns Verlag, München, 1911.)

Lymphatic Vessels

The lymphatic vessels are so profuse and intricate that if one were to dissolve all the tissues of the human body save the lymphatics, one would be left with something that still resembled a human (Fig. 4.31). There are only a few areas in the body that are free or almost free of lymphatics: the epithelium of the skin, mucous membranes, most parts of the eye, central nervous system, placenta, inner ear, cartilage, and bone marrow. The skin and the digestive, respiratory, and genitourinary tracts are so rich in lymphatics that, when isolated, these vessels look like the extensive branches of a large, old tree (Fig. 4.32).

All lymphatic vessels begin as thin, blind capillaries with walls consisting of a single layer of flattened endothelial cells. Individual capillaries interconnect (anastomose) and form a rich braid (plexus) in the tissue. As they continue through a tissue or organ, they unite into larger vessels, which then unite into still larger ones, and so on. All the lymphatics eventually connect to one of two large lymphatic trunks—either the right lymphatic duct or the thoracic duct (Fig. 4.31). The *right lymphatic duct* drains the upper right part of the body, including the right side of the head, the neck, the heart, the lungs, and part of the diaphragm. It empties into the right subclavian vein. The *thoracic duct*, which starts in the lower part of the body trunk as a dilated structure called *cisterna chyli* (see below), drains everything else, emptying into the left subclavian vein (Fig. 4.33). En route to the large lymphatic ducts, each vessel passes through at least one—but often many—lymph nodes. In each node, the vessels open up into a system of sinuses that filter the lymph before allowing it to pass into the efferent vessels.

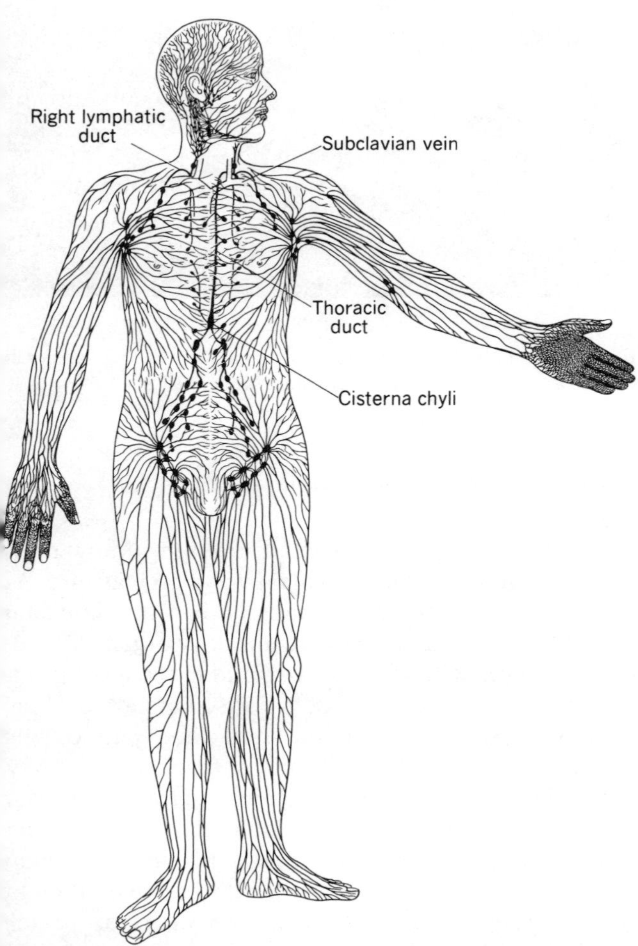

Figure 4.31. The lymphatic man. Main lymphatic vessels draining the human body.

The lymphatic system developed originally to carry fluids that had escaped from the blood. When the blood vessels (arteries) reach their destined tissues, they branch into arterial capillaries, which then connect with venous capillaries and veins. Because blood is pumped into capillaries under great pressure, some of it seeps into the adjacent tissue (Fig. 4.34). Most of this escaped fluid reenters the blood via venous capillaries; the remainder passes into the adjoining lymphatic vessels. Thus, the major part of the *lymph*, the fluid present in lymphatic vessels, is contributed by the blood. The remainder originates in the tissue fluid, which is produced by connective tissue cells and diffuses into the lymphatic capillaries. The composition of lymph varies, depending on the tissue in which it originated, so lymph from the liver is rich in proteins and lymph from the small intestines contains much fat. Fatty lymph is referred to as *chyle* (Gr. *chylos*, juice) and lymphatics containing chyle and originating in the villi of the small intestine are called *lacteals* (l. *lac*, milk; Fig. 4.35).

Lymphatic vessels develop in a manner similar to that of the blood vessels—that is, through continuous sprouting from the mesenchyme and through a subsequent coalescing of adjacent primitive vessels. Some of the vessels form local dilations—*lymph sacs*—which are later replaced by lymph nodes (Fig. 4.36). In human embryos, a closed system of lymphatics is established at the end of the second month. Parts of the lymphatic tissue (lymph nodes and nodules) undergo involution after puberty but when the need arises, these parts can enlarge again.

Blood Vessels

The vertebrate circulatory system consists of three types of blood vessel—*arteries* (arterioles), which

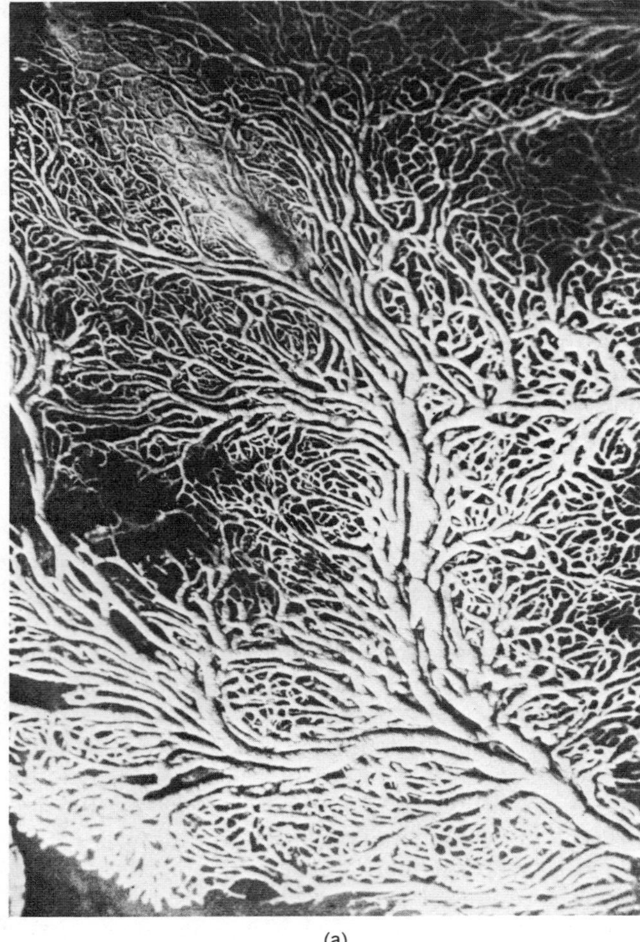

(a)

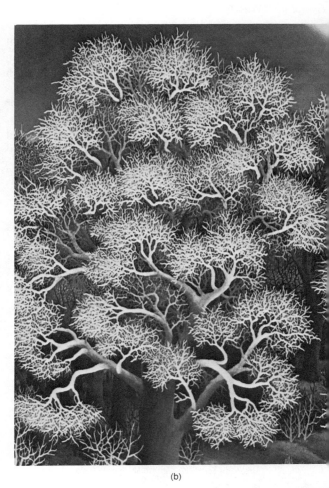

(b)

Figure 4.32. The liver's superficial lymphatics (*a*) look like branches of an old tree, and three branches in a painting by Ivan Generalić (*b*) look like lymphatics. (*a* from A. A. Sushko: *Morphology of Lymph Flow in the Human Liver,* Meditsina, Kiev, 1937.)

carry blood from the heart to the tissues; *veins* (venules), which return blood from the tissues to the heart; and *capillaries*, which connect arteries and veins. The capillary walls consist of a single layer of cells, the *endothelium*, continuous with the endothelial lining of arteries and veins. The arterial and venous walls are multilayered, consisting of an outer coat of connective tissue, a middle coat of smooth muscle, and an inner coat of endothelial and connective tissue. The main blood vessels of the human circulatory system are depicted in Figure 4.33.

4.3 EVOLUTION OF THE LYMPHOID SYSTEM

Since the evolution of the lymphoid organs was preceded by the appearance of circulatory systems, we shall consider these systems first.

4.3.1 Blood Circulatory Systems

Although circulatory (vascular) systems now serve several functions, their original evolution was directed primarily toward the distribution of digested food from the gut and oxygen from the respiratory organs to body tissues. In unicellular organisms and in the most primitive metazoa, with thin body walls, no such systems were necessary because digested food and oxygen could diffuse the short distances through the body. However, as multicellular organisms grew more complex in their bodily organization, the distances between the gut or respiratory organ and the remote parts of the body became too great to be overcome by simple diffusion, and so special channels or vessels developed in which food and oxygen are carried by circulating fluids. These fluids have also assumed the function of collecting and transporting wastes from the

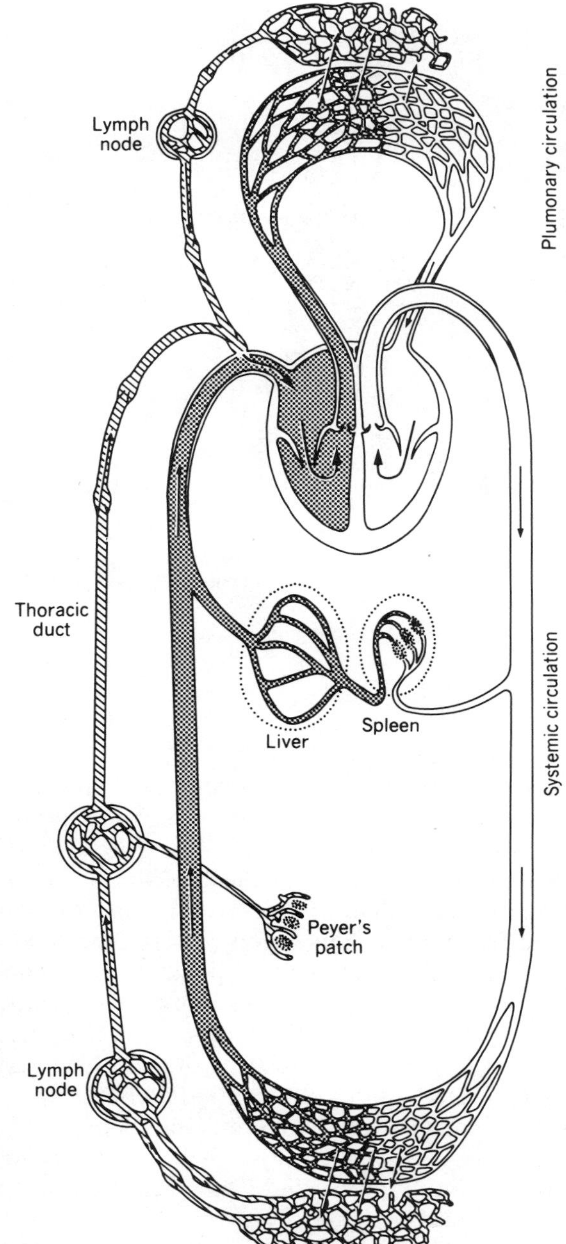

Figure 4.33. Relationship between the blood and lymphatic circulatory systems in the human. The heart pumps oxygenated blood through arteries and capillaries into tissues. Venous blood returns to the heart, is pumped into the lungs, where it is oxygenated, and is then returned to the heart. Some fluid seeps out of the blood capillaries into the tissue spaces, where it is collected by lymphatic vessels. The lymph thus formed is filtered through lymph nodes, collected by the lymphatic ducts, and returned to blood circulation via large venous vessels. While passing through lymph nodes, the lymph is enriched by lymphoid cells. [Redrawn and modified from H. S. Mayerson: *Sci. Am.* **208** (June):80–90, 1963.]

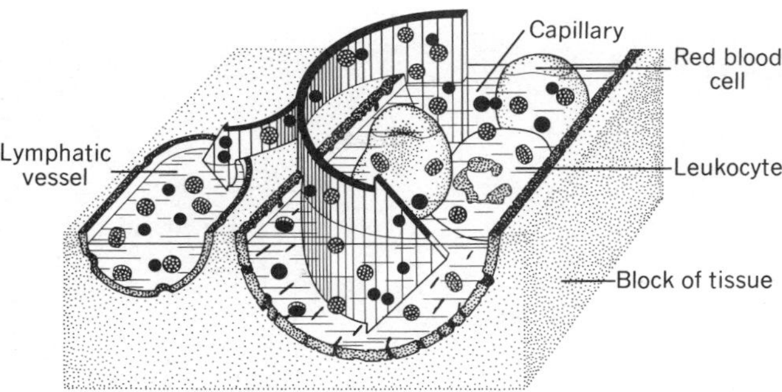

Figure 4.34. Lymph formation. Blood pressure forces some of the fluid from capillaries into tissue spaces. Most of the fluid reenters the capillaries, while the remainder drains into adjacent lymphatic vessels, where it becomes the lymph. (Redrawn from *The Rand McNally Atlas of the Body and Mind.* Rand McNally, Chicago, 1976.)

tissues. Only secondarily have vascular systems assumed additional functions, such as the distribution of defense elements through the body.

In animals, natural selection has produced at least three different solutions to the problem of how to distribute fluids rapidly to remote parts of the body (Fig. 4.37). Corresponding to these are three major types of vascular system, to which we shall refer here as gastrovascular, primovascular, and idiovascular.

The simplest distribution process that evolved was the use of the gut itself for fluid circulation. Such a *gastrovascular system* (Gr. *gaster*, stomach) can still be found in all coelenterates and in many flatworms. In simple coelenterates, such as *Hydra*, the gastrovascular system consists of the main saclike body cavity (gut) and channels extending into the tentacles. Fluids in the cavity move by bodily contractions and by beating of cilia on the surface of the lining cells. In more complex coelenterates, such as the jellyfish and some flatworms, the gastrovascular system has evolved into an intricate maze of channels extended to the farthest reaches of the body.

The *primovascular system* derives from the primary body cavity or blastocoele, and is clearly separated from the gut. In its most primitive form, seen in some nematodes (e.g., *Ascaris*), the primovascular system is the fluid-filled blastocoele itself. Food diffuses through the gut wall directly into this fluid, and circulation is accomplished by contractions of body muscles. Later in evolution, when the blastocoele becomes filled with mesenchymal tissue, the body fluids move through narrow, irregular spaces that are left unfilled. The spaces eventually coalesce into channels that extend the length of the body. In certain nemertines, this primovascular system consists of two vessels that run along the gut, have no branches, and are intercon-

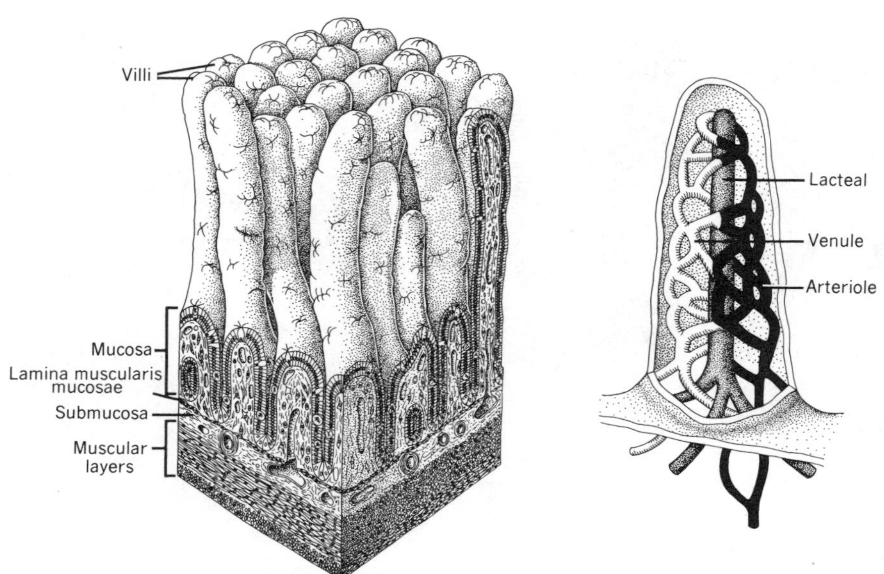

Figure 4.35. The wall of the small intestine with numerous villi (*a*) and a diagrammatic representation of one villus (*b*). (*a* from R. V. Krstić: *Die Gewebe des Menschen und der Säugetiere*. Springer-Verlag, Berlin, 1978; *b* from *The Rand McNally Atlas of the Body and Mind*. Rand McNally, Chicago, 1976.)

nected in the head and anal regions. In certain other nemertines, the system becomes more complicated by the development of a third vessel and ramification of the original two vessels. In many flatworms, the primovascular and gastrovascular systems coexist.

The origins of the *idiovascular system* (Gr. *idios*, one's own, distinctive) are still debated. Although the system appears first in animals that possess the coelom, the secondary body cavity seems to have contributed insignificantly to its genesis. The bulk of the system apparently arises in the mesoderm through a secondary formation of intercellular spaces, which then coalesce into channels and vessels. The degree of the system's complexity corresponds to the animal's evolutionary standing. Three examples of the idiovascular system are shown in Figure 4.37. The idiovascular system of *earthworms* consists of three long vessels (dorsal, ventral, and subneural) that run the entire length of the body, and numerous interconnecting lateral vessels. These form a closed system, some of them pulsating to propel the fluid circulating in them. The idiovascular system of *crustaceans* (for example, the crayfish), in comparison to that of the earthworm, exhibits two major innovations: it has a coelom-derived muscle organ (heart), the contractions of which propel the fluids in the vessels, and it has vessels divided into arteries (carrying blood rich in oxygen) and veins (carrying blood rich in carbon dioxide). However, in contrast to earthworms, the vascular system of crustaceans is an open one, so that the blood moves from the heart through arteries into intercellular spaces and is then drained from these by veins. In *vertebrates* (e.g., fishes) the idiovascular system is once again closed. Both the heart and the system of

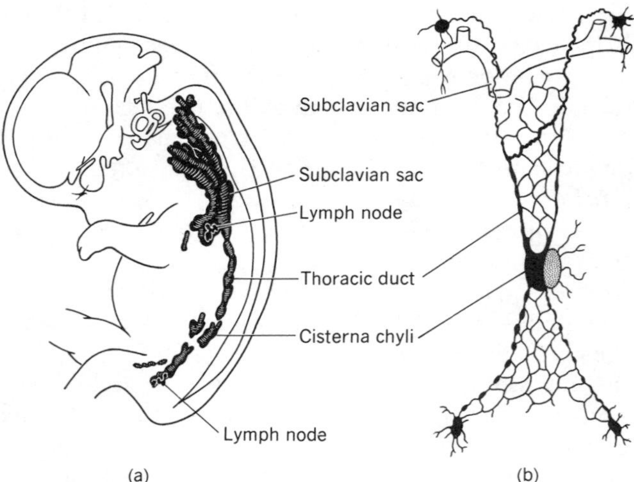

Figure 4.36. Development of lymphatic vessels in the human embryo. (*a*) Lymphatic system of a nine-week-old embryo. (*b*) Diagrammatic view of the developing thoracic duct. (After Arey from H. Wang: *An Outline of Human Embryology*. Williams and Wilkins, Baltimore, 1972.)

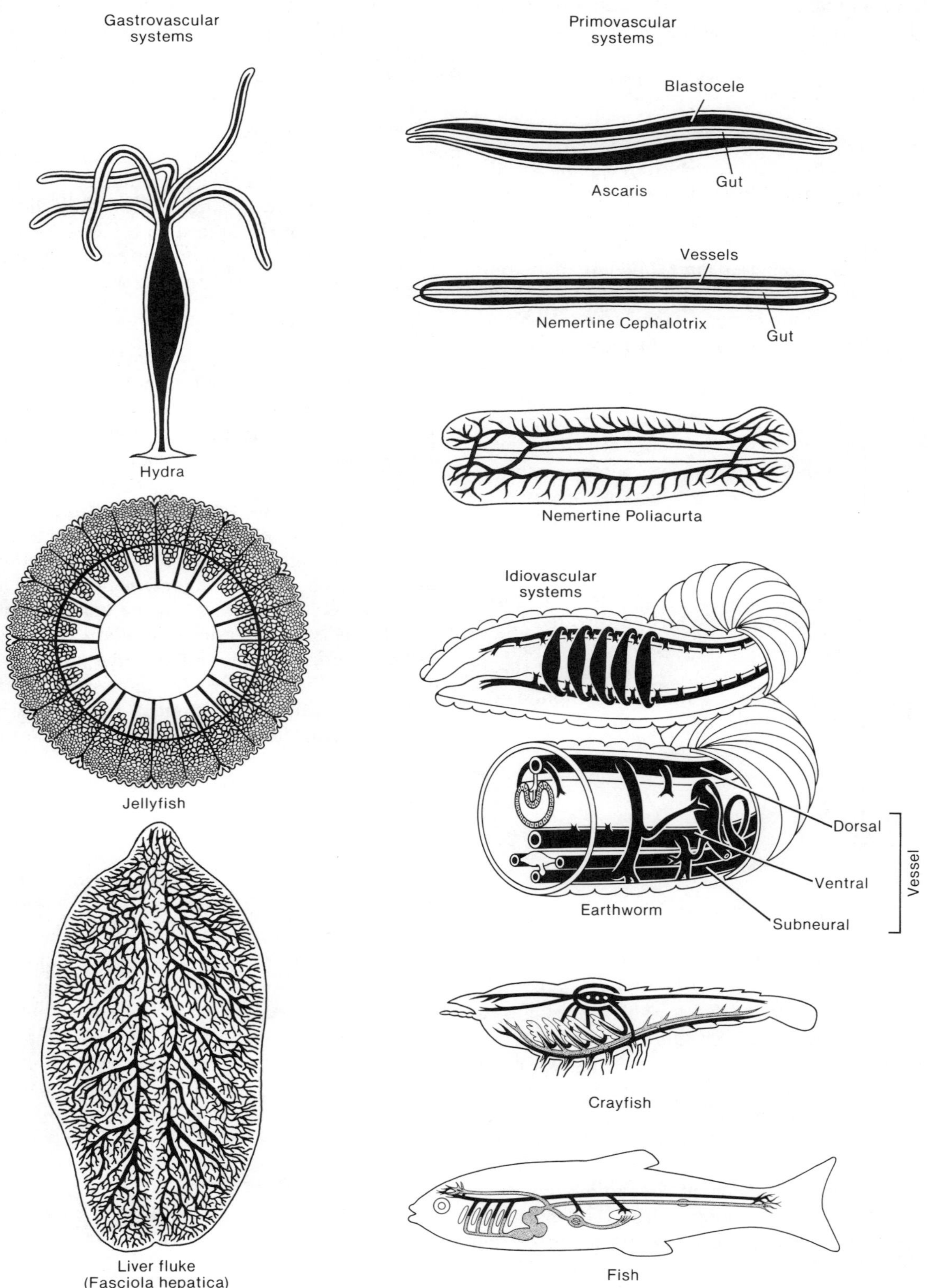

Figure 4.37. Examples of the three main types of vascular system.

vessels have increased in complexity, and arterial and venous blood are clearly separated.

4.3.2 Lymphoid System

Lymph is the fluid that seeps, because of high pressure from heart contractions, through closed capillaries into tissue spaces and is then drained by lymphatic vessels. Hence, lymphatic vessels appear only in organisms in which the heart exerts high pressure and in which rich systems of arterial capillaries have developed, an evolutionary step first taken by bony fishes. Lymphatic vessels have probably evolved in the same manner as the idiovascular system itself—from mesodermal intercellular spaces. They resemble veins except for the fact that they are not connected in any way with arteries. The increasing autonomy of the lymphatic system as evolution progresses is characterized by progressive reduction in the number of openings into the veins of the circulatory system (from many openings in fish to two in humans). The strongest stimulus for the elaboration of the lymphatic system was the change in vertebrate life from aquatic to terrestrial. This transition resulted in drastic reorganization of the respiratory and circulatory systems, which in turn led to an increase in blood pressure and seeping of more fluids from capillaries into tissue spaces. To drain all these extra fluids, vertebrates, beginning with amphibians, began to improve their originally primitive lymphatic systems.

4.3.3 Lymphoid Organs

Blood-Forming Organs

Invertebrates do not possess special blood-forming organs or even tissues. Whenever blood cells are present, they arise individually by transformation of certain mesodermal cells. In *vertebrates*, blood cells form at specific sites in the body at which specialized blood-forming tissues reside; in more advanced vertebrates the tissues organize themselves into two main special organs: spleen (in fish, amphibians, and reptiles) and bone marrow (in amphibians, reptiles, birds, and mammals). The transition from blood formation primarily in the spleen to blood formation primarily in the bone marrow thus occurs in amphibians. It is probably tied to the more general, drastic changes accompanying the transition from aquatic to terrestrial life. Among other things, terrestrial animals must have efficiently constructed bones, especially long bones, the most effective construction of which involves hollow bones. The newly acquired body space is then used for such other functions as depositing lipids and blood formation. Amphibians, in which bone marrow first appears, and most reptiles use bones for blood formation only transiently. In frogs, for example, bone marrow becomes most active during metamorphosis and during brief periods immediately following hibernation. For the rest of their lives, they, like all lower vertebrates, use the spleen as a blood-forming organ. Lizards comprise the first group that permanently uses bone marrow for blood formation.

Spleen

Phylogenetically (as well as ontogenetically; see section 4.2.1 of this chapter), spleen is derived from the gut. Its ancestor is the mesodermal tissue that envelops the gastrointestinal tract of the most primitive vertebrates, such as the hagfish, lamprey, and dipnoi. In the hagfish, this tissue contains masses of differentiating blood cells, organized into islets and cords around the venous channels. In the lamprey, an advance has been made in that the primordial spleen tissue is not so dispersed as in the hagfish, but concentrated largely in one area—the *spiral valve*, an epithelial, corkscrew-shaped organ in the gut (Fig. 4.38). In the dipnoi, the primitive splenic tissue is still embedded in the wall of the stomach but is clearly demarcated as a single body. The first clear separation of the

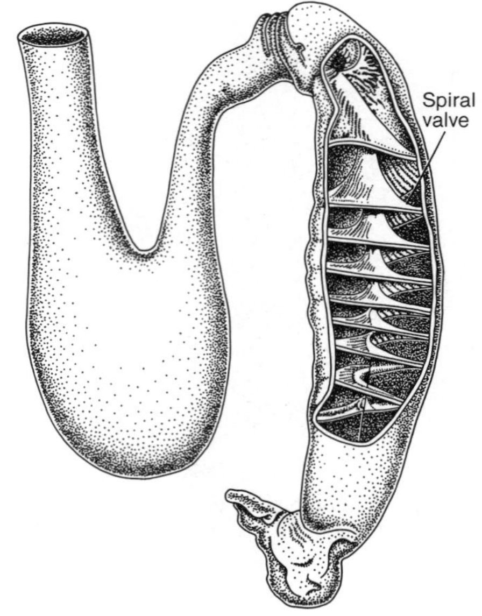

Figure 4.38. Spiral valve in the intestine of a shark.

spleen from the gut occurs in primitive bony fishes, such as the sturgeon, in which the blood-forming tissue forms a compact, discrete organ outside the gut, near the stomach-intestinal junction. From these fish upward, all vertebrates possess a spleen as a distinct organ. In the majority of fish, urodeles, and reptiles, the spleen is elongated in shape and runs a considerable length of the gut; in all other vertebrates, the organ has become much more compact. In fish and some amphibians, the spleen pulp is predominantly red; white pulp begins to appear in noticeable amounts only in certain other amphibians and in reptiles.

In addition to spleen, and later bone marrow, some vertebrates have also used certain other sites and organs for blood formation—for the formation of white blood cells, in particular. A common feature of these sites is that they lie near venous sinuses in which the stagnant blood current seems to provide the necessary stimulus for blood formation. These sites are the portal system in the kidney of lampreys, many bony fishes, and amphibians; subcapsular and framework (stromal) areas of the gonads in cartilaginous fishes; and the subcapsular region of the liver in bony fishes, amphibians, and turtles.

Thymus

Invertebrates do not possess any organized lymphoid tissue, only individual lymphoid cells scattered through the body. This condition probably also existed in ancestral vertebrates, but lymphoid cells later began to concentrate in the gut wall, probably because that was the place where they were most needed. At first, the cells moved freely through the tissues, but at later stages some of them began to assemble into lymphoid foci, particularly abundant in certain regions of the gut—the mouth and pharynx, the throat region, esophagus, and intestinal wall. Masses of lymphoid tissue are still found at these sites in virtually all vertebrates. In the next stage of development, portions of lymphoid tissue began to gain independence from the gut and to organize themselves into definite lymphoid organs—the thymus, spleen, and lymph nodes. The separation from the gut was gradual, and intermediate forms reflecting this stepwise achievement of independence can still be found among more primitive vertebrates.

The thymus is present in all but the most primitive vertebrates: it has so far not been identified in the hagfish and there is some doubt about its presence in lampreys. When present, it is derived—except in mammals—from the dorsal side of the embryonic gill pouches; in mammals, it is derived from the ventral side. Mammals also differ from other vertebrates in that a part of their thymus is derived from the skin on the neck of the embryo, rather than from the gill endoderm, which is the source of the rest of the organ and of the entire thymus of all other vertebrates.

The number of gill pouches involved in the derivation of the thymus, and consequently the thymus morphology as well, vary among the different vertebrate forms (Fig. 4.39). In higher fishes, every gill pouch produces a thymus bud, so the thymus consists of paired, irregular lymphoid masses situated above most of the gill slits. Of the amphibians, the *Apoda*, like the fishes, produce thymic tissue from every embryonic pouch; in urodeles the number of thymus buds is reduced, and in frogs, only the first pouch participates in thymus production. Correspondingly, the thymus of *Apoda* and urodeles is a rather diffuse, lobulated mass of tissue, whereas that of frogs is a single pair of compact oval bodies. Frogs, however, have, in addition to a definite thymus, a pair of *jugular bodies*, which are thymus-like structures derived from gill pouches (L. *jugulum*, throat). The thymus of young reptiles and of young and adult crocodilians derives from several embryonic pouches, and hence has the appearance of strands of tissue running the length of the animal's neck. In adult reptiles (with the exception of crocodilians), derivatives of all thymic pouches but two degenerate, and the definite thymus then consists of one or two pairs of more compacted bodies. The thymus of birds derives from the second and third embryonic

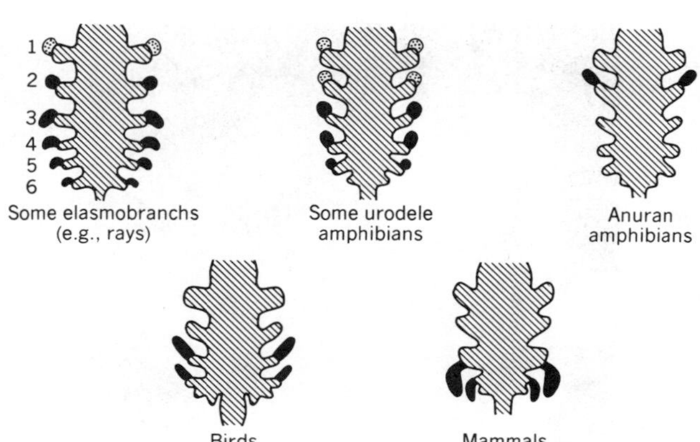

Figure 4.39. Origin of the thymus from pharyngeal pouches in different vertebrate classes. The paired pouches are numbered 1 through 6. The thymus is depicted as a black bud. The dotted buds indicate thymic rudiments that eventually disappear without contributing to the formation of the definitive thymus. (From J. J. Manning and R. J. Turner: *Comparative Immunobiology*. Halsted, New York, 1976.)

pouches and that of mammals from the second embryonic pouch.

Lymph Nodes

Although typical lymphatic vessels are present in all vertebrates upward from bony fishes, typical lymph nodes occur only in mammals. Accumulations of lymphoid tissues in conjunction with lymphatics have also been described in some amphibians, in crocodilians, and in some water birds, but these aggregates lack the characteristic structure of a definite lymph node.

4.4 CONGENITAL DEFECTS

Embryonic development of lymphoid organs, like that of any other organ, is a well-coordinated process, and any disturbance of this process may lead to the absence of a particular organ from birth—in other words, to a *congenital defect* (L. *congenitus*, born with). The more common congenital defects of lymphoid organs in the human and mouse are discussed briefly below.

4.4.1 Congenital Absence of Thymus in the Human

In 1965, Angelo M. DiGeorge described a child with the following defects (Fig. 4.40): abnormal face characteristics (low-set and notched ears, "fish-shaped" mouth, shortened jaw, eyes set wide apart and slanted in a direction opposite to that seen in mongoloids), innate heart disease, underdeveloped parathyroid gland, and underdeveloped thymus. When other physicians later observed a similar combination of defects in other children, they began referring to it as the *DiGeorge syndrome*.

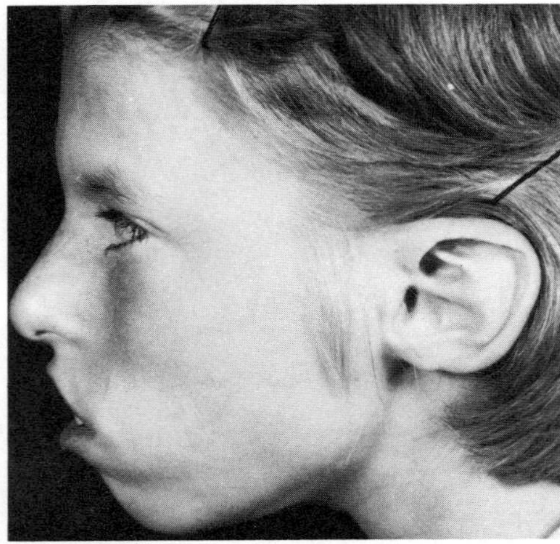

Figure 4.40. DiGeorge syndrome. Note the shortened philtrum (the groove in the midline of the upper lip) resulting in a fish-shaped mouth; low-set, notched ear-pinna; and shortened jaw. Not clearly visible are the eyes, set wide apart. (Photo: Dr. Fred S. Rosen.)

The combination of defects might seem at first to be purely coincidental, but a relatedness becomes obvious upon investigation. What the four defects have in common is that, in the twelfth week of gestation, the anlages of the affected organs (heart, parathyroid gland, and thymus) and of the face all happen to be located in the same region of the embryo. So one can explain the fourfold defect as the result of an intrauterine accident damaging this region. Infants with DiGeorge syndrome may die of heart failure or of so-called *neonatal tetany* shortly after birth. The cause of the latter is this: in normal individuals, the parathyroid gland secretes parathormone, which acts upon bones and causes them to release calcium into the blood. In children with DiGeorge syndrome, the parathyroid gland is underdeveloped, the level of parathormone is too low to release enough calcium needed for normal muscle function, and so the calcium shortage results in muscle spasms, or *tetany*. Children who do not succumb to either heart failure or tetany may die from fungal or viral infections, from which they cannot protect themselves because of the absence or underdevelopment of the thymus. (The precursors of T lymphocytes have nowhere to mature and the entire cellular arm of immunity is thus defective.) This defect can be corrected by transplantation of the fetal thymus.

Thymus development is also involved in *Nezelof syndrome*, bearing the name of the French pathologist who first described it in detail. Although present, the thymus in children with Nezelof syndrome remains relatively undifferentiated, embryonic in character, and incapable of sustaining normal T-lymphocyte differentiation. The affected children fail to thrive and suffer from recurrent, predominantly viral and fungal infections and from chronic diarrhea. In contrast to DiGeorge syndrome, Nezelof syndrome is inherited.

4.4.2 Congenital Absence of Thymus in the Mouse

In 1966, virologists in Glasgow discovered a mouse in their colony that, in contrast to its furry littermates, was completely *nude* (Fig. 4.41). The trait proved to be inherited, controlled by a recessive *nu* gene in chromosome 11; (*nu*/*nu* homozygotes are hairless; *nu*/+ are normal). Further study of the *nu*/*nu* mice revealed that they also lack the thymus, apparently because the differentiation pathway transforming pharyngeal pouches

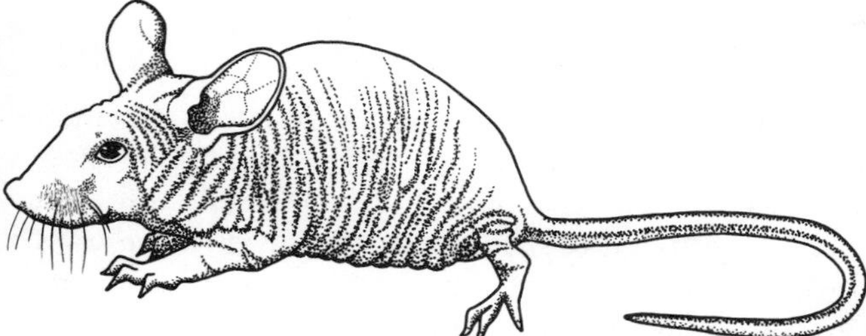

Figure 4.41. The athymic *nu/nu* (hairless or "nude") mouse.

into the epithelial thymus anlage is somehow genetically blocked. In the absence of the thymus epithelium, the precursors of T lymphocytes fail to mature and the mice have a greatly reduced ability to develop cellular immune reactions. (One consequence of this deficient cellular immunity is that the mice can accept and grow almost any kind of graft, be it fowl skin with feathers or a human tumor.) Whether the absence of hair and of the thymus are controlled by the same gene or by two closely linked genes has not yet been resolved. (Although hairless mice with thymuses are found occasionally among *nu/nu* animals, no athymic and haired mouse has ever been found; in other words, no recombination of the two traits has been observed. How the same gene—if there is only one—can affect hair growth and thymus differentiation simultaneously is a mystery.) The cellular immunity defect can be corrected by thymus transplantation but the transplant does not cause appearance of hair in *nu/nu* mice. Athymic mice are difficult to breed since they show reduced fertility and increased susceptibility to infections. Under normal conditions, the mortality of *nu/nu* mice is 100 percent within 25 weeks; 50 percent die within the first two weeks after birth. The nude mouse is an extremely important model for the study of many questions in immunology, virology, and oncology. (A mutation resembling *nu* is also known in the rat.)

4.4.3 Inherited Absence of the Spleen in the Mouse and Human

Like athymic mice, asplenic (spleenless) mice were also discovered in Great Britain, and, like the former, the latter were first detected because of another characteristic—hind-leg deformation (Fig. 4.42). The gene responsible for the deformity has been named *Dh*, for *dominant hemimelia*, because it acts in a dominant fashion and because it causes, among other things, limb shortening (Gr. *hemi*, half, *melos*, limb). Other defects expressed by *Dh*/+ heterozygotes are abnormal number of toes, small stomach, short intestine, and total absence of the spleen. *Dh/Dh* homozygotes die within a few days after birth with abnormalities similar to those of the heterozygotes, only much more severely expressed. The heterozygotes show age-dependent retardation of T-lymphocyte maturation as well as a decrease in total body B lymphocytes. By transferring the *nu* and *Dh* genes into the same mouse, geneticists produced athymic and asplenic animals that, under specific pathogen-free conditions, could survive for up to nine months.

In humans, absence (agenesis) of spleen has been observed in combination with certain other defects, of which the best known is the *Ivemark syndrome*, named after Biör I. Ivemark.

4.5 METHODS OF STUDY

The simplest way of learning how an organ functions is to remove it and then observe what effects this step has on the physiology of the organism. The removal can be accomplished by nature itself, as in the case of the congenital defects described in the preceding section, or by the experimenter through artificial excision (extirpation).

Removal of the spleen, *splenectomy* (Gr. *ektome*, excision), can be accomplished surgically. When properly done, the operation has little effect on the organism. At worst, it merely lowers or modifies the or-

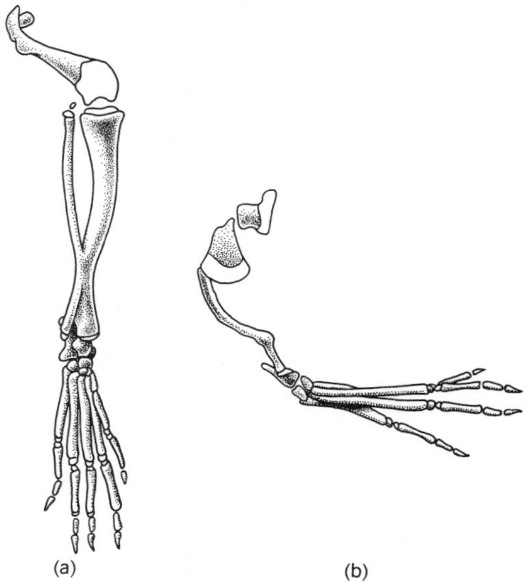

Figure 4.42. Skeletons of right hind limbs of a normal mouse (*a*) and a mouse carrying the dominant hemimelia gene (*Dh*/+) (*b*). (Based on A. G. Searle: *Genet. Res. Camb.* **5**:171–197, 1964.)

ganism's defense reactions. Extirpation of the thymus (*thymectomy*) can also be accomplished surgically, and the effects of the operation vary, depending on the age of the animal. Adult thymectomy has little, if any, effect on the organism's defense reactions. Neonatal thymectomy, on the other hand, often results in the total absence or drastic reduction of cellular immune reactions, in wasting of the animal, and death. Extirpation of the Fabrician bursa (*bursectomy*) can be done surgically or chemically, since immunologists discovered that injecting early fowl embryos with testosterone suppresses bursal development. Bursectomized fowl fail to develop humoral immune reactions. Complete extirpation of lymph nodes is not possible since they are so plentiful and scattered throughout the body. Surgical removal of major lymph nodes and tonsils (*tonsilectomy*) has little effect on the animal's physiology.

4.6 APPENDIX 4.1: RECAPITULATION OF BASIC HISTOLOGY

As was mentioned earlier (in Chapter 1), the vertebrate body is a "tube within a tube," with the digestive tract and its derivatives forming the inner tube. According to this extremely simplistic view, the body consists of two main tissue types: that of the body surface (outer and inner) and that between the surfaces. The outer or inner body surface is covered by *epithelium* (Gr. *epi*, upon, *thēlē*, nipple), and the space between the body walls is occupied by the *connective tissue*.

4.6.1 The Epithelium

The epithelium consists of polyhedral cells that adhere tightly and form continuous sheets (Fig. 4.43). There is practically no intercellular substance separating these cells, but they are covered by the *glycocalyx* (Gr. *glykys*, sweet, *kalyx*, husk, shell), a thin layer of glycoproteins believed to glue them together. According to their height, epithelial cells are defined as *squamous* (formed by relatively flat cells; L. *squama*, a scale), *cuboid*, or *columnar* (Fig. 4.43). Epithelium can consist of a single cell layer (*simple epithelium*) or multiple layers (*stratified epithelium*). The border between the epithelium and the underlying connective tissue is occupied by the *basal* or *basement lamina*, a thin, acellular plate secreted by the epithelial cells and used by them as a supportive base. In most tissues, the basal lamina is visible only with the electron microscope; it consists of an amorphous protein-polysaccharide substance with a delicate network of fine collagenous fibers embedded in it. In some tissues, the basal lamina is so thick that it is visible—after appropriate staining—with the light microscope. It is then referred to as the *basal* or *basement membrane*, but many histologists use the terms *lamina* and *membrane* interchangeably. The connective tissue layer directly underlying the basal lamina or membrane (*lamina propria*, Fig. 4.43) is usually rich in blood vessels, nerves, and muscle bundles. The blood vessels of the lamina propria provide nutrients for the epithelium, which is completely without vessels. The nutrients diffuse freely through the basal lamina and membrane.

Embryologically, epithelium can derive from any of

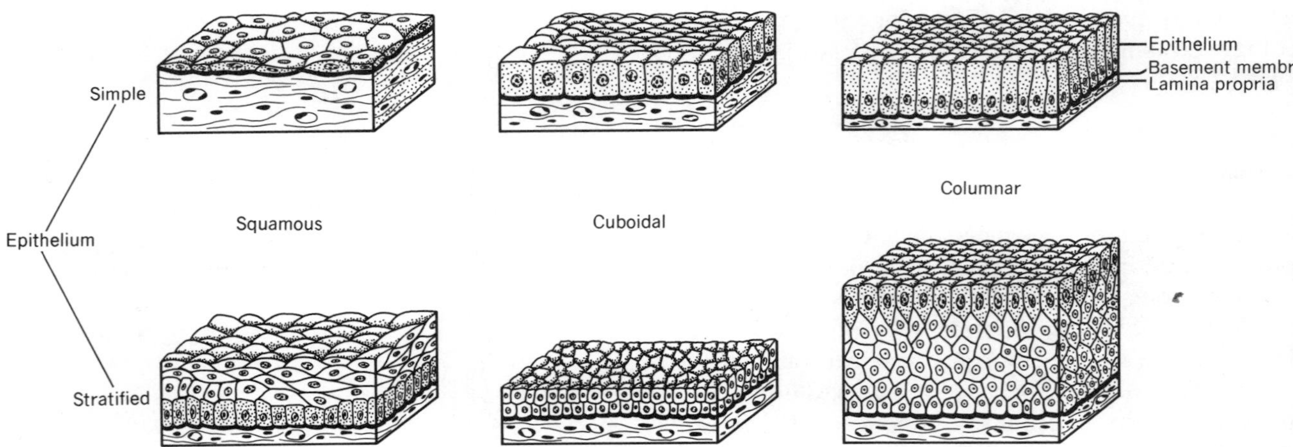

Figure 4.43. Types of epithelium.

the three germ layers. Most of the epithelium forming the outer body surface (skin) originates from the ectoderm, most of the epithelium lining the digestive tract derives from the endoderm, and the epithelium lining other internal organs (the kidneys, for example) is of mesodermal origin.

4.6.2 The Connective Tissue

In contrast to epithelium, in which cells are compacted tightly into sheets, connective tissue cells are separated by intercellular material and form a three-dimensional spongelike mesh. The connective tissue of embryos is referred to as the *mesenchyme* (Gr. *mesos*, middle, *enchyma*, infusion) because it first appears as a third layer (mesoderm), pushing itself in between the ectoderm and endoderm. The mesenchyme has irregularly shaped stellate cells (cells with many processes; Fig. 4.44) embedded in abundant amorphous, intercellular material secreted by the mesenchymal cells. These can differentiate into precursors of various specialized cells such as osteoblasts (bone-forming cells), odontoblasts (dentin-forming cells), lipoblasts (precursors of fat cells), mast-cell precursors, hematopoietic stem cells, endothelial cells, blood vessel-lining endothelial cells, macrophages, and fibroblasts (Fig. 4.45). Whether some of these undifferentiated, pluripotent mesenchymal cells persist in adult connective tissues is not known; however, adult connective tissues do contain cells that can differentiate into bone-forming cells, cartilage-forming cells, fat cells, and so on.

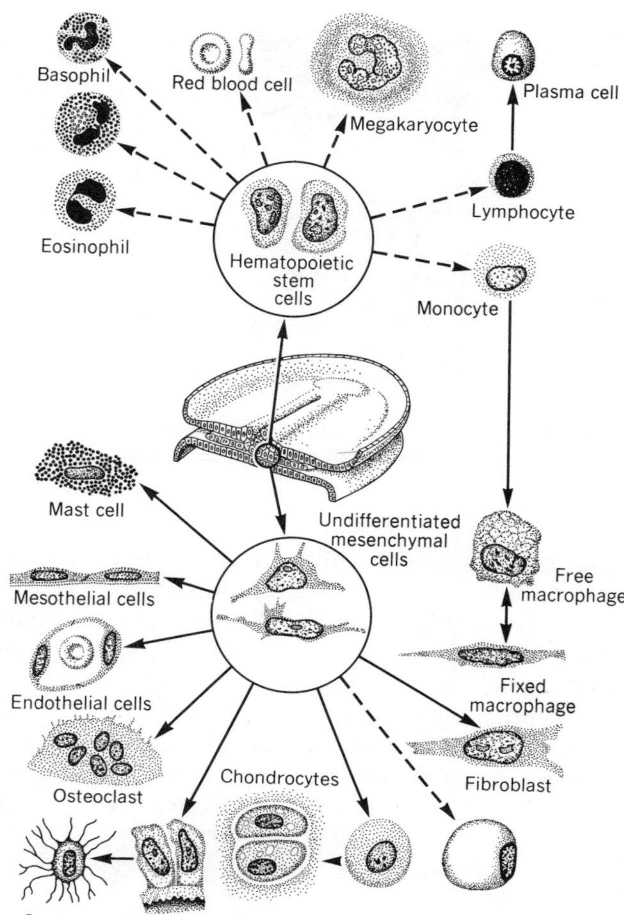

Figure 4.45. Cell types derived from undifferentiated or partially differentiated mesenchymal cells. Broken arrows indicate the existence of intermediate cell types between the progenitor and the end cell. (Not drawn in proportion to actual size. Modified from L. C. Junqueira, J. Cameiro, and A. Contopoulos: *Basic Histology*. Lange, Los Altos, California 1977.)

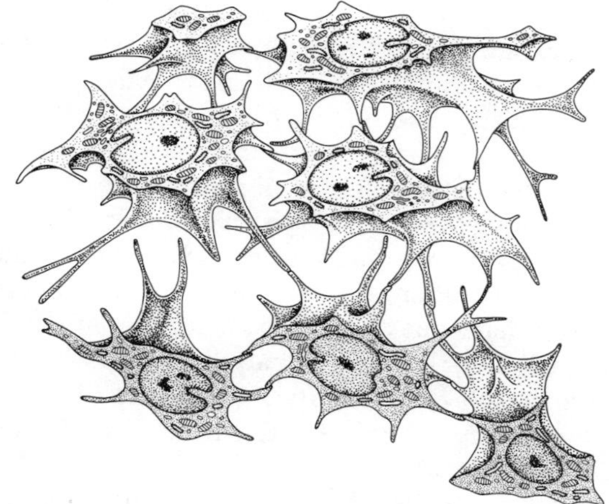

Figure 4.44. Embryonic mesenchyme. Only mesenchymal cells are depicted; intercellular substance is omitted.

Adult connective tissue consists of cells, an amorphous intercellular substance, intercellular fibers, and tissue fluids (Fig. 4.46). Of the great variety of connective tissue cells, the reticular cells, fibroblasts, and macrophages have preserved most of the original mesenchymal properties.

Reticular cells (Fig. 4.47) are found mostly in blood-forming organs such as the spleen and bone marrow. These cells send out long cytoplasmic processes that are interconnected, forming a spongelike network (L. *rete*, network). Attached to the external surface of reticular cells, and often following their outline, are thin fibers that strengthen the reticular network. Of the

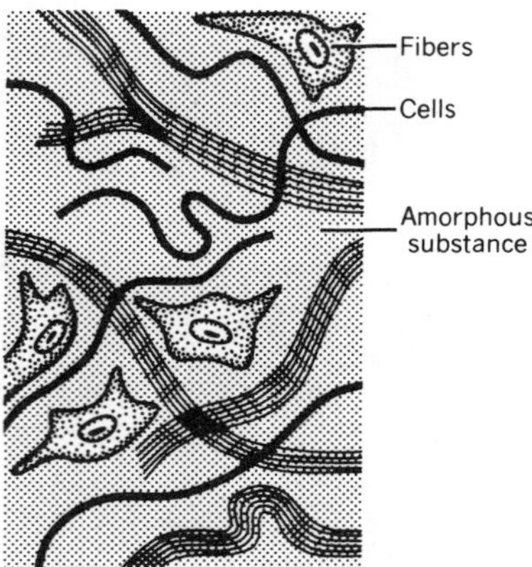

Figure 4.46. One of many types of adult connective tissue, with cells, fibers, and intercellular substance.

three mesenchymelike cells, the reticular cells are the most primitive and the least differentiated.

Fibroblasts (Fig. 4.48) are the most commonly found connective tissue cells. Young fibroblasts are irregularly shaped, with abundant cytoplasmic processes. They synthesize and intensively secrete protocollagen, which polymerizes into collagenous fibers, and mucopolysaccharides of the intercellular substance. The more mature fibroblasts, sometimes referred to as *fibrocytes* (Fig. 4.48), are far less active, smaller, have fewer processes, and often are spindle-shaped (L. *fibra*, fiber).

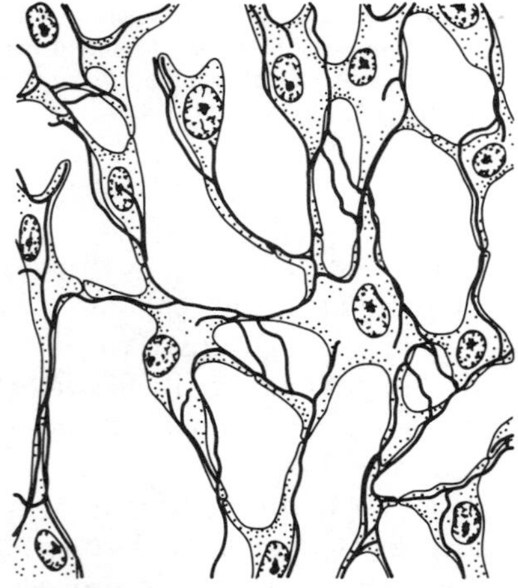

Figure 4.47. Reticular cells of connective tissue. Only cells and their fibers are depicted; intercellular substance is omitted. The cells must be imagined to form a three-dimensional mesh resembling a sponge. The fibers are in close contact with the cells, sometimes enveloped by them, but always separated from them by the plasma membrane. (From L. C. Junqueira, J. Cameiro, and A. Contopoulos: *Basic Histology*. Lange, Los Altos, California 1977.)

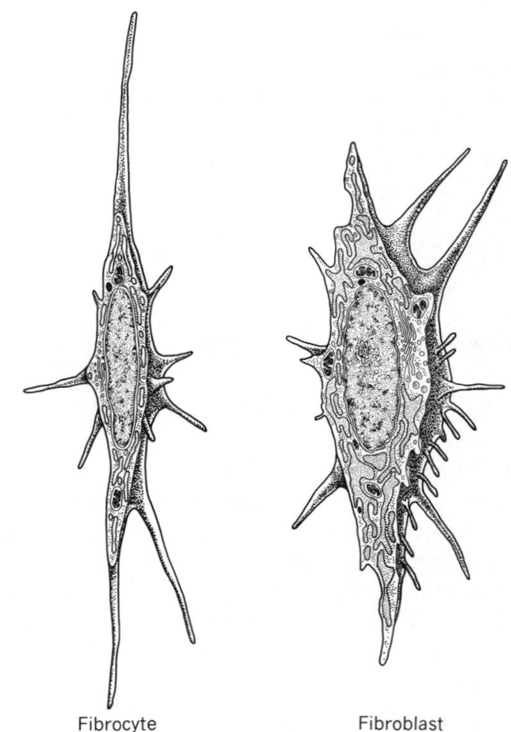

Figure 4.48. Fibrocyte and fibroblast.

The *macrophages* (see Fig. 5.14) are cells that come in different sizes, shapes, and functional states, but have at least one common characteristic—they phagocytose particles. Macrophages are scattered throughout the body, either wandering through tissues and bodily fluids or settled at a particular location. We shall learn more about macrophages in the next chapter.

The *intercellular material* consists of fibers embedded in an amorphous substance, and bodily fluids. Connective tissue fibers are of three basic types: collagenous, elastic, and reticular (Fig. 4.49). *Collagenous fibers,* as the name implies, are composed of collagen, a protein with a high glycine, proline, and hydroxyproline content. They assemble into parallel, thick, white bundles that can branch in a treelike fashion and show a longitudinal striation. *Elastic fibers* are much thinner than the collagenous ones, show no striation, and have a yellowish color. They not only branch out, but also interconnect, forming an irregular network. Their main constituent is the protein elastin. Both the collagenous and elastic fibers are produced by fibroblasts. *Reticular fibers* are even thinner than elastic ones and are visible only through a special staining procedure based on silver salts (they appear black after binding the silver).

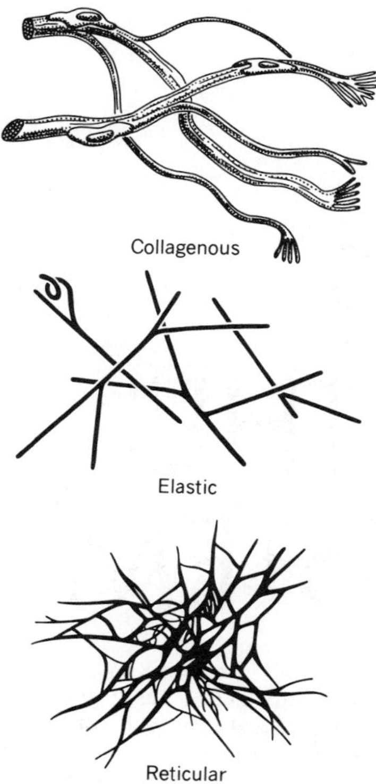

Figure 4.49. Three types of connective tissue fiber.

Like the collagenous fibers, the reticular fibers are made of collagen, but are synthesized by reticular cells rather than by fibroblasts. Like elastic fibers, reticular fibers form an intricate three-dimensional network.

The intercellular, amorphous *ground substance* is a viscous, transparent, colorless material consisting mostly of proteoglycans (polysaccharides with proteins attached to them and with the sugar component, in contrast to glycoproteins, dominant). The ground substance completely fills the space between cells and fibers of the connective tissue.

The *tissue fluid* of the connective tissue resembles blood plasma in that it contains ions and diffusible substances. It also contains a small percentage of low-molecular-weight plasma proteins.

REFERENCES

General

Balinsky, B. I.: *An Introduction to Embryology*, 4th ed. W. B. Saunders, Philadelphia, 1975.

DiFiore, M. S. H., Mancini, R. E., and De Robertis, G. D. P.: *New Atlas of Histology*. Lea and Febiger, Philadelphia, 1977.

Hamilton, W. J.: *Textbook of Human Anatomy*, 2nd ed. C. V. Mosby, Saint Louis, 1976.

Junqueira, L. C., Cameiro, J., and Contopoulos, A.: *Basic Histology*. Lange, Los Altos, California, 1977.

Kampmeier, O. F.: *Evolution and Comparative Morphology of the Lymphatic System*. Charles C. Thomas, Springfield, Illinois, 1969.

Krstić, R. V.: *Die Gewebe des Menschen und der Säugetiere. Ein Atlas zum Studium für Mediziner und Biologen*. Springer-Verlag, Berlin, 1978.

Langman, J.: *Medical Embryology*, 3rd ed. Williams and Wilkins Co., Baltimore, 1975.

Wang, H.: *An Outline of Human Embryology*. Williams and Wilkins, Baltimore, 1972.

Weiss, L.: *The Cells and Tissues of the Immune System: Structure, Functions, Interactions*. Prentice-Hall, Englewood Cliffs, New Jersey, 1972.

Weiss, L. and Greep, R. G.: *Histology*, 4th ed. McGraw-Hill, New York, 1977.

Yoffey, J. M. and Courtice, F. C.: *Lymphatics, Lymph and the Lymphomyeloid Complex*. Academic, London, 1970.

Original Articles

Aschoff, A. L.: Das reticulo-endotheliale System. *Ergeb. Inn. Med. Kinderheilkd.* **26**:1–118, 1924.

DiGeorge, A. M.: Congenital absence of the thymus and its immunologic consequences: concurrence with congenital hypoparathyroidism. *Birth Defects* **4**:116–118, 1968.

CHAPTER 5

CELLS OF THE IMMUNE SYSTEM

5.1 THE FAMILY TREE OF IMMUNOLOGICALLY IMPORTANT CELLS

A tour of a European castle often includes a visit to the portrait gallery, where the guide points out the *Stammbaum*, the family tree of the local nobility, explains the often complex relationships between the individual family members, and then leads you down a corridor decorated with portraits of the people who played a role in the history of the estate and sometimes of the country. In this chapter I shall be the guide who takes you through the gallery of the immunological nobility. We shall first examine the ontogenic relationships among the different branches of the family, say a few words about the family's founders, and then describe the individual branches and the individual cells.

The family of immunologically important cells (Fig. 5.1) is founded by *hematopoietic stem cells*, the relatively undifferentiated cells from which all other cells of the blood are derived. The stem cells give rise to *progenitor cells*, which constitute the basis of several cell lineages. In each lineage the *differentiating cells* undergo a series of divisions and differentiation steps, followed by maturation without further division, and the lineage then culminates in *mature cells*. Some mature cells are end cells, unable to differentiate further and committed to die after a short life. Other mature cells can be stimulated to undergo additional division and differentiation.

There are six main lineages, each derived from a different progenitor cell, but all sharing a hematopoietic stem cell. Named according to their mature (end) cells, they are erythrocytic, thrombocytic, granulocytic, monocytic, T-lymphocytic, and B-lymphocytic. (The corresponding mature cells are erythrocyte, thrombocyte, granulocyte, monocyte, T lymphocyte, and B lymphocyte, respectively.) Cells of the first (erythrocytic) lineage have nothing to do with immunity; they are concerned with gas transport. Cells of the second (thrombocytic) lineage are only peripherally involved in defense in that they play a role in blood clotting. Cells of the granulocytic and monocytic lineages play a role in certain nonspecific forms of defense and, in addition, carry out other functions not directly related to immunity. Cells of the two lymphocytic lineages are involved exclusively in immunity.

All mature cells of the six lineages are, at one time or another, present in the blood—in other words, they are *blood cells*. For this reason, their genesis is referred to as *hematopoiesis* or *hemopoiesis*, and the cells differentiating into mature blood cells are known as *hematopoietic cells*. Since the two lymphocytic lineages differ in many respects from the remaining four lineages, they are sometimes referred to as *lymphoid*, in contradistinction to *myeloid* cells (Gr. *myelos*, marrow), which include the erythrocytic, thrombocytic, granulocytic and monocytic lineages. (To confuse things a bit more, some hematologists use the term "myeloid" as a synonym for the granulocytic-

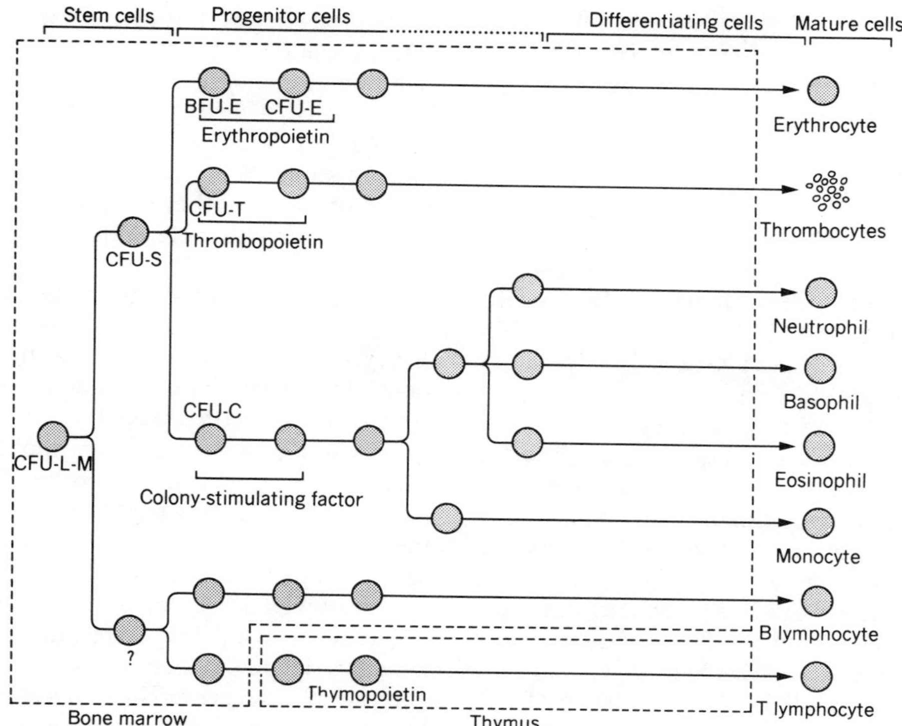

Figure 5.1. Scheme of hematopoietic cell differentiation. BFU, burst-forming unit; CFU, colony-forming unit; –C, culture; –E, erythroid; –L–M, lymphoid-myeloid; –S, spleen; –T, thromboid.

monocytic lineage.) Granulocytes, monocytes, and lymphocytes are referred to as *white blood cells* or *leukocytes* (Gr. *leukos*, white, *kytos*, cell).

5.2 HEMATOPOIETIC STEM CELLS

5.2.1 Definition

Stem cells are unspecialized cells characterized by an ability to proliferate extensively (they divide throughout life), self-renewal (they produce more cells of their own kind), and differentiating capacity (they evolve into more specialized cells). An adult organism needs stem cells as a reservoir for the replenishment of short-lived mature cells. In mammals, for example, stem cell reservoirs exist for intestinal epithelial cells, epidermal cells, and germ cells, as well as for blood cells.

Stem cells that give rise to mature blood cells (*hematopoietic stem cells*) are *pluripotent*, which means that they are able to differentiate into more than one cell type (in contradistinction to *unipotent* cells, which are able to differentiate into only one cell type). But they are able to differentiate into only certain cell types (in contradistinction to *totipotent* cells, which are able to give rise to all differentiated cells of a given individual). For example, hematopoietic stem cells can give rise to erythrocytes or monocytes, but not to neurons or to epidermal cells.

5.2.2 Differentiation Potential

To determine the type of cells into which a stem cell can differentiate, immunologists use the *spleen colony assay* (Fig. 5.2*a*), developed by James E. Till and Ernest A. McCulloch in 1961. This assay consists of irradiating a mouse with a dose of X-rays that kills all its blood-forming cells, and then inoculating into it a low number of stem cells from a genetically identical mouse. Some of the inoculated cells migrate into the spleen, where they settle down and begin to divide and differentiate. Because the recipient's own blood cells have been destroyed by irradiation so that only the scaffolding of the reticular cells remains in the spleen, and since the donor cells have been inoculated in a low number so that they populate the scaffolding only sparsely, the descendants of each stem cell form a spherical colony, or nodule (Fig. 5.2*b*). Seven to 10 days after the inoculation, the colonies bulge out at the spleen surface and can be counted with the naked eye. Alternatively, one can make sections of the spleen and study the colonies histologically. In the latter study, one can identify four kinds of colony—erythrocytic, granulocytic, thrombocytic, and mixed—each containing cells differentiated along one or several of the corresponding hematopoietic pathways. The frequency of the individual colony types varies according to the time of sampling: four days after inoculation, the colonies are either erythrocytic or granulocytic; two days later, some thrombocytic colonies begin to appear, in addition to mixed erythrocytic-granulocytic colonies; and, 12 days after the inoculation, about half the colonies are of the mixed type. Colonies of hematopoietic cells also form in the bone marrow of the irradiated mice, but these are difficult to demonstrate. Marrow colonies differentiate primarily into granulocytes.

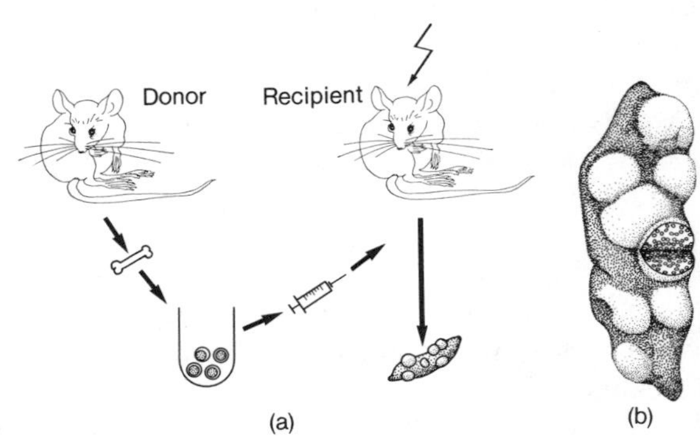

Figure 5.2. The spleen colony assay (*a*) and spleen with colonies of hematopoietic cells (*b*). One nodule in *b* is dissected. The sign ↯ in this and subsequent figures indicates that the animal has been irradiated by ionizing radiation. (The mouse is from a drawing by the Czech artist Ota Janeček.)

To determine the origin of cells within a colony, Alan M. Wu, James E. Till, Louis Siminovitch, and Ernest A. McCulloch used a neat trick: before inoculation into the irradiated recipient, they irradiated the stem cells, but with a dose (about 650 R) that induces chromosomal abnormalities without killing the cells. The abnormalities can be of many different kinds: the irradiation can, for example, break a chromosome and the broken portions can then attach to other chromosomes so that abnormally long and abnormally short chromosomes arise; or it can join two telocentric chromosomes at their centromeres and generate a metacentric one. Since the probability of the same aberration's occurring in two different cells is very low, each abnormal chromosome serves as a marker, unique for a given cell, and distinguishes it from other cells. When the stem cell divides and differentiates, all of its progeny inherit the marker as a kind of coat of arms.

Experiments with chromosomally marked spleen colonies revealed that whenever a single colony contained erythrocytic, granulocytic, and thrombocytic cell types, the different cells possessed the same marker. One must conclude, therefore, that cells of these three lineages all derive from the same stem cell, called *colony-forming-unit-spleen*, or *CFU-S*.

With lymphoid cells, the situation is complicated by the fact that one does not normally find these cells in colonies but scattered throughout the spleen, suggesting that they derive from a different, as yet unidentified stem cell. However, since the individual cells often share chromosomal markers with cells in the colonies, one can conclude that the unidentified lymphoid stem cells and the CFU-S derive from a common, more primitive stem cell, the *colony-forming-unit-lymphoid-myeloid*, or *CFU-L-M*.

5.2.3 Regulation of Stem Cell Behavior

At a certain moment in its life cycle, each stem cell must decide between two options—to remain a pluripotent stem cell or to differentiate toward mature cells. Since the number of stem cells in a normal adult remains constant, and since only as many cells as are needed for the replenishment of the aging mature blood cells differentiate, a mechanism must exist to regulate stem cell behavior and determine how many cells, at any point, will renew themselves and how many will differentiate. Theoretically, the regulation can be achieved by one of the following three mechanisms. First, the determination process might be totally random (stochastic). If each cell were to have a certain probability of either remaining a stem cell or differentiating, then, although one could not predict the behavior of an individual cell, one could predict fairly precisely the behavior of the entire population. In this respect, the situation would be analogous to the disintegration of radioactive atoms wherein the time when a particular atom disintegrates cannot be determined, but the half-life of a given isotope is a well-known constant. Second, the behavior of individual stem cells could be determined by their life histories. For example, one can imagine a system in which a cell that has undergone a high number of divisions has a higher probability of entering the differentiation pathway than a cell with a history of only a few divisions. Third, stem cell behavior might be determined by the cell's microenvironment. For example, some immunologists speculate that a cell remains in the stem cell pool only when it is in a certain niche—a certain place in an organ, surrounded by certain other cells. Since the number of these niches in a hematopoietic organ is fixed, there is also a fixed number of stem cells, and cells that do not find a niche for themselves enter the differentiation pool. Which of the three possible explanations of stem cell behavior is correct is not known; perhaps all three hypotheses have a grain of truth in them.

5.2.4 Kinetics of Stem Cell Proliferation

The life cycle of a cell—a stem cell or other type—can be divided into four phases, referred to as G_1, S, G_2, and M (Fig. 5.3). In the G_1 phase the cell performs its functions; in the S phase it duplicates its DNA; in G_2 it prepares itself for division; and in the M phase it undergoes mitosis. Some cells, however, can leave this active cycle and enter, for an extended period, a resting phase referred to as G_0. When the cell leaves the resting phase, it reenters the cycle at the beginning of the S phase.

To estimate the frequency of hematopoietic stem cells entering the S phase, immunologists feed the cells with high doses of highly radioactive ^{3}H-thymidine, a precursor necessary for DNA synthesis. The S-phase cells incorporate the precursor with its isotope into their DNA, and the isotope irradiates and kills the cells. (In a way, the cell commits suicide by using the dangerous isotope.) Cells that do not synthesize DNA do not incorporate the isotope, so they survive. By determining the effect of S-cell suicide on the function of the surviving cells, one can estimate the number of cells in the S phase. The number turns out to be surprisingly low—between 5 and 20 percent. This finding implies that most stem cells are in the resting G_0 phase and only a minority are in the active cycle.

5.2.5 Location and Origin

In adult mice, most hematopoietic stem cells (at least those of the CFU-S type) are located in the bone marrow, a few reside in the spleen (there are approxi-

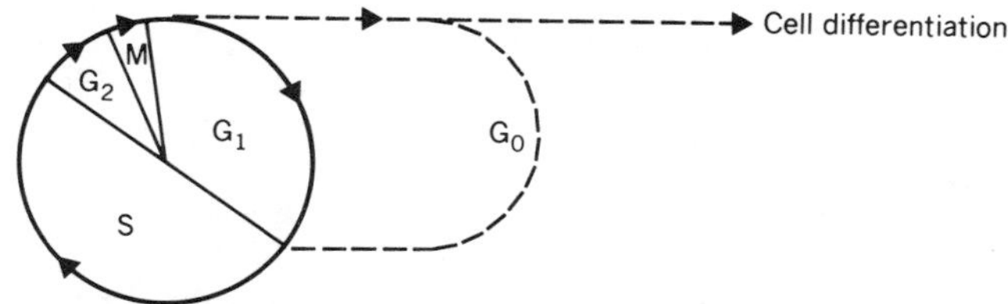

Figure 5.3. Cell cycle of a stem cell. G_0, G_1, G_2, M, and S are phases of the cell cycle.

mately 50 times as many marrow CFU-S as splenic CFU-S), and a very small number in the blood. In embryos, however, stem cells are also found in the spleen, liver, and yolk sac. The odyssey of a stem cell, up to its final refuge in the bone marrow, can be summarized as follows (Fig. 5.4). The fertilized egg (zygote) and its immediate progeny are totipotent cells and hence can be considered ultimate stem cells. Beginning with certain divisions (around the 64-cell stage in the mouse), restriction of the differentiation potential sets in. By day $3\frac{1}{2}$ in the mouse embryo (corresponding to the 64-cell stage), the original totipotent cells have differentiated into two pluripotent cell types—inner cell mass (ICM) and trophectoderm, neither of which can give rise to the other (ICM cells cannot be converted into trophectoderm and vice versa). Later, the ICM cells differentiate again into two cell types—primitive ectoderm and primitive endoderm—and again, the two types are not interconvertible. The primitive ectoderm forms the three germ layers of the embryo proper—the ectoderm, mesoderm, and endoderm. Hematopoietic stem cells are derived from the region of the mesoderm underlying the primitive streak (see Fig. 4.7). From this region, the future stem cells migrate into the yolk sac, where they form the blood islands (see Fig. 4.8). What happens next is not clear. Some embryologists believe that the yolk sac becomes the exclusive source of all hematopoietic stem cells in the developing embryo; others claim that the yolk sac is only a transient source of stem cells and that most stem cells in the fetal organs derive directly from the mesoderm. Whatever the case, stem cells from one of these sources first colonize fetal liver, then fetal spleen and thymus, and finally bone marrow. In adult mammals, small numbers of stem cells continually leave the marrow, enter the blood, and head for the spleen or thymus.

5.2.6 Morphology

Despite numerous attempts to identify stem cells visually, no one can claim with certainty to have actually

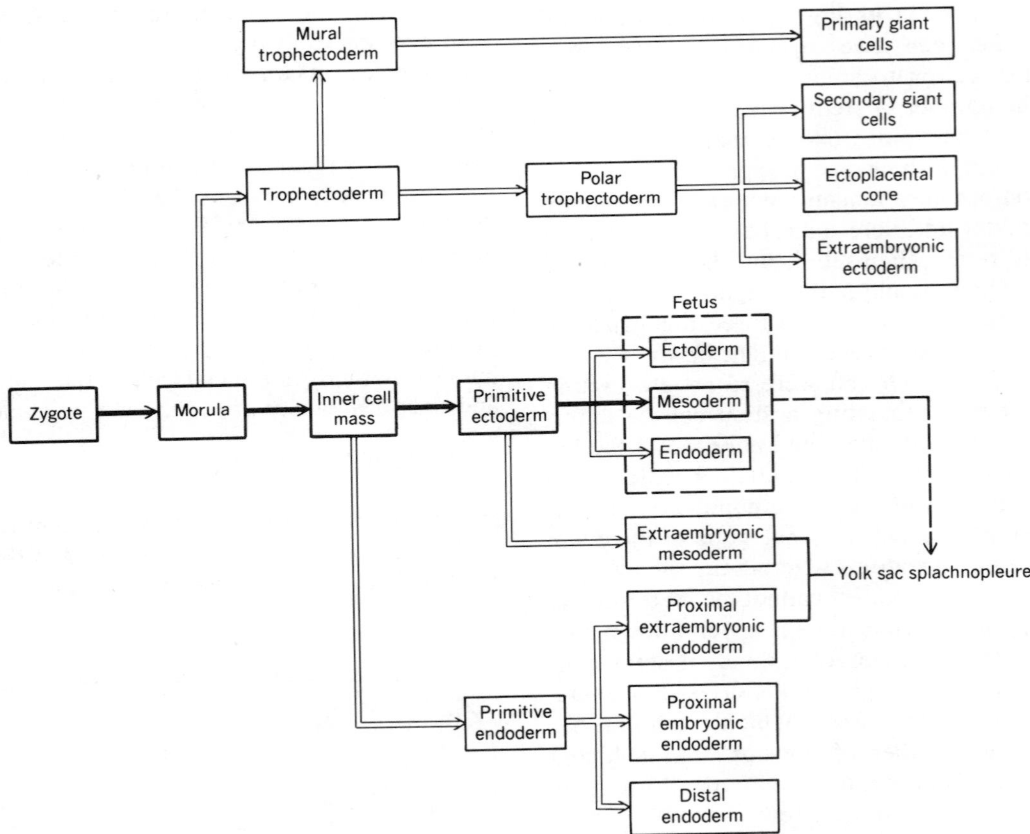

Figure 5.4. Restriction of differentiation potential during the development of mouse embryo. A germ layer or tissue can develop only into the layers or tissues indicated by the arrows. Heavy-line rectangles indicate the lineage leading to hematopoietic stem cells.

seen them. There are no reliable stem cell markers known, and some immunologists even wonder whether the lack of markers might not, in fact, be the identifying characteristic of these cells. Using what is primarily an elimination method (when one succeeds in identifying all cells but one in a preparation known to contain stem cells, one is justified in assuming that the unidentified cell is the stem cell), some immunologists have come to the conclusion that stem cells are relatively small cells with scanty cytoplasm, resembling small lymphocytes. Other immunologists believe that stem cells are large, blastlike cells with abundant cytoplasm. It is also possible that both opinions are correct and that stem cells form a heterogeneous, morphologically variable population. Evidence suggesting that stem cells vary in their self-renewing potential, adherence, size, density, and differentiation potential has, in fact, been obtained. In part, this variability undoubtedly reflects the division of stem cells into CFU-L-M, CFU-S, and the unidentified lymphoid stem cells, but additional stem cell types may also exist.

5.3 PROGENITOR CELLS

5.3.1 Definition

Progenitor cells are the progeny of stem cells committed to differentiation along a single pathway. They differ from stem cells in the following characteristics: they are unipotent; they have only limited, if any, capacity for self-renewal; they are in an active cell cycle, the majority synthesizing DNA; and they are responsive to inducers of differentiation (see below).[1]

5.3.2 In Vitro Assays for Progenitor Cell Detection

Much of our knowledge about progenitor cells is due to in vitro studies by Donald Metcalf, Malcolm A. S. Moore, and their co-workers, in which the authors grew cells in a semisolid (agar) medium in the presence of certain soluble substances (inducers). When an inducer is present, the progenitor cells differentiate along one of the five or six principal differentiation pathways, forming a colony that can be studied microscopically. Which of the five pathways a stem cell chooses depends to a large degree on the nature of the inducer. When a substance called erythropoietin is added, the cells differentiate along the erythrocytic pathway; differentiation of progeny cells along the thrombocytic pathway is thought to be driven by a largely hypothetical substance called thrombopoietin; addition of a colony-stimulating factor leads to the appearance of granulocytic colonies; 2-mercaptoethanol induces differentiation along the B-lymphocyte pathway; and differentiation of T lymphocytes is dependent upon the presence of thymopoietin.

Erythropoietin is a glycoprotein with an estimated molecular weight ranging from 27,000 to 61,000 daltons. It is produced mainly by the kidney; only about 5 to 10 percent appears to be of extrarenal origin. The amount of erythropoietin released by the kidney is controlled by the level of oxygen in the renal tissue: a decrease in oxygen level (hypoxia) leads to increased erythropoietin production and vice versa. The *colony-stimulating factor* (CSF) is a regulator of granulocyte-monocyte-macrophage production. It is present in biological fluids (e.g., plasma and urine) and can be extracted from most tissues of all mammalian species studied so far. It is produced by macrophages, monocytes, lymphocytes activated by exposure to antigen or mitogen, and by endothelial cells. *Thymopoietin* is one of the thymic hormones to be discussed later in this chapter.

5.3.3 Hematopoietic-Inducing Microenvironment

The in vitro data, as well as limited in vivo observations, suggest that, in a live animal, the differentiation of progenitor cells requires conditions fulfilled only by a certain *hematopoietic-inducing microenvironment* (HIM)—a term introduced by John J. Trentin, to whom we owe much of our present knowledge about the effects of microenvironment on hematopoiesis. The effect of the local environment is apparent, for example, from the distribution of the spleen colonies in the X-irradiated, bone marrow-injected mice. About half the colonies are located on the spleen surface and 80 percent of these are erythrocytic or of mixed composition. Some erythrocytic colonies also form in the red pulp. Granulocytic colonies, on the other hand, grow along the splenic trabeculae or in subcapsular sheets; thrombocytic colonies usually form beneath the capsule. These observations suggest that the location of colony-forming cells within the spleen determines the differentiation pathway along which these cells develop. The two principal conditions of a HIM are the presence of certain supportive cells at a given anatomical site (in addition to the presence of progenitor cells) and the availability of inducing factors. HIM for the

[1] Not all immunologists use the terms "stem cell" and "progenitor cell" in the sense defined here. For example, some extend the term "stem cell" to include what is here meant by "progenitor cell," while others reserve this term for the CFU-L-M.

differentiation of T lymphocytes is provided by the thymus, and for B lymphocytes by the bursa of Fabricius in birds and the bone marrow in adult mammals; HIM for all other hematopoietic lineages is provided by the bone marrow.

5.3.4 Morphology and Differentiation Potential

Progenitor cells represent a heterogeneous population both physiologically and morphologically. However, most progenitor cells are large (diameter of about 20 μm), with abundant, ribosome-rich cytoplasms and nuclei that show signs of synthetic activity (loose chromatin, conspicuous nucleoli).

Progenitor cells can differentiate along one of the six principal pathways, each of which has a separate progenitor cell, but how all these cells derive from the common stem cell is not known.

The *erythrocytic lineage* has at least two separate classes of progenitor cell, a more primitive progenitor cell called the *erythroid burst-forming unit*, or *BFU-E*, and a more differentiated *erythroid colony-forming unit*, or *CFU-E*. In the in vitro assays, the BFU-E gives rise to large clusters of erythroid cells (hence the name) in the presence of high erythropoietin levels; the CFU-E gives rise to small clusters and requires relatively small amounts of erythropoietin. There may be several intermediate classes of progenitor cell between BFU-E and CFU-E and between CFU-E and the *proerythroblast*, the earliest morphologically recognizable precursor cell of the erythrocyte (see below).

The *thrombocytic lineage* begins with an as yet undefined progenitor cell presumably responsive to a hypothetical hormone-like substance—the thrombopoietin. This progenitor cell probably passes through several stages before it becomes the immediate precursor of the *megakaryocyte*, the polyploid cell that eventually fragments into platelets (thrombocytes).

The *granulocytic* and *monocytic lineages* stem from a common progenitor cell called the *colony-forming unit-culture*, or *CFU-C*, because it is this cell that gives rise to granulocytic colonies in vitro. The cell is responsive to the colony-stimulating factor and probably also to several other agents produced by granulocytes, monocytes, and macrophages. There is probably more than one CFU-C class but the individual cells have not been identified. At what stage the progenitor cells of the two lineages arise from the common progenitor is not known. At some point beyond this stage, the granulocyte progenitor differentiates further into three different cells that are the precursors of the three granulocyte classes—the neutrophils, basophils, and eosinophils.

The *lymphocytic lineage* develops from a stem cell different from that giving rise to the myeloid compartment. This stem cell then gives rise to two progenitor cells—one for the T-lymphocytic and the other for the B-lymphocytic pathway. At what point these two lineages separate is not known.

5.4 DIFFERENTIATING AND MATURE CELLS

5.4.1 The Erythrocytic Lineage

The main consequence of a cell's commitment to the erythrocytic lineage is the synthesis of hemoglobin by the differentiating cells (Fig. 5.5). Hemoglobin synthesis begins in erythroblasts (normoblasts), which are the immediate progeny of erythrocytic progenitor cells (*proerythroblasts*, or pronormoblasts). Proerythroblasts are large cells (about 20 μm in diameter) with most of the intracellular space occupied by the nucleus. The narrow rim of cytoplasm is rich in ribosomal RNA (needed for hemoglobin synthesis) and so has a dark blue color in Giemsa-stained preparations. (Histologists refer to such a cytoplasm as basophilic; see below.) The proerythroblasts divide four times in a row and each produces 16 cells: one proerythroblast gives rise to two basophilic *erythroblasts I* (E_1), which then divide into four basophilic *erythroblasts II* (E_2); the latter produce eight *polychromatophilic erythroblasts* (E_3), and these give rise to 16 *acidophilic erythroblasts* (E_4). The time elapsed between two subsequent divisions in the human erythrocytic lineage is about 20 hours. During this differentiation, the cells become progressively smaller (the nucleus usually decreasing in size faster than the cytoplasm); the cytoplasm gradually loses most of its ribosomes, and its color therefore changes from blue (proerythroblasts and basophilic erythroblasts) to mixed (polychromatophilic erythroblasts) to pink (acidophilic erythroblasts); the nucleus loses its nucleoli and its chromatin becomes more compact.

The differentiation phase is followed by a maturation period in which the acidophilic erythroblasts expel their nuclei and turn into *reticulocytes* (cells which, when treated with certain stains, form an artifactual network, or reticulum, of precipitated ribosomes in their cytoplasm; hence, the name has nothing to do with the reticular cells described in the preceding chapter).

The entire differentiation and maturation process

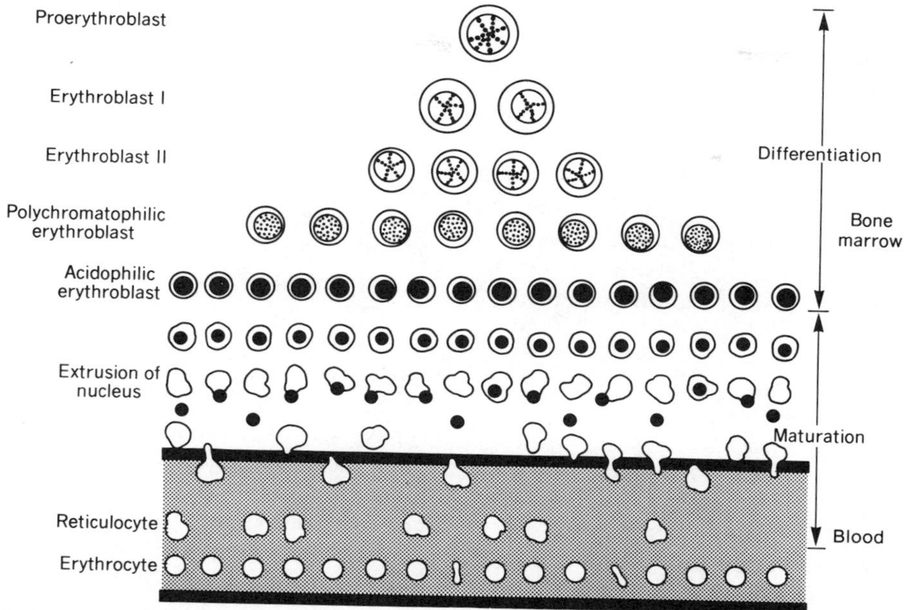

Figure 5.5. Erythropoiesis: differentiation of a progenitor cell into erythrocytes. (Based on M. Bessis: *Blood Smears Reinterpreted*. Springer International, Berlin, 1977.)

takes place in the bone marrow. The reticulocytes then enter the blood stream, and in the blood mature into *erythrocytes*, or red blood cells—small (8 μm in diameter), doughnut-shaped cells filled with hemoglobin. Erythrocytes of the human, mouse, and most other mammals lack the nucleus; nucleated erythrocytes are present in some mammals (e.g., the camel) and in most lower vertebrates. Human erythrocytes live for about 120 days and then are phagocytosed.

5.4.2 The Thrombocytic Lineage

In the thrombocytic lineage (Fig. 5.6), the progenitor cell gives rise to a *megakaryocyte*, which, as the name implies, is a cell with a large nucleus. During megakaryocyte differentiation, only the chromosomes—but not the cell itself—divide, a process referred to as *endoreduplication*. Since the chromosomes duplicate four times, the resulting cell has 16 times the number of chromosomes present in the progenitor cell (or 32 times the number of chromosomes present in the gamete). The cytoplasm of the differentiated megakaryocyte then accumulates granules and compartmentalizes by dividing into small, membrane-enveloped clumps, so that it soon looks like a honeycomb. The cell then fragments, each lump becomes an independent particle called a *thrombocyte*, or platelet, and the nucleus is phagocytosed and de-

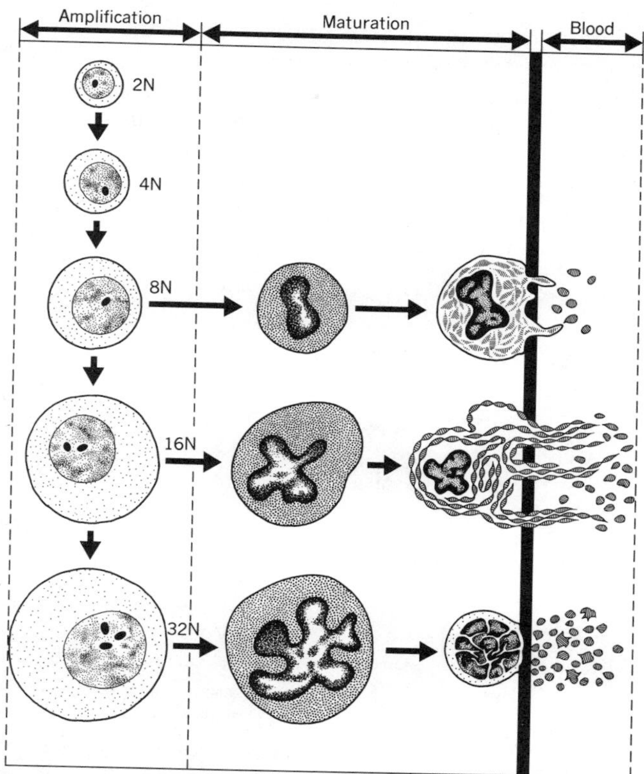

Figure 5.6. Thrombopoiesis: differentiation of a progenitor cell into thrombocytes (platelets). N indicates ploidy (number of haploid chromosomal sets) of the nucleus. (Modified from M. Bessis: *Blood Smears Reinterpreted*. Springer International, Berlin, 1977.)

stroyed. (One megakaryocyte gives rise to some 4000 platelets.) Thrombocytes, which are approximately one-third the size of erythrocytes, are involved in blood clotting (Gr. *thrombos*, clotting). When a wound occurs, it attracts large numbers of platelets, which release clotting substances and help to seal off small leaks in blood capillaries. The entire differentiation and maturation phase of a megakaryocyte takes place in the bone marrow; the liberated platelets then enter the blood stream, where they live for about seven to 10 days.

5.4.3 The Granulocytic Lineage

The differentiation phase of a granulocyte precursor (Fig. 5.7) consists of four successive cell divisions, which produce sequentially from each M_1 *myeloblast* (the immediate derivative of the progenitor cell) two *promyelocytes* (M_2), four *myelocytes I* (M_3), eight *myelocytes II* (M_4), and 16 *metamyelocytes* (M_5); these 16 then mature into 16 *granulocytes*. In the granulocytic lineage, as in the erythrocytic lineage, differentiation is accompanied by a progressive decrease in cell size, a change in nucleus-to-cytoplasm ratio in favor of the cytoplasm, increasing compaction of the nucleus, and, in most cases, a change in the staining properties of the cytoplasm. The granulocytic lineage has, in addition, two characteristic features that are absent in all other hematopoietic lineages. First, the nucleus of a differentiating granulocyte becomes oddly shaped and may assume different forms. For this reason, granulocytes are also known as *polymorphonuclear cells*, *polymorphonuclear leukocytes* (when referring to cells in the blood), or *polymorphs* (Gr. *poly*, many, *morphos*, form; having nuclei of varied forms). Second, starting with the promyelocyte, the Golgi apparatus begins to synthesize large quantities of certain enzymes and other active proteins, and packages them into small vesicles or *granules*, which fill the cytoplasm (hence the name "*granulocyte*," meaning "cell with granules").

Depending on the content (and thus also on the staining properties) of the granules, hematologists distinguish three types of mature granulocyte—*neutrophils*, *eosinophils*, and *basophils*. The stain commonly used to distinguish the different granulocyte types—*Giemsa* (named after Gustav Giemsa, the pharmacist and chemist who developed it for staining malarial parasites in blood preparations)—is a mixture of positively charged (cationic, basic) *methylene blue* and negatively charged (anionic, acidic) *eosin* (Gr. *ēōs*, dawn), a sodium salt of tetrabromofluorescein. The positively charged dye is capable of reacting with negatively charged compounds in the cell, attaching to them and thus staining them blue. (Such compounds are said to be *basophilic*, since they attract a basic dye; Gr. *philē*, to love.) The negatively charged eosin reacts with positively charged cellular constituents and stains them red or orange. (The constituents attract acidic dye and are therefore said to be *acidophilic*.) The basophilic and acidophilic granulocytes are so designated because their granules stain with the basophilic (blue) or acidophilic (red) component of the Giemsa stain, respectively. The name of the neutrophils derives from the fact that their granules contain a mixture

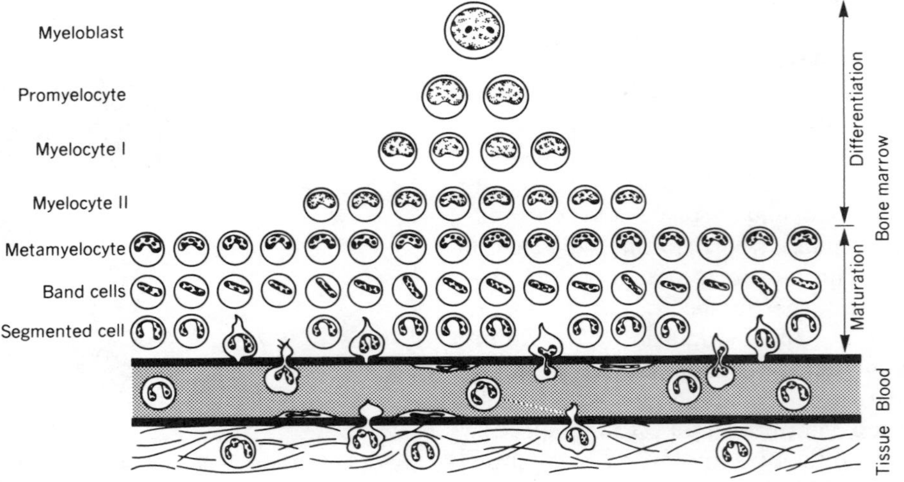

Figure 5.7. Granulopoiesis: differentiation of a progenitor cell into granulocytes (neutrophils). (Modified from M. Bessis: *Blood Smears Reinterpreted*. Springer International, Berlin, 1977.)

of positively and negatively charged compounds and hence assume a greyish-purple color, which is a neutral mixture of the basic blue and acidic red components of the dye. It is not known just when in the differentiation phase the granulocytic lineage separates into the neutrophilic, basophilic, and acidophilic branches, but this event must occur quite early, since the myelocytes can already be differentiated according to the granules they contain. A description of the three granulocyte types follows.

Neutrophils

Morphology. There are two main types of neutrophil—band cells (M_6) and segmented cells (M_7)—distinguished primarily by the shape of their nuclei (Fig. 5.8). In the younger *band cells*, the nucleus is indented, so that it resembles a kidney or a sausage, but the indentation is never deep enough to split the nucleus into distinct lobes: individual sections of the nucleus always remain connected by a broad band (hence the name). In the more mature *segmented cells*, the nucleus consists of from two to five lobes (segments), connected by thin filaments of chromatin. Some hematologists believe that the older a neutrophil grows, the more segments it develops in its nucleus, but there is no direct evidence to support this notion. The chromatin of the nucleus is coarsely clumped, suggesting that most of the genome is inactive and that the neutrophil is a dead-end cell that can neither divide nor differentiate further; nucleoli are absent. The cytoplasm contains numerous granules and electron-dense particles composed of glycogen, an important source of energy released by glycolysis.

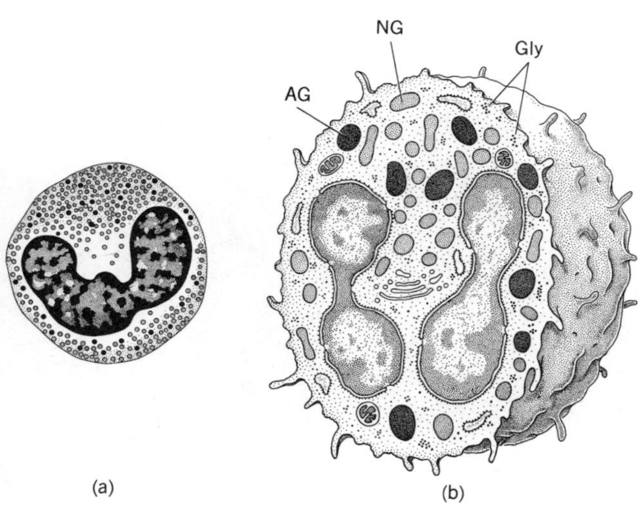

Figure 5.8. Blood cell gallery: neutrophil, as seen with a light (*a*) and electron (*b*) microscope. AG, azurophilic granule; Gly, glycogen particle; NG, neutrophilic granule. (*a* modified from M. Bessis: *Blood Smears Reinterpreted*. Springer International, Berlin, 1977; *b* modified from T. L. Lenz: *Cell Fine Structure*. Saunders, Philadelphia, 1971.)

Granules. Neutrophils contain two types of granule, primary (azurophilic) and secondary (specific). *Primary granules* (so designated because they develop early in granulocyte differentiation) stain purplish with the Giemsa stain (hence the name "azurophilic," derived from "azure"—the blue color of a clear sky), have a diameter of about 0.5 μm, and compose from 10 to 20 percent of the total granule population. They are typical lysosomes—that is, vesicles containing enzymes necessary for intracellular digestion. The vesicles also contain a rich mixture of compounds possessing antibacterial (bactericidal) activity. Some of these compounds are listed below (see also Chapters 11 and 13).

Hydrolases (e.g., nuclease, lipase, phospholipase, α-amylase, elastase, and collagenase) have an optimum of activity at pH 5.0. These enzymes break down organic molecules—such as those present in bacterial cell walls—into their building blocks (amino acids, sugars, and nucleotides).

Lysozyme is an enzyme complex that hydrolyses glycosides of bacterial cell walls.

Myeloperoxidase is an enzyme capable of binding hydrogen peroxide (H_2O_2) and thus causing the production of activated oxygen, which has bactericidal properties (see Chapter 11). Tests for peroxidase are often used for identification of primary granules.

Cationic proteins are so designated because they are rich in the positively charged amino acids arginine and lysine.

Secondary granules are only about 2 μm in diameter, stain faintly pink with Giemsa, and constitute from 75 to 80 percent of the total granule population. They contain *lysozyme* and *lactoferrin*, a protein originally found in milk and carrying an iron-containing heme group (L. *lac*, milk, *ferrum*, iron). The antibacterial effect of lactoferrin results from the fact that it binds iron and thus makes it unavailable to bacteria, which need it for their normal physiology.

Distribution and Cell Movement. In the blood of adult humans, neutrophils constitute from 45 to 70 percent of all leukocytes. Some neutrophils are also present in the connective tissue. Neutrophils are constantly on the move, from tissue to tissue, from one area to another. When placed on a flat glass or plastic surface, the cell immediately spreads out, retaining its nucleus in a central elevated area so that it resembles Smokey

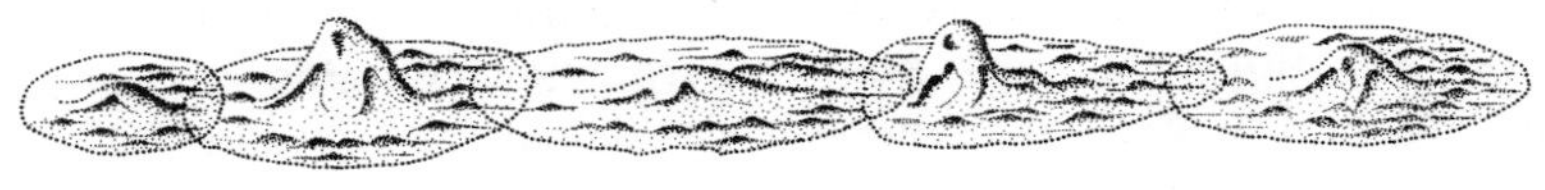

Figure 5.9. Movement of a neutrophil on a flat surface. A single cell shown in successive stages of locomotion. Direction of movement indicated by the arrow.

the Bear's hat (Fig. 5.9). It then flattens even more and attaches to the surface (it is one of the stickiest cells in the body). Next, it sends out a cytoplasmic projection (*protopod*; from Gr. *protos*, first, *pous*, foot) in one direction, detaches itself from the substratum at a region of its body (*uropod*; from Gr. *oura*, buttocks) opposite this projection, and moves this region forward, while the front region remains fixed. And in this manner it continues—it grips the surface at the front and then pulls its rear end forward. Normally, the direction of movement is random, with the cell now moving to the right, now to the left, now forward, now backward. When, however, the medium surrounding a neutrophil delivers a signal originating from, say, bacteria, the cell movement becomes directed toward the signal source. The cell still changes direction, but chooses a direction away from the signal less frequently than toward the signal. The capacity of a cell to move toward (or away from) a signal source is termed *chemotaxis* (Gr. *taxis*, orderly arrangement).

Function. The main function of neutrophils is to kill bacteria and other infectious agents. The main mechanism by which neutrophils fulfill this function is phagocytosis. We shall have a lot more to say about the activities of neutrophils in Chapter 11.

Eosinophils

Eosinophilic leukocytes, or eosinophils (Fig. 5.10), are round cells, 11 to 15 μm in diameter, with a bilobed nucleus and cytoplasm filled with eosin-binding granules. (Sometimes there are so many granules in the cell that they obscure the nucleus.) Eosinophils constitute from 1 to 5 percent of all peripheral white blood cells; however, like other granulocytes, they are also found in the connective tissue, particularly under epithelia with large bacterial populations, such as the intestinal, vaginal, and nasal mucosae. Eosinophilic granules, which are up to 1.5 μm in diameter, contain acid phosphatase, glucuronidase, cathepsins, ribonuclease, arylsulphatase, peroxidase, and other enzymes. The proteins of a granule often form one or two crystals embedded in an electron-dense matrix (Fig. 5.10*b*). Eosinophils, like neutrophils, are mobile phagocytic cells. Their function is not known, but since their numbers increase dramatically during parasitic infections, immunologists believe that these cells play a role in antiparasitic immunity. In addition, eosinophils might be involved in anaphylactic and allergic phenomena (see Chapter 13).

Basophils

Basophilic leukocytes are the smallest of all granulocytes, measuring about 10 to 12 μm in diameter (Fig. 5.11). They are characterized by spherical or ovoid granules, which stain dark violet or purple with Giemsa. The internal structure of the granules varies, depending on the histological treatment; sometimes it appears to be crystalloid, but at other times it reveals concentric lamellar structures that look like scrolls of parchment; at still other times it seems to be uniformly dense. The granules contain large amounts of heparin, a sulfated mucopolysaccharide that causes smooth-muscle contractions and prevents blood clotting, and histamine, a compound derived by decarboxylation

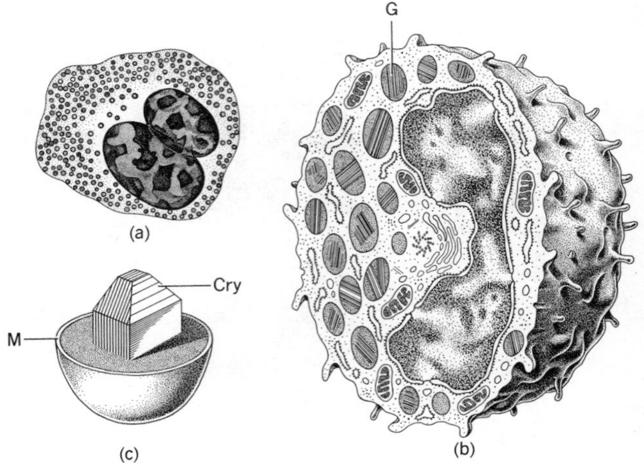

Figure 5.10. Blood cell gallery: eosinophil, as seen with a light (*a*) and electron (*b*) microscope. (*c*) Magnified granule with crystal. Cry, crystal; G, granule; M, membrane. (*a* redrawn from M. Bessis: *Blood Smears Reinterpreted*. Springer International, Berlin, 1977; *b* and *c* based on R. V. Krstić: *Die Gewebe des Menschen und der Säugetiere*. Springer-Verlag, Berlin, 1978.)

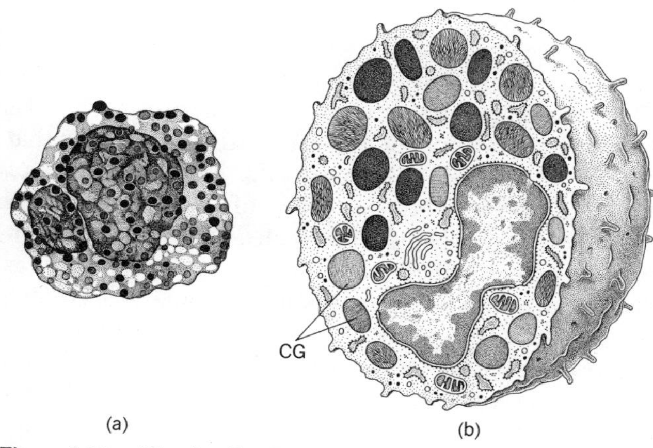

Figure 5.11. Blood cell gallery: basophil, as seen with a light (*a*) and electron (*b*) microscope. CG, crystalloid granule. (*a* modified from M. Bessis: *Blood Smears Reinterpreted*. Springer International, Berlin, 1977.)

from the amino acid histidine and capable of inducing increased blood vessel permeability. Heparin has many anionic, uniformly spaced sulfate groups that bind molecules of cationic dyes, such as *toluidine blue*, electrostatically. The aggregated toluidine blue molecules absorb light at a lower wavelength than the nonaggregated molecules and so appear red rather than blue. This change in the color of a dye after binding to tissue components is termed *metachromasia* (Gr. *meta*, after, *chrōma*, color). In addition to heparin and histamine, basophilic granules also contain numerous enzymes, such as decarboxylase, histidine dehydrogenase, and diaphorase (= lipoamide dehydrogenase). In contrast to neutrophils and eosinophils, basophils usually do not contain peroxidase in their granules.

The nucleus of a basophilic granulocyte, often masked by opaque granulation, is segmented into two or three lobes joined by strands of chromatin. Basophils occur in the blood, where they constitute approximately 1 percent of all leukocytes; in connective tissue of the skin; in hair follicles; and in adipose tissues. They show little phagocytic activity, their main function being to serve as targets for certain antibodies in anaphylactic and allergic reactions, and in antiparasitic immunity (see Chapter 13).

5.4.4. The Monocytic-Histiocytic Lineage

The early stages of monocyte differentiation are poorly understood. Many immunologists and histologists believe that monocytes and granulocytes have a common progenitor cell, but unequivocal proof for this contention is lacking. After branching off from this common progenitor, the monocytic lineage is believed to pass through at least three differentiation stages, referred to as monoblast, promonocyte, and monocyte (Fig. 5.12), but the first two cell types are not well defined. The number of cell divisions required for passing from one stage to the next and the duration of the individual stages are not known. The *monoblast* resembles corresponding cells (blasts) of other hematopoietic lineages (large cell; round nucleus with a fine chromatin network and several nucleoli; basophilic, ribosome-rich cytoplasm), and no stain or marker is available that would identify it specifically. The *promonocyte* resembles the monoblast, the main difference between the two being that the latter has a more abundant cytoplasm than the former. The promonocyte stage probably embraces several cell generations that are morphologically indistinguishable.

The differentiation phase of monocyte development takes place in the bone marrow; maturing monocytes then move into the blood circulation, where they remain for only a short period. From the blood, monocytes enter various tissues and there they transform into histiocytes (macrophages; see Fig. 5.12).

The Monocyte

The mature monocyte (Fig. 5.13) is a spherical cell, ranging in size from 10 to 40 μm. (Some hematologists

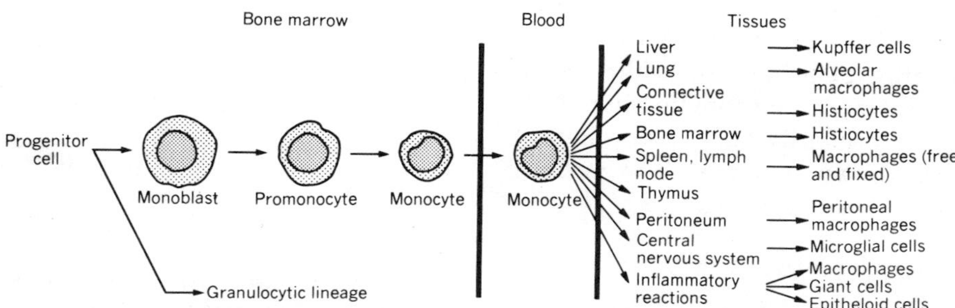

Figure 5.12. Development of monocytes, macrophages, and histiocytes from progenitor cells.

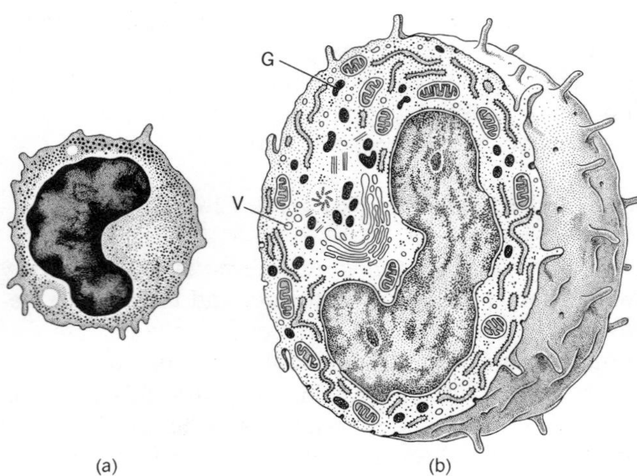

Figure 5.13. Blood cell gallery: monocyte, as seen with a light (*a*) and electron (*b*) microscope. G, granule; V, vesicle. (*a* modified from M. Bessis: *Blood Smears Reinterpreted*. Springer International, Berlin, 1977; *b* modified from R. V. Krstić: *Die Gewebe des Menschen und der Säugetiere*. Springer-Verlag, Berlin, 1978.)

distinguish two types of monocyte—small, with a diameter of up to 30 μm, and large, with a diameter greater than 30 μm.) The cell surface of a resting monocyte is smooth except for a few fingerlike projections (microvilli); the surface of an active monocyte is pimpled and wrinkled. The nucleus is characteristically horseshoe- or bean-shaped, with condensed chromatin close to the nuclear envelope and lacy loose chromatin in the center. Nucleoli are usually not visible, at least not in blood monocytes. Abundant cytoplasm contains Golgi apparatus (positioned in the nuclear indentation), a modestly developed rough endoplasmic reticulum, a large number of azurophilic lysosomes, and several vacuoles.

Monocytes are present in the peripheral blood, where they constitute from 2 to 8 percent of all leukocytes, and in various tissues. They are mobile cells with principally the same mode of locomotion as that of granulocytes. Monocytes also resemble granulocytes in that they adhere to a surface and spread themselves on it. They are actively phagocytic, devouring not only antigen-antibody complexes, viruses, and bacteria, but also entire cells, red or white. Small monocytes are usually more phagocytic than large ones. Monocytes serve primarily as a reservoir from which histiocytes are drawn, but they also perform many of the functions of macrophages.

Histiocytes and Macrophages

Morphology. In Greek mythology, Poseidon, the god of the sea, was attended by Proteus, a creature who had the power of changing his appearance at will. A Proteus—that is how the macrophage appears to histologists. Many a histologist has been fooled by this cell's changing appearance and described what he thought to be a new cell type, only to realize later that it was just another form of the old macrophage. Histological literature is full of exotic names—clasmatocytes, rhagiocrine cells, polyblasts, lymphoconnective cells, leukocytoid cells of the vascular adventitia, polymorphous histiogenic migratory cells, to list just a few—that all mean the same thing: the macrophage. Even now the cell has two legitimate names—*macrophage*, usually reserved for the forms that are on the move, and *histiocyte* (Gr. *histon*, tissue, *kytos*, cell), usually used to designate a cell that has settled down, temporarily or permanently. In actuality, however, there is no difference between a macrophage and a histiocyte.

The size and shape of a macrophage (Fig. 5.14) vary, depending on the environment and on its functional activity. The size ranges from 10 to 40 μm; the shape can be spherical, elongated, stellate, or just plain irregular. The cell surface is often richly differentiated into fingerlike and spherical projections or into folds and sheets, which make the cell look like a head of lettuce.

The nucleus is centrally located and is spherical or oval, often with a deep indentation; it has one nucleolus. The cytoplasm of a mature, functionally active macrophage contains a prominent endoplasmic re-

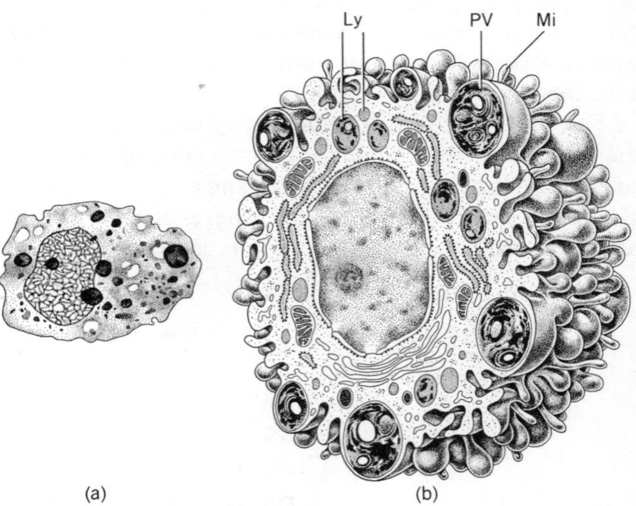

Figure 5.14. Blood cell gallery: histiocyte (macrophage), as seen with a light (*a*) and electron (*b*) microscope. Ly, lysosomes; Mi, microvillus; PV, phagocytic vacuole. (*a* modified from M. Bessis: *Blood Smears Reinterpreted*. Springer International, Berlin, 1977; *b* modified from R. V. Krstić: *Die Gewebe des Menschen und der Säugetiere*. Springer-Verlag, Berlin, 1978.)

ticulum, well-developed Golgi apparatus, colorless vacuoles, bundles of tubules and filaments, and abundant mitochondria and granules. The size and content of the granules vary considerably. The list of enzymes found in macrophages is a whole page long; in general, its granules contain everything necessary to digest almost any living matter devoured by this cell. In a nonfunctional or less active macrophage all the features just described are much less prominent.

Distribution. As has already been mentioned, there are two types of macrophage—migratory, which moves from tissue to tissue, and the *histiocyte*, which remains fixed at a particular site. The latter cells often bear different names, a holdover from the times when they were regarded as distinct entities. Some of the sites and the names of the histiocytes present in them are listed below (see also Fig. 5.12).

Liver. Kupffer cells, named after the German anatomist Karl W. Kupffer, are stellate cells with long projections, lining the trabecular liver cells.
Kidney. Mesangial cells (see Chapter 14).
Lung. Alveolar macrophages.
Connective tissue (intestine, ovary, testes). Histiocytes.
Bone marrow. Histiocytes (cells lining sinuses).
Spleen. Macrophages (cells in the white pulp and cells lining sinuses in the red pulp).
Lymph nodes. Macrophages (scattered cells and cells lining medullary sinuses).
Thymus. Macrophages (scattered cells).
Peritoneum. Peritoneal macrophages (cells in the peritoneal fluid).
Central nervous system. Microglial cells.

Many macrophages are situated along capillaries, where they have easy access to foreign particles invading the body. In the presence of foreign bodies that are difficult to digest (e.g., oil particles, *Mycobacteria* of tuberculosis or leprosy), macrophages fuse to form *giant cells* that can contain 20 or more nuclei. In chronic granulomas (inflammatory reactions resulting in the appearance of granular or nodular tissue), macrophages may become connected by tight junctions, become less phagocytic, contain fewer lysosomes, and thus transform into *epithelioid cells* (Gr. *eidos*, resemblance), which wall off the inflammatory site. All macrophages are derived from monocytes, and the one can transform into the other.

Life Span. Macrophages are long-lived cells with a life span of from two to three months. Normally they are nonproliferating cells, but under certain pathological conditions they can divide for as long as three months.

Locomotion and Adherence. Migratory macrophages are highly mobile cells, but their movements decrease after ingestion of large quantities of foreign material (not unlike a person who has eaten too much). The locomotion can be random or directed toward certain substances (chemotactic stimuli). The mechanism of the movement is apparently the same as that of granulocytes and its hallmark is the formation of a *cytoplasmic veil* (an undulating membrane). When isolated, macrophages stick easily to glass or plastic surfaces and spread out on them.

Function. Macrophages are involved in a great number of functions, both nonimmune and immune, some of which are listed below. (For a more complete discussion of macrophage functions, see Chapter 11.)

Nonimmune Functions. Synthesis of complement components (C2, C4, and others), transferrin (an iron-binding blood protein), pyrogen (fever-inducing protein), certain interferons (antiviral agents), colony-stimulating factors, enzymes (lysozyme, elastase, and collagenase), clotting factors (plasminogen activator, prothrombin, and proconvertin), and probably many other substances.

Participation in fatty acid and cholesterol synthesis.

Ingestion of chylomicrons (microscopic fat particles).

Degradation of certain proteins (globulins and albumins) and polysaccharides.

Elimination of necrotic cells and foreign bodies during the healing process. (Remember Metchnikoff's rose thorn experiment from Chapter 1?)

Transfer of iron to erythrocyte precursors.

Immune Functions. Phagocytosis. Macrophages are chronic eaters of foreign material. They swallow entire cells (often several at a time), bacteria, protozoa, and inorganic substances.

Involvement in antibody synthesis. Macrophages do not synthesize antibodies, but are involved in some important way in antigen processing and presentation.

Involvement in delayed-type hypersensitivities.

Involvement in tumor immunity.

Methods of Isolation. Purified macrophages can be obtained by one of the following methods:

Centrifuging whole anti-coagulant-containing blood and collecting the white ''buffy coat'' from the top of the red blood cell sediment.

Injecting thioglycolate (a salt of thioglycolic acid used in bacterial media) into the peritoneal cavity of an animal, harvesting the peritoneal fluid, and separating cells by centrifugation. (Twenty-four hours after the injection, this peritoneal exudate contains mostly neutrophils, but four days later it consists almost exclusively of macrophages.)

Rinsing lungs with physiological saline solution and thus detaching alveolar macrophages from alveoli (terminal saclike widenings of lung ducts).

Injecting animals intravenously with fine iron particles, perfusing the liver, and placing the perfusion fluid in a magnetic field. The Kupffer cells in the liver ingest the iron particles and can be pulled out of the suspension by the force of the magnetic field.

Adhering macrophages to a glass or plastic surface and so separating them from nonadherent cells in a cell suspension.

Macrophages can be cultured in vitro for up to two or three months without proliferation. However, permanent, proliferating, macrophage-derived cell lines are also available.

5.4.5 The Lymphocytic Lineage

Studies of cell differentiation along the lymphocytic pathway have revealed about as much detail as the famous painting by Claude Monet, *Impression*, *Sunrise*. In this painting we recognize rather precisely the fisherman's boat in the foreground, but we can only guess the contours of the harbor in the background through the veils of morning mist. In the lymphocytic lineage, we have a pretty good idea of the lineage's final stages, but almost everything else we can only surmise through the fog of ignorance. We *assume* that there is a common stem cell for the T and B lineages—a stem cell distinct from that giving rise to other blood cells; we *assume* further that T and B lineages each have a set of progenitor cells, but we know almost nothing about these progenitors; and we have accumulated bits and pieces of information about the intermediate stages of the lymphocytic differentiation pathway, but we are a long way from replacing the *impression* of the harbor with a photograph. The little we do know about T- and B-lymphocytic lineages is summarized in the following two sections.

5.5 THE T-LYMPHOCYTIC LINEAGE

5.5.1 What Is a Lymphocyte?

A *lymphocyte* (Fig. 5.15) is a round cell, 7 to 12 μm in diameter, with scanty cytoplasm, a round nucleus, and chromatin arranged in coarse masses. A number of stimuli will induce its transformation into a larger cell (*transformed lymphocyte* or *blast*; Fig. 5.16) and its division. There are two major classes of lymphocyte, T and B. *T lymphocytes* (T cells, thymus-processed lymphocytes) derive their name from the fact that they (and their precursors) spend a certain amount of time in the thymus. The letter *B* in the designation of *B lymphocytes* can mean one of three things—"bursa-derived," when referring to avian lymphocytes, "bursa equivalent-derived" or "bone marrow-de-

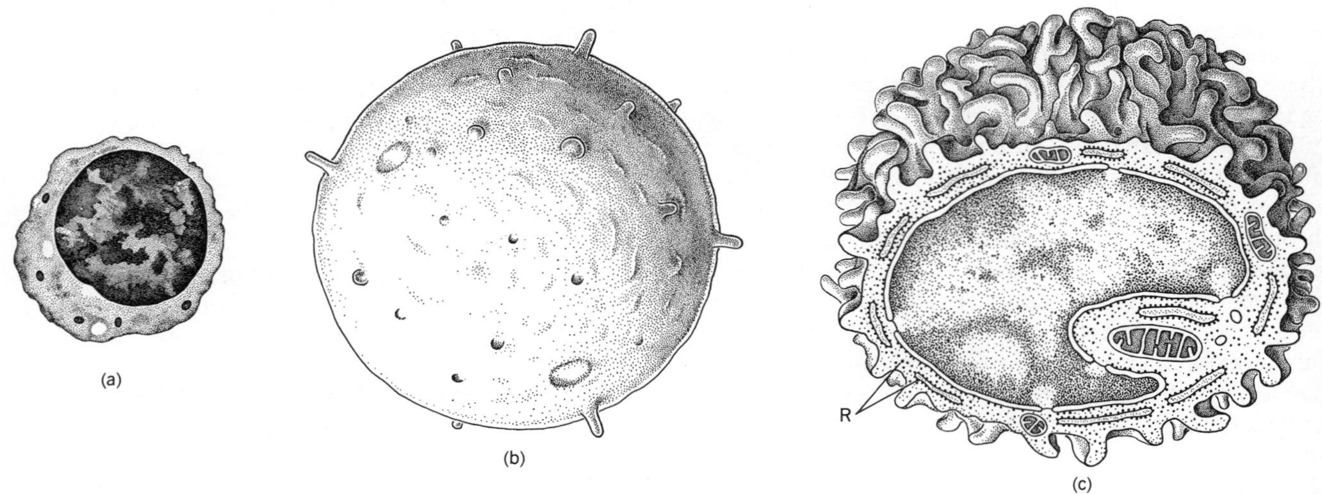

Figure 5.15. Blood cell gallery: lymphocyte, as seen with a light (*a*) and electron (*b*, *c*) microscope. R, ribosomes. Two functional states of lymphocyte surface—smooth (*b*) and rich with microvilli (*c*)—are shown.

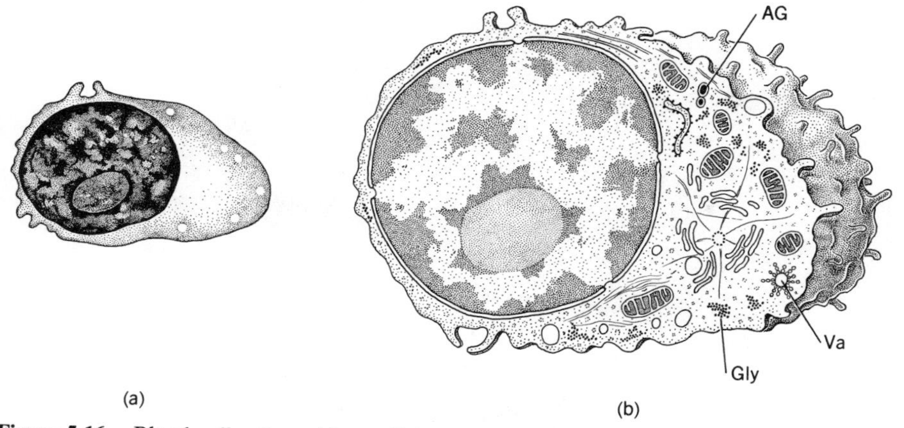

Figure 5.16. Blood cell gallery: blast cell (transformed lymphocyte) as seen with a light (*a*) and electron (*b*) microscope. AG, azurophilic granules; Gly, glycogen particles; Va, vacuole. (Modified from M. Bessis: *Blood Smears Reinterpreted.* Springer International, Berlin, 1977.)

rived,'' when dealing with mammals. The reason for this nominal ambivalence is that no equivalent of the avian bursa of Fabricius has been found in mammals. The designation ''bone marrow-derived,'' although commonly used, is nevertheless the most ambiguous of the three since T lymphocytes, too, as we shall see, are ultimately derived from bone marrow.

5.5.2 Life History of a T Lymphocyte

T lymphocytes originate from the same *stem cells* that give rise to all other blood cells. These stem cells produce *progenitor cells*, which move into the thymus and differentiate into *thymic lymphocytes* (*thymocytes*). These then leave the thymus, mature into immunologically competent *T lymphocytes*, and begin the life of circulating cells. When a circulating cell encounters a stimulating agent (an antigen, for example), it enters an active functional phase. If it is not stimulated, it remains in the body for a certain period and is then eliminated. One can thus divide the life of a T lymphocyte into four phases—prethymic, thymic, post-thymic unstimulated, and post-thymic stimulated.

The Prethymic Phase

In the prethymic phase, lymphocyte progenitors migrate into the thymus. Most of the migration takes place during embryonic and early post-natal life; in an adult, the number of progenitor cells entering the thymus declines gradually with age.

Evidence for Extrathymic Origin of Lymphocyte Progenitors. The most convincing evidence that thymocytes are derived from migrant cells, rather than from mesenchymal or epithelial elements of the thymus itself, comes from studies by John J. T. Owen and Malcolm A. S. Moore on fowl embryos. One can take fowl eggs after four days incubation, cut small windows in their shells, expose the yolk sacs beneath the shells, and join the exposed areas in pairs with paraffin wax (Fig. 5.17*a*). As the juxtaposed yolk sacs in the eggs fuse, a common circulatory system develops, and the two embryos exchange blood cells freely. If the embryos in a given pair are of opposite sexes, the blood cells carry either male or female chromosomes, depending upon their origin (Fig. 5.17*b*). Hence by analyzing dividing thymocytes in situ, one can tell whether the thymus has been settled by immigrating or indigenous cells. The experimental finding is that as many as 50 percent of the thymic lymphocytes in a given embryo are derived from the partner, indicating that lymphocyte progenitors are brought into the thymus by the blood stream.

Can T Lymphocytes Differentiate Outside of the Thymus? Experiments with chromosomally marked cells indicate that the thymic immigrants arrive first from fetal liver and fetal spleen, then from bone marrow. As we already know, fetal liver, fetal spleen, and bone marrow are true hematopoietic organs that not only harbor hematopoietic stem cells but also sustain differentiation of these cells into erythrocytes, platelets, granulocytes, and monocytes. (The yolk sac definitely sustains erythropoiesis; to what degree it allows thrombopoiesis, granulopoiesis, or monocytopoiesis is not known.) But what about lymphocytes? Can they, too, at one time or another, differentiate in the hematopoietic organs without making

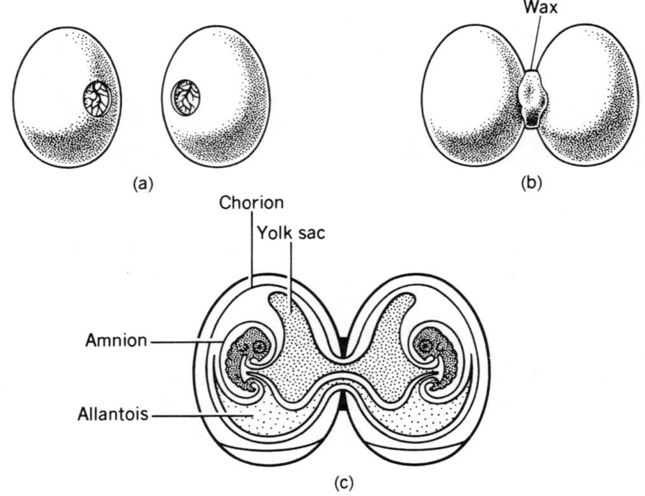

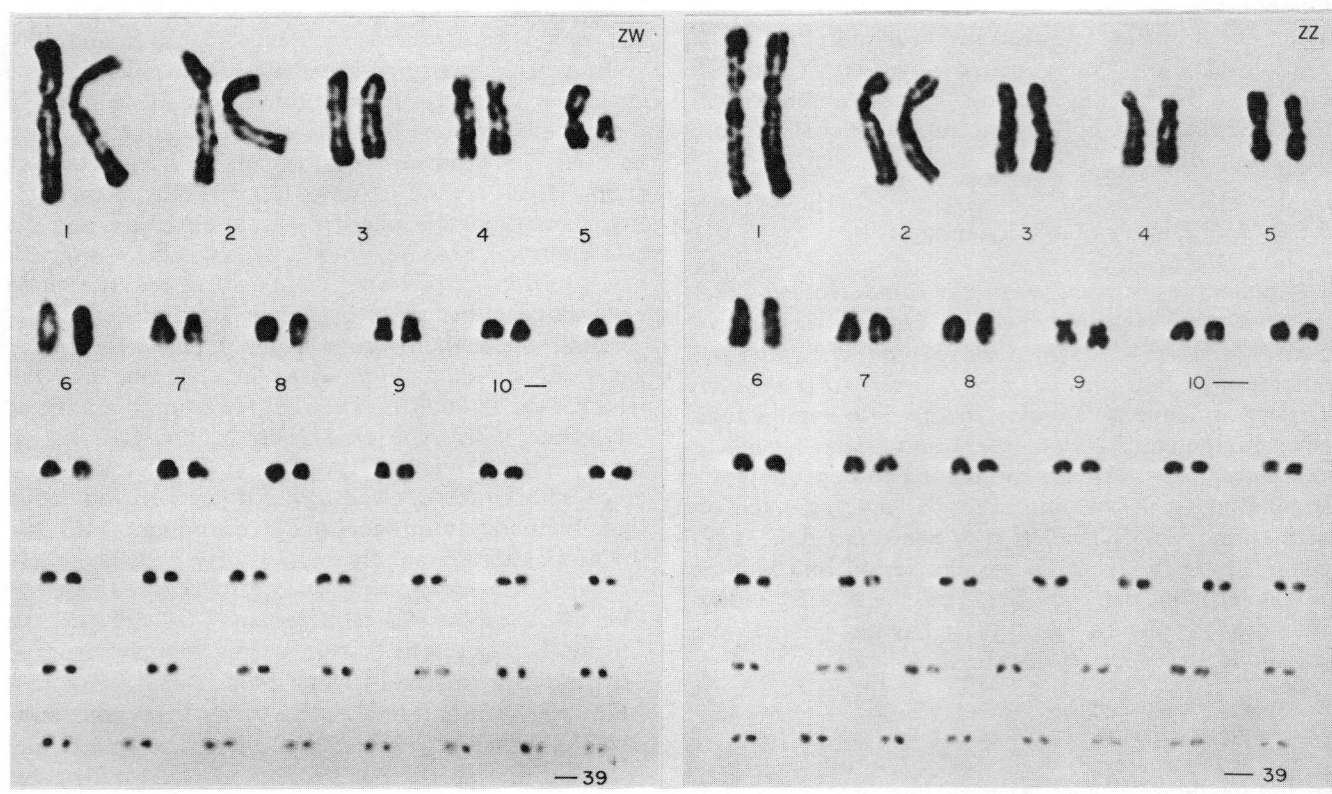

Figure 5.17. Technique for parabiosis in the domestic fowl. (*a*) Fertile eggs between six and 11 days of incubation are transilluminated. The most vascular regions of the chorioallantoic membrane are identified and a small hole is then cut through the shell there. (*b*) Matching holes are brought together and the pair of eggs is joined with wax. (*c*) Vascular anastomosis (connected blood vessels) develops between the chorioallantoic blood vessels, and hematopoietic cell chimerism is established. Markers of the chimera are the sex chromosomes: metaphase spreads of female chicken cells contain one large Z and one small W chromosome (*e*); those of the male cell contain two morphologically identical Z chromosomes (*d*). (*d* and *e* courtesy Dr. J. J. T. Owen.)

the thymic pilgrimage? Some authors claim that cells obtained from the yolk sac, fetal liver, or fetal spleen perform functions normally attributed to mature T lymphocytes. However, these authors have not excluded the possibility that the purported T lymphocytes got into these organs secondarily, after their sojourn in the thymus. Such a possibility is likely, since T lymphocytes (identified by characteristic cell-surface antigens) have been detected in mouse fetal liver only *after* the thymus has begun to function and to send out differentiated lymphocytes into circulation. Also, one does not find T lymphocytes in cultured fetal liver if the liver has been taken out of the embryo before the onset of thymus function. However, when one eliminates thymus-processed lymphocytes from a suspension of fetal liver or adult spleen cells, one can induce in some of the remaining cells the expression of antigens characteristic of mature T cells. One can accomplish such an induction in vitro by exposing the cells to agents that elevate levels of cyclic adenylmonophosphate (cAMP) or to thymic hormones. Furthermore, athymic (*nu*/*nu*) mice, with a defect in the thymus-anlage differentiation, possess cells expressing low levels of T cell-characteristic antigens. Yet these cells cannot perform typical T-cell functions, and probably represent precursors that have begun to differentiate—perhaps because of some abnormal stimulus—along the T-lymphocytic pathway, but which, in the absence of a normal thymus, are unable to complete the differentiation. In summary, there is no convincing evidence for an alternative pathway of T-lymphocyte differentiation, bypassing the thymus, or for extrathymic development of mature, functional T lymphocytes.

What Kinds of Cells Migrate into the Thymus? Experiments on the induction of T-cell antigens in fetal liver and spleen cells and observations on the presence of such antigens in athymic mice suggest that the thymic immigrants are not stem cells, but progenitor cells already committed to differentiation along the T-lymphocytic pathway. These experiments and observations, however, should not be interpreted to mean that progenitor cells, under physiological conditions, already express T cell-characteristic antigens. On the contrary, other experiments indicate that when one eliminates all cells expressing these antigens from bone marrow, the marrow's ability to supply thymic migrants remains unaffected. One can reconcile the two sets of observations by postulating that T-cell progenitors have the *ability* to express T-cell antigens, but normally do not express them outside the thymus or express them only at low concentrations. They can express these antigens, however, under abnormal conditions, such as those provided by the exposure to agents that increase cAMP levels or those that exist in athymic mice.

Morphologically, the T progenitors resemble cells referred to by hematologists as *lymphoblasts* when seen in blood smears. Lymphoblasts (Fig. 5.16) are from 12 to 20 μm in diameter and have a round or oval nucleus, with one pale blue-staining nucleolus, and a variable amount of basophilic cytoplasm. In contrast to that of other types of progenitor cell, the finely distributed chromatin network in the T-cell progenitors is only faintly visible. How far along the T-cell pathway the progenitors differentiate before they enter the thymus is not known.

The Thymic Phase

Entry of T-Progenitor Cells into the Thymus. Progenitor cells arrive in the thymus by way of the blood, initially from fetal liver and then from bone marrow. They enter the thymus by crawling between endothelial cells of postcapillary venules in the medulla and the corticomedullary junction. This port of entry is selective (no other blood cells are allowed to enter), unidirectional (progenitor cells get into the thymus but cannot get out), and dynamic (it can close temporarily, even to progenitor cells).

Proliferation of Progenitor Cells. In the mouse, the first wave of progenitor cells—a fairly uniform population of large and medium-sized lymphocytes—arrives in the epithelial thymus anlage on the eleventh or twelfth day of gestation. The cells distribute themselves throughout the thymus and settle down into the spaces of the three-dimensional epithelial mesh. This process takes several days, during which no new cells are allowed to enter the thymus. Then, on about the sixteenth day of gestation, a wave of mitotic activity sweeps through the thymus, starting in the subcapsular region and moving through the future cortex into the medulla. (It is only one or two days later that the cortex and medulla become clearly demarcated.) The proliferation is accompanied by a dramatic decrease in cell volume so that, within a few days, the embryonic thymus becomes populated predominantly by small lymphocytes. The proliferation period lasts about three days, during which the progenitor cells divide from six to eight times, with a mean generation time of approximately nine hours. It is only when the wave of proliferation reaches the medulla that new progenitor cells are admitted into the thymus. By then the wavelike character of the proliferation process is lost and proliferation foci become randomly distributed throughout the thymus. How many times a cell must divide before it is ready to leave the thymus and what differentiation steps it must pass through is not known. In fact, most cells do not leave the thymus at all, but die instead.

Differentiation Markers. During differentiation from progenitor cells to thymocytes, cells progressively change their properties, which can then be used as markers identifying various differentiation stages. A description of some of these markers of mouse or human lymphocytes follows. (See also Table 5.1.)

*Alloantigens Controlled by Thy-*1, *Lyt*, *and Tla Loci.* Thy-1, Lyt, and Tla alloantigens are cell-membrane molecules, reacting with antibodies produced in mice of certain strains after the injection of thymocytes from other strains. Binding of Thy-1, Lyt, or Tla antibodies to the corresponding antigens activates complement, which then kills the antigen-bearing cells. Alternatively, one can identify the antigen-bearing cells by tagging the antibodies with a visible label. There are several *Lyt* loci, of which *Lyt-*1 and *Lyt-*2 are the most useful as markers. Only one *Thy-*1 and one *Tla* locus are known. The *Lyt-*1, *Lyt-*2, and *Thy-*1 loci each have two alleles, each controlling a different antigen, so that some mouse strains carry one antigen and others carry another. All of these antigens are absent on progenitor cells; Lyt and Tla antigens are expressed only on lymphocytes (or their subpopulations), whereas the Thy-1 antigens are present on lymphocytes and certain other (e.g., epidermal) cells. What role, if any, these antigens play in lymphocyte differentiation is not known. The Tla antigens are described in more detail in Chapter 14.

Alloantigens Controlled by the Major Histocompatibility Complex (MHC). Like the Thy-1, Lyt, and Tla antigens, the MHC alloantigens, too, are cell-membrane molecules identifiable with antibodies produced by mouse-to-mouse or human-to-human immunizations. They fall into two classes—I and II. Class I antigens are present on most somatic cell surfaces of an adult organism, but in different quantities. Since the quantity of class I antigens in a given cell is genetically determined, it serves as a marker to identify the cell. Class II antigens are present only on certain cell types, including subpopulations of lymphocytes, which they help to identify. We shall learn more about MHC antigens in Chapter 8.

Xenoantigens. When one immunizes a rabbit (or some other animal) with a purified suspension of mouse thymocytes, one usually obtains, in addition to thymocytes, a mixture of antibodies reacting with many different cells. (Mouse thymocytes share with other cells certain antigens that the rabbit lacks, so the rabbit produces antibodies against these antigens.) When one adds to this mixture a suspension containing all kinds of cells except thymocytes, all antibodies except the thymocyte-specific ones bind to these cells and can be removed with them from the antibody mixture. An antiserum absorbed in this way then identifies thymocyte-specific xenoantigens—that is, antigens shared by all members of a given species (in contrast to alloantigens present in only some members of the species).

Table 5.1 Expression of Alloantigens on Cells of the T Lineage in the Mouse

	Relative Concentration of Alloantigens on Cell Surface of			
Antigen	Thymocyte Progenitors	Cortical Thymocytes	Medullary Thymocytes	Peripheral T Cells
H-2[a]	+++[b]	+	++	+++
Tla	−	+++	−	−
Thy-1	−	+++	++	+
Lyt-1	−	+++	++	+
Lyt-2	−	+++	++	+

[a] Mouse major histocompatibility complex antigens

[b] Arbitrary units: +++, high concentration; ++, intermediate concentration; +, low concentration; −, undetectable

Enzymes. Terminal deoxynucleotidyl transferase (TdT) is a DNA-polymerizing enzyme that catalyzes the assembly of monodeoxyribonucleotides in the absence of a template. A high concentration of this enzyme has been found in thymocytes of all species thus far tested; other lymphocytes contain only a low level of TdT.

Responses to Lectins. Lectins are proteins or glycoproteins that bind specifically to cell-surface receptors, thereby agglutinating or activating the cell. Lymphocytes belonging to the T lineage respond to certain lectins (e.g., concanavalin A, or ConA, and phytohemagglutinin, or PHA) more readily than do lymphocytes of the B lineage. The reason for the difference in the T- and B-cell response to ConA and PHA is not known. (Both T and B cells have the same number of ConA and PHA receptors, so that the simplest explanation for the difference—lack of receptors—does not apply.) For additional information on lectins see Chapter 10.

Response to Hormones. When one injects into mice hydrocortisone (steroid hormone produced by the cortex of the adrenal gland), one observes a selective depletion of thymic lymphocytes: the majority of the thymocytes are lysed by the hormone, while a minority remain viable. Cortisone-resistant and cortisone-sensitive thymocyte subpopulations also exist in the rat, rabbit, and hamster. In these species, corticosteroid hormones in lower doses affect lymphocyte migration, redistribution, and proliferation, in addition to causing cytolysis of thymocytes. Lymphocytes of humans, monkeys, guinea pigs, horses, and domestic fowl are unaffected by corticosteroid hormones. Thymocytes also interact, via specific receptors, with other hormones and other biologically active substances, such as insulin, histamine, β-catecholamines, and prostaglandins.

Radiosensitivity. Lymphocytes in general are much more sensitive to ionizing radiation (X- or γ-rays) than are most other nondividing somatic cells. Thus, when one X-irradiates a whole animal, using a dose of several hundred rads, most lymphocytes are killed, while other somatic cells survive. (To kill fibroblasts, nerve cells, macrophages, or muscle cells, a dose of several thousand rads is required.) The reason for this extreme radiosensitivity of lymphocytes is not known. Since certain lymphocytes are more radiosensitive than others, this property can be used to distinguish lymphocyte subpopulations. (For further details concerning the effect of ionizing radiation on the immune system, see Chapter 12.)

Receptor for Sheep Erythrocytes. When one mixes human thymocytes with sheep red blood cells, one observes, after prolonged incubation at 4°C, aggregation of the erythrocytes around individual thymocytes. Since the groups consisting of one thymocyte surrounded by multiple erythrocytes resemble small roses, they are referred to as erythrocyte rosettes (E-rosettes, for short; see Fig. 5.18; see also Fig. 5.26*a*). The grouping of cells into a rosette results from an interaction between specific receptors on thymocytes and certain surface molecules on sheep red blood cells. Receptors for sheep erythrocytes are present on thymocytes of humans and other primates; they are absent on thymocytes of the mouse and of many other species.

In addition to the markers listed above, subpopulations of thymocytes can also be distinguished on the basis of cell size, buoyant density, and electric charge (mobility in an electric field).

Heterogeneity of Thymic Lymphocytes. Thymocytes of an adult mouse can be divided into two major subpopulations—cortical and medullary (Table 5.2)—and one minor subpopulation.

Cortical thymocytes are small cells, located, as the name implies, in the thymus cortex and characterized by the presence of TdT in their cytoplasm and membranes. They have a high Thy-1 and Lyt content and a relatively low class I MHC antigen content, and they are highly sensitive to cortisone and irradiation.

Medullary thymocytes differ from cortical ones in that they are medium-sized cells, located primarily in the medulla, and in that they lack TdT and Tla, have a low Thy-1 and Lyt content but a high class I MHC

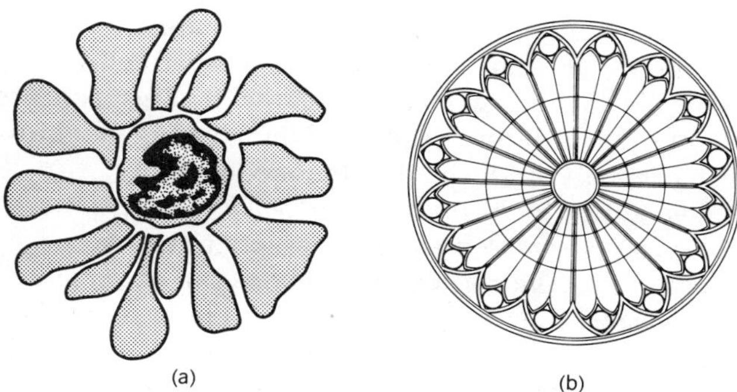

Figure 5.18. Two kinds of rosette. (*a*) E-rosette seen under electron microscope and consisting of a human T lymphocyte in the center surrounded by sheep red blood cells. (*b*) Rose window of a Gothic cathedral (Strasbourg).

Table 5.2 Distinguishing Properties of Cortical and Medullary Thymocytes

Property	Cortical Thymocytes	Medullary Thymocytes
Physical and metabolic properties		
Buoyant density	high	low
Cell size	small	medium
Mitotic index	high	low
Terminal deoxynucleotidyl transferase	+	−
Electrophoretic mobility	low	high
Alloantigens		
Tla antigens in the mouse	+	−
Thy-1, Lyt-1, and Lyt-2 antigens in the mouse	high	low
Class I major histocompatibility antigens	low	high
Xenoantigens		
Rat masked thymocyte antigen	−	+
Rat bone marrow lymphocyte antigen	+	−
Functional properties[a]		
Sensitivity to cortisone and irradiation	high	low
Responsiveness to phytohemagglutinin	−	+
Responsiveness to concanavalin A	weak	strong
Ability to recirculate from blood to lymph	−	+
Cytotoxic cells in cell-mediated immunological reactions	?	+
Helper cells in antibody responses to thymus-dependent antigens	−	+

Source. Modified from I. Goldschneider and R. W. Barton, *in* G. Poste and G. L. Nicolson (Eds.): *The Cell Surface in Animal Embryogenesis and Development*. Pp. 599–695, Elsevier/North-Holland, Amsterdam, 1976.
[a] To be discussed in later chapters

antigen content, and are relatively resistant to cortisone and irradiation.

Lymphocytes in the *minor subpopulation*, constituting only from 5 to 10 percent of all thymocytes, resemble mature T cells. However, it is certain that they are not immigrants from the outside because they carry thymocyte antigens not found on mature T cells. They are cells that have matured in the thymus and are about to leave it for peripheral lymphoid organs. Most of these cells are located in the medulla.

In addition to the *macroheterogeneity* just described, one also finds *microheterogeneity* within the two major populations. The cortical thymocytes can be separated into at least four subpopulations on the basis of their buoyant density, size, antigenic markers, and mitotic activity. Similarly, one can distinguish several subpopulations of medullary thymocytes on the basis of their participation in various forms of cellular immunity.

Ontogenetic Relationships among Thymic Lymphocytes. It should be clear from the preceding discussion that the thymus contains a great variety of lymphocytes, only some of which have been identified; many more thymocyte subpopulations will probably be identified when additional markers become available. However, identification of individual cell types is only the first step in attempting to comprehend what goes on in the thymus. The next step is to find out how these cells relate to each other. Is there more than one pathway of thymocyte differentiation? If so, do the different pathways all derive from a common progenitor cell? How many differentiation steps constitute each pathway? What are the intermediate forms of the different lineages? What role does the thymus anatomy play in differentiation? These are some of the questions that future immunologists will have to answer to understand thymus function in lymphocyte differentiation. As things stand now, we do not even know with certainty how the cortical and medullary thymocyte subpopulations relate to each other. Until recently, the most popular view was that cortical thymocytes were precursors of medullary thymocytes, and that differentiation proceeded in an orderly fashion from the cortex toward the medulla, from cells expressing Tla and a high content of Thy-1 and Lyt toward cells that had lost Tla, reduced their Thy-1 and Lyt contents, and were ready to leave the thymus. But this view is almost certainly wrong, since immunologists now know that both medullary and cortical thymocytes can leave the thymus. Three alternative views of the relationship between cortical and medullary thymocytes are depicted in Figure 5.19. Which of these is the correct one, nobody seems to know.

The Role of Epithelial Cells in Thymocyte Differentiation. Epithelial cells play a much more active role in thymocyte differentiation than just providing a scaffold to keep these cells in place. The absence of mature T cells in *nu*/*nu* mice and in children with DiGeorge syndrome indicates that lymphocyte precursor cells cannot differentiate without epithelial cells. The observation that a thymic rudiment explanted from an embryo before the arrival of lymphocyte precursors degenerates in tissue culture suggests that the epithelial cells cannot exist without lymphocytes. So there appears to be a functional interrelationship between the two principal elements of the thymus in that one cannot function without the other.

Epithelial cells play a double role in thymocyte differentiation: they secrete humoral factors (thymic hormones) necessary for the initiation and maintenance of differentiation, and they interact directly with thymocytes through cell-to-cell contacts and thereby influence their antigen specificity (see below). Membrane contacts between the cytoplasmic processes of epithelial cells and thymocytes have been documented by electron microscopists, and epithelial cells have been seen engulfing and releasing thymocytes, presumably as part of the interaction process between the two cell types.

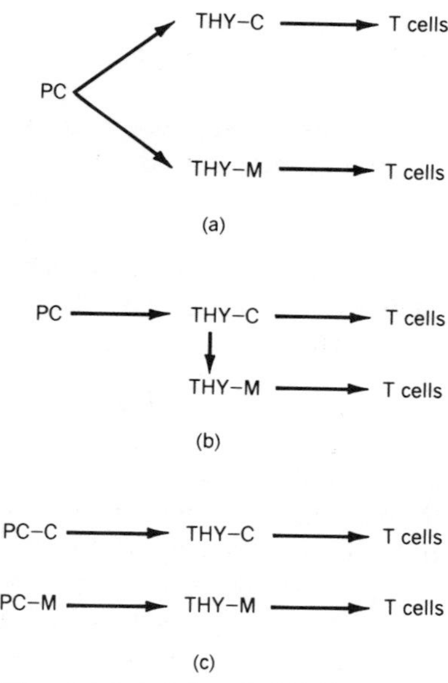

Figure 5.19. Three views of the relationship between cortical and medullary thymocytes. (*a*) The same progenitor cells move into either the cortex or medulla and differentiate independently into T cells. (*b*) Progenitor cells move into the cortex and some mature there into T cells; others move from the cortex and complete maturation in the medulla. (*c*) There are two kinds of progenitor cell, one for cortical thymocytes and another for medullary thymocytes. PC, progenitor cell; PC-C, progenitor cell of a cortical thymocyte; PC-M, progenitor cell of a medullary thymocyte; THY-C, cortical thymocyte; THY-M, medullary thymocyte. [Modified from I. Goldschneider and R. W. Barton: Development and differentiation of lymphocytes. *In* G. Poste and G. L. Nicolson (Eds.): *The Cell Surface in Animal Embryogenesis and Development*, pp. 599–695, North-Holland, Amsterdam, 1976.]

The Role of Thymic Hormones in Thymocyte Differentiation. Removal of the thymus at birth results, as we already know, in a severe reduction of the animal's immune potential. This defect can be corrected by placing a thymus from another animal in the kidney or in some other site of the thymectomized host. The immune potential is restored even when the thymus graft is enclosed in a *diffusion chamber*, consisting of a ring covered on both sides by semipermeable membranes (Fig. 5.20). The pores in the membranes are such that they allow molecules, but not cells, to pass through. Since the thymus graft in the chamber can neither receive nor send out cells, it must exercise its influence on thymocyte differentiation via soluble factors—

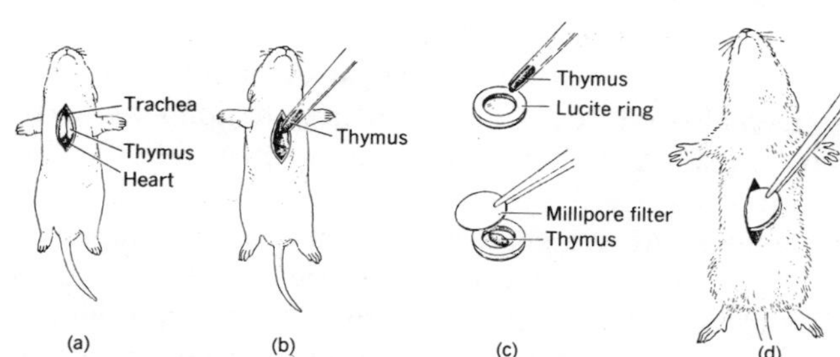

Figure 5.20. Grafting of thymus in diffusion chamber. Incision in the thorax of a newborn mouse exposes the thymus (*a*). The thymus is removed (*b*) and placed into a diffusion chamber consisting of a plastic ring and two millipore filters (*c*). Closed chamber with thymus is inserted into the peritoneum of an adult mouse (*d*). [From R. H. Levey, *Sci. Am.* **211** (July):66–77, 1964.]

presumably thymic hormones. This experiment indicates that thymocyte differentiation can occur without direct contact between the differentiating and the epithelial cells. However, it is not known whether T lymphocytes that have differentiated under the sole influence of thymic hormones are functionally completely equivalent to T cells that have had the opportunity of interacting with epithelial cells. There might be subtle but important differences between the two T-cell types—differences not detected by the crude methods of T-cell testing used in these experiments.

Several laboratories have succeeded in isolating from the thymus soluble factors capable of inducing differentiation of progenitor cells in the direction of thymus-derived lymphocytes. At least 12 such factors have been reported, but some of them are probably duplicates. All of these factors, with one exception, are proteins or polypeptides. The one exception is the so-called *thymosterin*, which appears to be a steroid. The two best-characterized thymic factors are thymosin and thymopoietin. *Thymosin*, a protein with a molecular weight of 12,600 daltons, has been isolated from saline extracts of calf thymus. When added to bone marrow cells, it causes their differentiation into cells biochemically and functionally indistinguishable from thymus-derived lymphocytes. *Thymopoietin* is an even smaller protein (molecular weight, 7000 daltons) that produces an effect similar to that of thymosin. Both thymosin and thymopoietin have been detected in the cytoplasm of thymic epithelial cells.

Surprisingly, several nonspecific factors, such as endotoxin or poly A : U (see discussion of adjuvants in Chapter 10), also induce differentiation of thymocyte progenitors. All these factors have one common property—they raise intracellular levels of cyclic AMP. This finding raises the question of how specific the role of thymic hormones is.

The Role of the Major Histocompatibility Complex (MHC) in Thymocyte Differentiation. When a T lymphocyte recognizes an antigen, it does not "see" the antigen alone; it recognizes it in conjunction with MHC molecules. A T lymphocyte thus possesses double specificity—one for the antigen and another for MHC molecules. As we shall discuss further in Chapter 8, MHC molecules occur in many forms, differing in their primary structure and carried by different individuals. A given T lymphocyte, however, recognizes an antigen preferentially in conjunction with one of these forms—that expressed by the epithelial cells of the thymus. As a part of their differentiation, lymphocytes are thought to learn, largely in the thymus, how to recognize the antigen in conjunction with the individual's own (self) MHC molecules. More about this learning process in Chapters 7 and 12.

The Post-Thymic Phase: Unstimulated Lymphocytes

Exit of Cells from the Thymus. Maturing T lymphocytes leave the thymus by way of blood vessels (veins) and lymphatics. To enter the vessels, they slip between cytoplasmic processes of the epithelial-cell mesh, cross the connective tissue spaces surrounding the vessels, and then pass between the endothelial cells of postcapillary venules into the vessels' lumen. Most lymphocytes exit the thymus in the medulla or in the corticomedullary junction. Like the entry of cells into the thymus, the exiting, too, is selective (only cells at a certain differentiation stage can leave) and unidirectional (the emigrating cells cannot return into the thymus).

Two Populations of Emigrating Cells. Two kinds of cell leave the thymus—spleen-seeking T lymphocytes and lymph node-seeking T lymphocytes (Fig. 5.21). *Spleen-seeking lymphocytes* are short-lived, rapidly dividing, cortisone-sensitive cells that home selectively for the red pulp of the spleen; they are presumably derived from cortical thymocytes (Fig. 5.21*b*). Upon reaching splenic sinuses, they exit from the blood into the pulp by passing between the lining endothelial cells. *Lymph node-seeking lymphocytes* are long-lived, cortisone-resistant cells, presumably derived from medullary thymocytes; they home selectively for the paracortex of the lymph nodes and the white pulp of the spleen (Fig. 5.21*c*).

Fate of Thymus Emigrants. The number of cells emigrating each day from the thymus is four times greater than the total number of lymphocytes in the blood. The thymus thus produces more cells than there is room for in the body. The majority of the emigrating lymphocytes apparently die shortly after reaching peripheral lymphoid organs, and only a few cells become long-lived. How does the organism decide which cells should live and which should die? One possibility is that the decision is actually made not by the organism but by an antigen: when the emigrant encounters an antigen for which it carries a receptor, it is stimulated and transformed into a long-lived cell; when it fails to meet the corresponding antigen within a certain period, it dies. According to this hypothesis, most long-lived lymphocytes found in the body are, in fact, memory cells that have already had their first encounter with the antigen. The surviving emigrants then undergo additional changes in their cell-surface properties before they become mature T lymphocytes.

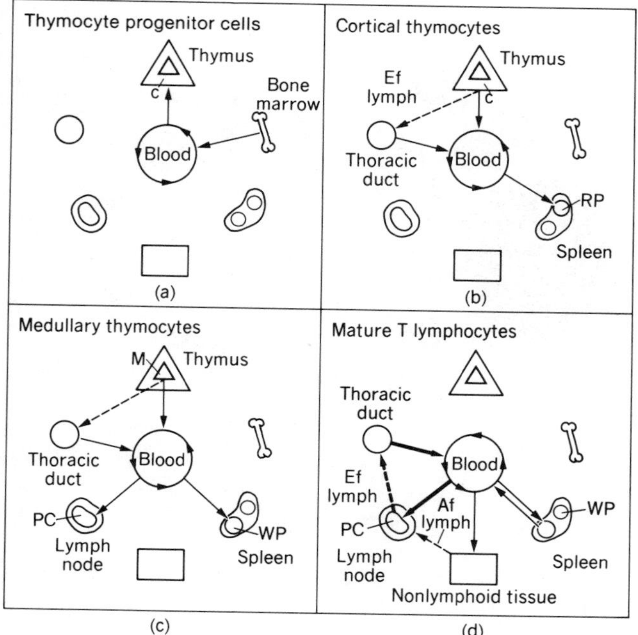

Figure 5.21. The lymphocyte odyssey. (*a*) Migration of progenitor cells from bone marrow via the blood into the thymus. (*b*) Migration of cortical thymocytes via the blood or lymph into the red pulp of the spleen. (*c*) Migration of medullary thymocytes via the blood or lymph into the paracortex of lymph nodes or the white pulp of the spleen. (*d*) Circulation of mature T cells. Af, afferent; C, cortex (of the thymus); Ef, efferent; M, medulla (of the thymus); C, paracortex (of the lymph node); RP, red pulp (of the spleen); WP, white pulp (of the spleen). Solid arrows indicate circulation via blood vessels, broken arrows via lymphatic vessels. Boldface arrows indicate the major pathway of lymphocyte circulation. [Modified from I. Goldschneider and R. W. Barton: Development and differentiation of lymphocytes. *In* G. Poste and G. L. Nicolson (Eds.): *The Cell Surface in Animal Embryogenesis and Development,* pp. 599–695, North-Holland, Amsterdam, 1976.]

Recirculation of Mature T Lymphocytes. Once they have matured, most of the surviving thymus emigrants enter the pool of *recirculating lymphocytes*—a collection of cells that run the same circuit over and over. The circuit, depicted in Figure 5.21*d* and elucidated mainly through the work of James L. Gowans, William L. Ford, and their associates, follows this pattern. Lymphocytes brought into a lymph node by a blood vessel leave the blood by crossing the walls of the postcapillary venule and migrate toward their respective domains—B cells to the lymphoid follicles and T cells to the interfollicular areas and the paracortex. After a short stay in these domains, the lymphocytes begin to migrate again, this time toward the medulla, where they are collected by the medullary sinuses, from which they are collected by the lymph and carried passively via efferent lymphatics into the thoracic duct. When the thoracic duct empties its contents into the great veins, the lymphocyte finds itself once more in the blood, and can then do one of three things: it can travel back into the lymph node and run the same circuit again; be carried by the blood into the white pulp of the spleen and leave the blood there, only to reenter it later (see below); or enter, with the blood, a nonlymphoid tissue, leave the blood, and be collected by afferent lymphatics and brought into the lymph node. Occasionally, the lymphocyte can take up a short residence in the lymph node or spleen before it enters the circuit again. In a normal individual, about half the blood lymphocytes enter lymph nodes; the other half go into the spleen. Only about 3 percent of blood lymphocytes are shunted into nonlymphoid tissues.

The question of how lymphocytes leave the blood in the lymph node is controversial. According to some investigators, lymphocytes are engulfed by specialized endothelial cells that line the postcapillary venules, enclosed in a membrane bag, transported in this bag through the cytoplasm, and released on the other side of the endothelial cell wall into the cortex (Fig. 4.23, inset on the extreme right). But other investigators believe that lymphocytes pass through special junctions between endothelial cells. Whatever the mechanism, the passage is restricted to lymphocytes and is a one-way process. (Migration of lymphocytes from the cortex into the blood vessel has never been observed.) Endothelial cells and lymphocytes must, therefore, somehow recognize each other, probably by cell-to-cell contacts, perhaps via specific receptors on the lymphocyte cell surface. (Treatment of lymphocytes with trypsin and neuraminidase, an enzyme splitting chemical bonds between neuraminic acid and other sugars, inhibits their migration through lymph nodes, as if through the loss of certain cell-surface molecules, the cells also lost their way.) Transport of lymphocytes is the endothelial cell's main function, and when lymphocytes are not around (e.g., after neonatal thymectomy or in athymic mice), the cells degenerate.

In the spleen, lymphocytes leave the blood by crossing the walls of the marginal sinus between the white pulp and the marginal zone, and once outside the sinus, they migrate toward their respective domains—the B cells to the lymphoid follicles and the T cells to the periarteriolar lymphoid sheath. What attracts lymphocytes toward the white pulp is not known; perhaps there is a gradient of some substances in this region of the spleen and lymphocytes just follow this gradient. From the white pulp, both the T and B lymphocytes migrate across the marginal zone toward the red pulp, where they are collected by the venous sinuses and carried away from the spleen by splenic veins. In the spleen, therefore, most of the lymphocytes enter and leave the organ by way of the blood. The entire process of T-lymphocyte migration—from progenitor cells in the bone marrow to the pool of recirculating lymphocytes—is summarized in Figure 5.21 (see also Chapter 4).

Two important techniques have enabled immunologists to elucidate this migration pattern. The first consists of introducing marked cells into an animal and following their fate by looking for the marker in various tissues. One of the best-known markers is a chromosome translocation number six, or *T*6. The marker arose from an exchange of segments between two nonhomologous chromosomes that resulted in two abnormal chromosomes, one of which is considerably shorter than the shortest pair of autosomes and has a marked constriction near the centromere (Fig. 5.22*b*). The chromosome is easily identifiable in dividing somatic cells (Fig. 5.22*a*). Since congenic lines that differ only in the translocation and are otherwise genetically identical and hence tissue-compatible exist, one can transfer cells from marked to unmarked animals without the complications of allograft reaction.

In the second technique, used extensively by James L. Gowans in his lymphocyte-traffic studies, the lymphocyte circuit is interrupted by cutting the thoracic duct, tying one of the loose ends, and inserting a plastic tube into the other end (Fig. 5.23). The process is called *cannulation*, from the Latin *cannula*, a diminutive of reed. In this way, the lymph flowing through the duct can be drained away into a test tube over several weeks. One can also label the drained cells with a radioactive isotope, introduce them back into the duct, and follow their distribution into the various tissues.

Locomotion. Lymphocytes are actively moving cells that can crawl through tissue spaces almost as rapidly as granulocytes. During movement, a lymphocyte assumes a hand-mirror shape, with the protopod portion (containing the nucleus and the centrosome) corresponding to the mirror and the uropod to the handle (Fig. 5.24). In contradistinction to granulocytes, T lymphocytes do not adhere to glass surfaces, do not spread on them, and do not phagocytose.

Life Span. Recirculating lymphocytes are long-lived cells with a life span of several months in small animals (mouse, rat) and several years in larger mammals, such as the human. There are reports in the immunological literature of human lymphocytes surviving for at least 10 years. The reports describe patients who were irradiated with a relatively high dose of X-rays (as a therapeutic measure in cases of cancer or certain spinal diseases). When the blood of these patients was examined 10 years after the irradiation, lymphocytes were found that carried unique chromosomal aberrations that were, in all likelihood, induced by the therapeutic treatment. The aberrations consisted, for exam-

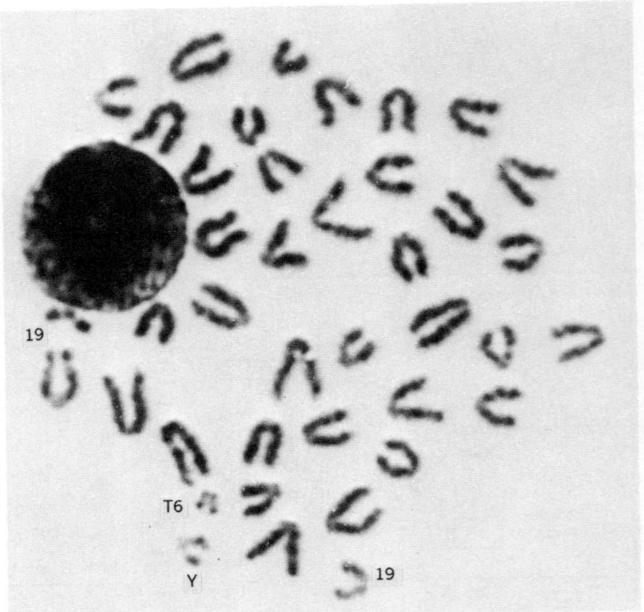

(a)

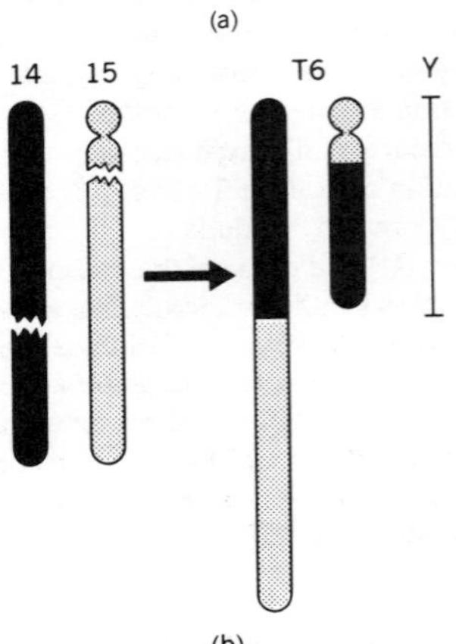

(b)

Figure 5.22. The *T*6 marker. (*a*) Chromosomes of a dividing lymph node cell, obtained from a male *T*6 + mouse. (*b*) Presumed mechanism (translocation) by which the *T*6 chromosome arose from chromosomes 14 and 15. The two chromosomes broke at indicated positions and the centromeric segment of chromosome 14 reunited with the telomeric segment of chromosome 15, and vice versa. The longer translocated chromosome is still shorter than the longest normal mouse chromosome, but the shorter translocated chromosome is shorter than the shortest normal chromosome (19 and Y; relative length of the latter is indicated by the segment) and is thus easily identifiable in mitotic preparations. (*a* courtesy Dr. David E. Harrison.)

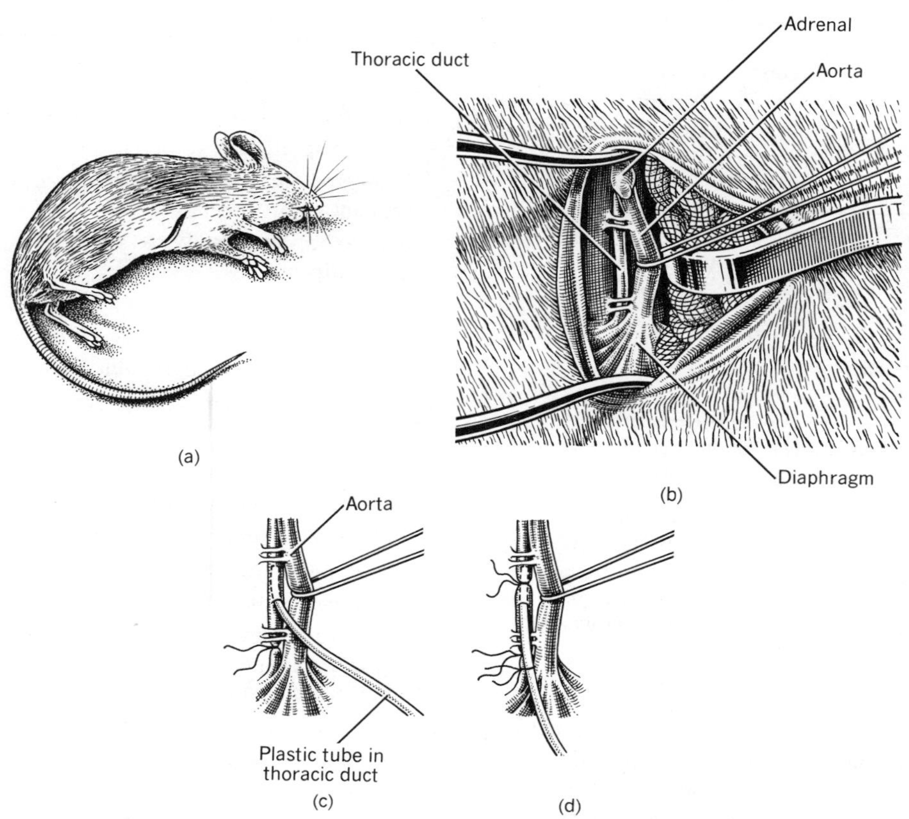

Figure 5.23. Cannulation of the thoracic duct in rats, showing successive phases of the operation. (*a*) A section is made in an anesthetized rat, as indicated. (*b*) The thoracic cavity is opened and the aorta pulled to the side. (*c*) The thoracic duct is tied and cut, and a plastic tube is inserted into it. (*d*) The tube is tied to hold it in place and the wound is closed. (Based on Bolman et al., *J. Lab. Clin. Med.* **33**:1349, 1948.)

ple, of a chromosome joined by its ends into a ring, and a chromosome with two centromeres. A lymphocyte carrying such aberrations cannot divide because the chromosomes cannot separate during mitosis. Cells with this kind of chromosomal aberration cannot, therefore, be the progeny of cells that divided in the postirradiation period; they must be cells that survived the entire period without cell division.

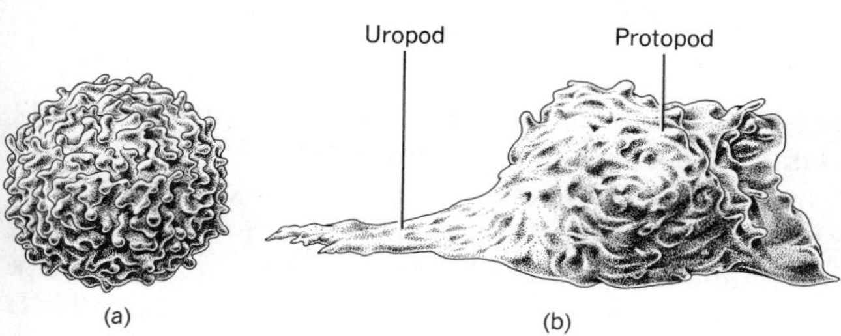

Figure 5.24. A lymphocyte in motion. (*a*) Stationary lymphocyte. (*b*) Moving lymphocyte assuming a hand-mirror shape.

Tissue Distribution. One finds mature T lymphocytes mainly in the thoracic duct and other lymphatics, in the blood, and in peripheral lymphoid organs (Table 5.3). In the last, T lymphocytes concentrate in discrete anatomical locations—the *thymus-dependent areas* (i.e., interfollicular and paracortical regions of lymph nodes, periarteriolar lymphoid sheath of the spleen, and interfollicular areas of Peyer's patches)—which become depleted of cells after thymectomy. Few mature T lymphocytes are present in the bone marrow and in nonlymphoid tissues. The frequency of T lymphocytes in individual organs varies according to the physiological state of an organism and to the species, but the hierarchy of organs in terms of decreasing T-cell numbers is always the same: thoracic duct > lymph nodes > blood > spleen > Peyer's patches.

Morphology. The T lymphocyte is a spherical cell, from 3.5 to 8 μm in diameter, covered with randomly distributed microvilli (see Fig. 5.15). The density of

Table 5.3 Organ Distribution of T and B Lymphocytes

Organ	Percent Lymphocytes	
	T	B
Thymus	>99	<0.5
Lymph node	60–80	20–40
Spleen	40–65	30–40
Blood	60–80	30–40
Thoracic duct lymph	85	10–15
Bone marrow	1–7[a]	40[b]

[a] In the mouse less than 1 percent; in humans up to 7 percent. In the avian bursa of Fabricius virtually all lymphocytes are of the B type.
[b] More than half of bone marrow cells with lymphocyte morphology bear neither T- nor B-cell-specific markers. A small percentage of such negative cells may also occur in other organs, so that the percentage of T and B cells does not always add up to 100.

Table 5.4 Distinguishing Properties of T and B Cells

Properties	T Cells	B Cells
Surface properties		
T cell-specific alloantigens and xenoantigens	+	−
B cell-specific alloantigens and xenoantigens	−	+
Readily detectable immunoglobulin	−	+
Receptor for C3 complement component	−	+
Receptor for immunoglobulin Fc region	−	+
Receptor for sheep erythrocytes	+	−
Negative charge	+	−
Adherence to artificial surfaces	−	+
Retained on antigen-coated columns	−	+
Retained on allogeneic monolayers	+	−
Migration and anatomical distribution		
Germinal centers and lymphoid follicles	−	+
Lymph-node interfollicular cortex and paracortex; spleen periarteriolar sheath; interfollicular areas in Peyer's patches	+	−
Rapid recirculation from blood to lymph	+	−
Functional properties[a]		
Killing of target cells	+	−
Antibody-forming cell precursors	−	+
Regulator cells in antibody- and cell-mediated immunological responses	+	−
Carrier specificity	+	−
Hapten specificity	−	+
Activated or tolerized at lower antigen concentrations	+	−
Proliferative response in mixed-lymphocyte reaction	+	−
Proliferative response to phytohemagglutinin and concanavalin A	+	−
Proliferative response to endotoxin	−	+

Source. Modified from I. Goldschneider and R. W. Barton, *in* G. Poste and G. L. Nicolson (Eds.): *The Cell Surface in Animal Embryogenesis and Development,* pp. 599–695, Elsevier/North-Holland, Amsterdam, 1976.
[a] To be discussed in later chapters

microvilli on the lymphocyte surface varies, depending upon the cell's functional state. Nine-tenths of the cell volume is occupied by a round, slightly indented nucleus (the indentation results from the pressure on the nuclear envelope by the rather rigid centrosome located nearby), filled with dense, heavily staining chromatin (with blocks of heterochromatin adhering to the nuclear envelope). A nucleolus is present but not visible on standard preparations examined by light microscopy. The scanty, often barely visible cytoplasm contains many free ribosomes, and hence assumes, on hematological preparations, a light blue color.

Markers. In the mouse, T lymphocytes are identified by their reactivity with anti-Thy-1 serum; in humans, they are distinguished from other cells by the E-rosetting technique; in the fowl, an antiserum detecting Thy-1-like antigens is also available. In all three species, T lymphocytes can also be identified by xenoantisera absorbed so as to react specifically with T cells, and by functional tests (participation in one of several cellular immunity reactions). Furthermore, the maturation of T lymphocytes is also accompanied by changes in expression of several alloantigens (see Table 5.1). The markers and properties distinguishing T cells from B cells are summarized in Table 5.4.

Heterogeneity. T lymphocytes can be divided into subclasses according to their function and to the cell-surface molecules they express. The functional classification distinguishes three main subclasses of T lymphocyte: helper, suppressor, and cytotoxic lymphocytes. *Helper T lymphocytes* (Th), constituting about one-third of the mature T-cell population, are programmed to amplify the function of other cells (B lymphocytes, other T lymphocytes, or macrophages). To carry out their helper function, they must be stimulated by an antigen in association with a particular class II MHC molecule. Helper T lymphocytes are also activated by class II molecules in mixed lymphocyte culture. Stimulated T-helper cells produce a variety of soluble substances (factors; see Chapter 7).

Cytotoxic T lymphocytes (Tc), also referred to as *killer* or *effector* cells, kill other cells (e.g., other lymphocytes) by changing the permeability of their membranes. To perform the killer function, Tc precursor cells must be stimulated by an antigen in association with class I MHC molecules; allogeneic class I MHC molecules can activate cytotoxic T cells in the absence of other antigenic differences.

Suppressor T lymphocytes (Ts) suppress, directly or via *suppressor factors*, the function of other cells (for example, helper T cells). Precursors of suppressor T cells are activated by antigens in association with a particular type of class II MHC molecule. Like Tc, Ts constitute only a small fraction of the mature T-cell population.

Parenthetically, we should mention an earlier functional classification of T lymphocytes into T_1 and T_2 subclasses. The classification was based on an observation that a mixture of spleen and lymph node lymphocytes gave a higher response in graft-versus-host reactions (a form of cellular immunity described in Chapter 12) than did either of the two cell populations alone. The observation was explained by the assumption of two T-cell populations, T_1 and T_2, acting in a synergistic manner. T_1 cells, present in the spleen and thymus, are rapidly dividing, noncirculating, cortisone-sensitive cells with moderately high concentrations of Thy-1 antigens; they are probably immature T cells of recent thymic origin. T_2 cells, present in lymph nodes, thoracic duct, and blood, are long-lived, recirculating, cortisone-sensitive cells with low concentrations of Thy-1 antigens.

Of the many antigens present in the lymphocyte cell membrane, the most useful for T-cell classification have proved to be antigens of the Lyt series, especially those controlled by the *Lyt-1* and *Lyt-2* loci, described by Edward A. Boyse and his co-workers. Depending on the expression of these two loci, Harvey Cantor and Boyse classified T lymphocytes into three subclasses—Lyt-1^+Lyt-2^-, Lyt-1^-Lyt-2^+, and Lyt-1^+Lyt-2^+. According to the current dogma, most helper T cells are Lyt-1^+Lyt-2^-, most cytotoxic and suppressor cells are Lyt-1^-Lyt-2^+, and not fully differentiated T lymphocytes are Lyt-1^+Lyt-2^+ (and correspond to the T_1 cells of the earlier classification). This classification is almost certainly an oversimplification of the true situation since cases have been described that do not fit in. We shall have more to say about it in Chapter 12. The ontogenic relationship of the T-lymphocyte subclasses is uncertain. There is some evidence indicating that Lyt-1^+Lyt-2^+ cells are precursors of both the Lyt-1^+Lyt-2^- and the Lyt-1^-Lyt-2^+ cells, but an alternative possibility—that the three cell types develop as separate lineages—has not been completely ruled out.

Another level of T-lymphocyte heterogeneity also exists. As we shall discuss in Chapter 7, T lymphocytes possess receptors with which they recognize antigens, and different groups of T cells possess receptors for different antigens. Hence, the T-cell pool consists of thousands of lymphocyte species, each displaying receptors of different binding specificity.

Function of T Lymphocytes. The two main functions of T lymphocytes are destruction of self cells which—for whatever reason—have altered their surface characteristics to the extent that they are thenceforth recognized as nonself, and regulation of immune reactions by their enhancement or suppression. T cells carry out these functions either directly, by cell-to-cell contact, or indirectly, through substances (factors) they secrete. The secreted factors can act on different cells—macrophages, neutrophils, basophils, eosinophils, B cells, and other T cells—and effect different kinds of function (recruitment of granulocytes and macrophages, keeping granulocytes at the reaction site, enhancement of granulocyte function, production of tissue damage, and inhibition or enhancement of T-cell and B-cell activities). These factors are described in Chapter 7; T-lymphocyte functions will be dealt with in Chapter 12.

The Post-Thymic Phase: Stimulated Lymphocytes

An unstimulated lymphocyte leads a rather monotonous life: it breathes, nourishes itself, moves around a bit, and makes its rounds over the same circuit. All this *dolce far niente* (sweet doing-nothing) changes dramatically when the lymphocyte encounters an antigen or becomes stimulated in some other way. Then it enters into an active phase characterized by lymphocyte transformation and proliferation. In the *transformation phase*, the lymphocyte synthesizes DNA, RNA, and proteins, and enlarges into a *transformed lymphocyte* (a *blast cell*), a large cell, 20 to 30 μm in diameter, with abundant basophilic cytoplasm and a nucleus containing finely reticulated chromatin and several nucleoli (see Fig. 5.16). In the *proliferative phase*, the large transformed lymphocyte divides repeatedly, but with each division the progeny become progressively smaller so that at the end the cells become small lymphocytes again.

The encounter with an antigen also changes the lymphocyte migration pattern. When the encounter takes place in the nonlymphoid tissue, the lymphocyte heads for the nearest (regional) lymph node, settles down there, and begins to transform. The progeny of the activated lymphocyte may migrate to more centrally located lymph nodes and proliferate in them. The small lymphocytes derived from the activated cells then enter the circulation again. When the encounter takes place in the blood, the lymphocyte usually settles and proliferates in the spleen. From there the lymphocyte progeny may migrate into the gut and localize primarily in the Peyer's patches. Therefore, the encounter with the antigen removes, for a short time, all cells capable of recognizing this antigen from the circulation. The removal is so effective that for this period the remaining circulating cells are unresponsive to the particular antigen (apparently because there are no more specifically reactive cells left in circulation). The mechanism responsible for the accumulation of activated lymphocytes in peripheral lymphoid organs is not known. One possibility is that the binding of an antigen changes the lymphocyte plasma membrane and because of this alteration, the lymphocyte is then not allowed to pass through the organ. In addition to the specific recruitment after the antigen encounter, there is also a certain nonspecific removal of cells from circulation. Apparently, the stimulated lymphocytes release substances that attract (trap) other lymphocytes in the peripheral lymphoid organs. The trapped lymphocytes help to amplify the immune reaction nonspecifically.

5.6 THE B-LYMPHOCYTIC LINEAGE

The main characteristic of cells belonging to the B-lymphocytic lineage is their preoccupation with immunoglobulin (Ig) synthesis. The synthesized Ig molecules may remain in the cytoplasm (cytoplasmic or cIg), may be incorporated into the plasma membrane (surface or sIg), or may be secreted into bodily fluids as antibodies. There are five immunoglobulin classes, referred to as IgM, IgG, IgA, IgE, and IgD. (The origin and meaning of these designations are explained in Chapter 6.) The form of Ig (cytoplasmic, surface, or secreted) and the Ig class are important markers in delineating different stages in the B-lymphocyte differentiation pathway. These stages can be studied most easily during embryogenesis, when the differentiation is synchronized in the sense that relatively large numbers of cells pass simultaneously through the same stage. In an adult organism the synchrony is lost, so that cells in different differentiation stages are present at any one time.

5.6.1 Models of B-Lymphocyte Differentiation

Ontogenetic studies by Max D. Cooper, Fritz Melchers, Benvenuto Pernis, and others have revealed the existence of at least five different cells in the B-lymphocyte differentiation pathway—pre-B cell, virgin B cell, mature B cell, memory cell, and effector cell.

The earliest cell identifiable as belonging to the B-lymphocyte lineage is the *pre-B cell*, characterized by the presence of cIgM and lack of sIg. Morphologically, pre-B cells resemble large or small lymphocytes. *Virgin (immature) B cells* differ from pre-B cells in that they express not only cytoplasmic but also surface IgM. Functionally, virgin B cells are characterized by their high susceptibility to tolerance induction (to becoming immunologically unresponsive). By exposing these cells to anti-IgM serum, one can block IgM expression irreversibly on their cell surfaces. *Mature (activated, committed) B cells* are cells that are set on a course leading eventually to the secretion of a particular Ig class. The sign of this commitment is the expression of this Ig class in the cell membrane. Cells committed to IgM synthesis express only sIgM; cells committed to IgG express sIgM and sIgG; cells committed to IgA express sIgM and sIgA; and cells committed to IgE presumably express IgM and IgE. Some of the class-committed B cells also express sIgD, so that one finds B lymphocytes with two or three types of receptor: cells committed to IgM synthesis express sIgM and sIgD; cells committed to IgG synthesis express sIgM, sIgG, and sIgD; cells committed to IgA synthesis express sIgM, sIgA, and sIgD; and cells committed to IgE synthesis presumably express sIgM, sIgE, and sIgD. *Memory B cells* are defined functionally by their ability to respond to specific stimuli in an accelerated fashion. The surface characteristics of these cells remain controversial. The *effector cells* are cells that have begun to secrete immunoglobulins and are on the way to becoming *plasma cells*.

The ontogenetic relationships among these major B-cell types are unclear. The differentiation sequence is assumed to be pre-B cell, virgin B cell, mature B cell, and effector cell, with memory cells arising, according to one hypothesis, directly from virgin B cells or, according to another hypothesis, from committed mature B cells (Fig. 5.25). The major unresolved question is which part of the differentiation sequence is antigen-driven and which is antigen-independent. According to one model, antigen is necessary to drive the virgin cells toward mature Ig class-committed cells; according to another model, this commitment arises independently of antigen but antigen is needed in later differentiation steps, particularly those leading to memory cells. The sequence in which different Ig classes are expressed on the maturing cells is thought to be IgM alone, IgM + IgG (IgA or IgE), IgM + IgG (IgA or IgE) + IgD, and IgG (IgM, IgA, or IgE), but this interpretation has not been proved to everyone's satisfaction either. In addition to antigen, the B-cell differentiation pathway is also influenced by regulatory T lymphocytes (see Chapter 13).

5.6.2 B-Cell Development in Embryos

In birds, represented by the domestic fowl, differentiation of B cells takes place in the bursa of Fabricius. As we already know from the previous chapter, the epithelial anlage of the bursa forms during the fourth and fifth day of embryonation. The anlage is seeded by B-progenitor cells (stem cells?) migrating from the yolk sac via the blood stream. Most of the progenitor cells arrive in the bursa sometime between the eleventh and fourteenth day of embryonic life, but according to some investigators, the actual seeding has already begun in seven- to eight-day-old embryos. The large, strongly basophilic progenitor cells enter the bursal epithelium by transitting through the surrounding basement membrane, and settle down in the bursal medulla. Soon afterwards they begin to divide, with a mean generation time of from seven to nine hours. Although progenitor cells probably continue arriving in the bursa over an extended period, they contribute only negligibly to the rapid increase in the cell number of the embryonic bursa; the main reason for this increase is rapid proliferation of the resident cells. At about 12 days of embryonation, the first cells containing cytoplasmic IgM appear; IgG-bearing cells appear at about hatching time, and IgA cells can be detected

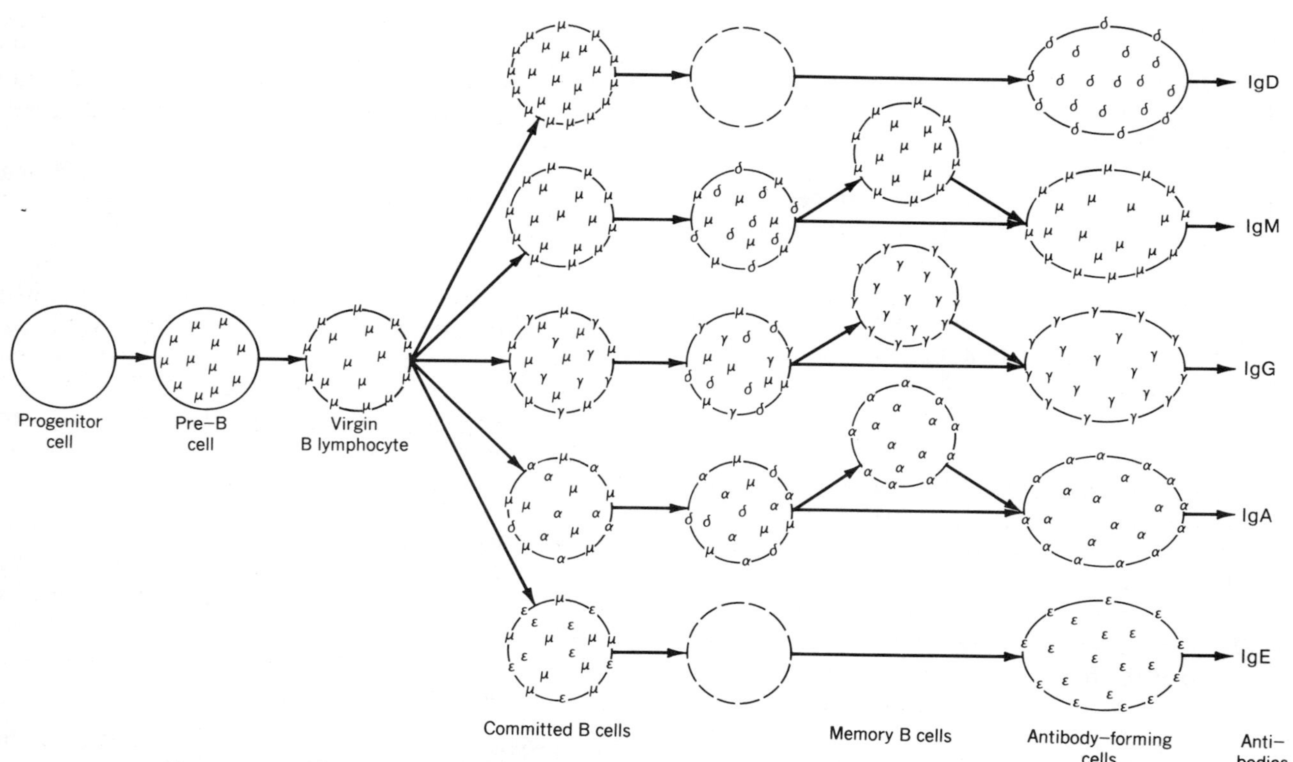

Figure 5.25. Model of B-lymphocyte differentiation. The diagram depicts, in a simplified way, isotype differentiation of a single B-cell clone. In real life many more cells and cell divisions are involved and the γ lineage is further divided into four ($\gamma1$ through $\gamma4$) in this process. The Greek letters indicate Ig isotypes (heavy-chain type), the broken circles uncertainties about the particular B-cell type.

only after hatching. At the time of hatching, lymphocytes also appear in the bursal cortex; whether they are descendants of medullary cells or come from outside the bursa is not clear.

In mammals, exemplified by the mouse, most embryonic B-cell development takes place in the liver. The sequence of events in the fetal liver is this.

Day 11. Entrance of progenitor (stem) cells into fetal liver.

Day 13. $cIgM^{+}sIgM^{-}$ cells appear; they persist in the liver up to birth. They are also found in fetal spleen and adult bone marrow but not in adult spleen or in lymph nodes.

Day 16. Cells bearing membrane IgM appear.

Birth. IgG- and IgA-bearing cells appear.

One to two weeks after birth. IgD-bearing cells appear.

5.6.3 B-Cell Development in Adults

In birds, the bursa of Fabricius continues to function as the B-cell source throughout life, although its activity gradually declines with age. In mammals, the site of B-lymphocyte production is eventually transferred from fetal liver and fetal spleen to fetal and adult bone marrow. In an adult mammal, bone marrow seems to be the only place where B-lymphocyte precursors are processed to the stage where they express Ig molecules on their cell surfaces. The Ig-positive cells are then exported in large numbers (about 10^8 cells per day in a young adult mouse) from the bone marrow to the spleen and lymph nodes. It is not known at what differentiation stage B cells depart from bone marrow; most immunologists believe that the departing cells are still relatively immature and that the completion of the maturation process occurs in the spleen.

5.6.4 Bursa Equivalent in Mammals

The predominant role of the bursa of Fabricius in avian B-cell development and the conspicuous absence of this organ in mammals has launched immunologists on a long search for a mammalian bursa equivalent. Some immunologists even hoped to discover a mysterious new organ, overlooked by the anatomists, that would be a unique place for B-lymphocyte maturation, as the thymus is for T-lymphocyte maturation. In this respect, the search failed, since there is no single organ in the mammalian body that does nothing but produce B lymphocytes. The mammalian bursa equivalent may be located multifocally in various hematopoietic tissues—the fetal liver, fetal spleen, and fetal and adult bone marrow. The most convincing evidence for this contention results from experiments in which explants were made from fetal liver, spleen, and bone marrow at the time when no Ig-bearing cells were present in these organs. When these explants were then grown in vitro, a gradual appearance of Ig-positive cells could be demonstrated.

5.6.5 Characteristics of Mature B Lymphocytes

Morphologically, B cells look the same as T cells. At one time immunologists thought that B lymphocytes were "hairier" (had more microvilli on their surfaces) and T cells were smoother, but it was later found that the number of microvilli depended on the physiological state of the cell, and that when one compared T and B lymphocytes in the same state, there was no morphological difference between them. B and T lymphocytes can, however, be distinguished by various other markers: B lymphocytes lack many of the T-lymphocyte markers and, in addition, possess some of their own. The most important B-lymphocyte markers are discussed below (see also Table 5.4).

Immunoglobulin Receptors. The most characteristic B-lymphocyte markers are immunoglobulin molecules, which are detectable with anti-Ig sera. Although it has been claimed that T lymphocytes express Ig molecules of the same class and specificity as B lymphocytes, most immunologists find that their anti-Ig sera react with B, but not with T lymphocytes. A mature B lymphocyte has been estimated to bear approximately 10^5 Ig molecules on its surface. The class distribution of cell-surface immunoglobulins varies, depending upon the species, age, and physiological condition, but usually sIgM is predominant, followed by sIgG, sIgA, and sIgD. sIgD is the most variable class in terms of cell-surface representation: frequency of sIgD-bearing cells ranges from 50 percent of the total Ig-bearing lymphocytes in umbilical cord blood to 2 percent of the peripheral blood lymphocytes in adults.

Alloantigens. Class II antigens controlled by the major histocompatibility complex (Ia antigens in the mouse, DR antigens in humans) are expressed preferentially on B lymphocytes and a few other cell types; they are either absent or expressed only on a minor subpopulation of T lymphocytes.

Xenoantigens. B lymphocytes of a given animal species share certain cell-surface molecules that are absent on T lymphocytes and are detectable by antisera produced in another species. To make such antisera specific for B lymphocytes, one must absorb them by a cell mixture from which B cells have been removed.

Complement Receptors. Complement is a system of serum proteins (complement components) activated by antigen-antibody complexes in a definite sequence (see Chapter 9). Some of the components (e.g., C3), once they have been activated, bind to receptors on lymphocytes. To detect this binding, one uses an *EAC-rosette assay*, in which sheep erythrocytes (E) are coated with specific xenoantibodies (A) and complement (C), and then mixed with lymphocytes (Fig. 5.26*b*). The bound antibodies activate the complement cascade, the activated C3 components attach to the erythrocyte membrane, and the bound C3 molecules then interact with the complement receptors of the lymphocytes. The result of these interactions is an erythrocyte rosette around each lymphocyte. Complement receptors are present on only a subpopulation of lymphocytes (the so-called *complement receptor-bearing lymphocytes*, or CRL), which largely overlaps with the population of Ig-positive cells; there is, however, a small percentage of Ig-negative and CR-positive cells.

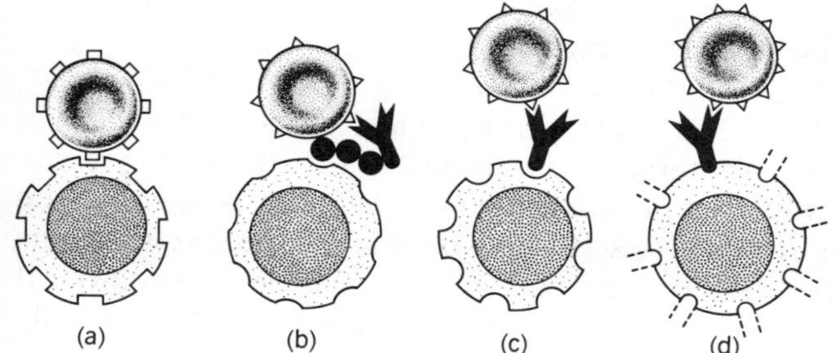

Figure 5.26. Four types of rosette formed between erythrocytes (small cells) and lymphocytes (large cells). (*a*) Spontaneous erythrocyte (SE) rosettes. Human peripheral blood lymphocytes have a receptor for an unidentified structure in the plasma membrane of sheep erythrocytes. (*b*) Erythrocyte-antibody-complement (EAC) rosettes. Sheep erythrocytes injected into rabbits form xenogeneic antibodies that bind to the corresponding red blood cell antigens and the first complement component binds to the antibodies. Additional complement components bind to the first one and, at the same time, attach to the erythrocyte membrane. Erythrocyte-bound complement components are recognized by a receptor in the lymphocyte membrane and thus a bondage between erythrocyte and lymphocyte forms. (*c*) Erythrocyte-antibody (EA) rosettes. Antibodies made against sheep erythrocytes react with the corresponding antigens and the Fc portion of the bound antibody is then recognized by an Fc receptor of a lymphocyte. (*d*) B cell-receptor-erythrocyte rosette. Immunoglobulin receptors in B lymphocyte membrane bind to erythrocyte antigens.

Fc Receptors. The complement-binding region of the Ig molecule (the Fc fragment) also binds to the so-called Fc receptors on certain lymphocytes. The binding of free Ig molecules to Fc receptors is rather inefficient; the efficiency increases, however, following interaction of Ig with an antigen or aggregation of free Ig molecules—after mild heating, for example. The reason for this increase in reactivity is not known; perhaps antigen binding and aggregation better expose the binding site in the Fc region. The binding can be detected in one of three ways. First, erythrocytes can be coated with specific antibodies and mixed with lymphocytes to form *erythrocyte-antibody* (*EA*) *rosettes* (Fig. 5.26*c*). Second, an antigen (for example, bovine serum albumin) can be labeled with a radioactive isotope and reacted with the specific antibody, and the antigen-antibody complexes attached to lymphocytes. Third, the Ig molecules can be labeled with fluorescein, aggregated, and then reacted with lymphocytes. Fc receptors are not particularly good markers of B lymphocytes because there are minor populations of B cells that lack the receptor and of T cells that possess it. Furthermore, Fc receptors are probably a heterogeneous family of molecules, with each molecular species having slightly different properties. The results of a test can therefore vary, depending upon the molecular species one is detecting primarily.

Reactions with Mitogens. B lymphocytes are stimulated specifically by certain substances referred to as *mitogens* (which stimulate cell division or mitosis). The best-known B-cell mitogen is lipopolysaccharide (LPS), isolated from the bacterium *Escherichia coli* (see Chapter 10). However, since LPS does not stimulate human peripheral B lymphocytes, it is not suitable for human studies. Other B-cell mitogens are purified protein derivative (PPD; see Chapter 2), dextran sulfate, and pneumococcal polysaccharide III. B lymphocytes can also be stimulated by the interaction with anti-Ig sera (see Chapter 6).

5.6.6 Tissue Distribution

In an adult organism, B lymphocytes are found in the bone marrow (bursa of Fabricius in birds), blood, peripheral lymphoid organs, and, in small quantities, in the thoracic duct lymph (see Table 5.3); they are absent in the thymus. In the peripheral lymphoid organs, B lymphocytes are concentrated in the follicles of the lymph node cortex, follicles of the splenic white pulp, splenic marginal zone, and follicles of the gut-associated lymphoid tissues. Since these locations remain populated by lymphocytes even after neonatal thymectomy, they are referred to as *thymus-independent areas*. A summary of B and T regions in peripheral lymphoid organs is presented in Table 5.5.

5.6.7 Migration and Life Span

In birds and mammals, the antigen-independent phase of B-lymphocyte differentiation occurs in the bursa of Fabricius and the bone marrow, respectively. From these organs, the virgin B cells move into the thymus-independent areas of the peripheral lymphoid organs—in particular, into the primary follicles. They reside there for a while, and unless stimulated, die. If stimulated (by an antigen, mitogen, or antibody), they differentiate further in one of two ways: either they convert into antibody-secreting plasma cells, or they enlarge into blasts, divide, and then transform back into small lymphocytes, in a process resembling T-lymphocyte transformation. The cells produced by the latter differentiation pathway are termed *memory B lymphocytes*, since they are believed to possess the capacity of an accelerated response on a second encounter with an antigen. The ontogenetic relationship between the plasma-cell and memory-cell differentiation pathway is not known: the two cells may be derived from the same virgin cell (the more likely alternative), or they may originate from different virgin cells (less likely). Depending on the site of residence of the original virgin cells, the differentiating plasma cells move into a medulla of a lymph node, red pulp of the spleen, or the submucosa and lamina propria of the gastrointestinal and respiratory tracts. The memory cells accumulate in the central portion of the lymphoid follicle, form the germinal center, and thus transform this follicle into a secondary one. (In animals maintained artificially in incubators under germ-free and, therefore, also antigen-free conditions, germinal centers and secondary follicles do not develop.) After a short residence in the germinal center, the memory cells exit from the lymph node (spleen or the GALT) through the mantle of the secondary follicle and enter the migratory circuit. Those exiting from the lymph node are picked up by the lymph and carried by efferent lymphatics into the thoracic duct and from there into the blood circulation. Memory cells exiting from the spleen join the blood directly, and then are carried back into lymph nodes and spleen, or into nonlymphoid tissues, from which they are collected by afferent lymphatics (Fig. 5.27). The migration of memory B lymphocytes is thought to be slower and their life span shorter than those of T cells.

Table 5.5 Distribution of T and B Lymphocytes in Various Regions of Peripheral Lymphoid Organs

Organ	Region	T Cells	B Cells
Lymph node	Follicles of the cortex	−	+
	Interfollicular cortex	+	−
	Paracortex	+	−
	Medulla	±[a]	+
Spleen	Follicles of the white pulp	−	+
	Periarteriolar lymphoid sheath	+	−
	Marginal zone	±[a]	+
	Red pulp	±[a]	+
Gut-associated lymphoid tissue	Follicles	−	+
	Interfollicular areas	+	−

[a] These areas are dominated by B cells and their progeny (plasma cells), but T cells also pass through them on their way to other locations in the body.

5.6.8 Heterogeneity and Function of B Lymphocytes

Several types of B cell can be distinguished, based on the type of Ig molecules they carry: $cIgM^+sIgM^-$ (pre-B cells), $cIgM^+sIgM^+$ (virgin B cells), $sIgM^+sIgG^+$, $sIgM^+sIgA^+$, $sIgM^+sIgD^+$, $sIgM^+sIgG^+sIgD^+$, $sIgM^+sIgA^+sIgD^+$, $sIgG^+$, and $sIgA^+$. Using functional criteria, one can distinguish those B lymphocytes that do from others that do not cooperate with T lymphocytes (B_1 and B_2 cells, respectively), virgin B lymphocytes of primary follicles, memory B cells of germinal centers, and plasma cells. The only known function of B lymphocytes is to produce immunoglobulins.

5.6.9 The Plasma-Cell Differentiation Pathway

The B lymphocyte differentiates into a *plasmablast* and then into a *plasma cell* by enlarging itself and developing its rough endoplasmic reticulum, ribosomes, and Golgi apparatus. The mature Ig-secreting plasma cell is an oval cell (diameter along the longer axis between 12 and 20 μm), characterized by the following features (Fig. 5.28): oval, eccentrically located nucleus, oriented with its longer axis at a right angle to the longer axis of the cell; heterochromatin arranged into evenly distributed chunks that adhere to the nuclear envelope and give the nucleus a cartwheel appearance;

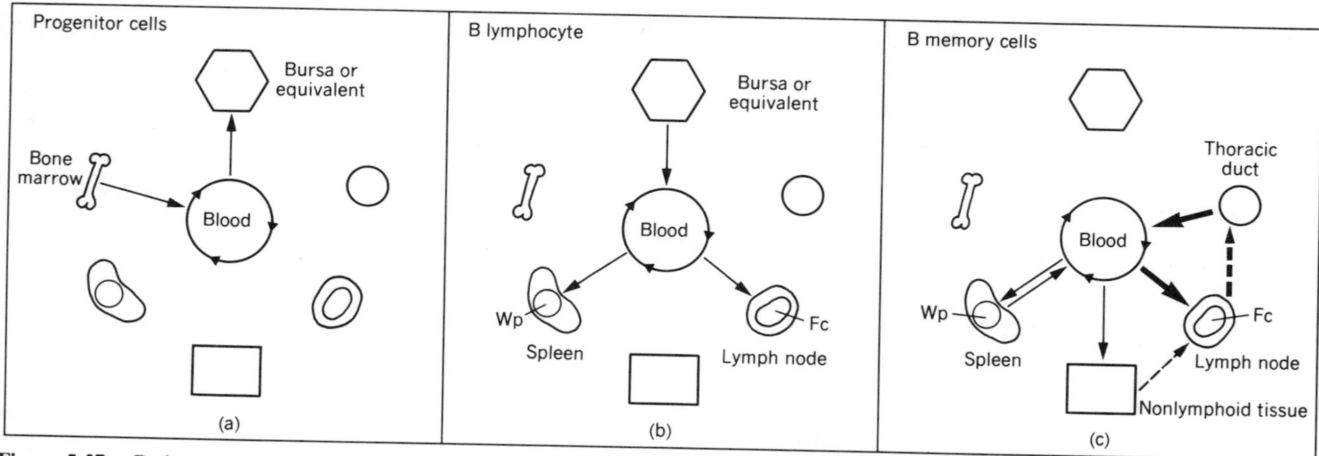

Figure 5.27. Pathways of B lymphocyte migration. (*a*) Migration of progenitor cells from bone marrow via the blood into the bursa of Fabricius or its equivalent. (*b*) Migration of maturing B lymphocytes from the bursa of Fabricius (or its equivalent) via the blood to follicles of lymph nodes and white pulp of the spleen. (*c*) Circulation of memory B cells. Af, afferent; Ef, efferent; Fc, follicular cortex; Wp, white pulp. Solid arrows indicate circulation via blood vessels, broken arrows via lymphatic vessels; boldface arrows indicate the major pathway of lymphocyte circulation. [Modified from I. Goldschneider and R. W. Barton: Development and differentiation of lymphocytes. *In* G. Poste and G. L. Nicolson (Eds.): *The Cell Surface in Animal Embryogenesis and Development*, pp. 599–695, North-Holland, Amsterdam, 1976.]

well-developed centrosome, visible on stained preparations as a colorless area near the cytoplasm (the nucleus is eccentrically located because the rigid centrosome pushes it to the side); and intensely basophilic cytoplasm, rich in rough endoplasmic reticulum and ribosomes. Mouse plasma cells carry a characteristic antigenic marker controlled by the plasma-cell antigen-1 (*Pca*-1) locus.

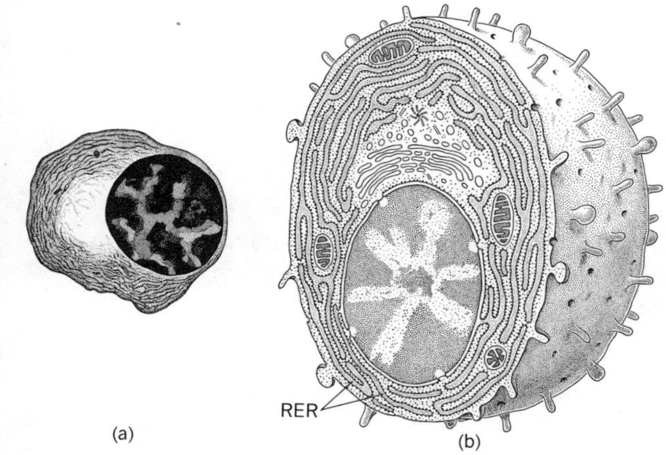

Figure 5.28. Blood cell gallery: plasma cell, as seen with a light (*a*) and electron (*b*) microscope. RER, rough endoplasmic reticulum. (*a* modified from M. Bessis: *Blood Smears Reinterpreted*. Springer International, Berlin, 1977; *b* modified from R. V. Krstić: *Die Gewebe des Menschen und der Säugetiere*. Springer-Verlag, Berlin, 1978.)

Plasma cells have a wide tissue distribution, being particularly abundant in lymphoid tissues (lymph node medulla, splenic red pulp, bone marrow) and in those connective tissues that tend to be exposed to foreign material (for example, the skin and the connective tissue beneath the absorptive epithelium of the intestine). Plasma cells live for a few weeks—secreting antibodies intensively the whole time—and then die.

5.6.10 Methods of Separating T and B Lymphocytes

To determine T- and B-lymphocyte function, immunologists often work with cell suspensions, or even whole animals, containing only one of the two cell types. The fanciest method of cell separation is based on the use of the *fluorescence-activated cell sorter* (FACS) developed by Leonard H. and Leonore H. Herzenberg and their colleagues. In this apparatus, droplets are generated by ultrasonic vibration in a small nozzle in such a way that each droplet contains a single cell tagged with a fluorescent label. As the droplets pass one by one through a laser beam, each cell is "interrogated" about the intensity, color, and polarization of its fluorescence. The characteristic signals from individual cells are then analyzed to determine whether the cell meets certain preselected criteria. If it does, the droplet containing the cell is electrically charged and then deflected and separated from the main stream as it passes through an electric field. By attaching appropriate fluorescent antibodies to either T or B cells, one can separate one or the other cell population from a cell suspension.

Most other methods of T- and B-cell separation are based on selective removal of one or the other lymphocyte type. Some of the methods of selective T- and B-cell depletion are described below.

Selective Depletion of T Lymphocytes

In Vivo. Animals having greatly reduced numbers of T lymphocytes can be obtained by exploiting one of the following experimental situations.

Congenitally Athymic Animals. As was discussed in Chapter 4, *nu/nu* mice fail to develop the epithelial thymus anlage and so fail to provide conditions for T-lymphocyte differentiation. However, they do possess immature T cells, which can differentiate partially under the influence of certain nonspecific factors.

Neonatal Thymectomy. This procedure removes the T-lymphocyte differentiation site at a time when most of the T cells are normally produced. However, at birth, some long-lived T lymphocytes are already present in the circulation, and these are, of course, not affected by the operation.

Adult Thymectomy. Removal of the adult thymus alone, without additional measures, has little effect since, shortly after birth, many T-lymphocyte progenitors have already differentiated into mature cells. To remove the latter cells, one must combine thymectomy with a lethal dose of total body X- or γ-irradiation. However, the ionizing radiation kills not only lymphocytes but other hematopoietic cells and stem cells as well. To keep the irradiated animals alive, one must, therefore, provide stem cells that will regenerate the recipients' hematopoietic tissues. The source of stem cells can be adult bone marrow or fetal liver, from which all mature T lymphocytes have been removed. The removal can be accomplished by using one of the in vitro methods described below (usually anti-Thy-1 + complement treatment).

Treatment with Antilymphocyte serum (ALS). This xenoantiserum, produced by immunization of one species (rabbit, horse) with thymocytes or thoracic duct lymphocytes of another species (mouse, human), often reacts preferentially with T lymphocytes. Repeated injection of ALS into animals results in depletion of T lymphocytes in the thymus-dependent areas. The mechanism of the depletion is unknown, but complement does not seem to play a major role in it, since the serum acts even in animals deficient in certain complement components. ALS treatment is a rather crude method of T-lymphocyte depletion that is neither completely specific nor completely effective. Using this procedure, one achieves only a transient T-cell depletion, at most.

Thoracic Duct Cannulation. Continuous draining of lymphocytes from the thoracic duct depletes primarily T cells, but this depletion, too, is usually incomplete and only temporary.

In Vitro. To remove T cells from a suspension of lymphoid cells, one incubates the suspension with an anti-T cell serum in the presence of complement. The antibody and complement bind to the cells and the latter kills them. The two reagents commonly used for T-cell depletion are the allogeneic anti-Thy-1 serum and a xenogeneic anti-T serum.

Selective Depletion of B Lymphocytes

In Vivo. To deplete animals of B lymphocytes is more difficult than to deplete them of T cells. The two procedures available are bursectomy and treatment with anti-Ig sera.

Bursectomy. In birds, removal of the bursa early in life results in a severe B-lymphocyte depletion. Bursectomized chickens are therefore essentially T-birds—that is, birds possessing only T lymphocytes.

Treatment with Anti-IgM Sera. Repeated injection of relatively large quantities of anti-IgM sera into embryos or newborn animals inhibits the development and maturation of B cells. This technique is applicable to both birds and mammals.

In Vitro. The removal of B lymphocytes from a population of lymphoid cells can be accomplished in one of the following ways.

Treatment with Anti-Ig Sera and Complement. Since all B lymphocytes, except the least differentiated ones, carry Ig molecules in their membranes, they can be killed with an anti-Ig serum and complement.

Filtration through Ig Columns. B lymphocytes can also be removed by passing the cell suspension through a column of beads to which anti-Ig molecules have been attached: B lymphocytes are retained by the column (their Ig receptors react with the anti-Ig molecules on the beads), while all other cells pass through it (Fig. 5.29). The retained B cells can then be eluted from the column.

Treatment with Antisera to B Cell-Specific Antigens. Exposure of a lymphoid cell suspension to a xenogeneic antiserum specific for B-cell antigens, in the presence of complement, selectively kills B lymphocytes.

Filtration through Nylon-Wool Column. This technique is based on the finding that B lymphocytes adhere more to nylon wool than do T lymphocytes. So a column packed with nylon wool retains most of the B lymphocytes and allows most of the T lymphocytes to pass through. The separation, however, is not complete, since the column also retains some T lymphocytes, especially the more immature ones.

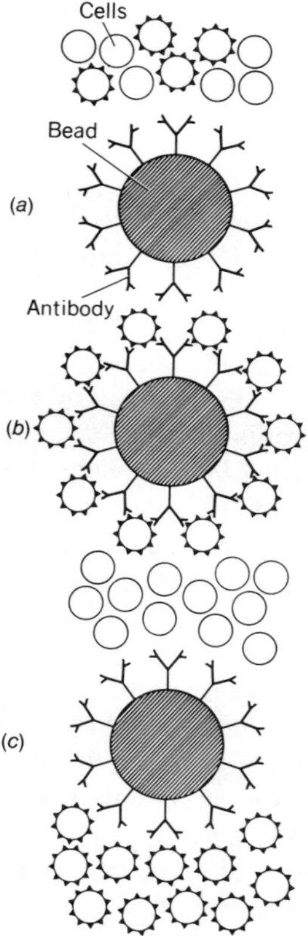

Figure 5.29. Cell separation by filtration through immunoadsorbent (Ig) columns. (*a*) Cells are applied to a column consisting of sepharose beads coated with specific antibody (only one bead shown). (*b*) Cells carrying antigen toward which coating antibody is directed bind via the antibodies to the beads; cells lacking this antigen pass through the column and can be collected. (*c*) By changing pH condition in the column, the antigen-antibody bondages are broken and the bound cells released and collected.

5.7 CELLS OF UNCERTAIN ORIGIN

The cells described thus far are all members of the same family, related by their origin from a common stem cell. The cell types that we are going to discuss now are like orphans, whose family relationships are unknown.

5.7.1 Mast Cells

Origin

Mast cells, or mastocytes (G. *Mast*, fattening material), so much resemble basophils that, for a long time, the former were regarded as tissue-borne, and the latter as blood-borne forms of the same cell. But two observations argue against such a relationship between basophils and mast cells. First, tissue basophils are clearly distinct from mast cells. Second, certain diseases selectively affect basophils but not mast cells, and vice versa.

Other cells considered as precursors of mast cells are reticular cells, fibroblasts, and lymphocytes, but no experimental evidence has ever been provided to document these relationships. The most likely possibility is that mast cells derive as a separate lineage directly from hematopoietic stem cells.

Morphology

The two conspicuous features that mast cells (Fig. 5.30) and basophils (Fig. 5.11) have in common are the heparin- and histamine-containing cytoplasmic granules and the basophilic cytoplasm. Mast cells differ from basophils in that their plasma membrane is less regular and their nucleus rounder, and in that they contain many small granules, while basophils contain a few large granules.

Tissue Distribution and Function

Mast cells are abundant in lymphoid organs (lymph nodes, spleen, and bone marrow), in connective tissues (particularly around blood vessels, nerves, and glands), and in the skin. They are absent in the blood and lymph. Like the basophils, mast cells possess receptors for a specific class of immunoglobulin molecule (IgE); these receptors are the initiators of anaphylactic and allergic reactions (see Chapter 13).

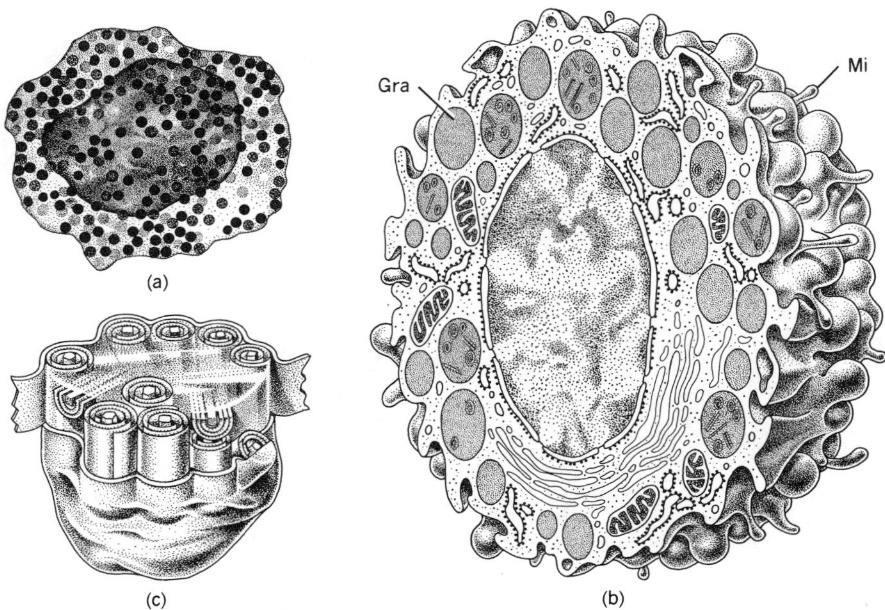

Figure 5.30. Mast cell, as seen with a light (*a*) and electron (*b*) microscope. (*c*) Granule (Gra in *b*). Mi, microvilli. (*a* modified from M. Bessis: *Blood Smears Reinterpreted.* Springer International, Berlin, 1977; *b* and *c* from R. V. Krstić: *Die Gewebe des Menschen und der Säugetiere.* Springer-Verlag, Berlin, 1978.)

5.7.2 Natural Killer Cells

Discovery

Evidence for the existence of natural killer cells came from two lines of research, one concerned with a phenomenon called hybrid resistance and the other dealing with host resistance to tumor cells. In 1958, George D. Snell observed that lymphomas of strain-X origin grew better in strain-X mice than in F_1 hybrids obtained by crossing the X strain with another strain. The poor growth in F_1 hybrids was manifested by a low death rate of the tumor recipients and long periods between inoculation of tumor cells and the appearance of detectable tumors. This *F_1 hybrid effect* went against both the theory and practice of tissue transplantation, since, according to the genetic rules of histocompatibility, an F_1 hybrid should not resist grafts from either of its parents (see Chapter 12 for the derivation of this rule). The effect could not be abrogated by irradiation of the F_1 host prior to transplantation, nor was it influenced by pretreatment of the host with parental cells. A similar effect was later observed by several other investigators with various other tumors and even some normal cells. However, an important condition for demonstrating the effect was the use of a relatively small number of cells for transplantation; when large cell doses were used, the cells seemed to grow equally well in the strain of tumor origin and in the F_1 hybrids.

The most extensive analysis of the hybrid effect was carried out by Gustavo Cudkowicz and his colleagues, who used normal cells instead of tumor cells. Cudkowicz lethally irradiated adult mice and injected them two hours later with 1,000,000 bone marrow cells. Five days after the irradiation, he injected the recipients with 5-fluoro-2′-deoxyuridine (FUdR) and one hour later with 5-idio-2′-deoxyuridine (IUdR) labeled with ^{125}I. The FUdR blocks the incorporation of thymidine into the DNA of DNA-synthesizing cells, and thus assures the incorporation of the labeled IUdR. Seventeen hours after the injection of the isotope, at the time when most of the incorporated isotope is excluded from circulation, the recipient is killed, its spleen is removed, the radioactivity of the whole organ is counted, and the results are expressed as the percentage of injected isotope retained in the spleen. The assay is based on the assumption that some transfused bone marrow cells migrate into the spleen, settle there, and begin to proliferate. The proliferating cells actively synthesize DNA, and this synthesis is measured by incorporation of the radioactive precursor. Cells that fail to proliferate do not incorporate the isotope. Irradiated mice that have not been inoculated with incompatible bone marrow cells show less than 0.1 percent incorporation; irradiated mice that have been inoculated with syngeneic bone marrow cells show between 0.3 and 1 percent incorporation. Using this assay, Cudkowicz and his colleagues demonstrated that strain C57BL/10 bone marrow cells grew poorly in (A × C57BL/10)F_1 hybrids as compared with their growth in syngeneic C57BL/10 or even allogeneic A mice. This *hybrid resistance* is caused by a host antigraft reaction in which the transplanted cells are killed within a few days of grafting. The cells responsible for the graft destruction differ from cells mediating orthodox tissue-transplant rejection in several characteristics: in addition to being able to recognize parental graft cells when they themselves are of F_1 hybrid origin, they are able to kill their target cells without previous exposure to these cells, they appear relatively late in ontogeny, and they retain their activity even after they have been X-irradiated with doses that inactivate other killer cells. In fact, so esoteric was the hybrid resistance phenomenon that, for a while, Cudkowicz had a hard time convincing other immunologists of its existence.

Independently of the studies on hybrid resistance, immunologists became aware of the natural killer cell's existence while investigating the role of T lymphocytes in tumor cell destruction. One of the assays for demonstrating immune T cells directed against tumor cells is the cell-mediated lymphocytotoxicity (CML) reaction, in which cell lysis is determined by the release of ^{51}Cr from the labeled target cells. These investigators frequently observed that a certain amount of the label was released in control experiments in which tumor cells were mixed with nonimmune lymphoid cells, and they attributed this "background" release to nonspecific factors that were beyond the investigator's control. Eventually, however, several immunologists—notably Ronald B. Herberman and his colleagues and Rolf Kiessling and George Klein—realized that lymphoid tissues contained naturally occurring cells capable of attacking tumor cell targets without prior sensitization. These cells clearly differed from T lymphocytes, which kill tumor cells only after previous immunization, and hence represented a new kind of cell, which immunologists began to refer to as *natural killer,* or *NK cells*. Later, when they had characterized these cells, immunologists realized that they were most likely identical with cells responsible for the hybrid resistance phenomenon.

Characteristics

Natural killer cells resemble granulocytes superficially and are probably identical with the so-called *large granular lymphocytes* (LGL) identified by histologists. They are larger than the small lymphocytes and contain a characteristically indented nucleus and azurophilic cytoplasmic granules. They are derived from bone marrow and are probably related to T lymphocytes, possibly representing one of the prethymic stages of the T-lymphocyte differentiation pathway. Their relatedness to T cells is indicated by the presence of a low concentration of Thy-1 molecules on the surface of the natural killer cell. In addition to this marker, mouse natural killer cells are also characterized by the presence of receptors for the Fc portion of IgG molecules; NK1 molecules thought to be specific markers for the natural killer-cell plasma membrane; Qa-4 and Qa-5 molecules, which may also be NK-cell specific; Ly-5 molecules (also known as T200); Ly-10 antigens; and a glycolipid ganglio-N-tetraosylceramide (asialoGM_1, which is a Galβ1 → 3GalNAcβ1 → 4Galβ1 → 4Glcβ1 → 1ceramide). Human NK cells carry low-affinity receptors for sheep erythrocytes. (NK cells rosette sheep erythrocytes at 4°C but not at 29°C, in contrast to T lymphocytes, which rosette erythrocytes at both temperatures.)

NK cells have been isolated from the spleen, lymph nodes, peripheral blood, and peritoneum. They have been demonstrated in primates, rodents, and birds. In mice, they have been detected in all strains, but some strains (e.g., C3H, CBA, and C57L) have considerably higher NK-cell levels than other strains (e.g., A). The cells appear during the third to fourth week of life, peak through the third month, and then decline in number continually with age. In addition to low levels of "endogenous" NK cells, there are also "induced" NK cells, which are produced in large numbers by a variety of viral, cellular, and chemical agents. All these agents have one thing in common: they stimulate the production of interferon, the cellular protein normally interfering with virus multiplication in host cells (see Chapter 14). Whether interferon acts on NK cells directly or indirectly by stimulating other cell types is not known. NK cells can be induced even in irradiated mice, indicating that proliferation is not necessary for their activation. The generation of high levels of antitumor NK activity is controlled genetically, with some of the regulatory genes possibly residing in the major histocompatibility complex. Similarly, the generation of NK cells responsible for hybrid resistance to bone-marrow transplants is controlled by loci that

Cudkowicz designated *Hh* for *hybrid histocompatibility* and mapped in the vicinity of the major histocompatibility complex. NK cells are relatively radioresistant, nonadherent, and nonphagocytic. What target-cell molecules they recognize and the method of recognition are not known. At first immunologists thought that the targets were virus-encoded cell-surface molecules because the NK cells seemed to kill virus-transformed cells exclusively. But there are now too many exceptions to this observation to sustain the validity of the original hypothesis. The strongest argument against the viral-antigen hypothesis is the observation that NK cells also kill bone marrow cells and a few other normal cells. However, for some reason NK cells do have a predilection for tumor cells and tumor-cell lines transformed by a virus. In contrast to T lymphocytes, killing by NK cells does not require matching of major histocompatibility complex molecules of the effector and the target cell (see Chapter 12).

The degree of specificity of NK cells still remains to be clarified. A given population of NK cells can kill a variety of tumor targets, but since it is not known what the cells recognize, this observation does not mean that the NK activity is not specific. Indeed, cloning of NK cells indicates that different clones display a different pattern of lysis and hence at least some degree of specificity. The matter is complicated by the observation that target cells themselves vary considerably in their sensitivity to NK-cell lysis. It is therefore often unclear whether the specificity of a given NK-cell clone reflects a difference in the target cell's ability to respond to NK-cell lytic signals or a failure of the NK cell to recognize the target.

The function of NK cells is not known. Because of their preoccupation with tumor cells and because of their activation by interferon, they are thought to play a role in the body's natural resistance to tumors, but direct evidence for this contention is not available.

5.7.3 K Cells

These cells were discovered by Peter Perlmann and Göran Holm in 1968. These investigators labeled chicken red blood cells with ^{51}Cr, attached an antigen—for example, the purified protein derivative (PPD)—to the erythrocytes, coated the red cells with guinea pig antibodies to PPD, and then mixed them with normal guinea pig lymphocytes obtained from the blood or spleen. The mixing resulted in the lysis of the erythrocytes, as revealed by the release of radioactive chromium. Apparently, normal guinea pigs possess cells in their blood and lymphoid organs that can kill antibody-coated target cells without the participation of complement and without the requirement of a previous exposure to the targets. This killing is referred to as *antibody-dependent cell-mediated cytotoxicity*, or ADCC, and the cells responsible for it are *K cells* (from "killer") or *null cells* (because for a while no markers could be detected on their surfaces). ADCC can also be obtained by coating red blood cells with antibodies to erythrocytic cell-surface antigens and by replacing erythrocytes as target cells with other cells derived, for example, from the liver. K cells resemble natural killer cells and comparative experiments indicate that a single cell can mediate both ADCC and the NK function. Very likely the K-NK system represents a heterogeneous population of cells in which some cells are more inclined to carry out ADCC and others tend toward NK activity. Like NK cells, K cells carry receptors for the Fc fragment of the IgG molecule and it is by means of this receptor that they bind the antibody-coated target cells. The binding occurs only at 37°C and the reaction progresses rapidly by an unknown mechanism with significant lysis occurring as early as the second hour of incubation. The K cells are thought to play a role in antitumor and antigraft immunity.

5.7.4 Dendritic Cells

Nineteenth century histologists made such a thorough job of investigating the mammalian body that it might seem foolish to try to improve on them. Yet, from time to time, investigators still do come across not only some interesting details that their predecessors missed, but even a totally new cell type. One such rare event occurred in 1973 when Ralph M. Steinman and Zanvil A. Cohn placed a suspension of mouse spleen cells into tissue culture and then had a closer look at the cells attached to the glass or plastic surface. When they realized that not all the adherent cells were either macrophages or lymphocytes, they decided to investigate the unidentified third cell type further. This investigation led them to the description of a new cell type, which they called *dendritic cells*, in reference to the morphology of these cells, which is characterized by long, cytoplasmic processes (Gr. *dendron*, tree). The processes, which often contain large, spherical mitochondria, are continually elongating, retracting, and reorienting themselves, leading to a wide variety of cell shapes and a random distribution of the cells over the glass surface. Both the cytoplasm and the large, contorted, refractile nucleus stain weakly with basic dyes. In some respects, the cells resemble the splenic reticular cells; they differ from these, however, in that they do not synthesize collagen. In contrast to macrophages, dendritic cells are incapable of phagocytosis.

Dendritic cells are present in the spleen, where they comprise about 1 percent of the total nucleated cell population, and in smaller numbers in lymph nodes and Peyer's patches. They are absent from bone marrow, thymus, liver, intestine, and the peritoneal cavity (including both resident and exudate cells). In the spleen, they are located in the white pulp follicles.

Dendritic cells lack the following markers—Thy-1, C3 receptors, cell-surface immunoglobulins, and Pc-1—but they carry molecules controlled by both the class I and class II loci of the major histocompatibility complex. They stimulate mixed lymphocyte reactions (see Chapter 12) at least 100 times more strongly than other cell types. Curiously, in tissue culture they also stimulate the proliferation of syngeneic T lymphocytes and often can be seen clustering around T cells. They are bone marrow-derived but no further details of their origin are known. It is thought that they play a role in presenting antigens to T lymphocytes (see Chapter 12).

5.7.5 Langerhans Cells

The German histologist Paul Langerhans discovered two cell types that now bear his name—islet cells of the pancreas and dendritic cells of the skin. Of these two, only the latter will interest us here. Langerhans discovered the dendritic cells in 1868 after staining sections of human skin by the gold chloride method of his teacher, Julius F. Cohnheim. The cells appeared as blackened stellate forms scattered throughout the epidermis and were clearly distinct from keratinocytes and melanocytes, the other two cell types of the stratum germinativum. Cells resembling Langerhans cells occur in the thymus, lymph nodes, and in certain proliferative disorders of histiocytes (e.g., histiocytosis X, malignant histiocytosis, and hairy-cell leukemia), in addition to the upper layers of epidermis. The cells have a clear cytoplasm with characteristic rod- or racquet-shaped granules, highly irregular, convoluted nuclei, and slender, branched processes extending far into the surrounding epithelium. On their surfaces they bear receptors for the C3 complement component and molecules controlled by the class I and class II loci of the major histocompatibility complex; they lack cell-surface immunoglobulin receptors. They are derived from bone marrow and appear to be related to cells of the monocyte-macrophage lineage. Morphologically, they resemble the dendritic cells of Steinman and Cohn but differ from these in their cell-surface markers and distribution. Langerhans cells, like dendritic cells, are capable of inducing antigen-specific and allogeneic T-cell proliferation. They are believed to function in the immune response of the skin by taking up antigens and presenting them to T lymphocytes.

5.8 PHYLOGENY

Table 5.6 summarizes the current knowledge of the distribution of the different blood-cell types among animal phyla and classes. Although this summary gives us certain hints about the blood cells' evolutionary origins, its use for the construction of phyletic trees for these cells is limited by two considerations.

First, cells of the different animal phyla have been identified almost solely on the basis of their morphological (often superficial) resemblance to cells of human blood. For example, the conclusion that eosinophils are present in almost all phyla is based on the detection of acidophilic granules in the cytoplasm of these cells. It is possible, however, that in some vertebrates acidophilic granules may also be present in non-eosinophilic cells and that these cells may resemble true eosinophils only superficially. To draw firm conclusions about evolutionary homologies of cells in different phyla, biologists will have to analyze these cells thoroughly, not only by morphological, but also by biochemical and functional methods. Second, even if all the cells were truly homologous to the corresponding cells in mammals, the possibility would still remain that at least some of the homologies could be the result of evolutionary convergence—that is, of an independent development of the same trait in two phyla. For example, erythrocytes of some annelids look very much like mammalian erythrocytes—to the extent that they too, in the final maturation step, expel their nuclei. Nevertheless, annelid erythrocytes cannot be immediate evolutionary ancestors of vertebrate red blood cells, for the two phyla are not on a direct evolutionary line. To distinguish between true evolutionary relatedness and evolutionary convergence of the individual blood cells, therefore, one must take into account all the knowledge about the origins of the individual phyla. If we apply these two considerations to the data in Table 5.6, not much remains to be said about the table. Perhaps all that the summary suggests is that most blood cells have a long evolutionary history, going back to the most primitive of the *Metazoa*.

Table 5.6 Distribution of Various Blood-Cell Types among Animal Phyla and Classes

Phylum or class	Presence (+) or Absence (−) of Blood Cell								
	Erythro-cytes	Thrombo-cytes	Neutro-phils	Eosino-phils	Baso-phils	Macro-phages	Lympho-cytes[a]	Plasma Cells	Hemo-blasts[b]
Porifera	−	−	·	+	·	−?	+	−	+
Cnidaria	−	−	·	+	·	−?	−?	−	−?
Platyhelminthes	−	−	·	+	·	−?	+	−	+
Annelida	− or +	·[e]	·	+	·	+	+	−	+
Sipunculida	− or +	·	·	+	·	+	+	−	+
Arthropoda	−	·	·	+	+?	+?	+	−	+
Mollusca	−	·	+?	+	·	+	+	−	+
Echinodermata	+	·	+?	+	·	+	+	−	+
Hemichordata	−	−	−	−	−	+	−	−	+
Urochordata	−	−	+	+	+	+	−	−	+
Cephalochordata	−	−	−	−	−	+	−	−	+
Agnatha	+	+	+	+	+	+	+	−	+
Chondrichthyes	+[c]	+	+	+	+	+	+	− or +	+
Chondrostei	+	+	+	+	+	+	+	+	+
Teleostei	+[c]	+	+	+	+	+	+	+	+
Dipnoi	+	+	+	+	+	+	+	+	+
Urodela	+[c]	+	+	+	+	+	+	+	+
Anura	+[c]	+	+	+	+	+	+	+	+
Reptilia	+	+	+	+	+	+	+	+	+
Aves	+	+	+	+	+	+	+	+	−
Mammalia	+[d]	+	+	+	+	+	+	+	−

[a] At some point during evolution, lymphocytes split into T and B cells; when this splitting occurred is not known. The interpretation of lymphocyte evolution is complicated by the fact that thymocytes of less advanced vertebrates (e.g., amphibians) carry easily detectable immunoglobulins on their surfaces, just as B cells do in mammals. One is therefore at a loss as to what criteria to apply for the distinction of T and B lymphocytes in nonmammalian and nonavian vertebrates.

[b] Hemoblasts are large cells resembling large lymphocytes of mammals. Biologists consider them to be pluripotent cells with the capacity to give rise to other cells. In flatworms, for example, they also give rise to germ cells.

[c] Most species have nucleated erythrocytes, but a few have anucleated erythrocytes.

[d] Most species have anucleated erythrocytes, but a few have nucleated erythrocytes.

[e] Unknown.

5.9 GENETIC DEFECTS ARRESTING DIFFERENTIATION OF HEMATOPOIETIC CELLS

The differentiation of stem cells into blood cells is genetically controlled. Like that of other cells, the differentiation of blood cells can be envisioned as a sequential switching on of some genes and turning off of others in an orderly sequence. A mutation at one of these genes can arrest the differentiation at a given stage and thus cause a defect in blood-cell formation. By studying various developmental defects, one can obtain information about the mechanism of differentiation and about the individual steps of the differentiation pathway. The most important hematopoiesis-affecting mutations discovered in the mouse and in humans are described briefly below, arranged according to the affected cell type, with the latter listed in the same order in which we dealt with them in the first part of this chapter.

5.9.1 Defects of Erythrocytic Differentiation

Stem-Cell Defects

Two mutations, both occurring in the mouse, have been particularly helpful in studies of stem-cell behavior. One of these, *W*, is an intrinsic stem-cell mutation, while the other, *Sl*, affects stem-cell behavior indirectly by changing the environment in which stem cells function.

The W Mutation. In 1915, Clarence C. Little discovered a mouse that—instead of being solid grey (agouti), as were most of his mice—had white spots all over its body. Genetic tests revealed that the spotting was controlled by a gene, *W*, which was lethal in a homozygous state: *W/W* mice died in the uterus or shortly after birth; the few surviving animals had solid white coats and black eyes. Later it was discovered that the main cause of death of the *W/W* animals was a subnormal number of erythrocytes in the blood (anemia).

Subsequently, other investigators discovered eight more mutations at the *W* locus, some of which had a less drastic effect than the original *W*. One, in particular (W^v; *v* for viable), permitted the survival of most of the homozygotes, so this mutation, often in combination W/W^v, was frequently used in *W* studies. The W^v homozygotes are usually sterile, since both males and females fail to produce germ cells.

In summary, the *W* mutation affects three traits simultaneously: coat color (absence of pigment-bearing cells, or melanocytes, in the hair follicles), hematopoietic cell differentiation (reduction in the number of erythrocytes), and fertility (absence of germ cells in both males and females). How can a single locus control three such diverse functions? One possible answer to this question is that melanocytes, hematopoietic stem cells, and germ cells all derive from a common mesenchymal cell, and that the genetic lesion at the *W* locus has already occurred in this cell. The problem with this explanation is that since all the blood cells are presumably derived from the same stem cell, they should all be affected by the *W* mutation—and they are not. One must, therefore, argue that the *W* mutation has a quantitative (regulatory) effect and that the degree of the effect is determined by other factors, independent of the *W* locus. According to this interpretation, the erythrocytic lineage of differentiation is simply more susceptible to the effects of the mutation than other hematopoietic lineages.

The Sl Mutation. The *Sl* mutation, too, was discovered originally because of its effect on coat color. The *Sl* homozygotes have black eyes and a white coat, and in the heterozygotes the *Sl* gene dilutes the normal color so that it acquires a steel tinge—hence the symbol. And like *W*, it was later shown to cause anemia and sterility. As in *W*, in the *Sl/Sl* mice, the three effects are caused by the absence of melanocytes, reduction of erythrocyte numbers, and absence of germ cells, respectively. The genetics of *Sl*, too, is quite similar to that of *W*: the *Sl* gene is dominant, there are several mutant alleles at the *Sl* locus (over 30 at the latest count), and the different alleles can be arranged into a series, according to the increasing severity of their effects, with a viable allele (Sl^d; *d* for Dickie, the geneticist who discovered it) at one end of the spectrum. Yet, the *W* and *Sl* are clearly distinct, since *W* is in chromosome 5 and *Sl* is in chromosome 10. The lesions caused by mutations at these two loci are also different, as is demonstrated by grafting experiments. When one transplants Sl^d/Sl bone marrow (stem cells) into W^v/W mice, one cures the anemia of the latter. By the same token, one cures the anemia of the Sl^d/Sl mice by transplanting W^v/W spleen or whole bone into them. These experiments suggest that the reason that many *W/W* stem cells fail to differentiate into erythrocytes lies in the cells themselves, whereas the reason that *Sl/Sl* cells do not differentiate lies in the hematopoietic environment. In other words, in the *W/W* mice, the hematopoietic environment is normal but the stem cells are defective, while in the *Sl/Sl* mice the environment is defective and the stem cells are normal. What, specifically, is wrong with the hematopoietic microenvironment in the *Sl/Sl* animals is not known.

Progenitor Cell Defects

Mutations of genes controlling the differentiation of progenitor cells into erythrocytes may lead to reduction in the number of red blood cells—a condition known as *anemia* (Gr. *an*, negative, *haima*, blood). However, anemia can also be caused by other factors that need not be genetic in nature—for example, sudden blood loss, increased red blood cell destruction, or nutritional deficiencies. Depending on the size of erythrocytes in the afflicted individuals, anemia can be *microcytic* (erythrocytes are smaller than usual), *macrocytic* (erythrocytes are larger than usual), or *normocytic* (erythrocytes are of normal size).

Of the large number of known genetic lesions affecting the erythrocytic lineage, we shall mention only one here—the *f* mutation in the mouse. The *f* gene in a homozygous state causes transient anemia at the stage of fetal liver erythropoiesis. Once the *f/f* embryos pass beyond this stage, the signs of anemia disappear. Apparently, the *f* mutation manifests itself only under conditions of rapid expansion of hematopoietic tissue. The gene is believed to act in erythropoietin-sensitive cells at a stage of erythropoiesis prior to the initiation of hemoglobin synthesis—that is, at the level of the progenitor cells. It may influence the size of the progenitor cell population or the rate at which the progenitor cells can enter the proerythroblast stage. The mutation also causes flexed tail (hence the designation, *f*) and sometimes white belly spots.

5.9.2 Defects of Thrombocytic Differentiation

A mutation in one of the genes controlling thrombocyte differentiation may cause an abnormal decrease in the number of blood platelets, a condition known as *thrombocytopenia* (Gr. *penia*, poverty). However, as in the case of anemia, thrombocytopenia can be caused by genetic and nongenetic defects. Several genetic defects leading to the condition have been reported in humans, but since these are genetically and mechanistically poorly defined and since they are not directly relevant to the topic under discussion here, the interested reader is referred to a hematology textbook for a fuller description.

5.9.3 Defects of Granulocytic and Monocytic Differentiation

Complete or almost complete absence of granulocytes is referred to as *agranulocytosis*; conditions involving a lowered number of granulocytes are termed *granulocytopenia* or *neutropenia*. (Although the latter designation refers specifically to neutrophils, it is often used as a synonym for granulocytopenia since neutrophils are the most frequent of all granulocytes in the blood.) Genetic lesion is only one of the many causes of this condition; transient granulocytopenia can also be induced by a variety of drugs, for example. The three main forms of human, genetically controlled granulocytopenia are infantile genetic agranulocytosis, familial neutropenia, and cyclic neutropenia.

Infantile genetic agranulocytosis (IGA; also known as chronic infantile agranulocytosis) leads to a severe reduction in the number of granulocytes; the few that are formed seem to be structurally and functionally normal. The question of inheritance of this disease is controversial. The defect has been described only in newborns, who, shortly after birth, become extremely susceptible to various bacterial infections and often die.

Familial neutropenia defines a group of diseases affecting not only granulocytes but other blood cells—in particular, monocytes. The diseases can be either of a *milder* (benign) or *severe* type. They occur in newborns and young children and lead to increased susceptibility to bacterial infections.

Cyclic neutropenia leads to a regular fluctuation in the number of granulocytes in the peripheral blood. In the phase of reduced granulocyte numbers, the patient becomes more susceptible to infections; in the phase of normal numbers, the afflicted person is healthy.

The nature of the lesions in these three neutropenias is unknown. A likely interpretation is that the lesions occur at the progenitor-cell level and disturb the regulation of granulopoiesis.

There is also a group of diseases in which the number of granulocytes is normal but the structure of these cells is altered so that they cannot function properly. Here we shall mention only one of these, the *chronic granulomatous disease* (CGD). This X-linked disorder appears to be a mutation in a gene controlling an enzyme necessary for the killing of certain bacteria (*Staphylococcus aureus, Serratia marcescens, Pseudomonas,* and others). The bacteria are phagocytosed, but then remain inside the granulocyte cytoplasm, protected from the action of antibodies. The granulocytes transport the ingested bacteria into various organs, where they cause the formation of firm, focal, granulated lesions (granulomas). Other characteristics of the disease are inflammation and enlargement of the lymph nodes, enlargement of spleen and liver, and attacks of pneumonia. Most children with CGD die at a young age.

5.9.4 Defects of Lymphocytic Differentiation

Disturbances of lymphocyte differentiation lead to defects in the animal's immune response—defects that, in humans, are referred to as *immunodeficiency diseases*. The first such disease was described in 1952 by Ogden C. Burton; since then, hundreds of other cases have been reported by other clinicians. Considering the complexity of lymphocyte differentiation, it is unlikely that any two of these cases are exactly the same. Nevertheless, there are enough similarities among certain cases to allow their grouping into individual diseases, such as those described below. The diseases are arranged according to the differentiation level at which the underlying defect has occurred. But since the nature of the defect is not known with certainty in any of the diseases, this arrangement must be considered tentative.

Stem-Cell and Progenitor-Cell Defects

Once a stem cell has committed itself to differentiation, it still has several options as to which particular differentiation pathway to choose. The choice, apparently, is made gradually, during a series of cell divisions, so that certain cells lose the ability to differentiate along certain pathways while retaining the ability to differentiate along those remaining. This is the only explanation for the fact that the defects described under this heading can affect two or three pathways simultaneously, while leaving others undisturbed. Diseases probably caused by defects of the stem cell shared by the T- and B-lymphocytic lineages are reticular dysgenesis, Swiss-type agammaglobulinemia, and severe combined immunodeficiencies.

Reticular dysgenesis (Gr. *dys*, bad, *genesis*, development) is a rare disease, characterized by the total, or almost total, absence of T and B lymphocytes, granulocytes, and monocytes; erythrocytes and thrombocytes are present. The defect responsible for this disease must, therefore, occur at the level of a stem cell common to the lymphocytic and granulocytic lineages. Children suffering from reticular dysgenesis die shortly after birth.

Swiss-type agammaglobulinemia belongs to a complex of *severe combined immunodeficiencies* (SCID), so called because they are among the most severe of all immunodeficiency states and because they usually affect both humoral and cellular immunity. "Swiss-type" refers to the fact that the defect was first described by a Swiss physician (W. H. Hitzig) in a Swiss patient, and "agammaglobulinemia" to the fact that one of the characteristics of the disease is a drastic reduction of the gamma globulin level in the patient's serum. The defect is inherited as an autosomal recessive trait and results in the absence of both T and B lymphocytes. The fact that patients have normal numbers of other blood cells, including granulocytes, indicates that the lesion occurs at the level of a stem cell common to the T- and B-lymphocytic lineages, one or more steps away from the stem cell affected in reticular dysgenesis. Patients with Swiss-type agammaglobulinemia, or with other forms of SCID, suffer from severe infections, notably viral and fungal, and fail to thrive. The disease breaks out shortly after birth and can be corrected by transplantation of bone marrow from a suitable normal donor.

SCID with ADA deficiency is another disease included in the complex of severe combined immunodeficiencies. Its clinical features resemble those of Swiss-type agammaglobulinemia but it differs in that it often leads to bone abnormalities and is associated with an identifiable enzyme defect. The afflicted enzyme is adenosine deaminase (ADA), which catalyzes the conversion of adenosine to inosine (Fig. 5.31). ADA-deficient patients carry a homozygous mutation at the ADA structural locus in chromosome 20. Although the heterozygotes for the mutation have half the normal ADA level, they remain clinically normal; the homozygotes lack the enzyme completely. The role of the enzyme deficiency in the pathogenesis of the disease is not yet known. ADA deficiency also occurs without an immunodeficiency, and vice versa. For example, in the Kung tribe of the Kalahari desert, the defective ADA gene is present without SCID in 1 percent of the population; ADA deficiency with or without immunodeficiency is also relatively frequent in Arabian horses. What role ADA deficiency plays in SCID is not known, but some immunologists speculate that the accumulation of intracellular adenosine caused by the absence of ADA leads to the inhibition of pyrimidine synthesis (pyrimidine starvation) and to cell death. Others believe that the accumulation of adenosine leads to an increase of cyclic AMP, a molecule believed to inhibit many lymphocyte functions. ADA is indeed found in lymphocytes, but it also oc-

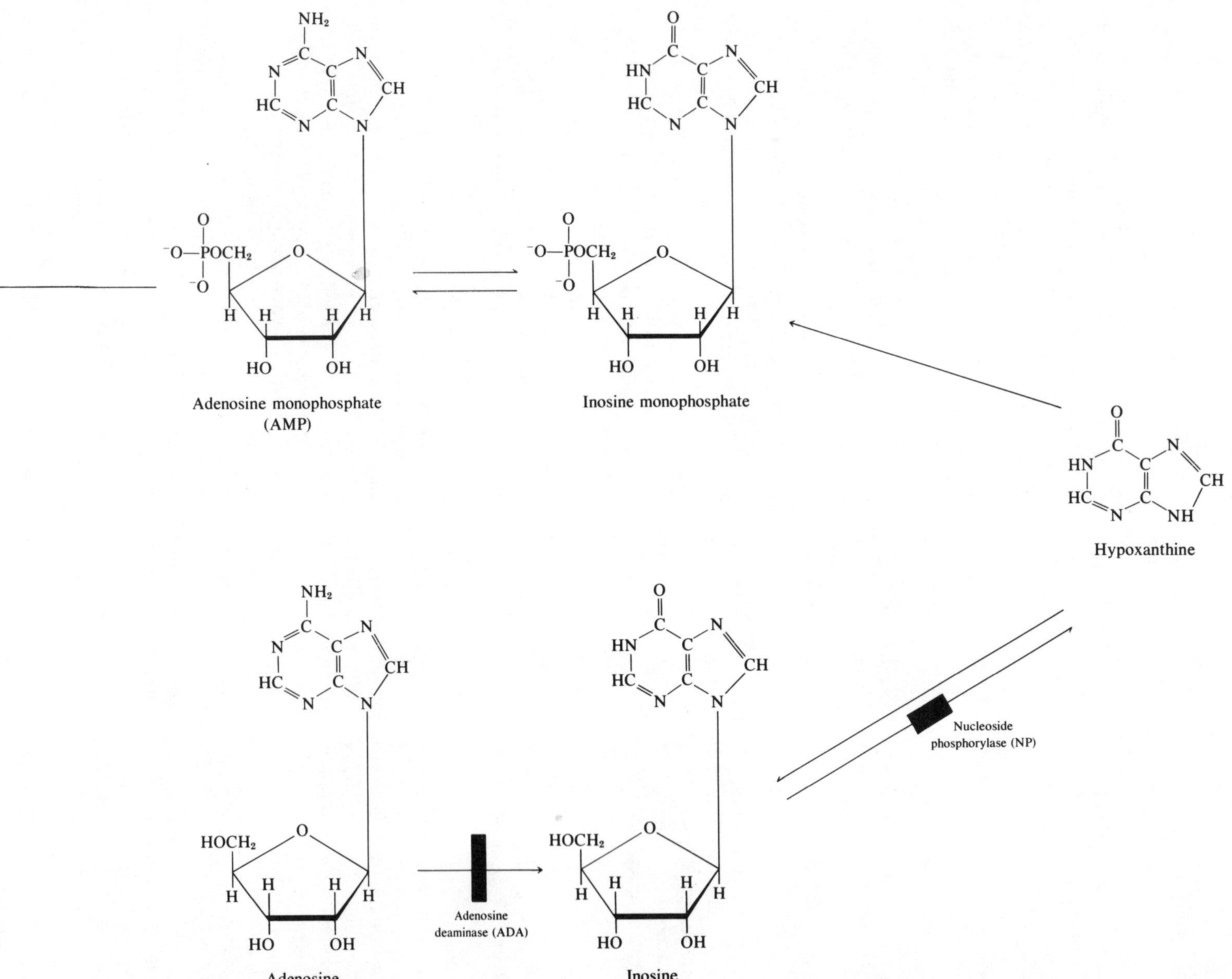

Figure 5.31. Adenosine metabolism and the sites of specific blocks in ADA and PNA deficiencies (indicated by black rectangles).

curs in erythrocytes and other cells. Why it should affect only lymphocytes is one of many unanswered questions about immunodeficiencies.

SCID with B lymphocytes differs from the previous two SCID diseases in that it affects only T, not B or any other blood cells. (B-lymphocyte levels are normal, whereas T lymphocytes are usually completely absent.) One can speculate that the lesion occurs still another step away from the stem cell, perhaps at the level of the T-progenitor cell. Although B cells are present, the patient's serum contains only low levels of immunoglobulin (some IgM and very little IgG and IgA). The reason for the Ig deficiency is apparently the unavailability of T-cell help necessary for the differentiation of B lymphocytes into Ig-secreting plasma cells. Supporting this notion is an observation that when the patient's B lymphocytes are cultured in vitro in the presence of normal T lymphocytes, they synthesize Ig normally.

T-Cell Defects

These deficiencies are assumed to affect different stages of T-lymphocyte differentiation. Some of the better-known defects are PNP deficiency, common variable hypogammaglobulinemia, and Wiskott-Aldrich syndrome.

PNP deficiency is another immunodeficiency with a well-characterized enzyme defect—the absence of purine nucleoside phosphorylase (PNP). The enzyme catalyzes the conversion of inosine to hypoxanthine (Fig. 5.31), a step following the one in which ADA is involved. The defect is caused by a mutation at a locus in chromosome 14, and the homozygotes for this mutation either lack the enzyme completely or produce normal levels of an inactive enzyme. The heterozygotes have half the normal enzymatic activity. PNP deficiency affects only T lymphocytes, and perhaps only a subpopulation of T lymphocytes, since there are reports that T helper functions remain normal. T-cytotoxic cells, however, are clearly affected in that they cannot provide the necessary protection against viral and other infectious diseases. The onset of the disease occurs at between four months and two years of age. The mechanism of PNP involvement in immunity is not known.

Common variable hypogammaglobulinemia (CVH) is a group of diseases that all have at least one characteristic in common—reduced levels of gamma globulin in the patient's sera (hence the name: Gr. *hypo*, under). The individual diseases differ in many other characteristics, including the nature of the defect. The primary lesion seems to occur in T lymphocytes and leads either to hyperproduction of suppressor cells or to hypoproduction of helper cells. B lymphocytes are affected only secondarily in that they are either prevented from completing or not given the necessary stimulus for their differentiation into plasma cells. CVH patients, therefore, have normal numbers of immature B cells but are deficient in plasma cells. The onset age of CVH is variable (hence the "variable" in the name), ranging from a few months to several years after birth. The most common problems of CVH patients are infections and gastrointestinal disorders, the latter presumably caused by the decreased IgA levels (see Chapters 6 and 13).

Wiskott-Aldrich syndrome (WAS), named after pediatricians A. Wiskott and Robert A. Aldrich, is a defect that nobody seems to know how to classify. Several observations suggest that it has something to do with T lymphocytes, but where in the T-differentiation pathway it acts is not known. The interpretation of the syndrome is complicated further by the fact that, in addition to its effect on immunity, it also causes reduction in the platelet and neutrophil numbers, increase in the eosinophils, and eczema. The T-cell defect results in slowing down of cellular immunity reactions (graft rejection, delayed-type hypersensitivity, and cutaneous hypersensitivity), despite the fact that the T-lymphocyte number is only slightly reduced. The patients have normal total serum Ig levels, but the class distribution is abnormal: levels of IgE, and often also of IgA and IgD, are elevated, the IgG level is normal, and the IgM level is reduced. The increased IgE (IgA, IgD) level is caused by an increased synthetic rate, which, in turn, may be a response to an increased rate of Ig destruction. The IgM level remains low because of an increased degradation and normal synthetic rate. Both T and B lymphocytes of WAS patients can be stimulated nonspecifically (for example, by mitogens), but they respond poorly to specific antigenic stimuli. For this reason, some immunologists believe that the WAS defect occurs in antigen recognition and processing. The cause of the thrombocytopenia seems to be some intrinsic defect in the last stages of platelet differentiation. (The patients have normal or even increased numbers of megakaryocytes in the bone marrow.) The cause of the eczema might, perhaps, be related in some way to the thrombocytopenia. The gene causing the Wiskott-Aldrich syndrome is X-linked and the affected boys rarely survive beyond the first decade of life; they die of overwhelming infections, bleeding, or lymphoid tumors.

B-Cell Defects

Examples of B-cell defects are X-linked agammaglobulinemia and IgA, IgM, or IgG deficiencies. *X-linked agammaglobulinemia* (XLA), when it was described in 1952 by Ogden C. Bruton, was the first human immunodeficiency disease recognized. It is characterized by sharply reduced levels of circulating immunoglobulin; however, in spite of the name, immunoglobulin is rarely completely absent in XLA patients. The defect occurs at the pre-B-cell level and apparently prevents the differentiation of these cells into mature B lymphocytes; XLA patients thus have normal pre-B-cell numbers but drastically reduced numbers of B lymphocytes. Boys with XLA are protected during the first six months of their lives by antibodies transferred passively from their mothers; but as these immunoglobulins gradually disappear from the circulation, the disease begins to set in in the form of frequent bacterial (especially pneumococcal and streptococcal) infections. Since the T-cell system and cellular immunity are largely unimpaired, XLA children display normal resistance to most viral and fungal infections. The disease can be treated by repeated gamma globulin injections.

An X chromosome-linked B-lymphocyte defect has also been discovered in *CBA/N strain mice*. The defect was originally described as an inability to mount a humoral immune response to pneumococcal polysaccharide, but later other abnormalities were also identified—unresponsiveness to certain thymus-independent antigens, lowered responsiveness to some B-cell mitogens and complete unresponsiveness to others, deficient antibody-dependent cell-mediated cytotoxicity responses, inability to produce B-cell colonies in vitro, reduced number of splenic B lymphocytes, increased density of surface IgM molecules on B lymphocytes, a reduced ratio of IgD to IgM molecules on B cells, absence of cells bearing surface antigens characteristic of B-lymphocytes, and low levels of circulating IgM. The defect is thought to result from an arrest of B lymphocyte maturation, and appears to be age-dependent rather than absolute. Spleen cells from 12-month-old CBA/N mice respond well to a number of immunological stimuli to which three-month-old mice are refractory. However, the mice do not acquire complete reactivity, since some responses remain below normal levels or even negative throughout their lives. The changes in the surface characteristics of the CBA/N B lymphocytes reflect a delayed B-cell maturation; in terms of B-lymphocyte differentiation, the three-month-old CBA/N mice are equivalent to newborn mice of other strains.

The *IgA deficiency* (IAD) is a state of almost complete absence of this single immunoglobulin class. It is the most common immunodeficiency, affecting approximately one in every 800 to 3000 persons, and while it is apparently controlled genetically, the mode of inheritance has so far not been elucidated. Many people with IgA deficiency are completely healthy, but others show symptoms related to the function of IgA molecules. IgA differs from other immunoglobulin classes in that it is present not only in the serum, but also in the body's secretions (see Chapters 6 and 13), where it plays a role in neutralization of infectious agents at their port of entry, and in absorption of noninfectious antigens introduced into the body by breathing or with food. All five symptoms of IgA deficiency—frequent infections of paranasal sinuses and pulmonary airways, gastrointestinal problems, allergies, autoimmune reactions, and lung and gastrointestinal tumors—may be the consequence of a breakdown in these IgA functions. In the absence of IgA on the mucosal surfaces of the lungs, sinuses, and gastrointestinal tract, these organs become easy prey to the pathogens introduced into them by breathing or with food. Antigens normally bound by IgA bind, instead, to mast-cell IgE and cause allergic reactions. Among the accumulating antigens, no longer cleared by IgA, could be some that resemble the body's own molecules, so when the body begins to mount immune reactions against these antigens, it also unleashes an attack against its own determinants (a state termed *autoimmunity*). Finally, the antigen accumulating in the lungs and gastrointestinal tract is a source of constant irritation, which can lead eventually to cancer. The actual site of the defect responsible for the IgA deficiency is not known. It could be either in the IgA-committed B lymphocyte, or in a T lymphocyte that regulates the differentiation of the IgA B cell into a plasma cell.

The *IgM deficiency*, one of the rarest immunodeficiencies, is characterized by almost complete absence of IgM in the serum and normal levels of other immunoglobulin classes. Patients with IgM deficiency can mount normal antibody responses to some antigens but are unable to cope with certain bacteria, in particular pneumococci and meningococci. The patient's ability to mount T-cell reactions is unimpaired. It would be particularly interesting to know the site of the defect responsible for this deficiency, since one is hard-pressed to explain how the synthesis of an Ig class can be suppressed without the concurrent suppression of other Ig classes when the expression of this class in the differentiation pathway precedes the expression of other immunoglobulins.

The *IgG deficiency* affects IgG selectively without influencing other immunoglobulin classes. The IgG class is known to consist of four subclasses (see Chapter 6), and the deficiency can affect various combinations of these. The symptoms of the disease are relatively mild, consisting mainly of frequent bacterial infections, and the ailment is often diagnosed relatively late in life.

Finally, we shall mention one disease, *ataxia telangiectasia*, that is difficult to classify, and in which immunodeficiency may be a secondary consequence of some basic systemic developmental defect. Ataxia telangiectasia is an autosomal recessive disorder characterized by a loss of ability to coordinate muscles controlled by the cerebellum (cerebellar ataxia, from Gr. *a*, negative, *taxia*, order), dilation of capillaries in facial skin and eyeballs (oculocutaneous telangiectasia, from Gr. *telos*, end, *angeion*, vessel, *ektasis*, a stretching out), lung infections, increased incidence of certain tumors, reduced number of T cells, and low levels of certain immunoglobulin classes in the serum. Some of these features are caused by an underdevelopment of the thymus, which remains embryonic in appearance. Ataxia telangiectasia is also associated with a defect in DNA repair, a translocation involving chromosome 14 in the peripheral leukocytes, and a prevalence of antibodies to an early antigen of the Epstein-Barr virus (see next section) in the patient's sera. The primary defect in ataxia may be in endoderm differentiation, or in the endodermal-mesodermal interaction of the developing fetus.

5.9.5 NK-Cell Defects

A defect in humans called the *Chédiak-Steinbrinck-Higashi syndrome*, after Moisés Chédiak, W. Steinbrinck, and O. Higashi, was once thought to be primarily an abnormality of granulocyte differentiation, but more recent studies indicate that it also involves an impairment of natural killer-cell function. At the base of this disorder may be a mutation in one of the genes controlling the formation of membranous vesicles—such as the lysosomal granules in granulocytes and the melanosomes (pigment granules) in the melanocytes. The defective vesicles enlarge to an abnormal size, making the cell more rigid and slowing its locomotion. The abnormal granulocyte granules are slow in carrying out their normal function, the killing of the phagocytosed bacteria is delayed, and the infection goes on, unchecked. The abnormal melanocyte granules are responsible for the partial albinism of the Chédiak-Steinbrinck-Higashi patients characterized by fair skin, silvery hair, and abnormal sensitivity to light. The patients also have profoundly depressed NK-cell activity and defective antibody-dependent cell-mediated cytotoxicity. The NK-cell defect may be responsible for the lymphoproliferative disorder accompanying this syndrome. Patients with this syndrome either die of bacterial infections or succumb to lymphoreticular tumors. A defect resembling the Chédiak-Steinbrinck-Higashi syndrome also occurs in mice carrying a mutation at the *beige* locus on chromosome 13. This mutation, too, affects both melanocytes, causing a characteristic change in coat color, and the NK cells.

5.10 DISORDERS CAUSED BY INCREASED PROLIFERATION OF HEMATOPOIETIC CELLS

In the preceding section, we discussed disorders in which cells, upon reaching a certain differentiation stage, failed to proliferate and differentiate further. In most instances, the cause of this *reduced ability to proliferate* and differentiate was a defect in a gene that should normally have been functioning at that stage. Since this gene is transmitted through germ cells and is therefore present in all somatic cells, any cell reaching this stage and activating the gene becomes defective. As a result, the individual becomes sick, because it lacks or is deficient in certain cells of a given differentiation pathway.

In this section we shall describe disorders in which a single cell and its progeny become unresponsive to the normal regulatory mechanisms and begin to proliferate in an uncontrolled manner. This *increased proliferation* is the consequence of a genetic change, transmitted to the progeny of the original cell but to no other somatic cell and to no germ cell; in other words, the disorder is restricted to a single clone. The uncontrolled proliferation is referred to by various names (see Chapter 4), of which we shall use only one, *neoplasia* (L. *neo*, new, Gr. *plasma*, thing formed), here; we shall refer to the product of neoplastic growth as the *neoplasm*. Neoplasia can be incited by a variety of agents, such as certain viruses, certain chemicals, and certain forms of radiation (for further details, see Chapter 14). Neoplastic cells cause disease by flooding the organism and displacing normal cells spatially and functionally.

Neoplasms of the lymphoid system have traditionally been grouped into two classes—leukemias and lymphomas. *Leukemia* (Gr. *leukos*, white, *haima*, blood), first described in 1845 by the German pathologist Rudolf Virchow (who introduced the term in 1856) and the English physician John H. Bennett, refers to a neoplastic condition marked by an increased number of circulating leukocytes (white cells) in the blood. *Lymphoma* (the Greek ending *-oma* is used to designate a neoplastic form of a given tissue), first described by the English physician Thomas Hodgkin in 1832, refers to an abnormal proliferation in a lymphoid organ—a lymph node, spleen, or thymus. (In this last instance the neoplasm is termed *thymoma*.) There is no sharp dividing line between leukemias and lymphomas and the two terms are often used interchangeably. Both conditions concern lymphoid cells, but in a leukemia, neoplastic leukocytes dominate the blood, whereas in a lymphoma, the leukocytes are confined largely to lymphoid organs.

Depending on the type of cell from which the neoplastic clone arose, the properties of the neoplastic cells, and symptoms accompanying the disease, pathologists distinguish several forms of leukemia and lymphoma. We shall describe them according to the species in which they occur, dealing first with human, then mouse, and finally with avian neoplasms.

5.10.1 Human Lymphoid Neoplasms

Leukemias

Human leukemias occur in two basic forms—acute and chronic. *Acute leukemia* is characterized by a sudden onset and rapid progress of the disease, which, if unchecked, ends fatally within a few weeks. It occurs most frequently in young children and can result in a more than 50-fold increase of leukocytes in the blood. *Chronic leukemia* has an insidious onset, can run its course over several years, is characterized by milder symptoms, and need not be fatal, even in untreated patients. The chronic phase, however, may suddenly change into an *acute blastic crisis*, resembling acute leukemia and characterized by the appearance of more immature leukocytes. The disease occurs in persons over 35 years of age.

The major signs of leukemia are fever, malaise, and prostration, spontaneous bleeding in the skin or subcutaneous tissues, frequent infections, and enlargement of lymph nodes and spleen (the latter are particularly frequent in the chronic form of the disease). Microscopic examination of the blood reveals an increase in the number of leukocytes, the presence in the circulation of abnormal, often immature cells of either the lymphocytic or granulocytic-monocytic lineage, and a decreased number of erythrocytes (anemia) and platelets (thrombocytopenia). Depending on the predominance of cells of one or the other lineage, leukemias are classified as lymphocytic, granulocytic, or monocytic. The susceptibility to infection is the consequence of the displacement of normal leukocytes by neoplastic, nonfunctional cells; the bleeding results from a shortage of platelets. The treatment of leukemia consists of radiation therapy, chemotherapy (both aimed at elimination of the rapidly dividing neoplastic cells), and bone-marrow transplantation (aimed at replacing losses of normal hematopoietic cells). The cause of human leukemia is unknown. Based on analogy with animal leukemias, viruses are suspected to be the inciting agents, but direct evidence of their involvement is not available.

A brief description of the main forms of human leukemia follows. The presumed target cells of various leukemias are depicted in Figure 5.32.

Acute Lymphoblastic Leukemia (ALL). The most frequent neoplasm in children, ALL is characterized by the presence in the blood of immature lymphocytes (blasts). It is divided into four groups, according to the phenotype of the neoplastic cells. Markers used to differentiate among these four forms are listed below.

Membrane Markers

cALL A common antigen of all acute lymphoblastic leukemias;

DR Human class II MHC antigens;

T T cell-specific antigen;

Ig Immunoglobulins in cytoplasm (cIg) or in the plasma membrane (sIg);

E A receptor responsible for the formation of rosettes with sheep erythrocytes.

Enzyme Markers

Tdt Terminal deoxynucleotidyl transferase;

He Hexosaminidase allozymes;

Ap Acid phosphatase.

The four forms of ALL are O-ALL, T-ALL, Pre-B-ALL, and B-ALL.

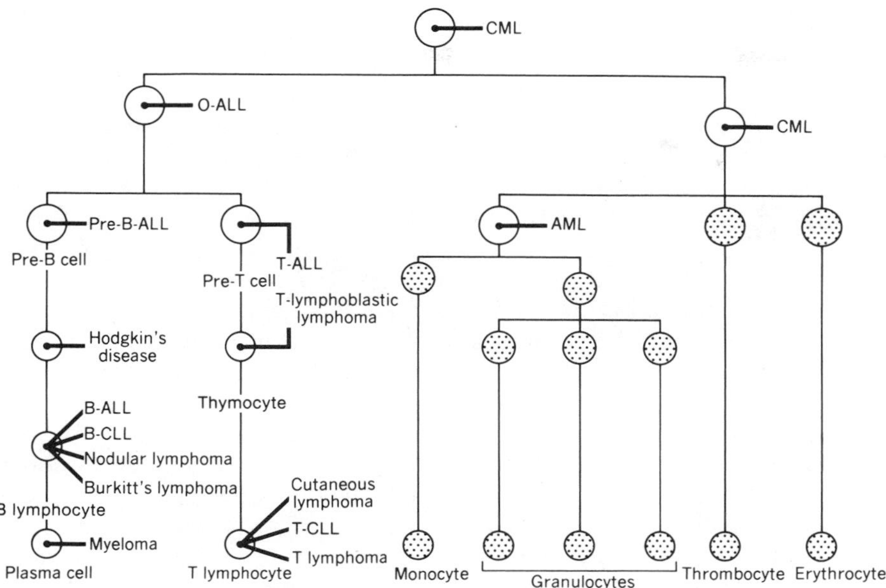

Figure 5.32. Presumed target cells of neoplastic transformation in various human leukemias. ALL, acute lymphoblastic leukemia; AML, acute myeloid leukemia; CLL, chronic lymphocytic leukemia; CML, chronic myeloid leukemia.

O-ALL is characterized by the absence of both T and B lymphocyte markers in the neoplastic cells and is also referred to as non-T, non-B ALL, or null-ALL. The phenotype of the leukemic cell is $cALL^+$, DR^+, T^-, E^-, Ig^-, Tdt^+, He^-, Ap^-. O-ALL is the most common type of ALL, representing almost two-thirds of acute lymphoblastic leukemias. The leukemic cells presumably derive from progenitor cells of the lymphocytic lineage before their commitment to either the T- or B-differentiation pathway.

T-ALL is characterized by the expression of T-lymphocyte markers. The phenotype is $cALL^-$ (a few are, however, positive), DR^-, T^+, E^+, Ig^-, Tdt^+, He^-, Ap^+. It occurs with a frequency of from 15 to 20 percent of all ALLs and is presumably derived either from a progenitor cell committed to the T-differentiation pathway or from a thymocyte.

Pre-B-ALL is a rare leukemia, expressing cytoplasmic IgM; surface IgM is absent. The phenotype is $cALL^+$, DR^+, T^-, E^-, Ig^+ Tdt^- (but a few are Tdt^+). The leukemic cells apparently arise by transformation of pre-B lymphocytes.

B-ALL is also a rare form of leukemia with a phenotype $cALL^-$, DR^+, T^-, E^-, sIg^+, Tdt^-, He^-, Ap^-. It is thought to derive from maturing B lymphocytes.

Chronic Lymphocytic Leukemia (CLL). In most cases, this is a mild disease, but in some patients it may progress to *acute blastic crisis*. It is known in two forms, the more common B-CLL and a rare T-CLL.

B-CLL constitutes more than 90 percent of all CLLs. In the chronic phase, the patient's blood contains an increased number of small B lymphocytes with the phenotype $cALL^-$, DR^+, T^-, E^-, sIg^+, Tdt^-, Ap^-. The membrane Ig is either of the IgM or IgM + IgD type. In the acute crisis, the blast cells flooding the blood carry the same Ig as the small neoplastic lymphocytes, indicating that both cell types belong to the same clone. The neoplastic transformation leading to CLL probably occurs in a cell of the B-lymphocytic lineage.

T-CLL is known in only a few cases. The neoplastic small lymphocytes carry T-cell markers and lack B-cell markers. The target for T-CLL neoplastic transformation is probably a cell within the T-lymphocytic lineage.

Acute Myeloid Leukemia (AML). This is a heterogeneous group of diseases characterized by an increase of immature myeloid (granulocytic or monocytic) cells in the blood. The two main forms are acute monocytic and acute myelomonocytic leukemias.

Acute monocytic leukemia (also called *histiocytic* or *Schilling leukemia*) is characterized by the appearance in the blood of immature monocytes with a phenotype $cALL^-$, DR^+, T^-, E^-, Tdt^-, He^-, Ap^-, and M^+ (an antigen common to cells of the monocytic series). The target of neoplastic transformation is probably the monocyte progenitor cell.

Acute myelomonocytic (*Naegeli*) *leukemia* constitutes about 4 percent of all leukemias and is characterized by the dominance of neoplastic monocytes or monocytes with the participation of granulocytes. It probably arises by transformation of a myeloid progenitor cell.

Chronic Myeloid Leukemia (CML). CML is characterized by an overproduction of granulocytes and, in 90 percent of all cases, also by the appearance of the *Philadelphia* (Ph^1) *chromosome*. This is a shortened version of chromosome 22 from which approximately half of the longer arm has been translocated to chromosome 9. The Ph^1 chromosome is present not only in cells of the monocytic and granulocytic series, but also in cells of the erythrocytic and thrombocytic series; it is absent in lymphocytes. Sporadically, Ph^1 also occurs in other leukemias and in healthy persons. Patients with CML progress within a few years to an acute blastic crisis that resembles acute leukemia. The crisis can be either lymphoid, resembling ALL, or myeloid, resembling AML. (Blasts in lymphoid and myeloid crises share antigenic markers and other characteristics with ALL or AML blasts, respectively.) The target cell of the neoplastic transformation in CML is either a hematopoietic stem cell or a progenitor cell committed to nonlymphocytic proliferation.

Hairy-Cell Leukemia (Also Called Leukemic Reticuloendothelosis). This is an uncommon chronic leukemia characterized by the proliferation of adherent, phagocytic cells with prominent cytoplasmatic projections (hence the name), extensive spleen enlargement, and pronounced reduction of all blood cells in circulation. The origin of the hairy cells is unknown. The cells share some characteristics (expression of surface Ig) with B lymphocytes, and other characteristics (phagocytosis, high-affinity Fc receptors) with monocytes. Some investigators believe that hairy cells are neoplastic counterparts of a new, as yet unidentified cell type normally present in the reticuloendothelial system (hence the synonym).

Lymphomas

In contrast to leukemias, in which neoplastic cells disseminate from the earliest stages, in lymphomas the disease often remains localized for a long time in lymphoid organs, and disseminates throughout the body only in the final stages. Human lymphomas can be divided into two groups—Hodgkin's disease and lymphomas of non-Hodgkin type.

Hodgkin's Disease. This disease was named for Thomas Hodgkin, an English pathologist who described it in 1832. Hodgkin reported seven cases with enlargement of the spleen and lymph nodes; however, only two of these were what would be considered Hodgkin's disease today, while the others apparently were tuberculosis and leukemias. Hodgkin's disease is characterized by a painless enlargement of lymph nodes, often accompanied by fever, generalized itching or eruptions on the skin, and anemia. The enlargement usually begins in one side of the neck and then spreads to other lymph nodes. Microscopic examination of the enlarged lymph nodes reveals the presence of characteristic cellular elements, referred to as *Hodgkin cells*. In their most characteristic form, Hodgkin cells measure 40 μm or more in diameter and have a single, bilobed, vesicular nucleus with one large, eosinophilic nucleolus. (The vesicular appearance of the nucleus is caused by the accumulation of the chromatin on the periphery.) Hodgkin cells give rise to giant *Reed-Sternberg cells* (named after the American pathologists Dorothy R. Reed and George M. Sternberg), which have multiple nuclei and conspicuous nucleoli. Originally, pathologists thought the Hodgkin and Reed-Sternberg cells were neoplastic reticulum cells; more recently, however, evidence has been accumulating that suggests they might be of B-lymphocyte origin. According to one hypothesis, the original stimulus favoring the development of Hodgkin's disease comes from a prolonged, ineffective (virus-induced?) T-cell proliferation in a local lymph node. The proliferating T lymphocytes then stimulate monoclonal proliferation of B lymphoblasts and their transformation, first into Hodgkin and then into Reed-Sternberg cells. The proliferation is first confined to a single lymph node, but then spreads into other lymph nodes, and finally into other organs of the body (spleen, liver, kidney, and lungs). In support of this hypothesis is the observation that Hodgkin patients invariably have a reduced ability to manifest delayed-type hypersensitivity, impaired ability to reject allogeneic skin grafts, and increased susceptibility to certain infections—for example, tubercle bacilli. According to this interpretation, the early stages of Hodgkin's disease are not neoplastic; neoplasia develops only later, after the transformation of B lymphoblasts.

The frequency of Hodgkin disease is about one in 100,000. The disease can develop at almost any age but the incidence is highest in early adult life. Boys and men are approximately four times more susceptible to it than girls and women. When untreated, the disease is fatal with survival of less than 1 year from the time of diagnosis. The treatment consists of surgical excision of enlarged lymph nodes, X-irradiation, and chemotherapy.

Non-Hodgkin Lymphomas. These neoplasms often form fleshy outgrowths in lymph nodes and are therefore also referred to as *lymphosarcomas* (Gr. *sarx* or *sarc*, flesh). Since they apparently can arise in any lymphoid tissue and from any lymphoid cell, they form a heterogeneous group of neoplasms. The most frequently affected lymphoid tissues are lymph nodes of the neck, armpits, and groin, followed by tonsils and lymph nodes of the mediastinum (the median dividing partition in the chest cavity) and abdomen; less frequently affected are the thymus and Peyer's patches. The neoplastic transformation always begins in one lymph node and then spreads into neighboring nodes and other organs. Externally, the disease manifests itself by a localized swelling of one or more lymph nodes. Microscopic examination of these lymph nodes then reveals the presence of neoplastic cells, the characteristics of which vary according to the type of disease. Each disease has a different name, presumably reflecting its most conspicuous feature. Unfortunately, pathologists do not agree among themselves as to what the most important characteristics of the individual diseases are, and so some of them have several names—more than a dozen, in some instances.

We shall divide the non-Hodgkins lymphomas into those of T-lymphocyte and those of B-lymphocyte origin. Of the T-cell lymphomas, we shall mention two cutaneous lymphomas (Sézary syndrome and mycosis fungoides), the T-lymphoblastic lymphoma, and the T lymphoma; of the B-cell lymphomas we shall describe the Burkitt's lymphoma and the nodular lymphoma. We shall acquaint ourselves with the important category of plasma-cell neoplasms in the next chapter.

Sézary syndrome, a disease named after A. Sézary, who described it in 1938, and *mycosis fungoides* are characterized by the appearance of the so-called *Sézary* or *mycosis cells*, which are attracted to epithelial tissues and are therefore abundant in the skin. For this reason, the two diseases are grouped together into a category of cutaneous lymphomas (L. *cutis*, skin). The Sézary and mycosis cells are morphologically indistinguishable and may, in fact, be identical. They are large cells with a characteristically deformed nucleus, which looks humped or rolled together (convoluted). Their phenotype (ALL^-, DR^-, T^+, Ig^-, E^+, Tdt^-) indicates their T-cell origin. Some Sézary cells produce a soluble factor potentiating immunoglobulin synthesis by B lymphocytes in vitro. The neoplastic cell could, therefore, be derived from post-thymic T lymphocytes, perhaps from helper cells. The attraction of Sézary and mycosis cells to skin could reflect some special relationship between skin and T lymphocytes. Such a relationship is also suggested by the fact that epithelial cells and T lymphocytes share the Thy-1 antigen, and that the *nu* gene affects a lymphoid organ and a skin derivative. Alternatively, this attraction could result from some chronic antigenic stimulation of T lymphocytes by cutaneous antigens. The infiltrating Sézary (mycosis) cells cause skin lesions characterized by reddish coloration (erythroderma), swelling (edema), and intense itching (pruritis). Sézary cells are also found in the blood and eventually infiltrate lymph nodes, bone marrow, and other organs, so that the condition resembles leukemia more than it does a lymphoma.

Mycosis fungoides (Gr. *mykés*, fungus, *-osis*, a condition, L. *fungus*, a mushroom; *fungoid* refers to an exuberant growth on the bodily surface) is so similar to the Sézary syndrome that some pathologists consider the two diseases identical, or one a variant of the other. Mycosis fungoides differs from the Sézary syndrome only in that the skin lesions often develop into skin neoplasms. Both Sézary syndrome and mycosis fungoides are rare diseases. In the United States, for example, only 70 patients with mycosis fungoides are recorded every year. They have, however, a grave prognosis: approximately 50 percent of patients die within four years of diagnosis.

T-lymphoblastic lymphoma, also called leukosarcomatosis, is characterized by the appearance of mediastinal (thymic) neoplasms at the onset of the disease. At later stages, neoplastic cells also infiltrate lymph nodes and cause their enlargement. These cells can be of two types (thus distinguishing two kinds of T-lymphoblastic lymphoma)—cells with convoluted nuclei (the more frequent type) and cells with round nuclei (less frequent). They are derived either from progenitor T lymphocytes or from thymocytes, and differ from typical lymphocytes in their larger size, the finely dispersed chromatin in their nuclei, and positive acid-phosphatase reaction. The disease occurs with a frequency of less than 1 percent of all lymphomas.

T lymphoma is a rare disease discovered relatively recently and characterized by selective proliferation of neoplastic cells in thymus-dependent regions of lymph nodes. The neoplastic cells arise from T lymphocytes in these regions and bear most of the T-lymphocyte markers.

Burkitt's lymphoma is named after Denis Burkitt, who described it in 1958 during his field studies in Uganda. However, his was not the first description of the disease: the condition had already been recorded in Africa in 1904. But only after Burkitt's studies did the lymphoma begin to attract the attention of many investigators. The disease manifests itself in young children (peak at the age of five years) as a large neoplasm in the jaw or abdomen. The African form of the disease occurs only in central Africa and New Guinea. The fact that the lymphoma incidence is influenced by temperature and rainfall suggests that a biological agent, such as a virus, is involved in neoplasm induction. A virus closely associated with Burkitt's lymphoma has indeed been found. It belongs to a category of herpes viruses and is named, after its discoverers, Epstein-Barr virus (EBV). The involvement of EBV in Burkitt's lymphoma induction is supported by several observations. First, Burkitt's lymphoma patients have a high level of EBV antibodies in their blood. Second, every lymphoma cell carries the virus genome integrated into its chromosomes. Third, EBV transforms normal human cells in vitro into continually growing, presumably neoplastic lines, and induces neoplasms in subhuman primates. Fourth, children with high levels of EBV antibodies run a high risk of developing Burkitt's lymphoma. However, EBV cannot be acting alone in the induction process because the virus occurs throughout the world, while the neoplasms occur endemically in a small region with particular climatic conditions. Apparently, some climate-related factor—now thought to be malaria—must also participate in the induction.

Immunological studies have revealed that Burkitt lymphoma cells bear immunoglobulin on their surfaces and so are of B-lymphocyte origin. This observation also fits with the virus hypothesis, since only B lymphocytes have receptors for EBV in their membranes. How malaria comes into the picture is not clear, but one possibility is that a persistent malarial infection causes prolonged, continual B-cell proliferation and thus produces a high supply of lymphoid cells susceptible to virus infection.

However, even EBV and malaria do not tell the whole story of Burkitt lymphoma induction. In central Africa almost everyone is infected by EBV at an early age, and more than half the children have malaria. Yet, of these doubly infected individuals, only a small percentage develop the lymphoma. There must, therefore, be additional factors involved in the induction—perhaps a genetic predisposition, an early infection, or a particular sequence and timing of infections by the two agents.

In addition to the African form of Burkitt's lymphoma, there is also another form, occurring in America and Europe. The two forms are histologically indistinguishable, but in the non-African form, EBV is often absent from the neoplastic cells.

Burkitt's lymphomas have a characteristic histological appearance, referred to as "starry-sky" pattern. The name refers to the fact that in a histological section one sees a uniform dark background of lymphoid cells sprinkled with lightly staining phagocytic cells, presumably macrophages.

The *nodular* (*follicular*) *lymphoma* is characterized by a specific pattern of growth in the lymph node. The neoplastic cells are arranged in multiple cohesive aggregates (nodules), which expand and destroy the normal lymph node architecture. The neoplastic nodules are rather uniformly distributed over the cortex and the medulla. The neoplastic cells arise by transformation of B lymphocytes, sometimes referred to as centroblasts and centrocytes (and hence, the lymphoma is also termed centroblastic, or centrocytic). The nodular variant is one of the most common non-Hodgkin's lymphomas. It affects older people primarily and almost never occurs in persons under 20 years of age.

5.10.2 Murine Lymphomas (Leukemias)

At the beginning of this century, several investigators noticed that mice of certain families developed lymphomas more frequently than others, suggesting that predisposition to neoplasia might be controlled genetically. Inspired by this observation, Jacob Furth and others initiated the development of inbred lines with high incidence of spontaneous lymphomas. To this end, they selected for brother-to-sister matings only animals whose close relatives developed the disease, and they eliminated descendants of mice that remained disease-free from breeding. After many years of tedious work, Furth ended up with an AKR strain that developed spontaneous lymphomas in 90 percent of mice less than a year old. (The designation refers to the fact that the ancestors of the strain were *a*lbino; that, of the Aa, Ab, Ac, Ad, etc., families into which the original matings were split, the A*k* family was used for further breeding; and that the strain was maintained at the *R*ockefeller Institute in New York.)

The existence of high-lymphoma strains proves that one of the principal factors in lymphoma development is an individual's genetic make-up. However, since some 10 percent of the AKR mice remain disease-free, despite the fact that they are genetically identical to and live under the same conditions as their brothers and sisters who develop lymphomas, it is clear that genetic factors alone cannot be responsible for the lymphoma induction.

In 1951, Ludwik Gross prepared a cell-free filtrate from an AKR lymphoma and inoculated it into newborn mice of the C3H strain, which has a low incidence of spontaneous lymphomas. When the majority of the inoculated mice developed lymphomas, he concluded that the second most important factor in lymphoma induction is a *virus*. Later, other investigators isolated other lymphoma-inducing viruses and demonstrated that they all belong to the same group, referred to as *murine leukemia viruses*, or *MuLV*. (Although the murine lymphoid neoplasms usually remain localized in lymphoid organs and may disseminate into the blood circulation only in late stages of development, thus behaving like lymphomas or lymphosarcomas, they are often referred to as leukemias.) Each virus bears the name of its discoverer, so that there is a Gross virus, a Tennant virus, a Bittner virus, an Abelson virus, a Friend virus, and so on. We shall learn more about MuLVs in Chapter 14. Here it suffices to state that they are recognized in electron micrographs of infected tissues as the so-called *C-particles*, characterized by their spherical shape, their RNA-containing and electron-dense center (nucleoid), and two or three concentric membranes.

MuLV-induced lymphomas are of four kinds—T, B, myeloid (granulocytic), and erythroid. A brief description of these follows; the presumed target cells of the individual MuLVs are depicted in Figure 5.33.

T-cell lymphomas arise in the thymus, apparently from thymocytes. The thymic origin of these lymphomas (*thymomas*) is indicated, for example, by the observation that thymectomy drastically reduces their incidence in high-lymphoma mouse strains. Thymoma development proceeds in four stages. The first is an *atrophy* of the thymus, when lymphocytes begin to disappear, first from the cortex and then from the medulla as well. The morphologically definable border between the cortex and medulla disappears and the thymus diminishes in size. The second stage is marked by *regeneration* of the wasted thymus—that is, the appearance of what seem to be normal lymphoid and reticular cells, and the restoration of thymic weight to approximately normal value. In the third phase, *focal lymphomas* begin to develop from large, lymphoblast-like, Thy-1^+ Ig^- cells in the cortex. The individual foci rapidly coalesce and then grow inward, completely filling the medulla. The developing lymphoma spreads to the

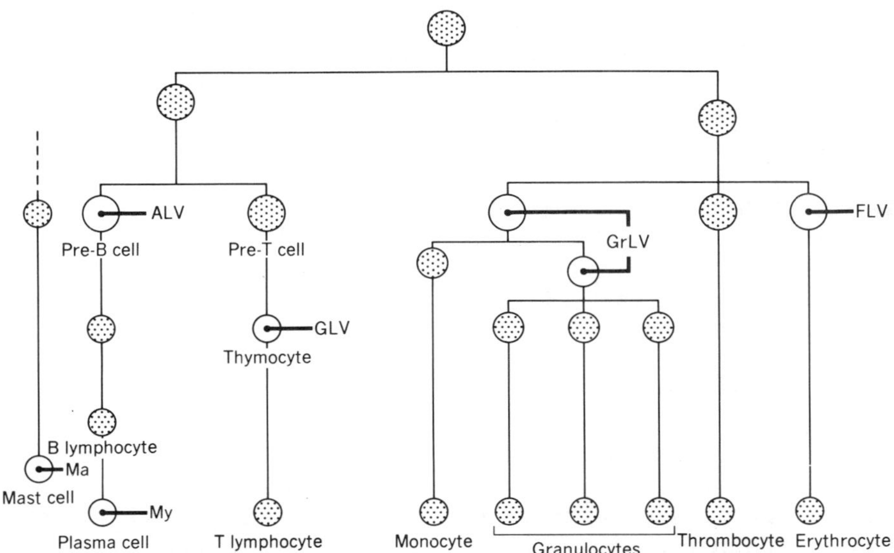

Figure 5.33. Presumed target cells of neoplastic transformation in mouse lymphomas. ALV, Abelson leukemia virus; FLV, Friend leukemia virus; GLV, Gross leukemia virus; GrLV, Graffi leukemia virus; Ma, mastocytoma; My, myeloma.

second lobe (it always starts in one lobe) and greatly enlarges the thymus. In the fourth stage, the neoplastic cells disseminate into other organs—neighboring lymph nodes, spleen, liver, bone marrow, and blood. The entire process, from the beginning of thymus atrophy to neoplastic cell dissemination, takes several months. The majority of the known MuLVs (Gross, Moloney, Tennant, and other viruses) induce this type of lymphoma.

B-cell lymphomas are much less frequent than T-cell lymphomas. A virus that induces B-cell lymphomas was isolated in 1970 by Herbert T. Abelson and Louise S. Rabstein, and is referred to as *Abelson MuLV*. When injected into newborn mice, the virus causes depletion of lymphocytes in the medullary cords and germinal centers, followed by the appearance of neoplastic, lymphoblast-like cells in the bone marrow, and finally formation of solid neoplasms in lymph nodes and in the membranes covering the brain. The neoplasm-bearing mice begin to die within one month from the time of inoculation. The neoplastic cells are Thy-1^-Ig$^+$ and are probably derived by transformation of cells in the early stages of B-lymphocyte differentiation. The mechanism of the neoplasm induction is not known. According to one hypothesis, the virus changes the surface properties of lymphocytes so that they are not retrieved from circulation by the medullary cords, leading to depletion of the cords and their collapse. In an effort to generate usable cells, the cords stimulate abnormal stem-cell proliferation in the bone marrow, thus increasing the chances of neoplastic transformation of these cells or of their progeny. Neoplastic cells then move into the lymph nodes and form solid lymphomas there. In contrast to T-lymphoma formation, the thymus in Abelson virus-infected mice is completely excluded from the neoplastic process and neoplastic cells are almost never found in the blood.

Myeloid (granulocytic) lymphomas only rarely occur spontaneously but they can be induced by the inoculation of Rich or Graffi MuLV into thymectomized mice. (In nonthymectomized mice the virus induces either lymphoid or lymphoid and myeloid lymphomas.) The first detectable sign of lymphoma formation is the loss of lymphocytes from the lymph node medullary cords and their replacement by mature neutrophils. Somewhat later, neoplastic, myeloblast-like cells appear in the lymph node and begin to replace the neutrophils. At about the same time, neoplastic cells also appear in the spleen, where they proliferate extensively and enlarge the organ. In the final stages, neoplastic cells invade liver and bone marrow, and also begin to circulate in the peripheral blood. The target cells of the neoplastic transformation process are probably progenitors of the granulocytic pathway.

Erythroid leukemia is inducible by the Friend or Rauscher form of the MuLV. Upon inoculation into a mouse, the Friend virus (FV) enters erythropoietin-sensitive progenitor cells committed to differentiation along the erythrocytic pathway, and transforms these cells within about 30 hours after the infection. As a result of this transformation, erythrocytic differentiation becomes independent of erythropoietin and the life spans of the differentiated cells are shortened. The transformation, however, does not make the cells self-maintaining (they either differentiate into erythrocytes or die), so they cannot be considered neoplastic. The neoplastic transformation occurs at some later stage when the virus enters more primitive cells of the erythrocytic pathway. *Friend neoplastic cells* are the result of the second transformation; they are characterized by immortality, ability to produce subcutaneous tumors, ability to produce permanent cell lines when grown in tissue culture, and restriction of their ability to differentiate along the erythrocytic pathway. However, they can be induced to differentiate in vitro by exposure to certain chemicals, such as dimethylsulfoxide (DMSO) or butyric acid. The massive proliferation of neoplastic cells in the spleen leads to its enlargement to a point where it ruptures and the animal dies. This event occurs within from one to three months after the infection.

There are at least two variants of the Friend virus, FVA and FVP. The FVA variant causes a *reduction* of the number of erythrocytes (*a*nemia), probably by shortening their life spans; in contrast, the FVP variant induces an *increase* of erythrocytes in the blood (*p*olycythemia), probably by overproduction of cells committed to the erythrocytic pathway. Of the two, only the FVP variant is independent of erythropoietin.

The FV itself is complex, consisting of two viruses—the *spleen focus-forming virus* (SFFV), so designated because it produces characteristic foci of rapidly proliferating cells (erythroblasts) in the spleen, and the MuLV-F, which acts as a helper for both the formation of foci in the spleen by the defective SFFV and for the development of erythroleukemia (it supplies factors necessary for SFFV maturation).

5.10.3 Avian Lymphomas

The two most common neoplastic diseases of the domestic fowl are Marek's disease and leukosis. Both can attack a large number of birds at one time and cause major losses to the poultry industry.

Marek's disease, named after Joseph Marek who described it in 1907, is caused by a herpes virus (Marek's disease virus, or MDV). Upon infection, the virus enters T lymphocytes and transforms them into neoplastic cells, which then lodge in internal organs such as the spleen, gonads, liver, and heart, and form solid neoplasms (lymphomas). The virus is also carried (whether by lymphocytes or by some other means is not known) to at least two other sites of the body—the nerve trunks and the feather-follicle epithelium. In the peripheral nervous system, the virus causes degenerative lesions that paralyze the legs and wings. Whether the lesions are induced by multiplication of the virus or by lymphocytes reacting against the infected cells is not known, but lymphocytes are always associated with the lesions. In the feather-follicle epithelium, the virus multiplies, lyses the infected cells, and is shed with dander. Inhalation of the contaminated dander by other birds spreads the infection through the flock. The disease can be prevented by vaccination of the birds with an attenuated virus. It is so far the only neoplasm that can be prevented by vaccination.

Avian leukosis complex is a group of diseases caused by RNA-containing *avian leukosis viruses* (AVLs), which are related to the C-type viruses responsible for mouse leukemias. There is a large number of these viruses, each causing a somewhat different type of *leukosis*, a disease characterized by abnormal proliferation of lymphopoietic tissues. Depending on the type of tissue affected, one can distinguish *lymphoid leukosis* (with multiple neoplasms forming primarily in internal organs such as spleen and liver), *myelocytomatosis* (a disease involving myelocytes and leading to neoplasms of bone surfaces), *osteopetrosis* (or a "big bone disease," with enlargement of leg bones), and *myeloblastosis* and *erythroblastosis* (affecting progenitor cells of the granulocytic and erythrocytic series, respectively).

Avian leukosis viruses can be divided into two groups—nondefective, which can complete their replication without any help from other viruses, and defective, which are dependent upon products of other viruses for some specific step in their replication. The nondefective viruses induce lymphoid leukosis after long latency periods; the defective viruses induce myeloblastosis or erythroblastosis after short latency periods. The targets of nondefective viruses are the B lymphocytes that reside in the bursa of Fabricius—lymphocytes in early stages of maturation. The targets of the defective viruses are progenitor cells of the erythrocytic and granulocytic lineages (Fig. 5.34).

The main characteristic of neoplastic cells is their unlimited ability to proliferate. But proliferation is also a feature of normal lymphocytes, and experiments have demonstrated that, in tissue culture, lymphocyte proliferation can be maintained over long periods by repeated antigenic stimulation. Furthermore, many

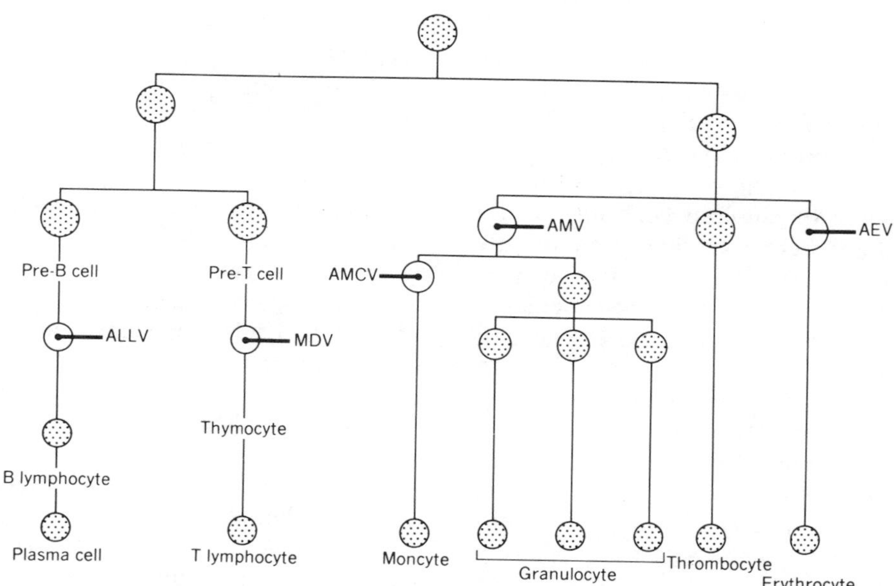

Figure 5.34. Presumed target cells of neoplastic transformation in avian lymphomas. AEV, avian erythroblastosis virus; ALLV, avian lymphoid leukosis virus; AMCV, avian myelocytomatosis virus; AMV, avian myeloblastosis virus; MDV, Marek's disease virus.

lymphoid neoplasms probably begin because of prolonged lymphocyte stimulation and pass through a preneoplastic stage in which they express some, but not all of the neoplastic properties. Thus, there is no sharp dividing line between normal and neoplastic development; the two states merely represent the extreme ends of a continuous spectrum.

5.11 LYMPHOID CELL LINES

For many studies, it is advantageous to maintain lymphocytes and other white blood cells in tissue culture. However, when not stimulated, normal lymphocytes die in culture within a few days. To obtain a *permanent* (*established*) *cell line*—that is, a line that consists of indefinitely dividing cells—lymphocytes must be transformed (altered in their properties). Although this transformation into established cell lines occasionally occurs spontaneously, one must induce transformation chemically or by a virus to obtain high frequencies of transformed cells. The most conspicuous of the cellular changes accompanying transformation are changes in the manner of cell growth and in the number of chromosomes. Nontransformed cells grow to a certain density and then stop dividing. The growth arrest occurs at the point where cells begin to contact each other and establish a single, confluent sheet or *monolayer*—a phenomenon referred to as *contact inhibition*. Following transformation, contact inhibition may become inoperative and cells may show a disorganized, multilayered growth pattern. The chromosomal changes are from diploidy to *heteroploidy*, which can be of two kinds—aneuploidy, which is addition or subtraction of a few chromosomes, or polyploidy, which is multiplication of entire chromosomal sets.

The most reliable test for the occurrence of transformation is inoculation of cultured cells into a histocompatible animal and demonstration of neoplasms at the inoculated site. Human cells, of course, cannot be tested in this manner, but they can be inoculated into athymic (*nu*/*nu*) mice, which tolerate the growth of almost any transplant.

A transformed culture often represents a heterogeneous mixture of cells, from which one can obtain homogeneous cultures by cloning, which involves isolating individual cells or colonies of cells and growing new cultures from them. The ease with which cells grow into colonies is termed *plating efficiency*. Cells in culture have a generation time of about 24 hours. Before they reach their maximum density and stop growing, one must *passage* them by subdividing the culture and starting fresh cultures from each aliquot.

Permanent cultures of lymphoid cells can be obtained either from neoplasms or from normal white blood cells. The first human long-term lymphoid cultures were initiated from the blood of patients with Burkitt's lymphoma or with infectious mononucleosis, a disease characterized by the presence of abnormally large numbers of mononuclear leukocytes in circulation. Since both Burkitt's lymphoma and the tissues of patients with infectious mononucleosis possess the Epstein-Barr virus, this virus is believed to be involved in the in vitro neoplastic transformation process. Indeed, the addition of a cell lysate containing EBV to cultures of normal leukocytes significantly increases the frequency of transformation.

There are more than 1000 permanent human lymphoid (lymphoblast) lines available. Most of the lines have B-cell characteristics (they are DR^+, T^-, E^-, they carry cell-surface immunoglobulins, and some also secrete Ig into the culture fluid), but a few T-cell lines have also been established. In the mouse, most of the existing lines have been derived from lymphomas and so display T-lymphocyte characteristics. Permanent macrophage-like cell lines have been derived either from some murine lymphomas, or by transformation of mouse peritoneal macrophages in vitro with simian virus 40 (SV 40). The characteristics of the lines include phagocytosis of carbon particles or opsonized sheep erythrocytes, production of lysozyme, staining for acid phosphatase, and presence of C3 complement receptors.

5.12 APPENDIX 5.1: REVIEW OF CELL STRUCTURE

The times are long gone when a cell was regarded as a mere bag filled with liquid *cytoplasm* and a grain called a *nucleus*. Transmission electron microscopy has revealed a staggering complexity in the cytoplasm once believed to be homogeneous, and scanning electron microscopy has disclosed a bizarre array of shapes on the cell surface. What the light microscope sometimes shows as a simple ball is often revealed by the electron microscope to resemble some odd creature out of Tolkien's Mirkwood. Figure 5.35 depicts a cell that resembles a lymphocyte and is filled with specialized structures (*organelles*), each concerned with a specific function. The structure and function of the main organelles are described briefly below.

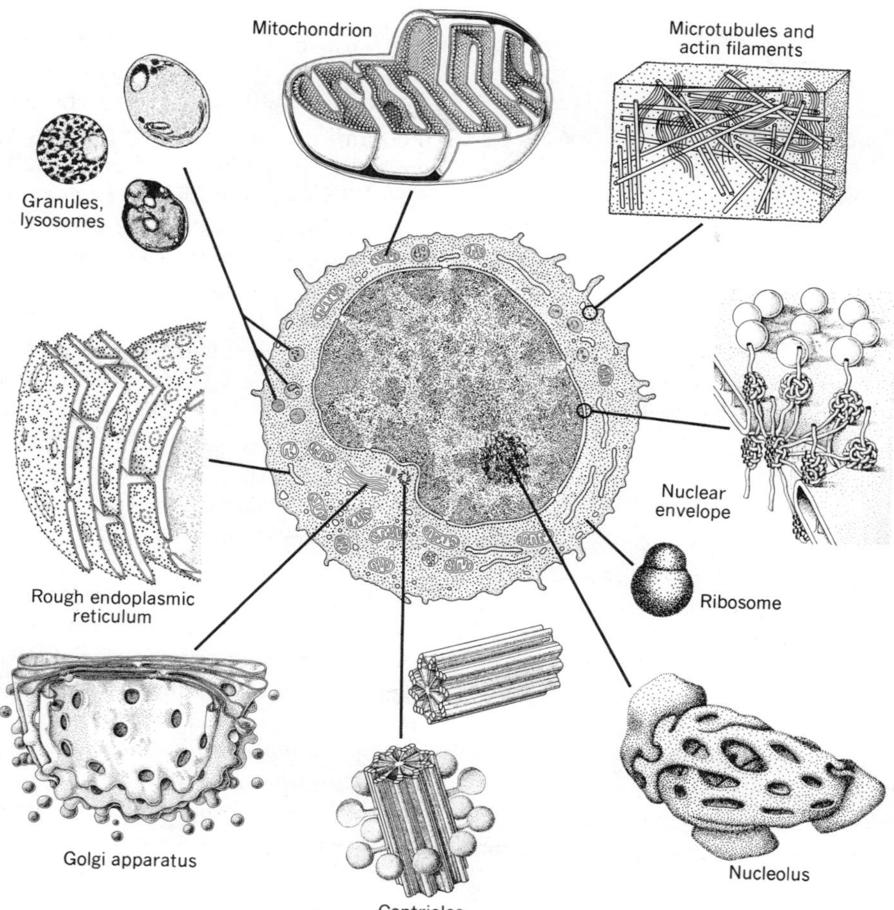

Figure 5.35. The cell and its organelles.

The plasma (cell) membrane envelops the surface of all cells, forming a barrier that determines what can enter or leave the cell. Transmission electron microscopy shows it to have a "butter sandwich" organization, consisting of two densely staining parallel sheets (the two "slices of bread," which, in cross section, look like two parallel lines; cf. Fig. 5.36), separated by a faintly staining inner core (the "butter").

The membrane is composed of lipids and proteins in an approximately 1 : 1 ratio. The two major classes of membrane lipids are cholesterol and phospholipids. *Phospholipids* derive from either *glycerol*, a three-carbon alcohol (and are then referred to as *phosphoglycerides*), or from *sphingosine,* a more complex alcohol (and are then termed *sphingolipids*). The derivation of phosphoglycerides is accomplished by the replacement of two hydroxyl (OH) groups with long-chain fatty acids, and the third group with phosphorylated alcohol:

```
FATTY ACID – G
             L
FATTY ACID – Y
             C
             E
             R
             O – PHOSPHATE + ALCOHOL
             L
```

Diversity of phosphoglycerides is achieved through a variation of the fatty acids and through the attachment of additional groups to the phosphate (Fig. 5.37). The two *fatty acid chains*, each of which contains an even number of carbon atoms (usually between 14 and 24), project from the glycerol backbone in a direction opposite that of the phosphate group. The structure thus

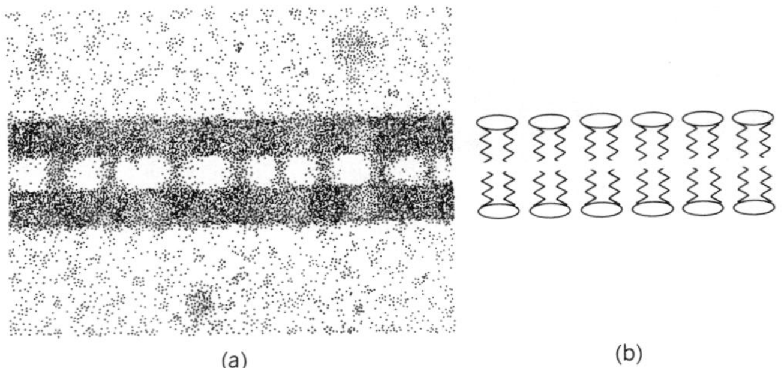

Figure 5.36. Cross section through plasma membrane. (*a*) Sandwichlike structure, as seen through the electron microscope. (*b*) Molecular interpretation of the picture on the left (lipid molecules forming a bilayer).

resembles a tuning fork, the fatty acid chains constituting the prongs and the phosphate group the handle.

The *sphingolipids* are based on the sphingosine molecule, which is an unsaturated aminoglycol with two hydroxyl groups and one amino group (Fig. 5.37). This molecule, too, is shaped like a tuning fork, but only one of the two prongs (15-carbon fatty acid) is constant, while the second prong is variable. The latter can be of several fatty acids attached to the sphingosine backbone through the amino group. The handle of the spingolipid molecule may be phosphate and cholin (*sphingomyelin*), a simple hydroxyl (*ceramids*), a simple sugar (*cerebrosides*), or a complex polysaccharide (*gangliosides*).

Cholesterol (Fig. 5.37), a steroid, is abundant in membranes of erythrocytes, liver cells, and myelinated nerve cells.

When separated, the prongs and handles behave differently. The prongs mix freely with (are soluble in) organic solvents such as ether or chloroform but do not mix with (are insoluble in) water; the handles, on the other hand, are insoluble in organic solvents, but dissolve readily in water. The difference in solubility is explained by the electrical properties of the two fragments. In the phosphate groups, the negatively charged electrons are asymmetrically distributed in relation to the positively charged nuclei, so that the whole group is *polar*: one region carries a negative and the other a positive charge. Because water molecules are also strongly polarized, they are attracted to the polar phosphate groups (the groups are water-loving, or *hydrophilic*, from Gr. *hydōr*, water, *philos*, fond). In the fatty acid chains the electrons are symmetrically distributed around the nuclei so that the chains are *nonpolar* and repel water (they are water-abhorrent, or *hydrophobic*, from Gr. *phobos*, fear). A molecule with one hydrophilic and one hydrophobic end is termed *amphipathic* (Gr. *amphi*, two-sided).

When a lipid comes into contact with an aqueous medium, the hydrocarbon tails try to avoid the water, while the polar heads of each molecule show affinity for it. To satisfy both preferences, the lipid molecules arrange themselves in one of two structures. A small number of lipid molecules form a *micelle* (L. *micella*, small morsel, grain), a spherical aggregate in which the hydrophobic tails are directed inward and the polar heads outward toward the aqueous environment (Fig. 5.38*a*). A large number of lipid molecules aggregate into a *bilayer* (Fig. 5.38*b* and *c*), in which lipid molecules form two sheets. In each sheet the hydrophilic heads are on the outside and the hydrophobic tails are facing each other on the inner surface of the bilayer. It is this arrangement that constitutes the basic structure of the plasma membrane and gives the membrane its characteristic appearance in cross section. In electron-microscopic preparations, the polar groups in the lipid bilayer combine easily with heavy, strongly electron-scattering metal atoms of the fixative, and produce the typical densely stained double line.

The *membrane proteins* fall into two categories, integral and peripheral. The *integral proteins* (Fig. 5.39) are usually amphipathic, and their hydrophobic portions penetrate deeply into the hydrophobic part of the lipid bilayer. Because of this characteristic, they can be liberated from the membrane by reagents that disrupt hydrophobic interactions (e.g., detergents or organic solvents). The hydrophilic moiety of an integral protein usually protrudes into the aqueous medium surrounding the membrane. The *peripheral proteins* (Fig. 5.39) do not penetrate the membrane, but are held at the membrane surface by predominantly electrostatic interactions, and can therefore be isolated, using reagents that disrupt these interactions (e.g., a high ionic-strength solution of NaCl).

In the *fluid mosaic model* of the plasma membrane, the lipids are visualized as constituting a "sea," with protein "icebergs" floating in it (Fig. 5.39). According to this model, cell membranes are dynamic structures, in which both lipids and proteins are in constant motion. The rapidity of this motion depends on the composition of the fatty acid chains (the chain length and degree of saturation: the longer the chains and the more saturated, the more strongly they interact with one another and the more they decrease the fluidity of the bilayer), temperature (with increased temperature the lipids become more viscous and the membrane more fluid), and other factors.

Bilayers resembling the plasma membrane can also

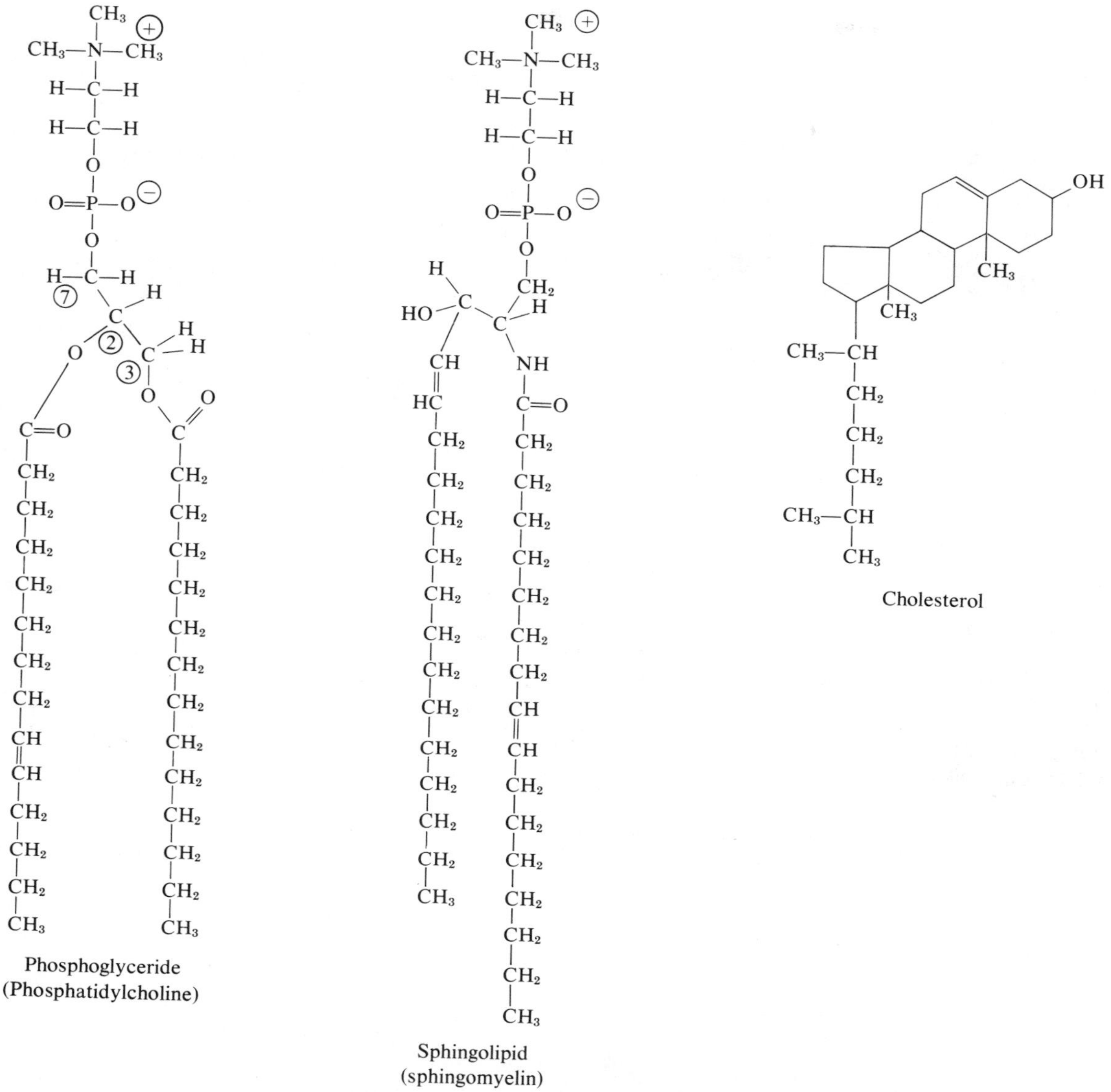

Phosphoglyceride
(Phosphatidylcholine)

Sphingolipid
(sphingomyelin)

Cholesterol

Figure 5.37. Lipids of the cell membrane.

be generated artificially in the form of *liposomes* (lipid vesicles). Liposomes are small (several hundred Ångström units in diameter), spherical or slightly elongated pouches, consisting of a lipid bilayer and enclosed aqueous compartment (Fig. 5.38*d*). They can be produced by dispersing a lipid in an aqueous solution (for example, by sonication[1] or by injection through a fine needle). By dispersing other molecules, in addition to the lipids, in the solution, one can incorporate them into the aqueous compartment or even into the lipid bilayer of the liposome. Antigen-containing liposomes are increasingly used in a variety of immunological studies.

The cytoskeleton is a network of fine cables and

[1] Ultrasound passing through a solution induces several complex phenomena, the most important of which is *cavitation*. As the sound wave passes through the liquid, the succession of positive and negative pressures produces cavities, which become filled with gas dissolved in the liquid. The cavities expand and then collapse violently, producing surface changes that result in disperson of the lipid (or other substances) in the solution. This dispersion by ultrasound is referred to as *sonication*.

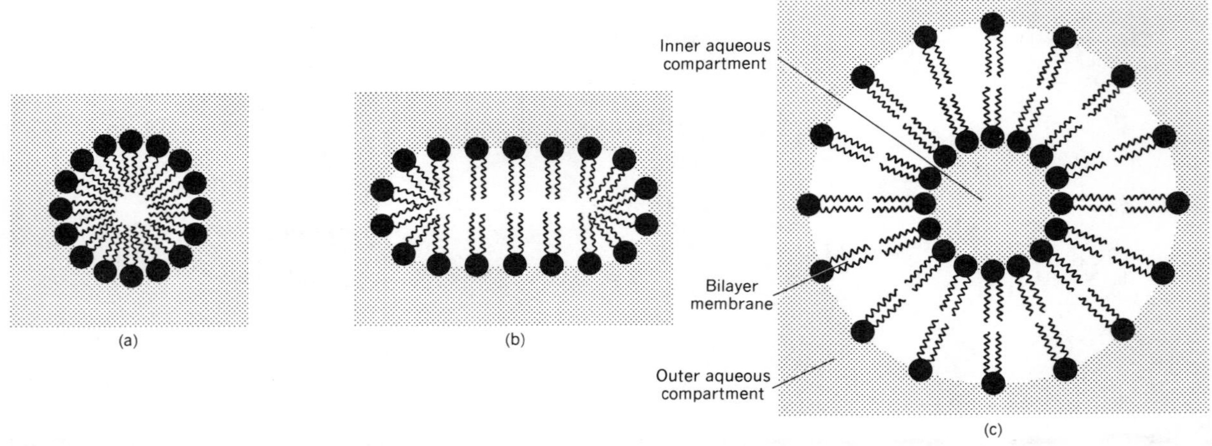

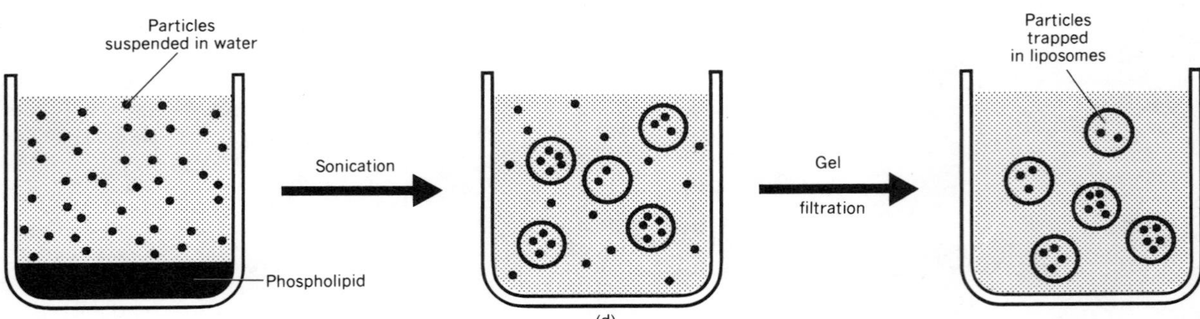

Figure 5.38. Formation of micelles and liposomes. Micelles (*a*, *b*), liposome (*c*), and preparation of liposome-containing particle (*d*). (*d* modified from L. Stryer: *Biochemistry*. Freeman, San Francisco, 1975.)

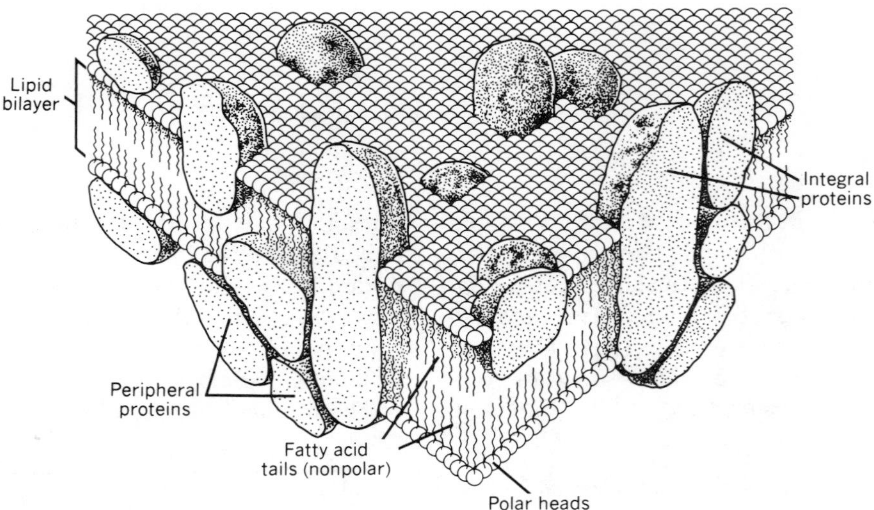

Figure 5.39. The fluid mosaic model of the cell membrane. In the sea of phospholipids and cholesterol float icebergs of proteins. (Modified from R. V. Krstić: *Ultrastruktur der Säugetiere*. Springer-Verlag, Berlin, 1976.)

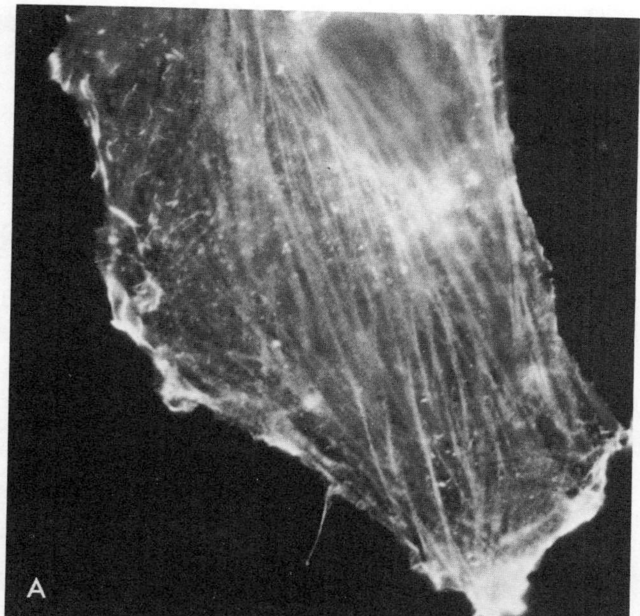

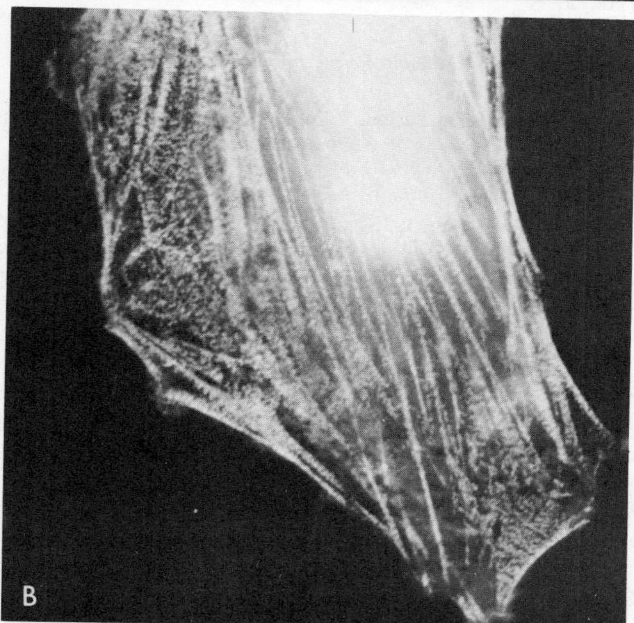

Figure 5.40. The cytoskeleton. A normal rat kidney fibroblast stained with fluorescein-labeled antibodies to actin (*a*) and myosin (*b*). (Courtesy of Drs. M. H. Heggeness, J. F. Ash, and S. J. Singer; magnification ×1000.)

fibers traversing the cell interior (Fig. 5.40). The cables are of two kinds—actin filaments and microtubules. The basic subunit of the *actin filaments* is *actin*, a water-soluble, small-molecular-weight (42,000 daltons) protein that polymerizes to form filaments in the presence of salt. The polymerization involves adenosine triphosphate (ATP) and divalent cations such as Ca^{2+}. (One molecule of ATP is split for each actin bond, and in the polymerized form, each actin monomer has one adenosine-diphosphate group bound to it.) Pairs of filaments then associate into double helical cables. The basic subunit of the *microtubules* is *tubulin*, a protein with molecules consisting of two different monomers (the basic molecule is a heterodimer), each with a molecular weight of about 55,000 daltons. Polymerization of heterodimers into microtubules involves splitting of guanosine triphosphate (GTP) and binding of guanosine diphosphate groups to subunits. Both actin filaments and microtubules grow by self-assembly. The cytoskeleton maintains the shape of the cell and is essential for the cell's motility. (Microtubules are also required for the motility of cilia and flagella.)

The nucleus is one of the most conspicuous and constant cell organelles. It is bound by a *nuclear envelope*, consisting of two membranes separated by a *perinuclear space*. The two membranes are continuous with the membranes of the endoplasmic reticulum (see below) and are perforated by relatively large (600 Å in diameter) openings called *nuclear pores*. These consist of membranous cylinders that pierce the envelope and an inner complex structure of threads woven into several knots (Fig. 5.35). The pores are the gates through which material flows between the nucleus and the cytoplasm. Most of the inner nuclear space is taken up by *chromatin*, consisting of partially or completely uncoiled chromosomal fibers. There are two kinds of chromatin—the more coiled, more darkly staining, genetically inactive *heterochromatin*, and the less coiled, faintly staining, genetically active *euchromatin*. The spaces between the chromatin fibers are filled with a fluid component called *nuclear sap* (nucleoplasm). Each nucleus contains one or more *nucleoli* (plural of nucleolus), which are the sites of ribosomal RNA synthesis. In the electron microscope the nucleolus appears as a knot of granular strands (*nucleolonema*, from Gr. *nema*, thread) embedded in an amorphous substance (*pars amorpha*). The nucleolus is connected to the chromatin of one or more chromosomes—the *nucleolus organizer region*.

The *endoplasmic reticulum* is a maze of membrane-bound lamellae, cisternae, flattened sacs, vesicles, and intricate passageways embedded in the cell's cytoplasm. It was so named because originally it was believed to exist only in the inner portion of the cytoplasm (endoplasm); when later studies proved it to be present in the outer ectoplasm as well, it was too late to change the designation. It exists in two forms—the ribosome-studded *rough endoplasmic reticulum* (RER) and the ribosome-free *smooth endoplasmic reticulum* (SER). The extent of ER development varies from cell to cell, depending on the cell's functional status. The RER represents the channel system for intracellular transport, and is the site of protein synthesis and secretion and the anchoring site of many enzymes involved in cellular metabolism. The SER is believed to be involved in steroid and glycogen metabolism.

The Golgi apparatus, named after the Italian microscopist Camillo Golgi, is a highly variable cell organelle concerned with secretion. It consists of several membrane-bound, perforated lamellae, stacked upon one another like the leaves of a book. At the "margins," vesicles containing various secretions are constantly pinched off. The cuplike Golgi apparatus usually lies near the nucleus, which it faces with its concave side and with which it is connected via the endoplasmic reticulum. The extent of Golgi-apparatus development depends on the cell's synthetic and secretory activity. Some cells have only one apparatus, others have several such organelles, interconnected by complicated channel systems.

Lysosomes are vesicles filled with enzymes. They come in different sizes and with varying content, depending on their function. The enzymes are synthesized on the rough endoplasmic reticulum and then packaged into lysosomal bags. The main function of lysosomes is intracellular digestion.

Ribosomes are small organelles consisting of ribosomal RNA and protein, organized into two subunits—a large and a small particle. They exist either freely in the cytoplasm, or attached to the outer surface of the rough endoplasmic reticulum. They are the main chemical factories of protein synthesis, a process during which they line up in single file on the string of messenger RNA, forming *polyribosomes* (polysomes).

Centrioles are cylindrical organelles, located in the vicinity of the nucleus, often in the concave region of the Golgi apparatus. Each cell has two, positioned at right angles to each other. The wall of the centriole cylinder consists of nine parallel microtubule triplets interconnected by lamellae of an electron-dense substance; individual triplets are also connected, by the same substance with the center of the cylinder (like spokes of a wheel; see Fig. 5.35). The cylinder is closed at one end and open at the other. Centrioles are relatively autonomous organelles that contain their own DNA and are self-replicating. During mitosis, the centrioles migrate to opposite poles of the cell and organize the *mitotic spindle*—the array of microtubular *spindle fibers* that pulls chromosomes apart into the forming daughter cells. The region of cytoplasm that contains the centrioles is called the *centrosome* or the *cytocentrum*.

Mitochondria are membrane-bound, oblong organelles concentrated primarily in those regions of the cytoplasm where there is a high energy demand. Their main function is to trap and release chemical energy. They have a complex, compartmentalized, highly variable structure; they contain their own DNA, and they can replicate independently of cell division.

Inclusions of other types—granules, crystals, vacuoles, fat globules, and others—are also present in many cells. Some of these we have already mentioned; others will be discussed in subsequent chapters.

REFERENCES

General

Bessis, M.: *Blood Smears Reinterpreted.* Springer International, Berlin, 1977.

Goldschneider, I. and Barton, R. W.: Development and differentiation of lymphocytes. In G. Poste and G. L. Nicolson (Eds.): *The Cell Surface in Animal Embryogenesis and Development*, pp. 599–695. North-Holland, Amsterdam, 1976.

Greaves, M. F., Owen, J. J. T., and Raff, M. C.: *T and B Lymphocytes: Origins, Properties and Roles in Immune Responses*. Excerpta Medica, Amsterdam, 1973.

Hayward, A. R.: *Immunodeficiency*. Arnold, London, 1977.

Katz, D. H.: *Lymphocyte Differentiation, Recognition, and Regulation*. Academic, New York, 1977.

Krstić, R. V.: *Die Gewebe des Menschen und der Säugetiere*. Springer-Verlag, Berlin, 1978.

Lennert, K.: *Malignant Lymphomas Other Than Hodgkin's Disease.* Springer-Verlag, Berlin, 1978.

Lenz, T. L.: *Cell Fine Structure*. Saunders, Philadelphia, 1971.

Metcalf, D. and Moore, M. A. S.: *Haemopoietic Cells*. North-Holland, Amsterdam, 1971.

Quesenberry, P. and Levitt, L.: Hematopoietic stem cells. *New Engl. J. Med.* **301**:755–760, 1979.

Twomey, J. J. and Good, R. A. (Eds.): *The Immunopathology of Lymphoreticular Neoplasms*. Plenum, New York, 1978.

Original Articles

Bruton, O. C.: Agammaglobulinemia. *Pediatrics* **9**:722–728, 1952.

Burkitt, D.: A sarcoma involving the jaws in African children. *Br. J. Surg.* **46**:218–223, 1958.

Cantor, H. and Boyse, E. A.: Functional subclasses of T lymphocytes bearing different Ly antigens. I. The generation of functionally distinct T-cell subclasses in a differentiative process independent of antigen. *J. Exp. Med.* **141**:1376–1389, 1975.

Cantor, H. and Boyse, E. A.: Functional subclasses of T lymphocytes bearing different Ly antigens. II. Cooperation between subclasses of Ly^+ cells in the generation of killer activity. *J. Exp. Med.* **141:**1390–1399, 1975.

Ford, C. E.: Traffic of lymphoid cells in the body. *In* G. E. Wolstenholme and R. Porter (Eds.): *The Thymus. Experimental and Clinical Studies. Ciba Foundation Symposium*, pp. 131–152, Churchill, London, 1966.

Ford, W. L., Gowans, J. L., and McCullagh, P. J.: The origin and function of lymphocytes. *In* G. E. Wolstenholme and R. Porter (Eds.): *The Thymus. Experimental and Clinical Studies. Ciba Foundation Symposium*, pp. 58–79, Churchill, London, 1966.

Gowans, J. L. and Knight, E. J.: The route of recirculation of lymphocytes in the rat. *Proc. R. Soc. Lond.* (*Biol.*) **159:**257–81, 1964.

Gross, L.: A filterable agent, recovered from A K-leukemic extracts, causing salivary gland carcinomas in C_3H mice. *Proc. Soc. Exp. Biol. Med.* **83:**914–2121, 1953.

Hodgkin, T.: On some morbid appearance of the absorbent glands and spleen. *Med. Chir. Trans.* **17:**68–114, 1832.

Langerhans, P.: Ueber die Nerven der menschlichen Haut. *Virchow Arch. Pathol. Anat. Physiol.* **44:**325–337, 1868.

Moore, M. A. S. and Owen, J. J. T.: Chromosome marker studies on the development of the haemopoietic system in the chick embryo. *Nature* **208:**989–990, 1965.

Moore, M. A. S. and Owen, J. J. T.: Experimental studies on the development of the thymus. *J. Exp. Med.* **126:**715–725, 1967.

Owen, J. J. T. and Ritter, M. A.: Tissue interaction in the development of thymus lymphocytes. *J. Exp. Med.* **129:**431–437, 1969.

Perlman, P. and Holm, G.: *In* P. Miescher and P. Grabar (Eds.): *Mechanisms of Inflammation Induced by Immune Reactions*, p. 325–341, Schwabe, Basel, 1968.

Steinman, R. M. and Cohn, Z. A.: Identification of a novel cell type in peripheral lymphoid organs of mice. I. Morphology, quantitation, tissue distribution. *J. Exp. Med.* **137:**1142–1162, 1973.

Till, J. E. and McCulloch, E. A.: A direct measurement of the radiation sensitivity of normal mouse bone marrow cells. *Rad. Res.* **14:**213–219, 1961.

Wu, A. M., Till, J. E., Siminovitch, L., and McCulloch, E. A.: A cytological study of the capacity for differentiation of normal hemopoietic colony-forming cells. *J. Cell Physiol.* **69:**177–184, 1967.

Wu, A. M., Till, J. E., Siminovitch, L., and McCulloch, E. A.: Cytological evidence for a relationship between normal hematopoietic colony-forming cells and cells of the lymphoid system. *J. Exp. Med.* **127:**455–463, 1968.

CHAPTER 6

IMMUNOGLOBULINS AND B-CELL RECEPTORS

We have now reached the last of the Chinese boxes we have been opening, one after another, in this second movement of the book: having discussed organisms, organs, and cells, we have only the molecules to deal with. Immunologically important molecules, like all other molecules of the body, are manufactured by cells and either secreted into bodily fluids or displayed on cell surfaces. In this chapter, we shall discuss molecules called immunoglobulins, which are manufactured by B lymphocytes or their differentiated progeny, the plasma cells. But before we do so, we have to learn a few things about the blood, the fluid in which most immunoglobulins are dissolved. In the next chapter, we shall deal with molecules manufactured by T lymphocytes.

6.1 INTRODUCTION

6.1.1 Blood, Plasma, Serum, Antibodies

Blood consists of cells and a fluid phase, *plasma*, in which the cellular elements are suspended (Fig. 6.1). When drawn into a test tube, blood changes within six minutes from a liquid to a semisolid gel, a *clot*, which later shrinks and squeezes out a straw-colored fluid—the *serum*. The clotting (coagulation), is initiated by the interaction of blood with the glass or plastic surface of the test tube; when the surface is covered with paraffin, clotting does not occur. Since the clotting reactions require calcium ions, clotting can be prevented by the addition to the blood of chelating agents such as ethylenediaminetetraacetic acid (EDTA) or of soluble citrates, oxalates, and fluorides, which bind calcium or change it to a nonionized form. The relationship among blood, plasma, and serum can be summarized as follows:

plasma = blood minus cells
serum = plasma minus clotting factors.

Plasma constitutes slightly more than half the blood's total volume. It consists mostly of water (more than 90 percent), the rest being proteins (7 percent), carbohydrates, lipids, and mineral salts. Plasma plays a role in defense reactions, transports digested food from the small intestine to the tissues, transports wastes from the tissues to the kidneys, and delivers hormones to target tissues. It contains several hundred proteins, and sorting out such a diversified mixture of molecules is a formidable task that can be accomplished only by combining the variety of biochemical and immunological techniques described in the appendices of this chapter and of Chapter 10. The crudest separation of

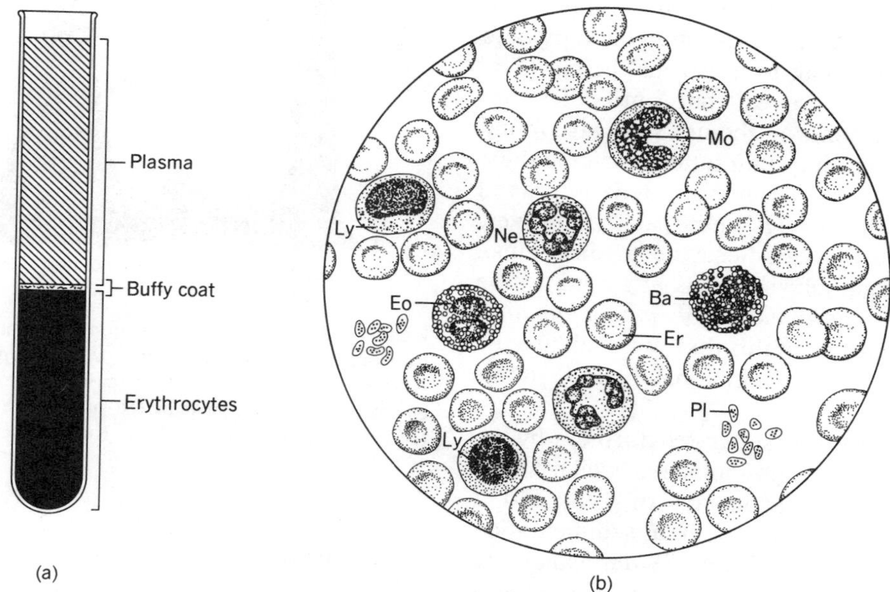

Figure 6.1. Composition of blood. (*a*) Blood drawn into a test tube containing an anti-clotting agent (after centrifugation): the plasma separates from the cellular components (erythrocytes and white cells in the buffy coat). (*b*) Cellular elements as seen on a blood smear under the microscope. Ba, basophils; Eo, eosinophils; Er, erythrocytes; Ly, lymphocytes; Mo, monocytes; Ne, neutrophils; Pl, platelets.

plasma proteins is achieved by the addition to the plasma or serum of neutral salts, such as ammonium or sodium sulfates. The salt precipitates out (renders insoluble) one fraction of plasma proteins, *globulins*, while leaving another fraction, *albumins*, in solution.

Albumins and globulins differ not only in their solubility but also in their net charges, and this latter property can be used for further protein fractionation. The introduction of an electric current into the plasma (*electrophoresis*) separates globulins into three main fractions, denoted α, β, and γ, in order of their decreasing mobility in the electric field (Fig. 6.2*a*). When more than three globulin fractions are resolved, they are referred to by numbers added to the Greek letter (e.g., $\alpha 1$, $\alpha 2$, $\beta 1$, $\beta 2$, and so on). After the injection of an antigen into an animal (*immunization*), the electrophoretic profile of the recipient's serum may change in a manner depicted in Figure 6.2*b*: the γ-globulin peak, normally only slightly higher than the α and β peaks, increases disproportionately. Such a serum can be shown, by one of the many techniques discussed in the appendix to Chapter 10, to react specifically with the immunizing antigen, while no such reactivity can be demonstrated in the serum obtained prior to immunization. The antigen-reactive substance in the serum is referred to as *antibody* and the antibody-containing serum as *antiserum* (in contradistinction to *normal serum*, which does not contain antibody to a given antigen). The addition of the antigen to the antiserum—as first demonstrated by Tiselius and Kabat (see Chapter 2)—removes antibody activity and reduces the γ-globulin peak to its normal height (Fig. 6.2). This experiment proves that antibodies are γ-globulins. Although some antibodies were also found later in the slowly migrating subfraction of β-globulins, the overwhelming majority of antibody activity proved to be associated with the γ-globulin peak. However, not all γ-globulins are antibodies, and to distinguish antibody-containing globulins from other globulins, the former are referred to as *immune globulins* or *immunoglobulins* (abbreviated Ig). In this text, we shall use the terms "antibody" and "immunoglobulin" interchangeably.

Immunoglobulins can be separated further, by ultracentrifugation, into a high-molecular-weight fraction with a sedimentation constant of 19S, and a low-molecular-weight fraction with a sedimentation constant of 7S. The terms *19S* and *7S antibodies* are often used in reference to these fractions. Sometimes one can also distinguish a third fraction with a sedimentation constant falling somewhere between those of the first two fractions.

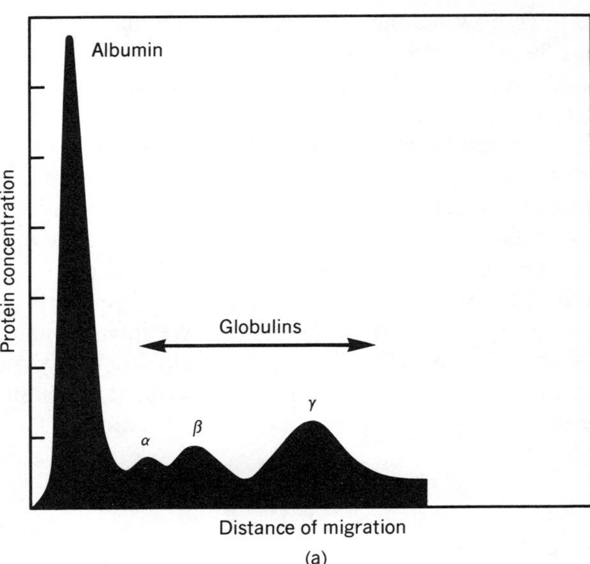

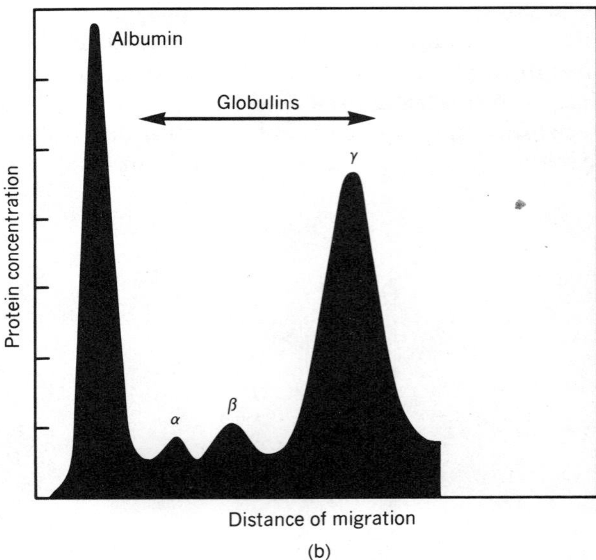

Figure 6.2. Serum fractionation by moving-boundary electrophoresis. (*a*) Normal serum. (*b*) Immune serum (antiserum). After absorption of the antiserum by the immunizing antigen, the electrophoretic pattern depicted in *b* changes to that seen in *a*. (Based on A. Tiselius and E.A. Kabat: *J. Exp. Med.* **69**:119–131, 1939.)

6.1.2 Homo- and Heterogeneity

There are some 10^{16} immunoglobulin molecules in each milliliter of normal serum. Were all these molecules of one kind, biochemists would have little trouble in studying them; but since they constitute a heterogeneous mixture, their analysis is a complicated matter. How many kinds (species) of Ig molecule are in the serum is not known, but a figure of 1×10^6 is probably not an unreasonable estimate (see section 6.8). Were the different kinds of molecule equally represented (which they are not), there would be about 100 molecules of each kind in one milliliter of serum. Even if one were to use liters of serum, the number of molecules of one kind would still be too small for any biochemist to work with. Fortunately, there are ways of increasing the concentration of a single kind of Ig so that it becomes a predominant, easily purifiable component of the serum, referred to as *homogeneous antibody* (immunoglobulin). The three main sources of homogeneous antibodies are sera (or urine) of patients (animals) with plasma-cell neoplasms, sera from certain immunizations, and hybridomas.

Homogeneous Antibodies Produced by Plasma-Cell Neoplasms. Plasma-cell neoplasms occur in both humans and certain animals. While normal plasma cells produce a certain amount of immunoglobulin and then die, neoplastic plasma cells (myeloma cells) may proliferate and synthesize antibodies indefinitely. The products of myeloma cells are referred to as *myeloma proteins* when found in the serum, and as *Bence-Jones proteins* when detected in the urine. The former are often normal immunoglobulins with antigen-binding ability; the latter are Ig fragments (so-called light chains). We shall describe both the myeloma and the Bence-Jones proteins in more detail in section 6.12.

Homogeneous Antibodies Produced by Immunization. In most immunizations, the antigen stimulates many different B-lymphocyte clones, each capable, after differentiation into plasma cells, of producing a different kind of antibody. The result is a heterogeneous mixture of immunoglobulins with different specificities. When one subjects an antiserum produced by such an immunization to zone electrophoresis (see Appendix 6.1), a broad, diffuse band, typical of heterogeneous protein mixtures, forms in the γ-globulin region. Occasionally, however, immunization with a certain antigen either stimulates a single B-cell clone or creates conditions for the predominance of one or a few clones that produce antibodies with restricted heterogeneity. When electrophoresed, such antibodies form a sharp band similar to that formed, for example, by the homogeneous albumin. Why most immunizations stimulate multiple clones while some activate only a few is not known. The conditions leading to the production of homogeneous antibodies must, therefore, be found by trial and error. Because homogeneous antibodies are often produced after immunization with polysaccharides consisting of repeating determinants, some immunologists believe that determinant homogeneity is one of the factors that sways immune response toward monoclonality. This explanation, however, fails in those instances where homogeneous antibodies arise against relatively complex and heterogeneous antigens. The tendency toward monoclonal antibody response must be controlled genetically, since rabbits, for example, can be bred for homogeneous antibody production, and since certain inbred mouse strains produce homogeneous antibodies when immunized with certain antigens, while others do not. Some of the best-known examples of homogeneous antibodies are rabbit antibodies produced to heat-killed, pepsin-digested streptococci, or rabbit and mouse antibodies to various haptens such as p-azobenzoate, p-azobenzenarsonate or dinitrophenyl. Work on homogeneous antibodies has been pioneered by Richard M. Krause, Klaus Eichmann, and Alfred Nisonoff.

Monoclonal Antibodies Produced by Hybridomas. The most promising means of homogeneous antibody production was developed by George Köhler and César Milstein in 1975. In this method, one fuses (hybridizes) two somatic cells, one belonging to a neoplastic myeloma cell line and the other representing a normal B lymphocyte obtained from an immunized animal. The resulting *hybridoma* inherits the capacity for continuous growth from the neoplastic parent and the ability to secrete antibodies to the immunizing antigen from the B cell. Since the hybridoma is derived from a single B lymphocyte, it produces only one kind of antibody, which is equivalent to that produced by a single clone and is hence referred to as *monoclonal antibody*. The procedure for producing antibody-secreting hybridomas is described in the Appendix 6.15.2.

6.1.3 Isolation of Immunoglobulins

There are many ways of separating 7S immunoglobulins from other globulins and from albumins. One of the more frequently used methods is a combination of salt fractionation and ion-exchange chromatography (for a description of these techniques, see the Appendix 6.14.2). The method consists of three steps. First, one adds ammonium sulfate (or some other neutral salt) to the serum, precipitating the globulins while leaving the albumin in solution. In the second step, one separates the precipitate by centrifugation, redissolves it, and dialyzes the solution against a phosphate buffer, removing all small-molecular-weight contaminants. In the third step, one passes the redissolved globulins through a DEAE-cellulose column equilibrated with phosphate buffer. The pH and ionic strength of the column can be adjusted by pre-equilibration so that all the globulins in the solution bind to the cellulose except immunoglobulins, which pass through the column and are collected in a relatively pure form. However, not all the immunoglobulins pass through, so the method is good only for the isolation of some Ig classes.

6.1.4 Unraveling of the Basic Immunoglobulin Molecule

Working with purified 7S immunoglobulins, Rodney R. Porter demonstrated in 1959 that papain, an enzyme isolated from the latex of *Carica papaya*, splits the basic molecule into three pieces, of approximately equal size (molecular weight of about 45,000 daltons; Fig. 6.3). Two of these pieces retain the antibody's ability to combine with an antigen and are therefore referred to as *Fab fragments* (for "fragment antigen binding"). Since these fragments can bind but cannot precipitate the antigen, they must be univalent—they possess only one *combining site* each. (At least two combining sites are needed for precipitation, presumably to bridge two antigen molecules; see Chapter 10 for further details.) The unfragmented basic Ig molecule, which can both bind and precipitate an antigen, is *bivalent*—it contains two combining sites.

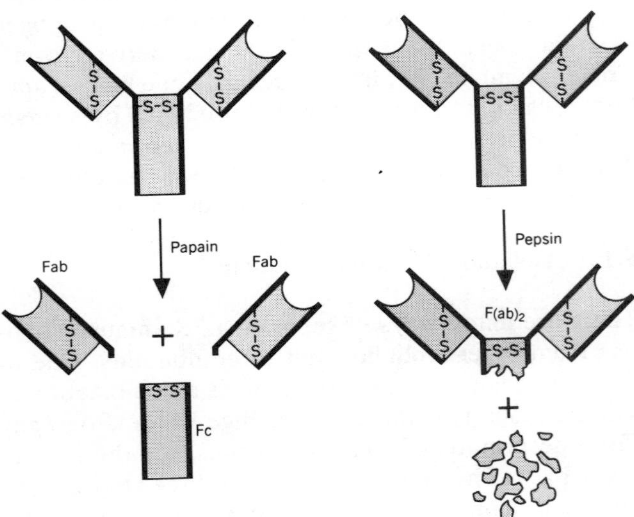

Figure 6.3. Fragmentation of rabbit IgG molecules by proteolytic enzymes.

The third fragment produced by papain digestion differs from the two Fab fragments in that it can be crystallized from a solution. Porter therefore referred to it as *Fc* (for "fragment crystalline"). Since crystals form easily only from identical molecules, the crystallization of Fc fragments suggests that the fragments do not vary much from antibody to antibody. By the same token, the inability to crystallize Fab fragments (or the whole Ig molecule, for that matter) indicates that they are responsible for most of the antibody variability and heterogeneity.

Treatment with pepsin, another proteolytic (peptide bond-splitting) enzyme, breaks the part of the basic Ig molecule corresponding to the Fc fragment into several small pieces and leaves the rest of the molecule intact (Fig. 6.3). The remaining large fragment has a molecular weight approximately double that of one Fab fragment; it also has the ability to bind and precipitate an antigen, indicating that it possesses two combining sites. Because it consists of two Fab fragments joined by a covalent bond, it is referred to as $F(ab)_2$. The two enzymes thus act on approximately the same region of the Ig molecule, but one (papain) splits the molecule on one side and the other (pepsin) on the other side of the bond that holds the two Fab fragments together.

In 1959, Gerald M. Edelman demonstrated that treatment of the basic Ig molecule with mercaptoethanol, an agent that breaks disulfide (—S—S—) bridges, reduces the size of the molecule, apparently by dissociating it into its subunit chains. Subsequent studies revealed the existence of four such chains in each molecule, two with molecular weights of about 53,000 daltons each and another two with molecular weights of about 22,000 daltons each. The two larger chains have been denoted as *heavy* (H) and the two smaller as *light* (L).

Mercaptoethanol treatment of Fab fragments yields two chains from each fragment—one that has the molecular weight of an L chain, and another (referred to as the *Fd fragment* simply because d is the next letter in the alphabet after a, b, and c) that is slightly heavier than the L chain.

On the basis of this information, Porter proposed, in 1962, a model of the basic Ig molecule that proved to be essentially correct. According to this model (Fig. 6.4), the molecule consists of four polypeptide chains—two identical H chains and two identical L chains—held together by disulfide bridges. The molecule has two combining sites, each carried by one of

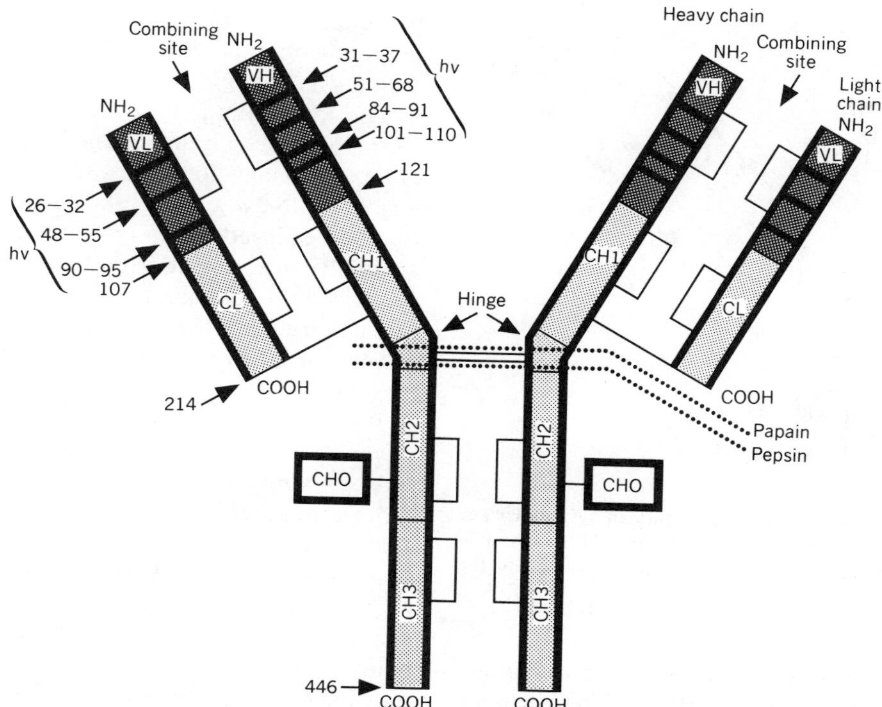

Figure 6.4. Diagram of human immunoglobulin G molecule. Thick lines indicate polypeptide chains, thin lines indicate positions of disulfide bridges, dotted lines indicate positions of enzymatic cleavage, and numbers indicate amino acid residues. C, constant region; CHO, carbohydrate; COOH, carboxyl terminal; H, heavy chain; L, light chain; NH_2, amino terminal; V, variable region.

the two Fab fragments, each of which consists of one complete L chain and approximately half the H chain (the Fd fragment).

The first Ig polypeptide to be sequenced completely was an L chain of a Bence-Jones protein. A comparison of the sequence of two different L chains by Norbert Hilschmann and Lyman C. Craig revealed that the two chains were identical starting with the amino acid in position 107 at the C terminal of the molecule, and totally different from the N terminal to the residue in position 106. The L chain could thus be divided into two segments—a *variable* (*V*) *region*, showing wide variation in amino acid sequence from one molecule to another, and a *constant* (*C*) *region*, which is unvarying except for minor inherited differences. Edelman and his co-workers demonstrated that similar regions existed in the heavy chain. To distinguish them, those in the light chain are designated VL and CL and those in the heavy chain VH and CH. Following the sequencing of an entire Ig molecule by Edelman and his co-workers in 1969, Edelman and W. Einar Gall noticed that each Ig polypeptide chain could be divided into *homology regions* or *domains*, each domain consisting of approximately 110 to 120 amino acids (molecular weight of 10,000 to 12,000 daltons). When one aligns the different domains so as to show maximum homology with one another, one discovers that any two of them share up to 30 percent of their amino acids. Each light chain contains two domains—one in the V region (VL) and the other in the C (CL)—whereas each heavy chain consists of four domains—one VH and three CH (CH1, CH2, and CH3).

Papain is an enzyme with relatively broad specificity for peptide bonds. The fact that it splits only one peptide bond of several hundred in the four Ig polypeptide chains indicates that most bonds are inaccessible to enzymatic digestion, probably because the chains are folded into globular structures. Each domain is believed to be folded into one such globule so that the entire molecule consists of 12 globules (Fig. 6.5). The folding occurs around intrachain disulfide bridges, of which each homology region contains at least one. The region in which disulfide bridges form *between* the two heavy chains (the site of the papain and pepsin attack)

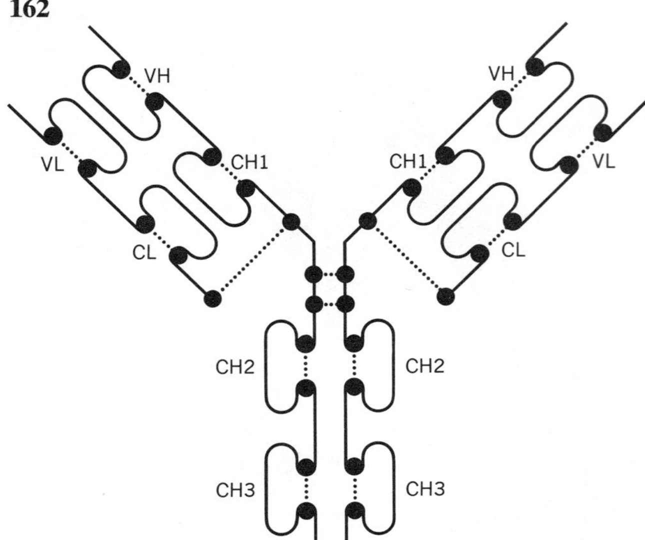

Figure 6.5. Schematic representation of a human IgG molecule, showing looping out of the polypeptide chains around the disulfide bridges (indicated by dotted lines). Thick black dots indicate the position of half-cystine residues.

is relatively unfolded and highly flexible, an arrangement that allows the arms formed by the Fab fragments to move in space in relation to each other, rather like butterfly wings. Because of this "swivel" function, the unfolded segment is termed the *hinge region*.

6.1.5 Discovery of Human Immunoglobulin Classes and Subclasses

Shortly after Tiselius had separated serum globulins in an electric field into the α, β, and γ fractions and Tiselius and Kabat had found antibody activity in the γ fraction, ultracentrifugation studies revealed that most of the antibody that contained γ-globulins had a sedimentation constant of 7S. Two characteristics, the migration rate in an electric field and the sedimentation rate in a gravity field, thus defined the first group or *class* of immunoglobulin molecules, referred to as IgG (Latin *G* corresponds to the Greek γ).

The discovery of the second immunoglobulin class came about as follows. In 1937, Michael Heidelberger and K. O. Pedersen discovered that sera of horses immunized to pneumococcus polysaccharide contained about 10 percent γ-globulin that had a much higher sedimentation constant (approximately 19S) than the other γ-globulins. In 1944, J. Waldenström found large amounts of this heavy-molecular-weight γ-globulin in the sera of patients with a malignant disease of the lymphoid cells (see section 6.12). When, in 1956, H. F. Deutsch and his co-workers found similar γ-globulin fractions in normal human sera too, it became apparent that there was, in addition to IgG, a group of larger immunoglobulins, and these were referred to as *macroglobulins*, or IgM.

The third immunoglobulin class was discovered in 1953 by Pierre Grabar and C. A. Williams, Jr., two immunologists who found antibodies in serum proteins migrating between β- and γ-globulins. These antibodies differed from IgM in their size (they were smaller than IgM) and from IgG in their migration in an electric field. Grabar and Williams originally named this new Ig class β_x-globulin, but this designation was later changed to β_{2A}-globulin; still later, the new class was named IgA.

By taking advantage of the relatively large physicochemical differences among IgG, IgM, and IgA, immunochemists have been able to isolate the three immunoglobulin classes in a relatively pure form. The purification was further simplified by the use of sera from patients with myelomas that contained highly elevated levels of a single immunoglobulin species (and hence also of a single Ig class). One of the many uses to which immunologists have put the purified preparations is the production of class-specific antisera. For example, one injects purified human IgG into rabbits (or goats or horses), and repeats the immunization until one detects antibodies to the immunizing immunoglobulin in the recipient's serum. The production of such an anti-Ig serum is possible because rabbit and human IgG differ biochemically (e.g., in their amino acid sequences) and some of these differences are recognized as antigens by the rabbit. However, the rabbit anti-IgG serum produced in this manner often reacts not only with IgG, but also with IgM and IgA. The reason for this crossreactivity is that the antiserum contains antibodies to light chains shared by molecules of the three classes. To remove these crossreacting antibodies one absorbs the antiserum with purified IgM or IgA preparations: one mixes the antiserum with these preparations and removes the resulting precipitate by centrifugation. The absorption removes all antibodies except those reacting specifically with the IgG preparation. In a similar way, one can also produce antisera specific for IgA or IgM molecules. Availability of such antisera has made possible the identification of two other immunoglobulin classes, IgD and IgE.

In 1965, David S. Rowe and John L. Fahey isolated a myeloma protein that did not react with the anti-IgG, anti-IgM, or anti-IgA sera. In turn, antiserum made by immunization with this protein did not react with purified preparations of IgG, IgM, or IgA, but did react with normal human serum. The protein thus belonged to a new immunoglobulin class, which Rowe and Fahey designated IgD.

The existence of the fifth class, IgE, was suspected for some time but the immunoglobulin was not positively identified until 1967, when Kimishige and Teruka Ishizaka fractionated sera from allergic patients and demonstrated that allergic reactions were mediated by an immunoglobulin that was serologically and physicochemically distinct from all previously identified classes.

In summary, there are five classes of human immunoglobulin—IgG, IgM, IgA, IgD, and IgE. They differ in their physicochemical and serological properties, as well as in the primary structure of their constant regions. The monomeric molecules of all classes have the same basic structure, consisting of two heavy and two light chains. In the IgM and IgA classes, these monomers are linked to form larger polymers, whereas in IgG, IgD, and IgE, each molecule consists of only one monomeric unit.

Serological analysis of proteins belonging to the same class revealed an additional heterogeneity and resulted in the division of classes into *subclasses*. The first three subclasses of IgG were described in 1964 by Howard M. Grey and Henry G. Kunkel. These two investigators obtained sera from several patients with IgG myelomas, isolated the myeloma proteins, and injected them separately into rabbits. They then tested (by the diffusion method in agar gel; see Chapter 10) the individual antisera thus obtained against their entire collection of IgG myeloma proteins, but found that each antiserum reacted with almost all the proteins. They therefore absorbed the antisera with selected proteins (other than the immunizing ones) and then tested them again against the entire panel. This time, each antiserum reacted with only a limited number of proteins, and the entire collection could be divided, according to the reactivity pattern, into three groups, which Grey and Kunkel designated We, Vi, and Ge (the names of prototype proteins in each group; see Table 6.1). These designations were later changed to γG2a, γG2c, and γG2d, respectively, and still later to IgG1, IgG3, and IgG4 (the fourth group, IgG2, was discovered somewhat later). Since the antisera also reacted with normal human sera, Grey and Kunkel concluded that they had identified normal subclasses of IgG. Later, other investigators discovered, in a similar manner, subclasses of other human (and animal) Ig classes.

In humans, there are four known IgG subclasses (IgG1, IgG2, IgG3, and IgG4), two IgM subclasses

Table 6.1 Reactivity of Absorbed Rabbit Anti-Human Myeloma Protein Antisera with a Collection of IgG Myeloma Proteins Obtained from Different Patients

Myeloma Protein	Reactivity of Antiserum						Subclass
	Anti-Vi[a] (absorbed by Sp)	Anti-Fe (absorbed by Ke)	Anti-Zu (absorbed by Ke)	Anti-Sp (absorbed by Vi)	Anti-Ci (absorbed by We)	Anti-Ge (absorbed by We)	
Vi	+	+	+	−	−	−	Vi(IgG3)
Fe	+	+	+	−	−	−	
Zu	+	+	+	−	−	−	
We	−	−	−	−	−	−	
Sp	−	−	−	+	−	−	We(IgG1)
Le	−	−	−	+	−	−	
Ku	−	−	−	+	−	−	
Ke	−	−	−	+	−	−	
Cu	−	−	−	+	−	−	
Br	−	−	−	+	−	−	
Ge	−	−	−	+	−	−	
Ci	−	−	−	−	+	+	Ge(IgG4)
Ro	−	−	−	−	+	+	
				−	+	+	

Source. Based on H. M. Grey and H. G. Kunkel: *J. Exp. Med.* **120**:253–266, 1964.
[a] Vi, Fe, Zu, and so on are abbreviations of patients' names.

Table 6.2 Immunoglobulin Classes and Subclasses in Various Vertebrates

Species	Class and Subclass				
Human	IgG1, IgG2, IgG3, IgG4	IgA1, IgA2	IgM1, IgM2	IgD	IgE
Ape	IgG	IgA	IgM	IgD	IgE
Monkey	IgG	IgA	IgM	IgD	IgE
Mouse	IgG2a, IgG2b, -[a], IgG1	IgA1, IgA2	IgM	IgD	IgE
Rat	IgG2a, IgG2b, IgG2c, IgG1	IgA	IgM	?	IgE
Guinea pig	IgG2, -, -, IgG1	IgA	IgM	?	IgE
Rabbit	IgG2, -, -, IgG1	IgA1, IgA2	IgM	?	IgE
Dog	IgG2a, IgG2b, IgG2c, IgG1	IgA	IgM	?	IgE
Cattle	IgG2, -, -, IgG1	IgA	IgM	?	?
Horse	IgGa, IgGb, IgGc, IgGT	IgA	IgM	?	?
Fowl	IgG	IgA	IgM	?	?
Reptile	IgG	?	IgM	?	?
Amphibian	IgG	?	IgM	?	?
Fish	?	?	IgM	?	?
Lamprey	?	?	IgM	?	?

Source. From A. C. Wang, *in* H. H. Fudenberg et al. (Eds.): *Basic and Clinical Immunology*, Lange, Los Altos, California, 1976.
[a] Indicates the absence of an additional subclass corresponding to that in the human.

(IgM1 and IgM2), and two IgA subclasses (IgA1 and IgA2); no subclasses of the IgD and IgE classes have yet been demonstrated convincingly. Classes and subclasses known in nonhuman species are listed in Table 6.2.

The difference between classes and subclasses is one of degree: subclasses of the same class show greater relatedness (in terms of amino acid sequence) than do different classes. At the genetic level, as we shall see shortly, the distinction between classes and subclasses is unnecessary. However, the distinction does have a meaning when one considers the complete Ig molecule, for there are important physicochemical and chemical characteristics that differentiate classes, but not subclasses. For example, all IgM molecules, no matter what subclass they belong to, have the same pentameric structure, not found in other Ig classes. It is because of these characteristics that the class-subclass division is maintained. The properties of human Ig classes and subclasses are described in section 6.5.

6.2 FROM Ig GENES TO Ig MOLECULES

6.2.1 Organization of Ig Genes

The basic genetic unit (*gene*)[1] involved in the synthesis of Ig molecules is a stretch of DNA containing a sequence of about 330 nucleotide pairs and coding for a polypeptide chain about 110 amino acids long. This polypeptide forms a *domain*—the principal structural element of the Ig molecule. Each Ig molecule is made up of several such domains.

A haploid genome contains several hundred copies of the basic unit (the exact number is not known). The copies are not the same but are sufficiently similar that one can assume they all derive from a single ancestral gene. They are grouped into three *families*—κ, λ, and H (the origin of the designations will be explained later in this chapter), each family carried by a different chromosome. In the mouse—which we shall use as a model animal since most of the work on the molecular genetics of immunoglobulins has been done in this species—the κ family is carried by chromosome 6, the H family by chromosome 12, and the λ family by chromosome 16. (In the human the H family is on chromosome 14 and the location of the other two families is not known.) The κ and λ families can each be divided into three *groups*—V, J, and C; the H family can be divided into four groups—V, J, D, and C (Fig. 6.6).

[1] In immunoglobulin genetics, the concept of the gene breaks down completely. Here, one is dealing with a hierarchy of structural elements of the DNA supermolecule, any one of which can be called a gene. In this book, we shall reserve the term *gene* to denote the shortest contiguous stretch of nucleotide pairs coding for a portion of a polypeptide chain. Occasionally, we shall also refer to this stretch as a *coding sequence* or *exon* and contrast it with *noncoding sequences* or *introns*, which can be transcribed into mRNA but are not translated into polypeptides.

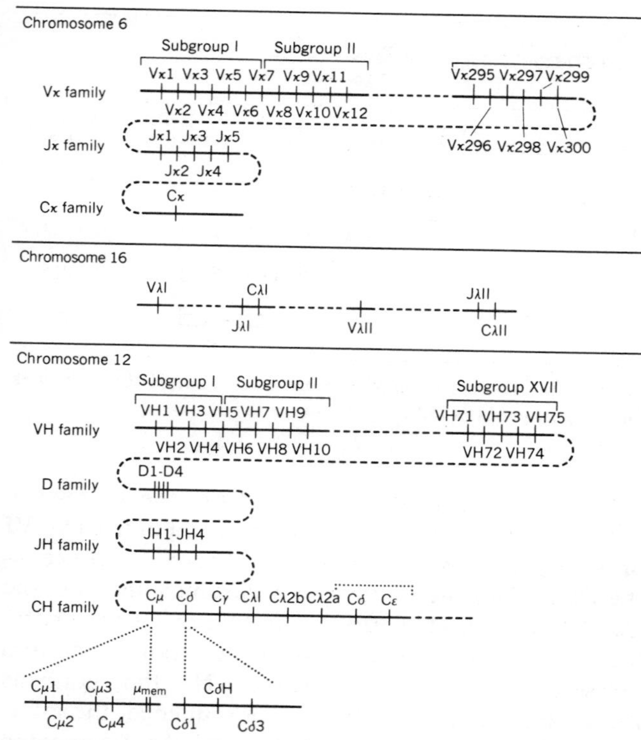

Figure 6.6. Organization of Ig-encoding genes in the mouse. Broken lines indicate an unknown number of genes separating the genes on the solid lines.

The V κ *group* consists of some 300 genes (the estimates vary from 100 to 600) but each gene is 39 nucleotide pairs shorter than the basic coding unit (it is only about 291 nucleotide pairs long, instead of the usual 330). The genes are arranged in tandem so that neighboring genes are separated by a noncoding sequence of several thousand nucleotide pairs. The 300 or so genes can be divided into about 50 *subgroups*, each composed of about six genes; genes in each subgroup are related to one another more closely than genes in different subgroups. The *Jκ group* consists of five genes (Jκ1 through Jκ5), each 39 nucleotide pairs long and separated from the next gene by some 300 to 350 nucleotide pairs. A single J gene represents the 39 nucleotide pairs missing from a single Vκ gene (together, Vκ and Jκ give the full length of the basic coding unit). Of the five J genes probably only four are functional. The *Cκ group* consists of a single, untruncated basic unit (the *Cκ gene*), separated from the last J gene by some 2500 nucleotide pairs.

The λ *family* of the mouse consists of only three genes—one V, one J, and one C—although this complex is probably duplicated so that, all together, there are two V genes (VλI and VλII), two J genes (JλI and JλII), and two C genes (CλI and CλII). The arrangement of these genes in the chromosome is not known but that depicted in Figure 6.6 appears to the most likely. In other species, the λ family is more complex, containing multiple copies of V genes and perhaps also of the J genes.

The *H family* is the most complex of the three, consisting of four gene groups—V, D, J, and C—arranged in this order in the chromosome (Fig. 6.6). The *V*H *group* is comprised of at least 75 genes divided into at least 17 subgroups with four to six genes per subgroup. Each VH group is probably 297 nucleotide pairs long and the individual genes are separated by noncoding sequences, each sequence about 14,000 nucleotide pairs long. The *D group* consists of four very short (a few nucleotide pairs long) coding sequences separated by short stretches of noncoding DNA. The *J group* also consists of four coding sequences, each sequence from 45 to 51 nucleotide pairs long. The individual JH genes are again separated from each other by short noncoding sequences. The *C group* is comprised of eight gene complexes designated μ, δ, γ3, γ1, γ2b, γ2a, α, and ε[2], arranged in this order (although the position of the ε complex is not certain) and spanning a DNA stretch of about 150,000 to 250,000 nucleotide pairs. The γ complexes are designated by the same letter because they are more similar to one another than they are to the other C-gene complexes. The *Cμ complex* is separated from the J group by about 8300 nucleotide pairs. It consists of four genes, designated Cμ1 through Cμ4, each about 330 nucleotide pairs long. The noncoding stretches separating neighboring Cμ genes are from 100 to 300 nucleotide pairs long. The *Cδ complex*, which is separated from the Cμ complex by about 4500 nucleotide pairs, consists of at least three genes—Cδ1, CδH, and Cδ3; a fourth, Cδ2, may also exist somewhere in the chromosome. The Cδ1, CδH, and Cδ3 genes are 285, 104, and 320 nucleotide pairs long, respectively. Each of the three *Cγ complexes* is believed to consist of four genes—Cγ1, CγH, Cγ2, and Cγ3; the *Cα complex* is thought to consist of four genes—Cα1 through Cα4; and the *Cε complex* of another four genes, Cε1 through Cε4. However, the postulated composition of the Cγ, Cα, and Cε complexes is yet to be proved.

6.2.2 Expression of Ig Genes

A diploid B lymphocyte that has two editions of each chromosome, and therefore has a total of six (three pairs) Ig-encoding chromosomes, expresses Ig genes in only two of these: genes of either the κ or λ chromosome (but never both) and genes of the H chromo-

[2] Alternative designations for the γ2a, α, γ2b, γ1, δ, and μ complexes are *Igh-1*, *Igh-2*, *Igh-3*, *Igh-4*, *Igh-5*, and *Igh-6*, respectively; see section on allotypes.

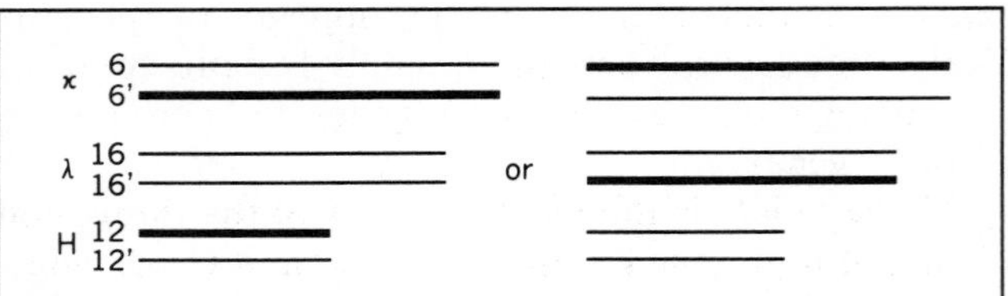

Figure 6.7. Expression of mouse Ig chromosomes in a single B lymphocyte. Numbers indicate Ig-bearing chromosomes. Heavy lines indicate expression of Ig genes in a given chromosome; thin lines mean that the Ig genes in this chromosome are silent.

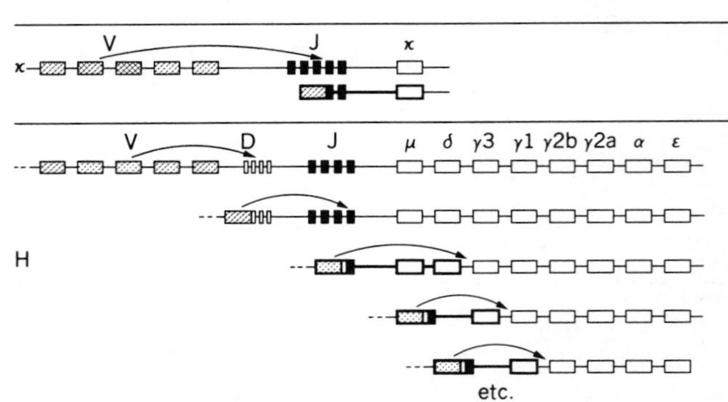

Figure 6.9. Transposition of Ig genes in L(κ) and H chromosomes. Shuffling of genes is indicated by arrows.

some. In each pair of active chromosomes, only one expresses its Ig genes, while its partner remains inactive; thus, in each lymphocyte, only two of the six chromosomes express Ig genes (one κ or λ and one H chromosome; see Fig. 6.7). Each of the two active chromosomes expresses only one gene (or gene complex) in each group (Fig. 6.8)—that is, one V, one J, one D (in the case of the H chromosome), and one C gene—although at a certain stage of its development, a lymphocyte may express two or even three C-gene complexes transiently. Which of the numerous V, J, or D genes are selected for expression is determined largely by chance, so different lymphocytes express different genes. In preparation for the expression, the selected V gene is moved to a position next to the J gene (in the κ or λ chromosome), or first next to the D and then next to the J gene (in the H chromosome; see Fig. 6.9). This transposition restores the original size of the basic coding unit. (Remember, the J and D sequences were probably derived from the original V gene by splitting off pieces from one end of it.) The VJ or VDJ segments and one of the C-gene complexes—the Cκ or Cλ gene in the κ or λ chromosome, and the Cμ, Cδ, Cγ3, Cγ1, Cγ2b, Cγ2a, Cα, or Cε gene complex in the H chromosome—are then transcribed into messenger RNA. The messenger RNA thus contains the contiguous VJ or VJD coding sequence, the interconnecting noncoding sequence, and the fragmented coding sequence of one of the C-gene complexes.

In the next stage, all the noncoding sequences are excised from the messenger and an RNA molecule is formed with a contiguous VJC or VDJC coding sequence (Fig. 6.10). This molecule is then translated into a single, contiguous polypeptide chain. The

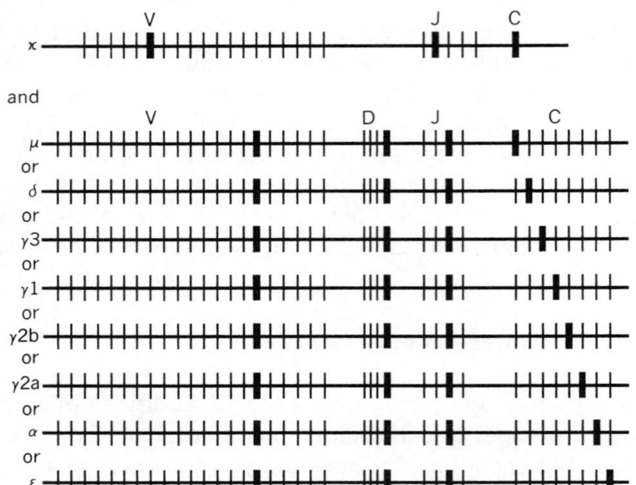

Figure 6.8. Expression of mouse Ig genes in a single B lymphocyte. Each vertical line represents a gene in a V, J, D, or C family, as indicated. A heavy vertical line means that the gene is expressed; a thin line indicates a gene that is not expressed.

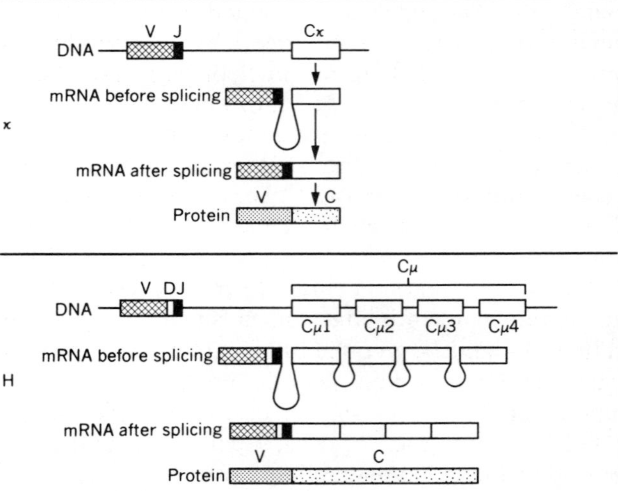

Figure 6.10. Splicing of messenger RNA transcribed from Ig chromosomes. Looped-out segments are presumably cut off and the coding sequences joined as indicated. The spliced mRNA is then transcribed into an Ig polypeptide chain.

polypeptide encoded by either the κ or λ chromosome is derived from only two basic coding units (VJ and C) and, therefore, has only two domains, V and C. The polypeptide encoded by the H chromosome, with the possible exception of some of the δ-encoded chains, is derived from five basic coding units (VDJ, C1, C2, C3, and C4, or VDJ, C1, CH, C2, and C3, where CH is only a fragment of the basic unit), and therefore contains five domains—V, C1, C2, C3, and C4, or V, C1, CH, C2, C3 (where CH, again, is a fragment of a domain called the *hinge region*). The κ or λ chromosome-encoded polypeptide is therefore shorter (it constitutes the *light chain*) than the H chromosome-encoded polypeptide (which constitutes the *heavy chain*). Because there are two light chain-encoding gene families, κ and λ, there are also two light-chain *isotypes*, Lκ and Lλ. Although a single cell, as already mentioned, activates either the κ or the λ family but never both, and hence produces either Lκ or Lλ chains, different cells produce different L chains so that every individual always has some cells producing Lκ and other cells producing Lλ chains.

The expression of the heavy chain-encoding genes follows a somewhat different route. As in the case of L-chain production, the lymphocyte presumably starts the process of H-gene expression by moving a selected V gene next to a selected D gene and transposing the VD segment next to a selected J gene. It then transcribes the contiguous VDJ segment together with the nearest C-gene complex—the μ and probably also the δ complex—and with everything that is between VDJ and μ. The transcript is probably spliced in two different ways, one producing a molecule that is translated into the μ heavy chain, and another producing a molecule that is translated into the δ heavy chain. As the cell then differentiates further and divides, it moves the same VDJ segment to the next C gene complex in the tandem, the $\gamma3$ complex, transcribes this new gene arrangement (VDJ + $\gamma3$), and produces $\gamma3$ heavy chains. Next it may move the VDJ segment into the vicinity of the $\gamma1$ complex, then to the $\gamma2b$ complex, and so on. Thus, by transposing the same VDJ segment sequentially to different C-gene complexes in the tandem and always transcribing the segment with the nearest C complex, the original cell gives rise to progeny, each containing different Ig-encoding mRNA molecules. Although individual cells apparently pass through a stage in which they contain two or three mRNA types at one time (e.g., VDJ + μ, VDJ + δ, and VDJ + $\gamma3$), each cell eventually commits itself to the production of only one of these types (e.g., either VDJ + μ, VDJ + δ, or VDJ + $\gamma3$). In the end, therefore, each differentiated cell synthesizes only one heavy-chain isotype, μ, δ, $\gamma3$, $\gamma1$, $\gamma2b$, $\gamma2a$, α, or ϵ. However, the different chains produced by the progeny of a single precursor cell carry the same V domain encoded by the VDJ segment that the precursor cell selected. Theoretically, therefore, a single precursor B lymphocyte can give rise to progeny cells, some of which synthesize μ chains, others δ chains, still others $\gamma3$ chains, and so on. Whether it always realizes this full potential and produces in its progeny the entire assortment of heavy chains is doubtful. More likely it channels large-scale production to only a few selected chains that best fit the activating stimulus.

Since each lymphocyte always activates two Ig chromosomes—κ or λ and H—it simultaneously produces L and H chains that combine post-synthetically and intracellularly to form the L_2H_2 tetramers so characteristic of the Ig molecules. These basic molecules may then associate to form more complex structures. The H-chain isotype (μ, δ, $\gamma3$, $\gamma1$, $\gamma2a$, $\gamma2b$, α, and ϵ) determines the class or subclass of the Ig molecule (IgM, IgD, IgG3, IgG1, IgG2a, IgG2b, IgA, and IgE, respectively). IgM, IgD, IgG, IgA, and IgE are regarded as different immunoglobulin *classes*; IgG3, IgG1, IgG2a, and IgG2b are regarded as *subclasses* of the IgG class. The distinction between classes and subclasses was originally introduced because the subclass molecules within a given class resemble one another more closely than they resemble molecules of different subclasses (e.g., IgG3 is more related to IgG1 that it is to IgM or IgA). However, there is no *principal* difference between classes and subclasses since both the class- and subclass-determining regions of the Ig molecule are encoded by separate and equivalent gene complexes (i.e., there are separate gene complexes for the corresponding regions of IgG3, IgG1, IgG2a, and IgG2b, which are subclasses of the IgG class, as there are separate complexes for the corresponding regions of IgM, IgD, IgA, and IgE, which are molecules of different classes). Nonetheless, an important fact to remember is that, at the end of its differentiation pathway, a B cell opts for one of the eight CH complexes and that the choice of the complex determines the class or subclass of the Ig molecules produced.

In each class or subclass the molecule can be of either the κ or λ type, depending on whether the cell has chosen the activation of the κ or the λ chromosomes. Since the decision between κ and λ is made early in the ontogeny of a B lymphocyte and since the decision, once made, is permanent, hybrid Ig molecules containing one κ and one λ chain each do not normally arise.

Because in different lymphocyte precursors the same Cκ gene is joined with different Vκ and Jκ genes, when one compares a series of κ light chains produced by different B-lymphocyte clones, one finds that the chains have a virtually identical amino acid sequence in the region encoded by the C gene but different sequences in the region encoded by the VJ segment. In other words, the light chain can be resolved in a *constant (C)* and a *variable (V) region*. Each of the two regions consists of only one domain encoded by the corresponding basic genetic unit (VJκ and Cκ). Similar joining of different VDJ segments with the same μ, δ, γ3, γ1, γ2b, γ2a, α, or ε gene complexes also occurs in the H-gene family, so that the heavy chains, too, can be divided into variable and constant regions. The VH region, like that of the Lκ chain, is comprised of only one domain, but the CH region consists of four domains, one of which, however, may be reduced to hinge region.

Until now we have treated the Ig genes as if they were monomorphic, that is, as if each gene existed in only one form (allele) shared by all individuals of a given species. However, different mice may *not* have the same gene at a given locus. For example, the genes of the γ1 complex have an identical nucleotide-pair sequence in all mice except at one position. As a result of this difference, there are two types of γ1 chain differing by an amino acid substitution at a position corresponding to the variant site in the DNA sequence. This allelic variation at the same locus in a given complex is called *allotypy* and the variants are referred to as *allotypes*. Since the variation can occur at any of the Ig-encoding loci, there are allotypes associated with κ, μ, γ1, γ3, γ2a, and other chains. In the mouse, all allotypic variation described occurs in the constant region of the Ig chains. V-region allotypes undoubtedly exist but are difficult to detect because, in the V-gene group, it is not easy to distinguish products of allelic genes from products of different loci. However, V-region allotypes have been detected in the rabbit. (V genes, being derived presumably from the same ancestral gene, share portions of their DNA sequences, and it is in these common segments that the allotypic variation has been discovered.) The unique DNA sequences distinguishing individual V genes, and the corresponding unique amino acid sequences distinguishing individual V polypeptides constitute the basis for the so-called *idiotypy*—the occurrence of individually specific markers (*idiotypes*) on V-gene products. Both allotypes and idiotypes are recognized as antigenic determinants by antibodies and are therefore most commonly detected by serological methods.

The human Ig genes are probably organized in a fashion similar to that of the mouse genes, although there are some characteristic differences. For example, humans, in contrast to the mouse, have four Cλ genes (λ1 through λ4) and hence four different Lλ chain isotypes (like the mouse, however, the human has only one Cκ gene). Furthermore, humans have ten rather than eight CH gene complexes: μ1, μ2, δ, γ1, γ2, γ3, γ4, α1, α2, and ε. Thus there are two subclasses of human IgM (IgM1 and IgM2) and two subclasses of human IgA (IgA1 and IgA2), in addition to the four subclasses of IgG also found in the mouse.

6.3 PRIMARY AND SECONDARY STRUCTURE OF Ig MOLECULES

Now that we have learned the basics, we can proceed to a more detailed account of immunoglobulin structure and genetics. We shall begin by discussing the individual structural features of the molecule one by one, and then describe in detail the formal genetics of immunoglobulins.

6.3.1 Fragments

Treatment with agents capable of cleaving peptide bonds breaks up Ig molecules into *fragments*. The agents commonly used are various proteolytic enzymes, such as papain, pepsin, trypsin, and subtilisin, and nonenzymes, such as cyanogen bromide (CNBr). Under defined conditions (certain pH, presence of certain cofactors), virtually all proteolytic enzymes cleave Ig molecules preferentially in the more accessible interdomain regions and leave the globular portions of the domains intact. When the conditions are not defined, an uncontrollable digestion of the entire molecule may occur.

Ig fragments produced by various enzymes are listed in Table 6.3. The fragments are referred to by F symbols to which either an abbreviation of the fragment's full name (Fab, Fc, etc.) or a meaningless letter (Fd, Fb) is added. Since fragments can be produced from any Ig class, in situations where confusion might arise the origin of the fragment is indicated by subscript isotype designation (e.g., Fc_{α} or Fab_{μ}). Some fragment designations also carry an abbreviation of the enzyme that produced them [e.g., Fab(p) and Fab(t) are Fab fragments produced by papain and trypsin, respectively].

6.3.2 Chains

Dissociation, Separation, Reassociation

The basic Ig molecule consists of four chains, two heavy and two light. In an intact molecule, the chains

Table 6.3 Fragments of the IgG Molecule

Fragment Designation	Domains Retained by the Fragment	Fragmenting Enzyme
Fab	VL—CL VH—CH1	Papain
Fc	CH2—CH3 CH2—CH3	Papain
$F(ab)_2$	VL—CL VH—CH1 VH—CH1 VL—CL	Pepsin
Facb	VL—CL VH—CH1 CH2 VH—CH1 CH2 VL—CL	Plasmin
Fd	VH—CH1	Papain
Fc′	-CH3 -CH3	Papain, pepsin, subtilisin
Fv	VL- VH-	Pepsin

are held together by covalent (disulfide) and noncovalent bonds. To break the bonds and separate the heavy from the light chains, one exposes the molecule to a reducing agent (e.g., 2-mercaptoethanol) in the presence of an agent (e.g., iodoacetamide) that alkylates the reduced S–S bonds and prevents their reassociation when the reducing agent is removed (see Appendix 6.1). One then separates the free H and L chains by gel filtration chromatography (e.g., on a Sephadex G-200 column). However the reduction of most Ig molecules under these conditions is only partial, and the chains continue to be held together by noncovalent bonds. To achieve complete chain dissociation, one must denature the Ig molecules by adding urea or guanidine hydrochloride to the reaction mixture. Following denaturation and reduction, the chains lose their native conformation and acquire the configuration of a random coil.

One can then mix the separated H- and L-chain fractions again and achieve a partial chain *reassociation*. The degree of reassociation depends largely on the harshness of the reducing conditions. Completely denatured chains reassociate only through noncovalent interactions, but gently dissociated chains can reassociate even by forming disulfide bridges between correctly juxtaposed sulfhydryl groups. In the products of the latter type of reassociation, the native configuration can be largely restored, including the reformation of four-chain molecules. The dissociation-reassociation techniques have played an important role in determining the contribution of individual chains to antigen-binding activity. Surprisingly, even after a complete loss of ordered structure, the chains regain some antibody activity upon reassociation.

Classification

Biochemists distinguish two main chain types, light (L) and heavy (H), according to chain length; geneticists, however, distinguish three types, Lκ, Lλ, and H, encoded by three different gene families on three nonhomologous chromosomes (Fig. 6.7). The λ and H chains are distinguished further into different *isotypes*[3] according to what gene or gene complex of the C-gene group they are coded for. Since both the mouse and the human have only one Cκ locus, there is only one κ isotype in these species. The mouse has two Cλ loci and correspondingly two λ isotypes, λI and λII; the human has four Cλ loci and hence four λ isotypes, λ1 through λ4. As for the H chain, there are eight CH loci and so eight isotypes in the mouse (μ, δ, γ3, γ1, γ2b, γ2a, α, and ε), and ten CH loci and ten isotypes in the human (μ1, μ2, δ, γ1, γ2, γ3, γ4, α1, α2, and ε). Three of the four human λ isotypes were originally referred to as KERN(−)Oz(−)(=λ1), KERN(−)Oz(+)(=λ2), and KERN(+)Oz(−)(=λ3), where KERN and Oz are antigenic determinants detected by specific antisera and "+" or "−" indicates the presence or absence of the determinant. Oz(+) differ from Oz(−) chains in that the former have lysine and the latter arginine at position 188; KERN(+) and KERN(−) chains have glycine and serine, respectively, at position 157. [Incidentally, the fourth combination, KERN(+)Oz(+), has never been found.] A summary of Ig chain classification is given in Table 6.4.

Since any H chain can associate with any L chain, molecules of a given class or subclass can occur in several forms differing in their L chains: each can be of the κ, λ1, λ2, λ3, or λ4 type. Hybrid molecules of the κλ or λxλy type do not occur, nor do molecules that have neither κ nor λ. The ratio of the κ and λ types varies from class to class, subclass to subclass, and species to species. For example, in mice, most of the

[3] The term *isotype* was originally introduced as a counterpart to *allotype* and *idiotype* and was meant to designate antigenic determinants shared by all individuals of a given species (Gr. *isos*, the same) but absent in individuals of other species (in contrast to *allotypes*, antigenic determinants carried by only some individuals of a given species, and *idiotypes*, individual-specific antigenic determinants). However, the definitions of all three terms were later broadened to include any markers, not just serologically detectable ones, that distinguish chains or molecules.

Table 6.4 Classification of Immunoglobulin Chains

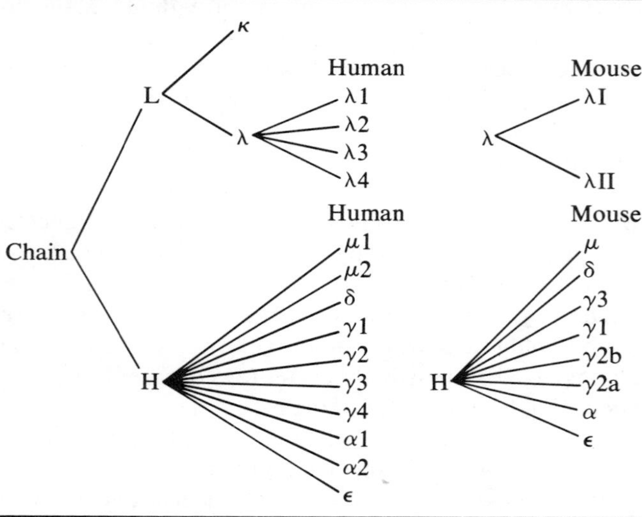

immunoglobulin (over 95 percent) is of the κ type, while the overall κ : λ ratio in humans is 6:4. In the horse, more than 95 percent of immunoglobulin is of the λ type. The ratio can also change during immunization, apparently because of the changes in class representation in the different stages of the immune response.

Amino Acid Sequence

Each light chain of an immunoglobulin molecule is composed of some 200, and the heavy chain of some 400, amino acids. There are 20 kinds of amino acid, arranged in the linear polypeptide chain in a particular sequence that characterizes a given protein and distinguishes this protein from other molecules. This *primary structure* reflects the protein's evolutionary history, function, tertiary structure, and genetic control. Therefore, by deciphering its amino acid sequence, a biochemist can learn a great deal about a molecule. However, determining the complete amino acid sequence of polypeptide chains as long as those composing an immunoglobulin molecule is not an easy task, and many a biochemist spends months, or even years, working out the primary structure of one polypeptide. Sequencing of the entire H chain, in particular, is a formidable task, since the polypeptide must first be cleaved into smaller peptides, each peptide must be isolated and sequenced, and the peptides must be ordered (see Appendix 6.1). Owing to the effort of Norbert Hilschmann, Gerald M. Edelman, Frank W. Putnam, Lee Hood, J. Donald Capra, Michel Fougereau, and others, amino acid sequences of several Ig chains or chain segments are now known. In humans, complete sequence has been determined for 34 light chains (20 κ and 14 λ) and five heavy chains (one γ1, two μ, one α1, and one ε). A few complete or semicomplete sequences are also known for the mouse and the rabbit. Partial sequences are available for many light and heavy chains in humans and other species.

For easier reference, the amino acid residues are numbered, starting from the N terminal of the molecule and proceeding toward the C terminal. When several proteins of a similar kind are sequenced, it is desirable, for comparative purposes, to designate homologous residues in different chains by the same number using the molecule sequenced first as a reference. This practice, however, presents problems when the second molecule proves to be longer than the first one, for example, or when additional amino acids are found to be inserted in the middle of the second chain. In such situations, biochemists use small letter designations for the extra positions.

In humans, the two types of light chain (κ and λ) are of the same length, each consisting of 214 amino acid residues. Several other mammalian species (e.g., mouse, rabbit) possess light chains of similar length. In these species, L chains are designated as κ or λ, according to their homology to human κ and λ chains, which were the first to be sequenced completely.

In contrast to light chains, the different heavy chains vary considerably in length. In humans, the shortest H chain is γ1, which is 446 residues long; the longest chain is μ, which is composed of 567 amino acid residues. Most of the "extra" amino acids (in comparison to γ chains) are at the carboxy terminal "tail" of the molecule. A similar tail, though somewhat shorter, is also present in the α chain. Since both IgM and IgA occur in polymeric forms, the tail is believed to play a role in the polymerization of the basic Ig molecules.

6.3.3 Domains

Figure 6.11 depicts a complete amino acid sequence of a human IgG1 molecule, as determined by Gerald M. Edelman and his co-workers. The molecule is broken down into segments, each about 100 to 110 amino acids long. The light chain, which is 214 amino acids long, is split into two segments, designated V_L and C_L; the heavy chain, which is 446 amino acids long, is partitioned into four segments, designated V_H, C_H1, C_H2, and C_H3. The segments are aligned so that identical or similar sequences are at corresponding positions. The alignment reveals two types of homology: the V_L segment is homologous to V_H, and the C_L, C_H1, C_H2, and C_H3 segments are homologous to one another. In con-

```
       1                 10                  20                  30
VL   D   I Q M T Q S P S T L S A S V G D R V T I T C R A S Q S I N T — — W L A W Y Q
VH   Pca V Q L V Q S G — A E V K K P G S S V K V S C K A S G G T F S R S A I I W V R

       110                 120                   130                 140
CL   T V A A P S V F I F P P S D E Q — — L K S G T A S V V C L L N N F Y P R E A K
CH1  S T K G P S V F P L A P S S K S — — T S G G T A A L G C L V K D Y F P E P V T
CH2  L L G G P S V F I F P P K P K D T L M I S R T P E V T C V V V D V S H E D P Q
CH3  Q P R E P Q V Y T L P P S R E E — — M T K N Q V S L T C L V K G F Y P S D I A

       40                  50                  60                  70
VL   Q K P G K A P K L L M Y K A S S — L E S G V P S R F I G S G S G T E F T — — — —
VH   Q A P G Q G L E W M G G I V P M F G P P N Y A Q K F Q G — R V T I T A D E S T N

             150                 160                 170                 180
CL   V — — Q W K V D N A L Q S G N S Q E S V T E Q D S K D S T Y S L S S T L T L S K
CH1  V — — S W N S — G A L T S G — V H T F P A V L Q S — S G L Y S L S S V V T V P S
CH2  V K F N W Y V D G — V Q V H N A K T K P R E Q Q Y — D S T Y R V V S V L T V L H
CH3  V — — E W E S N D — G E P E N Y K T T P P V L D S — D G S F F L Y S K L T V D K

                       80                  90                  100
VL   — — — L T I S S L Q P D D F A T Y Y C Q Q — Y N S D S K M F G Q G T K V E V K G
VH   T A Y M E L S S L R S E D T A F T F C A G G Y G I Y S P E E Y N G G L V T

             190                 200                 210
                                                                          Hinge region
CL   A D Y E K H K V Y A C E V T H Q G L S S P V T — K S F — — N R G E C
CH1  S S L G T Q — T Y I C N V N H K P S N T K V — D K R V — — E P K S C D K T H T C P P C P A P E
CH2  Q N W L D G K E Y K C K V S N K A L P A P I — E K T I S K A K G
CH3  S R W Q Q G N V F S C S V M H E A L H N H Y T Q K S L S L S P G
```

Figure 6.11. Complete amino acid sequence of a human IgG1 molecule (myeloma protein Eu). The sequence is aligned to show maximum homology among stretches of two polypeptide chains. The numbering system on the top of the first- and third-sequence rows refers to only V_L and C_L, respectively, and not to the other sequences. Hyphens indicate gaps introduced artificially into the sequence to maximize homology. (Based on G. M. Edelman, B. A. Cunningham, W. E. Gall, P. D. Gottlieb, U. Rutishauser, and M. J. Waxdal, *Proc. Natl. Acad. Sci. U.S.A.* **63:**78–85, 1969.)

```
       1                 10                  20                  30                  40
κ      — — — — — — — T V A A P S V P I F P P S — — D E Q L K S G — — T A S V — V C L L
λ      — — — Q P K — — — A A P S V T L F P P S — — S E E L Q A N — — K A T L — V C L I
γ1C1   — — A S T K — — — — G P S V F P L A P S S K S T — — S G G — — T A A L — G C L V
μC1    G S A S — — — — — — — — A P T L F P L V — S C E B S B P S S — — — T V A V — G C L A
α1C1   — — A S P — — — — T S P K V F P L S — L C — S T Q P D Q N — — — V V I — A C K V
εC1    G S — — — — — — T — T G P T V F P L T R C C K B I — P S — N A T S V T L — G C L A

γ1C2   — — — Q L — — — L G G P S V F L F P P K P K D T L M I — S R — T P E V — T C V V
μC2    V I A Z L — — — — — — P P K V S V F V P — P R D G F F G B P R K S — K L — I C Q A
α1C2   — — — H P R L S L H R P A L — — — — — — — — Z B — L L L G S Z — — A B L — T C T L
εC2    — — — — — — R B — F T P P T V K I L Z S S C — B G — — L G — H F P P T I Z L C L V

γ1C3   — — — Q P R — — — — E P Q V T T L P P S — R D — E L T K N Q — — V S L — T C L V
μC3    V P D Z — — B T — — A I R V F A I P P S F A S I F L T — — — K S T K L — T C L V
α1C3   — — — — — — — N T F — R P E V H L L P P — P — S Q Q L A L N Q L — V T L — T C L A
εC3    D S D — P R — — — — G V S A Y L S R P S P F D — L F I — — R K S P T I — T C L V

μC4    V — A — — — — — — L H R P D V Y L L P P A — R — E Q L N L — R E S A T I — T C L V
εC4    — — — — P R — — — A A P E V Y A F A — T P — — E W P — G S R D K R T L — A C L I
```

```
                         50                  60                  70                  80
κ      N N F Y P — — R E A K V Q — — W K — V D — N A L Q S G N — — S Q — — — — — E S V T
λ      S D F Y P — — G A V T V A — — W K — A D G S P V K A G V — — — — — — — — E T T T
γ1C1   K D Y F P — — Q P V T V S — — W N — — S G — A L T S G V — — — — — — H — — — — T F
μC1    Q D F L P — — D S I T F S — — W K Y — — — — — — K B N S D I S — S — T — — R G F
α1C1   Q G F F P — Q Q P L S V T — — W S — E S G Q — — — — G V — — — — — — — T — A R N F
εC1    T G Y F P — — E P V M V T — — W B — — T G S L — — N G — — — — — — — — — — — — T T L

γ1C2   V D V S H — — E D P E V K F N W Y — V D G V E V — — — — — — — — — — H — N A K T K
μC2    T G F S P — — R Q I Q V S — — W L R — E G K Q V G S G V — — — — — T — T N E — V Z
α1C2   T G L R D — — A S — G V T F T W T P S S G K — — — S A V — — — — — — — — — — Q G —
εC2    S G Y T P — — G T I N I T — — W L — Z B G — Z V M D — V D L S — — — — — — — — — —

γ1C3   K G F Y P — — S D I A V E — — W E — S B G E P — Z D — N Y — — — — — — — — — K T T
μC3    T D L T Y — — D S V T I S — — W T R Q D G E A V K T H T T B S Z S H P B A — T T
α1C3   R G F S P — K — D V L V R — — W L Q G S Q E L P R — E K Y L — — — — T W A S R Q
εC3    V B L A P S K G T V N L T — — W S R A S G K P — — — — — V B — — — H S — — — — —

μC4    T G F S P — — A D V F V Q — — W Q M Q R G Q P L S P E K Y V — — — — T S A — P M
εC4    Q N F M P — — E D I S V Q — — W L H N E V Q L P — — — — D A R — — H S — — T T Q
```

```
                   90                      100                    110                120
κ     — — Q Q D S K D S — — T Y S L S S T L T L S — K A — D Y — E K H K V — Y A C E V
λ     P S K — Q S — N N — — K Y A A S S Y L S L T — — P E Q W K S — H R S — Y S C Q V
γ1C1  P A   L Q S — — S G — L Y S L S S V V T V P S — S — — S L — G T Q T — Y I C N V
μC1   P S V L R G — — — G — K Y A A T S Q V L L P S K — — D V M Q G T N E H V V C K V
α1C1  P P S Q D A — — S G B L Y T T S S Q L T L P — — A T Q C L A G — K S — V T C H V
εC1   P A T T L T — L S G — H Y A T I S L L T V S G — A — — W A K — — Q M — F T C R V

γ1C2  P R E E Q Y — B S — — T Y R V V S V L T V L — — H Q D W L D G — K E — Y K C K V
μC2   A Z A K E S G P — — T T Y K V T S T L T I — — K E S B W L S Q — S M — F T C R V
α1C2  P P D R D — — L C G C — Y S V S S V L S G C — — A Q P W D H G — K T — F T C T A
εC2   T A S T E S E — — G E L A S T E S E L T L S Q K H — — W L S D — R T — Y T C E V

γ1C3  P P V K D S — D — G — S F F L Y S K L T V D — K S — R W Q Q G — N V — F S C S V
μC3   S A V G E A — — — — — — — — — — — — — — S I C — — E B B W N S G — E R — F T C T V
α1C3  Q P S Q — G T — — — T T F A V T S I L R V A — — A E D W K K G — D T — F S C M V
εC3   T R K E E K Q R N G — T L T V T S T L P V G T R — — B W I E G — E T — Y Z C R V

μC4   P — E P Q A — P — G — R Y F A H S I L T V S — — E E E W N T G — E T — Y T C V V
εC4   P R K T K K — — S G — — F F V F S R L E V — T R A E — W Q E K — D E — F I C R A


                   130                   140                    150                     160
κ     T H Q G — L S S P V T — K S F N R G E C —
λ     T H E G — — S T — V — E K T V A P T E C S
γ1C1  N H K P — S N T K V — D K K V E P K S C D K T H T C P P C P A P
μC1   Z H P — — B G B K — — E K D V — P L P — —
α1C1  K H Y T — B P S — — — Z B — V T V — P C — P V P S T P P T P S P S T P P T P S P — — — — S C C
εC1   A H T P — S S T B N — V K T F S V — — C S

γ1C2  S N K A — L P A P I — E K T I S K A K G —
μC2   D H R G — L — T F Q — Q B — — A S S M C —
α1C2  A Y P E — S K T P L T A — T L S K — S G —
εC2   T Y Z G — — H T F — — Z B S — T K — K C A

γ1C3  M H E A — L H N H Y T Q K S L S L S P G —
μC3   T H T D — L P S P L K Q — T I S R P K G —
α1C3  G H E A — L P L A F T Q K T I D R L A G K P T H V B V S V V M A E V D G T C T
εC3   T H P H — L P R A L — M R S T T K T S G —

μC4   A H E A — L P N R V T E R T V D K S T G K P T L Y B V S L V M S B T A G T C Y
εC4   V H E A A S P S Q T V Q R A V S V N P G K
```

Figure 6.12. Primary structure of L- and H-chain constant region domains. Numbers indicate amino-acid positions, Greek letters indicate chains, and C1 through C4 symbols represents domains. The sequences have been aligned to show maximum homology; hyphens indicate gaps introduced to maximize homology. (Compiled from different authors.)

trast, the two V segments show little homology to any of the C segments. The segments are referred to as *homology regions* or *domains*. Comparison of Figures 6.11 and 6.12 shows that the domains are centered on the intrachain disulfide bridges and that each domain consists of a disulfide-bonded loop, flanked on each side by a short stretch (about 45 amino acids long) of unlooped chain. An IgG molecule consists of 12 domains: four in the V region (two VL and two VH domains) and eight in the C region (two CL, two CH1, two CH2, and two CH3 domains; cf. Figs. 6.5 and 11). Twelve domains are also present in the basic subunit of the IgA molecule, whereas each of the IgM, IgD, and IgE molecules has one pair of extra domains (total of 14 domains; cf. Fig. 6.12) in the constant region. The extra domain is referred to as CH4.

The domain organization is not limited to the human, but appears to be a general feature shared by all immunoglobulin molecules so far studied. Domains of different chains, different Ig classes, and different vertebrate immunoglobulins vary slightly in length, but they are usually no shorter than 100 and no longer than 110 amino acid residues. The V are often slightly longer than the C domains. The amino acid sequence homology among various domains suggests that they are related in their origin, having all evolved by gene duplication from a single ancestral gene (see section 6.11). Different domains not only share amino acid sequences but also have a similar tertiary structure, with each domain folded into a half-globule (see section 6.4). At the DNA level the sequences coding for the different domains are separated by stretches of noncoding sequences. The coding sequences become contiguous only in the spliced mRNA molecule (see Fig. 6.10).

6.3.4 The Hinge Region

The hinge region is a short segment of the heavy chain between CH1 and CH2 domains. It is singled out as a separate region because it shows no homology to any of the known domains. A typical hinge region is present in the γ and α chains, and apparently absent in μ, δ, and ϵ chains. Its origin is obscure but some immunochemists believe that it might represent the remnants of a collapsed ancient domain, perhaps related to $C\mu1$ and $C\mu2$. Supporting this hypothesis is the observation that at the DNA level, the hinge region-coding sequence exists as a single block separated from C1- and C2-encoding sequences by noncoding introns. In all the γ and α chains the hinge region is about 10 to 15 amino acids long, but the regions of different chains show surprisingly little homology (Fig. 6.13). For example, while the corresponding domains of $\gamma1$,

Amino Acid at Position

Species	Chain	209						215					220					225					230					235					240
													l					Pap ↓	h			h					Pep ↓						
Human	$\gamma1$	T	K	V	D	K	R/K	V	E	P	K	S	C	D	K	T	H	T	C	P	P	C	P	A	P	E	L	L	G	G	P	S	V
												h	h						h			h	Pap ↓										
	$\gamma2$	T	K	V	D	K	T	V	E	R	K	C	C	—	—	—	V	Q	C	P	P	C	P	A	P	P	V	A	—	G	P	S	V
		h					h					Pap ↓	h						h			h											
	$\gamma3$	C	T	P	H	R	C	P	E	P	K	S	C	D	T	P	P	P	C	P	R	C	P	A	P	E	L						
																			h			h											
	$\gamma4$	T	K	V	D	K	R	V	E	S	K	Y	G	—	—	—	P	P	C	P	P	C	P	A	S	E	F	L	G	G	P	S	V
													Tryp ↓					Pap ↓	h								Pep ↓						
Rabbit	γ	T	K	V	D	K	T	V	A	P	S	T	C	S	K	P	—	T/M	C	P	P	—	—	—	P	E	L	L	G	G	P	S	V

Figure 6.13. Amino-acid sequences and sites of enzymatic cleavage in the hinge regions of human and rabbit γ chains. h and 1 designate disulfide bonds to heavy and light chains, respectively. Pap, papain; Pep, pepsin; Tryp, trypsin. The numbering system is that of the IgG1 protein Eu. The alternatives at 214 in human γ_1 and at 225 in rabbit γ are associated with allotypic variation. The sequences are aligned and gaps are introduced to maximize homology with $\gamma1$. The sequences shown also include segments bordering on the hinge regions; the exact length of the hinge region will probably be determined soon by recombinant DNA techniques. The hinge region proper is probably the segment between portions 220 and 235.

$\gamma2$, $\gamma3$, and $\gamma4$ show more than 90 percent homology to one another, the hinge regions of these chains share only about 40 percent of their amino acids.

The two predominant amino acids in the hinge region are cysteine and proline. The cysteine residues are involved in the formation of the inter-H-chain disulfide bridges, and the proline is believed to form the rigid part of the hinge since rotation of polypeptide chains around bonds adjacent to proline is not so free as that around other bonds. However, the region is not inflexible, since it permits the two arms of the Y-shaped molecule to open up and close. The number of interchain disulfide bridges in the hinge region varies from one to 15, depending on the chain isotype and on the species. The interchain bridges prevent folding of the hinge region and so, indirectly, are responsible for the high susceptibility of this portion of the Ig molecule to enzymatic attack. It is in this region that the fragmentation of IgG molecules by papain and pepsin begins (Fig. 6.13).

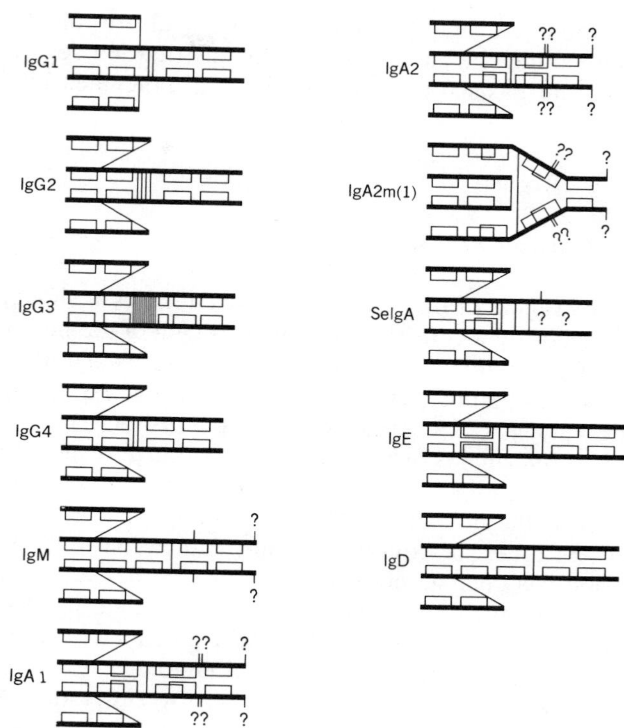

Figure 6.14. Distribution of disulfide bridges in human immunoglobulins of various classes and subclasses. For IgM and IgG, only monomeric units are shown. Heavy lines represent heavy and light chains; thin lines show disulfide bridges; "?" indicates position of bridges uncertain.

6.3.5 Disulfide Bridges

There are two kinds of disulfide bridge in normal Ig molecules—interchain (H to H or H to L) and intrachain. The interchain bonds are somewhat weaker than the intrachain ones and can, therefore, be selectively reduced without denaturing the chains.

Interchain Bridges

H–H Bridges. Most of the H–H bridges occur in the hinge region, but in some Ig classes (e.g., human IgM) disulfide bonds can also form at the C terminal of the heavy chain. The number of bridges in the hinge region varies from class to class and from subclass to subclass (Fig. 6.14). For example, human $\gamma1$ or $\gamma2$ chains are connected by two disulfide bridges, but in the IgG3 molecule one can count 15 bridges between the two $\gamma3$ chains.

H–L Bridges. In most Ig molecules, the light chain is attached to the heavy chain by one disulfide bridge. An exception is the human IgA2 molecule, which contains no disulfide bridge between H and L chains. When present, the bridge is between a cysteine in the H chain and the C-terminal cysteine of the κ or penultimate cysteine of the λ chain. The former can be positioned close to the middle of the H chain, as, for example, in mouse and human IgG1 molecules, or nearer to the N terminal, as in most other immunoglobulins.

L–L Bridges. Under pathological conditions, disulfide bonds can also occur between two light chains. For example, most Bence-Jones proteins are secreted as dimers with the two monomers connected by an S–S bridge.

Intrachain Bridges

The number of intrachain disulfide bridges varies, depending on the chain type (Fig. 6.14): all light chains have two intrachain S–S bridges; all human γ and α heavy chains have four, and human μ, ϵ, and δ heavy chains have five. In each chain, one of the bridges is always in the V region; all the others are in the C region. Since any two cysteines in either the heavy or light chain are separated by at least 40, and sometimes up to 70, amino acid residues (Fig. 6.11), they must be transposed next to each other to be joined by a disulfide bridge. The simplest way such a transposition can be accomplished is by looping out the intervening amino acid sequence (Fig. 6.5). The loops, which are about 55 to 75 amino acids long, alternate with shorter unlooped segments. The number of loops depends again on the chain and, in the case of heavy chains, its isotype: all light chains possess two loops; human γ and α heavy chains have four, and human μ, δ, and ϵ chains have five. The regularity of intrachain-bond distribution and the particular folding pattern of the polypeptide chains dictated by this distribution constitutes the basis for the division of Ig molecules into domains.

6.3.6 Regions

The Constant Region

The C region of the light chain is encoded by a single, contiguous gene; in contrast, the C region of the heavy chain is genetically determined by five pieces of coding sequences (exons, genes) separated from each other by intervening DNA sequences (introns). Each of the exons determines one CH domain or a hinge region. In the chromosome, the exons are arranged in the same order as the domains in the polypeptide chain. At the protein level, of course, the only indication that the region has been assembled from parts is the sequence homology of these parts: as was discussed earlier, the C region can be broken down into segments and when these are properly aligned, strong homology is apparent among them. This homology, in turn, suggests that the individual genes of the C region-encoding complex have a common origin. Except for allotypic variation, the C-region primary structure of all chains of a given isotype is the same in all individuals of a given species. It is this conservation of amino acid sequence that gave the C region its name.

The Variable Region

The V region of the light chain is put together from two pieces of genetic information, the V gene proper and the J gene. The V region of the heavy chain is controlled by at least three separate coding sequences—the V gene proper, the D gene, and the J gene. In contrast to the C region, which is always encoded by the same gene or gene complex in different chains of a given isotype, the V region of different chains derives from different V, D, and J genes. It is this origin from different genes that is mainly responsible for the chain-to-chain variability of the V region, although other mechanisms may also contribute (see section on Antibody Diversitv).

The chain-to-chain variability of the individual positions in the V-region sequence is not the same. Tai Te Wu and Elvin A. Kabat defined the *variability* of each position by using the ν ratio:

$$\nu = \frac{\text{number of different amino acids observed at a given position}}{\text{frequency of the most common amino acid at that position}}$$

Figure 6.15 depicts ν values for the individual positions (the so-called *Wu-Kabat plots*) of the human VL and VH regions. The plots show certain positions to vary considerably and others far less. The positions with high variability form the *hypervariable regions*, and the others form the *framework regions*.

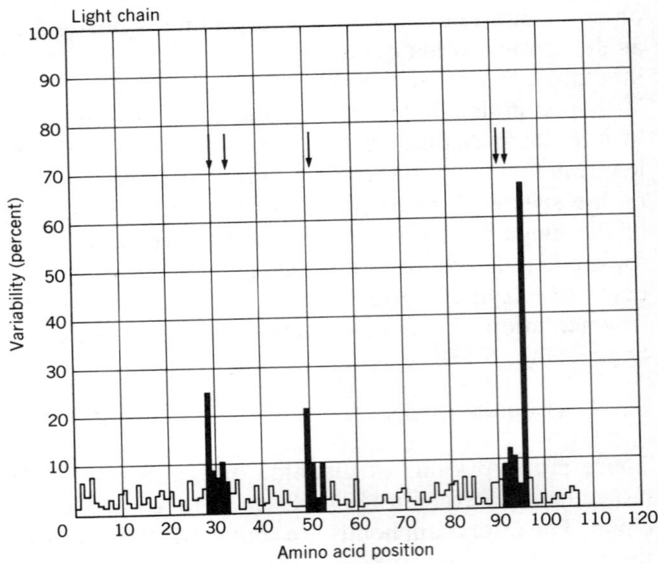

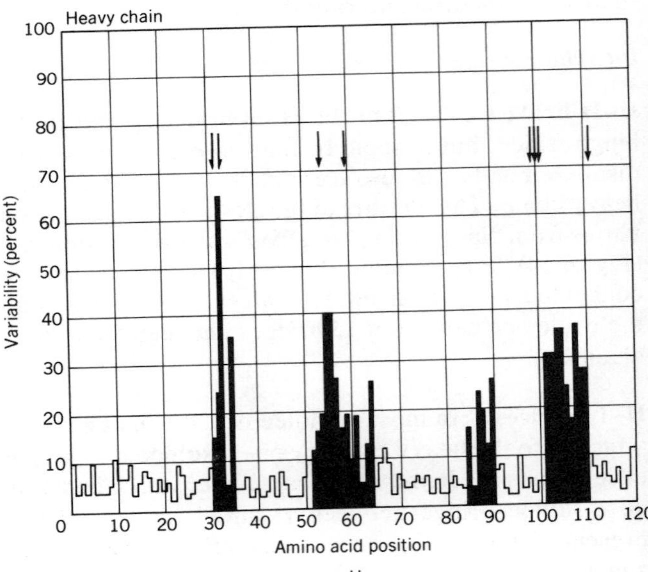

Figure 6.15. (*a*) Plot of amino acid variability in the V region of immunoglobulin light and heavy chains. Hypervariable regions are indicated by solid bars. (*b*) The VH sequences of nine human heavy chains. Solid lines indicate identity with protein Tie. Hyphens in brackets indicate deletions of residues present in protein Tie. Hypervariable regions are shaded. E* denotes pyrrolidine carboxylic acid. [*a* from J. D. Capra and A. B. Edmundson: *Sci. Am.* **236** (January):50–59, 1977. *b* from J. D. Capra and J. M. Kehoe: *Proc. Natl. Acad. Sci. U.S.A.* **71**:4032–4036, 1974.]

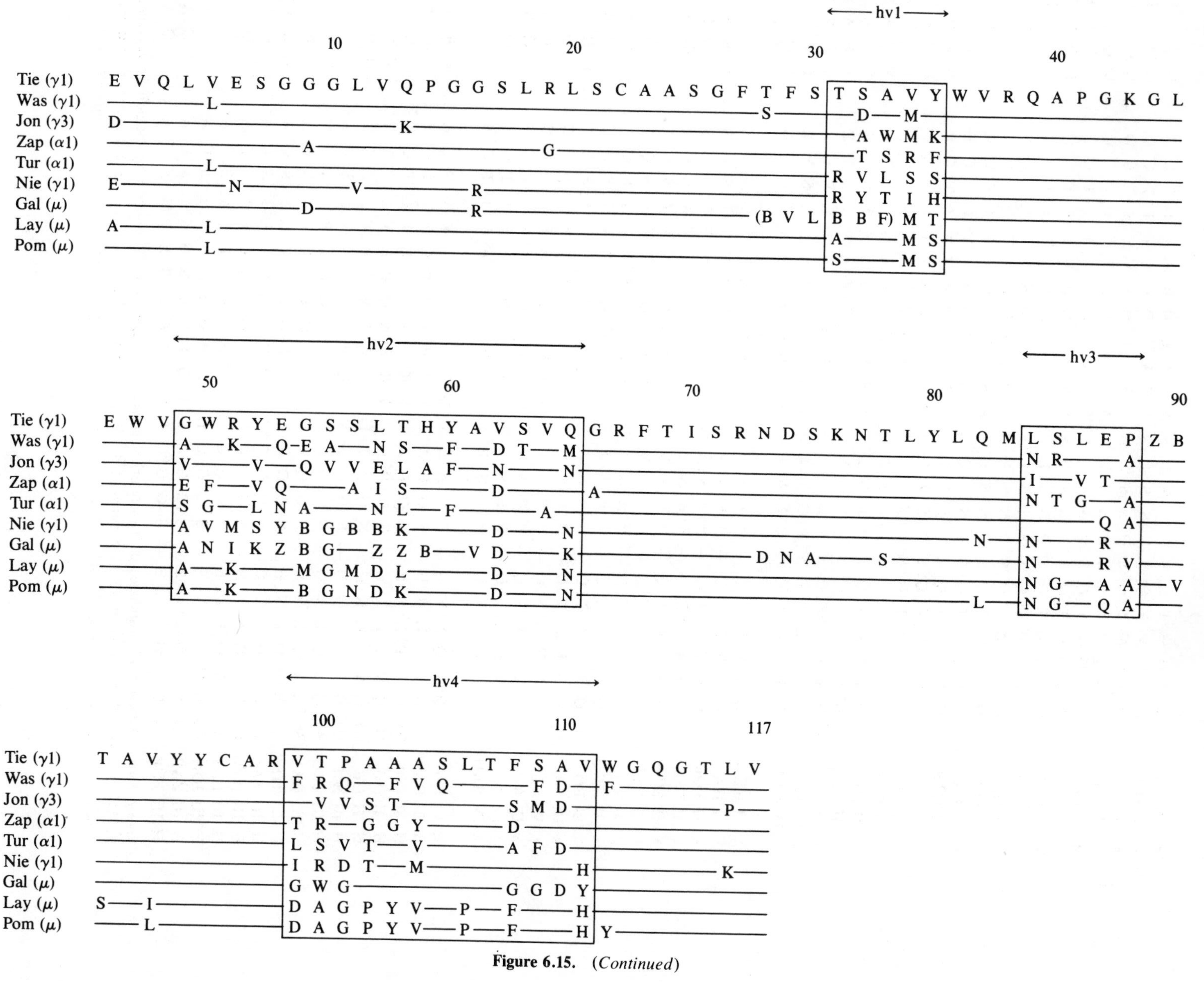

Figure 6.15. *(Continued)*

	0					5					10					15					20							80		
κ I ROY		D	I	Q	M	T	Q	S	P	S	S	L	S	A	S	V	G	D	R	V	T	I	T	C	Q	...	L	Q	P	E	D
κ I REI		D	I	Q	M	T	Q	S	P	S	S	L	S	A	S	V	G	D	R	V	T	I	T	C	Q	...	L	Q	P	E	D
κ I AU		D	I	Q	M	T	Q	S	P	S	S	L	S	A	S	V	G	D	R	V	T	I	T	C	Q	...	L	Q	P	E	D
κ I AG		D	I	Q	M	T	Q	S	P	S	S	L	S	A	S	V	G	D	R	V	T	I	T	C	Q	...	L	Q	P	E	D
κ I BI		D	I	Q	M	T	Q	S	P	S	S	L	S	A	S	V	G	D	S	V	T	I	T	C	Q	...	L	Q	P	E	D
κ I SCW		D	I	Q	M	T	Q	S	P	S	S	L	S	A	S	V	G	D	R	V	T	I	T	C	Q	...	L	Q	P	E	D
κ I DEE		D	I	Q	M	T	Q	S	P	S	S	L	S	A	S	V	G	D	R	V	T	I	T	C	R	...	L	L	P	E	D
κ I HAU		D	I	Q	M	T	Q	S	P	S	S	L	S	A	S	V	G	D	R	V	T	I	T	C	R	...	L	Q	P	E	D
κ I GAL		D	I	Q	M	T	Q	S	P	S	S	L	S	A	S	V	G	D	R	V	T	I	I	C	R	...	L	Q	P	E	D
κ I OU		D	I	Q	M	T	Q	S	P	S	S	L	S	A	S	V	G	D	R	V	T	I	T	C	R	...	L	Z	P	Z	B
κ I KA		D	I	Q	M	T	Q	S	P	S	T	L	S	V	S	V	G	D	R	V	T	I	T	C	E	...	L	Z	P	Z	B
κ I CAR		D	I	Q	M	T	Q	S	P	S	T	L	S	A	S	V	G	D	R	V	A	I	T	C	R	...	L	Z	P	Z	B
κ I EU		D	I	Q	M	T	Q	S	P	S	T	L	S	A	S	V	G	D	R	V	T	I	T	C	R	...	L	Q	P	Q	D
κ I NI		D	I	Q	M	T	Q	S	P	S	S	L	S	A	T	V	G	D	R	V	T	L	L	C	E	...	L	Z	P	Z	B
κ II CUM	E	D	I	V	M	T	Q	T	P	L	S	L	P	V	R	P	G	E	P	A	S	I	S	Y	R	...	V	Q	A	E	D
κ II MIL		D	I	V	L	T	Q	S	P	L	S	L	P	V	R	P	G	E	P	A	S	I	S	Y	R	...	V	Z	A	Z	D
κ II TEW		D	I	V	M	T	Q	S	P	L	S	L	P	V	T	P	G	E	P	A	S	I	S	Y	R	...	V	E	A	E	D
κ III TI		E	I	V	L	T	Q	S	P	G	T	L	S	L	S	P	G	E	R	A	T	L	S	C	R	...	L	E	P	E	D
κ III B6		Z	I	V	L	T	Z	S	P	G	T	L	S	L	S	P	G	Z	R	A	A	L	S	Y	R	...	L	Z	P	E	D
κ IV LEN		D	I	V	M	T	Q	S	P	N	S	L	A	V	S	L	G	E	R	A	T	I	N	C	K	...	L	Q	A	E	D
λ I NEW		Q	S	V	L	T	Q	—	P	P	S	V	S	A	A	P	G	Q	K	V	T	I	S	C	S	...	L	R	T	G	D
λ I HA		Q	S	V	L	T	Q	—	P	P	S	V	S	G	T	P	G	Q	R	V	T	I	S	C	S	...	L	R	S	E	D
λ I VOR		Q	S	V	L	T	Q	—	P	P	S	A	S	G	T	P	G	Q	R	V	T	I	S	C	S	...	L	Q	S	E	D
λ II TRO		Q	S	A	L	T	Q	—	P	R	S	V	S	G	S	P	G	Q	S	V	T	I	S	C	T	...	L	R	A	D	D
λ II BOH		Q	S	A	L	T	Q	—	P	R	S	V	S	G	S	P	G	Q	S	V	T	I	S	C	A	...	L	Q	A	E	D
λ II NEI		Q	S	A	L	T	Q	—	P	A	S	V	S	G	S	P	G	Q	S	I	T	I	S	C	T	...	L	Q	V	E	D
λ II VIL		H	S	A	L	T	Q	—	P	A	S	V	S	G	S	L	G	Q	S	I	T	I	S	C	T	...	L	Q	A	E	D
λ II MCG		Q	S	A	L	T	Q	—	P	P	S	A	S	G	S	L	G	Q	S	V	T	I	S	C	T	...	L	Q	A	E	D
λ II BO		Q	S	A	L	T	Q	—	P	P	S	A	S	G	S	P	G	Q	S	V	T	I	S	C	T	...	L	R	A	E	D
λ III SH		—	S	E	L	T	Q	—	D	P	A	V	S	V	A	L	G	Q	T	V	R	I	T	C	Q	...	A	Q	A	E	D
λ VI DEL		—	Y	V	L	S	Q	—	P	P	S	V	S	V	A	P	G	Q	T	A	R	I	T	C	Q	...	V	E	A	G	D
λ IV KERN		—	Y	A	L	T	Q	—	P	P	S	V	S	V	S	P	G	Q	T	A	V	I	T	C	S	...	A	Q	S	V	D
λ IV X		—	Y	D	L	T	Q	—	P	P	S	V	S	V	S	P	G	Q	T	A	S	I	T	C	S	...	T	Q	A	M	D
λ IV BAU		—	Y	G	L	T	Q	—	P	P	S	L	S	V	S	P	G	Q	T	A	S	I	T	C	S	...					
H I EU		Q	V	Q	L	V	Q	—	S	G	A	E	V	K	K	P	G	S	S	V	K	V	S	C	K	...	L	R	S	E	D
H II DAW	G1	Q	V	T	L	R	E	—	S	G	P	A	L	V	R	P	T	Q	T	L	T	L	T	C	T	...	V	G	P	G	D
H II COR	G1	Q	V	T	L	R	E	—	S	G	P	A	L	V	K	P	T	Q	T	L	T	L	T	C	T	...	—	D	P	V	D
H II OU	M	Q	V	T	L	T	E	—	S	G	P	A	L	V	K	P	K	Q	P	L	T	L	T	C	T	...	V	N	P	V	D
H II HE	G1	Q	V	T	L	K	E	—	N	G	P	T	L	V	K	P	T	E	T	L	T	L	T	C	T	...	M	D	P	V	D
H III NIE	G1	Q	V	Q	L	V	Q	—	S	G	G	G	V	V	Q	P	G	R	S	L	R	L	S	C	A	...	L	R	P	E	D
H III TRO	A1	Q	V	Q	L	V	Q	—	S	G	G	G	L	V	K	P	G	G	S	L	R	L	S	C	V	...	L	R	T	E	D
H III GAL	M	E	V	Q	L	V	E	—	S	G	G	D	L	V	Q	P	G	R	S	L	R	L	S	C	A	...	L	R	V	E	D
H III TIE	G1	E	V	Q	L	V	E	—	S	G	G	G	L	V	Q	P	G	G	S	L	R	L	S	C	A	...	L	E	P	Z	B
H III WAS	G1	E	V	Q	L	L	E	—	S	G	G	G	L	V	Q	P	G	G	S	L	R	L	S	C	A	...	L	E	A	Z	B
H III POM	M	E	V	Q	L	L	E	—	S	G	G	G	L	V	Q	P	G	G	S	L	R	L	S	C	A	...	L	Q	A	Z	B
H III LAY	M	A	V	Q	L	L	E	—	S	G	G	G	L	V	Q	P	G	G	S	L	R	L	S	C	A	...	L	Q	A	Z	V
H III JON	G3	D	V	Q	L	V	E	—	S	G	G	G	L	V	K	P	G	G	S	L	R	L	S	C	A	...	V	T	P	Z	B
H III ZAP	A1	E	V	Q	L	V	E	—	S	G	G	A	L	V	Q	P	G	G	S	G	R	L	S	C	A	...	G	E	A	Z	B
H III TUR	A1	E	V	Q	L	L	E	—	S	G	G	G	L	V	Q	P	G	G	S	L	R	L	S	C	A	...	L	Q	A	Z	B

Figure 6.16. Amino acid sequences of framework residues in V regions of 49 human immunoglobulin residues in V the N terminal and the other at the C terminal of the V region. Greek letter indicates chain isotype, Roman numbers which the chain was obtained. Hyphens designate gaps introduced to maximize homology. Numbers at the top of

85 90 95 105
a b c d e f g h

I A T Y Y C Q Q F D N L P L T — — — — — — — — — — F G G G T K V D F K R
I A T Y Y C Q Q Y Q S L P Y T — — — — — — — — — — F G Q G T K L Q I T R
I A T Y Y C Q Q Y D Y L P W T — — — — — — — — — — F G Q G T K V E I K R
I A T Y Y C Q Q Y D T L P R T — — — — — — — — — — F G Q G T K L E I K R
F A T Y Y C Q Q Y Y N L P Y T — — — — — — — — — — F G Q G T K L E I K R
I A T Y Y C Q Q Y D N V P I T — — — — — — — — — — F G Q G T R V E N K G
F A T Y Y C Z Z S Y T T P Y T — — — — — — — — — — F G P G T K V E M T R
F A T Y Y C Q Q N Y I T P T S — — — — — — — — — — F G Q G T R V E I K R
F A T Y Y C L Q Q N S Y P R S — — — — — — — — — — F G Q G T K V E I K R
F A T Y Y C Z Z S Y S S P T T — — — — — — — — — — F G Z G T R L Z I K R
F A T Y Y C Q Z Y L D L P R T — — — — — — — — — — F G Q G T K V D L K R
F A T Y Y C Q Q Y N T F — F T — — — — — — — — — — F G P G T K V D I K R
F A T Y Y C Q Q Y N S D S K M — — — — — — — — — — F G Q G T K V E V K G
F A V Y Y C Q Z Y D T L P M T — — — — — — — — — — F G V A S K V E S K R
V G V Y Y C M Q R L E I P Y T — — — — — — — — — — F G Q G T K L E I R R
V G V Y Y C M Q A L Q T L L T — — — — — — — — — — F G G G T N V E I K R
V G V Y Y C M Z A L Q A P I T — — — — — — — — — — F G Q G T R L E I K R
F A V Y Y C Q Q Y G S S P S T — — — — — — — — — — F G Q T T K V E L K R
F A V Y Y C Q Q Y G S S P F T — — — — — — — — — — F G Q G S K L E I K
V A V Y Y C Q Q Y Y S T P T S — — — — — — — — — — F G Q G T K L E I K R

E A D Y Y C A T W D S S L N A — — — — — — — — V V F G G G T K V T V L G
E A H Y H C A A W D Y R L S A — — — — — — — — V V F G G G T Q L T V L R
E A D Y F C A T W D D S L D G — — — — — — — — P V F G G G T K V T V L G
E A D Y Y C C S Y A G R Y S — — — — — — — — — V I F G G G T K L T V L G
E A H Y Y C C S Y A G R F T — — — — — — — — — T V F G G G T N L T V L G
E A D Y Y C C S Y A G B S T — — — — — — — — — R V F G G G T R V T V L S
E A D Y Y C S S Y T S S N S — - 001 — — — — — V V F G G G T K L T V L G
E A D Y Y C S S Y E G S D N — - — — — — — F V F G T G T K V T V L G
E A D Y Y C S S Y V D N N N — - — — — — — V V F G G G T K L T V L R
E A D Y Y C N S R D S S G K H - — — — — — V L F G G G T K L T V L G
E A D Y Y C E V W D D R T A H - — — — — — V V F G G G T K L T V L G
E A D Y F C Q T W D T O T — — — — — — — — — — A I F G G G T K L T V L S
E A D Y Y C Q A W D S M S — — — — — — — — — — V V F G G G T R L T V L S
T K L T V L G

T A F Y F C A G G Y G I — — — — — — — — — Y S P E E Y N G G L V T V S S
T A T Y Y C A R S C G S Q — — — — — — — — Y F D Y W G Q G I L V T
T A T Y Y C A R I T V I P A P A G — — — Y M D V W G K G T P V T
T A T Y Y C A R V V N S V M A G Y Y Y Y Y M D V W G K G T T V T V S S
T A T Y Y C V H R H P R T L — — — — — — — A F D V W G Q G T K V A V S S
T A V Y Y C A R I R D T A M — — — — — — — F F A H W G Q G T L V T V S S
T A V Y Y C A A T B B F B W S T F — — — S L N Y W G Q G N L V T V S S
T A L Y Y C A R G W G — — — — — — — — — — G G D Y W G Q G T L V T V S T
T A V Y Y C A R V T P A A A S L T — — — F S A V W G Q G T L V T
T A V Y Y C A R F R Q P F V Q — — — — — F F D V W G Q G T L V T
T A L Y Y C A R D A G P Y V S P T — — — F F A H W G Q G T L V T
S A I Y Y C A R D A G P Y V S P T — — — F F A H W G Q G T L V T
T A V Y Y C A R V V V S T — — — — — — — — S M D V W G Q G T P V T
T A V Y Y C A R T R P G G Y — — — — — — — F S D V W G Q G T L V S
T A L Y Y C A R L S V T A V — — — — — — — A F D V W G Q G T K V S

regions of 49 human immunoglobulin light and heavy chains. Only two stretches of the sequence are shown, one at subgroup, and abbreviations in capital letters names of the myeloma protein or Bence-Jones protein from the figure refer to positions in the first sequence. (Compiled from various authors.)

Hypervariable Regions. These regions are short stretches of extreme variability. No particular order can be made and no grouping into families of related sequences is apparent in these stretches; the variation seems to be completely random. Inspection of the hypervariable-region sequences does not indicate where these sequences have come from (what chain, what species, what vertebrate class).

Hypervariable sequences make up 25 of the 110 VL-region amino acids; in the VH domain, they constitute about 30 of the 120 amino acids.

The location of hypervariable regions in the V polypeptides is depicted in Figure 6.15*a* and *b*. Because of the variable length of different V domains and because of the different residue numbering systems used by different authors, the positions of the variable regions do not always fit exactly in the same areas (as can be seen by comparing the *a* and *b* portions of Fig. 6.15). There is also some uncertainty about the number of hypervariable regions. All immunochemists agree that there are at least three hypervariable regions in both VL and VH domains (hv1 through hv3); the question is whether the segment of the V domain encoded by the J chain should be considered as the fourth hypervariable region (hv4). Despite these uncertainties, the hypervariable regions always fall at homologous positions in V domains of all species so far studied.

Hypervariable regions contain residues that contact the antigen and bind to it on the basis of mutual complementarity (*complementarity-determining residues*, or CDR). Although the regions are discontinuous at the primary structure level, they converge at the level of the tertiary structure to form a continuous, highly contoured surface of the *combining site*. However, not all of the hypervariable-region amino acids are complementarity-determining (see below). In human heavy chains, only hv1, hv2, and hv4 line the combining site (see Fig. 6.15*a*); the function of the hv3 region is not known.

Framework Residues. Occupying positions outside the hypervariable regions, the framework residues constitute about 80 percent of the V region (Fig. 6.15*a* and *b*). In comparison to the hypervariable residues, the framework residues are less variable and more evolutionarily conserved, but the degree of conservation changes from position to position.

To illustrate the different degrees of variability at different positions, we shall consider a sample of about 49 human myeloma and Bence-Jones proteins (Fig. 6.16). The proteins have been sequenced in their entirety, but to make points about the residue variability in the framework regions, we shall consider only two stretches of the V-region sequence: positions 1 through 24 and 78 through 108. The first thing one notices in Figure 6.16 is the *invariable residues shared by all or nearly all chains in the sample*. For example, without exception, all chains have cysteine at positions 23 and 88, tyrosine at position 86, and with few exceptions, glycine at positions 16, 100, and 101, leucine at position 78, glutamine at position 81, aspartic acid at position 82, and alanine at position 84. More significantly, there are conserved short *sequences*—for example, at positions 86 through 88 and 99 through 102. This sharing of residues and sequences at homologous positions in all 49 chains suggests that all contemporary human V regions have evolved from a common ancestor. The exceptions to this sharing (a few chains with a residue different from the unvarying one at a given position) suggest that evolution has not stopped, but is still experimenting with new possibilities, even at the most conserved positions.

A second level of conservation is apparent from the fact that all 50 sequences can be divided into three *groups* corresponding to the κ, λ, and H chains; in other words, there are residues shared by all, or almost all, κ chains and absent in λ or H chains (e.g., glutamic acid at positions 89 and 90), others present only in κ but not in λ or H (e.g., proline at position 9, or glutamic acid at position 83), and still others specific for H chains (e.g., glycine at position 9 or leucine at position 19). The existence of chain-specific residues indicates that, after diverging from a common ancestor, the three sets of V-region (Vκ, Vλ, and VH) chains evolved independently of one another. It also reconfirms what we already know, namely that the three groups of V chain are controlled by three different sets of genetic loci.

A third level of residue conservation becomes apparent when one compares the sequences within each group. One then realizes that the groups are not homogeneous but can be split into several *subgroups*, each characterized by a series of subgroup-specific residues. For example, there are four subgroups in the Vκ group, designated I through IV (Fig. 6.16). All sequences in subgroup I have glutamic acid at position 3, serine at position 9, valine at position 15, and so on, while all other Vκ sequences have different residues at these positions. All sequences in subgroup II share leucine at position 9, proline at position 12, threonine at position 14, and so on; and again, Vκ sequences not belonging to this subgroup have different residues at these positions. The two sequences in subgroup III have glycine at position 9, leucine at positions 13 and

21, and so on. And finally, the one subgroup IV sequence is characterized by asparagine at position 9, alanine at position 12, leucine at position 15, and so on.

Human subgroups are designated by Roman numerals added to the chain designation. There are four subgroups of Vκ (VκI through VκIV), five subgroups of Vλ(VλI through VλV), and five subgroups of VH (VHI through VHV). The subgroups are identified by amino acid or DNA sequencing, although antisera have also been produced recently, allowing serological recognition. Each subgroup is defined by a certain prototype sequence consisting of the most common amino acids at individual positions. Individual sequences within a given subgroup differ from this basic sequence only at a small number of positions (Fig. 6.16)—excluding, of course, the hypervariable regions. Different subgroups of a given group differ in as much as 40 percent of their amino acid sequence; the homology within a subgroup is on the order of 75 percent.

The original system of *mouse subgroup* designation was similar to the human system, but recently—because of difficulties in subgroup definition—a new system has been introduced, and the term "subgroup" itself has been replaced by the term "isotype." The principle of the new system of grouping is this: all sequences available for a given chain are analyzed and a hypothetical prototype sequence is constructed for each position by selecting the most common of all amino acids found at the position. This prototype sequence is referred to as V_0. Since limited sequence data are available for most proteins, the prototype sequence is constructed only for the first 23 (κ) or first 27 (H) residues. Any sequence differing from the prototype sequence by three or more residues is assigned a Vn number and regarded as a separate isotype. Each isotype can be divided further, based on additional framework variation observed beyond residue 23 (or 27). The subdivisions are designated by letters (e.g., Vκ21A, Vκ21B, Vκ21C, etc.). At the time of writing, the following isotypes (groups and subgroups) have been identified for the three basic chains. *κ chain*—Vκ1 through Vκ25, with Vκ10 divided into Vκ10A and Vκ10B, and Vκ21 divided into Vκ21A, Vκ21B, and Vκ21C; a total of 28 isotypes. *λ chain*—Vλ1 through Vλ2 (two isotypes). Of 21 partially sequenced Vλ1 proteins, 12 had an identical sequence and nine differed from this prototype sequence by no more than three amino acids, all in the complementarity-determining regions. Vλ2, which is thus far represented by only one myeloma protein, differs from the prototype Vλ1 sequence in 14 residues in both framework and complementarity-determining regions. *H chain*—VH1 through VH11, with VH1 divided into A, B, C, and D, and VH4 divided into A, B, C, D, and E; a total of 17 isotypes.

The portion of the L or H chain where the variable domain joins the first constant domain is called the *V–C junction* (*switch point*). Where exactly the variable sequence ends and the constant sequence begins has, until now, been difficult to determine, for the transition from relative variability to relative constancy is gradual, rather than abrupt (Fig. 6.17). However, the new methods of Ig gene analysis at the DNA level make precise identification of the initial point possible (see section 6.7). The *intrasubgroup* grouping of amino acid sequences represents a *fourth level* of framework-residue conservation. How much further subgroups should be divided is debatable. It is not difficult to see that there are clusters with similar sequences within each subgroup: should they be considered as sub-subgroups, characterized by sub-subgroup-specific residues, and should the sub-subgroups then be divided further into sub-sub-subgroups, and so on? Or, should the clusters be considered as repeated occurrences of

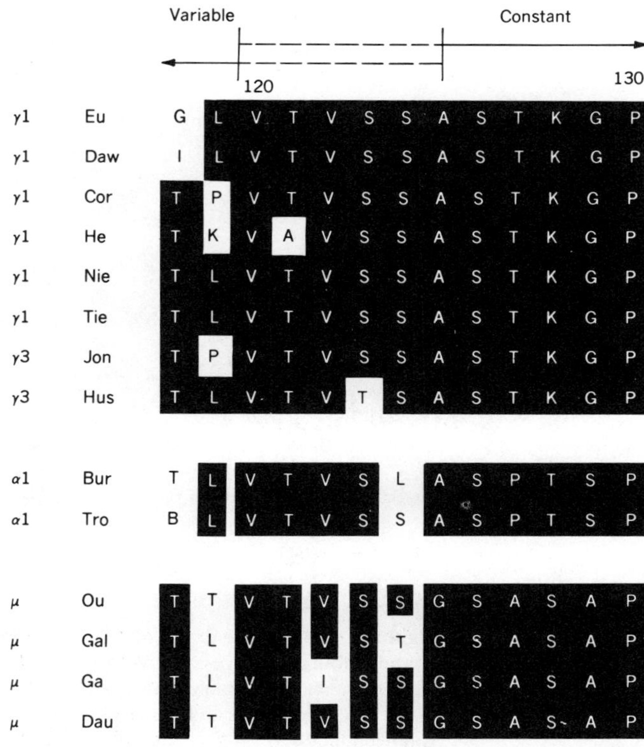

Figure 6.17. Amino acid sequences at the V–C junction of several heavy immunoglobulin chains. Homologies are indicated by shading. Notation the same as that in Figure 6.16. (Compiled from various sources.)

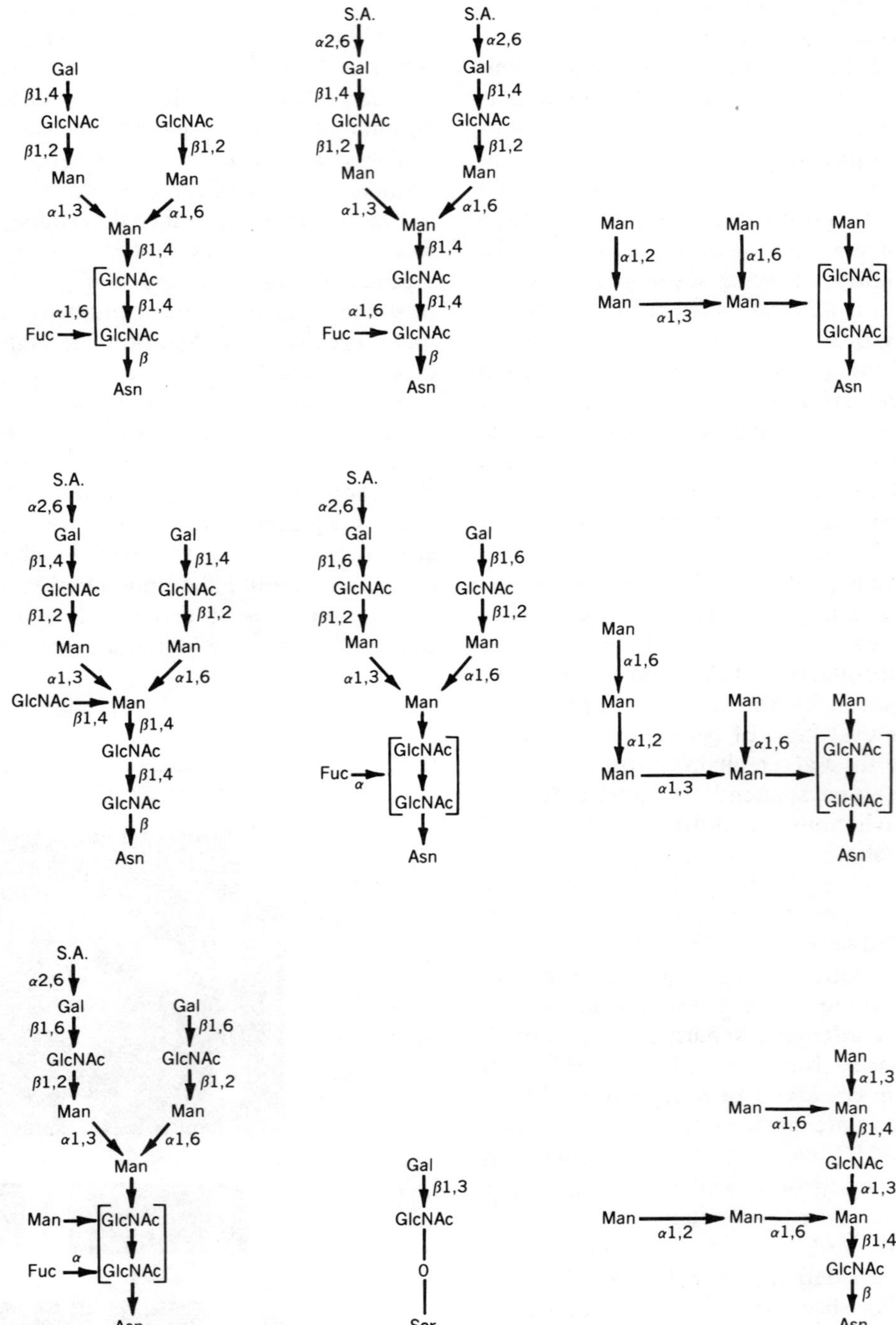

Figure 6.18. Carbohydrate moiety of the immunoglobulin molecule. Examples of oligosaccharides found in association with Ig polypeptide chains. Asn, asparagine; Fuc, fucose; Gal, galactose; GalNAc, N-acetylgalactosamine; GlcNAc, N-acetylglucosamine; Man, mannose; O, oxygen; S.A., sialic acid; Ser, serine. (From A.-C. Wang *in* H. H. Fudenberg, D. P. Stites, J. L. Caldwell, and J. V. Wells (Eds.): *Basic and Clinical Immunology*. Lange, Los Altos, California, 1976.)

the same unique sequence? Is there, perhaps, a continuous variability spectrum with unvarying residues at one end and hypervariable positions at the other end? Answers to these questions can be provided only by determining the complete organization of the V-gene family at the DNA level.

At present, the relationship between variability (conservation) at the protein level and gene organization at the DNA level is not completely understood. The simplest view is that there is a separate V gene proper for each defined framework sequence, but this view does not take into account the variability generated somatically during the differentiation of a progenitor cell into a mature B lymphocyte. Although most somatically generated variability occurs in the hypervariable regions, some may also affect the framework residues. We shall return to the question of how variability is generated in Section 6.8.

When one compares framework sequences of different species in terms of shared residues and similar overall chain organization, one finds evidence for common evolutionary origin of V regions of various phylogenetic groups (see also section 6.11). The most striking interspecies V-region homology thus far discovered is that between Vκ regions of the human and mouse. Some 60 percent framework Vκ positions are shared between these two species—a degree of homology equal to that seen between two human Vκ chains belonging to different subgroups. In other species, the homologies are less pronounced. The V-region residues shared by all individuals of a given phylogenetic group are referred to as *phylogenetically associated* or as *species-specific*. (The latter term, however, is somewhat misleading because it is virtually impossible to prove that the residues are restricted to a single species; although a given residue at a particular position may be found only in cats, for example, one cannot exclude the possibility that the same residue will be found later in all individuals of another species.)

6.3.7 The Carbohydrate Moiety

Immunoglobulins are almost always associated with carbohydrate chains of variable length and shape: some consist of only two sugar residues, but most contain a dozen or more units (Fig. 6.18). The chains can be either simple or branched. The number of carbohydrate chains attached to one Ig molecule varies, depending on the Ig class: IgG contains two carbohydrate chains per molecule, IgM 10, IgA 16, IgD six, and IgE 12. Sometimes even molecules of the same class and subclass vary in their carbohydrate contents.

Normally, carbohydrate chains attach to the Fc portion of the Ig molecule (to the CH2 domains), but under pathological conditions carbohydrates can also be found attached to L chains and to V regions of H chains. The most common bond linking the carbohydrate moiety to the polypeptide chain is that between the amino group of asparagine carbon number 1 and the sugar N-acetylglucosamine (Fig. 6.19). The bond formation is catalyzed by an enzyme, N-acetylglucosamine-asparagine transglucosylase, which recognizes a trio of amino acids consisting of asparagine in the first position, variable amino acid (X) in the second position, and serine or threonine in the third position. However, not all the asp-X-ser/thr trios in the immunoglobulin chains are acted upon by the enzyme; some—those in the V region, for instance—are apparently inaccessible because they are buried in the interior of the molecule. Occasionally, the enzyme attaches the sugar to the serine or threonine, instead of to asparagine. The function of the carbohydrate moiety is

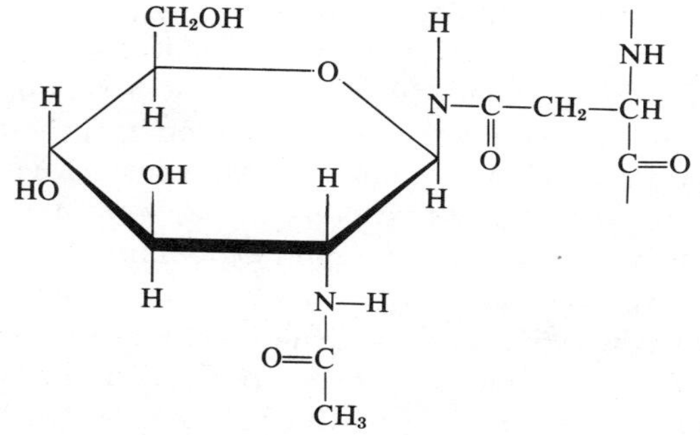

N-acetylglucosamine linked to an asparagine residue
(*a*)

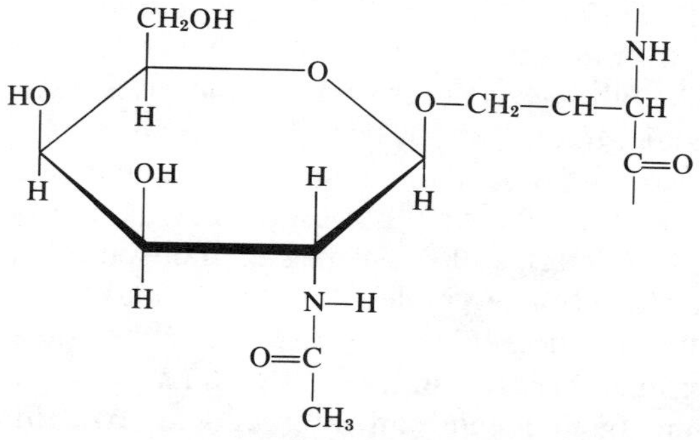

N-acetylgalactosamine linked to a serine residue
(*b*)

Figure 6.19. Two common bonds linking carbohydrates to polypeptide chains. (*a*) N-acetylglucosamine linked to an asparagine residue. (*b*) N-acetylgalactosamine linked to a serine residue.

unknown. It may play a role in Ig secretion by plasma cells or participate in Ig effector functions.

6.4 TERTIARY STRUCTURE OF Ig MOLECULES

6.4.1 The Overall Arrangement of Ig Molecules

Electron Microscopy

A specimen (molecule) is visible in an electron microscope only when it scatters incident electrons in a proportion different from that of the background—that is, when it shows sufficient contrast. To enhance contrast, the specimen is embedded in a medium ("stain"), such as sodium phosphotungstate, that scatters electrons in a high proportion, in comparison to the specimen. In this *negative staining technique*, the specimen appears as a light, electron-translucent footprint on a dark, electron-opaque background (Fig. 6.20*a*).

When electron microscopists looked at Ig molecules alone, without an antigen bound to them, they did not see much. The molecules appeared as irregular globular particles lacking any characteristic structure. To stretch out these molecules and see more of them, investigators combined them with antigens. Originally, large antigens, such as virus particles, were used, but in such preparations the immunoglobulins were difficult to see because they were obscured by the bulky antigens. In 1967, Robin C. Valentine and N. Michael Green found a solution to these problems in the *bifunctional hapten technique*, in which they replaced bulky antigens with two small haptens (molecules that can bind antibody but alone cannot induce antibody formation; see Chapter 10), separated by a spacer chain of eight or more carbon atoms (Fig. 6.20*c*). An example of such a bifunctional hapten is a polyethylenediamine chain with an immunologically active (functional) dinitrophenyl group at each end. The bifunctional hapten is so small that it cannot be seen in an electron micrograph (to be visible in the microscope, a molecule must be larger than 70 Å; the bifunctional hapten is only about 20 Å long), and so one has an unobscured view of the stretched-out Ig molecules. Since both the hapten and the Ig molecules have two binding sites, one bifunctional hapten can interact with two Ig molecules and one Ig molecule can interact with two different haptens, so that dimers and rings of three (Fig. 6.20), four, five, or more Ig molecules can form.

In an antigen-antibody complex, the IgG molecule is Y-shaped, with a variable angle between the two arms. The angle is always at least 90° and sometimes as large as 180°, so that the molecule assumes a T configuration. The T-shaped or "clicked open" form is frequently seen in crystals, in which the Ig molecules form a regular lattice. After trypsin digestion, the molecules become V-shaped.

IgM molecules look like starfish, with five arms stretching out from a central disk. Depending on the antigen bound to the IgM molecules, some or all of the arms may bend and the molecules may assume a variety of bizarre forms (Fig. 6.21).

X-Ray Diffraction Analysis

Information about the spatial arrangement of polypeptide chains within the Ig molecule is provided by the X-ray diffraction analysis of antibody crystals (see Appendix 6.14.2). Such an analysis is a difficult undertaking and the results, therefore, have been slow in coming. The two main obstacles facing an X-ray crystallographer are the heterogeneity of antibodies (to obtain crystals, one must use single-antibody solutions) and the large size of the Ig molecule. The former obstacle has been overcome by the use of myeloma and Bence-Jones proteins, the latter by cleaving the molecule into two types of fragment, Fab and Fc, and analyzing each separately. So far, most of the work has been done using crystals of papain-produced Fab fragments or Bence-Jones proteins, which are naturally occurring dimers of L chains; Fc fragments have proved to be difficult to work with, mainly because X-rays damage their crystals easily. Recently, work has also started on intact Ig molecules.

The analysis of both the fragments and the intact molecules has been carried out in phases, with each subsequent phase providing a picture of the molecule at a higher resolution than that of the preceding phase. Although at the time of writing, a resolution has not yet been reached at which all the atoms and their positions in the molecule can be identified, researchers in at least four laboratories—headed by David R. Davies, Allen B. Edmundson, R. Huber, and Roberto J. Poljak—are close to this goal.

Crystallographic studies have confirmed the domain-type organization of the IgG molecule previously deduced from amino acid sequence analysis. The domains are ovoid or cylindrical, with the longer and shorter axes measuring approximately 40 Å and 20 Å (C domains) or 24 Å (V domains), respectively (Figs. 6.22 and 23). All domains, regardless of their origin, have essentially the same three-dimensional organization. In each domain, the polypeptide chain is folded in a characteristic way, called the *immunoglobulin fold*

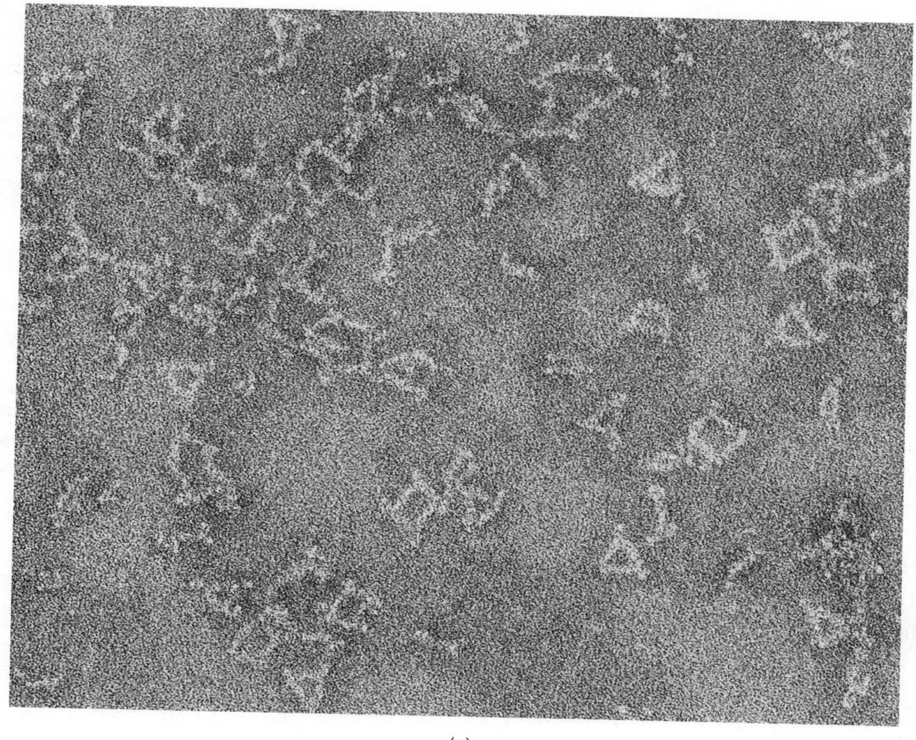

(a)

(b)

NO_2

NO_2

NH

H_2C

CH_2

H_2C

CH_2

H_2C

CH_2

H_2C

CH_2

NH

NO_2

NO_2

(*c*)

Figure 6.20. Bifunctional hapten technique for visualization of immunoglobulin molecules in electron microscope. (*a*) Electron micrograph of IgG molecules joined into multimolecular complexes. Magnification ×500,000. (*b*) Diagrammatic representation of one of the complexes seen in (*a*) (indicated by an arrow). (*c*) Structure of bifunctional haptens with dinitrophenyl (DNP) haptens at both ends. The antibodies in (*b*) and (*c*) have anti-DNP specificity. (*a* by Dr. N. M. Green.)

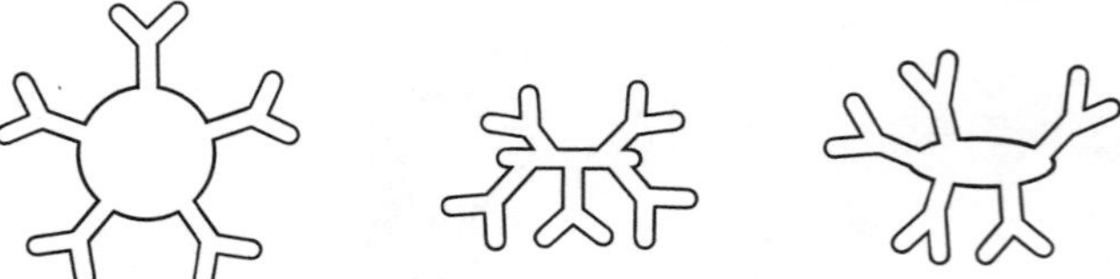

Figure 6.21. Diagram of some of the forms an IgM molecule can assume. Based on electron micrographs.

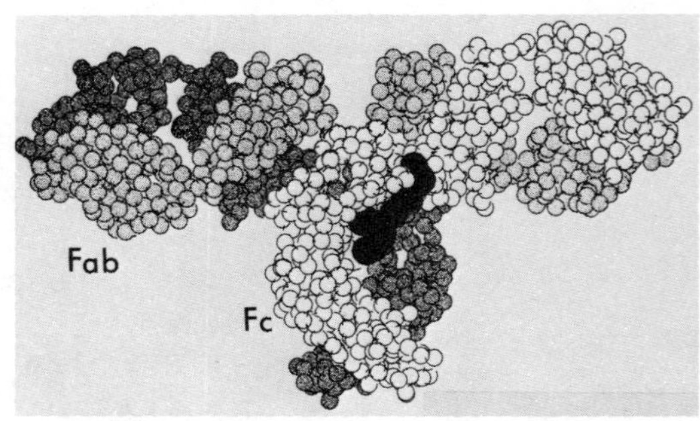

Figure 6.23. Space-filling model of an IgG molecule. One heavy chain is white, the other is dark grey. The two light chains are shaded; the carbohydrate moiety is black. (From E. W. Silverton, M. A. Navia, and D. R. Davies: *Proc. Natl. Acad. Sci. U.S.A.* **74**:5140–5144, 1977.)

(Fig. 6.24). More than 50 percent of the chain forms short, straight stretches that bend in a hairpin fashion; the rest of the chain is difficult to characterize, except to say that in the C domain, two short helical stretches (in C1 domains, residues 125–132 and 185–192) can be identified. Nearly all the hairpin bends contain glycine (essentially unvarying at these positions), often flanked on the N-terminal side by proline, serine, or threonine. The straight strands are organized into two parallel planes: one plane (face x) contains four straight stretches (in C_L, for example, the stretches span residues 116 and 120, 132 and 140, 160 and 169, and 173 and 182), and the other (face y) contains three stretches (in C_L, between residues 147 and 151, 193 and 199, and 202 and 208). The stretches are designated fx1 through fx4 in the x face, and fy1 through fy3 in the y face. The strands run in an antiparallel fashion (one strand runs in one direction and the adjacent strand in the opposite direction), and the entire arrangement is stabilized by hydrogen bonds between adjacent strands. This organization of strands held together in one plane is designated *β-pleated sheet* (see Appendix 6.1). The space between the two x and y faces is filled with hydrophobic side chains, so that the interior of each domain is inaccessible to water.

The two β-pleated sheets are connected by a single intrachain disulfide bridge, which runs approximately perpendicular to them. The two sulfur atoms of the bridge are located near the center of the domain, and are 18 Å apart in the more compact C domain and 24 Å apart in the more loosely organized V domain.

The V domains of both the H and L chains contain an extra loop (residues 43 through 61) that is absent from C domains; in the latter, the extra loop is compensated for by the somewhat greater length of the extended stretches.

The individual domains are paired at a particular angle and face. The two V domains (VL and VH) are paired in the form of a cross, with their N terminals relatively close together and C terminals more remote from each other, and they contact each other by their y faces. The CH1 and CL domains are also crossed but contact each other by their x faces. In the two CH2 domains, crossing is almost impossible because of the restriction imposed by the S–S-bridged hinge region. Consequently, the two domains are not in contact with each other, and the gap between them is filled with the carbohydrate moiety. The two CH3 domains are paired in a fashion similar to that of the CH1 and CL domains.

Two adjacent domains (VH and CH1, CH1 and CH2,

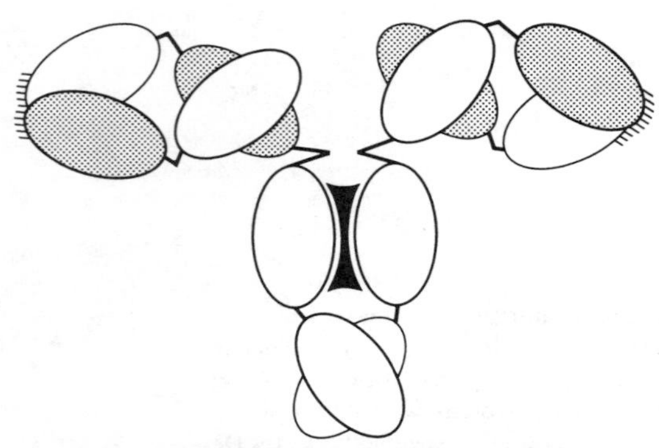

Figure 6.22. Model of an IgG molecule, showing the quaternary relationships of the individual domains.

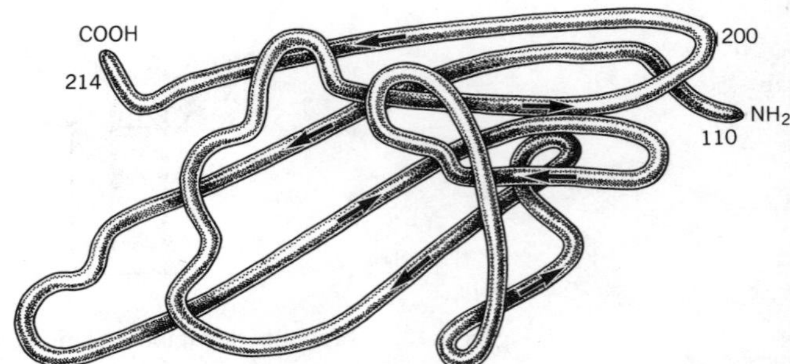

Figure 6.24. Basic folding pattern of the polypeptide chain in the constant domains of an immunoglobulin molecule. Arrows indicate orientation of strands; numbers indicate amino acid residues. (Based on A. B. Edmundson, K. R. Ely, E. E. Abola, M. Schiffer, and N. Panagiotopoulos: *Biochemistry* **14**:3953–3961, 1975.)

etc.) are connected by extended strands (Fig. 6.22), bent in such a way that the longitudinal axes of the two domains run at angles of approximately 130°. In addition, adjacent domains are arranged in such a way that one has its x face "up" and the y face "down," while the other has the y face "up" and the x face "down."

Interestingly, in Bence-Jones protein dimers, the two monomers, although identical in amino acid sequence, do not assume identical configurations. Instead, one monomer assumes the role of an H chain, while the other remains a normal L chain.

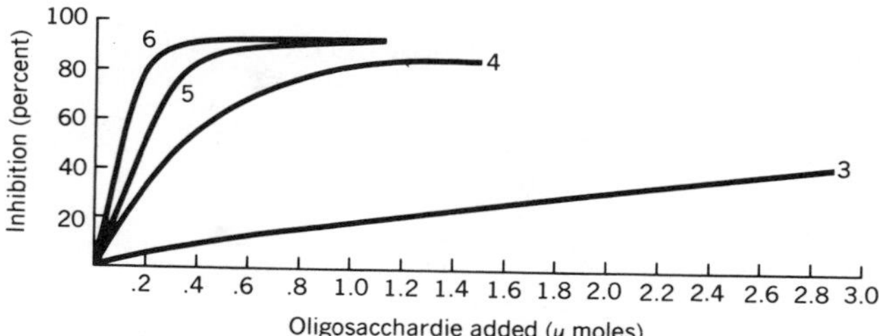

Figure 6.25. Inhibition by oligosaccharide of the dextran–antidextran precipitin reaction. The oligosaccharides are 3, isomaltotriose; 4, isomaltotetraose; 5, isomaltopentaose; 6, isomaltohexaose. They consist of 3, 4, 5, and 6 glucose monomers, respectively. (From E. A. Kabat: *J. Immunol.* **84**:82–85, 1960.)

6.4.2 Structure of the Combining Site

Size of the Combining Site

Electron micrographs reveal that antigens always attach to the tips of the two arms of the Y- or T-shaped molecule; the combining site of the Ig molecule must, therefore, be located in these two areas. The narrowness of the tips suggests that the combining site occupies only a small portion of the Ig molecule.

The actual size of the combining site was first determined by Elvin A. Kabat for a human antibody (Kabat's own) to dextran, a polymer consisting of many repeating glucose units arranged into long, branched chains. Kabat wanted to know how large a segment of the dextran molecule could fit into the combining site of an antidextran Ig molecule. To this end, he prepared a series of short chains (oligosaccharides), some containing only three glucose units (isomaltotriose), others four units (isomaltotetraose), still others five (isomaltopentaose) or six (isomaltohexaose) units. Since the antidextran Ig must recognize glucose units (there is nothing else in the dextran molecule), the short chains should combine with this antibody; but the chains are too small to be crosslinked by the antibody and thus precipitated out of the solution (as happens when the long dextran molecules combine with antibodies). When the oligosaccharides are smaller than the combining site, they attach only poorly to it, so that when dextran is added to the mixture, its reaction with antidextran, as measured by the amount of precipitate formed, is only partially inhibited. The longer the chain of the oligosaccharide, the better it inhibits the precipitate formation, until at a certain size—that at which it completely fills the combining site—a maximum of inhibition is achieved. Larger oligosaccharides then fail to increase the degree of inhibition.

In the actual experiment (Fig. 6.25), chains consisting of four glucose units inhibited better than those consisting of three units; five-unit chains inhibited better than four-unit chains; and maximum inhibition occurred with the six-unit chains. Since the dimensions of the six-unit chain (isomaltohexaose) are about 34 × 12 × 7 Å, Kabat concluded that this must also be the size of the antidextran combining site. Measurements with other antigens and antibodies indicated that the size of the combining site varies, but not very much.

Amino Acid Composition of the Combining Site

To determine which amino acids of the combining site actually bind the antigen, Jonathan S. Singer and his colleagues devised a method they called *affinity labeling*. The method consists of the following four steps. First, antibodies are produced against hapten H. Second, the hapten is combined chemically with a compound, X, which has a reactive group capable of forming a covalent bond with amino acids of a polypeptide chain. Third, radioactivity-labeled H–X complex is reacted with the anti-H immunoglobulin. (The attachment of X to H does not change the latter in terms of specificity, so that anti-H still recognizes the compound.) Once H–X is positioned in the combining site, the reactive group of X binds covalently to the nearest available amino acid (A), forming an H–X–A complex. Fourth, the antibody with the H–X–A complex is digested enzymatically and sequenced, and the amino acid to which H–X is attached is identified through the radioactive label.

Depending on the nature of X, one can distinguish several variants of the affinity labeling method. In the variant originally used by Singer and his colleagues, the source of the reactive group was a diazonium salt. The method was carried out as follows. First, rabbits were injected with hapten p-azobenzenearsonate (ABA) attached to ovalbumin to make the hapten immunogenic, and antibodies to ABA were produced. Second, ABA was diazotized and the resulting compound was stabilized with fluoroborate:

$$\underset{NH_2}{\overset{AsO_3H_2}{C_6H_4}} \xrightarrow[HCl]{NaNo_2} \underset{N{\equiv}N^+}{\overset{AsO_3H_2}{C_6H_4}} \longrightarrow \underset{N{\equiv}N^+(BFu)^-}{\overset{AsO_3H_2}{C_6H_4}}$$

(Fluoroborate is an anion that forms a stable salt with the positively charged diazonium group, $-N{\equiv}N^+$, but plays no role in the reaction.) The resulting *m*-nitrobenzene diazonium fluoroborate (NBDFB) was then labeled with tritium. Third, antibodies to ABA were reacted with NBDFB, and formation of covalent bonds at the combining site was allowed to occur. NBDFB can bind to the nearest tyrosine, histidine, or lysine. The reaction with tyrosine can be visualized as follows:

Polypeptide chain of the combining site

$$\underset{\text{Tyrosine}}{\overset{\sim\sim CH_2}{C_6H_4 - OH}} + \underset{\text{NBDFB}}{\overset{AsO_3H_2}{C_6H_4 - N{\equiv}N^+(BFu)^-}} \rightarrow$$

$$\rightarrow \underset{OH}{\overset{\sim\sim CH_2}{C_6H_3}}{-}N{=}N{-}C_6H_4{-}AsO_3H_2$$

Fourth, the position of the tyrosine to which NBDFB bound was determined by amino acid sequencing.

In other variants of the affinity labeling method, the diazonium group can be replaced by:

The Bromoacetyl Group, $-\overset{O}{\overset{\|}{C}}-CH_2-Br$, which forms covalent bonds with lysine and tyrosine; the group can be separated from the hapten by spacers of different length, and this arrangement allows the reactive group to reach amino acids further away from the site of actual hapten binding;

A Photoactivatable Group, for example, an azide, N_3, which is inert in the dark but is activated when exposed to light; it can then attach to any C–H bond in the polypeptide;

The Diazoketone Group, $-NH-CH_2COCHN_2$, which, when irradiated with ultraviolet light, forms a carbene $-NH-CH_2COCH$, and this radical then reacts with the C–H bond.

The two main conclusions drawn from affinity labeling studies were that, first, labeled amino acids derive from both H and L chains and so both participate in the formation of the combining site; second, all labeled amino acids derive from the V region, both the hypervariable and framework portions. Hence, C regions do not contribute in any way to the architecture of the combining site.

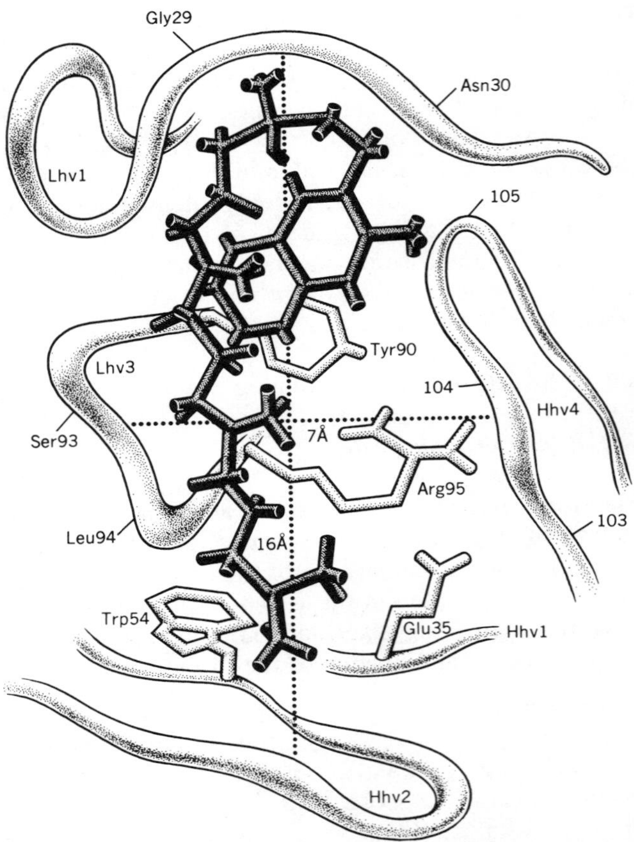

Figure 6.26. A view into the combining site of a human IgG molecule with a hapten, vitamin K_1OH, bound to it. Hapten drawn in black, Ig polypeptide in grey. Lh1, Lh3, Hhv1, Hhv2, and Hhv4 indicate the location of the hypervariable regions of the L and H chains. Numbers give the positions of the indicated amino acids. (Modified from L. M. Amzel, R. J. Poljak, F. Sank, J. M. Varga, and F. F. R. Richards: *Proc. Natl. Acad. Sci. U.S.A.* **71**:1427–1430, 1974.)

Spatial Arrangement of the Combining Site

Information about the actual tertiary structure of the combining site derives from X-ray diffraction studies. To carry out such studies on myeloma proteins, one must first screen a large number of antigens to find one that binds specifically to a given protein. One then allows this antigen to diffuse into the Fab crystals of the myeloma protein and to interact with the antibody. X-Ray diffraction analysis of such antigen-antibody complexes then not only determines the position and orientation of the antigen and of the contact residues in the combining site, but also provides information about the types of bond between the antigen and the antibody.

One of the first antigen-antibody complexes studied in this manner was that consisting of γ-hydroxyl derivative of vitamin K_1 (K_1OH) and human myeloma protein New (Fig. 6.26). Since then, other complexes have also been analyzed, revealing the combining site to be a crevice between the VL and VH domains on the tips of the Fab fragments (Fig. 6.27). The size and shape of the crevice can vary, depending on the particular antibody: it can be a shallow groove, 15 × 6 Å in size; a large, wedge-shaped, hollow space with dimensions 12 × 15 × 20 Å; or a deep, conical pocket, about 10 Å in diameter. The cavity is lined mainly or exclusively with residues from the hypervariable regions that come together at the N-terminal surface of the molecule (Fig. 6.27). In fact, the size and shape of the combining site varies mainly because of amino acid substitutions, deletions, or additions in the hypervariable regions.

Both H and L chains participate in and appear to be necessary for optimal antigen binding. Isolated L chains bind haptens with low affinity and this binding can be demonstrated only when highly sensitive detection methods are used. Isolated H chains are generally insoluble, but when solubilized, they bind haptens better than do isolated L chains, but far less than do intact Ig molecules; they can also discriminate between related antigens.

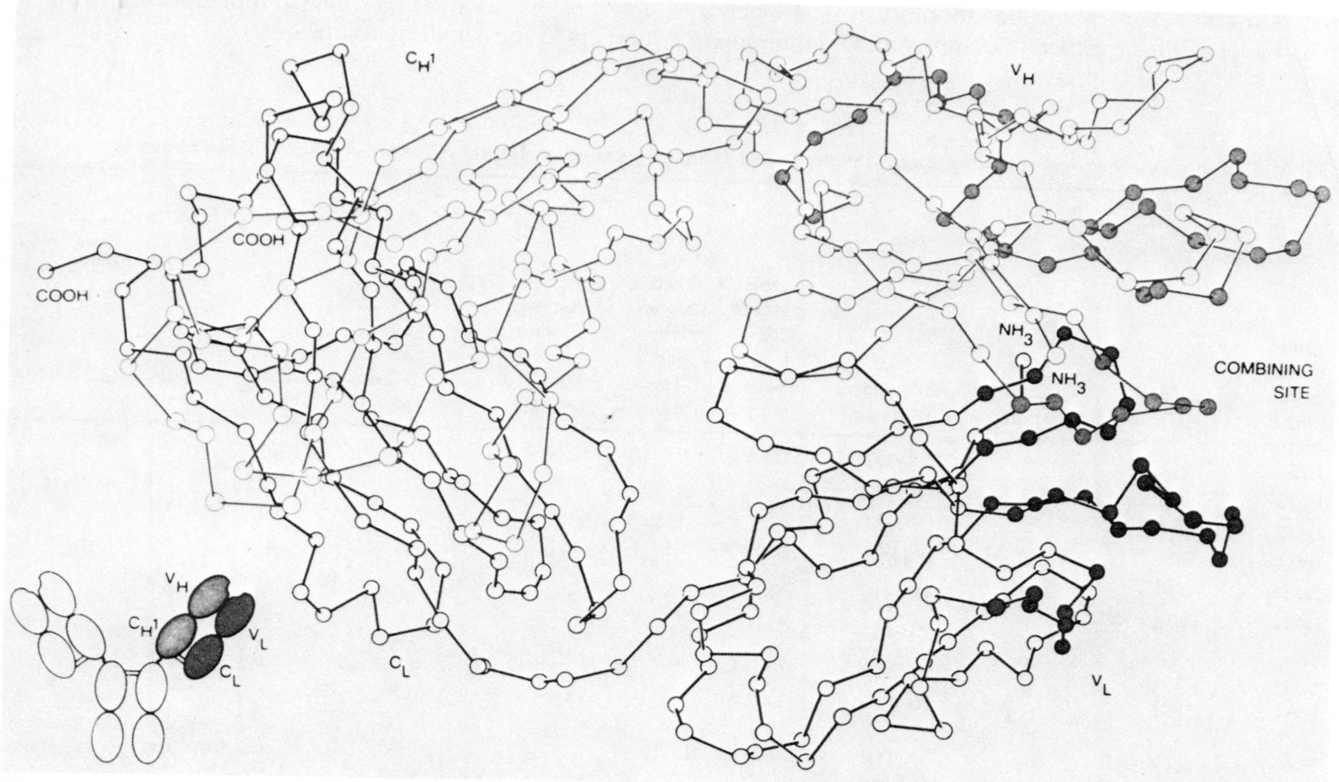

Figure 6.27. Carbon skeleton of a Fab fragment from mouse myeloma protein McPC603. The drawing shows how the amino acids of the hypervariable regions (triangles) come together in the combining site. Heavy line indicates H chain, light line L chain. [Redrawn from J. D. Capra and A. B. Edmundson: *Sci. Am.* **236** (January):50–59, 1977.)

6.5 PROPERTIES OF Ig CLASSES AND SUBCLASSES

From the description of the basic Ig molecule we now turn to discussion of the properties that distinguish individual Ig classes and subclasses. The overall properties are summarized in Table 6.5; the structural features of the polypeptide chains composing the different Ig molecules are depicted in Figure 6.28. The classes will be dealt with in the order of their decreasing concentration in normal human serum. The emphasis will be on human immunoglobulins, which have been studied most extensively, but animal immunoglobulins will also be mentioned when appropriate.

6.5.1 Immunoglobulin G

The IgG molecule has the structure of the basic H_2L_2 tetramer, and most of what we said about immunoglobulin structure in the preceding section referred to this molecule. In normal serum of most animals, IgG is the major immunoglobulin class, constituting about 75 percent of the total Ig. Human IgG has a molecular weight of 146,000 daltons and a sedimentation constant of 6.6S (or roughly 7S). At alkaline pH (8.6), IgG has the slowest electrophoretic mobility of all major plasma proteins except complement component C1q—a fact that facilitates its isolation by ion-exchange chromatography.

Human IgG falls into four subclasses—IgG1, IgG2, IgG3, and IgG4—that constitute 70, 20, 8, and 2 percent, respectively, of the total IgG. However, the proportion of each subclass varies from individual to individual and may be controlled genetically. IgG1 differs from all other IgG molecules in the position of the half-cystine linking the L and H chains: in IgG1 the half-cystine is at position 220; in other IgG molecules it is at position 131 (Fig. 6.28). The different subclasses also differ in the number of disulfide bridges (Fig. 6.14). Their number in the IgG3 molecule is controversial, with estimates varying between five and 15. The IgG3 molecule has an extra 95 amino acids in the γ chain and is therefore heavier than molecules of other IgG subclasses.

No subclasses have yet been found in the IgG of the rabbit. In this species, the two γ chains are held together by a single disulfide bridge; however, the $C\gamma1$ domain contains two intrachain disulfide bridges.

Four IgG subclasses are known in the mouse: IgG1, IgG2a, IgG2b, and IgG3. The two IgG2 subclasses are structurally similar to and difficult to isolate from one another. Of the total IgG, IgG2a represents the largest, and IgG3 the smallest fraction.

Table 6.5 Physicochemical and Metabolic Properties of Human Immunoglobulins (Compiled from Various Sources)

Immunoglobulin	Heavy Chain	Sedimentation Constant	Molecular Weight	Carbohydrate Content (percent)	Number of Oligosaccharides per H Chain	Average Electrophoretic Mobility (pH 8.6)	Serum Level (Mean, Adult, mg/ml)	Half Life (days)	Catabolic Rate[a]	Synthetic Rate (mg/kg day)
IgG1	$\gamma1$	7S	146,000	2–3	1	γ	9	21	7	33
IgG2	$\gamma2$	7S	146,000	2–3	1	γ	3	20	7	
IgG3	$\gamma3$	7S	165,000	2–3	1	γ	1	7	17	
IgG4	$\gamma4$	7S	146,000	2–3	1	γ	0.5	21	7	
IgM1	$\mu1$	19S	970,000	12	5	Fast γ to β	1.5	10	8.8	3.3
IgM2	$\mu2$									
IgA1	$\alpha1$	7S to 15S	160,000	7–11	8	Fast γ to β	3.0	6	25	24
IgA2	$\alpha2$		160,000	7–11		Fast γ to β	0.5	6		
SeIgA	$\alpha1$ or $\alpha2$	11S	385,000	7–11	?	—	0.05	—	—	—
IgD	δ	7S	184,000	9–14	3	Fast γ	0.03	3	37	0.4
IgE	ϵ	8S	188,000	12	6	Fast γ	0.00005	2	71	0.002

[a] Percent intravascular pool catabolized per day.

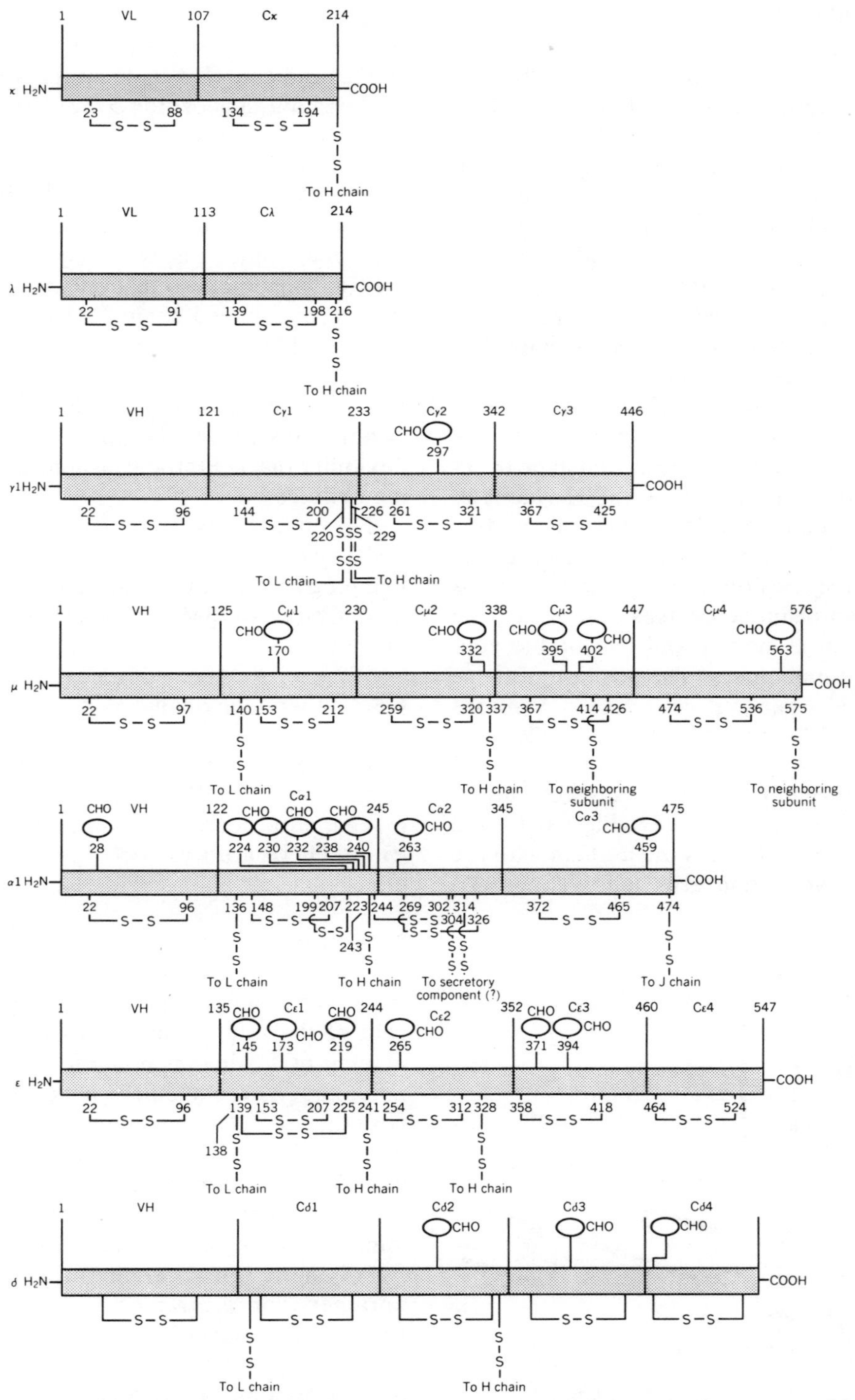

Figure 6.28. Main structural features of human immunoglobulin chains. The numbers indicate amino acid positions, with the numbering in all chains based on actual sequence, rather than homology. Details of δ-chain structure are unknown. CHO, carbohydrate moiety.

6.5.2 Immunoglobulin M

Human serum IgM has a molecular weight of 970,000 daltons and a sedimentation constant of 19S. Each IgM molecule is a pentamer composed of five subunits (monomers), each with a molecular weight of about 180,000 daltons (sedimentation constant 7.8S), and all joined by disulfide bridges and by an extra piece, the so-called *joining* or *J chain* (discussed under the IgA heading; see Fig. 6.29). The pentamer can be split into monomers by mild reduction, using, for example, 0.01 M 2-mercaptoethanol at neutral pH. Each subunit has the basic structure, which consists of two H (μ) and two L chains, so that the "monomer" is in fact itself a tetramer. The H chains are composed of five domains—one variable (VH) and four constant (Cμ1 through Cμ4), one domain more than the H chains of IgG (if one does not count the IgG hinge region as a separate domain). The molecule is rich in carbohydrate, containing five carbohydrate moieties per μ chain. There are two disulfide bridges connecting the two H chains of each monomer and one bridge connecting two adjacent monomers. The position of these bonds is controversial. Half-cystines occur at positions 22, 97, 140, 153, 212, 259, 320, 337, 367, 414, 426, 474, 536, and 575; of these numbers 140, 337, 414, and 575 are known to be involved in interchain bond formation, while the rest form intrachain bonds (Figs. 6.14 and 28). Half-cystine number 140 links the μ chain with the L chain, so the controversy concerns half-cystines 337, 414, and 575. Originally, the monomer-linking cystine was reported to be at position 414, but more recent studies indicate that its location is probably at the end of the chain, at position 575. (The μ chain consists of 576 amino acids, so the monomer-linking cystine is at the penultimate position.)

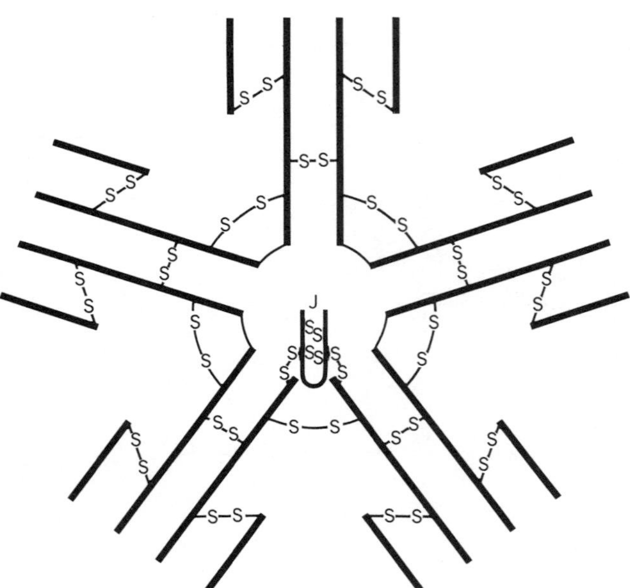

Figure 6.29. The clasp model of the pentameric IgM molecule.

The linkage of the J chain with the monomers is also controversial. According to the *clasp model* (Fig. 6.29), the J chain functions as a clasp that closes the circle of the five monomers so that only two of the five attach to the hairpin-shaped chain.

The IgM molecule has ten antigen-combining sites (two in each monomer), but it often uses only five of these (at least for strong binding). Why this should be so is not known, but one possibility is that the lack of flexibility of the F(ab)$_2$ arms limits the molecule's binding abilities.

Two subclasses of human IgM have been reported but they have so far been distinguished only by peptide mapping and not by the more usual serological method of analysis. No IgM subclasses are known in the rabbit or mouse.

6.5.3 Immunoglobulin A

IgA is present not only in the serum, but also in various bodily fluids, such as saliva, intestinal and bronchial mucus, nasal secretions, sweat, breast milk, and colostrum. There are thus two IgA types—serum and secretory.

Serum IgA

In humans, serum IgA constitutes from 15 to 20 percent of the total immunoglobulin pool. More than 80 percent of it is in a monomeric form; the rest occurs as polymers. The monomers have the typical four-chain structure (α_2L_2), a molecular weight of some 160,000 daltons (the α chain, like the γ chain, consists of four domains), a sedimentation constant of 7S, and a relatively high carbohydrate content. The two chains are joined by a single disulfide bridge.

Polymeric IgA occurs in the form of dimers, trimers, tetramers, or pentramers, in which the two, three, four, or five monomeric units are held together by disulfide bridges and by the J chain (always one J chain per molecule). The polymers can be reduced to monomers, by a thiol treatment, for example.

Human serum IgA falls into two subclasses, IgA1 and IgA2, the former occurring at a higher concentration than the latter. The two subclasses differ in electrophoretic mobility (the α2 chains are more negatively charged than the α1 chains); carbohydrate content (α1

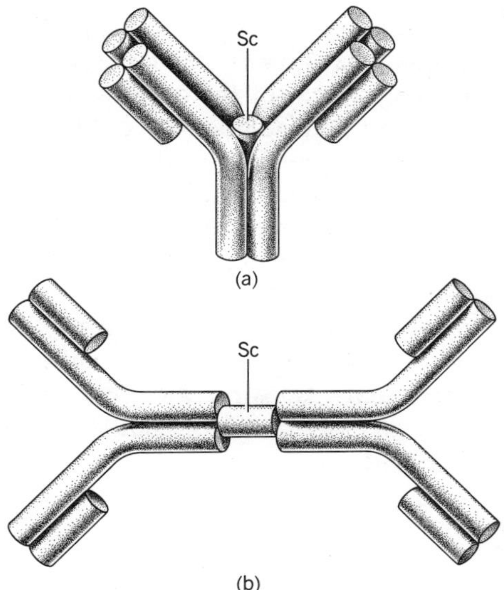

Figure 6.30. Two forms of IgA dimer. (*a*) Monomers are stacked upon each other. (*b*) Monomers are joined by the C termini of their H chains. Sc, secretory component.

but not $\alpha 2$ chains have galactosamine-containing carbohydrates attached to them); molecular weight (the $\alpha 2$ chain is slightly heavier than the $\alpha 1$ chain; where the amino acids responsible for this difference are located is not known); and amino acid sequence (12 amino acids present in the hinge region of $\alpha 1$ are deleted in $\alpha 2$, and the $\alpha 1$ hinge region contains a duplicated stretch of seven amino acids that is absent in the $\alpha 2$ chain hinge region). The IgA2 subclass occurs in two forms: in A2m(1), the two L chains, instead of being bonded to H chains, are joined by disulfide bridges; in A2m(2), normal H-L chain disulfide bonds occur.

The $\alpha 1$ chain contains 17 half-cystines (Fig. 6.28), of which one forms a disulfide bridge with the L chain, one with the H chain, one with the J chain, and two with the so-called *secretory component* (only in secretory IgA, see below); the remaining half-cystines participate in the formation of intra-H-chain disulfide bridges. There is one such bridge in the VH domain, one in the Cα3 domain, and two each in the Cα1 and Cα2 domains.

Secretory IgA

Most secretory IgA molecules consist of two IgA monomers (each having the basic four-chain Ig structure), one J chain, and one secretory component. The molecule has a molecular weight of from 380,000 to 390,000 daltons and a sedimentation constant of 11S. The two monomers can either be stacked on top of each other (less frequent form) or joined by their Fc ends (more prevalent form; Fig. 6.30). The precise organization of the molecules is not known, but in the currently favored model (Fig. 6.31) the J chain forms a disulfide bridge with the penultimate half-cystine of the α chain, and the secretory component forms similar bonds with the half-cystines in positions 304 and 314. A minority (10 to 20 percent) of secretory IgA occurs in the form of higher polymers (tetramers and hexamers); another 10 percent is of the 7S type, derived in part from serum, and in part, perhaps, from secreted products of dissociated 11S IgA.

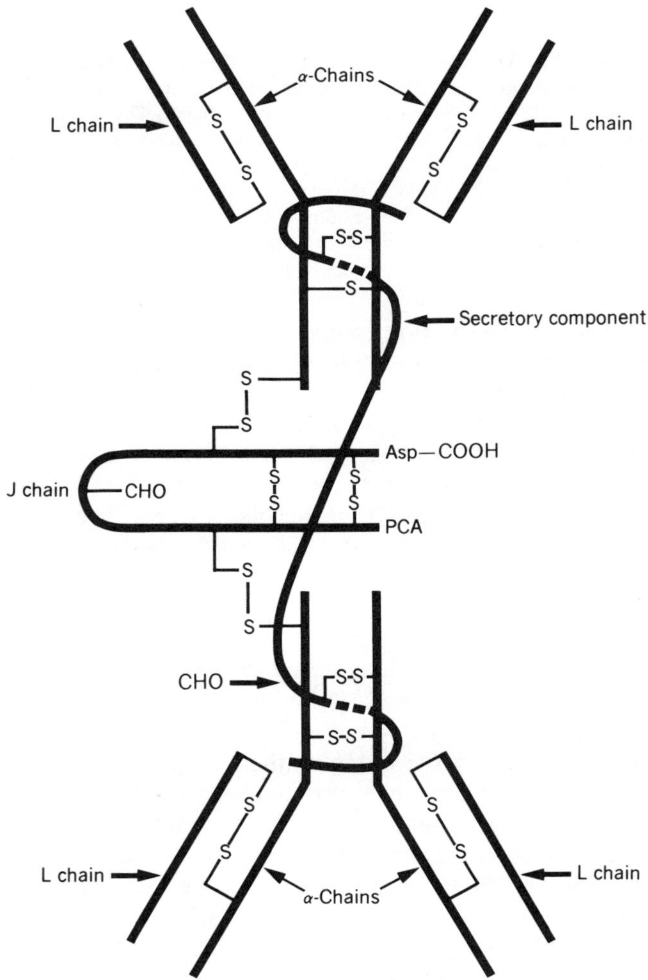

Figure 6.31. Diagram of human secretory IgA molecule, showing the postulated arrangement of IgA monomers, secretory component, and J chain. (From M. W. Turner *in* L. E. Glynn and M. W. Steward (Eds.): *Immunochemistry: An Advanced Textbook*. Wiley, Chichester, 1977.)

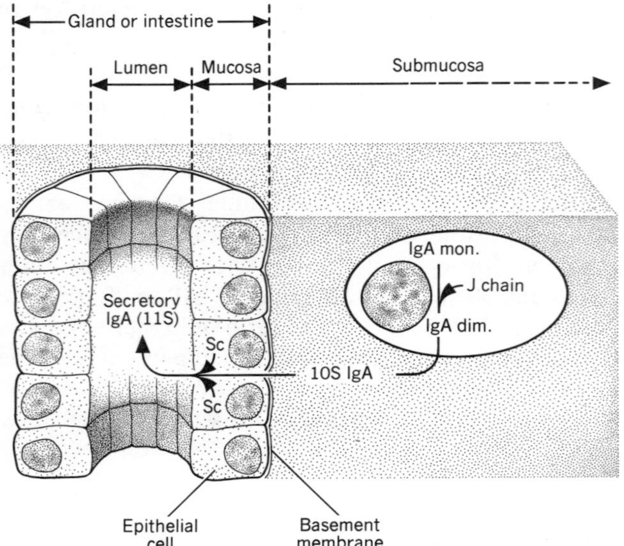

Figure 6.32. Diagram of secretory IgA synthesis in the gastrointestinal tract or in an exocrine gland. Plasma cells in the submucosa synthesize IgA monomers (IgA mon) and J chains. The latter connect monomers into IgAdimers (IgA dim), which have the sedimentation constant of 10S. During the passage of IgA dimers through epithelial cells of the mucosa, the secretory component (Sc) is added and the completed seIgA molecule, which now has the sedimentation constant of 11S, is secreted into the lumen.

The secretory IgA monomers are synthesized by plasma cells present under mucosal surfaces and then pass through epithelial cells, where they acquire the secretory component (Fig. 6.32). The addition of the secretory component is presumably catalyzed by a cytoplasmic enzyme in the epithelial cells. The J chain is added to IgA already in the plasma cell. The complete molecule is then secreted into the body fluids.

Secretory Component

The component was discovered in 1965 by Thomas B. Tomasi and his co-workers and was formerly referred to as the secretory "piece" or the transport (T) chain. It is secreted by the lining epithelial cells of exocrine glands[4], in which it can exist either free or bound to secretory IgA. The component is a nonimmunoglobulin glycoprotein, containing from 16 to 23 percent carbohydrate. The molecular weight of the free secretory component is about 80,000 and that of the bound component about 50,000 to 60,000 daltons. N-terminal amino acid sequence analyses of secretory components from different species reveal a high degree of homology (Fig. 6.33) and indicate evolutionary conservation of the component in most mammals. The bound component is covalently attached by way of disulfide bridges to each of the two monomers in the IgA dimer, but the precise manner of this attachment has not yet been discovered. A possible model of the linkage between the secretory component and the secretory IgA is shown in Figure 6.31. The free secretory component contains one intrachain disulfide bridge, which probably breaks when the component attaches to IgA. The presence of bound secretory component promotes the resistance of IgA to enzymatic cleavage. The component may also serve as a receptor for IgA, directing the transport of the immunoglobulin molecules through epithelial cells.

The J Chain

The joining chain was discovered simultaneously in 1966 by J. Rejnek and G. Cederblad and their co-workers. Unlike the secretory component, the J chain is synthesized by plasma cells and attached to the Ig molecule either before or at the time of secretion. It is a highly conserved glycoprotein with a molecular weight of about 14,000 to 15,000 daltons and is thus similar in size to L chains. It contains seven or eight half-cystines per molecule, and is quite hydrophilic (in addition to half-cystine, it is rich in arginine, isoleucine, and aspartic acid).

The J chain is covalently bound to H chains of IgA and IgM. It connects to the tails of 19 extra amino acids at the carboxyl termini of the α and μ chains. More specifically, the bondage is between the penultimate half-cystine in the H chain and the half-cystine of the J chain. As has already been indicated, in the IgA, the J chain attaches to both monomers of the dimer via two disulfide bridges; in IgM it seems to serve as a clasp joining monomeric units number one and five.

6.5.4 Immunoglobulin D

The concentration of serum IgD is variable, but generally low. Because of this fact and because of its sus-

	Amino Acid Position														
Species	1				5					10					15
Human	K	S	P	I	F	G	P	E	E	V	D	S	V	E	G
Bovine	K	S	P	I	F	G	—	—	D	V	D	S	V	D	G
Canine	K	S	P	I	F	G	P	E	E	V	N	I	V	E	G

Figure 6.33. N-terminal amino acid sequences of secretory components from different species. Presumed homologies are indicated by boxes.

[4] Exocrine glands are glands that secrete outwardly through excretory ducts.

ceptibility to proteolysis by serum plasmin, IgD is difficult to isolate. Like IgG, and IgD molecule is a four-chain ($L_2\delta_2$) monomer, with a molecular weight of from 175,000 to 185,000 daltons and a sedimentation constant of 7S. In comparison to IgG, the molecular weight of IgD is higher but the sedimentation constant is lower, indicating that the IgD molecule must be less compact than the IgG molecule. The H (δ) chain consists of five domains (although recent DNA-cloning experiments indicate that molecules containing only three domains plus the hinge region in their H chains also occur), and the two H chains are linked by a single disulfide bridge. The molecule is rich in carbohydrates and, like IgA1, contains N-acetylgalactosamine. There are indications that several subclasses of IgD might exist, but because of the low IgD concentration in serum, these are difficult to analyze.

6.5.5 Immunoglobulin E

Of all the immunoglobulins, IgE occurs in the serum at the lowest concentration. The IgE molecules are monomers with molecular weights of from 188,000 to 196,000 daltons, a sedimentation constant of 8S, and the electrophoretic mobility of fast γ-globulins. Like those of other immunoglobulins, the IgE monomers consist of two L chains and two H (ϵ) chains. Each ϵ chain consists of five domains (VH and Cϵ1 through Cϵ4) and contains 15 half-cystines (Fig. 6.28)—one participating in the disulfide bridge with the L chain, two in the two H–H disulfide bridges, and the rest in intrachain bonds. An unusual feature of the IgE molecule is the separation of the two inter-H-chain disulfide bridges by one complete domain. (One bridge is located between Cϵ1 and Cϵ2 and the other between Cϵ2 and Cϵ3.) There is also an extra intra-H-chain disulfide bridge in the Cϵ1 domain. No subclasses of IgE have yet been detected.

6.6 FORMAL GENETICS OF IMMUNOGLOBULINS

Not so long ago the only source of information about mammalian, and in particular human, Ig genes was *recombinational analysis*, in which one makes conclusions about gene organization from the way traits segregate among the progeny of a given cross, mating, or marriage. Recombinational analysis is the basis of *formal genetics*, in which one treats genes as formal, abstract units rather than as concrete, chemical entities. Although the formal genetic approach to the question of Ig gene organization has now largely been superceded by new techniques of molecular genetics—in particular, techniques of recombinant DNA analysis—formal genetics remains an important tool in certain areas of study, of animal and human populations, for example. In addition, formal genetics played an important role in the past in establishing the principles of immunoglobulin inheritance. It is therefore appropriate that we devote a section of this chapter to the achievements of formal genetics.

To study the segregation of genes among progeny, one needs markers at the phenotype level that allow one to extrapolate on the behavior of these genes. These markers must be present in some and absent in other individuals of a given species, for if they were present in all individuals—as isotypes are, for example—one would not be able to follow their segregation. The two most useful markers in immunoglobulin genetics are allotypes and idiotypes. So, before we acquaint ourselves with the accomplishments of formal Ig genetics, we shall first review what is known about these two markers.

6.6.1 Allotypes

Introduction

Definition and Discovery. The term *allotypy* was introduced in 1966 by Jacques Oudin to designate proteins existing in two or more forms, or *allotypes*, each form being present in some but absent from other individuals of a given species. In this broad sense, the term is used only infrequently; more commonly, by allotypy immunologists mean genetically determined antigenic differences in serum proteins, specifically in immunoglobulins. We shall use this restricted definition.

Immunoglobulin allotypes were discovered simultaneously in 1956 by Jacques Oudin (in rabbits) and R. Grubb (in humans). Later, other investigators discovered allotypes in the mouse, monkey, cattle, rat, and domestic fowl.

Methods of Detection. Allotypes are defined serologically by reactions of specific antibodies with antigenic determinants on immunoglobulin molecules (i.e., by antibodies reacting with antibodies). Allotypic antisera are produced by the immunization of an individual with immunoglobulins (normal serum, purified Ig fraction, myeloma proteins) of another individual. Of course, antibodies in this situation form only when the selected recipient is negative and the donor is positive for a given allotype. When one starts searching for an allotype, one does not know which individuals are positive and which are negative, so one must often test several donor-recipient combinations before finding a suitable one. Once an allotype has been defined, one establishes the right immunizing combination by typing available individuals with the antiallotypic serum. In animals, the immunization is almost always deliberate, whereas in humans one is dependent on antibodies produced incidentally by such circumstances as disease, pregnancy, or blood transfusion. Theoretically, one should also be able to detect allotypic differences by xenoantisera, but in practice this procedure rarely works. Apparently, the allotypic differences are too small for another species to recognize them in the presence of large interspecies differences.

The allotypic antibody reacts with only a portion of the immunoglobulin molecule, and since this portion determines the molecule's antigenic specificity, it is referred to as the *allotypic determinant*, or simply, determinant. (Some other names are antigenic specificity, specificity, allotypic marker, or factor.) An antiserum produced in an inbred-strain combination can be produced by anyone possessing the strains involved. In contrast, identity of reagents produced by crossimmunization of outbred individuals can be established only by exchange of the antisera among the investigators concerned.

Since both the antibody and antigen are in a soluble form, theoretically, the allotype-antibody reaction should result in the formation of a measurable precipitate. Often, however, it does not, apparently because the antigenic difference is too small and the lattice necessary for the precipitate formation too unstable (see Chapter 10). Therefore, methods other than those based on direct measurement of precipitate formation must usually be used. One such method will be described later in this chapter.

Once an allotypic determinant is defined, its mode of inheritance must be determined. The *genetic analysis* of an allotypic determinant is carried out in three stages. In the first stage, the locus coding for the determinant is identified either by a breeding test (in animals) or family studies (in humans). In the second stage, the relationship of the identified locus to other known loci is established by genetic linkage analysis. In the third stage, the population behavior of the newly defined gene (the frequency with which it occurs in different populations, the gene combinations in which it is found most frequently, the zygosity status) is defined.

Simultaneously with the genetic analysis, *immunochemical studies* are also carried out, the purpose of which is to identify the class and subclass, chain, region, and position of the antigenic determinant. The basic assumption underlying these studies is that when a difference is found at a single position between allotype-positive and allotype-negative chains or fragments, this position is the site of the allotypic determinant.

Nomenclature. The discoverer of a new allotypic determinant has the privilege of naming it so that the determinant can be referred to simply and without ambiguity. Although there are certain rules for this naming, there is no authority to enforce them, and a scientist can choose to ignore them. Furthermore, since it often happens that two or more laboratories discover an allotypic system independently and simultaneously, two or more names for the same system appear in the literature. One would think that in such cases, the scientists concerned would get together, toss a coin, and accept the nomenclature of the one who wins. But this rarely happens. To resolve the problem of multiple names, a nomenclature committee is formed, and after long discussions, it reaches some kind of acceptable compromise. But even then, some scientists refuse to go along; they stubbornly insist on their own nomenclature, so that instead of reducing two names to one, one ends up with three. Fortunately, more and more scientists realize that one—in their view, perhaps, imperfect—name is better than two perfect ones, and accept the recommendations of a nomenclature committee. No committee, however, has succeeded in imposing common nomenclature rules for the different animal species: the mouse, human, rabbit, and fowl allotypes are all named differently.

In general, two types of symbol are necessary, one for the locus (gene, allele—these symbols should always be printed in italics) and one for determinants encoded by this locus (printed in Roman type). The latter are usually designated either by small letters or by numbers. The numbering system is superior to the letter system, if for no other reason than because it is open-ended—one cannot run out of numbers but one can run out of letters. The specific nomenclature systems will be described when we deal with allotypes of the different species—human, rabbit, and mouse.

Human Allotypes

Discovery. The first human allotype was discovered by chance during an analysis of sera from patients with lower than normal γ-globulin levels. To determine the γ-globulin levels, the Swedish immunologist R. Grubb used an indirect method based on inhibition of hemagglutination. He first coated human erythrocytes, positive for Rh(D) blood group antigen, with a special kind of Rh antibodies that bound to the red cells but did not agglutinate them (the so-called "incomplete" antibodies; see Chapter 10). To achieve agglutination, Grubb added to the coated and washed red blood cells a xenogeneic (rabbit) antiserum to human γ-globulin, which also reacted with red cell-bound antibodies and glued individual erythrocytes together into a clump. The reaction could be inhibited by the addition of normal human serum, which competed with the coated antibody for combining sites of the xenogeneic antibodies. Since inhibition was greater the more γ-globulin the added serum contained, the method provided a means of quantitating the γ-globulin concentration.

The method worked well for Grubb with a single exception: one serum, when mixed with the coated erythrocytes, caused agglutination even in the absence of the xenogeneic antiserum. Upon analyzing it further, Grubb discovered that the agglutinating factor reacted not with the erythrocytes themselves, but with the antibodies coating them. He then screened sera from several hundred donors, both normal and with various diseases, and found the hemagglutinating factor with particularly high frequency (some 15 percent) in sera from patients with rheumatoid arthritis (see Chapter 14). Later studies demonstrated the hemagglutinating factor to be an autoantibody formed under pathological conditions against the patient's own immunoglobulins. To find out what kind of immunoglobulin the autoantibody reacted with, Grubb modified his assay system by mixing coated erythrocytes with the hemagglutinating factor and adding human serum from another individual to the mixture. If the individual carried the antigenic determinants that the autoantibody specifically recognized on his Ig molecules, the hemagglutination would be inhibited; if not, normal agglutination would occur. By testing a large panel of individuals, Grubb found the determinant to be present in the immunoglobulins of 60 percent of Swedes, and the presence or absence of the determinant to be controlled by alleles at a single genetic locus. Since the determinant was present in *gam*maglobulins, Grubb designated the controlling locus *Gm*. Later studies by Grubb and by many other investigators revealed the existence not only of additional Gm determinants, but also determinants encoded by loci other than *Gm*.

Method of Detection. The most widely used method for human allotype detection is Grubb's original *hemagglutination inhibition assay* (Fig. 6.34). The three principal reagents of this assay are human erythrocytes, allotype-positive human immunoglobulin used for erythrocyte coating, and antibody recognizing the allotype of the coating immunoglobulin. The most frequently used coating immunoglobulin is antibody to the Rh(D) antigen (in this instance, the erythrocytes must be Rh-positive). However, since this antibody is heterogeneous and this heterogeneity complicates the allotype analysis, methods have been devised in which it is replaced by allotype-positive homogeneous myeloma proteins linked artificially to erythrocytes by chemical means. The antiallotypic reagent can be derived from one of the following sources: patients with rheumatoid arthritis, multiply transfused patients, multiparous women, and rabbits. *Sera of rheumatoid*

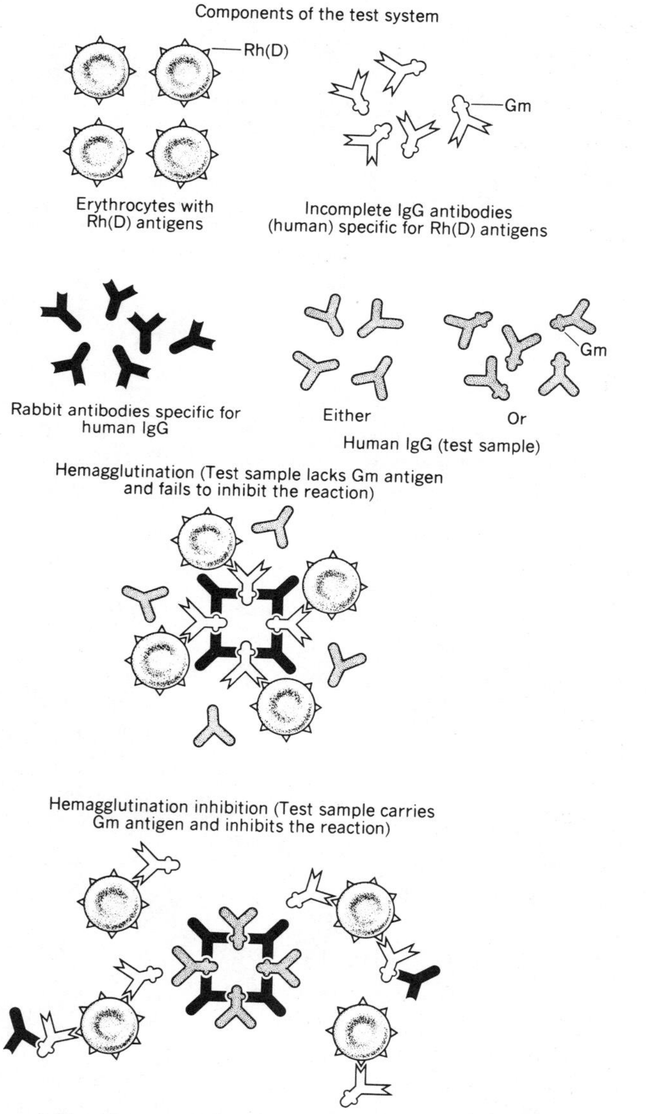

Components of the test system

Rh(D)

Gm

Erythrocytes with Rh(D) antigens

Incomplete IgG antibodies (human) specific for Rh(D) antigens

Rabbit antibodies specific for human IgG

Gm

Either

Or

Human IgG (test sample)

Hemagglutination (Test sample lacks Gm antigen and fails to inhibit the reaction)

Hemagglutination inhibition (Test sample carries Gm antigen and inhibits the reaction)

Figure 6.34. Hemagglutination inhibition assay for the detection of human Gm allotypes. Explanation in the text.

patients, or so-called "rheumatoid agglutinators" ("Raggs"), were originally used almost exclusively in human allotype studies. However, when later studies revealed that normal sera, or "normal agglutinators" ("Snaggs"), discriminated allotypes better than did "rheumatoid agglutinators," the use of the latter was discontinued. *Sera of multiply transfused patients* often contain allotype-specific antibodies induced by the transfused serum globulins. *Sera of women after multiple pregnancies* can contain antibodies to fetal Ig that has crossed the placenta and immunized the mother. The antibodies are directed against allotypes that the child inherited from the father. For unknown reasons, alloantibodies to human Ig are almost always of the IgM class. *Xenoantisera* are produced by the immunization of rabbits or primates with human Ig or myeloma proteins. Before use, such antisera must be absorbed with human sera negative for the studied allotype. The disadvantage in using xenoantisera is their relatively low discriminating power.

In the assay, inhibition of the hemagglutination by the tested serum sample means that immunoglobulins in the sample share allotypic determinants with the coating antibody. Absence of inhibition (that is, presence of agglutination) indicates absence of a given allotypic determinant in the studied sample.

Nomenclature. There are two nomenclature systems in use for human allotypes—the original one, proposed by the discoverers of the individual allotypes, and a new one, recommended in 1974 by the International Committee on Immunoglobulin Allotypes at the World Health Organization (WHO). In the original nomenclature, most allotypic determinants were designated by small letters; in the new, they are designated by numbers. In the WHO nomenclature, the loci are designated according to the Ig isotype (class and subclass) carrying the allotype. Thus, *Gm*, *Mm*, *Am*, and *Km* symbols designate loci encoding IgG, IgM, IgA, and κ-type L-chain allotypes, respectively. Reference to a subclass is indicated by the subclass number preceding the letter m. Thus, *G1m*, *G2m*, and *G3m* are loci coding for IgG1, IgG2, and IgG3 allotypes, respectively. The allotypic determinant is then given in parentheses [e.g., G1m(1), G1m(2), G1m(3), etc.] and alleles at a given locus are indicated by the determinant written as a superscript. For example, $G1m^1$, $G1m^2$, and $G1m^3$ are alleles at the *G1m* locus encoding determinants G1m(1), G1m(2), and G1m(3), respectively. The numbering of determinants present in different Ig classes always starts from 1.

Allotypic Systems. Human allotypes have been found only in the C region; none has so far been detected in the V region. Six allotype loci have been identified—*G1m*, *G2m*, *G3m*, *Mm*, *A2m*, and *Km*, encoding allotypes present in $\gamma1$, $\gamma2$, $\gamma3$, μ, $\alpha2$, and κ chains, respectively. No allotype associated with the δ and ϵ chains has yet been found (Table 6.6). The 33 determinants described are distributed among the individual systems as follows: 27 Gm, one Mm, two Am, and three Km. However, some of the determinants [e.g., G1m(3) and G1m(4), G3m(10) and G3m(13)m, G3m(5) and Gm(12)] are apparently identical. (The *Gm* symbol without a number preceding the letter *m* indicates that the determinant has not yet been assigned to a subclass.) In population studies, the *Gm*, *Mm*, and *Am* genes are closely linked in a tight cluster that segregates independently from the *Km* gene. A specific combination of alleles at the individual loci in the cluster is called a *haplotype* (phenogroup, allogroup). An example of a haplotype is a gene combination—$G1m^4$, $G2m^{23}$, $G3m^{5,11,13,14}$, *Mm*, *A2m*—the components of which are all genes carried by a single chromosome (Table 6.7).

Rabbit Allotypes

Discovery. The first rabbit allotypic determinant was discovered in 1956 by Jacques Oudin, who immunized rabbits with ovalbumin, isolated the antiovalbumin-ovalbumin precipitate, and injected it into another rabbit. The antibodies thus produced reacted with normal sera of some, but not all rabbits tested. Later, Oudin, Sheldon Dray, Stanislaw R. G. Dubiski, A. S. Kelus, and others discovered and analyzed a whole series of additional allotypic determinants.

Methods of Detection. Rabbit allotypic determinants are usually detected by alloantisera, and less often by xenoantisera produced in goats or fowl. As the immunizing antigen one can use immune precipitate (of the type originally used by Oudin) emulsified in the so-called Freund's adjuvant, which enhances the antibody response (see Chapter 10); complexes of rabbit antibodies with bacteria (e.g., *Proteus vulgaris*); or Ig fraction of the donor's serum.

Rabbit allotypic antibodies are usually of the precipitin type and can therefore be used in a direct precipitation assay. A common method of carrying out this test is letting the antibody diffuse in agar gel against normal rabbit serum or purified Ig fraction, and taking the formation of a precipitin line as a sign of

Table 6.6 Human Ig Allotypes

Chain	Locus Designation		Determinant Designation		Location	Amino Acid at Position
	Recommended	Original	Recommended	Original		
$\gamma 1$	*G1m*	*Gm*	1	a	$C\gamma 3$	Asp 356 Leu 358
			−1	Non-a	$C\gamma 3$	Glu 356 Met 358
			2	x	$C\gamma 3$	
			4(3)	$f(b^{w},b^{2})$	$C\gamma 1$	Arg 214
			7	r	C_H	
			17	z	$C\gamma 1$	Lys 214
			18	Rouen 2	C_H	
			20	San Francisco 2	C_H	
$\gamma 2$	*G2m*		23	n	$C\gamma 2$	
			−23	Non n	$C\gamma 2$	
			5(12)	$b,b^{1}(b^{\gamma})$	$C\gamma 2$	
$\gamma 3$	*G3m*		−5	$\text{Non-b},b^{1}$	$C\gamma 2$	
			6	$c(c^{3})$	$C\gamma 3$	
			11	$b^{\beta}(b^{0})$	$C\gamma 3$	Phe 436
			−11	$\text{Non-}b^{\beta}(\text{non } b^{0})$	$C\gamma 3$	Tyr 436
			13(10)	$b^{3}(b^{\alpha})$	$C\gamma 3$	
			14	b^{4}	$C\gamma 3$	
			15	s	$C\gamma 2$	
			16	t	$C\gamma 2$	
			21	g	$C\gamma 2$	Tyr 296
			−21	Non-g	$C\gamma 2$	Phe 296
			24	c^{5}	C_H	
			25	Bet	C_H	
			26	u	C_H	
			27	v	C_H	
$\gamma 4$	*G4m*		Not assigned	4a	$C\gamma 2$	Leu 309
			Not assigned	4b	$C\gamma 2$	Gap 309
Unclassified	*Gm*	*Gm*	7	γ	C_H	
			8	e	C_H	
			9	P	C_H	
			12	$b\gamma$	C_H	
			18	Ro^{2}	C_H	
			19	Ro^{3}	C_H	
			20	z(S.F.)	C_H	
$\alpha 2$	*A2m*	*Am*	1	1	C_H	131 No bridge to L chain
			2	2	C_H	131 Bridge to L chain
μ	*Mm*	*Mm*	1	1	C_H	
κ	*Km*	*Inv*	1	1	$C\kappa$	Val 153 Leu 191
			2	2	$C\kappa$	
			3	3	$C\kappa$	Ala 153 Val 191

Table 6.7 Common Human Ig Haplotypes in Various Ethnic Groups

Alleles at Loci				
G1m	*G2m*	*G3m*	*G4m*	*A2m*
Caucasians				
4,−1[a]	23	5,11,13,14,25,−21	4b	1
4,−1	23−	5,11,13,14,25,−21	4a	1
1,17	23−	21,−5	4a	1
1,2,17	23−	21,−5	4a	1
Melanesians				
1,4		5,13,14		
1,17		5,13,14		
1,17		21		
1,2,17		21		
Mongolians				
1,4	23	5,11,13,14,25	4a	1
1,17	23−	21	4a	1
1,17	23−	11,13,25		
Bushmen				
1,17		5,13,14		
1,17		21		
1,17		5		
1,17		13		
Blacks				
1,17	23−	5,11,13,14		
1,17	23−	5,6,11		
1,17	23−	5,6,11,14		
1,17	23−	11,13		
Ainu				
1,17		21		
1,2,17		21		
2,17		21		
1,17		13		

Source. From A. Nisonoff, J.E. Hopper, and S.B. Spring: *The Antibody Molecule*, Academic, New York, 1975.

[a] A minus sign preceding a number indicates a nonmarker; following a number it indicates the absence of that marker. The nonmarkers are indicated only for Caucasians.

positive reaction. Alternatively, one can label the Ig fraction with ^{125}I and use the formation of a radioactive precipitate as a measure of the antigen-antibody reaction. (The precipitate can be separated from the solution by centrifugation.) If the number of determinants per molecule is too small to form an insoluble precipitate, the reaction can be enhanced by the addition of either unlabeled Ig or xenogeneic anti-Ig serum (e.g., goat anti-rabbit). Some investigators also prefer a hemagglutination assay to the precipitation test. They coat rabbit erythrocytes with rabbit Ig that carries a given allotypic determinant, use antiallotypic serum to agglutinate the red cells, and detect the presence or absence of the allotypic determinant in a test serum by determining whether the serum does or does not inhibit the reaction.

Nomenclature. Originally, all rabbit allotype loci were designated by the prefix "A," for allotype (or "Ms," in the case of certain μ-chain allotypes), and the individual loci were denoted by small italicized letters (*a*, *b*, *c*, etc.). Determinants were designated by nonitalicized small letters and numbers (a1, a2, a3, b4, b5, etc.); the numbers were assigned consecutively in the order of discovery of the determinants, regardless of the loci coding for the determinants. Only determinants discovered in wild, as opposed to domesticated, rabbits were numbered, starting with the numeral 100. In current nomenclature, the prefixes A and Ms are omitted, except for determinants that have not yet been assigned to a particular locus.

Allotypic Systems. Rabbit allotypes (Table 6.8) have been detected in the C region of κ (*b*) and λ (*c*) light chains, and the C regions of γ (*d* and *e*, which are probably identical), α1 (*f*), α2 (*g*), and μ (*n*) heavy chains; a few have also been detected in the V region (*a*, *x*, *y*). The V-region allotypes are present in all Ig classes and molecules.

Mouse Allotypes

Most of the work on mouse allotypes was done by Leonard A. Herzenberg, Rose Lieberman, and Michael Potter. Combining the two original nomenclature systems (Herzenberg's, and Lieberman's and Potter's), Rose Lieberman and Margaret C. Green have attempted to come up with a third, compromise system, which will be used in this text. The recommended system designates the immunoglobulin-coding loci by *Igh* or *Igl* symbols (*h* and *l* for heavy- and light-chain loci, respectively) appended with a serial number, assigned in the order of discovery (*Igh*-1, *Igh*-2, *Igh*-3, etc.). The allotypic determinants are also designated consecutively in the order of discovery, regardless of the coding locus, and are separated from the locus symbol by a period (Igh-1.1, Igh-1.2, Igh-1.3, etc.).

Table 6.8 Rabbit Ig Allotypes

Chain	Locus	Determinant	Location	Amino Acid at Position
γ	*de*[a]	d11	Cγ1 hinge	Met 215
		d12	Cγ1 hinge	Thr 215
		e14	Cγ1 Fc	Thr 309
		e15	Cγ1 Fc	Ala 309
	Not assigned	A8	Cγ1 Fc	
		A10	Cγ1 Fc	
μ	*n*	n81		
		n82		
	Not assigned	Ms1		
		Ms2		
		Ms4		
		Ms5		
		Ms6		
α1	*f*	f69	Cα	
		f70	Cα	
		f71	Cα	
		f72	Cα	
		f73	Cα	
α2	*g*	g74	Cα, Fc and Fab	
		g75	Cα, Fc and Fab	
		g76	Cα, Fc and Fab	
		g77	Cα, Fc and Fab	
VH	*a*	a1	VH	Multiple
		a2	VH	
		a3	VH	
		a100	VH	
		a101	VH	
		a102	VH	
		a103	VH	
	x	x32	VH	
	y	y33	VH	
κ	*b*	b4	Cκ (Vκ?)	Multiple
		b5	Cκ (Vκ?)	
		b6	Cκ (Vκ?)	
		b9	Cκ (Vκ?)	
λ	*c*	c7		
		c21		

[a] The d and e determinants were once thought to be controlled by separate loci, *d* and *e*, respectively. Now it appears that, although distinct, they are controlled by the same locus, *de*.

Mouse allotypic determinants (Tables 6.9 through 6.11) have been detected in the C region of heavy chains γ1 (*Igh*-4), γ2a (*Igh*-1), γ2b (*Igh*-3), μ (*Igh*-6), α (*Igh*-2), and δ (*Igh*-5), and the light chain λ (*Igl*-1). A total of 43 determinants encoded by these *Igh* loci have been described, most of them controlled by the *Igh*-1 and *Igh*-4 loci. All five *Igh* loci are closely linked. Specific combinations of alleles at the five loci (haplotypes) are designated by the same superscript letters as the alleles at the *Igh*-1 loci. The *Igl*-1 locus, which segregates independently of the *Igh* gene cluster, is thus far known in two allelic forms, one coding for the presence and the other for the absence of an allotypic determinant. No serologically detectable allotypic variation has yet been found in the κ light chains, but intraspecies V-region variants of κ have been detected, using such other techniques as isoelectric focusing and peptide mapping. Two of the three markers detected by isoelectric focusing have the same strain distribution as the peptide mapping marker, whereas the third isoelectric focusing marker has a different distribution.

Allotype-Isotype Relationship

Most allotypic determinants are restricted to a single Ig class and subclass. For example, the human G1m(1) determinant is present only in IgG1 molecules of some individuals and is absent in all IgG2, IgG3, IgG4, IgM1, IgA1, IgD, and IgE molecules. This finding is not surprising, since the amino acid sequence in the region where the determinant maps is often very different in different classes. For example, the sequence in the G1m(1)-determining region of the different heavy chains is this.

γ1	Glu	Glu	Leu	Thr	Lys
μ	Ser	Ile	Phe	Leu	Thr
α	Ser	Gln	Gln	Leu	Ala
ε	Asp	—	Leu	Phe	Ile

No wonder the anti-Glm(1) serum does not react with IgM, IgA, and IgE molecules.

There are, however, exceptions to this class-restricted specificity of allotypic reagents. For instance, in the mouse, determinant 4 is shared by IgG2a and IgG2b molecules, which is not too surprising since the two subclasses of IgG are closely related. Another determinant (8) is shared by IgG1 and IgG2a; the biochemical basis for this sharing is not understood.

The statement about the restriction of determinants does not apply to those present in the light chains (C or V regions) and in the heavy-chain variable region.

Table 6.9 Mouse Igh Allotypes

Chain	Locus	Alleles	Determinants
γ1	*Igh-4*	*a,b*	8,19,42
γ2a	*Igh-1*	*a,b,c,d,e,f,g,h,j,k,l,m,n*	1,2,3,4,5,6,7,8,26,27,28,29,30
γ2b	*Igh-3*	*a,b,d,e,f,g*	4,9,11,16,22,23,31,32,33,34
α	*Igh-2*	*a,b,c,d,f*	12,13,14,15,17,35
μ	*Igh-6*	*a,b,e*	38,39,40,41
δ	*Igh-5*	*a,b,e*	36,37
Unassigned	Unassigned	Unassigned	10,18,20,21,24

Since a given L chain can presumably combine with any H chain, and since classes and subclasses are determined by H chains, L-chain allotypes can be shared by different classes and subclasses.

Another special case in terms of class-subclass distribution is the group of so-called *nonmarkers* (isoallotypes)—determinants that are genetic variants (allotypes) in one subclass but isotypes in another (they are present in all Ig molecules of this other class, and are absent in other classes and subclasses). An example of a nonmarker is the human Glm(-) determinant. When one prepares a peptide map of a G1m(1)-positive IgG1 molecule, one finds the G1m(1) determinant associated with a certain peptide, to which we shall refer as peptide a. In a G1m(1)-negative IgG1 molecule, one finds a corresponding but slightly different peptide, which we shall designate non-a. So IgG1 molecules are either a or non-a. Peptide mapping of IgG2 and IgG3 molecules reveals that they are *all* of the non-a type.[5] Hence non-a is an allotypic variant in IgG1, but not in IgG2 and IgG3. Since non-a is present in all IgG2 and IgG3 molecules and since all individuals have these molecules, no normal individual can make antibody to it—the peptide is a nonmarker. However, under pathological conditions, individuals apparently can produce autoantibodies against the non-a peptide, and such antisera then react with sera of all tested individuals because all individuals possess the non-a peptide. The only way to study these antibodies is by testing them against myeloma proteins, which, since each represents a single molecular type, can be distinguished into a and non-a types. The determinant so distinguished is referred to as Glm(-1), since it does not represent an allotypic marker in the true sense of the word. Other examples of human nonmarkers are G3m(-5), G3m(-11), and G3m(-21), which are present only in some IgG3 but in all IgG1 molecules; G4m(4a), which is present in some IgG4 but in all IgG1 and IgG3 molecules; and G4m(4b), which is present in all IgG2 and absent from all IgG1 and IgG3 molecules.

[5] In IgG4 and other Ig classes, neither the a nor the non-a peptide can be found. In these molecules the corresponding amino acid sequence is so different from IgG1 that the peptide can no longer be identified as one type or the other:

γ1 (a)	Arg Asp Glu Leu
γ1, γ2, or γ3 (non-a)	Arg Glu Glu Met
γ4	Glu Glu Glu Met.

Structural Basis of Allotypic Variation

Amino acid sequencing has revealed that there are several ways in which allotypic differences arise (Tables 6.6 and 6.8). The simplest is the replacement of an amino acid at a given position by another residue, as in the case of the human Glm(4) determinant, for example. In other allotypes, the generation of a new determinant requires a change of two amino acids, either in the same region [e.g., the human determinant Glm(1)], or in two separate regions of the unfolded chain (e.g., the human Km determinants 1, 2, and 3; here, presumably, the native chain is folded in such a way that positions 153 and 191 are sterically close to each other on the surface of the Ig molecule and the amino acids at these positions can be recognized by a single antibody). Still other allotypic variants apparently involve changes in the carbohydrate moiety or in the tertiary structure of the Ig molecule.

The so-called *complex allotypes*, the two best known examples of which are the rabbit *a* and *b* systems, constitute a special case. The *b* system controls a series of four determinants—b4, b5, b6, and b9—in the constant region of the light κ chains. When chains carrying different determinants were sequenced, no allotype-specific residue could be identified. Instead, a multitude of amino acid residues associated with a given determinant was found. When one compares

Table 6.10 Distribution of Alleles of the *Igh* Loci in the *Igh* Haplotypes

Igh Haplotype	Prototype Strain	Locus (chain)					
		Igh-1 (γ2a)	*Igh*-2 (α)	*Igh*-3 (γ2b)	*Igh*-4 (γ1)	*Igh*-5 (δ)	*Igh*-6 (μ)
a	BALB/c	*a*	*a*	*a*	*a*	*a*	*a*
b	C57BL	*b*	*b*	*b*	*b*	*b*	*b*
c	DBA/2	*c*	*c*	*a*	*a*	*a*	.[a]
d	AKR	*d*	*d*	*d*	*a*	*a*	.
e	A	*e*	*d*	*e*	*a*	*e*	*e*
f	CE	*f*	*f*	*f*	*a*	*a*	.
g	RIII	*g*	*c*	*g*	*a*	*a*	.
h	SEA	*h*	*a*	*a*	*a*	*a*	.
j	CBA/H	*j*	*a*	*a*	*a*	*a*	*a*
k	KH-1[b]	*k*	*c*	*a*	*a*	.	.
l	KH-2[b]	*l*	*c*	*a*	*a*	.	.
m	Ky[b]	*m*	*b*	*b*	*b*	.	.
n	NZB	*e*	*d*	*e*	*a*	*a*	*e*

[a] Not tested.
[b] Wild mouse.

polypeptides carrying different determinants (Fig. 6.35), one finds that, for instance, b4 and b6 differ in 15 of 54 analyzed residues. A similar situation exists in the a allotypes, but they are located in the V region.

How can such large differences among allotypes be explained? In two principal ways. The first possibility is that *b*4, *b*5, *b*6, and *b*9 are alleles at a single locus, which, for some reason, is highly prone to mutational diversification. (The reason could be either that the diversification is favored by natural selection, or that

Table 6.11 *Igh* Haplotypes of the Mouse

Prototype Strain	*Igh* Haplotype	Allotypic Determinants Encoded by Loci (Ig Chain in Parentheses)					
		Igh-1 (γ2a)	*Igh*-2 (α)	*Igh*-3 (γ2b)	*Igh*-4 (γ1)	*Igh*-5 (δ)	*Igh*-6 (μ)
BALB/c	*a*	1,6,7,8,26,28,29,30	12,13,14	9,11,22,31,33,34	8,19	36	38,39
C57BL	*b*	2,27,29	15	9,16,22,33,34	42	37	40,41
DBA/2	*c*	3,8,29	35	9,11,22,31,33,34	8,19	36	?
AKR	*d*	4,6,7,8,26,29	13,17	4,23,31,32,33,34	8,19	36	?
A	*e*	4,6,7,8,26,28,29,30	13,17	4,23,31,32,33	8,19	36	39,41
CE	*f*	5,7,8,26,30	14	9,11,31,32	8,19	36	?
RIII	*g*	3,8,26	35	9,11,31	8,19	36	?
SEA	*h*	1,6,7,8,28,29	12,13,14	9,11,22,31,33,34	8,19	36	38,39
CBA	*j*	1,6,7,8,28,29,30	12,13,14	9,11,22,31,33,34	8,19	36	38,39
KH-1[a]	*k*	3,5,7,8	35	9,11,25	8,19	?	?
KH-2[a]	*l*	3,5,8	35	9,11,22	8,19	?	?
Ky[a]	*m*	1,2,6,7,8	15	9,16,22	8,19	?	?
NZB	*n*	4,6,7,8,26,28,24,30	13,17	4,23,31,32,33	8,19	36	39,41

[a] Wild mouse.

		110										120											130	
b4	D	P	V	()	A	P	T	V	L	I	F	P	P	A	A	D	Q	V	A	T	G	T	V	T
b6				G	A	P	T	V	L	L	F	P	P	?	?	S	E	L	A	T	G	T	A	T
b9	D	P	P	I	A	P	T	V	L	L	F	P	P	S	A	D	Q	L	T	G	Z	T	V	T
b5																								

		150										160									170			
b4	V	D	G	T	T	Q	T	T	G	T	Q	D	S	K	T	P	Q	D	S	A	D	C	T	Y
b6															T	P	Q	D	G	S	G	C	T	
b9	V	D	D	E	I	Q	Q	S	G	I	E	N	S	T	T	P	Q	S	P	E	D	C	T	Y
b5															T	P	Q	N	S	D	D	C	T	

		190										200												
b4	H	K	E	Y	T	C	K	V	T	Q	G	T	T	S	V	V	Q	S	F	N	R	G	D	C
b6																				S	R	K	S	C
b9	H	S	()	Y	T	C	Q	V	H	N	S	A	G	S	I	V	Z	S	F	N	R	G	N	C
b5			E	Y	T	C	K																	

Figure 6.35. Amino acid sequence of short stretches of rabbit κ chains carrying different *b*-locus allotypes. (From A. D. Strosberg: *Immunogenetics* **4**:499–513, 1977.)

the diversification is permitted because it does not seriously affect the gene's function.) The second possibility is that *b*4, *b*5, *b*6, and *b*9, in fact, represent loci in a tightly linked cluster. If so, the observed large number of amino acid substitutions would simply reflect evolutionary diversification of related but distinct loci. The illusion of allelism (and *b*4, *b*5, *b*6, and *b*9 do, indeed, behave like alleles most of the time) would be the result of some regulatory mechanism that would normally permit the expression of only one locus in the cluster. Hence, if *b*4 were expressed in one chromosome and *b*5 in another, they would appear as alleles even though they might be physically separated from each other on the genetic map by other loci. The main reason immunogeneticists have come up with this second explanation is that in most other cases known, polypeptides controlled by alleles of a single locus differ by only one or a very few residues. (A notable exception to this rule is the alleles of the major histocompatibility loci; see Chapter 8.) Furthermore, complex allotypes are associated with a host of irregularities not observed in the case of simple allotypes. Some of the irregularities are these.

Multiallelic Rabbits. If *b*4, *b*5, *b*6, and *b*9 were alleles, a single individual should not possess more than two of them, and this is normally the case. Occasionally, however, rabbits are found expressing three alleles—for example, *b*4, *b*5, and *b*6. The third allele is often expressed in a transitory and unpredictable fashion.

Transitory Allotypes. The use of sensitive techniques revealed that some 50 percent of normal rabbits express low levels of group-*a* allotypes that were not anticipated by breeding data.

Latent Allotypes. After hyperimmunization with ovalbumin, extremely low amounts of a1 allotype-bearing molecules have been found in animals previously identified as *a*2/*a*3 heterozygotes. It should be mentioned, however, that transitory and latent alotype phenomena have also been observed with simple allotypes.

Pecking Order. Heterozygotes for the *a* and *b* loci might be expected to contain equal quantities of allotypes controlled by allelic genes. Instead, one finds that in a normal rabbit, certain alleles are preferred. One can arrange the *a* and *b* alleles in a pecking order of preference: a101 > a1 > a3 > a2 > a100, and b4 > b6 > b5 > b9. The order may change after immunization with different antigens.

All these phenomena—so the proponents of the cluster hypothesis argue—can best be explained as a result of regulatory genes variously affecting the expression of structural genes in the cluster. Thus, the information for the third allele in multiallelic rabbits and for the transitory and latent allotypes is already present in the gene cluster, but becomes expressed only when the regulatory genes provide the necessary signal. These phenomena, however, can also be explained in an orthodox way, so the issue remains unresolved.

6.6.2 Idiotypes and Fine-Specificity Markers

Discovery and Definition

Individual Ig species (groups of identical molecules) differ in their variable regions, and theoretically these differences should be recognizable as antigens by other antibodies. If so, one should be able to produce anti-Ig sera reactive specifically with one Ig species and unreactive with all other immunoglobulins. The first indication of the existence of such individually specific antigenic determinants came from studies of myeloma proteins. In the 1950s, several immunologists noticed that, when properly absorbed, anti-myeloma protein sera reacted only with the immunizing protein and no other. For example, in 1955 R. J. Slater and his colleagues immunized rabbits with myeloma proteins from 21 patients and demonstrated that after absorption with nonimmunizing proteins, the antisera retained reactivity against only the immunizing myeloma. At that time, myeloma proteins were still regarded as abnormal immunoglobulins, and the antigenic determinants recognized in this manner were, therefore, thought to be somehow related to the neoplastic origin of the molecules bearing them. After eight years Henry G. Kunkel and his co-workers realized the implications of this finding. To demonstrate antigenic determinants restricted to a given Ig species, Kunkel and his colleagues purified, from normal human serum, natural antibodies to the blood-group substance A, immunized rabbits with the purified fraction, and demonstrated that the antiserum, when absorbed with normal human serum, reacted only with the purified antibodies of the original donor and not with anti-A immunoglobulins from other individuals or with a variety of other antibodies and normal human sera.

Simultaneously with Kunkel and his colleagues, though independently of them, Jacques Oudin and M. Michel made a similar observation using rabbit antisera to rabbit immunoglobulins. Oudin and Michel immunized rabbit X with *Salmonella typhimurium*, coated the bacteria with the antibodies thus obtained, and then injected the bacteria-antibody complexes into rabbit Y. After a prolonged immunization, they obtained a second antiserum that reacted with the anti-*Salmonella* immunoglobulins of the first antiserum but did not react with normal serum of rabbit X (obtained by bleeding prior to the immunization) or with anti-*Salmonella* sera of 17 other rabbits.

Kunkel termed the entities detected by the absorbed anti-myeloma protein sera *individually specific antigenic determinants*, whereas Oudin designated the determinants recognized by the rabbit anti-rabbit Ig sera as *idiotypic* and the property of antibodies to possess idiotypic determinants as *idiotypy*. For a while, immunologists made the distinction between individually specific determinants as defined by xenoantisera and idiotypic determinants recognized by alloantisera, but later they came to the conclusion that the difference between the two types was trivial, if it existed at all, and dropped the former term. At present, the term *idiotypic determinant* (*idiotype*) refers to a unique antigenic determinant restricted to antibodies of a single or of only a few related species. Some immunologists, however, use the word "idiotype" to designate the population of Ig molecules reacting with a given anti-idiotypic serum. Much of the current knowledge of idiotypes is due to Jacques Oudin, Henry G. Kunkel, Klaus Eichmann, and Alfred Nisonoff.

Methods of Study

Idiotype-detecting antisera can be produced in an animal of a different species (xenoantisera), in an animal of the same species (alloantisera), in an animal of the same inbred strain (syngeneic antisera), or in the same individual that provides the immunizing antibodies (autoantisera). In addition to idiotypic antibodies, xenoantisera also contain isotypic and allotypic antibodies, but these can be absorbed out with pooled Ig. Alloantisera, when produced in allotype-matched donor-recipient combinations, can be used unabsorbed; otherwise they, too, must be absorbed with pooled Ig. Syngeneic antisera and autoantibodies need no absorption but are difficult to produce. As immunizing antigen, purified antibody fractions, antigen-antibody complexes, myeloma proteins, proteins of patients with macroglobulinemia, Bence-Jones proteins, or monoclonal antibodies may be used.

Idiotypic antibodies (i.e., antibodies specific for a particular idiotype) can be detected by a variety of serological methods, of which direct or indirect precipitation and the radioimmunoassay (see Chapter 10) are the most commonly used.

Specificity of Idiotypic Antibodies

Originally, immunologists believed idiotypic antibodies to be absolutely specific and idiotypic determinants to be restricted to a single Ig species in a single individual. Later studies, however, proved that this concept applied only to some idiotypic antibodies and idiotypic determinants referred to as *minor*, *individual* (IdI), or *private*, and that other idiotypic antibodies were crossreactive and the corresponding determinants were shared by more than one Ig species. The latter type of determinant is referred to as *major*, *shared*, *crossreactive*, *cross-specific* (IdX), or *public*. Major idiotypes are extremely rare among outbred animals (e.g., humans or rabbits) but somewhat more frequent among inbred individuals (e.g., inbred mouse strains). They are usually inherited from generation to generation and so are the only idiotypes accessible to experimentation. (An experimenter, particularly a geneticist, has little use for a trait expressed only in a single individual.) The degree of crossreactivity of the major idiotypes varies from case to case. Some idiotypes are restricted to members of a single inbred strain or a single group of genetically related individuals; others may be shared by several strains or be associated with related V_H and V_L isotypes. In fact, a continuous scale of shared determinants—from V-region allotypes through crossreactive idiotypes to individual idiotypes—may exist. However, even if an idiotype is shared by a group of individuals (e.g., members of an inbred strain), not all individuals of this group necessarily express it.

There are many reasons why individuals differ in their idiotypes. The most obvious is the absence of an idiotype-encoding gene in some individuals and the presence of this gene in other individuals. While the genetic information for many idiotypes, particularly the major ones, is known to exist in the germ line, some idiotypes may be generated somatically. In this instance, differences in idiotype expression may arise even among individuals of an inbred strain, for these individuals are identical in their germ-line genes but need not be identical in their somatic genes. Somatic differences among individuals may explain why it is sometimes possible to produce idiotypic antibodies by immunization between individuals of the same inbred strain. However, even individuals with the right gene need not *express* this gene.

Relationship between Idiotype and Antigen Specificity

As a rule, a given idiotype is associated with antibody molecules of one specificity—that is, with antibody reacting with a single antigen. However, there are exceptions to this rule, the most notable being the so-called *Oudin-Cazenave paradox*, originally discovered during a study of fibrinogen, a human plasma protein known to be cleaved by plasmin into two fragments, D and E. Jacques Oudin and Pierre-André Cazenave immunized rabbits with complete fibrinogen and then separated D- and E-specific antibodies from the antisera thus obtained. As expected, these antibodies did not crossreact, indicating that the D and E fragments have no antigenic determinants in common, but most surprisingly they shared the same idiotype. Similar observations were made with certain other proteins. The paradox remains unexplained but presumably reflects a phase in determination of idiotypic specificity in which an antigen is recognized as a whole, rather than as a series of individual determinants.

Location of Idiotypic Determinants

All idiotypic determinants are located in the V region. Some determinants are close enough to the combining site to be blocked by the combination of antibodies with antigens (*site-associated determinants*), while others are not affected by antigen binding (*determinants not associated with the combining site*). Since idiotypes reflect different degrees of Ig molecule uniqueness, they are presumably associated with residues known to vary—most of them with complementarity-determining residues (*hypervariable regions*), but some with the variable framework residues. The degree of residue variability determines the degree of idiotype crossreactivity (cross-specificity): combinations of residues occurring in only one Ig species (produced by a single B-cell clone) form the structural basis of individual (minor) idiotypes. V-region stretches shared by several molecular species are the sites at which the major determinants reside. Most idiotypic determinants (about 90 percent) result from the interaction of H and L chains: a few are borne by H chains and still fewer by L chains.

Inheritance of Idiotypes

As was mentioned earlier, some major idiotypes are inherited from generation to generation and so can be used as markers in genetic studies. Most of these studies have been carried out in the mouse, a species in which certain inbred strains respond to certain antigens by producing antibodies with one predominant idiotype. There are over 20 major idiotypes known in the mouse; the most extensively studied are described below.

The T15 Idiotype. Antibodies to phosphorylcholine and myeloma proteins that bind it (e.g., TEPC15) share an idiotype, T15, detected by alloantisera prepared against TEPC15. The T15 idiotype is found in BALB/c mice and other strains that carry the *Igh-*1^a allele. The T15-controlling gene is termed *Igh-Pc*.

The J558 Idiotype. BALB/c antibodies to the α-1,3 dextran, a storage polysaccharide of many bacteria and yeasts (see Chapter 10), and α-1,3 dextran-binding BALB/c mice and other strains that carry the *Igh-*1^a MOPC104E (IgM, λ) share an idiotype, J558, encoded by an *Igh-Dex* gene and detected by J558 alloantisera. The idiotype is also present in many other *Igh-*1^a-bearing mouse strains.

The S117 Idiotype. BALB/c antibodies to the N-acetylglucosamine of group-A streptococcal carbohydrate (A-CHO) share with the N-acetylglucosamine-binding myeloma protein S117 (IgA, κ) an idiotype, S117, which is also present in A-CHO antibodies of several other *Igh-*1^a strains, but not in A-CHO antibodies of other strains. The S117 idiotype, encoded by the *Igh-Sa*3 gene (Sa for streptococcal A carbohydrate), is detected by guinea pig anti-S117 sera.

The A5A Idiotype. A/J-strain mice immunized against group-A streptococcal carbohydrate produce antibodies, the majority of which carry a common idiotype, A5A. (The designation is derived from the name of an A5A antibody-producing lymphocyte clone obtained by cloning spleen cells of A/J mice immunized with group-A streptococci.) The A5A idiotype has been found only in the *Igh-*1^e strains A/J and A/He, and is detected by guinea pig antisera to A-CHO antibodies. The A5A-encoding gene is termed *Igh-Sa*1.

The ARS Idiotype. Antibodies produced in A/J mice immunized with p-azophenylarsonate (for the formula, see Chapter 10) share an idiotype, ARS, detected by a xenoantiserum (rabbit anti-mouse antibodies to p-azophenylarsonate). Like A5A, ARS is found only in *Igh-*1^e-bearing mouse strains. The ARS-encoding gene is referred to as *Igh-Ars*.

Idiotypes behave as if controlled by single Mendelian genes, the expression of which ranges from codominance to incomplete dominance, apparently depending on the action of modifying genes. All the major idiotype genes known in the mouse are linked to one another, and as a group they are linked to the *Igh* genes coding for the C regions of H chains. The individual idiotype genes are referred to by the *Igh* symbol, followed by an abbreviated symbol of the particular idiotype (examples were given above).

In breeding experiments in which segregation of more than one marker can be followed, the parental marker combinations usually remain together among the segregants, but new combinations also appear. Most of the latter result from the unreliability of typing individual mice for idiotypes, but some can be shown to be true genetic recombinants. From a study of over 30 such recombinants, a genetic map has been constructed, indicating the position of the idiotype-encoding genes with respect to one another and in relation to C region-encoding loci (Fig. 6.36).

Isoelectric Focusing and Fine-Specificity Markers

V-region variability can be detected by means other than serological analysis—for example, by isoelectric focusing or by fine-specificity characterization. In *isoelectric focusing*, an electric current is applied across a continuous pH gradient, causing proteins in a mixture to move and to concentrate as narrow bands at

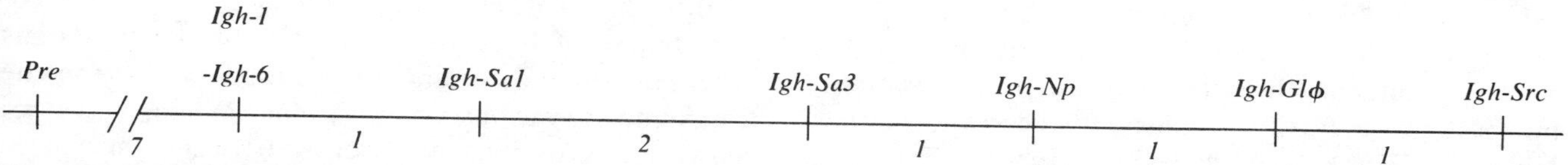

Figure 6.36. Linkage map of mouse idiotype-encoding genes. Numbers indicate approximate distances in centimorgans. Glø, poly-(L-Glu, L-Lys, L-Phe); Igh, immunoglobulin heavy chains; Np, 4-hydroxy-3-nitrophenyl; Pre, prealbumin; Sa1, A5A idiotype of anti-Strep-A-CHO; Sa3, S117 idiotype of anti-Strep-A-CHO; Src, extra antigens on sheep red blood cells. (Based on M. Weigert and R. Riblet: *Springer Sem. Immunopathol.* **1**:133–169, 1978.)

their isoelectric point, the pH at which their net charge is zero (see Appendix 6.1). The resolution power of isoelectric focusing is so high that even a single myeloma protein can often be separated into from two to five bands, representing molecular species altered post-translationally. Isoelectric focusing is therefore useful for distinguishing Ig species with different variable regions and different charge distributions. The problem with the technique is that when a serum contains too many molecular species, the isoelectric spectrum or spectrotype (i.e., series of bands appearing after staining for proteins) becomes uninterpretable. Nevertheless, major isotypes often appear on a spectrotype as dominant bands that can be used as markers in the same way that antigenic determinants are used in serological analysis.

Another way to distinguish individual species of Ig molecule is determining their *fine specificity* which, presumably, reflects differences in the V region. A measure of specificity is the *affinity*, or binding strength, of an antibody and the stability of the bond between antibody and antigen (see Chapter 10). Most antibody populations are too varied to be dissected into individual species that differ from one another in their affinities, but antibodies to certain simple haptens have been analyzed successfully for fine specificity by Olli Mäkelä and other immunologists. Particularly useful fine-specificity markers are the so-called *heteroclitic antibodies*, which, paradoxically, bind more strongly to a nonimmunizing hapten than to the immunizing one. For example, mice of the C57BL strain group, when immunized with 4-hydroxy-3-nitrophenylacetyl (NP), produce NP antibodies with higher affinity for the related hapten, 4-hydroxy-5-iodo-3-nitrophenylacetyl (NIP; for formulas see Chapter 10) than for the immunizing hapten, NP. Since other strains produce NP antibodies that are not heteroclitic, the affinity of these antibodies for NIP can be used as a marker in genetic studies.

6.6.3 Recombinational Analysis

Using allotypes and idiotypes as markers, researchers have screened thousands of progeny in the mouse and rabbit but have found no recombinants between Ig genes. In humans, the search has been more successful. Extensive family studies by Jacob B. Natvig, Henry G. Kunkel, Arthur G. Steinberg, Erna van Longhem, Claude Ropartz, and others have yielded not only regular recombinations (Fig. 6.37*a*), but also several abnormal chromosomes (Fig. 6.37b through d). A description of these rare chromosomal events follows.

Regular, Intergenic Crossingover. Figure 6.37*a* shows two examples of this event. In one, the $\gamma 2$- and $\gamma 3$-encoding gene complexes remained together and were separated from the $\gamma 1$-encoding complex; in the other, the $\gamma 2$ complex was separated from $\gamma 3$ and $\gamma 1$. This result suggests that the three γ-encoding loci are arranged in the order shown in Figure 6.37 ($\gamma 2$ . . . $\gamma 3$ . . . $\gamma 1$).

Gene Duplication (Fig. 6.37*b*). In normal meiosis, the two homologous chromosomes bearing the $\gamma 2$, $\gamma 3$, and $\gamma 1$ gene complexes pair in such a way that $\gamma 2$ in one chromosome is exactly opposite $\gamma 2$ in the other, $\gamma 3$ is opposite $\gamma 3$, and $\gamma 1$ is opposite $\gamma 1$. Occasionally, however, the two chromosomes mispair in the way shown in Figure 6.37*b* through *d*: $\gamma 3$ pairs with $\gamma 2$ and $\gamma 1$ with $\gamma 3$. Such mispairing is possible because of the considerable homology among the γ genes (all three gene complexes share large segments of identical nucleotide-pair sequences). When crossingover occurs in such mispaired chromosomes in the way shown in Figure 6.37*b*, the resulting recombinant chromosome inherits two $\gamma 1$ complexes instead of one. The crossingover between mispaired chromosomes is termed *unequal*, and the event resulting in gene doubling is called gene duplication.

Gene Deletion (Fig. 6.37*c*). If, in the same mispaired chromosome, unequal crossingover occurs in the way shown in Figure 6.37*c*, the resulting recombinant chromosome loses one of the three gene complexes ($\gamma 3$). The event resulting in gene loss is termed gene deletion.

Gene Fusion (Fig. 6.37*d*). In the three situations discussed so far, crossingover occurred *between* genes. On rare occasions, it can also occur within a gene, and it is then called *intragenic* (as opposed to *intergenic*). Intragenic crossingover between properly paired chromosomes may recombine determinants encoded by this gene. This event has not been observed in families, but must have occurred in natural populations where allotypic determinants encoded by a given gene are found in various combinations. When, however, intragenic crossingover occurs between mispaired chromosomes in the way shown in Figure 6.37*d*, a new gene that consists partly of one ($\gamma 3$) gene and partly of another ($\gamma 1$) is generated. This event is referred to as

a Regular, intergenic crossingover

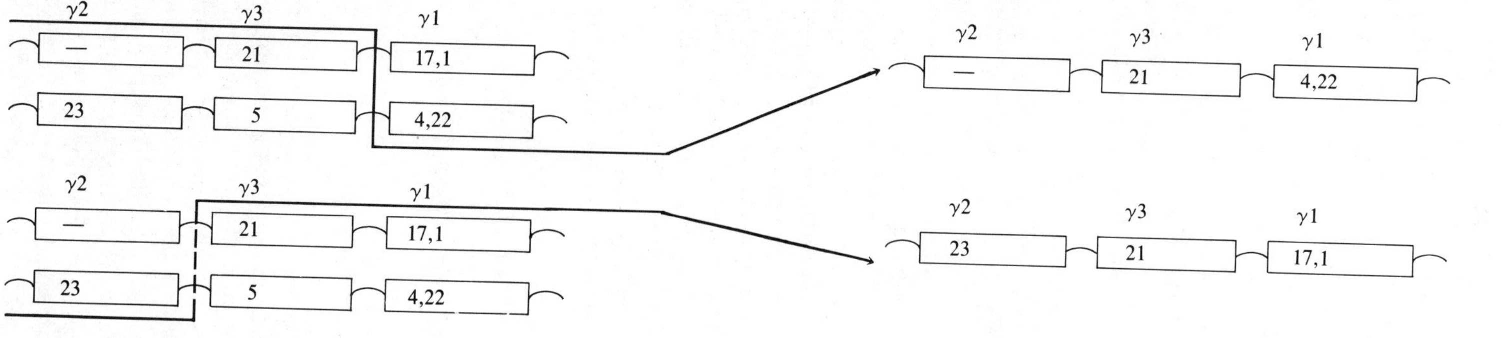

b Unequal intergenic crossingover resulting in gene duplication

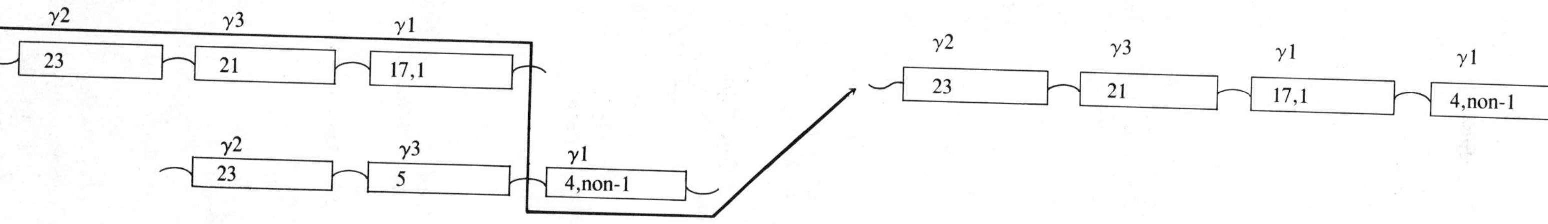

c Unequal intergenic crossingover resulting in gene deletion

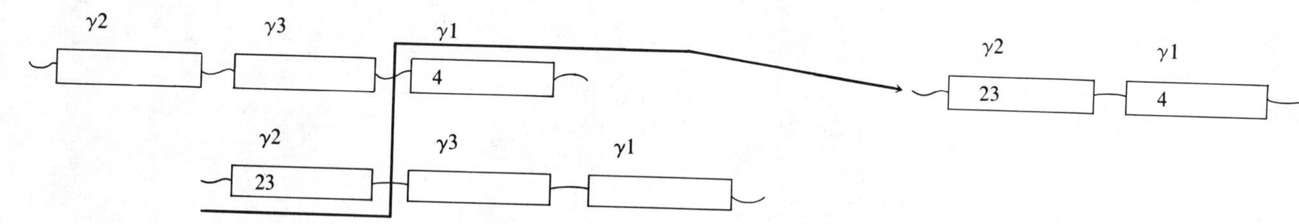

d Unequal, intragenic crossingover resulting in gene fusion

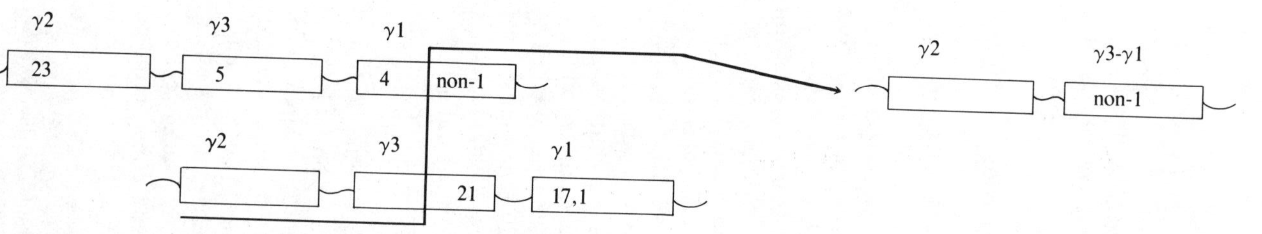

Figure 6.37. Various types of crossingover within the human gene cluster encoding CH regions of IgG1, IgG2, and IgG3 molecules. Numbers inside rectangles indicate allotypic determinants of the Gm system. Left panel, parental chromosomes; right panel, recombinant chromosomes of the progeny. Arrows indicate direction of crossingover.

gene fusion, or *Lepore-type recombination* because the fused gene product was first recognized in hemoglobin Lepore. Another recorded case of gene fusion involved the $\gamma 4$ and $\gamma 2$ complexes and suggested the following order of the γ loci: $\gamma 4 \ldots \gamma 2 \ldots \gamma 3 \ldots \gamma 1$.

The type of recombinational analysis just described for the human γ loci can also be carried out for CL and all other CH loci. However, since the allotypic markers outside the γ system are scarce, the knowledge of non-γ loci is limited. A summary of what we do know is presented in the genetic maps in Figure 6.38. Because of our limited knowledge, the order of some loci must be considered tentative. The definite order will probably be established soon by recombinant DNA techniques and DNA sequencing, just as it has already been established for mouse Ig genes.

6.6.4 Population Genetics of Ig Loci[6]

The first thing one notices while studying Ig genes in human populations is that different ethnic and geographical groups differ in their genetic composition. Caucasians carry genes somewhat different from those of blacks, Melanesians, or Mongolians; Swedes differ from Hungarians, French, or Italians. For a population geneticist, differences in gene and haplotype[7] frequencies are most informative.

Let us consider, as an example, the group of loci coding for the human CH polypeptide chains. Of the 10 or so loci in this group, five (*G1m*, *G2m*, *G3m*, *G4m*, and *Am2*) are accessible to population genetics analysis because they code for defined allotypic differences. A total of 20 alleles is known at these five loci—five at the *G1m* locus, nine at the *G3m* locus, and two each at the remaining three loci. However, not all of these alleles occur in all of the ethnic groups and populations (Table 6.7). Among Caucasians, only three alleles at the *G1m* locus ($G1m^{4,-1}$, $G1m^{1,17}$, and $G1m^{1,2,17}$) and two at the *G3m* locus ($G3m^{5,11,13,14,25,-21}$ and $G3m^{21,-5}$) are present in appreciable frequencies. Although other alleles may occasionally be found, they are usually extremely rare and often exist in the population only transiently. However, even the common alleles do not occur with equal frequencies. For example, in Europe there is a gradation of decreasing frequency of the $G1m^{1,17}$ allele from north to south and from west to east. (In some Scandinavian countries, the frequency of $G1m^{1,17}$ reaches 100 percent; in the south and east it declines below 45 percent.) Alleles that are common in one ethnic group (population) may be rare in or absent from another. The $G1m^{4,-1}$ allele of Caucasians does not occur in any other ethnic group, and the $G1m^{1,2,17}$ allele occurs in Caucasians, Melanesians, and among the Ainus of northern Japan, but not in blacks or Mongolians.

Similar considerations also apply to haplotype frequencies (Table 6.7). From the number of alleles known at the five Ig loci in the CH group, one can calculate the number of theoretically possible allelic combinations as 360. Of these, only a very small fraction (18) actually occur in the human population (approximately four different haplotypes in each ethnic group). Like the gene frequencies, the haplotype frequencies may vary from ethnic group to ethnic group, and within each ethnic group; the common haplotypes of the different ethnic groups are listed in Table 6.7.

All these observations are an important source of information about a population—its origin, composition, and dynamics. In addition, however, they can also be used to draw certain conclusions about the organization of genetic complexes. For example, the $G1m^{1,4}$ allele of the Mongolians and Melanesians, as was already mentioned, probably arose by intragenic crossingover from alleles $G1m^{-1,4}$ and $G1m^{1,17}$ present among Caucasians. Similar considerations can be used to trace the origin of other alleles and haplotypes.

6.7 MOLECULAR GENETICS OF Ig LOCI

6.7.1 DNA Rearrangements Preceding Gene Expression

Demonstration of Gene Transposition

The most stunning discovery in the molecular genetics of the immunoglobulin genes was that genes are moved around (transposed) before they are expressed. The transposition of Ig genes was first predicted on theoretical grounds and was then demonstrated experimentally in a spectacular way. The first observation that led to the formulation of the transposition hypothesis was made in 1953 by Charles W. Todd, who reported that, in the rabbit, the same pair of *a*-locus allotypic determinants (a1 and a3) occurred in immunoglobulins of two different classes, IgG and IgM. Subsequently, Arnold Feinstein also demonstrated the presence of a1

[6] A student not familiar with the theory of population genetics should first consult the Appendix to Chapter 8 and only then return to this section.

[7] *Haplotype* is a combination of alleles of a gene complex carried by a single chromosome.

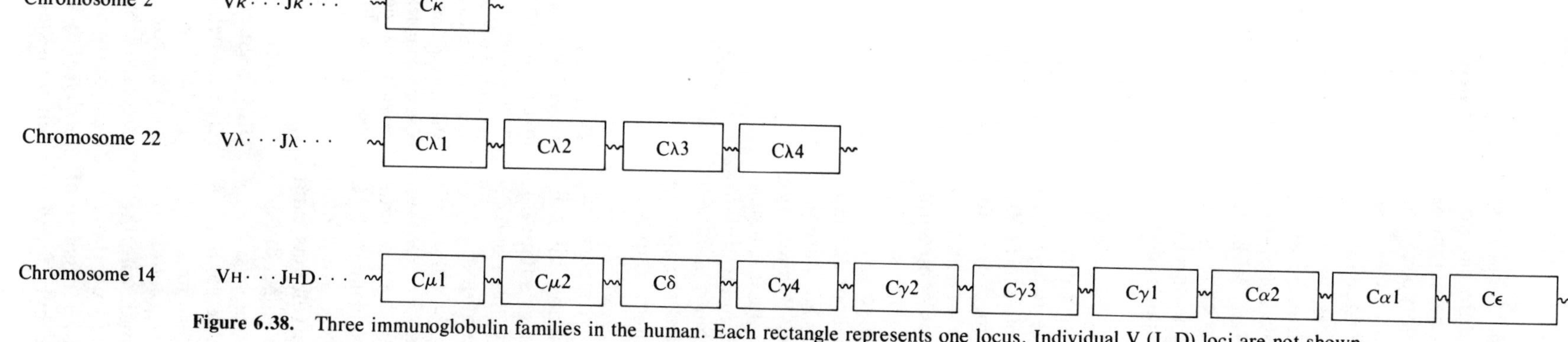

Figure 6.38. Three immunoglobulin families in the human. Each rectangle represents one locus. Individual V (J, D) loci are not shown.

and a3 on IgA molecules. The implication of this *Todd phenomenon* was that genes coding for different immunoglobulin classes (different heavy chains) must share the information coding for the a allotypes. The full impact of this finding became clear when Marian E. Koshland and her co-workers demonstrated in 1969 that the a allotypes were located in the V region. Since the determinants specifying immunoglobulin isotype (class) reside in the C region, the inevitable conclusion was that different C regions can associate with the same V region. This conclusion was supported by genetic studies that demonstrated that the gene coding for the V-region allotype a is linked to a gene, *d*, coding for a C-region allotype.

The genetic consequences of the Todd phenomenon were formulated explicitly in 1965 by William J. Dreyer and J. Claude Bennett, who came to the conclusion that the immunoglobulin polypeptide was encoded by two genes—one containing information for the V region, the other for the C region—and that a given VH gene can associate with C genes controlling H chains of different immunoglobulin classes. This conclusion was supported by the amino acid sequence analysis of Hilschmann and Craig and by peptide mapping analysis of Koiti Titani and Frank W. Putnam, published in the same year as the Dreyer-Bennett hypothesis. The complete sequences of three human Bence-Jones proteins proved to be very similar in their C-terminal halves and very different in their N-terminal halves, which again suggested the joining of two genes in the production of a single immunoglobulin (L chain).

Ig gene transposition was then demonstrated at the molecular level by Susumu Tonegawa and his colleagues (Fig. 6.39). These investigators isolated L chain-encoding mRNA from a mouse myeloma and divided it into two aliquots. They left one aliquot intact so that it contained information in single chains for both the V- and C-region polypeptides (V-C probe), and digested the second aliquot enzymatically so that only the C region-encoding sequences remained (C probe). They then isolated total DNA from two sources, mouse embryos and mouse myelomas, and cleaved it with restriction enzymes (see Appendix 6.2) into pieces of different sizes. After separation of different-sized DNA fragments by electrophoresis, they unwound the DNA helices and determined which of the fragments had hybridized (see Appendix 6.2) with the RNA of the V-C probe and which with the C probe. They observed that, when tested on the embryonic DNA, the C probe hybridized to a fragment of a certain size, whereas the V-C probe hybridized to this fragment and to another of a different size. In contrast, when tested on myeloma-cell DNA, both the C and V-C probes hybridized to a single DNA fragment.

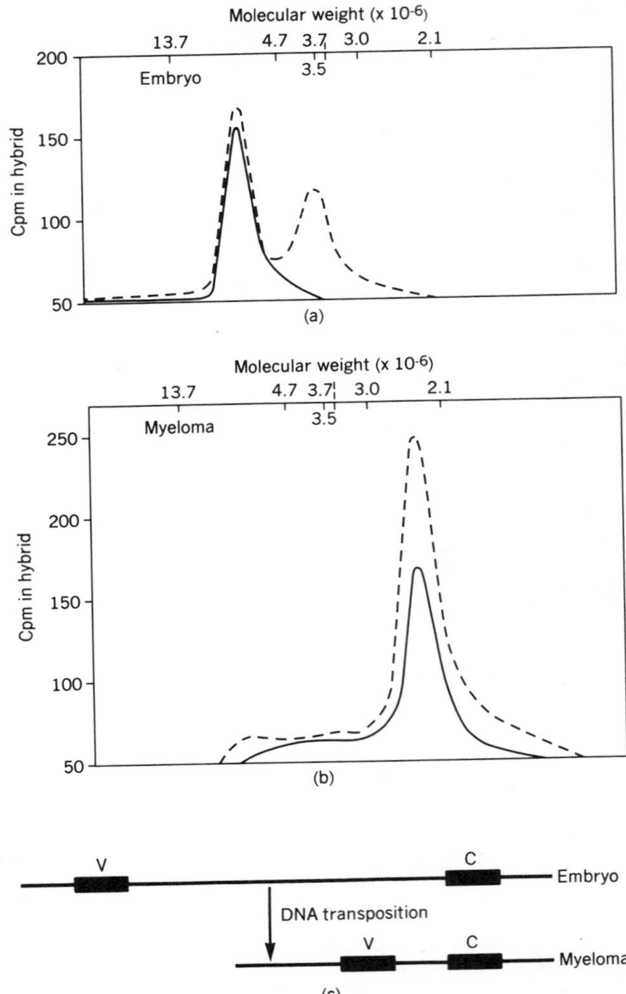

Figure 6.39. Experiment demonstrating V-gene transposition to the vicinity of a C gene. The *a* and *b* panels show hybridization of DNA fragments from mouse embryo (*a*) or mouse myeloma (*b*), with immunoglobulin mRNA carrying information for only the C (solid line) or both the V and C polypeptide (broken line). Explanation in the text. The *c* panel indicates the interpretation of the experiment: in the mouse embryo, a given V gene is widely separated from the C-gene complex: during B-cell differentiation, the V gene is transposed to the vicinity of the C gene. Cpm, counts per minute. (Modified from S. Tonegawa, N. Hozumi, G. Matthyssens, and R. Schuller: *Cold Spring Harbor Symp. Quant. Biol.* **41:**877–899, 1976.)

One can conclude from this experiment that in embryonic DNA, the V- and C-region sequences are present on two different fragments, and hence that physically, they are widely separated from each other in the chromosome, whereas in the myeloma cell representing a differentiated B lymphocyte, the V and C genes are carried by a single DNA fragment, and so are relatively close to each other in the chromosome. In other words, the widely separated V and C genes of the undifferentiated cell are moved closer to each other during B-lymphocyte differentiation (Fig. 6.39*c*).

Studies by Susumu Tonegawa, Philip Leder, Leroy Hood, Jerry M. Adams, Tosuku Honjo, and others have demonstrated the existence of two principal kinds of gene transposition, the so-called V-J joining, which occurs in both light and heavy chain-encoding chromosomes, and the heavy-chain switch, which occurs in heavy chain-encoding chromosomes only.

V-J Joining

In this form of transposition, one of the many V genes is moved to the vicinity of a J gene (in κ- and λ-encoding chromosomes), or first to the vicinity of a D gene and then the VD segment is transposed to the vicinity of a J gene (in H chain-encoding chromosomes). The available data indicate that a crucial role in the transposition process is played by short, highly conserved, noncoding sequences flanking the V, D, and J genes. Two such sequences exist—a heptamer consisting of seven nucleotide pairs, and a decamer consisting of 10 nucleotide pair. The two sequences always occur together, with the heptamer immediately adjacent to the V, D, or J gene and the decamer separated from the heptamer by either 11 or 22 essentially random nucleotide pairs. The prototype sequences of the segments flanking the V_L or V_H genes are CACAGTG for the heptamer and ${}^{A}_{G}ACA{}^{A}_{T}AAACC$ for the decamer. The prototype sequences of the segments flanking the J_L and J_H genes are CACTGTG for the heptamer and GGTTTTTGTA for the decamer. The sequences flanking the D genes have not been identified at the time of writing but are presumed to be the same as those flanking the J genes (see Fig. 6.40). The deviations from the prototype sequences in individual Ig chromosomes are only slight, and most of them occur in the V gene-associated sequences (Table 6.12). The sharing of sequences by all three Ig-gene families suggests that the common ancestor of these sequences already existed before the Ig genes separated into families—that is, some 500 million years ago (see section 6.11).

In the V-gene groups, the conserved sequences are always on the 3′ end of each gene; in contrast, in the J group, they are on the 5′ end of each gene. When one folds the DNA strand back on itself, one can see that the J-associated sequences are inversely complementary to the V-associated sequences:

V gene — CACAGTG — GACAAAAACC —
J gene — GTGTCAC — ATGTTTTTGG —

This fact undoubtedly plays a role in V-J joining. The D-associated sequences are believed to flank the gene on both sides.

As was already mentioned, the heptamers and decamers are separated either by 11 ± 1 or 22 ± 1 nonconserved nucleotide pairs. The only exception is the sequence flanking one of the $J\kappa$ genes but this gene is believed to be nonfunctional anyway. Within each gene group, the nonconserved spacer is of uniform length—22 nucleotide pairs in the V_H, $V\lambda$, J_H, and $J\kappa$ groups, and 11 nucleotide pairs in the $V\kappa$, $J\lambda$, and

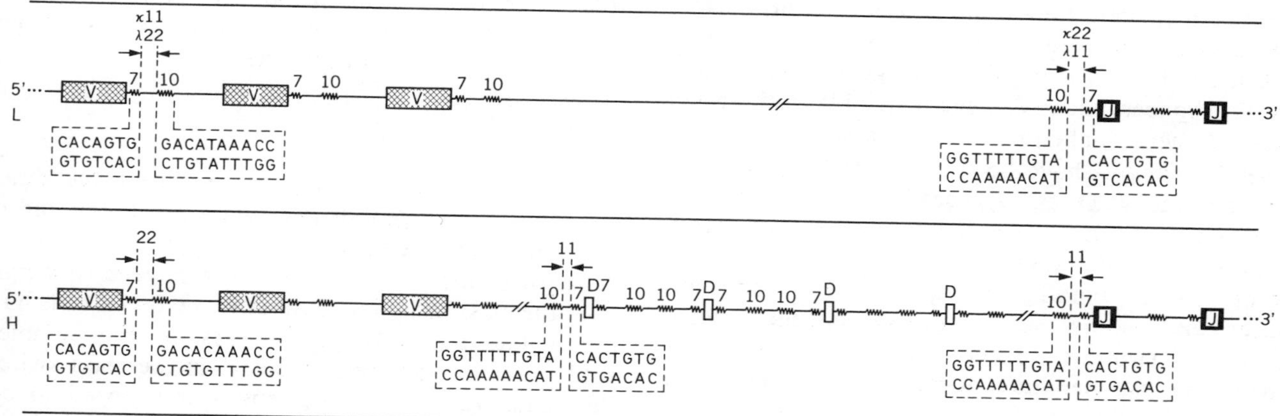

Figure 6.40. Arrangement of noncoding heptamers and decamers believed to play a role in joining of V and J genes. Numerals indicate the number of nucleotide pairs in each DNA segment.

Table 6.12 Noncoding Nucleotide Sequences Flanking V and J Genes

Gene	Nucleotide Sequences	Number of Nucleotides Separating Conserved Sequences
Vκ41	*CACAGTG* ATACAAATCAT*AACATAAACC*	11
Vκ2	*CACAGTG* ATTCAAGCCAT*GACATAAACC*	11
Vκ3	*CACAGTG* ATTCAAGCCAT*GACATAAACC*	11
Vκ21	*CACAGTG* CTCAGGGCTG*AACAAAAACC*	10
VH107	*CACAGTG* AGAGGACGTCATTGTGAGCCCA*GACACAAACC*	22
Vλ1	*CACAATG* ACATGTGTAGATGGGGAAGTAG*ATCAAGAACA*	22
Jκ1	*GGTTTTTGTA* GAGAGGGGCATGTCATAGTCCT*CACTGTG*	22
Jκ2	*GGTTTTTGTA* AAGGGGGGCGCAGTGATATGAAT*CACTGTG*	23
Jκ3	*GGGTTTTGTG* GAGGTAAAGTTAAAATAAAT*CACTGTA*	20
Jκ4	*AGTTTTTGTA* TGGGGGTTGAGTGAAGGGACAC*CAGTGTG*	22
Jκ5	*GGTTTTTGTA* CAGCCAGACAGTGGAGTACTAC*CACTGTG*	22
JH107	*AGTTTTAGTA* TAGGAACAGAGGCAGAACAGA*GACTGTG*	21
JH315	*GGTTTTTGTA* CACCCACTAAAGGGGTCTATGA*TAGTGTG*	22
Jλ1	*GGTTTTTGCA* TGAGTCTATAT*CACAGTG*	11

Source. From P. Early et al.: *Cell* **19**:981–992, 1980.
Conserved sequences are italicized.

probably in the D groups. Since one turn of the DNA helix requires about 10.4 nucleotide pairs, the heptamers are separated from the decamers by either one or two turns of the helix. This regularity of spacing means that the relative orientation on the DNA helix of the conserved sequences is much the same as if they formed a continuous stretch of 17 conserved nucleotide pairs. In other words, if one were to cut out the spacers, the heptamers would connect almost exactly to the decamers on the helix. Another important fact is that, in the joining process, a gene flanked by a one-turn spacer is always connected with a gene flanked by a two-turn spacer: a VH gene with a two-turn spacer joins a JH gene flanked by a one-turn spacer; a Vκ gene with a one-turn spacer joins a Jκ gene flanked by a two-turn spacer; and a Vλ gene with a two-turn spacer joins a Jλ gene flanked by a one-turn spacer.

Several models have been proposed for the actual joining of the V, D, and J genes. In the one depicted in Figure 6.41, the conserved sequences are recognized by sets of hypothetical joining proteins, one set of proteins binding to sequences by a one-turn spacer, and another set binding to sequences separated by a two-turn spacer. Each protein probably consists of two separate domains or subunits, one binding to the $\genfrac{}{}{0pt}{}{\text{CACAGTC}}{\text{GTGTCAG}}$ sequence, and the other to the $\genfrac{}{}{0pt}{}{\text{TACAAAAACC}}{\text{ATGTTTTTGG}}$ sequence. The proteins for the V- and J-associated sequences may be the same, but since the sequences show inverse complementarity, the proteins must bind in opposite orientation to the V and J genes.

A joining protein bound across a two-turn spacer may then interact with a protein bound across a one-turn spacer to form a complex that brings the two selected genes together by looping out the entire intervening DNA segment. Once complexing has occurred, the proteins may excise the looped-out segment enzymatically and bind the loose ends of the chromosome. The available evidence does, indeed, suggest that V-J joining is accompanied by the deletion of the DNA which, in the embryo, separates the genes joined in the differentiated lymphocyte.

Class Switch

The V-J and V-D-J joining occurs during the differentiation of a progenitor cell into a pre-B cell and always precedes the synthesis of free μ chains in pre-B cells. In contrast, the second form of gene transposition, the class switch, occurs after the pre-B cells have differentiated into B lymphocytes bearing complete IgM molecules on their surfaces. In the class switch, the same VJ or VDJ segment is transposed to one of the C-gene complexes—in the mouse to the γ3, γ1, γ2b, γ2a, α, or ϵ complexes. (Transposition to the δ complex probably does not occur, although this point

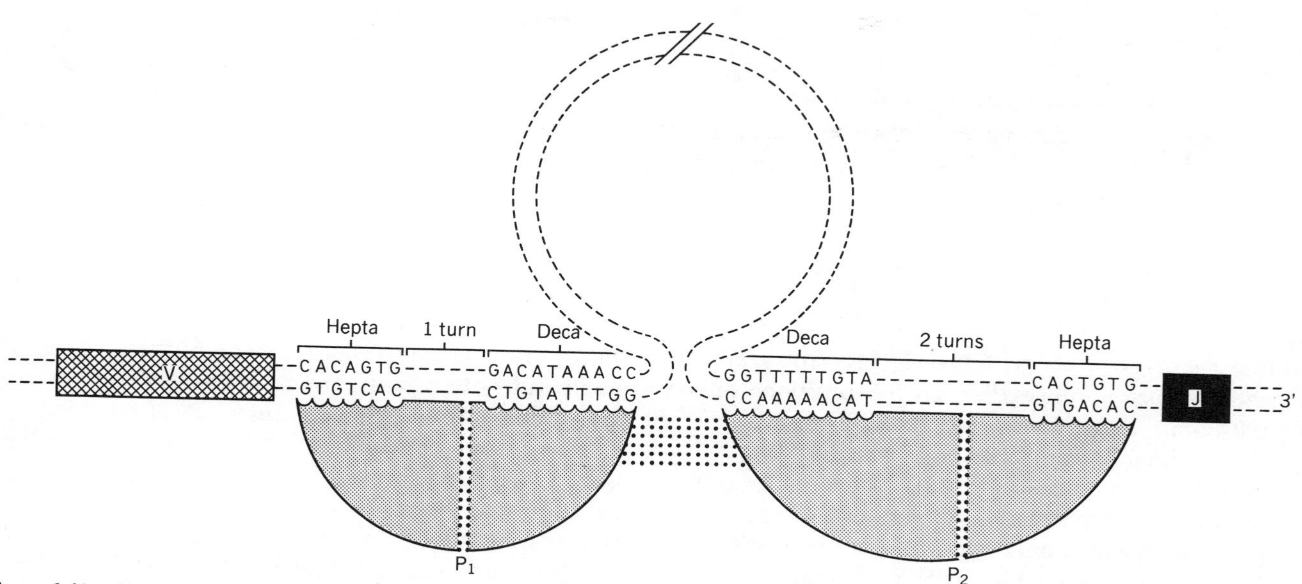

Figure 6.41. Hypothetical joining proteins (P_1 and P_2) believed to recognize conserved nucleotide sequences in the vicinity of V and J genes. Dotted lines between proteins indicate bondages.

has yet to be established.) The transposition is thought to be sequential, so that in the same cell clone, a VJ segment is first moved to the $\gamma3$ complex, then to the $\gamma1$ complex, and so on, but again there is an alternative possibility—that in different clones the VJ segments are moved to different C-gene complexes—that has not yet been ruled out. In contrast to V-J joining, in the class switch the transposed VJ or VDJ segment is not joined with the C gene—it is only moved closer to it, and the two coding sequences remain separated by a long noncoding segment.

The basic mechanism responsible for the class switch is believed to be the same as that operating during V-J joining, namely the recognition of short, conserved noncoding sequences by specific switch proteins. However, the switch proteins are different from the joining proteins, and moreover, the class-recognition sites (S) to which the switch proteins bind do not lie adjacent to the genes they help transpose, but are scattered through the intron separating the coding sequences. The sites appear to be class-specific, so presumably there is one set of sites (Sγ3) in the intron between the δ and $\gamma3$ complexes, another set (Sγ1) in the intron between $\gamma3$ and $\gamma1$, and so on. In addition, there is one set of recognition sites (Sμ) in the intron separating VJ or VDJ from the μ complex. Corresponding to these different sites there are presumably different switch proteins (Pμ for Sμ, Pγ3 for Sγ3, Pα for Sα, etc.), each recognizing the nucleotide-pair sequence specifically at a given site. The switch is thought to occur when one protein binds to an Sμ site and another binds to, say, an Sγ3 site. The two proteins then interact to form a heterodimer that places the VDJ segment next to the $\gamma3$ complex, looping out the intervening sequence. The loop may then be excised or held inactive (it is not yet clear which) while the juxtaposed genes are transcribed into a single mRNA molecule. The juxtaposition site may vary, depending on the sites in the two introns to which the switch proteins have attached. It is this variation in the point of attachment that is responsible for the variable length of the intron between the transposed VJ or VDJ segment and the C-gene complex. The overall exon-intron organization of the chromosomal region affected most by Ig-gene rearrangements is depicted in Figure 6.42.

6.7.2 Transcription

Once rearranged, the Ig genes are transcribed into single-stranded messenger RNA (mRNA) molecules that pass the genetic information from the DNA in the nucleus to proteins in the cytoplasm. In the case of the κ- and λ-encoding DNA, the transcript consists of the VJ segment, the VJ-C intron, and the C gene (Fig. 6.10). The composition of the transcripts made of the H-encoding DNA is uncertain; it probably varies, depending on the occurrence and type of the class switch. Lymphocytes in which the class switch has not yet occurred probably transcribe the VDJ and VC intron segments together with the μ- and δ-encoding sequences. Mouse lymphocytes in which the switch has occurred probably transcribe the VDJ and the V-C in-

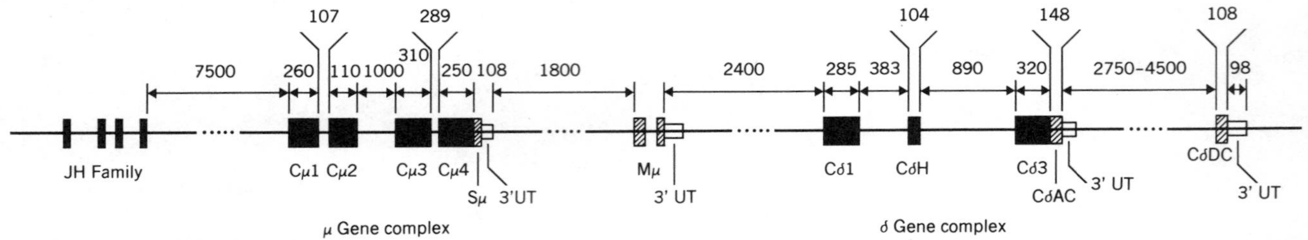

Figure 6.42. Organization of mouse Cμ and Cδ gene complexes. Numerals indicate number of nucleotide pairs in each DNA segment.

tron segments together with the γ3, γ1, γ2b, γ2a, α or ϵ gene complexes, depending on the positions of the switch point.

The primary transcript is subject to post-transcriptional modifications. The transcript of the L chain-encoding DNA, a large 40S RNA molecule, exists in the nucleus only fleetingly and is quickly degraded into an intermediate 24S RNA molecule (Fig. 6.43). Still in the nucleus, this intermediate molecule is subject to a process called *splicing*, because it resembles the joining of two pieces of tape or film. In the splicing phase, all the introns, including the large one separating the J- and C-encoding sequences, are excised and all the coding sequences are joined into one continuous strand. The mechanism of splicing is not known, but it is assumed that the process consists of looping out of the introns and cutting off the loops (Fig. 6.10). The splicing signals appear to be the GT and AG doublets at the beginning and end of each intron, respectively. However, the post-transcriptional modification consists not only of removal, but also addition of nucleotides to the transcript. The largest segment added consists of 200 nucleotides, all of one kind (A). This poly-A sequence is attached by the enzyme poly-A polymerase to the 3′ end of the RNA strand. Its function may be to facilitate the strands' movements through the nuclear-membrane pores.

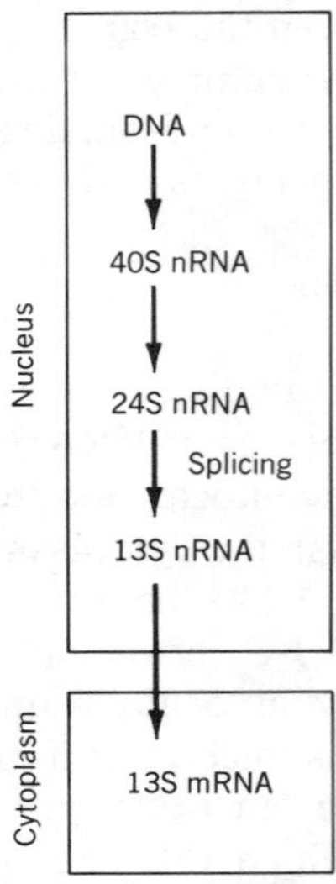

Figure 6.43. Processing of the RNA molecule carrying the message for mouse Lκ chain. mRNA, messenger RNA; nRNA, nuclear RNA.

The processed L chain-encoding mRNA has a sedimentation constant of 13S and consists of six segments (Fig. 6.44). At the 5′ end it has about 150 untranslated nucleotides, followed by about 50 nucleotides coding for the so-called signal sequence (see below). The bulk of the message consists of about 320 V chain- and another 320 C chain-coding nucleotides. At the 3′ end are another 200 untranslated noncoding nucleotides and the poly-A tail. The origin and function of the two untranslated segments are unknown. The 13S RNA passes from the nucleus through the nuclear membrane into the cytoplasm, where it becomes immediately involved in the translation process.

The H-chain RNA is presumably organized and modified in a way similar to that of the L-chain RNA, except that its C-encoding portion is larger and more complex.

6.7.3 Translation

The conversion of the information contained in the nucleotide sequence of RNA into a sequence of amino acids of the polypeptide chain is called *translation*.

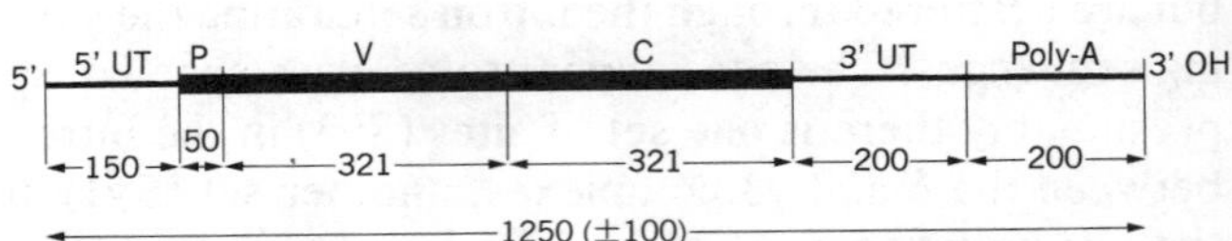

Figure 6.44. Organization of the 13S mRNA coding for murine Lκ chain. C, constant region; P, precursor (signal) sequence; UT, untranslated segment; V, variable region. Coding sequences are indicated by heavy lines, noncoding sequences by light lines. Numbers indicate the length of individual segments in nucleotides. (Based on C. Milstein, G. G. Brownlee, E. M. Cartwright, J. M. Jarvis, and N. J. Proudfoot: *Nature* **252**:354–359, 1974.)

During this process, ribosomes attach, one by one, to the 3′ end of mRNA, travel along the RNA strand toward the 5′ end, and during this journey translate nucleotide triplets sequentially into corresponding amino acids. Hence, as the ribosome travels along the RNA, it assembles a progressively longer polypeptide chain, and when it reaches the end of the coding sequence, it has a complete polypeptide chain dangling from it. Since the L and H chains are encoded by separate mRNA molecules, they are also synthesized separately. The synthesis of a complete L chain takes about one minute, that of an H chain about two minutes.

L-chain RNA can accommodate four to eight ribosomes on one strand; H-chain RNA accommodates 11 to 20 ribosomes. Polyribosomes (the complexes of ribosomes and RNA) are attached to the membranes of the rough endoplasmic reticulum (RER), where protein synthesis takes place. The synthesized H and L chains are somewhat (about 15 amino acids) longer than the corresponding chains in the assembled Ig molecule. The difference results from a short N-terminal extension called the *signal sequence*, encoded by the P segment of RNA. The P segment, in turn, is encoded by the so-called *leader (L) DNA sequence*, which is separated from the main body of each V gene by a short intervening sequence. The leader sequences are located at the 5′ ends of the individual V genes.

What exactly happens with the synthesized polypeptide chain is not known, but according to the signal hypothesis (Fig. 6.45), the synthesis is initiated by free ribosomes, starting at the N-terminal signal sequence. The hydrophobic signal peptide attaches to the RER membrane, passes through it toward the lumen of the RER channels, and thus also attaches to the membrane the large (60S) subunit of the ribosome. The completed polypeptide is released into the lumen, the signal sequence is cleaved off and degraded, the free chain folds, and the heavy and light chains assemble into H_2L_2 molecules. The assembly occurs so rapidly that there are virtually no free H chains detectable in the cytoplasm at any time; the existence of a small pool of free L chains suggests that slightly more of these chains are synthesized than H chains, perhaps to help the H chains get off the ribosomes. The manner of H- and L-chain assembly probably depends on the H-chain isotype. The principal pathways are these.

(1)
$$H + L \rightarrow HL$$
$$HL + HL \rightarrow H_2L_2$$

(2)
$$H + L \rightarrow HL$$
$$HL + H \rightarrow H_2L$$
$$H_2L + L \rightarrow H_2L_2$$

(3)
$$H + L \rightarrow HL$$
$$HL + L \rightarrow HL_2$$
$$HL_2 + H \rightarrow H_2L_2$$

(4)
$$H + H \rightarrow H_2$$
$$H_2 + L \rightarrow H_2L$$
$$H_2L + L \rightarrow H_2L_2$$

(5)
$$L + L \rightarrow L_2$$
$$L_2 + H \rightarrow HL_2$$
$$HL_2 + H \rightarrow H_2L_2$$

The γ and α chains assemble predominantly through H_2 and then H_2L intermediates, whereas μ chains assemble primarily through HL half-molecules.

The assembled immunoglobulin molecules travel through the channels and cisternal spaces of the RER into the Golgi apparatus, where most of the carbohydrate moieties are attached to them. The completed molecules are believed to be enclosed in a small vesicle, which travels from the Golgi apparatus to the cell surface, where it fuses with the plasma membrane and releases its contents into the cell's external milieu (Fig. 6.46).

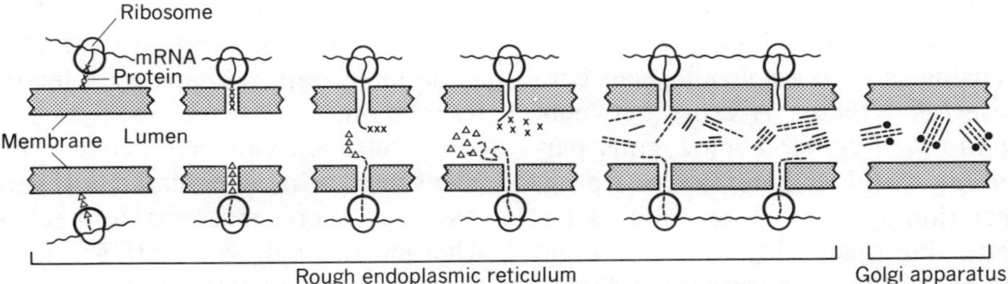

Figure 6.45. The signal hypothesis of protein synthesis. The diagram depicts successive stages (from left to right) of ribosome attachment to the membranes of the rough endoplasmic reticulum, penetration of the polypeptide chain through the membrane, and release and folding of the polypeptide chain in the lumen of the RER and Golgi apparatus. Full circles represent carbohydrate.

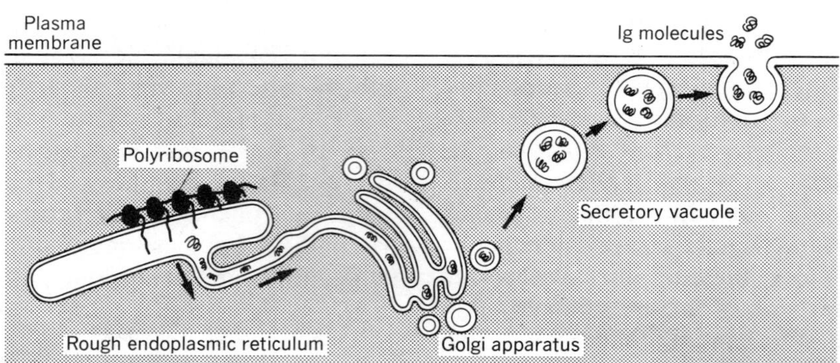

Figure 6.46. Diagram of Ig molecules' passage from the site of protein synthesis on the rough endoplasmic reticulum through the Golgi apparatus and secretory vacuoles to the extracellular space.

6.7.4 Regulation of Ig-Gene Expression

All diploid organisms possess two gene copies at any given locus, one in each chromosome of the homologous pair. As a rule, organisms express both these genes (the genes are said to be codominant) so that, in a heterozygote, two gene products are detected. Often, however, one of the products is nonfunctional or its effect is masked by another product, so that at the phenotype level, a trait controlled by one gene (allele) may appear dominant over the trait controlled by the second, recessive gene. An exception to this codominancy rule is the group of loci carried by the sex chromosomes. In mammals, the X chromosome in the XY male does not have a partner chromosome, so all the X-linked loci are present in a single dose. The female, though it has two X chromosomes, also expresses only one set of X-linked genes; the other set is inactivated by some still unknown genetic mechanism. The X-chromosome inactivation occurs randomly so that some loci (or loci in some cells) are inactivated in one X chromosome, while others (or the same loci in other cells) are inactivated in the other chromosome.

The second major exception to the codominancy rule comprises the immunoglobulin loci. We shall explain this exception using as an example allotypes controlled by the mouse *Igh*-1 locus. A cross between, say, *Igh*-1^a/*Igh*-1^a and *Igh*-1^b/*Igh*-1^b homozygous parents should produce *Igh*-1^a/*Igh*-1^b heterozygous progeny, and this expectation appears to be fulfilled because sera of the offspring react with both anti-a and anti-b reagents. However, when one tests individual Ig molecules, one finds that they are either a^+b^- or a^-b^+, but never a^+b^+. Moreover, a single plasma cell secretes only a^+b^- or a^-b^+ antibodies, never both. So at the cell level, only one of the two alleles is expressed—either *a* or *b*. Because of the exclusion of one allele from expression, the phenomenon is referred to as *allelic exclusion*. But since, in each cell, each of the two alleles has an equal chance of being expressed, half the cells express the *a* and the other half the *b* allele; the individual possesses an equal mixture of a and b immunoglobulin molecules and so is phenotypically heterozygous at the *Igh*-1 locus.

What might be the mechanism of allelic exclusion? This question may have been answered by the time this book is published, but so far one can only choose between the number of hypotheses. According to the *restricted rearrangement hypothesis*, each lymphocyte produces only one or very few protein molecules necessary for the initiation of gene rearrangement, and once this molecule has bound to one of the two chromosomes, it is inactivated and hence unable to rearrange and activate the other chromosome. According to the *abortive rearrangement hypothesis*, many rearrangements are aberrant and so nonfunctional; since the probability that both chromosomes in a single cell will rearrange correctly is low, most cells express only one allele. Finally, according to the *post-rearrangement hypothesis*, both homologous chromosomes rearrange but the expression of alleles is restricted at some later step, perhaps by selective transcription or translation.

In addition to allelic exclusion, the expression of Ig genes must also be regulated at several other levels: for instance, there must be a mechanism determining whether the cell will activate genes in the κ or λ chromosomes or restrict V-gene transposition in each chromosome to one of the many genes. While information about the organization of Ig genes is beginning to fill blackboards in many laboratories and classrooms, the regulation of these genes remains a *tabula rasa*.

6.8 ANTIBODY DIVERSITY

6.8.1 Estimates of Antibody Diversity

How many different antibodies can an individual produce? At first, immunologists believed that immunoglobulins were absolutely specific and that there were as many different antibodies as there were antigens. But gradually this belief became untenable, as evidence indicating the number of antigens to be astronomical accumulated. The human body contains about 2×10^{12} lymphocytes, of which roughly half are B cells. If every B cell carried a receptor for a different antigen (which we know is not true), a single individual would be able to recognize about 10^{12} different antigens. There is thus a physical upper limit to the number of different antibodies any individual can theoretically produce, while there seems to be no limit to the number of antigens existing in the universe.[8] Does this conclusion mean that there is a large number of antigens to which the body is unable to produce specific antibodies? Probably not. Although an individual is unable to respond to some antigens, in most instances this failure is caused by a defect in the function of supportive and accessory cells, not by a lack of B lymphocytes with receptors for these antigens. We seem to be in a paradoxical situation, in which an almost infinite number of antigens exists, and yet an individual is able to form specific antibodies to all these antigens, despite the fact that it can make a maximum of 10^{12} different antibodies (and probably, as discussed below, far fewer than that). The paradox has been resolved by the finding that antibodies are not absolutely specific and that a single antibody species can react with more than one antigenic determinant. The extent of this crossreaction will become apparent shortly.

Niels K. Jerne compared the immune system to a glove factory. Rather than taking measurements of individual customers and manufacturing gloves to specific orders, the factory makes a certain number of gloves of each size so that each person will find gloves that fit. And the fit is usually good despite the fact that no two pairs of hands are identical. Antibodies, too, may be constructed in such a way that they differentiate the gross, but not the finest, morphological features of the antigenic molecule; or, to continue the glove analogy, they are made to fit fingers of different sizes but do not distinguish different fingerprint patterns. The number of theoretically possible gross patterns of an antigenic molecule—in contrast to the total number of antigens—is apparently limited. In this way, the body manages to have in store antibodies to all possible antigens, even to those it will never encounter.

[8] Of course, lymphocytes do not remain the same throughout the life of an individual, so the lymphocyte repertoire may, theoretically, be greater than 10^{12}. But the point of this discussion is that *at any one time* a great number of antigens would pass unrecognized if antibodies were absolutely specific.

We stated that the maximum number of antibody species a human body can theoretically produce is 10^{12}. (Analogous numbers would be 10^9 for the mouse and 10^6 for the tadpole.) But does the body indeed produce so many different antibodies? There are several ways of answering this question, though none is sophisticated enough to provide us with a reliable figure. We shall mention here only one of these ways—one based on determination of antibody species elicited by a single hapten.

H. W. Kreth and Alan R. Williamson immunized mice of one strain with the hapten 4-hydroxy-5-iodo-3-nitro-phenacetyl (NIP) conjugated to a carrier protein (see Chapter 10), took out the recipient's spleen, made a highly diluted spleen cell suspension, and then injected the cells into irradiated syngeneic mice in a quantity that had a high probability of sustaining proliferation of only one antibody-producing clone in each new recipient. They then challenged the new recipients with the same hapten and determined the spectrotype of the produced—presumably monoclonal—antibodies. Most of the inoculated mice produced antibodies of different spectrotype, but five of the 337 monoclonal antibodies had the same spectrotype. From this frequency of repeats, the authors calculated that a mouse can produce between 2700 and 16,000 different NIP-binding antibodies. From other studies it is known that these antibodies are not absolutely specific, and Kreth and Williamson estimated that one NIP-reacting antibody may bind to some 100 different haptens. From these figures, the authors estimated that a mouse can produce on the order of 10^6 different antibodies.

6.8.2 Generation of Antibody Diversity

What ways does the body use to generate so many protein species? Many papers attempting to answer this question have been published, long textbook passages have been devoted to the various hypotheses put forward to explain generation of antibody diversity, and arguing at meetings about the merits of the various proposals has long been a favorite pastime of many immunologists. Not much has come out of all these discussions, published or unpublished, thus confirming William Blake's dictum that:

. . . Art and Science cannot exist but in
minutely organized Particulars
And not in generalized Demonstrations
of the Rational Power.

Only recently have procedures permitting experimental dissection of the problem become available. A major advance has been achieved mainly by the application of DNA cloning and sequencing techniques, allowing a direct comparison of the genetic material in the germ-line (embryonic) and differentiated (somatic) cells.

The principal possibilities of how antibody diversity is generated are these: either the information for different antibodies is already present in the germ line (*germ-line hypothesis*), or this information is generated somatically during lymphocyte differentiation (*somatic hypothesis of antibody diversification*).

An extreme form of the germ-line hypothesis says that, for each antibody species, there is a separate V gene already present in the germ cell. An extreme form of the somatic hypothesis maintains that there are very few V genes in the germ line and that these mutate during lymphocyte proliferation into the different alleles necessary for the production of the 10^6 or so antibody species. Since no other somatic cell but the lymphocyte undergoes such a vast genetic diversification, and since the diversification affects only the V and not the C genes, there would have to be a special *generator of diversity* (GOD) operating on V genes in lymphocytes. There are also many possible compromise hypotheses allowing the participation, in varying degrees, of both the germ line and the somatic line, and there are, of course, many possible GODs in the somatic version of the diversification hypothesis.

As the controversy now nears its resolution, it is becoming evident—as so often happens when lines are drawn too sharply in a discussion—that both sides have been partly right. Three mechanisms have been identified that contribute to the generation of antibody diversity: numerical diversification, combinatorial diversification, and somatic mutation.

Numerical V-Gene Diversification

One solution to the problem of antibody diversity would be to have one gene coding for the V region of each antibody species. Simple gene counting should, then, provide at least part of the answer to how antibody diversity is generated. Unfortunately, gene counting is anything but simple. Some of the ways one can attempt to determine the number of V genes and the result these methods have produced are discussed briefly below.

Idiotype Mapping. As described earlier, idiotypes can be used as markers for V-region genes, which can then be mapped with respect to one another. Idiotypes, however, provide information only about mouse VH loci, for no major mouse VL idiotypes are known and major idiotypes in noninbred species are rare. The murine VH idiotype map currently contains 15 genes and this number must, therefore, represent the absolute minimum of VH loci in the mouse genome.

Amino Acid Sequence Analysis. We already know that VH, Vκ, and Vλ chains can be divided into subgroups, based on their primary structure, with chains in each subgroup resembling one another more than chains belonging to different subgroups. The intersubgroup differences in amino acid sequence are so large that the existence of separate loci coding for the individual subgroups can safely be assumed. There should, therefore, be at least as many VH, Vκ, and Vλ loci as there are VH, Vκ, and Vλ subgroups. But since it is unlikely that we know all the subgroups, the V-locus count cannot be made directly. Instead, one must determine how often a given V-region sequence repeats itself in a sample of randomly chosen proteins and then use this figure to estimate how many subgroups still remain to be detected. The estimate is further complicated by the fact that complete amino acid sequence is known for only a few V-region chains, and so the comparisons are based mostly on incomplete sequences.

In the murine Vκ system, 25 subgroups have been described, based on sequence comparisons of the first 23 N-terminal residues. From the frequency of repeated sequences, immunochemists have estimated that another 25 subgroups still remain to be detected, thus raising the total count of Vκ subgroups to 50. However, nucleic acid hybridization experiments suggest that each Vκ subgroup is encoded not by one but by approximately six loci, so that the total number of Vκ loci is 6 × 50, or 300. In a similar way, immunochemists estimated the total number of murine VH loci at 50 to 150 and the number of Vλ loci at two.

RNA-DNA Hybridization. Isolated L- or H-chain messenger RNA (or DNA obtained by copying RNA, using viral reverse transcriptase) reanneals with Ig genes in denatured DNA preparation (see Appendix 6.2). The rate of reannealing will be slow if the DNA contains only one or a few Ig genes and faster in the presence of multiple copies with which the RNA can hybridize. (In the latter instance, the RNA strands will find the complementary DNA strands more easily.) By comparison with the rate of RNA-DNA hybridization of a standard containing a known gene number, one can then estimate the number of Ig genes (C and V), but the method is prone to many technical problems that could influence the estimates. Impure RNA, low specific activity of the RNA, and a low degree of homology between the RNA and the individual V genes—all these factors may adversely affect the result and lead to misleading interpretations of the data. Because of these technical difficulties, data obtained in one laboratory are often at variance with those from other laboratories. Although all laboratories agree that there is only a low number of Vλ genes—perhaps only one or two copies per haploid genome—the estimates for Vκ genes range from 50 to several hundred.

Recombinant DNA Studies. In these studies, the Ig-encoding genes are excised from the rest of the genome, inserted into bacterial plasmids, cloned, and then analyzed (see Appendix 6.2). In the future, this technique will provide direct means not only of counting the V genes, but also of determining their organization in the chromosomes.

Combinatorial Diversification

The fragmentation of the basic V-gene unit and the separation of short sequences (D and J) from the main V-gene body constitute the basis for combinatorial diversification of the V-gene repertoire. This diversification occurs at two levels. First, the fact that in the mouse any one of the four functional Jκ genes can combine with any one of several hundred V genes gives a fourfold increase in the total number of possible V regions. The same also applies to VH and JH genes, but here the number of possible combinations is increased further by the fact that any of the VH genes can combine with any of the D genes prior to joining with one of the JH genes. At this level, therefore, several thousand different V regions of both the light and heavy chains can be generated. The association of L and H chains, the V regions of which are controlled by different gene families, may contribute further to the combinatorial assortment of antibody molecules.

A second level of combinatorial diversification is achieved by the inaccuracy of V-J, V-D, and VD-J joining. Consider, as an example, the joining of Vκ to Jκ in the mouse. Although the joining always occurs in the same general area (that coding for residue number 95—a proline in most κ chains), there may be some variation with respect to the precise site of the cut; this variation may result in the generation of different triplet codons at the recombination site and insertion of different amino acids at the corresponding positions in the polypeptide chain. A hypothetical example of this variation is given in Figure 6.47, where recombinations numbers 1 and 2 would result in the sequence Pro-Trp, recombination number 3 in the sequence Pro-Arg, and recombination number 4 in the sequence Pro-Pro.

This imprecision of joining accounts for much of the variability in the third hypervariable region of the light chains (V-J joining), and the third and fourth hypervariable regions of the heavy chains (V-D and V-J joining, respectively). It also explains the variable length of the V regions discussed earlier in this chapter. Attempts have also been made to explain other hypervariable regions on the same principle, the assembly of the V-gene body from several *minigenes*, but experimental evidence in support of this explanation is lacking.

Diversification by Somatic Mutations

There is no doubt that genes can mutate not only in the germ line but also in somatic cells. During lymphocyte differentiation, many cell divisions occur (in humans about 10^6 new lymphocytes arise every second), and at each division the DNA has a certain probability of mutation. Somatic mutations can, therefore, also be expected—and have, in fact, been demonstrated—to occur in the genes coding for the V regions of the Ig molecules. The most direct evidence for the occurrence of somatic mutation has been obtained in the mouse Vλ system. Here, nucleotide-sequence comparisons of the Vλ genes in myelomas (differentiated B cells) and embryos (germ line) have revealed several

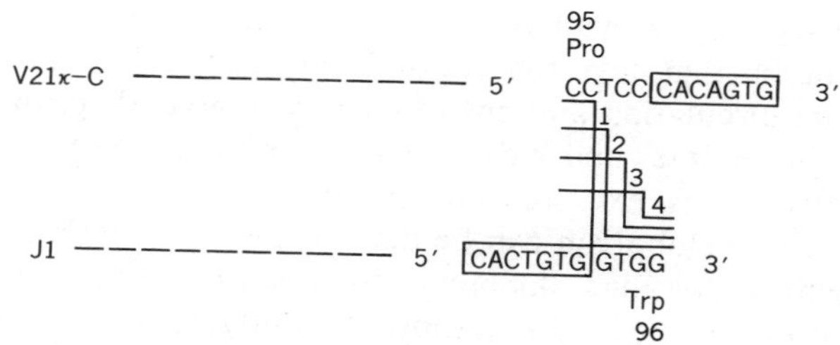

Figure 6.47. Diagram depicting how cutting and rejoining the DNA strands of a given pair of V and J genes at slightly different positions can lead to the reconstitution of different triplet codons at the recombination site and thus to insertion of different amino acids at positions 95 and 96 of the V-region polypeptide. See text for further details. (From H. Sakano, K. Hüppi, G. Heinrich, and S. Tonegawa: *Nature* **280**:288–294, 1979.)

base changes, most of them in the hypervariable regions.

A mutation in the DNA molecule may be such that—because of the degeneration of the genetic code—it does not change the meaning of a given codon and does not lead to amino acid replacement in the corresponding polypeptide chain; or it may generate a codon that controls a different amino acid. Preliminary data suggest that the latter type of mutation may be more frequent in V genes than in other genes. This observation does not necessarily mean that replacement mutations are more frequent in V than in other genes; it probably means that replacement mutations are selected against in most genes other than V genes.

In summary, the available data indicate that all three mechanisms contribute to the diversification of V genes: there is a large number of V genes in the germ line, and V genes are further diversified somatically by combinatorial assortment and by somatic mutations. However, the relative contribution of these three mechanisms is not yet completely understood. Particularly unclear is the role of somatic mutation in the overall antibody diversification.

6.9 METABOLISM OF IMMUNOGLOBULINS

Molecules are like individuals: they are born, they live to serve their function, and they perish and are degraded. So the metabolism—the life history of a molecule—can be divided into two phases: the biosynthetic or *anabolic* phase (Gr. *anabolē*, a raising up) and degradation or the *catabolic* phase (Gr. *catabolē*, a casting down). In a healthy individual, the sum of the biosynthetic and degradation rates of a given protein is zero and the concentration of the protein in the body fluids remains stable. In certain diseases, this steady state may be disturbed and biosynthesis may prevail over degradation, or vice versa. Proteins that have run out their life spans are removed from circulation and enzymatically degraded, primarily in the liver and kidney; from there the degradation products are excreted into the urine.

The metabolism can be determined by isolating the immunoglobulins, labeling them with a radioactive isotope, reinjecting them into the body, and determining their fate by periodically sampling bodily fluids (blood and urine). The initial amount of radioactivity injected—measured after a certain time, allowing mixing and equal distribution of the label through the body—is taken as 100 percent (or one), and the percentage (fraction) of radioactivity remaining in a fixed volume of blood at different times after this first sampling at time zero is calculated from the data. Plotting of the obtained values on a semi-logarithmic scale (the percent or fraction on the logarithmic scale and the time in days on the nonlogarithmic scale) gives a straight decay line with a certain slope. The time corresponding to a point exactly halfway between the starting point and a point where the line intercepts the ordinate is termed the *half life* of the molecule. By using formulas, the derivation of which is not always simple, one can calculate several other parameters characterizing the molecules' metabolism (Table 6.5).

Different Ig subclasses have strikingly different half lives. The human IgG is one of the longest-lived proteins, with a half life of some 22 days, whereas IgE and IgD are among the shortest lived, with half lives of only 2.4 and 2.8 days, respectively. Fab fragments and L chains have half lives of less than 24 hours, whereas the half life of the Fc fragment is comparable to that of the intact molecules.

The concentration of immunoglobulin in the serum does not always correspond to the rate of Ig biosynthesis. For example, IgA is synthesized at a rate similar to that of IgG, yet the concentration of the former in the plasma is five times lower than that of the latter because IgA is cleared from the serum five times more rapidly than IgG. On the other hand, the concentration of human serum IgD is $\frac{1}{500}$ of the total immunoglobulin because IgD is synthesized at $\frac{1}{100}$ the rate of IgG and cleared six to eight times faster. In disease, some of these metabolic Ig parameters may change drastically.

6.10 FUNCTION OF IMMUNOGLOBULINS

Immunoglobulins are two molecules in one, not only in the way they are constructed but also functionally. The two major functions of immunoglobulin molecules are antigen recognition, executed by the Fab portion of the molecule, and effector functions, executed by the Fc portion.

6.10.1 Antigen Recognition

Antibodies recognize and bind antigens via the combining sites of their V regions. Although combining sites are designed to bind almost any kind of antigen specifically, even antigens that do not exist in nature, the main targets of antibody recognition in the body are antigens carried by bacteria and their products; other important targets are viral antigens and those carried by protozoal and metazoal parasites. The mere binding of antibody to antigen only rarely protects the body from a parasite. (An example of such direct protection is the neutralization, through antibody binding, of the harmful effects of bacterial toxins.) More often, the binding serves to identify the foreign matter and to single it out for destruction by other agents. For further discussion of the role of antibodies in defense, see Chapters 13 and 14.

6.10.2 Effector Functions

The Fc portion of an immunoglobulin molecule serves to bind complement, to bind immunoglobulins to various cell receptors, and to transfer immunoglobulins across membranes.

Complement Binding

An antibody bound to an antigen is recognized by a plasma protein called complement. There is more than one way in which this recognition occurs, but in the one that is best understood, the C1q component of the complement's system binds to a specific site in the CH2 domain of the Ig molecule. This binding initiates a chain of enzymatic reactions that first produces soluble factors capable of participating nonspecifically in the destruction of foreign matter, and then perforates plasma membrane and thus destroys cells identified by antibodies as foreign. We shall learn more about complement and its binding to antibodies in Chapter 9.

Binding to Cells (Cytotropism)

In its complement-activating function, an antibody attaches first to an antigen via the Fab region and then binds a complement component via the Fc region. The process can also be reversed, so that an antibody synthesized by one cell attaches via the Fc region to another cell and then binds antigen via the Fab region. Reaction of the passively attached antibody with an antigen activates the cell, which then carries out a particular defense function. There are apparently several ways in which membrane receptors can interact with the Fc portion of the antibody molecule; here we shall mention only two.

IgE Binding by Basophils and Mast Cells. Basophils and mast cells carry cell-surface receptors capable of binding IgE in the absence of antigen. Since the binding is species-specific (i.e., mouse IgE can bind to mouse but not to human basophils, and vice versa), it is referred to as *homocytotropic* (Gr. *homos*, the same, *kytos*, cell, *tropē*, a turning toward). The interaction of the passively adsorbed immunoglobulin with the antigen results in the release, by the basophils and mast cells, of substances capable of mediating allergic reactions. (For more details, see Chapter 13.)

Cytophilic Antibody Binding by Macrophages. The Fc portion of some IgG molecules may be recognized by a specific Fc receptor on certain phagocytic cells. The attachment of these *cytophilic antibodies* (Gr. *cytos*, cell, *philos*, fond) occurs, again, in the absence of antigen but the passively attached antibody binds antigen secondarily. Macrophages activated by the combination of cytophilic antibodies with antigen then carry out the effector functions described in Chapter 11.

Transfer of Immunoglobulins across Membranes

Antibodies are often needed at sites to which antibody-synthesizing cells do not have easy access (e.g., digestive, respiratory, and reproductive tracts), or where such cells have not yet developed (i.e., in the fetus and newborn). Antibodies must reach such sites by passing through tissues and membranes, and the Fc portion of the immunoglobulin molecule is specifically adapted to facilitate this passage. We shall discuss immunity at these special sites in Chapter 13. Functions of the individual immunoglobulin classes and subclasses are summarized in Table 6.13.

6.11 EVOLUTION OF IMMUNOGLOBULINS

Immunoglobulins are vertebrate proteins, for although their origin must be rooted in advanced invertebrates, the track of immunoglobulin evolution disappears in the cyclostomes, the most primitive vertebrates. As was mentioned in Chapter 1, invertebrates possess glycoproteins that, like antibodies, are able to bind antigens, but no structural evidence is available to suggest evolutionary relationship between the two. Here we shall first describe the immunoglobulins in the individual vertebrate classes and then speculate on immunoglobulin evolution.

6.11.1 Immunoglobulins of Various Vertebrates

Cyclostomes

The living representatives of these round-mouthed, jawless vertebrates are the hagfish and the lamprey—two eel-like fish parasites. Upon immunization, both species produce antibodies that resemble immuno-

Table 6.13 Major Effector Functions of Human Immunoglobulins

Immunoglobulin	Classical Pathway Complement Fixation	Alternative Pathway Complement Activation	Placental Transfer	Binding To Mononuclear Cells	Binding To Mast Cells and Basophils	Reactivity with Staphylococcal Protein A
IgG1	++	−	+	+	−	+
IgG2	+	−	+	−	−	+
IgG3	+++	−	+	+	−	−
IgG4	−	−[a]	+	−	(?)	+
IgM	+++	−	−	−	−	−
IgA1	−	+	−	−	−	−
IgA2	−	+	−	−	−	−
SeIgA	−	−	−	−	−	−
IgD	−	−	−	−	−	−
IgE	−	−[a]	−	−[b]	+++	−

Source. From M. W. Turner, *in* L. E. Glynn and M. W. Steward (Eds.): *Immunochemistry: An Advanced Textbook.* Wiley, Chichester, 1977.
[a] Aggregated molecules may activate complement by alternative pathway.
[b] Human IgE has been reported to bind to macrophages.

globulins in that each molecule consists of four chains, two small and two larger ones. These antibodies are thought to be related to IgM, but their precise structure is controversial. The fact that so important a problem as the structure of immunoglobulins in the most primitive vertebrates has yet to be resolved is a sad testimony to the vogues and trends in immunological interests. Areas of obvious significance too often lose out to areas of transient popularity.

Cartilaginous Fishes

The most intensively studied group of *Chondrichthyes* (cartilaginous fishes) is the sharks. Two types of immunoglobulin have been found in sharks, one with a sedimentation constant of 7S and molecular weight of between 160,000 and 180,000 daltons, and another with a sedimentation constant of 18S and molecular weight of between 800,000 and 900,000 daltons. Both types belong to the same Ig class, related to mammalian IgM. The 7S component consists of H_2L_2 monomers, and the 18S type of $(H_2L_2)_5$ pentamers, in which the monomers are joined by the J chains. Both the H and L chains consist of a V and C region, with the V region showing sequence homology with the corresponding mammalian V region. The 7S and 18S molecules are related to each other antigenically and structurally, and apparently belong to a single class of primitive IgM.

Bony Fishes

The class of *Osteichthyes* (bony fishes) is divided into two subclasses—*Actinopterygii* (ray-finned fishes), represented by the carp, goldfish, and gar, and *Sarcopterygii* (fleshy-finned fishes), represented by the lungfish. All bony fishes possess a high-molecular-weight immunoglobulin (sedimentation constant of 14 to 16S, molecular weight of 600,000 to 700,000 daltons) related to IgM and existing in the form of $(H_2L_2)_4$ tetramers. Some bony fishes, in particular the *Sarcopterygii*, have, in addition, a low-molecular-weight immunoglobulin with a sedimentation constant of 6 to 7S and a molecular weight of about 120,000 daltons. The H chain of this poorly characterized, low-molecular-weight component is believed to consist of only three domains—one V and two C.

Amphibians

Of the amphibians, the anurans—represented by *Rana, Xenopus* and other frogs—are thought to be more advanced than the urodeles, represented by newts. Urodeles are believed to possess only a high-molecular-weight, IgM-like immunoglobulin, while the evidence for the presence of a low-molecular-weight class in at least some urodelian species is controversial. The anurans, on the other hand, clearly possess two immunoglobulin classes—a high-molecular-weight immunoglobulin (900,000 daltons) with a sedimentation constant of 18 to 19S, and a low-molecular-weight immunoglobulin (180,000 daltons) with a sedimentation constant of 7S. The high-molecular-weight component is related antigenically and structurally (presence of J chains) to mammalian IgM. It may exist in a pentameric $(H_2L_2)_5$ form in some species (e.g., *Rana*) and a hexameric $(H_2L_2)_6$ form in others (e.g., *Xenopus*). The low-molecular-weight component is probably related to the low-molecular-weight component of bony fishes, but is clearly distinct antigenically and structurally from the IgM-like component. Some immunologists believe the low-molecular-weight immunoglobulin is related to mammalian IgG, but there are important differences between the H chains of the two classes in size, migration rate, and amino acid composition. The anuran 7S Ig could, therefore, be a class distinct from IgG.

Reptiles

In some reptiles (e.g., turtles), three immunoglobulin types have been found—one IgM-like, high-molecular-weight (18S) type, and two low-molecular-weight types (7.5S and 5.7S). The H chains of the 7.5S and 5.7S types are antigenically related in that the larger chain has all the antigenic determinants present in the smaller chain, but it also has some additional determinants. It is unlikely, however, that the 5.7S immunoglobulin is a degradation product of the 7.5S component; the two may represent distinct but closely related immunoglobulin classes. The 7.5S immunoglobulin is probably homologous to the low-molecular-weight immunoglobulin of the anurans on the one hand, and mammalian IgG on the other.

Birds

There are at least three immunoglobulin classes present in birds: high-molecular-weight immunoglobulin (17S, 890,000 daltons), the H chain of which shares antigenic determinants with the human μ chain; low-molecular-weight immunoglobulin (7S, 170,000 daltons), probably related to mammalian IgG; and a component antigenically related to human IgA. The IgA-like molecules are present in intestinal secretions in 11S to 16S forms, and in the serum in a 175,000 dalton form. Some birds (e.g., ducks) possess, in addition, a 5.7S immunoglobulin that may be related to similar forms in turtles.

Mammals

Spot checks of several species indicate that probably all mammals possess the five immunoglobulin classes found in humans and in the mouse (IgM, IgG, IgA, IgD, and IgE).

6.11.2 Evolution of Immunoglobulin Classes

The knowledge of immunoglobulins in different vertebrate groups is still too fragmentary to permit any firm conclusions about the evolution of individual immunoglobulin classes. In particular, there is a need for amino acid or nucleotide sequence data that would allow conclusions about the homologies of the different Ig types. From the available data, one can reconstruct immunoglobulin evolution as follows.

From the first vertebrate, the immunoglobulin molecules have existed in the characteristic four-chain structure, so that the steps leading to this structure must have taken place in the ancestors of contemporary vertebrates. The most primitive class is IgM, which probably appears first in cyclostomes and persists all the way to mammals. The IgM molecules can exist in various degrees of polymerization—as monomers in sharks, tetramers in bony fishes, hexamers in some anuran amphibians, and pentamers in most other vertebrates.

Starting with some bony fishes, particularly the *Sarcopterygii*, a second immunoglobulin class makes its appearance. It is of low molecular weight but its size may vary, apparently according to the number of C domains its H chains contain: it may possess two C domains and then its sedimentation constant is around 5.7S; or it may have three C domains, when its sedimentation constant increases to about 7S or more. The main unanswered question is whether this low-molecular-weight immunoglobulin is related to mammalian IgG. Some immunologists argue that this class has evolved independently of IgG and persisted up to mammals, where IgG replaced it.

The IgA class has so far been found only in mammals and birds, but considering its low serum concentration, it is possible that it might have been missed in studies of other vertebrates. A few less advanced vertebrates were tested for the presence of IgA in their secretions, but the results were negative.

The IgE class has so far been found only in mammals. Although in some birds (e.g., pigeons, ducks) the presence of homocytotropic antibodies has been demonstrated, no evidence is available to prove that these antibodies are of the IgE class. (Homocytotropism—the ability of proteins to bind to cell surfaces—has also been demonstrated for immunoglobulins that do not belong to the IgE class.)

No data are available on the presence of IgD molecules outside the few mammalian species thus far tested.

The emergence of different immunoglobulin classes probably reflects the progressive specialization of protein groups in carrying out various functions. Precisely what these functions were can only be inferred indirectly from fragmentary observations. Thus, IgM possesses a combination of characteristics—good complement-binding ability, efficient agglutination, and predominant localization within blood vessels—that predisposes it to handle bacterial and protozoal parasites. Molecules of IgG are adapted for the transfer from mother to young and for the protection of the fetus and newborn. Also, owing to its smaller size, IgG can leave blood vessels and enter tissue fluids and perform its function at sites that IgM molecules cannot enter. Increasing demands to handle antigens that entered the body orally or nasally, or that were concentrated in the gut led to the appearance of the third immunoglobulin class, IgA, which, owing to the presence of the secretory component, can cross epithelial membranes more easily than IgG. IgE is suited primarily to inducing inflammatory lesions and thus to dealing with metazoal parasites. IgD is specialized for membrane-receptor function. Changing demands on these various functions probably provided strong selective pressure in the evolution of the individual classes.

Little is known about the evolution of the antigen-binding function. No differences in antibody heterogeneity and binding ability (affinity) have been found among the various vertebrate classes. It seems, therefore, that the antibody repertoire developed early in immunoglobulin evolution, probably before the emergence of present-day vertebrates. However, differences have been found in the way affinity changes during immunization. In all vertebrates, antibodies with low affinity appear first and are later replaced by high-affinity antibodies, but this replacement takes longer in less advanced vertebrates.

6.11.3 Evolution of Immunoglobulin Chains

Individual immunoglobulin chains and the domains within each chain appear to have a common evolutionary origin. The main source of information for tracing this origin has been the primary structure—the amino acid sequence—of these chains.

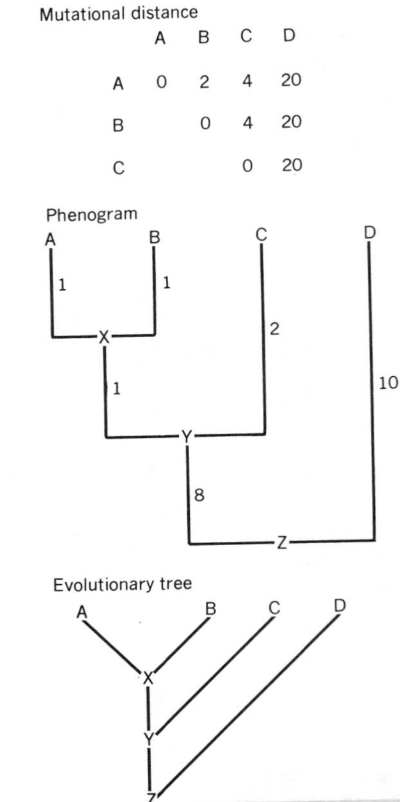

Figure 6.48. Construction of a phylogenetic tree from mutational differences among four proteins—A, B, C, and D. Explanation in the text. (Based on N. Arnheim *in* M. Sela (Ed.): *The Antigens*, Vol. 1, pp. 377–416, Academic, New York, 1973.)

The evolution of a protein can be envisioned as a gradual accumulation of mutations in the DNA, resulting in step-by-step replacement of amino acids at different positions in the protein. The rate of this replacement is thought to be constant by some, though not all, geneticists, so that a protein evolves in a clocklike fashion. In different proteins, the clock runs at different speeds, so that some proteins evolve more rapidly than others. Hence, by determining the frequency with which corresponding positions in two different proteins are occupied by the same amino acid, or by calculating the minimum number of mutations necessary to change from one protein to another, one can estimate to what degree the two proteins are evolutionarily related. And by relating the speed of the protein's own clock to the time scale of biological evolution, one can also estimate how long ago two related proteins have had a common ancestor. One can then plot all this information in the form of a genealogical tree, with individual proteins shown branching off from a common trunk.

Figure 6.48 depicts such a tree. The first step in its construction is to determine the amino acid sequence of the proteins. The second step is to determine from the amino acid sequence the mutational differences between the proteins (the minimum number of genetic events required to change a gene coding for one protein into a gene coding for another). In the third step, the tree is constructed from the mutation distances among all three proteins. In the example shown, proteins A and B are the closest to each other of the four, with a mutational distance of 2 between them. Assuming common origin, the evolution of proteins A and B from an ancestor protein, X, requires one mutational event for A and one for B. Proteins A and B are equidistant from C, suggesting that X and C had a common ancestor, Y. Evolution from Y to X required one mutational event and evolution from Y to C two events, resulting in a mutational distance of 4 between A + B and C. Proteins A, B, and C are equidistant from D, suggesting that Y and D had a common ancestor, Z. Evolution from Z to D required 10 mutational events and from Z to Y eight events, resulting in a total distance of 20 between A + B + C and D. From these considerations, summarized graphically in the phenogram of the middle panel, one can deduce the evolutionary tree depicted in the lower panel.

Sequence comparisons of the various Ig chains and their regions reveal that the V and C regions are the most distant, with hardly any sequence homologies remaining between them. But a common origin of the V and C regions is suggested by their similar layout in terms of length, position of disulfide bridges, and tertiary structure. Apparently, the regions separated from each other early in immunoglobulin evolution, and each continued to evolve on its own.

The homology among the different C domains suggests that they (and the V regions) evolved from a common primordial gene, which probably carried information for some 110 amino acids—the present length of a single V or C domain. Among the acids were two cysteines positioned in such a way that formation of a disulfide bridge between them arranged the polypeptide chain into a single loop.

The second largest difference in terms of amino acid sequence exists between the L and H chains and between the two L chains (κ and λ), so these chains too—or rather, their C regions—must have separated early in the evolution of the immunoglobulin molecule. Of the H chains, relatively large differences exist between μ and γ and somewhat smaller differences are found between μ and α, μ and δ, and μ and ϵ. However, the data concerning δ and ϵ are limited and the conclusions drawn from them tentative. Hence, the μ chain appears to be the oldest, followed by the γ, α, δ, and ϵ. The separation from a common ancestor of the subclass-specific H and L chains occurred relatively recently. The presumed evolution of the immunoglobulin C and V genes is summarized in Figure 6.49.

6.11.4 Possible Mechanism of Ig Gene Evolution

The following is a hypothetical scheme of how the evolution of Ig genes might have proceeded at the molecular level (Fig. 6.50). At the beginning there was a

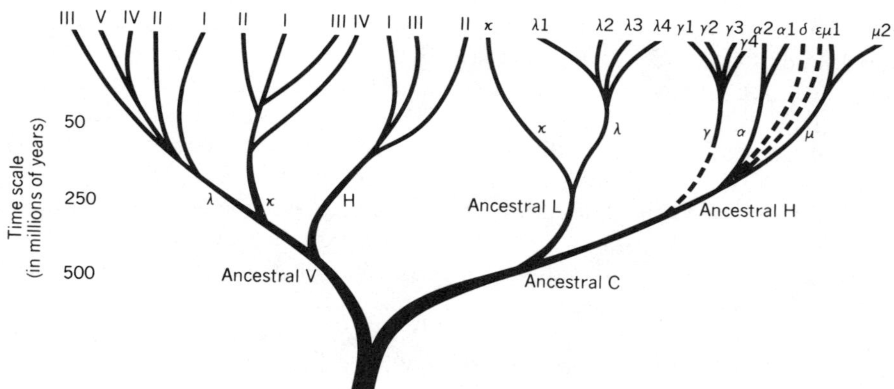

Figure 6.49. Genealogical tree of the human immunoglobulin gene families. Roman numerals indicate V-region subgroups.

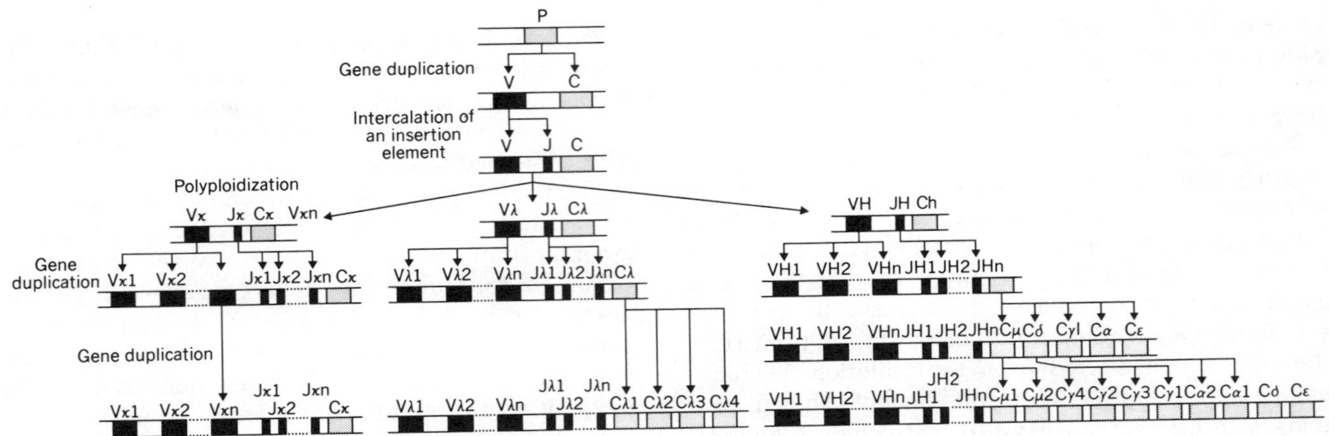

Figure 6.50. A hypothetical scheme of the human immunoglobulin gene evolution.

primordial gene, P, already described in the preceding section. The function of the P gene might have been related to some primitive form of defense reaction or might have been only distantly related to immunity. At an early stage, perhaps at the time when the most advanced invertebrates began to branch off into vertebrates, the P gene gave rise to two genes by a process known as gene duplication. The two genes remained closely linked but were separated by a segment of noncoding DNA—the primordial intron. They were transcribed as a unit into one messenger RNA and the two coding sequences were joined, at the RNA level, into one piece by splicing and elimination of the intron sequences. The duplication allowed the two genes to evolve separately and to assume different functions; one became the ancestor of all V genes and the other, the ancestor of all C genes. Both genes were under selective pressure—the V gene to diversify, and the C gene to assume additional functions such as interaction with complement, binding to cell-surface receptors, passing through epithelial membranes, and stabilizing the primitive immunoglobulin molecule. In response to these pressures, both genes duplicated further, mainly by the process of unequal crossingover. The duplicated C loci formed a unit that coded for the individual C domains; the duplicated V loci diversified by accumulating mutations, so that each locus coded for a V region of somewhat different specificity.

The whole complex of V + C loci was still transcribed as a unit and the transcript was tailored by splicing to the desired length. As the V genes duplicated further, the transcript grew too long for the cell to handle. Beyond this stage, no further duplication of the V genes was possible unless some radical new solution was invented to allow transcription of one V gene at a time and combination of this single V gene with the C-gene unit. The solution might have been found by chance when an episome, a genetic element that can exist freely in a cell or be incorporated into a chromosome, was accidentally inserted into one of the V genes.

Episomes are frequent in prokaryotes, the best-known example being the λ phage. In eukaryotes, too, certain viruses can, at a certain stage of their life cycle, be inserted into a chromosome and be treated by the cell as if they were the individual's own genes. Later they can again leave the chromosome and assume life as independent viruses (see Chapter 14). The insertion and excision is facilitated by noncoding sequences flanking the episome's main body. Often episomes have a noncoding sequence of 30 nucleotide pairs at one end, which is then repeated in an inverted fashion at the other end. These repeated inverted sequences are related to those found in the V-gene introns and are believed to function in both systems in the same way—by allowing recombination and excision of looped-out structures.

The intercalation of an episome into one of the V-region genes split the gene into the longer V gene proper and the shorter J gene. The V gene proper, flanked by the repeated sequences, was then able to duplicate independently of the J (and C) gene, since the whole complex did not need to be transcribed as a unit any longer. Since each V gene had its own promoter (region of DNA at which RNA polymerase binds and initiates transcription), and since a mechanism whereby the gene could be transposed next to the J-C gene complex evolved simultaneously, the transcription unit of one V gene (of many), one J gene (of several, since these genes, too, duplicated in at least some chromosomes), and one C-gene complex could be formed when the Ig genes were called upon to perform their function. With this arrangement, the number of duplicated V genes was limited only by the cell's physical possibilities. (The VH gene was probably split twice by episome insertions, first giving rise to the J gene and then producing the D gene.)

The next step in the evolution of the Ig-gene complex was the distribution of the original single complex to three different chromosomes. The simplest way this event could have taken place was by polyploidization of part of or the entire chromosomal set. Polyploidy, a condition of having multiples greater than two of a haploid set of chromosomes, is relatively frequent in plants and might have been frequent in the ancestral invertebrates; in present-day vertebrates, however, it is extremely rare. The duplicated chromosomes have the same advantage as duplicated genes—they can evolve independently. The triplication of the original V-C bigene established the three currently known Ig linkage groups, Lλ, Lκ, and H, which then evolved, mostly by gene duplication, into contemporary gene families. The size of the families varied, depending on the demands on Ig function in individual species, with the clusters expanding by gene duplication and contracting by gene deletion. This dynamic state of the multigenic system is probably maintained even in contemporary vertebrate species.

6.12 PATHOLOGY OF IMMUNOGLOBULINS

In a normal organism, immunoglobulin production is regulated by complex feedback mechanisms operating at both the level of Ig-producing cells and that of Ig molecules themselves. Disturbances of these controls may result in abnormal levels of normal immunoglobulins, normal levels of abnormal immunoglobulins, or abnormal levels of abnormal immunoglobulins. Examples of some such disturbances are given below, first for humans and then for the mouse.

6.12.1 Human Immunoglobulinopathies

Discovery

The first human immunoglobulinopathy (disease of immunoglobulin production) was described in London in the mid-nineteenth century. The story of this discovery has been told many times but, since a textbook would not be complete without it, we shall tell it here again.

In 1844, Mr. Thomas Alexander McBean, a 45-year-old London grocer, came to his physician, Dr. Thomas Watson (no relation to the famous companion of Sherlock Holmes), complaining of severe chest pains. When Dr. Watson analyzed his patient's urine, he observed a strange phenomenon about which he did not know what to think. So he dispatched the urine sample to Henry Bence Jones, pathologist at London's Saint George Hospital, with the following note:

> Dear Dr. Jones,
>
> The tube contains urine of very high specific gravity. When boiled, it becomes slightly opaque. On the addition of nitric acid, it effervesces, assumes a reddish hue, and becomes quite clear; but as it cools, assumes the consistence and appearance which you see. Heat reliquifies it. What is it?
>
> Dr. Watson.

Bence Jones, an acquaintance of Thomas Huxley, Charles Darwin, and Michael Faraday, identified the protein as "hydrated deutoxide of albumen" and concluded, also on the basis of the post-mortem on the patient, who had died, that the substance was the result of a hitherto-undescribed disease "essentially malignant in nature," affecting "osseous systems" (bones). The description of the disease published by Bence Jones in 1848 is acknowledged today as the first recorded case of a disease known as multiple myeloma; the "hydrated deutoxide of albumen" was identified more than a century later as free immunoglobulin light chains, but in honor of its discoverer, the substance is still referred to as Bence-Jones protein.

Classification

Mr. McBean's illness later proved to be one of a group of diseases affecting Ig levels, Ig structure, or both. There is no generally accepted classification of these diseases, and the individual diseases themselves are often referred to by different names so that the situation is quite confusing. Here we shall divide immunoglobulinopathies into *hyperglobulinemias*, leading to higher than normal immunoglobulin levels (Gr. *hyper*, above, over), and *hypoglobulinemias*, resulting in lower than normal immunoglobulin levels (Gr. *hypo*, under). We shall further divide the former subgroup into *generalized hyperglobulinemias*, causing elevated levels of several Ig species, and *monoclonal hyperglobulinemias*, causing elevated levels of one (rarely two) immunoglobulin species. The monoclonal immunoglobulin present in abnormally high levels is sometimes referred to as *paraprotein* and the condition causing the appearance of these proteins as *paraproteinemia* (Gr. *para*, alongside, near).

Description

Generalized Hyperglobulinemia. This condition may pertain to one Ig class, to several classes, or to total Ig. It may occur in a *primary* form, not obviously associated with any disease, or in a *secondary* form, accompanying known infections. Some of the primary forms may, in fact, not be diseases at all but genetically controlled conditions. For example, black Africans have higher immunoglobulin levels than Caucasians—a condition thought to be the result of high antigenic stimulation in the African countries until it was realized that the condition often continued when the wide range of stimuli was removed (e.g., in blacks living in Europe). The condition may, therefore, represent ethnic variation in immunoglobulin level rather than a disturbance in Ig production. Secondary generalized hyperglobulinemia, affecting one or more Ig classes, often occurs in patients with malaria, trypanosomiasis, or leishmaniasis (see Chapter 14).

Monoclonal Hyperglobulinemia. This condition may occur in a benign (mild) or malignant (severe) form. The *benign monoclonal gammopathy*, characterized by relatively large amounts of homogeneous IgM, IgG, or IgA proteins in the serum, occurs with a frequency of about 5 percent of all persons over 50 years of age. Some of these persons eventually develop Ig-producing neoplasms but many remain completely healthy. The high level of single Ig species is thought to be the result of an accidental extreme expansion of a single B-cell clone following specific antigenic challenge. The expansion, however, stops at a certain point without turning into uncontrolled growth (malignancy).

The severe forms of monoclonal hyperglobulinemia are referred to by various names—paraproteinemias, paraglobulinemias, paraproteinopathies, or plasma-cell dyscrasias. Depending on the Ig class they affect, the following diseases are distinguished: multiple myeloma (affecting IgG, IgA, IgD, or IgE), Waldenström's macroglobulinemia (affecting IgM), and H-chain disease (affecting heavy chains).

Multiple myeloma (myelomatosis) is a neoplastic disease of plasma cells manifested by invasive destruction of the skeleton and by the appearance of abnormal (myeloma) protein in the blood. The disease is believed to be induced by continual stimulation of the reticuloendothelial system, which accompanies chronic inflammation or chronic infection. The induction, however, seems to require a certain predisposition, and, at least in mice, seems to involve oncogenic viruses. The starting point of the disease is a neoplastic transformation of a single plasma cell or its precursor, leading to neoplastic cells capable of uncontrolled proliferation. This transformation very likely occurs in the bone marrow. The proliferating plasma cells disturb the dynamics of normal bone formation at multiple sites and cause multiple lesions (hence the name of the disease), which, as shown in X-rays, give the bone a moth-eaten appearance. Pain in the bones, particularly of the lower back, is usually the first sign of multiple myeloma.

The large quantities of salts, particularly calcium, released during bone destruction exceed the excretory capacity of the kidney, leading to the appearance of high calcium levels in the blood and impairment of renal functions.

In most myelomas, the proliferating plasma cells secrete immunoglobulins; nonsecreting neoplasms are rare (fewer than 1 percent of all myelomas). Most of the secreting myelomas (45 percent) secrete only complete Ig molecules; about 30 percent secrete complete Ig molecules and free light chains (*Bence-Jones proteins*); approximately 25 percent secrete only Bence-Jones proteins. Among the myelomas secreting complete Ig molecules, IgG secretors are about twice as frequent as IgA secretors; IgD- and IgE-secreting myelomas are rare (less than 1 percent of all the myelomas). Since neoplastic cells of a given myeloma represent a single plasma-cell (B-cell) clone, all the secreted immunoglobulins are of one kind. And since the proteins are produced in large quantities, they appear as a major band on electrophoresis of the patient's serum. When measured by densitometric tracing, the band appears as a sharp spike, the sharpness of the band indicating homogeneity of the constituting protein. Rare myelomas producing two or more immunoglobulin species are thought to arise by transformation in a single individual of two or more plasma cells belonging to two or more B-cell clones.

The quantity of protein produced is too large for the kidney to catabolize; as a consequence, proteins precipitate in renal tubuli and the precipitated cast blocks the tubuli. Some of the protein apparently also enters the cytoplasm of the kidney cells and thus interferes with normal tubular transport mechanisms. This kidney malfunction leads to dehydration and release of the Bence-Jones protein into the urine (proteinuria). High levels of myeloma protein also disturb feedback mechanisms controlling the rate of Ig synthesis and cause reduction of serum Ig levels.

The proliferation of neoplastic plasma cells disturbs

the differentiation of other hemopoietic cells in the bone marrow. Disturbances of erythropoiesis lead to less than normal erythrocyte counts (anemia), and lower erythrocyte counts result in imbalances of oxygen transport, which in turn lead to the patient's feelings of malaise and tiredness. Disturbances of thrombopoiesis result in lower platelet count, which in turn leads to defects in blood coagulation, and hence to bleeding, blood loss, and anemia. Disturbances of lymphopoiesis increase the patient's susceptibility to bacterial infections and further decrease normal serum Ig levels. At advanced stages of the disease, neoplastic cells spread from bone marrow to other organs and cause enlargement of spleen and liver. The tumors can be treated by X-irradiation and chemotherapy, but the treatment merely slows down, rarely stops, the progression of the disease.

Waldenström's macroglobulinemia, first recognized by a Swede, J. Waldenström, in 1944, originates by neoplastic transformation of an IgM-synthesizing cell. The exact identity of this cell is not known, but the fact that the neoplastic cells proliferate mostly in the spleen and lymph nodes and less in the bone marrow suggests that some basic difference exists between the targets of the transformation process in multiple myeloma and in Waldenström's macroglobulinemia (see below). The limited proliferation of the transformed IgM-secreting cells in the bone marrow does not cause bone lesions and pains. In the absence of bone destruction, the blood calcium levels remain normal and there is no kidney impairment. Instead, the proliferating cells cause spleen enlargement (splenomegaly), lymph node enlargement (lymphadenopathy), and abdominal pain. Secondarily, the cells also invade the liver and cause hepatomegaly. Disturbances of erythropoiesis in the spleen and bone marrow result in the reduction of red blood cell count and anemia—one of the most common symptoms of Waldenström's macroglobulinemia.

The mature transformed cells produce high quantities of pentameric IgM, which appears as a characteristic spike on serum electrophoresis. Only about 10 percent of patients with Waldenström's macroglobulinemia produce free L chains, along with complete IgM molecules, and have Bence-Jones proteins in their urine. About 80 percent of the patient's peripheral blood lymphocytes exhibit surface IgM identical to that in the serum spike. Since the IgM-positive cells are also IgD-positive, it seems that the target of the neoplastic transformation is an $IgM^{+}IgD^{+}$ B cell, which then matures into an IgM-secreting plasma cell.

The high concentration of IgM makes the plasma thicker, which slows blood circulation. The effects of the latter are particularly apparent in organs with rich nets of fine capillaries, such as the retina of the eye and the central nervous system. The rupture of capillaries in the eye results in internal bleeding, passages of fluids into tissues, and finally in sight impairment. Bleeding in the central nervous system may lead to transient loss of power of voluntary movements (paralysis), reflex abnormalities, deafness, and loss of consciousness. The viscous blood also means harder work for the heart and lungs and so leads to heart problems and breathing difficulties.

The superfluous IgM tends to form complexes with blood coagulation factors and thus contributes to clotting disturbances, bleeding, and anemia. Furthermore, IgM interferes with normal platelet function by causing spontaneous platelet agglutination; this effect then aggravates the patient's clotting problems. IgM also spontaneously agglutinates red blood cells, causing their premature destruction, which contributes to the anemia.

Waldenström's macroglobulinemia is a disease of advanced age, with the disease's first symptoms appearing in the fifth or sixth decade of life. The patient's clinical condition can often improve dramatically following removal of excess protein by plasmapheresis (Gr. *aphairesis*, a withdrawal)—a procedure whereby the blood is withdrawn from the body, and cells are separated from the plasma by centrifugation and returned, resuspended in salt solution, to the body. The proliferation of neoplastic cells can be slowed by chemotherapy and the patient's life expectancy prolonged by several years. However, the disease is incurable.

In the *H-chain diseases*, the defect probably occurs at the DNA or the post-transcription level, at the time when the Ig-coding sequences are put together. The defects result in the omission of some pieces of the H chain, so that those produced are shorter than normal. The defective H chains cannot associate with L chains and are therefore secreted in a free form in the serum (hence the disease's name). As in other paraproteinemias, the neoplastic transformation occurs in a single original cell, from which a malignant clone arises. H-chain fragments are occasionally also produced by non-neoplastic cells. The genesis of the H-chain disease thus requires two infrequent events: genetic lesion, leading to shortening of the gene product, and neoplastic transformation, leading to the generation of a malignant clone. The low probability of the occurrence of these two events in the same cell could explain the extreme rarity of the disease.

On electrophoresis, the band constituted by the abnormal protein is often relatively broad, probably because variable amounts of carbohydrates are added to the H chains and because the chains tend to polymerize into molecules of varying size. Sometimes the abnormal protein occurs in a form that is not easily identifiable, and in such instances, electrophoresis must be combined with immunodiffusion using anti-H chain-specific sera as test reagents. Depending on the isotype of the abnormal protein, three diseases—alpha, gamma, and mu—can be distinguished; their relative frequencies are 53, 33, and 12 percent, respectively.

In *alpha heavy-chain disease*, the defect occurs in B cells committed to the synthesis of α chains. Since these cells occur in high numbers in lymph nodes surrounding the posterior part of the digestive tract, the defect often leads to the development of malignant lymphoma in the small intestine. The developing neoplasms are sometimes called *Mediterranean lymphomas* in reference to the fact that they are frequent among persons living in the Mediterranean area. From lymph nodes, the neoplasms can spread to other lymphoid organs and the liver, causing their enlargement. In the intestine, the neoplasms cause severe malabsorption, leading to chronic diarrhea, weight loss, and overall weakness. The lymphoma is so aggressive that most patients die within four years of diagnosis.

All the abnormal α proteins studied have been of the $\alpha 1$ type; no $\alpha 2$ abnormal protein has so far been detected. The reason for this preference is unknown. The defective α chains have a molecular weight ranging from 36,000 to 56,000. All have normal hinge and Fc regions but carry a large deletion in the Fd region (V and CH1 domains; see Fig. 6.51). The extent of the deletion varies among the individual cases and among individual molecules, possibly because of varying degrees of postsynthetic degradation.

In the *gamma heavy-chain disease*, the defect occurs in the B cell committed to the synthesis of γ chains and residing in one of the many lymph nodes. The node is enlarged by the proliferating neoplastic cells and a typical lymphoma develops. The condition is often associated with chronic diseases such as tuberculosis or rheumatoid arthritis. $\gamma 1$-secreting lymphomas are more frequent than lymphomas secreting other γ subclasses. Four types of γ chain defect have been reported (Fig. 6.51).

Type 1 chains carry partial deletions in the Fd region but have normal hinge and Fc regions. The chains thus consist of a few N-terminal, V-region amino acids (the number varies from protein to protein) directly linked to the hinge region (at residue 216). This type is the most common of the four.

Type 2 chains carry a deletion of 15 amino acids in the hinge region (residue 216 through 232).

Type 3 chains have most of the Fd region and all of the hinge region deleted.

Type 4 chains are of variable length and apparently arise by enzymatic cleavage of types 1, 2, and 3.

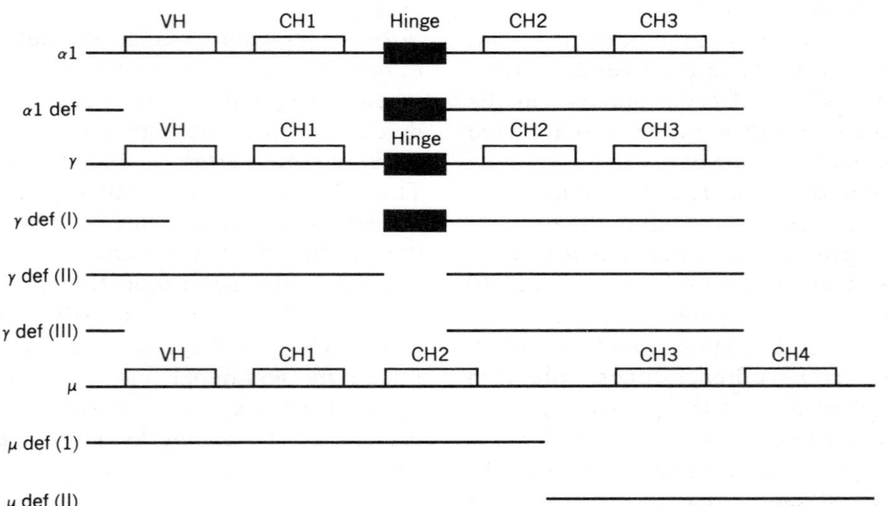

Figure 6.51. Human $\alpha 1$, γ, and μ chains and their fragments, produced in patients with various forms of heavy-chain disease. Deleted segments are indicated by the gaps in each line; in actuality, however, the protein-synthesizing apparatus "jumps over" these gaps and produces single fragments of each chain. Def, deficient chains; I, II, III, various types of deficient chain within a given class.

In *mu heavy-chain disease*, the defect occurs in a B cell committed to the synthesis of the μ chain. The neoplastic cells proliferate in the spleen and abdominal lymph nodes and cause a clinical picture resembling chronic lymphocytic leukemia. In contrast to the α and γ forms of the disease, in which the neoplastic cells secrete only free H chains, in μ-chain disease, the cells secrete both H and L chains. The abnormal μ protein has a molecular weight ranging from 180,000 to 300,000 daltons and occurs in the form of pentamers, in which the individual chains are often (but not always) connected by J chains. The deletion may occur in different regions of the molecule (Fig. 6.51): VH, CH1, and CH2 in some molecules, CH3 and CH4 in others.

Whether defects similar to those causing heavy-chain diseases also occur in L chains is not clear. In about one-third of patients with typical Bence-Jones proteinuria, fragments equal to about half an L chain can be demonstrated, but these may be the products of postsynthetic degradation rather than the results of genetic defects at the DNA or RNA levels.

Hypoglobulinemias

These conditions are characterized by reduction in the total Ig level, or reduction (absence) of certain Ig classes. These reductions occur as one of the symptoms accompanying T- or B-cell defects described in the preceding chapters: Bruton's agammaglobulinemia, selective IgA deficiency, ataxia telangiectasia, Wiscott-Aldrich syndrome, severe combined immunodeficiency, and common variable immunodeficiency.

6.12.2 Mouse Plasmacytomas

Discovery

Although mouse pathologists had come across plasma-cell neoplasms (myelomas, plasmacytomas) developing spontaneously in certain mouse strains from time to time, the use of these tumors as an important immunological tool became possible only after a way was found of inducing them with high frequency. Means of artificially inducing plasmacytomas were found by chance.

In 1959, Ruth M. Merwin and Glenn H. Algire studied the long-term survival of allogeneic tissues enclosed in a diffusion chamber (see Fig. 5.20) and implanted intraperitoneally into recipient mice. They observed that in one of the strains used (BALB/c), the abdomen of the recipient carrying the diffusion chamber for some six months became filled with large quantities of fluid (ascites), and the viscera were overgrown by neoplastic cells that they identified as plasmacytomas. Later studies established that the diffusion chamber alone, or just a piece of plexiglas, also induced plasmacytomas when implanted into the peritoneum of BALB/c mice. Apparently, the irritation produced by the foreign implant caused inflammation, and the chronic inflammatory reaction provided conditions for neoplastic transformation of plasma cells or their precursors.

One year later, Michael Potter and C. L. Robertson arrived at a similar conclusion from another end. Originally these two investigators did not want to produce plasmacytomas either; all they were interested in was getting a good antibody response to some mouse allotypic determinants they were studying. To boost the response, they used a trick long known to immunologists: they incorporated the antigen into the so-called adjuvant (see Chapter 10)—in their case, heat-killed bacteria suspended in mineral oil. They too noticed that some 40 to 60 percent of the immunized BALB/c mice developed plasmacytomas, and they later identified the mineral oil as the neoplasm-inducing agent. Injection of mineral oil has since become a standard way of inducing plasma-cell tumors in mice and other animals. Much of the pioneering work on mouse plasmacytomas has originated in the laboratory of Michael Potter.

Factors Playing a Role in Plasmacytoma Induction

Plasmacytomas can be induced in only two inbred mouse strains, BALB/c and NZB (and the hybrids of these); attempts to induce plasma-cell neoplasms in other inbred strains have failed. Thus, an important factor in plasmactyoma induction is the individual's genetic makeup: the BALB/c and NZB mice apparently carry genes that make them susceptible to such induction, while other strains lack them.

The second factor is the irritative inflammatory reaction initiated by the presence of mineral oil in the peritoneum. A detailed histological investigation revealed that the oil at first causes the development of an oil granuloma—a nodular or granular tissue consisting mostly of oil-laden histiocytes that adhere to one another and attach to the peritoneal surface; later, this tissue becomes vascularized from mesenterial vessels. Scattered among the histiocytes are some lymphocytes, and it is apparently from these cells that the plasma-cell neoplasms develop. However, oil alone does not seem to suffice for neoplasm induction, for oil-treated germ-free mice have only a low incidence of plasmacytomas. Apparently, another factor necessary for providing the right conditions for the neoplastic transformation is antigenic stimulation.

All plasmacytomas so far examined by electron microscopy have been found to contain intracisternal viruslike particles. Although no direct evidence is available to involve viruses in plasmacytoma induction, the presence of ubiquitous virus particles in these neoplasms makes such an involvement a likely possibility.

Nomenclature and Characteristics

The first plasmacytomas were designated by the letter X and a serial number. Later, other letters were used as prefixes before the serial designation: MOPC (*m*ineral *o*il-induced *p*lasma*c*ytoma), TEPC (*te*tramethylpentadecane-induced *p*lasma*c*ytoma), Adj.PC (*adj*uvant-induced *p*lasma*c*ytoma), and others.

Hundreds of BALB/c or NZB plasmacytomas have been induced by Michael Potter and Melvin Cohn. Most of the neoplasms are propagated as lines by serial transplantation: a piece of the neoplastic tissue is taken up into a large needle (trocar) and inoculated under the skin of a syngeneic recipient; as soon as the neoplasm grows to a certain size, a piece is transplated to a new recipient, and this procedure is repeated for as long as an investigator is interested in the neoplasm. Some neoplasms have been maintained in this way for more than 20 years. However, the plasmacytomas can also be frozen and stored at low (−75°C) temperatures. Some can also be adapted to growth in tissue culture and serially propagated in vitro.

Most plasmacytomas secrete immunoglobulins; the frequency of nonsecretors is about 12 percent. Of the secretors, the majority (62 percent) are IgA producers (this fact, perhaps, has something to do with the site—in the vicinity of the gut—at which these neoplasms arise); less frequent are IgG producers (22 percent); and IgM producers are rare (less than 1 percent), as are neoplasms that produce L chains only (3 to 4 percent). Rare also are biclonal plasmacytomas producing immunoglobulins of two classes or subclasses. Upon transplantation in vivo or in vitro, some secretors may become nonsecretors spontaneously.

Myeloma Proteins

The plasmacytoma products—the *myeloma proteins*—share many properties with human paraproteins. For some time after the discovery of myeloma proteins, some immunologists had doubts about whether they were dealing with normal immunoglobulin molecules. And even when biochemical studies revealed myeloma proteins to be structurally indistinguishable from immunoglobulins, doubts persisted as to whether myeloma proteins possessed functional properties characteristic of antibodies—in particular, antigen-binding capability. Much effort was spent on finding antigens that would bind specifically to individual myeloma proteins. Thousands of substances were screened (many by Melvin Cohn and his co-workers) until, at last, some molecules were found that interacted specifically with one or a few of the myeloma proteins (see section on idiotypes). The finding of antigens complementary to the combining regions of certain myeloma proteins established, once and for all, that these proteins belonged to the same category as normal monoclonal antibodies.

6.13 THE B-CELL RECEPTOR

6.13.1 The Clonal Selection Theory

To an immunologist, an organism looks like the drawing in Figure 6.52—a mosaic of lymphocyte clones with each clone committed, in terms of V-region specificity, to the synthesis of one antibody species. An indication of this commitment is the cell-surface (B-cell) receptors capable of binding complementary antigens so that one lymphocyte clone specifically binds antigen 1, another antigen 2, still another antigen 3, and so on. Upon interaction with an antigen, say antigen 1, the interacting cell divides rapidly and thus expands the clone carrying the anti-1 receptors. The progeny of the stimulated B lymphocyte eventually differentiate into plasma cells, secreting antibodies to antigen 1. This concept, advanced by F. Macfarlane Burnet and referred to as the *clonal selection theory*, predicts the presence, in the membrane of a B lymphocyte, of immunoglobulin molecules with the same antigen-binding specificity as the antibody molecules secreted by the cell's progeny after antigen stimulation. This prediction has been borne out fully by many experiments on antigen binding by B lymphocytes.

6.13.2 Antigen Binding by B Lymphocytes

Interaction of an antigen with a B cell can be demonstrated by several methods, of which techniques based

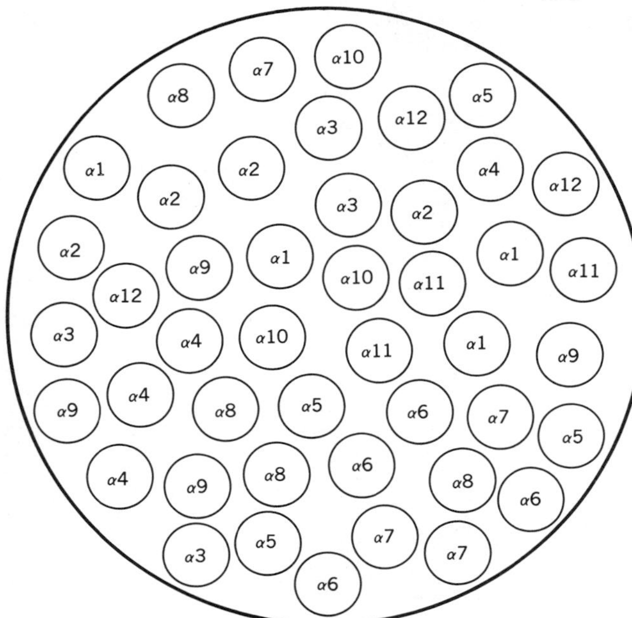

Figure 6.52. An immunologist's view of an organism: a mosaic of lymphocyte clones (small circles) with specificity for various antigenic determinants. Numerals indicate determinants; α indicates anti-.

on rosette formation and on binding of labeled antigen are frequently used. A mouse immunized with sheep red blood cells makes antibodies to antigens present in the erythrocyte membrane. If the clonal selection theory is correct, the pool of B lymphocytes should contain a few cells with receptors for these antigens. Upon mixing of B lymphocytes with sheep red blood cells, these few cells should find the erythrocytes, forming rosettes visible under the light microscope (see Fig. 5.26). The main difference between these *B-cell rosettes* and the T-cell rosettes discussed in Chapter 5 is that the receptor in the former is distributed clonally, while in the latter it is not. In other words, whereas most of the cells in a T-cell suspension form rosettes, only a few cells do in a B-cell suspension—presumably the few clones with receptors for the red blood-cell antigen. B-cell rosetting is not restricted to sheep red blood cells; it can be accomplished with almost any kind of red blood cells or with any particulate antigen attached artificially to red blood cells.

Antigen-binding cells (ABC) with specificity toward soluble antigens can be identified by a technique called autoradiography. In this technique, the antigen is labeled with a radioactive isotope (e.g., ^{125}I), the cells are mixed with the labeled antigen, the unbound antigen is removed by washing, the cells are fixed on a microscope slide, and the preparation is placed in contact with photographic emulsion. The decaying radioisotope emits electrons, which turn silver grains of the developed photographic emulsion into black spots. These indicate the position of ABCs in the fixed preparation.

Using these two techniques, immunologists have estimated that normal lymphoid tissues contain 0.001 to 0.01 percent of cells specifically reacting with a given antigen—which comes to about 25,000 cells per mouse spleen. Immunization raises the frequency of ABCs to from 1 to 3 percent.

6.13.3 Detection of Surface Immunoglobulins on B Lymphocytes

The first person who, without knowing it, detected immunoglobulins on cell surfaces was Göran Möller. In a study published in 1961, Möller described the tissue distribution of major histocompatibility complex (MHC) antigens in mouse lymphoid tissues. To detect these antigens, he first incubated cells with mouse anti-MHC sera and then with fluorescent goat antibodies to mouse immunoglobulin (see Appendix 10.1). As a specificity control of the antigen-antibody reaction, he incubated lymphoid cells with anti-Ig serum alone, without prior treatment by anti-MHC sera. He noticed that a fair number of cells in the control preparation stained with the fluoresceinated reagent, but he attributed this "nonspecific" staining to serum proteins attached passively to the lymphocytes. Ten years later, Benvenuto Pernis, Martin C. Raff, and others realized that the staining was not at all nonspecific, but resulted from the binding of the anti-Ig reagents to immunoglobulins in the cell membrane of lymphocytes, identifed as B cells.

Functional evidence for the existence of Ig-bearing cells was provided by Stewart Sell and P. G. H. Gell four years after Möller's observation. These two immunologists observed that when they added antiallotype sera to a culture of lymphocytes, a fraction of the lymphocytes underwent blast transformation. They concluded, therefore, that the anti-Ig sera reacted with immunoglobulin molecules on cell surfaces of some of the lymphocytes, and that the interaction activated these cells, setting them on a transformation course. Later studies revealed that $F(ab)_2$ fragments of the antibodies do activate lymphocytes, but Fab fragments do not, indicating that binding of the antibodies to more than one point on the membrane is required for the activation to occur.

6.13.4 Relationships among Receptors, Surface Immunoglobulins, and Antibodies

Evidence that the Antigen-Binding Receptor Is Immunoglobulin

The experiments just described established that lymphocytes carry antigen-binding receptors and that immunoglobulin molecules are present in the lymphocyte membrane. Although it seemed logical to put these two observations together and to conclude that immunoglobulins were the antigen-binding receptors, more convincing arguments were necessary to prove this contention. One such proof was the finding that preincubation of lymphocytes with anti-Ig sera blocked antigen binding by these cells. We shall mention other evidence that shows that the antigen receptor is identical to surface immunoglobulin (sIg) later.

Evidence that ABCs Are Precursors of Antibody-Secreting Cells

In 1969, Gordon L. Ada and Pauline Byrt linked antibody-secreting cells to ABCs by the following experiment (Fig. 6.53). They labeled antigen X with highly radioactive isotope ^{125}I, incubated normal splenocytes with the labeled antigen, and then injected the cells into syngeneic, lethally irradiated mice and immunized the mice with the same antigen as had been used for labeling. While control mice injected with cells exposed to unlabeled antigen produced antibodies to the antigen, the experimental mice did not. Ada and Byrt concluded from this result that the radioactivity of the antigen bound by the corresponding B-cell receptors specifically killed the antigen-reactive cells in the inoculum. Because of this *antigen suicide*, there were no cells left that could recognize antigen X and so no antibodies to antigen X could be formed, although the mice responded normally to antigen Y. Therefore, ABCs must be the precursors of antibody-secreting cells and must carry receptors with the same specificity for an antigen as the secreted antibody.

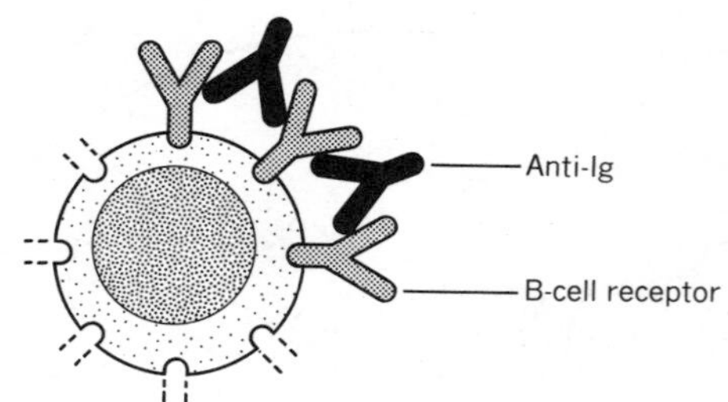

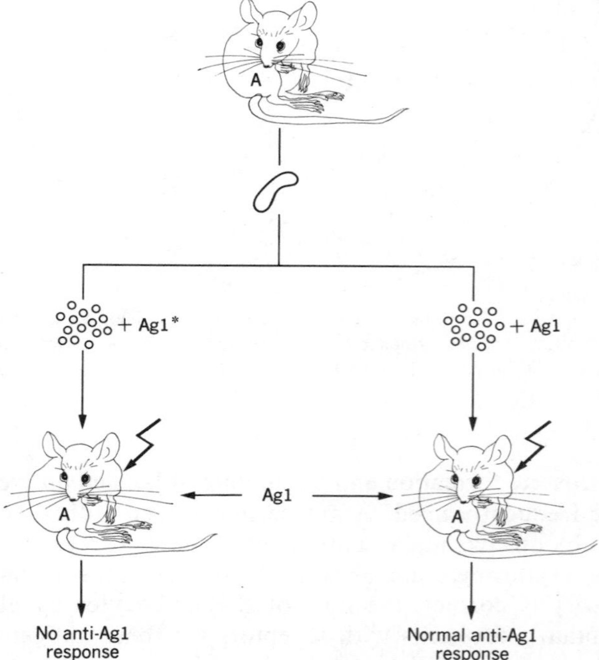

Figure 6.53. Antigen suicide experiment of Gordon L. Ada and Pauline Byrt, demonstrating binding of an antigen by a B-cell receptor. Highly radioactive antigen (Ag) indicated by asterisk.

6.13.5 Characteristics of B-Cell Receptors

How Many Different Receptors Does a Single B Cell Express?

At the moment that a cell commits itself to immunoglobulin synthesis, it also selects, from the large V-gene pool, one V_H and one V_L gene; these two genes then determine the antigen-binding specificity of the cell's immunoglobulins. This selection is final and permanent. From this moment on, all cells derived from the original progenitor express this same V region in both their surface receptors and in the antibody they might secrete. Hence, in terms of antigen-binding specificity, a given B cell or a B-cell clone expresses only one kind of receptor throughout its entire life history. However, in terms of a C-region isotype, a given cell may not only change its receptor during the differentiation process but may also express more than one type of receptor. As we already know, in the original pre-B cell, the V region is attached to a $C\mu$ polypeptide so that the first cell-surface receptor expressed by a differentiating cell is of the IgM type. Following this early stage, the B cell may attach the same V region to the $C\delta$, $C\gamma$, $C\alpha$,

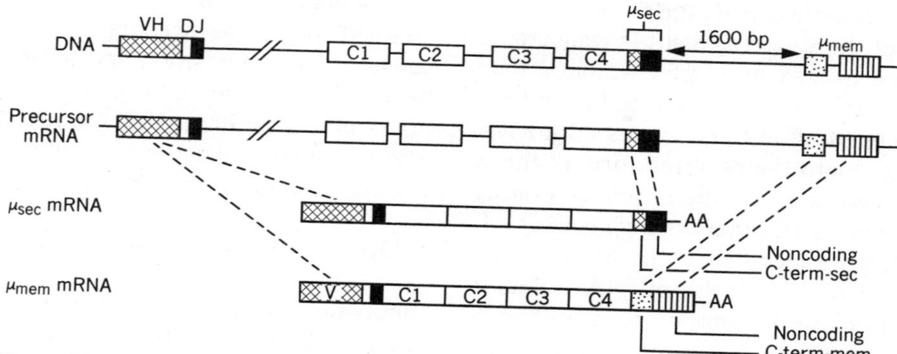

Figure 6.54. Synthesis of the membrane version of the mouse μ chain. μ_{sec}, genes coding for the secreted form of μ; μ_{mem}, genes coding for the membrane form of μ. (Modified from J. M. Adams: *Immunol. Today* **1**:10–17, 1980.)

or possibly Cϵ region and express two or three kinds of receptor—IgM and IgG, IgM and IgA, or possibly IgM and IgE, with or without simultaneous expression of IgD (see Fig. 5.25). As the cell then differentiates further, either toward a memory cell or toward a plasma cell, all but one kind of receptor are diluted out so that the differentiated B cell largely expresses one receptor of the same kind (in terms of V-region specificity and C-region isotope) as the secreted antibody.

Ig-Isotype Distribution among Ig-Positive Lymphocytes

Figure 6.54 compares the frequency of lymphocytes expressing different Ig isotypes with the frequency of different Ig classes and subclasses in the serum. The differences are striking. The two dominant classes expressed on lymphocytes are IgM and IgD (most lymphocytes react with both anti-μ and anti-δ sera and hence carry both receptors); the dominant class in the serum is IgG, followed by IgA and IgM, while serum IgD is barely detectable. The prevailing IgG subclass on human lymphocytes is IgG2; in the serum it is IgG1. These differences apparently reflect the succession of stages in B-lymphocyte differentiation and the functional demands imposed on surface and secreted immunoglobulins.

Chemical Properties of Membrane-Bound Immunoglobulins

Immunochemists have been aware for some time that the membrane-bound immunoglobulins are very similar, but not completely identical to secreted antibodies. The difference between the two forms of immunoglobulin has recently been elucidated by recombinant DNA techniques. Cloning of the μ chain-encoding genes has revealed the existence of two DNA regions responsible for the difference between membrane-bound and secreted μ chains. The region used for the synthesis of secreted chains (μ_{sec}) is contiguous with the gene coding for the Cμ4 domain and consists of a sequence coding for the C-terminal tail of the chain and of a short noncoding sequence (Fig. 6.54). The region used for the synthesis of the membrane version of the μ chain (μ_{mem}) is separated from the Cμ4 gene by an intron some 1600 nucleotide pairs long; it, too, consists of a coding and noncoding sequence.

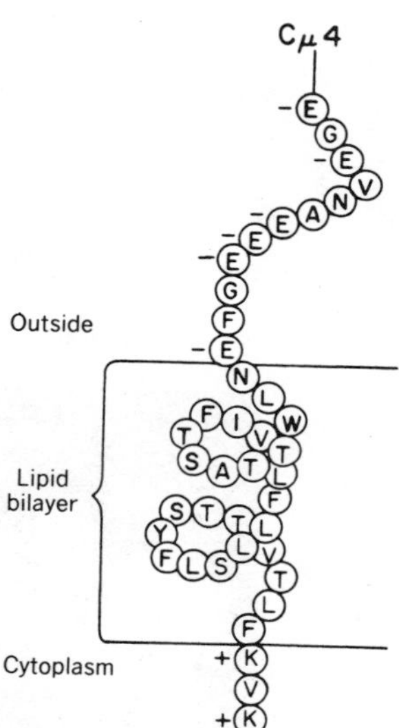

Figure 6.55. Postulated anchoring of the μ chain in the plasma membrane. The M segment encoded by the μ_{mem} sequence is envisioned as an α helix spanning the membrane. The transmembrane segment is flanked by positively and negatively charged residues. Letters indicate amino acids. (From J. Rogers, P. Early, C. Carter, K. Calame, M. Bond, L. Hood, and R. Wall: *Cell* **20**:303–312, 1980.)

The entire μ gene complex, from the 5′ end of the V gene to the 3′ end of the μ_{mem} segment, is transcribed as a unit into a long mRNA molecule, which is then spliced in two ways. In one, the sequence beyond the 3′ end of μ_{sec} is snipped off and the truncated mRNA molecule is translated into the secreted form of the μ chain. In the other, the μ_{sec} and the intron separating μ_{mem} from μ_{sec} (as well as all other introns) is excised, so that now the mRNA molecule has the μ_{mem} instead of the μ_{sec} segment at its 3′ end; this mRNA molecule is then translated into the membrane form of the μ chain. The membrane version of the μ chain is 21 amino acids longer than the secreted form. Most of the amino acids comprising the extra segment are uncharged and some are hydrophobic (Fig. 6.55). Because of its composition and location, the segment is believed to anchor the μ chain in the membrane. An arrangement similar to that found in the μ complex has also been detected in the δ complex and may exist in all H chain-encoding complexes.

6.13.6 Movement of Molecules in the Cell Membrane

Incubation of Ig-bearing B lymphocytes with anti-Ig serum causes redistribution of Ig receptors in the cell membrane. The redistribution can be followed, using

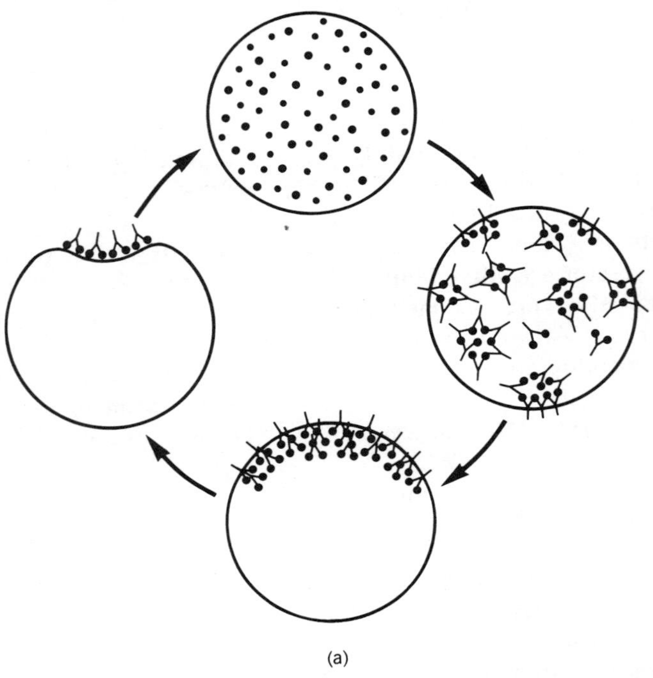

(a)

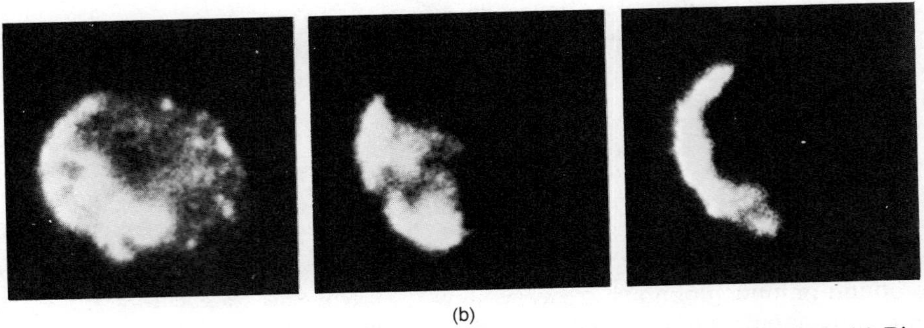

(b)

Figure 6.56. Patching and capping Ig molecules on the surfaces of B lymphocytes. (*a*) Diagrammatic representation of different stages of capping. (*b*) Photographs of capping cells with surface molecules visualized by fluoresceinated antibodies. (*b* courtesy Dr. Catherine Neauport-Sautes.)

fluorescein-labeled antibodies directed against the Ig receptors. It occurs in three successive stages, referred to as patch formation, cap formation, and pinocytosis (Fig. 6.56).

Patch formation (*patching*) is the stage when the originally diffusely distributed Ig molecules (seen in the fluorescent microscope as a continuous ring around the cell because one looks at a sphere projected into a circle; cf. Fig. 6.56) group into small aggregates or patches. Patching presumably occurs because each antibody molecule has two binding sites and so can attach to one sIg molecule with one site and to another molecule with the second (i.e., the antibody crosslinks two Ig molecules). Patching is a passive process that can occur even in the cold (i.e., at 0 to 4°C) and does not require energy (it cannot be blocked by metabolic inhibitors).

Cap formation (*capping*) is the stage in which all the Ig molecules congregate at one pole of the cell in a caplike structure. Since caps usually form at the uropod (over the Golgi apparatus), immunologists believe that the process is somehow related to the cell movement. This assumption is supported by the finding that capping does not occur in the cold (it proceeds best at 37°C), that it requires energy (it is blocked by metabolic inhibitors such as sodium azide), and that the region of the lymphocyte beneath the cap contains an accumulation of actin, myosin, and tubulin—all substances involved in cell movement. One possible way in which capping occurs is that the sIg in the patches attaches to the cytoskeleton beneath the cell membrane and is then in some way pulled by the actinomyosin fibers toward the Golgi pole of the cell.

Pinocytosis is the final stage, in which the cap disappears from the cell surface by being engulfed and interiorized. If the cells stripped of the cap are washed and incubated at 37°C, the surface Ig reappears within from six to 20 hours; the reappearing molecules are newly synthesized Ig reinserted into the membrane.

Capping is not restricted to Ig and lymphocytes: most other membrane proteins can be redistributed with the use of appropriate antibodies, and other cells—fibroblasts, for example—can also sustain capping. Capping of some proteins, however, requires a double layer of antibodies—the first consisting of antibodies to protein, and the second of antibodies to these antibodies. Cell-surface Ig, on the other hand, can also be capped by an exposure to a multivalent antigen. Redistribution of some membrane proteins may reach only the capping stage, without the subsequent pinocytosis of the cap. (The cap may, in some instances, fall off the membrane.)

The physiological role of Ig redistribution is not known. The phenomenon, however, is useful as a method for determining topological relationships of cell-membrane proteins. The principle of this determination is as follows (Fig. 6.57). Consider two different antibodies against cell-membrane proteins. Do these antibodies react with two antigenic determinants of the same protein, or with determinants of two different proteins? To answer this question, one incubates the cell with the first antibody and allows it to cap the corresponding antigen. One then reacts the same cell with the second antibody under conditions preventing further capping (for example, in the presence of sodium azide). If the two antibodies detect antigenic determinants on the same molecule, the second antibody reacts only with antigens in the cap. If, on the other hand, the two antibodies detect determinants on two different molecules, then after capping one molecule, the second molecule remains diffusely distributed throughout the membrane. To distinguish the two antibodies, one can label them with two different fluorescent stains.

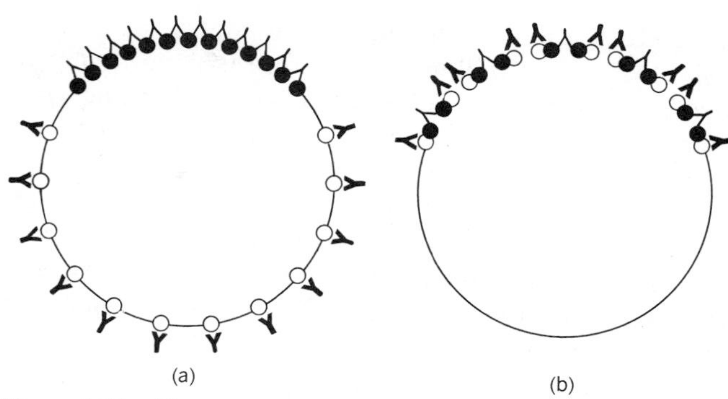

Figure 6.57. The use of capping to determine whether antigenic determinants detected by two different antibodies (X and Y) are carried by the same or different molecules. (*a*) After capping with the first antibody (X), molecules detected by the second antibody (Y) remain evenly distributed in the membrane outside the cap. Conclusion: the two determinants are carried by separate molecules. (*b*) After capping with the first antibody, molecules detected by the second antibody are found in the cap. Conclusion: the two determinants are carried by the same molecule.

6.13.7 Function of sIg Molecules

According to the clonal selection theory, the function of B-cell receptors is to bind antigens as a first step, leading to specific activation of B lymphocytes and eventually to antibody secretion. The presence of the different receptor isotypes merely reflects the different stages of B-lymphocyte differentiation that lead to the production of different antibody classes. This explanation may apply to all the immunoglobulin classes except sIgD, for there is no known function of serum IgD. Many immunologists therefore believe that sIgD plays a regulatory, rather than antigen-binding role. According to one hypothesis, antigen binding to sIg receptors leads to the release of sIgD from the surface. In the serum, the idiotype borne by the released IgD molecules is recognized by regulatory cells, which then act on lymphocytes that bear Ig molecules with the same V-region specificity. This action is thought to regulate lymphocyte proliferation.

6.14 APPENDIX 6.1: INTRODUCTION TO PROTEIN ANALYSIS

6.14.1 Protein Structure

Acid-Base Concepts

Molecules of water dissociate into hydrogen cations (H^+) and hydroxyl anions (OH^-) according to the equation

$$H_2O \rightleftarrows H^+ + OH^-$$

At a given temperature, the concentration of the three products of the equation is constant, so that

$$\frac{[H^+][OH^-]}{[H_2O]} = k_1$$

(The brackets indicate concentration.) Since, however, the concentration of nondissociated water (the denominator of this equation) is extremely large in comparison to the concentration of the H^+ and OH^- ions (the equation's numerator), it may be considered constant. Kleiner and Orten, in their biochemistry textbook, compare the situation to a leaking ship: the amount of water pouring into the ship's hull is of great consequence for the ship, but is totally inconsequential to the ocean. The latter, for all practical purposes, remains constant.[9] Therefore:

$$\frac{[H^+][OH^-]}{k_2} = k_1$$

$$[H^+][OH^-] = k_1 k_2 = k_w$$

At 25°C, the concentration of H^+ and OH^- ions is 0.000,000,000,000,01, or 1.0×10^{-14}. Since the concentration of H^+ in pure water must equal that of OH^-,

$$[H^+] = 1.0 \times 10^{-7}$$

In other words, pure water contains 1.0×10^{-7} grams of H^+ per liter. To avoid the use of negative numbers, Sven P. L. Sørensen suggested changing the sign of the negative exponent to positive and referring to it as "pH." Thus,

$$pH = \log_{10} \frac{1}{[H^+]} = -\log_{10} [H^+]$$

The pH of water (a neutral solution) is 7.0.

When one adds H^+ ions to water, the ratio of H^+ and OH^- will change, while the $[H^+][OH^-]$ product will remain the same: as the concentration of H^+ increases, the concentration of OH^- will decrease and the reverse situation will occur when one adds OH^- ions to water. The reciprocal relationship between H^+ and OH^- concentrations can be seen from the pH scale in Table 6.14.

A compound that releases hydrogen ions when dissolved in water is referred to as an *acid*; a compound that releases OH^- ions is termed a *base*. A solution that contains more than 1.0×10^{-7} grams per liter of hydrogen ions (has a pH of less than 7.0) is, therefore, termed *acidic*; one that has less than 1.0×10^{-7} grams per liter of hydrogen ions (has a pH of more than 7.0) is termed *basic* (*alkaline*); and one that has a pH equal to 7.0 is referred to as *neutral*.

Table 6.14 The pH Scale

$[H^+]^a$	pH	$[OH^-]^a$
1.0	0	10^{-14}
0.1	1	10^{-13}
0.01	2	10^{-12}
0.001	3	10^{-11}
0.0001	4	10^{-10}
0.00001	5	10^{-9}
10^{-6}	6	10^{-8}
10^{-7}	7	10^{-7}
10^{-8}	8	10^{-6}
10^{-9}	9	10^{-5}
10^{-10}	10	10^{-4}
10^{-11}	11	0.001
10^{-12}	12	0.01
10^{-13}	13	0.1
10^{-14}	14	1.0

[a] Concentration in grams per liter.

[9] Kleiner, I. S. and Orten, J. M.: *Biochemistry*, 6th ed. Mosby, St. Louis, 1962.

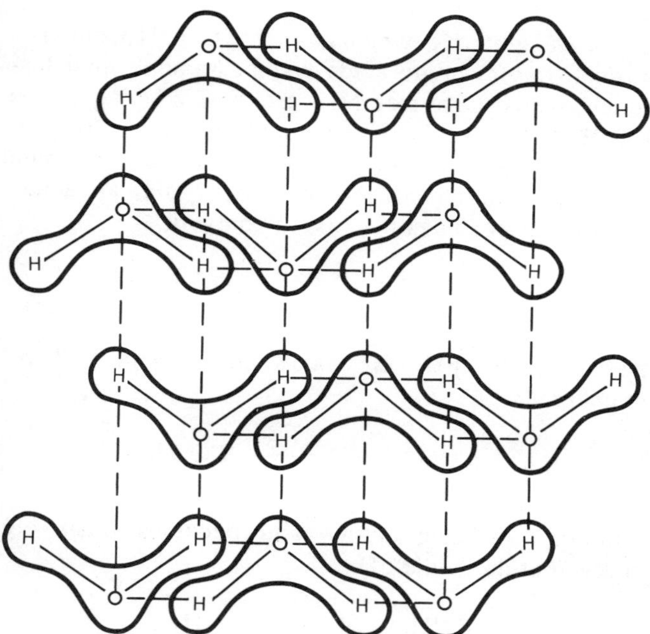

Figure 6.58. Polarization of water molecules and their cohesiveness through electrostatic interactions.

In nondissociated water molecules, the oxygen draws electrons away from the hydrogen nuclei so that the region about the oxygen atom becomes negatively charged and the regions about the hydrogen nuclei become electronegative (Fig. 6.58). The water molecule is thus a *polar structure*. In liquid water, the positively charged region of each molecule tends to orient itself toward the negatively charged regions of a neighboring molecule so that a partially ordered structure ensues (Fig. 6.58). Electrostatic interactions between neighboring molecules—the affinity of water molecules for one another—cause water to be highly *cohesive*.

Properties of Amino Acids

Proteins are composed of amino acids that have a general formula:

$$H_2N-\overset{\displaystyle H}{\underset{\displaystyle R}{\overset{|}{\underset{|}{C}}}}-COOH$$

where R is a side chain (radical), differentiating the individual acids. Two amino acids conjoin into a dipeptide by the union of carboxyl (COOH) and amino (NH_2) groups, with the elimination of one water molecule:

$$H_2N-\overset{\displaystyle H}{\underset{\displaystyle R}{\overset{|}{\underset{|}{C}}}}-\overset{\displaystyle O}{\overset{\|}{C}}-\boxed{OH + H}\!\!\begin{matrix}\searrow\\ \nearrow\end{matrix}\!\!\!\!\!\begin{matrix}\\ H\end{matrix}N-\overset{\displaystyle H}{\underset{\displaystyle R'}{\overset{|}{\underset{|}{C}}}}-COOH \longrightarrow$$

$$\longrightarrow H_2N-\overset{\displaystyle H}{\underset{\displaystyle R}{\overset{|}{\underset{|}{C}}}}-\overset{\displaystyle O}{\overset{\|}{C}}-\overset{\displaystyle H}{\overset{|}{N}}-\overset{\displaystyle H}{\underset{\displaystyle R'}{\overset{|}{\underset{|}{C}}}}-COOH + H_2O$$

A dipeptide can attach to a third amino acid and form a tripeptide, and by combination with additional amino acids, the growing chain can then become a tetrapeptide, a pentapeptide, a hexapeptide, and eventually a *polypeptide*, the constituent of a *protein*. The linkage between two amino acids

$$-\overset{\displaystyle O}{\overset{\|}{C}}-\overset{\displaystyle H}{\overset{|}{N}}-$$

is referred to as the *peptide bond* (see below). The polypeptide chain has a free NH_2 group at one end and a free COOH group at the other. The two ends are therefore referred to as amino or N terminal, and carboxyl or C terminal, respectively. The N terminal, the point of initiation of protein synthesis, is taken as the beginning of a polypeptide chain. The molecular weight of the amino acid residues ranges from 57 to 186 daltons, with the average about 110. Hence, a protein with a molecular weight of 44,000 contains approximately 400 residues.

At neutral pH, amino acids have negatively charged carboxyl groups and positively charged amino groups: they are dipolar ions or *zwitterions* (Gr. *Zwitter*, hermaphrodite, mongrel). In acid solution (e.g., pH 1), the carboxyl group is uncharged and the amino group is positively charged; in alkaline solution (e.g., pH 11), the amino group is uncharged and the carboxyl group is negatively charged:

$$\underset{\text{pH 1}}{H-\overset{\displaystyle NH_3^+}{\underset{\displaystyle R}{\overset{|}{\underset{|}{C}}}}-COOH} \underset{+H^+}{\rightleftharpoons} \underset{\text{pH 7}}{H-\overset{\displaystyle NH_3^+}{\underset{\displaystyle R}{\overset{|}{\underset{|}{C}}}}-COO^-} \underset{+H^+}{\rightleftharpoons} \underset{\text{pH 11}}{H-\overset{\displaystyle NH_2}{\underset{\displaystyle R}{\overset{|}{\underset{|}{C}}}}-COO^-}$$

The 20 amino acids commonly found in proteins are listed in Table 6.15. They are divided into four groups,

Table 6.15 Amino Acids and Their Symbols

Amino Acid	Three-Letter Symbol	One-Letter Symbol	Mnemonic Help for One-Letter Symbols
Hydrophobic (Nonpolar)			
Alanine	Ala	A	*A*lanine
Valine	Val	V	*V*aline
Leucine	Leu	L	*L*eucine
Isoleucine	Ile	I	*I*soleucine
Proline	Pro	P	*P*roline
Phenylalanine	Phe	F	*F*enylalanine
Tryptophan	Trp	W	T*W*o rings
Methionine	Met	M	*M*ethionine
Uncharged Polar			
Glycine	Gly	G	*G*lycine
Serine	Ser	S	*S*erine
Threonine	Thr	T	*T*hreonine
Cysteine	Cys	C	*C*ysteine
Tyrosine	Tyr	Y	t*Y*rosine
Asparagine	Asn	N	asparagi*N*e
Glutamine	Gln	Q	*Q*-tamine
Acidic			
Aspartic acid	Asp	D	aspar*D*ic acid
Glutamic acid	Glu	E	glu*E*tamic acid
Basic			
Lysine	Lys	K	before *L*
Arginine	Arg	R	a*R*ginine
Histidine	His	H	*H*istidine

Further three-letter symbols: Asx, Glx = either acid or amide. Further one-letter symbols: B = Asx, Z = Glx, X = undetermined or nonstandard amino acid residue.

according to the properties of their side chains. The *hydrophobic* (*nonpolar*) amino acids possess side chains that are neither polarized nor do they have the capacity to dissociate into ions. These amino acids are therefore poorly soluble in water (hence the name). The *polar* amino acids cannot dissociate either, but their side chains are polarized and can form hydrogen bonds with water (see below). These amino acids are therefore more soluble in water than the hydrophobic ones. The remaining amino acids can dissociate certain atomic groups in their side chains and so acquire an electric charge, either *negative* (*acidic* amino acids aspartic and glutamic, which have free COOH groups) or *positive* (*basic* amino acids lysine, arginine, and histidine, which have free NH_2 groups). Whether a free COOH or NH_2 group of an amino acid does or does not dissociate depends on the pH of the solution in which the acid is dissolved. At an alkaline pH, an acidic amino acid becomes negatively charged:

$$-COOH + OH^- \xrightarrow[\text{pH}]{\text{alkaline}} -COO^- + H_2O$$

At an acidic pH, the same amino acid will be uncharged:

$$-COO^- + H^+ \xrightarrow[\text{pH}]{\text{acidic}} -COOH$$

Similarly, a basic amino acid becomes positively charged at an acidic pH:

$$-NH_2 + H^+ \xrightarrow{\text{acidic}} -NH_3^+$$

and uncharged at alkaline pH:

$$-NH_3 + OH^- \xrightarrow[\text{pH}]{\text{alkaline}} -NH_2 + H_2O$$

Since different proteins have different numbers of charged amino acids, and since each protein has a unique amino acid sequence, each protein molecule has a characteristic distribution pattern of charged groups on its surface (Fig. 6.59). The actual *net charge* of a protein (that is, the sum of all the positive and negative charges) will vary, depending on the pH of the medium in which the protein is dissolved (Fig. 6.59). By varying the pH, one can vary the net charge of a protein over a considerable range. But there will always be a certain pH at which all the positive charges

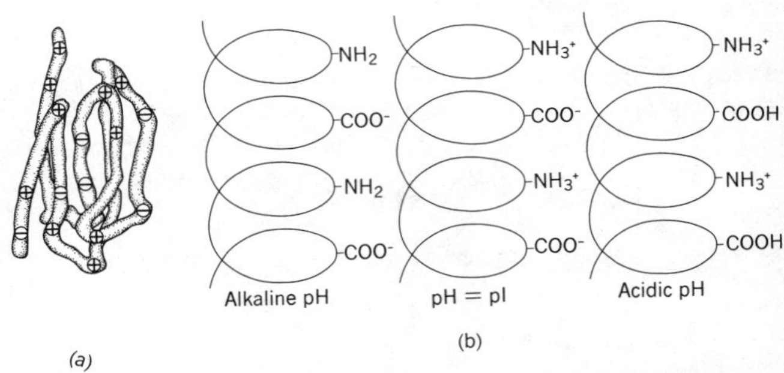

Figure 6.59. Charge distribution on a protein molecule. (*a*) An example of a protein molecule with particular spatial distribution of positive and negative charges. (*b*) Portion of a helical polypeptide chain; the diagram depicts how the net charge changes with the pH of the solution. At alkaline pH, the net charge is −2; at the isoelectric point, pI, the charge is O; and at acidic pH, the charge is +2.

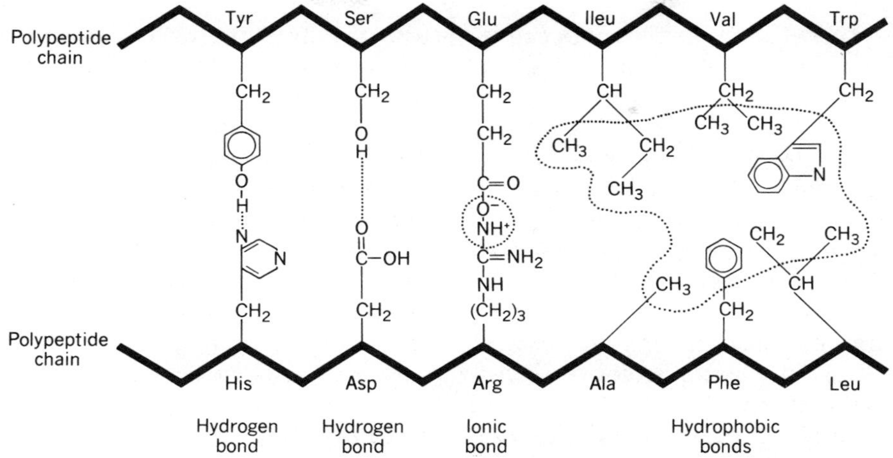

Figure 6.60. Noncovalent bonds between two polypeptide chains. Bonds indicated by dotted lines.

will cancel out all the negative charges and the molecule will be uncharged. This pH, at which the net charge of a protein is zero, is referred to as the protein's *isoelectric point*.

Bonds

There are two principal kinds of bond holding atoms together—covalent and noncovalent. In *covalent bonds*, two adjacent atoms share one or more electron pairs in their outermost energy levels (orbitals; see Fig. 6.60). Such sharing provides each atom with a stable octet of electrons in these levels. An example of a covalent bond is the *peptide bond*, which we mentioned earlier in this section; another example is the *disulfide bridge*, joining two atoms of sulfur (–S–S). A disulfide bridge is formed by the oxidation of two cysteines and their joining into one disulfide, termed *cystine*:

$$\underset{\text{Cysteine}}{H_2N-CH(COOH)-CH_2-SH} + \underset{\text{Cysteine}}{HS-CH_2-CH(COOH)-NH_2} \xrightarrow[-2H]{\text{Oxidant}} \underset{\text{Cystine}}{\overbrace{H_2N-CH(COOH)-CH_2-S}^{\text{Half-cystine}}-S-CH_2-CH(COOH)-NH_2}$$

One-half of the cystine molecule, corresponding to one cysteine, is sometimes referred to as a half-cystine.

To break the disulfide bridge, biochemists expose the protein to a large excess of a reducing agent such as 2-mercaptoethanol. To prevent spontaneous reformation of the broken bonds, the reduction must be followed immediately by alkylation by, for example, iodoacetic acid:

Reduction

$$\text{—Cys—S—S—Cys—} \xrightarrow[\text{2-mercaptoethanol}]{2(H_3CH_2CH_2OH)} 2\,(\text{—Cys—SH}) + 2(SCH_2CH_2OH)$$

Alkylation

$$2\,(\text{—Cys—SH}) \xrightarrow[\text{Idoacetic acid}]{2(ICH_2COOH)} 2\,(\text{—Cys—S—}CH_2COO^-) + 2HI$$

However, some proteins cannot be reduced readily by 2-mercaptoethanol unless they are partially unfolded by denaturing agents such as urea or guanidine hydrochloride:

$$\underset{\text{Urea}}{H_2N-C(=O)-NH_2} \qquad \underset{\text{Guanidine hydrochloride}}{H_2N-C(=NH_2^+Cl^-)-NH_2}$$

The denaturing agents are thought to disrupt noncovalent bonds (see below), unfold the protein, and so expose the disulfide bridges.

There are three major kinds of *noncovalent bond*—hydrogen, ionic, and van der Waals (Fig. 6.60). To explain these bonds, first we shall have to say a few words about the hydrogen atom, which consists of a single, negatively charged electron, and a nucleus with a single, positively charged proton. If hydrogen is covalently bonded with oxygen, as for example in the –OH group, it shares its electron with the oxygen atom. However, to speak of sharing is not quite correct because the oxygen atom, which itself has eight electrons circling its nucleus, tends to pull the lone hydrogen electron away from the hydrogen atom. Almost completely deprived of its electron, the hydrogen atom is then reduced to a nearly bare, positively charged nucleus. In this manner the –OH group becomes polarized, with the hydrogen atom expressing a positive, and the oxygen atom a negative charge. Should the polarized group happen to be close to another oxygen atom or to nitrogen (a hydrogen acceptor), the positive portion of the hydrogen atom will be attracted to the negative atom and a *hydrogen bond* will form between the two atoms. Another atom that has the capacity to take almost complete possession of hydrogen's electron is nitrogen, as in the –NH group. Thus, hydrogen bonds can occur in the following combinations of atoms: O–H . . . O, O–H . . . N, N–H . . . O, and H–H . . . N (where the ellipses indicate the bond). Two examples of hydrogen bonds are shown in Figure 6.60.

In the hydrogen bond, the oxygen atom does not fully possess the hydrogen's electron, the charges of the atoms are not fully expressed, and the atom is merely polarized. In certain groups of atoms (e.g., –COOH), and under certain conditions (i.e., certain pH), the hydrogen electron may be acquired completely by the oxygen atom and the hydrogen nucleus freed from the bond. Because of the extra electron in its oxygen, the group becomes negatively charged (i.e., $-COO^-$). The free hydrogen nuclei may be picked up by other groups (e.g., $-NH_2$), transforming these groups into positively charged ions (i.e., $-NH_3^+$). Whenever groups with the same charge come close, they repel each other; groups with opposite charges, on the other hand, attract each other, and this attraction is the basis for the *ionic bond* (Fig. 6.60).

For the explanation of the *van der Waals bond*, let us consider an atom as if it were composed of relatively concentrated positive charge (the nucleus) surrounded by negatively charged diffuse clouds (electrons). The distribution of the clouds around the atom is not always symmetrical, and when a transient asymmetry develops, charge differences arise between different regions of the atom. At this instant, the temporary dipole may influence electron distribution in an atom that happens to be nearby, and a weak attractive force between the two atoms is generated. Because of the weakness and the short range of the attractive forces, van der Waals bonds play a role in situations whereby many atoms simultaneously come close to many other atoms—for example, during complementary interaction of an antigen with a specific antibody.

Atoms, groups of atoms, or molecules can also be forced to stick together in the same way that two oil droplets are forced to fuse into a larger drop in water. Because of the polarization of its molecules, water is a highly cohesive substance. A nonpolarized (noncharged) molecule placed in water takes up space and separates water molecules, creating an unfavorable situation in terms of energy. When two nonpolarized molecules are placed in water, they take up two spaces and the situation becomes even less favorable. To improve this condition, water molecules push the two nonpolar molecules together so that they occupy as little space as possible. This tendency of water to cluster nonpolar molecules is termed *hydrophobic interaction*; here, nonpolar molecules stay together not because they form bonds between each other, but because they are driven together by the tendency of water to retain its cohesiveness.

The Conformation of Proteins

Each protein has a characteristic three-dimensional arrangement of atoms, referred to as its *conformation*. This arrangement can be studied at four levels—primary, secondary, tertiary, and quaternary. The term *primary structure* applies to the characteristic sequence of amino acids in a given polypeptide chain and to the location of disulfide bridges. *Secondary structure* refers to the spatial relationship of amino acids that are close to one another (i.e., to the distances between individual atoms, the distribution of noncovalent bonds, and the angles formed by the covalent bonds). *Tertiary structure* refers to the spatial arrangement of amino acids that are far apart in the polypeptide chain (i.e., to the way the chain bends, folds, and twists). There is no sharp separation between secondary and tertiary structures; the dividing line between them is arbitrary. The term *quaternary structure* is used for proteins composed of more than one polypeptide chain, and denotes the way these chains are arranged with respect to one another.

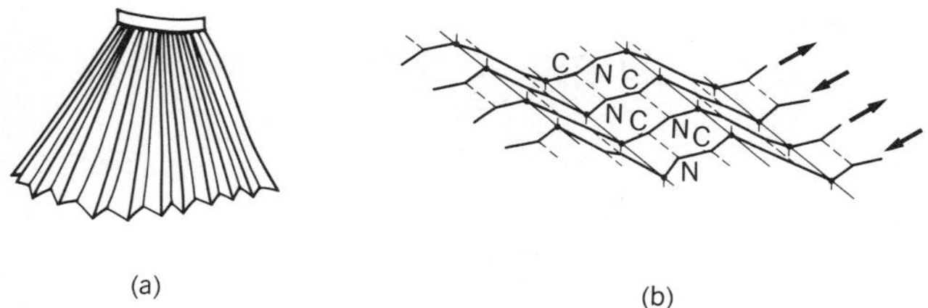

Figure 6.61. The β-pleated sheet. (*a*) A pleated skirt, which the sheet resembles. (*b*) Four anti-parallel polypeptide chains in a pleated arrangement.

Although each protein is arranged differently in terms of its secondary structure, certain structural "leitmotifs" are apparent in the construction of many different molecules. The two most common are the α helix and the β-pleated sheet (the Greek letters having the same functions that the designations "first" and "second" would). The *α helix* resembles a climbing plant where the polypeptide backbone is the stalk and the side chains are the outwardly extending leaves. The coil contains 3.6 amino acid residues per turn. The *β-pleated sheet* resembles a pleated skirt (Fig. 6.61). Here, the polypeptide chains are more extended than in the α helix and run in a zigzag form. Several of these chains are arranged into a simple, ruffled sheet, with the side chains projecting above and below it. Both the α helix and the β-pleated sheet are stabilized by hydrogen bonds between the side chains.

6.14.2 Methods of Protein Analysis

Isolation and Purification

Salt Fractionation. For a protein to dissolve and remain in solution, its charged groups must interact with the molecules of the solvent. When such interactions are prevented from occurring, protein molecules interact with one another, forming large aggregates that fall (precipitate) out of solution. A number of agents can bring about precipitation of proteins, but the most commonly used are inorganic salts, such as ammonium or sodium sulfate. When one gradually adds a salt—say, ammonium sulfate—to a protein solution, a large amount of water binds to each ammonium sulfate molecule. As the number of ammonium sulfate molecules in the solution increases, less and less water is available to interact with the proteins, until, at some point, there is not enough water present to maintain the proteins in solution and they precipitate. Since different proteins precipitate at different salt concentrations, the method can be used as a first step in protein-purification schemes.

Column Chromatography. The separation of chemical substances and particles by differential movement through a column or sheet of some suitable adsorbent is termed *chromatography* (Gr. *chroma*, color; *graphō*, to write; the name derives from the method's first use in separating plant pigments). More strongly adsorbed substances are retarded in their movement and emerge from the column (sheet) later than less strongly adsorbed substances. Of the numerous chromatographic procedures, we shall describe only two—exclusion chromatography and ion-exchange chromatography.

In *exclusion* (*gel-filtration*) *chromatography*, the adsorbents are small beads of a crosslinked carbohydrate polymer, such as Sephadex (a trade name for crosslinked polymeric dextran). The beads are full of threadlike filaments (see Fig. 6.62). When allowed to swell in water, buffer, or some other solution, they form a gel, which one packs in a column. One then applies the sample to the top of the column and percolates a buffer solution through the gel at a constant rate. The swollen beads that make up the gel

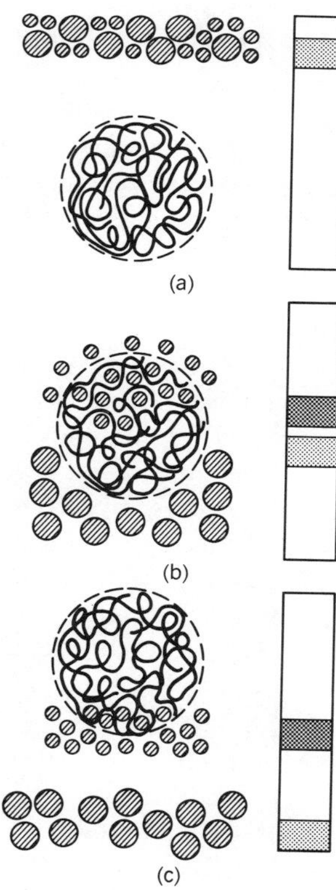

Figure 6.62. Principle of exclusion (gel-filtration) chromatography. The left-hand portion of the figure shows a single bead and the separating molecules of the sample; the right-hand portion shows the column with the separating fractions of the sample. (*a*), (*b*), and (*c*) represent three successive stages of protein separation.

function as thousands of little filters because of the intertwined threads inside them. The large molecules in the sample cannot enter the beads because they are larger than the interstices formed by the filaments; they pass down the larger spaces between the beads relatively quickly and without much resistance, and are then eluted from the column. Since this group of molecules is excluded from entering the beads, it is referred to as the *excluded fraction*.

The small molecules that enter the beads through the interstices are retarded in their movement, so they are separated from the more rapidly moving larger molecules. (They represent the *included fraction*.) The degree of retardation depends on how much time the molecules spend inside the beads—and this time is determined by the size of the molecules and the diameter of the openings between the filaments. By using polymers of different crosslinking degrees (Sephadex G10 through G200), one can manipulate the size of these openings and the resulting degree of separation of large from small molecules. The exclusion limit of a gel gives the size (and hence, also the molecular weight) of the smallest molecules incapable of penetrating the bead's openings. The eluate is collected in small fractions and the amount of protein present in each fraction is determined optically by its capacity to absorb light in the ultraviolet region.

In *ion-exchange chromatography*, the separation of molecules from a mixture occurs on an electrostatically charged adsorbent (ion exchanger), according to the molecule's net charge at a given ionic strength (Fig. 6.63). The ion exchanger consists of an insoluble matrix (a synthetic resin, a polysaccharide, or a protein) to which positive (in the case of an anion exchanger) or negative (in the case of a cation exchanger) functional groups are covalently bound. In the commonly used anionic exchanger diethyl aminoethyl (DEAE) cellulose, the insoluble matrix is cellulose and the charged functional groups are the DEAEs. The DEAE-cellulose is allowed to swell in a medium that can provide suitable counterions—in this instance, in a buffer containing NaCl. The chloride anions bind to the DEAE cations on the cellulose and establish an equilibrium:

$$\text{Cellulose-DEAE}^+ + \text{Cl}^- \rightleftarrows \text{Cellulose-DEAE}^+\text{Cl}^-$$

The swollen cellulose is packed into a column, and the protein sample, dissolved in a suitable buffer, is applied to the top and eluted with buffers of increasing or decreasing pH, or by keeping pH constant and varying ionic strength. Positively charged proteins and proteins bearing no net charge pass through the column unretarded. Negatively charged proteins compete with the Cl^- ions and displace them on the cellulose, the degree of displacement being dependent on the net protein charge, and on the pH and salt concentration of the eluting buffer. By changing the pH of the buffer and thus affecting the net charge of the proteins, or by increasing the molarity of the buffer and thus introducing more ions to compete with the proteins for the charged group, one can eventually release all the proteins from the exchanger. However, the interaction of proteins with the exchanger retards their movement down the column, and since some proteins are retarded more than others, the individual protein species separate from one another.

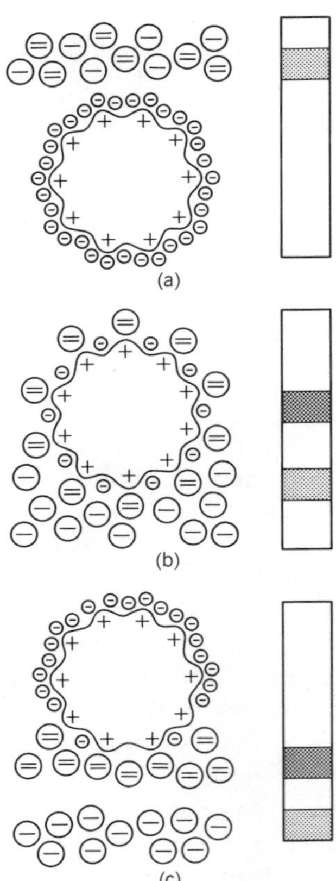

Figure 6.63. Principle of ion-exchange chromatography. The left-hand portion of the figure depicts the exchange of ions on a single bead; the right-hand portion depicts the column with the separating fractions of the sample. (*a*), (*b*), and (*c*) represent three successive stages of protein separation.

Electrophoresis. The process of separating charged particles by migration in an electric field is termed *electrophoresis* (electro + Gr. *phorēsis*, a carrying). The electric current is brought into the electrophoretic apparatus by two electrodes, a positively charged *anode* (Gr. *anodos*, a way up; an electrode toward which negatively charged anions migrate) and a negatively charged *cathode* (Gr. *cathodos*, a way down; an electrode toward which positively charged cations migrate). The protein sample is placed between these electrodes at a site referred to as the *origin*. The migration of protein particles occurs in a *medium*, which can be liquid (moving boundary or free electrophoresis), semisolid, or solid (zone electrophoresis). In *moving boundary electrophoresis*, the original form of electrophoresis invented by Arne Tiselius, a buffered protein solution is placed in a U-shaped tube and buffer is carefully layered over the sample (Fig. 6.64). When the current is turned on, the proteins in a sample, such as human serum, migrate toward the anode, but each migrates at a characteristic rate determined by its net charge. Thus they separate from one another with reasonably sharp boundaries between them. Since the refraction index of the solution changes sharply at these boundaries, the index provides information about the direction of migration and concentration of each protein.

In *zone electrophoresis*, which has almost completely supplanted the moving boundary method, the migration of charged particles occurs in a liquid-soaked solid or semisolid matrix, such as filter paper, cellulose acetate, agarose, or agar gel. (The ionized liquid—the electrolyte—is used to conduct the electric current.) The separated proteins are visualized with a suitable stain as individual zones or bands. In these techniques, the spongelike matrix possesses pores large enough for even the largest protein molecules to pass through. The separation is therefore almost exclusively on the basis of charge (electrophoretic mobility). However, there are also techniques in which charge separation is combined with a molecular sieving effect: the pores in the matrix are such that they allow smaller molecules to pass but hinder the movement of large molecules. In such a case, molecules separate not only according to their charge, but also according to their molecular weight. The two kinds of matrix used for molecular sieving are starch gel and polyacrylamide gel. The latter arises by the polymerization of a monomer acrylamide, $CH_2{=}CH{-}CO{-}NH_2$, crosslinked by a comonomer, usually N,N′-methylene-bis-acrylamide (Bis), $CH_2{=}CH{-}CO{-}NH{-}CH_2{-}NH{-}CO{-}CH{=}CH_2$. The advantage of polyacrylamide is that, by controlling the degree of polymerization, one can also control the pore size and so obtain gels with varying sieving capacities. Polyacrylamide gel electrophoresis (PAGE) has become one of the most commonly used electrophoretic methods.

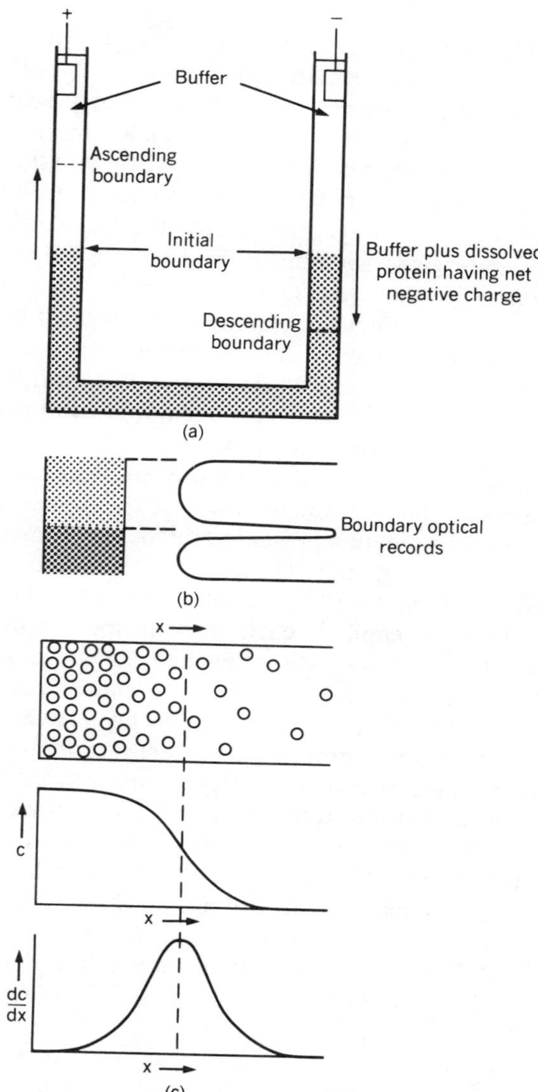

Figure 6.64. (*a*) Schematic view of Tiselius' moving boundary electrophoresis apparatus. (*b*) Optical record of moving boundaries. (*c*) Transformation of concentration-gradient curves.

A further improvement of the zonal techniques is *disc gel electrophoresis*, which is the PAGE method in principle but carried out in a discontinuous pH gradient (hence the name). The description of the method and its principle of separation is beyond this book's scope; the interested reader is referred to more specialized literature.[10] The net effect of the gradient—the

[10] An excellent description of disc gel electrophoresis and other biochemical methods appears in T. G. Cooper: *The Tools of Biochemistry*, Wiley, New York, 1977.

narrowing of the bands into sharp discs—improves the resolution power of PAGE considerably.

The sieving effect of the polyacrylamide gel can be used for estimating the molecular weights of proteins on the same principle as that of gel-filtration chromatography. For many reasons, however, these estimates turn out to be inaccurate unless one adds an anionic detergent, sodium dodecyl sulfate (SDS), to the system. In the presence of SDS, mobilities of proteins become a linear function of the logarithms of their molecular weights. The SDS changes the configuration of protein molecules into a uniform cigar shape and puts negative charge on proteins, thus producing a constant charge-to-weight ratio.

Another variant of PAGE, with even higher resolution power, is *two-dimensional gel electrophoresis*, which is a combination of isoelectric focusing and electrophoresis through the gel prior to the addition of the sample to establish a pH gradient. Then, when the protein sample is applied, each protein species moves through the gradient until it reaches a zone in which the pH corresponds to its isoelectric point. The protein stops in this zone (it is focused into it) because in it, its net charge becomes zero. Since different proteins have different isoelectric points, they focus into different zones of the gel and thus separate from one another. Once separated by isoelectric focusing according to their net charge, the proteins are subjected to SDS-PAGE and separated according to their molecular weight. If focusing is carried out in one direction and SDS-PAGE in another direction, perpendicular to the first, a two-dimensional array of spots is obtained.

Characterization

Centrifugation. The behavior of a particle during centrifugation depends on its size and density, as well as on the density and viscosity of the medium. The behavior can be described in terms of its *sedimentation constant*, S, defined as the velocity of the particle per unit of centrifugal field:

$$s = \frac{2r^2(P_p - P_m)}{9\eta}$$

where r is the radius of the particle and P_p its density; P_m is the density and η is the viscosity of the surrounding medium (all in egs units). The sedimentation can be expressed in seconds, or, as is more common, in svedberg units: $S = s \times 10^{13}$ sec. The above equation applies to spherical particles; particles of other shapes sediment more slowly because of higher friction.

Determination of Amino Acid Composition. To determine the types and relative frequencies of amino acids in a protein, all of the protein's peptide bonds are broken and the individual amino acids are freed. The cleaving of the peptide bonds is accomplished by hydrolysis—the addition of the H^+ and OH^- ions of a water molecule on either side of the bond. Complete hydrolysis is achieved by boiling the protein in HCl for 24 hours. The amino acids in the hydrolysate are then separated by ion-exchange chromatography. Since the individual amino acids differ in their charges, they emerge at different times from the column and can be identified by comparison with the chromatographic pattern of a standard amino acid mixture. The quantity of the amino acids is proportional to the optical absorbance of the eluted fractions.

Peptide Mapping. Inorganic acids, such as HCl, are totally nonspecific hydrolyzing reagents that, given enough time, cleave all peptide bonds in the entire protein molecule. But there are also reagents that are far more specific in their action on the polypeptide chain in that they cleave peptide bonds only between certain amino acids. Such a reagent is cyanogen bromide (CNBr), which cleaves the polypeptide chain only on the carboxyl side of methionine residues. Another example is proteolytic enzymes, such as trypsin or chymotrypsin, which also recognize only certain amino acids in the polypeptide chain and split the bond in which these acids are involved: trypsin splits polypeptide chains on the carboxyl side of arginine and lysine, chymotrypsin the peptide bonds of the three aromatic amino acids—tyrosine, tryptophan, and phenylalanine. Cleavage of a protein by specific reagents thus reduces the protein molecule into smaller fragments, termed peptides. The number and size of peptides produced from a given molecule depends on the number and position of amino acids that the reagent recognizes. For example, a protein that has seven methionine residues will be split by CNBr into eight peptides, a protein with eight methionine residues splits into nine peptides, and so on. Since different proteins have different numbers of amino acids of a given kind, the number and size of the peptides produced by specific hydrolytic reagents is as characteristic of the individual protein species as fingerprints are of individual people. One can therefore identify a protein by this peptide mapping, or fingerprinting. Following partial hydrolysis with one or two of the specific reagents, the individual peptides are separated by ion-exchange chromatography, in the same way that amino acids were in the preceding procedure.

Amino Acid Sequencing. The procedures used for the determination of a protein's primary structure consist of the following steps. First, the molecule is cleaved into large fragments, using cyanogen bromide. Second, the large fragments are cleaved into smaller peptides by proteolytic enzymes. Third, individual peptides are isolated and purified by a combination of ion-exchange chromatography and other biochemical methods. Fourth, the sequence of amino acids in the individual peptides is determined. Fifth, the entire procedure is repeated, using a different proteolytic enzyme (e.g., if trypsin was used in the first round, chymotrypsin can

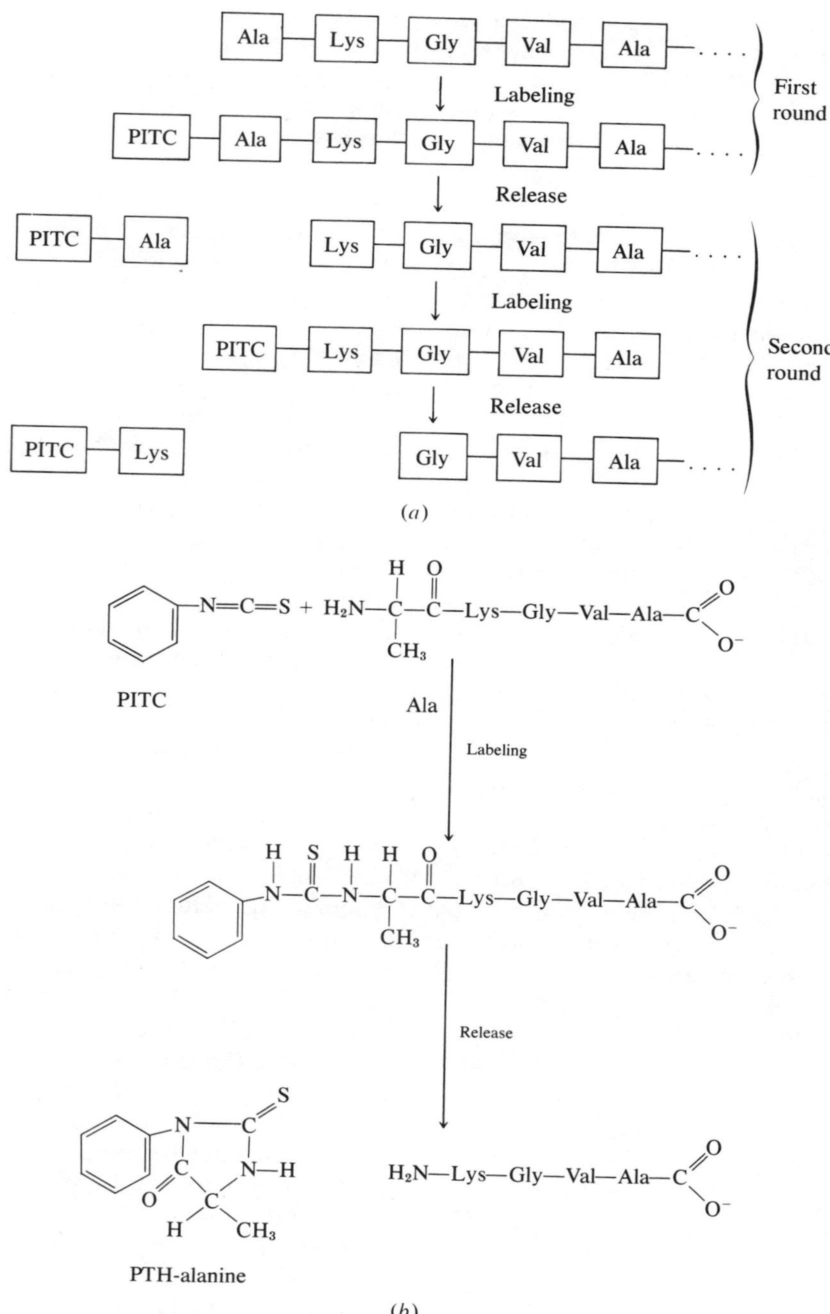

Figure 6.65. Principle of Edman degradation. (A) General scheme. (B) Chemical reactions. PITC, phenyl isothiocyanate; PTH, phenylthiohydantoin.

be used in the second round). Since different enzymes split the protein at different positions and produce different peptides, the order of the peptides in the molecule can be established by comparing the sequences of the two sets of peptide and searching for overlapping sequences. And sixth, from the ordered peptides, the sequence of the entire polypeptide chain is determined.

The sequencing of an isolated peptide is based on the so-called *Edman degradation* procedure, devised by Pehr Edman. The principle of the method is the stepwise removal of the individual amino acid, starting from the N terminal of the peptide, and isolation and identification of the amino acid in each step (Fig. 6.65). The removal of amino acids is made possible by a reagent called phenyl isothiocyanate. The stepwise degradation proceeds as follows. First, phenyl isothiocyanate reacts with the terminal amino group of the peptide and forms a phenylthiocarbamoyl derivative. Second, treatment of the peptide with mild acid, usually in an organic solvent, breaks the first peptide bond at the N terminal and releases the first amino acid linked to the phenylthiohydantoin (PTH) without disturbing the other bonds in the peptide. Third, the released amino acid is identified chromatographically. Fourth, the entire procedure is repeated, phenyl isothiocyanate is added to the second amino acid (now terminal), and PTH-amino acid is cleaved off, identified, and so on, until the entire sequence of the peptide is established.

In some proteins, the amino group of the N-terminal amino acid is bound covalently to another group—for example, N-acetylglycine of pyrrolidone carboxylate (Fig. 6.66). Such *blocked N termini* are inaccessible to identification by the Edman procedure.

A somewhat different approach to primary structure determination is exemplified by the newly developed *microsequencing procedures*. In these methods, cells are cultured in the presence of a radioactively labeled amino acid, and the isotope is allowed to be incorporated into the newly synthesized protein. The protein is then isolated and the positions at which the radioactivity appears along the polypeptide chain are determined by sequencing in an automatic sequenator. These positions are presumed to be occupied by the amino acid used in the culture for labeling.

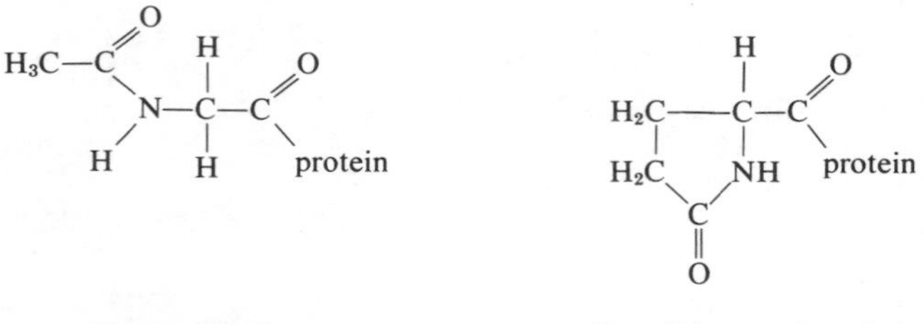

N-acetylglycine Pyrrolidone carboxylate

Figure 6.66. Blocked N-terminal amino acids.

X-Ray Diffraction Analysis. This method provides information on the tertiary and quaternary protein structure. Its prerequisite is the availability of crystallized proteins. A crystal is an ordered, three-dimensional lattice formed by repeated points (ions, atoms, molecules). When one aims a beam of X-rays at the crystal, the rays, which have a wavelength about the same size as the distance between neighboring points, penetrate the crystal and travel through it until they hit one of the points of the lattice. The collision with the electron clouds of the atoms in the lattice diffracts the rays at a certain angle, changing their amplitude proportionally to the number of electrons in the cloud. Waves diffracted by different points combine and either reinforce or cancel one another out, depending on whether they are in or out of phase. Behind the crystal, the diffracted rays form an abstract image of the three-dimensional structure—a kind of three-dimensional shadow of the crystals' internal organization. A photographic plate placed into this shadow will record a two-dimensional cut through the three-dimensional image. The record will appear as a regular array of spots of different intensities. Since the image depends on the angle of the incident rays, the crystal is slowly rotated and the changing patterns of the shadow recorded.

The abstract image can be transformed into a real one by a set of equations and complex calculations carried out by a computer. The calculations provide information about the density of electrons at the individual points in the crystal, which in turn identifies the points as individual atoms or ions. The electron density distribution in a single plane is traced by contour lines on a sheet of plastic in the same way that altitude contour lines are drawn on geological survey maps. By stacking sheets representing different sections on top of each other, one produces a three-dimensional image of the crystal. Although theoretically, from the best X-ray diffraction pictures one should be able to deduce the position of every atom in the molecule and thus the protein's primary structure, in practice the analysis is so complex that knowledge of the amino acid sequence beforehand makes determination of tertiary structure a considerably easier task to accomplish. Since proteins produce very complex X-ray diffraction patterns, the analysis is carried out stepwise. First, only spots with certain intensities are chosen and a rough model of the molecule is constructed. Then, additional spots are taken into account and more details are added to the model. And finally, all the spots are considered and the position of each atom in the molecule is determined.

6.15 APPENDIX 6.2: SELECTED METHODS OF SOMATIC AND MOLECULAR GENETICS

6.15.1 Somatic-Cell Hybridization

In the 1960s, cell biologists observed that cells grown in tissue culture can occasionally fuse, forming *somatic cell hybrids*. The frequency of these fusions (normally very low) can be increased by adding Sendai virus particles irradiated with ultraviolet light to the cultured cells. These particles attach to the cell surfaces (without being able to infect the cells) and cause some so far largely unidentified changes in the membrane; these changes enhance the probability of cell fusion. Sendai virus as a mediator of cell fusion is, however, gradually being replaced with polyethylene glycol (PEG), the effect of which is the same, but more reproducible. The fusion of membranes is followed by the fusion of cytoplasms, and, after a while, by the fusion of nuclei as well. The transient hybrid cell with unfused nuclei is termed a *heterokaryon* (Gr. *heteros*, other; *karyon*, nucleus).

Following fusion, hybrid cells must be separated and isolated from the parental cells. Such isolation is accomplished by using cell lines with certain genetic defects (i.e., resistance to 8-azaguanine and 5-bromodeoxyuridine) for fusion and by growing the cells in a medium that arrests the proliferation of the parental, but not the hybrid cells. The drug 8-*azaguanine* (8AzG) is an analog of one of the DNA bases that, when incorporated into DNA, interferes with normal replication and transcription, and thus prevents the cells from proliferating. However, by continually growing cells in the presence of high concentrations of this drug, one can select mutants that are resistant to the toxic effects of 8AzG. The mutation occurs in a gene coding for the enzyme *hypoxanthine-guanine-phosphoribosyl transferase* (HGPRT), which the cell uses to incorporate 8AzG into DNA. When this enzyme is inactivated by a mutation, the 8AzG can no longer be incorporated, and the mutant cell becomes resistant to 8AzG action. The inactive enzyme also fails to catalyze the incorporation of certain normal bases, but the cell overcomes this deficiency by synthesizing these bases internally from more basic constituents in the culture medium.

The drug 5-*bromodeoxyuridine* (5BUdR) is another base analog with an effect similar to that of 8AzG. Mutants resistant to the toxic effect of 5BUdR have a defect in a gene coding for the enzyme *thymidine kinase* (TK), which is used by normal cells for the incorporation of 5BUdR (and also of thymidine) into DNA.

Both the 8AzG-resistant and 5BUdR-resistant cell lines are sensitive to another drug, *aminopterin*, which is nontoxic to normal cells. Aminopterin blocks de novo synthesis of hypoxanthine and thymidine, and since the cells are unable to use these two DNA precursors from the medium, they die. (The 8AzG-resistant cells cannot use hypoxanthine because of the inactive HGPRT; and the 5BUdR-resistant cells cannot use thymidine because of the inactive TK.)

When one mixes 8AzG-resistant and 5BUdR-resistant cells in a medium containing *h*ypoxanthine, *a*minopterin, and *t*hymidine (the so-called *HAT medium*), only the hybrids will grow: the parental cells will die because they are sensitive to aminopterin, but the hybrid cells will survive because their 8AzG-resistant parent provides them with a normal, nondefective TK gene, and the 5BUdR-resistant parent provides them with a nondefective HGPRT gene. Hybrid cells are therefore capable of using both the thymidine and the hypoxanthine in the medium and so are resistant to the effects of aminopterin. Hence, the HAT medium provides a strong selective pressure for the growth of only hybrid cells.

If one of the parents is a cell with limited growth capacity, it can be fused and selected without first making it drug-resistant. However, the other parent must then be drug-resistant. For example, an 8AzG-resistant cell can be fused with a normal lymphocyte in the HAT medium. The nonhybridized 8AzG-resistant parental cells in the mixture die because of the aminopterin effect, and the nonfused lymphocytes will eventually die because they cannot survive in a culture without antigenic stimulation. So the only surviving cells will, again, be the hybrids.

For some time after the fusion, the hybrids are unstable, and gradually, in successive generations, they lose some of their chromosomes. To achieve homogeneity, the hybrids need to be cloned, but even when a clone is established, its stability is not guaranteed. A cell line derived from a somatic cell hybrid is referred to as a *hybridoma*.

6.15.2 Production of Antibody-Secreting Hybridomas

To obtain an antibody-secreting hybridoma, spleen cells from an immunized animal (mouse) are fused with

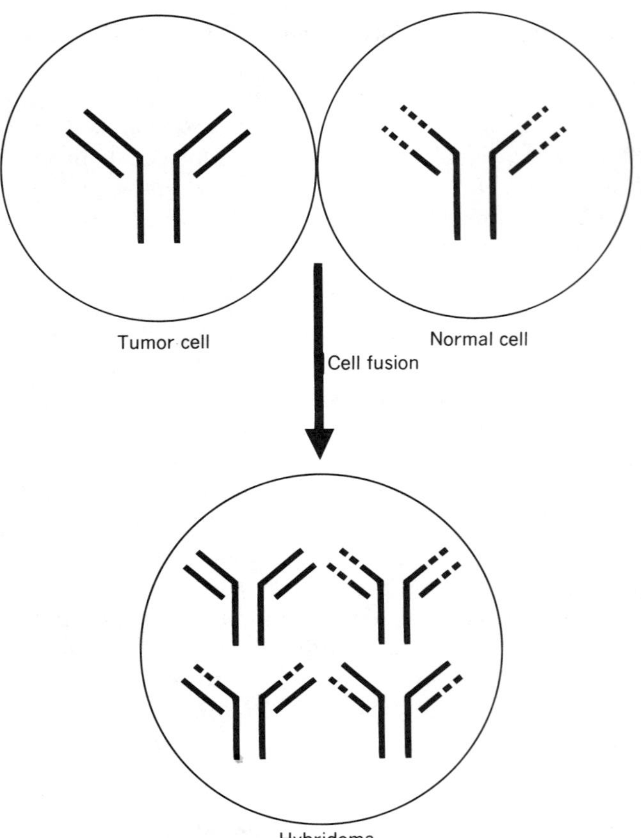

Figure 6.67. A hybridoma produced by fusion of a myeloma tumor cell with a normal antibody-producing cell. Since the heavy and light chains recombine freely in a single cell, the hybridoma can theoretically produce four types of Ig molecule differing in their V regions.

a drug-resistant plasmacytoma cell line (Fig. 6.67). The spleen cell brings the information for the synthesis of a single antibody species into the hybridoma; the plasmacytoma cell brings in immortality. The hybridoma thus produces monoclonal antibody against the antigen used for the immunization of the donor mouse. In addition, it secretes the myeloma protein secreted by the original plasmacytoma cell. However, plasmacytoma nonsecretors can also be used, and the hybridoma then produces only the induced antibody. The most difficult task in establishing antibody-producing hybridomas is keeping them active; many hybridomas suddenly stop producing antibodies, probably because they lose some of the chromosomes necessary for sustenance of antibody synthesis. The identity (in terms of differentiation stage) of the spleen cell that fuses with the plasmacytoma cell is not known.

6.15.3 RNA-DNA Hybridization

In the DNA, the two complementary strands are held together by hydrogen bonds between complementary bases (thymine is bonded with adenine and cytosine with guanine). Heating of a DNA solution beyond melting point breaks the bonds and causes the strands to separate from each other. During subsequent slow cooling, a single strand can often meet its complementary partner by chance, re-form the hydrogen bonds, and thus, to a certain degree, reconstitute the double helical structure (reanneal). When solutions of single-stranded DNA from two different sources are mixed, *hybrid molecules* may form by reannealing of segments with complementary base sequences. The extent of hybridization of DNA molecules will depend on the extent of homology between the two specimens: the more homologous segments the two DNA species share, the more extensive the hybridization will be. The degree of hybridization is thus a measure of relatedness between two DNA species.

During transcription, the cell uses one of the two DNA strands as a template for the assembly of the single-stranded messenger RNA, which then transfers genetic information from the DNA to proteins. Since the mRNA is complementary to one DNA strand, it can be hybridized with DNA of the corresponding gene. The rate of this RNA-DNA hybridization will depend on the number of gene copies in the particular genome. If an individual possesses only one locus coding for a given mRNA, the probability of this mRNA finding the complementary DNA segment is low and the hybridization slow. If, however, the individual carries several hundred gene copies that are not identical but sufficiently homologous so that mRNA of one gene may hybridize with any one of the other genes, the hybridization will be faster. Hence, from the RNA-DNA hybridization rate, one can determine the number of gene copies present in a genome. As an alternative to RNA-DNA hybridization, one can first replicate the mRNA, using the enzyme reverse transcriptase, obtain single-stranded complementary DNA, and perform a DNA-DNA hybridization.

There are many specific ways of carrying out RNA-DNA (or DNA-DNA) hybridization. One way is to use cells that synthesize large quantities of mRNA of a single kind (e.g., antibody-producing plasma cells). By culturing these cells in the presence of radioactively labeled precursors, one can specifically label this mRNA, and extract and purify it. (Contamination of the preparation by transcripts of other genes would lead to false estimate of gene number.) Simultaneously, one extracts total DNA, shears it into fragments, heat-dissociates the strands, and immobilizes them on a membrane filter. When one then passes the solution of labeled mRNA through the filter, one retains on the filter amounts of mRNA (radioactivity) proportional to the number of complementary DNA strands. By determining the radioactivity of the filters and comparing it with a known standard, one can estimate, in this *Southern blot technique* (named after the biochemist who invented it), the number of gene copies in the genome.

6.15.4 Gene Cloning

A bacterium such as *Escherichia coli*, a common inhabitant of mammalian intestine, contains, in addition to a circular chromosome, one or more small DNA rings that replicate independently of the chromosomal DNA. These circles, referred to as *plasmids* or *episomes*, can also integrate into the main bacterial chromosome and regularly move on and off it. Recently, geneticists have learned how to break a plasmid, insert a short segment of foreign DNA (gene) into it, reseal the ring, and reinsert the recombined DNA molecule into a bacterium. The chimeric plasmid replicates and the bacterium manufactures, in addition to its own DNA, foreign DNA and sometimes proteins encoded by the foreign DNA (Fig. 6.68).

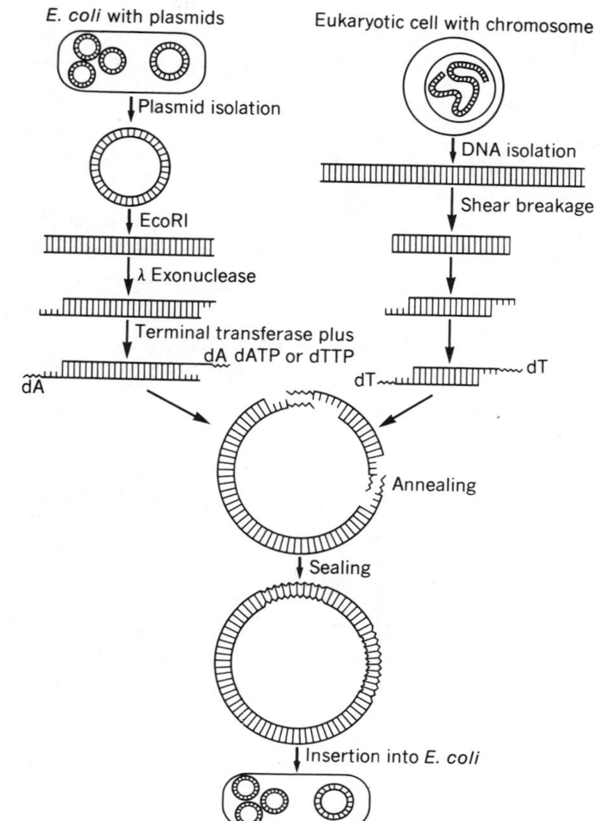

Figure 6.68. Construction of a recombinant plasmid, using the dA-dT tailing technique.

This *gene cloning* or *recombinant DNA analysis* has become possible because of the discovery of the so-called *restriction enzymes*, which recognize specific short sequences in the unmodified, double-stranded DNA, and then break both polynucleotide chains. The normal function of these enzymes is the degradation of foreign DNA infecting a cell. (Indigenous DNA is protected from their action by another enzyme, usually a methylase, that modifies the DNA.) There are two classes of restriction enzyme—class I, which recognize DNA at one site but cleave it at another, and class II, which recognize and cleave DNA at the same site. The recognition site of class II enzymes exhibits twofold symmetry about the central nucleotide pair, e.g.,

$$\begin{array}{ccc} \text{AAG} & \vdots & \text{CTT} \\ ||| & \vdots & ||| \\ \text{TTC} & \vdots & \text{GAA} \end{array}$$

In other words, at the recognition site, the two strands have the same nucleotide sequence, only running in opposite directions. It is because of this arrangement that the restriction enzyme can recognize and break *both* strands. The individual enzymes are referred to by symbols indicating, in an abbreviated form, their microbial origin (e.g., EcoRI is a restriction enzyme derived from *E. coli*, Hind I is derived from *Hemophilus influenzae* strain Rd, and so on). In addition to converting circular plasmids into linear molecules, restriction enzymes also chop long DNA molecules into fragments of defined length and nucleotide sequence. This observation is the basis of *restriction-enzyme mapping* which, in analogy to peptide mapping, allows the identification of individual DNA species through the characteristic assembly of fragments into which they break following the action of a given restriction enzyme. The individual fragments can be isolated and their nucleotide sequence determined—again, in a process analogous to sequencing of peptide fragments produced by the action of specific proteases.

In DNA cloning experiments, restriction enzymes are used to break open the plasmid ring. The insertion of the foreign DNA into the open circle can be accomplished in one of three principal ways—by dA-dT tailing, by the use of another set of restriction enzymes, or by the use of synthetic linkers. In the dA-dT tailing technique (Fig. 6.68), both the plasmid and the foreign DNA are cleaved by an exonuclease—an enzyme that preferentially attacks phosphodiester (nucleoside linking) bonds at the termini of the double-stranded DNA. One such enzyme—λ exonuclease—removes a few nucleotides at the termini, but only in one strand, leaving both ends of the DNA molecule single-stranded. The single strands are recognized by another enzyme—terminal transferase—which is used to attach short sequences to both ends (e.g., sequence of deoxyadenylate residues to the plasmid DNA and of deoxythymidylate residues to the foreign DNA). The plasmid DNA tails then pair with complementary tails of the foreign DNA and form a ring, which can be sealed covalently by the combining action of three enzymes—exonuclease III, polymerase I, and DNA ligase. These enzymes also fill the gaps in the molecules with complementary nucleotides.

The second method takes advantage of class II restriction enzymes that make staggered, single-stranded breaks, generating mutually cohesive "sticky" ends (Fig. 6.69; other class II enzymes generate fully base-paired ends). Combination of complementary cohesive ends of the plasmid and foreign DNA produces a ring that can then be sealed by the enzyme DNA ligase.

In the third method, one prepares synthetic linkers, which are a few nucleotides long and represent the sequence of a restriction enzyme site (e.g., EcoRI). One then attaches the linkers to both ends of the foreign single- or double-stranded DNA, using the enzyme DNA ligase (so-called blunt-ended ligation, since both the DNA and the linkers have blunt ends produced by nuclease S1 digestion). Treatment of the attached linkers and of the plasmid by a given restriction enzyme (in this case, EcoRI) produces sticky ends that allow the incorporation of the foreign DNA into the plasmid.

The main difficulty of all DNA cloning techniques is the insertion into the plasmid (*vector*) of the specific gene one is interested in studying. To isolate this gene, one must have a *probe* for its detection. The probe can be corresponding mRNA, cDNA transcribed from the mRNA, or an artificial messenger synthesized chemically, based on the knowledge of a protein's primary structure and of the genetic code.

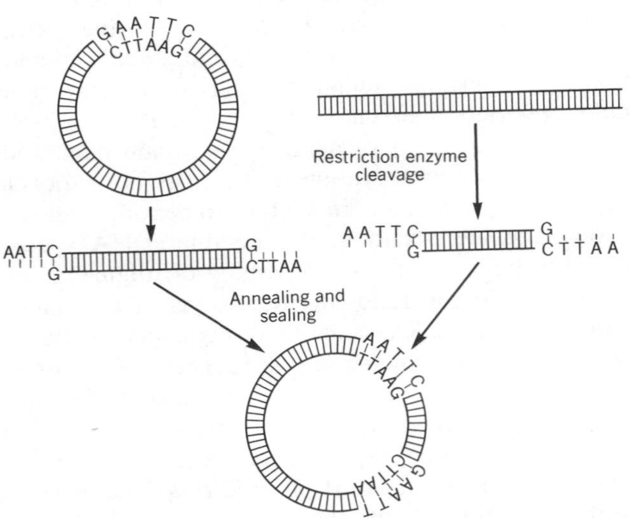

Figure 6.69. Construction of a recombinant plasmid by restriction-enzyme cleavage, resulting in "sticky ends."

REFERENCES

General

Cooper, T. G.: *The Tools of Biochemistry*. Wiley, New York, 1977.

Gally, J. A.: Structure of immunoglobulins. *In* M. Sela (Ed.): *The Antigens*, Vol. I, pp. 161–298. Academic, New York, 1973.

Glover, D. M.: Gene cloning: a new approach to understanding relationships between DNA sequences. *In* J. Paul (Ed.): *Biochemistry of Cell Differentiation II*, pp. 1–44. University Park Press, Baltimore, 1977.

Glynn, L. E. and Stewart, M. W. (Eds.): *Immunochemistry. An Advanced Textbook*. Wiley, Chichester, 1977.

Kabat, E. A.: *Structural Concepts in Immunology and Immunochemistry*, 2nd ed. Holt, Rinehart, and Winston, New York, 1976.

Kubo, R. T., Zimmerman, B., and Grey, H. M.: Phylogeny of immunoglobulins. *In* M. Sela (Ed.): *The Antigens*, Vol. 1, pp. 417–477. Academic, New York, 1973.

Lehninger, A. L.: *Biochemistry. The Molecular Basis of Cell Structure and Function*. Worth, New York, 1970.

Litman, G. W. and Good, R. A. (Eds.): *Immunoglobulins*. Plenum, New York, 1978.

Mage, R., Lieberman, R., Potter, M., and Terry, W. D.: Immunoglobulin allotypes. *In* M. Sela (Ed.): *The Antigens*, Vol. 1, pp. 299–376. Academic, New York, 1973.

Nisonoff, A., Hopper, J. E., and Spring, S. B.: *The Antibody Molecule*. Academic, New York, 1975.

Oudin, J.: Idiotypy of antibodies. *In* M. Sela (Ed.): *The Antigens*, Vol. 2, pp. 277–364. Academic, New York, 1974.

Poljak, R. J., Amzel, L. M., and Phizackerley, R. P.: Studies on the three-dimensional structure of immunoglobulins. *Prog. Biophys. Mol. Biol.* **31**:67–93, 1976.

Potter, M.: Immunoglobulin-producing tumors and myeloma proteins of mice. *Physiol. Res.* **52**:631–719, 1972.

Stryer, L.: *Biochemistry*. Freeman, San Francisco, 1975.

Turner, M. W.: The immunoglobulinopathies. *In* D. J. H. Brock and O. Mayo (Eds.): *The Biochemical Genetics of Man*, 2nd ed., pp. 633–685. Academic, London, 1975.

Weigert, M. and Riblet, R.: The genetic control of antibody variable regions in the mouse. *Springer Sem. Immunopathol.* **1**:133–169, 1978.

Original Articles

Ada, G. L. and Byrt, P.: Specific inactivation of antigen-reactive cells with ^{125}I-labeled antigen. *Nature* **222**:1291–1292, 1969.

Bence Jones, H.: On a new substance occurring in the urine of a patient with "mollities ossium." *Phil. Tr. Roy. Soc. Lond.* **138**:55–62, 1848.

Cederblad, G., Johansson, B. G., and Rymo, L.: Reduction and proteolytic degradation of immunoglobulin A from human colostrum. *Acta Chem. Scand.* **20**:2349–2357, 1966.

Deutsch, H. F., Morton, J. I., and Kratochvil, C. H.: Antigenic identity of hyperglobulinemic serum components with proteins of normal serum. *J. Biol. Chem.* **222**:39–51, 1956.

Dreyer, W. J. and Bennett, J. C.: The molecular basis of antibody formation: a paradox. *Proc. Natl. Acad. Sci. U.S.A.* **54**:864–869, 1965.

Edelman, G. M. and Gall, W. E.: The antibody problem. *Annu. Rev. Biochem.* **38**:415–466, 1969.

Edelman, G. M., Cunningham, B. A., Gall, W. E., Gottlieb, P. D., Rutishauser, U., and Waxdal, M. J.: The covalent structure of an entire γ-immunoglobulin molecule. *Proc. Natl. Acad. Sci. U.S.A.* **63**:78–85, 1969.

Feinstein, A.: Character and allotypy of an immune globulin in rabbit colostrum. *Nature* **199**:1197–1199, 1963.

Grabar, P. and Williams, C. A.: Méthode permettant l'étude conjuguée des propriétés électrophorétiques et immunochimiques d'un mélange de protéines. Application au serum sanguin. *Biochem. Biophys. Acta* **10**:193–195, 1953.

Grey, H. M. and Kunkel, H. G.: H chain subgroups of myeloma proteins and normal 7S γ-globulin. *J. Exp. Med.* **120**:253–266, 1964.

Heidelberger, M. and Pedersen, K. O.: The molecular weight of antibodies *J. Exp. Med.* **65**:393–414, 1937.

Hilschmann, N. and Craig, L. G.: Amino acid sequence studies with Bence-Jones proteins. *Proc. Natl. Acad. Sci. U.S.A.* **53**:1403–1409, 1965.

Köhler, G. and Milstein, C.: Continuous cultures of fused cells secreting antibody of predefined specificity. *Nature* **256**:495–497, 1975.

Koshland, M. E., Davis, J. J., and Fujita, N. J.: Evidence for multiple gene control of a single polypeptide chain: the heavy chain of rabbit immunoglobulin. *Proc. Natl. Acad. Sci. U.S.A.* **63**:1274–1281, 1969.

Kreth, H. W. and Williamson, A. R.: The extent of diversity of anti-hapten antibodies in inbred mice: anti-NIP (4-hydroxy-5-iodo-3-nitro-phenacetyl) antibodies in CBA/H mice. *Eur. J. Immunol.* **3**:141–147, 1973.

Merwin, R. M. and Algire, G. H.: Induction of plasma cell neoplasms and fibrosarcomas in BALB/c mice carrying diffusion chambers. *Proc. Soc. Exp. Biol. Med.* **101**:437–439, 1959.

Möller, G.: Demonstration of mouse isoantigens at the cellular level by the fluorescent antibody technique. *J. Exp. Med.* **114**:415–434, 1961.

Oudin, J.: The genetic control of immunoglobulin synthesis. *Proc. R. Soc. Lond.* (*Biol.*) **166**:207–219, 1966.

Porter, R. R.: *In* A. Gelhorn and E. Hirschberg (Eds.): *Symposium on Basic Problems in Neoplastic Disease*, pp. 177–181. Columbia University Press, New York, 1962.

Potter, M. and Robertson, C. L.: Development of plasma cell neoplasms in BALB/c mice after intraperitoneal injection of paraffin-oil adjuvant, heat-killed staphylococcus mixtures. *J. Natl. Cancer Inst.* **25**:847–861, 1960.

Rejnek, J., Kostka, J., and Kotynek, O.: Electrophoretic behavior of H and L chains of human serum and colostrum gammaglobulin. *Nature* (*Lond.*) **209**:926–928, 1966.

Rowe, D. S. and Fahey, J. L.: A new class of human immunoglobulins. I. A unique myeloma protein. II. Normal serum IgD. *J. Exp. Med.* **121**:171–199, 1965.

Sell, S. and Gell, P. G. H.: Studies on rabbit lymphocytes in vitro. I. Stimulation of blast transformation with an antiallotype serum. *J. Exp. Med.* **122**:423–440, 1965.

Slater, R. J., Ward, S. M., and Kunkel, H. G.: Immunological relationships among myeloma proteins. *J. Exp. Med.* **101**:85–108, 1955.

Titani, K. and Putnam, F. W.: Immunoglobulin structure: amino-terminal and carboxyl-terminal peptides of type I Bence-Jones proteins. *Science* **147**:1304–1305, 1965.

Todd, C. W.: Allotype in rabbit 19S protein. *Biochem. Biophys. Res. Commun.* **11**:170–175, 1963.

Tomasi, T. B., Tan, E. M., Solomon, A., and Prendergast, R. A.: Characteristics of an immune system common to certain external secretions. *J. Exp. Med.* **121**:101–124, 1965.

Valentine, R. C. and Green, N. M.: Electron microscopy of an antibody-hapten complex. *J. Mol. Biol.* **27**:615–617, 1967.

Waldenström, J.: Incipient myelomatosis or "essential" hyperglobulinemia with fibrinogenopenia—a new syndrome? *Acta Med. Scand.* **117**:216–247, 1944.

Wu, T. T. and Kabat, E. A.: An analysis of sequences of variable regions of Bence-Jones proteins and myeloma light chains and their implications for antibody complementarity. *J. Exp. Med.* **132**:211–250, 1970.

(See also references 12, 35, 37, 45, 51, 70, 71, and 95 in Chapter 2.)

CHAPTER 7

T-CELL FACTORS AND RECEPTORS

Leaving the B lymphocyte and entering the realm of T-cell products, we descend into the immunological Dark Ages. We find ourselves surrounded by blindness and ignorance, like Dante descending to the inferno:

> Midway in our life's journey, I went astray from the straight road and woke to find myself alone in a dark wood. How shall I say what wood that was! I never saw so drear, so rank, so arduous a wilderness![1]

We shall, therefore, want to make the trip through this immunological limbo as short as possible. We shall first deal with the products that the T cell secretes or sheds (factors, mediators), and then with the substances it displays on its surface (receptors).

7.1 FACTORS

Following activation, a lymphocyte manufactures and secretes soluble substances, variously referred to as factors, mediators, or lymphokines[2], that affect the behavior of other cells. The substances were originally thought to be exclusively T-cell products, but later studies have demonstrated that at least some of them can also be manufactured by other lymphocytes (i.e., B cells). One learns about the existence of these factors by adding a supernatant from a lymphocyte culture to the target cells and noticing how the target cells change. In the factor's presence, the cells may stop moving or accelerate their movement; they may be killed by the factor or be augmented in their function; they may be activated or inhibited. There are many ways one can search for soluble factors, and since most of them are successful, it appears that many different factors exist. Unless one succeeds in isolating a given factor, there is almost no way of comparing it to

[1] Dante Alighieri: *The Divine Comedy*, "The Inferno," Canto I. Translated by John Ciardi.

[2] The term *lymphokines* (lympho + Gr. *kinesis*, movement) is usually reserved for soluble substances produced by lymphocytes and *acting* on lymphocytes. The term *mediator* derives from the observation that the substances *mediate* cellular reactions. In this text, we shall use the terms *factor* and *mediator* indiscriminately.

factors described by other investigators using other experimental systems, and since it is extremely difficult to isolate and characterize a factor biochemically, the literature is full of factors of all kinds—at least 60 at the time of this writing. Which of them are the same and which different no one can tell: this Augean stable has not yet found its Hercules.

The known factors can be divided into four groups, according to the target cell they affect (macrophage, granulocyte, lymphocyte, or other); within each group, individual factors may be subdivided further, according to their effects (Tables 7.1 and 2).

7.1. Macrophage-Affecting Factors

The three main effects of factors on macrophages are inhibition of macrophage migration, macrophage activation, and macrophage chemotaxis. A description of the factors responsible for these effects follows.

Migration Inhibitory Factor (MIF)

MIF was the first mediator discovered. A. R. Rich and M. R. Lewis reported in 1932 that fragments of spleens taken from guinea pigs that had been immunized with tuberculi bacilli sent out cells in tissue culture, and that the migration of these cells could be inhibited by the addition of the immunizing antigen (the old tuberculin; see Chapter 2). However, it was not until 30 years later that this observation was followed up in a systematic manner. In 1962, M. George and J. H. Vaughan described a method that simplified the study of migration inhibition (Fig. 7.1). They isolated peritoneal exudate cells (PEC) from immunized guinea pigs, placed these cells in small glass capillary tubes, sealed the tubes at one end, centrifuged them, cut them at the cell-medium interphase, and placed the fragments in a chamber containing culture medium either with or without immunizing antigen. After some 18 to 20 hours' incubation at 37°C, they observed, at each capillary's opening, a fanlike spreading of the cells in cultures without the antigen and a bulbous accumulation of the cells in cultures exposed to the antigen (Fig. 7.1*e* and *f*). The peritoneal exudate cells (i.e., cells that pass or exude into the peritoneum or the abdominal cavity, particularly following inoculation of irritants, such as mineral oil) consisted of from 70 to 80 percent macrophages and 10 to 20 percent lymphocytes. Further studies—in particular, those by John R. David and Barry R. Bloom—demonstrated that both of these cells participate in the migration-inhibition reaction. It turned out that the immune lymphocytes, when restimulated in vitro by the immunizing antigen, produced a soluble substance that inhibited the migration of the macrophages out of the tube. In the absence of the antigen, the lymphocytes are not activated, MIF is not produced, and the macrophages move out freely from the tube. In the presence of the antigen, the MIF produced by the activated lymphocytes inhibits macrophage migration and the macrophages pile up at the tube's opening. The cell migration can be quantitated by tracing and measuring a magnification of the area of migration on a piece of paper. The effect of the MIF is usually expressed as the migration index (MI), which is the ratio of mean area of migration in the presence of antigen to that in the absence of antigen. The effect is considered significant when the migration index is less than 0.8 (20 percent inhibition or more). In addition to this direct method, in which macrophages and lymphocytes are cultured together, one can also assay the MIF indirectly by first culturing lymphocytes separately with antigen and then adding the supernatant from such culture to the macrophage culture.

Lymphocytes from normal (unimmunized) animals do not produce MIF in measurable quantities, apparently because they are not stimulated in sufficient numbers by the antigen. For a similar reason, lymphocytes immune to one antigen will not produce measurable amounts of MIF when exposed in culture to an-

Table 7.1 Factors Produced by Activated Lymphocytes

Factors Affecting Macrophages
Migration inhibitory factor (MIF)
Macrophage-activating factor (MAF)
Macrophage chemotactic factor (MCF)
Factors Affecting Polymorphonuclear Leukocytes
Leukocyte inhibitory factor (LIF)
Leukocyte chemotactic factor (LCF)
Factors Affecting Lymphocytes
T-cell growth factor (TCGF) or interleukin-2 (IL-2)
Factors affecting antibody production
Transfer factor
Factors Affecting Other Cell Types
Lymphotoxin
Growth inhibitory factor
Clonal inhibitory factor
Proliferation inhibitory factor
Interferon
Osteoclast-activating factor
Colony-stimulating activity

Table 7.2 Properties of Factors Produced by Activated Lymphocytes

Factor	Molecular Weight (Daltons)	Stability at 56°C	Disc Gel Electrophoresis[b]	Isopyknic Centrifugation in CsCl	Neuraminidase	Chymotrypsin
Migration inhibition factor	25,000 (H)[a]	Stable	Albumin (H)	Protein (H)	Resistant (H)	Sensitive
Macrophage-activating factor	35,000–55,000 (GP)		Prealbumin (GP)	Denser than protein (GP)	Sensitive (GP)	
Macrophage chemotactic factor	12,500 (H) 35,000–55,000 (GP)	Stable	Albumin	Protein	Resistant	Sensitive
Leukocyte inhibitory factor	68,000	Stable	Albumin	Protein	Resistant	Sensitive
T-cell growth factor (interleukin-2)	30,000–35,000	Stable		Protein		
T cell-replacing factor	25,000			Glycoprotein		
Specific helper factor	35,000–60,000					
Nonspecific suppressor factor	30,000					
Specific suppressor factor	35,000–60,000					
Transfer factor	4000	Labile				
Lymphotoxin	90,000 (H) 35,000–55,000 (GP)	Stable (H) Labile (GP)	Postalbumin (H) Albumin (GP)	Protein	Resistant	Sensitive
Interferon	25,000	Stable				

[a] H, human; GP, guinea pig.
[b] Migrates in the part of the gel associated with the individual protein.

other antigen. Normal lymphocytes, however, will produce MIF when activated by mitogens such as concanavalin A, for these substances activate a fair proportion of the lymphocyte population (see Chapter 10).

In vitro, MIF production can be demonstrated four to six hours after lymphocyte stimulation, and the stimulated cells continue to produce MIF for as long as four days, provided the stimulus persists. In vivo, the production of MIF—as well as that of most other mediators—is associated with delayed-type hypersensitivity (see Chapter 12). MIF has been demonstrated not only in guinea pigs, but also in other mammals, including humans. Its action is not species-specific: for example, MIF of human origin inhibits macrophages obtained from guinea pigs. This cross-reactivity occurs despite the fact that human and guinea pig MIFs differ in their properties. The guinea pig MIF molecules are larger (molecular weight of 35,000 to 55,000 daltons) than human MIF molecules (molecular weight of 25,000 daltons) and guinea pig MIF appears to be a neuraminidase-sensitive glycoprotein, whereas human MIF is a neuraminidase-resistant protein. The MIF is believed to act by making macrophage membranes stickier, causing macrophage clumping. It is apparently this clumping that causes the macrophages to pile up on one another at the opening of the capillary tube.

Macrophage-Activating Factor (MAF)

In 1974, George B. Mackaness and his co-workers demonstrated that macrophages of animals recovering from infections by intracellular parasites exhibit enhanced function in vitro. Such activated cells are more spread out on glass, more adherent, more phagocytic, more tumoricidal (they kill tumor cells), and more bactericidal (they kill microorganisms, even those antigenically unrelated to the ones that cause the original infection) than macrophages from uninfected animals. Similar activation of macrophages occurs by their exposure in vitro to supernatants from cultures of antigen-stimulated lymphocytes. Apparently, the stimulated lymphocytes produce a macrophage-

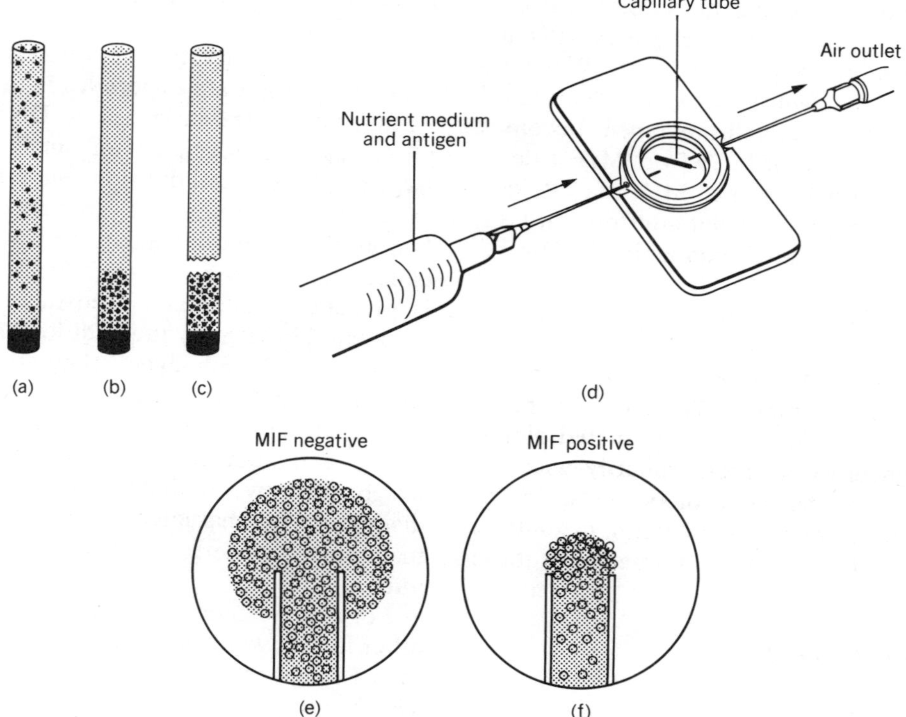

Figure 7.1. Method of assaying inhibition of macrophage migration in vitro. (*a*) Capillary tube filled with peritoneal exudate cells. (*b*) Capillary tube after centrifugation. (*c*) Breaking of capillary tube at the cell-medium interface. (*d*) Placement of the broken tube into a culture chamber. (*e*) and (*f*) Magnified unsealed tips of the capillary tube showing two patterns of macrophage migration—uninhibited (*e*) and inhibited (*f*).

activating factor (MAF) that enhances macrophage function both in vivo and in vitro.

In addition to the aforementioned signs of activation, there are others, such as increased ruffled-membrane activity, increased activity of membrane adenylate cyclase, increased incorporation of glucosamine into membrane components, an increased level of lactate dehydrogenase in the cytoplasm, an increased number of cytoplasmic granules, decreased electron-dense surface material, and decreased levels of certain lysosomal enzymes (acid phosphatase, cathepsin-D, β-glucuronidase). Measurement of these activities is used in some of the assays testing MAF effect.

Physicochemically, MAF is indistinguishable from MIF and the two might be the same. The difference between them might be only in the method of detection. The membrane stickiness produced by MIF (and the resulting migration inhibition) might be an early stage of macrophage activation; following this stage, the actual macrophage activation occurs, accompanied by many metabolic changes, and it is these changes that the MAF assays measure. Supporting this interpretation is the finding that while, in MIF assays, one observes an effect within 24 hours, one must wait three days to detect the activation in the MAF assay. The actual function of the MIF/MAF system in vivo is probably related to this late activation phase.

Macrophage (Monocyte) Chemotactic Factor (MCF)

To demonstrate this mediator, one uses a special culture chamber, consisting of two compartments separated by a micropore filter. One places a macrophage suspension in one chamber and supernatant from a culture of antigen-stimulated lymphocytes in the other. The mediator present in the supernatant diffuses into the cell chamber and establishes a concentration gradient that causes cells to move across the membrane into the supernatant chamber. Since the attraction of cells to chemical stimuli is referred to as chemotaxis (chemo + Gr. *taxis,* orderly arrangement), the mediator responsible for the macrophage movement in the chamber is termed *macrophage chemotactic factor*

(MCF). The direction of movement is determined by the direction of the gradient—the cells move toward the higher concentration of the mediator. When no gradient exists and the factor is evenly distributed throughout the chamber, the cell movement becomes chaotic. The distinctiveness of MCF from MIF is demonstrated by the observation that MIF placed in a chamber with macrophages does not interfere with the cell movement toward the MCF-containing chamber.

7.1.2 Factors Affecting Leukocytes

Leukocytes, as we already know from Chapter 5, are white blood cells present in the buffy coat—the upper, lighter cell layer of centrifuged, noncoagulated blood. Here, we shall concern ourselves primarily with the granulocytic portion of the white blood cells. Of the two known varieties of leukocyte-affecting mediators, one inhibits and the other heightens migration of these cells.

Leukocyte Inhibitory Factor (LIF)

To measure the effect of LIF, buffy-coat cells and lymphocytes are placed in capillary tubes. The lymphocytes can be derived from immune animals and restimulated in vitro by the addition of the immunizing antigen, or from normal animals and stimulated in vitro by the addition of a mitogen. The mediator released by the activated lymphocytes slows down the migration of leukocytes out of the capillary tube.

Leukocyte Chemotactic Factor (LCF)

There may be more than one factor affecting directed movement of lymphocytes. Some of these factors apparently act alone, while others seem to require an interaction with antigen-antibody complexes to become active. Whether there are separate factors for the three types of granulocyte (i.e., neutrophils, basophils, and eosinophils) is not known, although clearly, all three types are sensitive to LCF action. In vivo, LCF may play a role in chronic inflammation and delayed-type hypersensitivity reactions.

7.1.3. Lymphocyte-Affecting Factors

Several factors that are produced by and act on lymphocytes have been described. Their action results in lymphocyte activation, measured in terms of blast transformation, antibody synthesis, or induction of delayed-type hypersensitivity.

T-Cell Growth Factor (TCGF)

Mixing and cocultivation of lymphocytes derived from genetically disparate donors leads to lymphocyte activation, manifested in increased DNA synthesis, morphological transformation of small lymphocytes into large blasts, and cell division. Supernatants from such mixed lymphocyte cultures stimulate mitosis in normal lymphocytes, and this effect is ascribed to a mediator called the *T-cell growth factor* (TCGF). A similar factor is present in cultures of sensitized lymphocytes restimulated in vitro by the addition of an antigen and in cultures of T lymphocytes stimulated by mitogens and concanavalin A. The effect of TCGF can be measured by the incorporation of ^{3}H-thymidine into the DNA of the activated cells. The factor has a molecular weight of between 30,000 and 35,000 daltons and its distinguishing characteristic is that it promotes and maintains long-term cultures of T lymphocytes in vitro.

For completeness, we shall mention at this point one other factor, which is produced by *macrophages* rather than T lymphocytes, but which acts on T lymphocytes. This *lymphocyte-activating factor* (LAF) has a molecular weight of between 12,000 and 18,000 daltons and acts by promoting T-cell response to almost any kind of activating stimuli.

In a recent attempt to unify the nomenclature of lymphokines, the LAF and TCGF have been renamed *interleukins* (i.e., acting between leukocytes). LAF is now referred to as *interleukin*-1 (IL-1) and TCGF as *interleukin*-2 (IL-2). We shall have more to say about their functions in Chapter 12.

Factors Affecting Antibody Production

To produce antibodies, B cells require the presence of T cells. In 1971, Richard W. Dutton and his colleagues demonstrated that T cells can be replaced in this helper function by a soluble mediator, designated the *T-cell replacing factor* by Anneliese Schimpl and Eberhard Wecker, who described a similar mediator one year later. Schimpl and Wecker cocultured lymphocytes of mouse strain X with metabolically inactivated lymphocytes of strain Y in a mixed lymphocyte culture (Fig. 7.2; see Chapter 12). They then harvested the supernatant fluid from these cultures and added it, together with an antigen (sheep red blood cells), to a culture of spleen cells obtained from athymic mice. The addition of the supernatant caused the B cells in the culture to produce antibodies to the sheep red

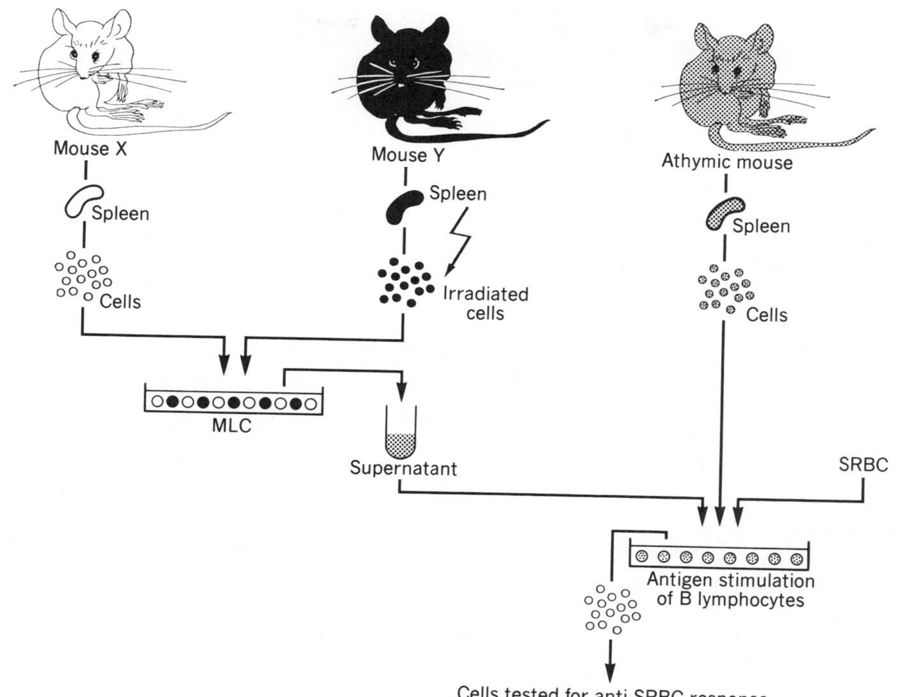

Figure 7.2. An experiment demonstrating the existence of the T-cell replacing factor. Explanation in the text. MLC, mixed lymphocyte culture; SRBC, sheep red blood cells.

blood cells in the absence of T lymphocytes. No antibodies were formed in cultures that did not contain the added supernatant or in cultures with supernatants from syngeneic mixtures of lymphocytes. The supernatant from the allogeneic mixed culture apparently contained the *T-cell replacing factor* (TRF), which performed the function of T helper cells (see Chapter 13). (Instead of mixed-lymphocyte-culture supernatants, one can use supernatants from mitogen-stimulated lymphocytes.) The T-cell replacing factor is nonspecific in that factors produced by lymphocytes of one strain act on B-cell cultures derived from the same or any other strain. The factor also lacks antigen specificity: the same factor promotes synthesis of antibodies to any antigen.

But there is also a second category of antibody synthesis-affecting factors that are antigen-specific. These have been described in several laboratories, and it is not clear just how many of them exist. As an example, we shall describe how the factor was produced by Michael J. Taussig (Fig. 7.3). He prepared bone marrow cells from an unimmunized donor mouse and injected them into three groups of syngeneic, irradiated recipients. The first group received no other cells (Fig. 7.3*a*); the second group received T cells prepared from mice immunized to an antigen, in this particular case the synthetic polypeptide (T,G)-A– –L (Fig. 7.3*b*); and the third group received a supernatant from a culture of syngeneic spleen cells incubated with (T,G)-A– –L and obtained from irradiated mice injected with hymus cells and (T,G)-A– –L (Fig. 7.3*c*). After the cell transfer, all three groups of mice were injected with (T,G)-A– –L and tested for the presence of (T,G)-A– –L-specific antibodies. As expected, the first group of mice, injected only with bone marrow cells and the antigen, failed to produce (T,G)-A– –L-specific antibodies (see Chapter 13); the second group, inoculated with both T and B cells, gave good antibody response; likewise, the third group, consisting of mice injected with B cells and the supernatant from a culture of antigen-activated, thymus-derived cells. also responded well to the injection of the same antigen. Apparently, the supernatant used in this third group contained a soluble factor that replaced the helper function of T cells. Further experiments demonstrated that the factor produced by (T,G)-A– –L-stimulated T cells acted on (T,G)-A– –L-binding B cells and had no effect when a different antigen was injected into the

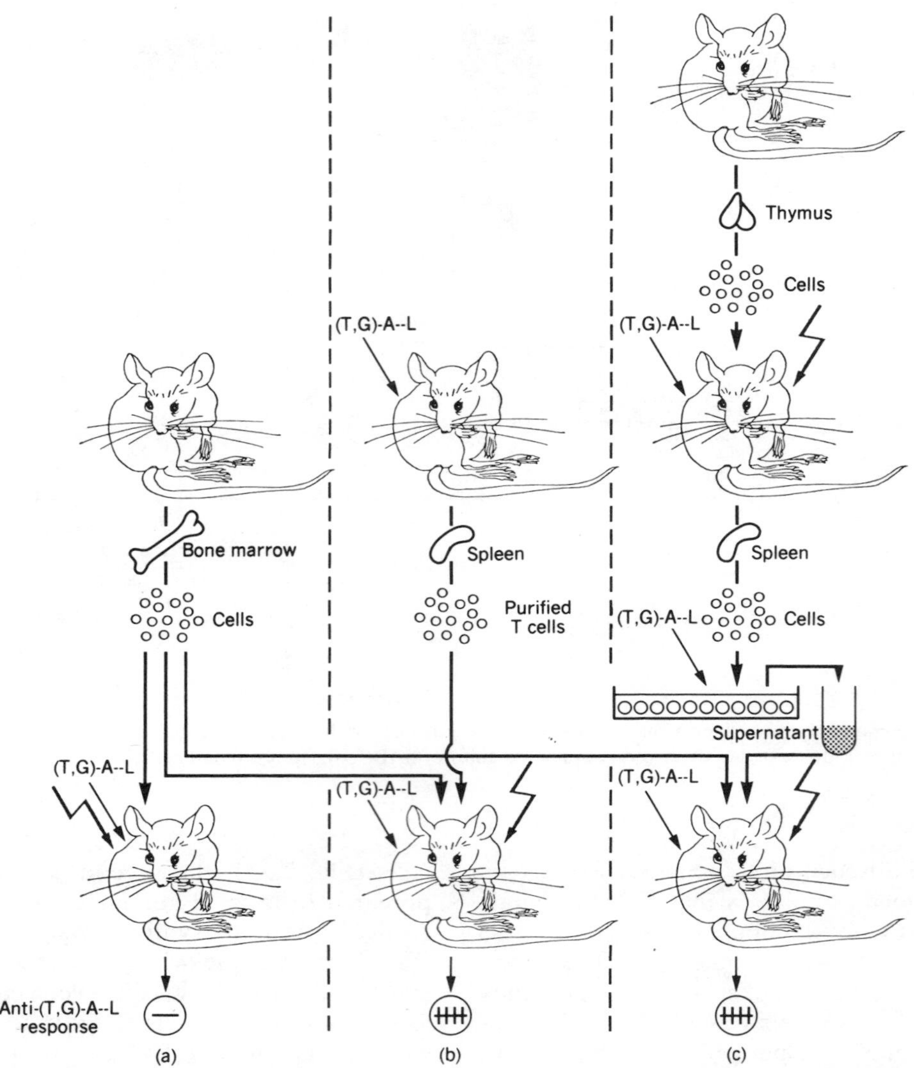

Figure 7.3. An experiment demonstrating the existence of antigen-specific T-helper factor. Explanation in the text. (T,G)-A--L, synthetic copolymer of tyrosine, glutamic acid, alanine, and lysine.

recipients in this third group of mice. In other words, the factor was antigen-specific.

Passage through a column of beads to which antibodies to class II major histocompatibility complex (MHC) molecules were covalently attached removed the factor from the supernatant. This observation is interpreted by many immunologists as evidence that the factor itself contains MHC molecules (see below).

Using somewhat different assay system, one can demonstrate that supernatants of antigen-activated T lymphocytes also contain factors that suppress, rather than enhance antibody response. These *suppressor factors*, like the helper factors, can be of either the nonspecific or specific variety. A nonspecific suppressor factor can be produced, for instance, by Con A stimulation of T lymphocytes in a tissue culture. As an example, we shall describe how a specific suppressor factor was produced by Tomio Tada and his colleagues (Fig. 7.4). Mice are immunized with protein X (e.g., keyhole limpet hemocyanin, KLH), and their T cells are injected into another mouse, together with a hapten (e.g., dinitrophenyl, DNP) coupled to protein X. While a control group of mice, injected only with the hapten-protein X conjugate, gives a normal antibody response to the hapten, the T cell-injected mice give almost no response. Apparently, in the new recipient,

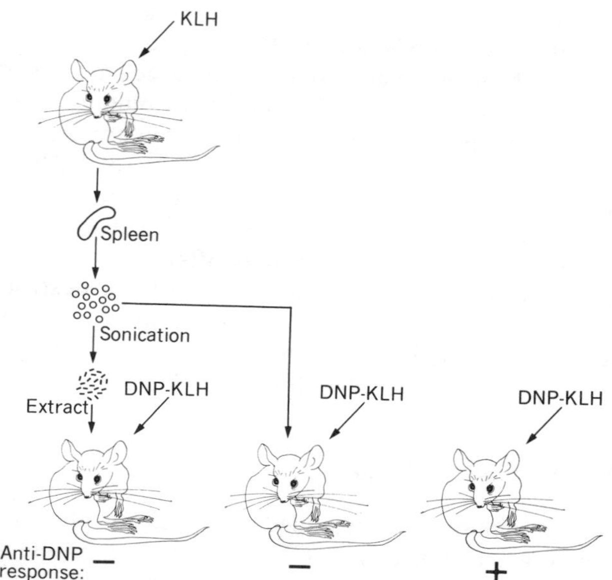

Figure 7.4. Generation of an antigen-specific suppressor factor. DNP, dinitrophenyl (hapten); KLH, keyhole limpet hemocyanin (carrier).

the T lymphocytes from the protein X-immunized mice act as suppressor cells that block the response to protein X and also to the hapten, since the hapten alone, without protein X (carrier), cannot immunize the host. Similar suppression can also be achieved by injecting an extract obtained from T lymphocytes disrupted by sonication, instead of viable T cells. The extract apparently contains a soluble factor responsible for the suppression of antibody response in the new host. A suppressor factor generated by immunization of mice with protein X suppresses response to a hapten conjugated to this protein and does not suppress the response in mice injected with the same hapten on a different protein. The suppressor factor is also removed by antibodies to class II MHC molecules.

The combination of these two properties—antigen specificity and reactivity with MHC antibodies—is the most puzzling thing about both the helper and suppressor factors, since size estimates indicate that both factors have a molecular weight of about 35,000 to 60,000 daltons. The complete MHC molecule of the type seemingly present in the helper factor alone has a molecular weight of about 60,000 daltons. Yet, when isolated from normal cells, the MHC molecules have no demonstrable antigen-binding activity, suggesting that the antigen specificity of the factor must be carried by some component other than the MHC. To allow for the factor's antigen specificity, one must postulate the antigen-binding component to be a reasonable size. (The smallest known antigen-binding immunoglobulin molecule has a molecular weight of about 150,000 daltons.) So one faces a dilemma that seems to be irreconcilable with present knowledge: one set of studies suggests the presence in the helper factor of two components, each of which has a molecular weight in excess of 35,000 daltons, while another set of studies indicates that the factor's molecular weight may not be greater than 35,000 daltons. There are several possible solutions to this conundrum. First, the factor may be a T-cell receptor (see below), which is not directly related to MHC molecules; the reactivity of anti-MHC sera with the factor would be an artifact caused by possible contamination of these sera with antibodies to the idiotype of the MHC antibodies. Since a similar idiotype can be expressed by T-cell receptors, the idiotypic antibodies may crossreact with the factor. A second possibility is that the factor may be composed of fragments of both the T-cell receptor and MHC molecules. As we shall see later, the T-cell receptor apparently recognizes antigens in conjunction with MHC molecules, and it may be that the factor is a degradation product of the complex formed by the T-cell receptor and the MHC molecule. Third, the MHC may contain a thus far unidentified class of genes coding for the T-cell receptor; antibodies to these hypothetical MHC molecules may contaminate antisera to known classes of MHC molecules. Finally, some of the known MHC molecules may—despite all the evidence to the contrary—possess an antigen-recognizing function.

I have listed these possibilities in what is, in my judgment, the order of decreasing likelihood. There may, of course, be a fifth explanation that no one has thought of yet.

Transfer Factor

In 1955, H. Sherwood Lawrence made an observation that to this day remains one of the most perplexing enigmas of modern immunology. He obtained leukocytes from the peripheral blood of a person who showed signs of moderate to strong delayed-type hypersensitivity to tuberculin or to diphtheria toxoid, disrupted the cells by repeated freezing and thawing, and injected the extracts into the skin of one arm of an unsensitized person. Twenty-four hours later, he injected the other arm of this recipient with the same antigen used for sensitization of the original cell-extract donor and observed a typical delayed-type hypersensitivity reaction at this second site. He concluded, therefore, that the extract contained a factor capable of transferring the delayed-type hypersensitivity reaction to an unsensitized person, and he designated this mediator the *transfer factor*. The puzzling thing about the transfer factor is that it is apparently of low molecular weight (less than 4000 daltons) and yet it appears to be antigen-specific: it confers on the treated person sensitivity only to the antigen used for the sensitization of the original donor and not to unrelated antigens. Immunologists are hard-pressed to come up with a substance that would contain so much information in so small a molecule. There is some evidence that the substance may be a single-stranded polynucleotide. The factor apparently acts by preparing normal lymphocytes so that they, too, are then able to respond to a given antigen by increased DNA synthesis and mediator production—the two phenomena characterizing the onset of delayed-type hypersensitivity. Success in using the transfer factor to correct immunodeficiencies has been claimed by some clinicians.

7.1.4 Mediators Affecting Other Cell Types

Lymphotoxin

The first mediator of this category was described in 1968 by Nancy H. Ruddle and Byron H. Waksman, who immunized rats to antigen X, cultured lymph node cells from the immunized animal in the presence of antigen X, and demonstrated that the cell-free supernatants from these cultures killed fibroblasts grown from rat embryos. The observation indicated that the stimulated lymphocytes produced a soluble toxin (hence the name *lymphocyte cytotoxic factor*, or *lymphotoxin*) that destroyed appropriate target cells. Later, similar lymphotoxins were demonstrated in mixed lymphocyte culture and in cultures of lymphocytes stimulated by mitogens. Lymphotoxin release can be demonstrated within hours following stimulation, and it continues for days at a uniform level. Although cells other than fibroblasts are also sensitive to the lymphotoxin action, many cells are resistant to it. Fibroblasts—in particular, the highly sensitive mouse cell line L—have remained the most convenient target in this type of study. Cell death caused by lymphotoxin can be ascertained through the change of cell morphology, the decrease in incorporation of labeled amino acids into the cell's cytoplasm, and the release of radioactivity by prelabeled cells. The action of lymphotoxin is nonspecific and independent of the species of origin (human lymphotoxin can act on mouse cells and vice versa). The binding of lymphotoxin to target cells probably occurs via specialized structures (receptors), and the presence or absence of these structures on a given cell type apparently determines this cell's susceptibility or resistance to the lymphotoxin.

It has been estimated that a single cell can bind about 600 lymphotoxin molecules. After binding, lymphotoxin triggers a series of events that injure the cell membrane and culminate in cell lysis. The role of lymphotoxin in vivo is unclear; the mediator may play a role in defense against emerging tumor cells. It acts over a short range, probably only after a lymphocyte has contacted a target cell and marked it for destruction. Inability to produce lymphotoxin may be one of the things wrong in patients with defective cell immunity (e.g., those afflicted with Hodgkin's disease or the Wiskott-Aldrich syndrome).

Growth Inhibitory Factors

Some mediators, when added to a culture of target cells (e.g., human HeLa cells), inhibit their proliferation and colony formation. The inhibitory action is ascribed to *proliferation inhibitory* and *clonal inhibitory factors*, respectively. However, since a low concentration of lymphotoxin can also inhibit growth rather than kill cells, it is possible that the three mediators are, in fact, identical.

Interferon

Many cells infected by a virus (they need not be lymphocytes) manufacture a soluble factor, *interferon*, which kills other virus-infected cells. We shall deal with interferon in more detail in Chapter 14.

There are several other mediators produced by lymphocytes that have no known immunological function (e.g., osteoclast-activating factor, procoagulant factor, colony-stimulating factor), and so will not be dealt with here.

7.1.5 Function of Mediators

Specific immune reactions begin by the binding of an antigen to the lymphocyte receptor. The initial number of antigen-binding cells is probably low, and so, to be effective, the reaction must be amplified rapidly. Such an amplification is probably the main function of factors produced by activated lymphocytes. The factors attract other cells to the site of the immune reaction, increase the activity of the immigrant cells, and activate other lymphocytes, which then produce more mediators, which stimulate more lymphocytes, and so on. At least some mediators also participate directly in the immune reaction in that they destroy cells identified by lymphocytes as being nonself.

7.2 THE T-CELL RECEPTOR

The T-cell receptor—the molecule in the T-cell membrane capable of specifically binding antigens—is the San Andreas Fault of immunology: here the plates rub against each other, shifting gradually and unnoticed, and a major "earthquake" may occur at any moment. One could probably write a book about this receptor—so much work has gone into its elucidation—but in the end, if one were to summarize the facts, the summary would not come to much more than the few pages that follow. What do we know about the T-cell receptor?

7.2.1 The T-Cell Receptor Does Exist

Because of the receptor's elusiveness, one may harbor some doubts as to whether T cells possess specific antigen receptors at all. The evidence for the receptor's existence comes from studies of antigen binding by T cells. To demonstrate antigen-binding T cells, one should, theoretically, be able to use the same methods as are used for the demonstration of B-cell receptors. But in practice, many of these methods—for unknown reasons—do not work easily with T cells. The one method that has consistently worked for most immunologists is the one in which the T cell commits suicide by binding highly radioactive antigens. When one incubates T cells in vitro with such a "hot" antigen, then washes the cells and injects them, together with B cells and an unlabeled antigen, into X-irradiated mice, the mice become specifically unresponsive to this antigen while retaining normal responsiveness to other antigens. The results of this experiment can be interpreted as evidence that high levels of radioactivity kill cells that bind the labeled antigen, so that after the injection into the animal, there are no T cells left to provide the necessary help for B cells capable of responding to the particular antigen. In addition, experiments demonstrating antigen-binding T cells by autoradiography, rosette formation, or retention of T cells on antigen-coated columns have worked in the hands of at least some investigators, so that there can be little doubt that T cells, like B cells, can bind antigens specifically.

7.2.2 Antigen Specificity of T Lymphocytes

How does the antigen specificity of T cells compare with that of B cells? Are T cells equally, more, or less specific than B cells? The answers to these questions depend on whom one asks. Some immunologists have reported experimental evidence demonstrating that there is no difference between T cells and antibodies in their crossreactivity patterns to a given set of antigens; others claim that T cells are more broadly crossreactive than antibodies. The problem with these comparisons is that they are not fair to the T cells, since the reactivity pattern of a T cell is measured following its activation by the antigen, whereas crossreactivity of antibodies is measured by their mere binding of the antigen. Since it is a long way from antigen binding to the fully activated lymphocyte, one is asking, in such experiments, much more from T cells than from antibody molecules. Also, T-cell receptors and antibodies may not always recognize the same set of determinants, so that failure of antibodies to bind with certain determinants does not necessarily imply narrower antibody crossreactivity. In all experiments in which the two objections were minimized, the outcome has always been that the discriminatory power of T-cell receptors is the same as that of antibodies.

7.2.3 The T-Cell Receptor Repertoire

The second question many immunologists have asked regarding the T-cell receptor is whether the receptor has the power to recognize the same range of antigens as the antibodies. There is an old observation that one can easily induce antibodies to a hapten (provided it is presented to B cells on an appropriate carrier), but one cannot stimulate cellular (T-cell) immunity to these simple compounds so easily. Some immunologists have used this observation to argue that the repertoire of the T-cell receptor is devoid of hapten-recognizing specificity and so is more limited than that of antibodies. Is it really true that T cells cannot be activated by haptens? Immunologists are once again split into two camps—one says yes, the other says no. Experiments supporting one or the other view have been reported, but it is probably a fair assessment of the situation to state that none of the experiments purporting T-cell activation by haptens is completely free of serious objections. The most difficult part of these experiments is proving that T-cell reactivity is indeed directed to the hapten itself and not to some other determinants generated by the hapten's attachment to the carrier molecule. On the other hand, B cells alone—without the help of T cells—cannot be activated by haptens either. Since T cells bind haptens, there is little reason to believe that the diversity of the T-cell receptor repertoire is different from that of the B lymphocyte.

7.2.4 The Preoccupation of the T-Cell Receptor with MHC Molecules

In 1974, Rolf M. Zinkernagel and Peter C. Doherty discovered a completely new and unexpected feature of the T-cell receptor—its preoccupation with the MHC molecules. The discovery stemmed from the following experiment (Fig. 7.5). Zinkernagel and Doherty inoculated a mouse of hypothetical strain X with a virus, which, for the sake of simplicity, we shall refer to as virus 1. After a few days, they killed the mouse and added its spleen cells to a culture of X-strain fibroblasts (target cells) infected with virus 1 and labeled with radioactive isotope. Lysis of the fibroblasts (manifested by the release of the cytoplasmically bound radioactive isotope) indicated that, in the mouse, cytotoxic (cytolytic, killer, effector) T cells were generated against the virus-infected cells, and that these cells were also able to destroy target cells in vitro. As expected from earlier studies done by other investigators, the cytotoxic cells were specific for the virus in the sense that they destroyed cells infected by virus 1, but not cells infected by another virus. Most surprisingly, however, the cytotoxic T lymphocytes also possessed a second specificity, one for the MHC molecules of the strain from which they originated. Thus, X-strain lymphocytes, immune to virus 1, killed virus 1-infected target cells of other strains, provided all these strains shared their MHC alleles with X. Virus 1-infected target cells derived from congenic lines that shared with X all genes except those belonging to the MHC were not killed by these cytotoxic T cells. T lymphocytes immune to a given virus thus display a dual specificity: they are specific for the infecting virus and for the MHC of the immunizing cell (normally the MHC of the mouse inoculated with the virus). They kill only target cells matched for these two specificities, cells infected with the same virus and expressing the same MHC molecule as the original donor of the cytotoxic cells. Evidence for this dual specificity of cytolytic T lymphocytes is summarized in Table 7.3.

Table 7.3 Reactivity of Cytotoxic T Lymphocytes with Different Normal or Virus-Infected Target Cells

Cytotoxic T Lymphocyte	Killing of Target Cells					
	a	*a*-v_1	*a*-v_2	*b*	*b*-v_1	*b*-v_2
a anti-v_1	−	+	−	−	−	−
a anti-v_2	−	−	+	−	−	−
b anti-v_1	−	−	−	−	+	−
b anti-v_2	−	−	−	−	−	+

a, *b*, alleles at the MHC loci; v_1, v_2, virus 1 and virus 2; *a* anti-v_1, cytotoxic T cells generated in mice carrying the *a* MHC allele and infected with virus 1; a-v_1, target cells carrying the *a* MHC allele and infected with virus 1 (*a* alone signifies uninfected cells); +, cell lysis; −, absence of cell lysis

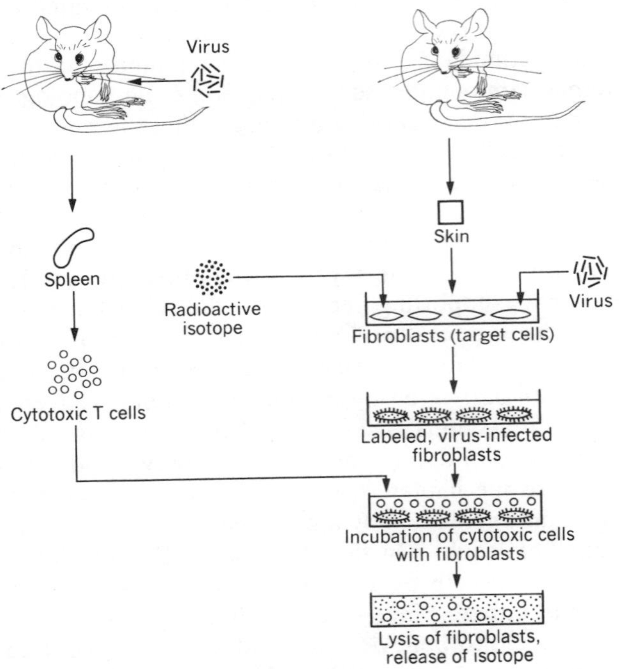

Figure 7.5. Experimental design for testing MHC restriction of cytotoxic cells generated against viral antigens.

Zinkernagel and Doherty explained their experiment by postulating that T lymphocytes recognize an antigen (in this instance, an antigen appearing as a consequence of a virus infection) together with the individual's own MHC molecules and become immune to a particular antigen-MHC combination. Such lymphocytes can then interact only with target cells carrying the same antigen-MHC combination; when one component in this combination changes (either the antigen or the MHC molecules), no reaction occurs. Since the MHC appears to restrict the specificity of T lymphocytes, the phenomenon is called *MHC restriction*. Studies by Michael J. Bevan, Gene M. Shearer, Elizabeth Simpson, and their collaborators have demonstrated that MHC restriction is not limited to viral antigens, but encompasses all sorts of other antigens. In fact, it appears that precursors of cytotoxic T cells cannot "see" antigens except in the context of MHC molecules. In this respect, the body adheres to the etiquette of a proper English home: a foreigner can be introduced only by a person known to the family.

Evidence that other T lymphocytes—helper and suppressor cells—also recognize antigens only in the context of MHC molecules will be discussed in Chapter 13.

7.2.5 Thymus as the Lymphocyte Training Center?

In normal circumstances, T lymphocytes recognize antigens in the context of the individual's own MHC molecules; that is, lymphocytes from individual X recognize antigens in the context of MHC-X molecules, lymphocytes from individual Y recognize antigens in the context of MHC-Y molecules, and so on. But where do the lymphocytes learn in which MHC context they should recognize antigens? The answer to this question is not available. Experiments done by Rolf M. Zinkernagel, Michael J. Bevan, and their colleagues suggest that the MHC specificity of T lymphocytes is determined in the thymus by the MHC molecules of the thymic epithelium. However, other investigators dispute the interpretation of these experiments or even contradict it with experimental data suggesting that the thymus plays either no role at all or only a limited role in determining the repertoire of the T-cell receptor.

7.2.6 One or Two Receptors?

There are two principal ways (and many variants of these) of explaining the dual specificity of T lymphocytes (Fig. 7.6). One hypothesis postulates that there is only one kind of T-cell receptor, which recognizes the antigen and MHC molecules (or more precisely, portions thereof) simultaneously. Such a hypothesis presupposes that the antigen either associates directly with the MHC or at least comes so close to it in the plasma membrane that the two are seen as one by the T-cell receptor. A variant of this hypothesis postulates that the antigen, by interacting with the MHC molecules, actually modifies the latter, and it is this *altered self* that the T-cell receptor recognizes. According to the second hypothesis, there are two kinds of T-cell receptor—one for antigen, and the other for MHC molecules. The two receptors may differ only in their specificity and belong biochemically to the same class of molecules, or they may be molecules of two different classes. There is some experimental evidence supporting the first and some other evidence supporting the second hypothesis. The current debate about the merits of the two hypotheses resembles a soccer game between two well-matched teams: now it is the blue team that is winning, and now the red, but the decisive goal has yet to be scored.

7.2.7 The Nature of the T-Cell Receptor

In the early 1970s, immunologists from several laboratories reported that their anti-Ig sera (i.e., sera reacting with class-specific determinants of the constant immunoglobulin region) reacted with T cells as easily as they reacted with B cells, implying that the T-cell receptor was an immunoglobulin. However, other immunologists, using the same reagents and the same assay system, found no trace of known immunoglobulins on the T-cell surface. Time has shown the latter investigators to be right: in carefully controlled experiments, available anti-Ig sera do not detect any significant amount of Ig on T cells; the earlier positive results must, therefore, have been artifacts.

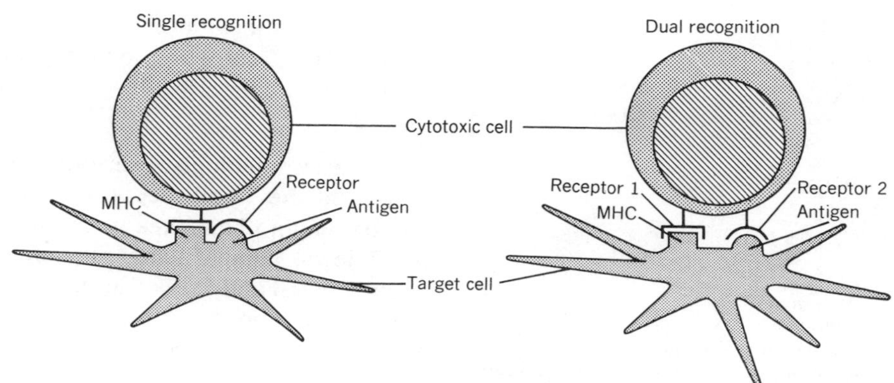

Figure 7.6. Two interpretations of dual T-lymphocyte specificity.

The observation that antisera to constant-region determinants of known immunoglobulin classes do not react with T cells does not, however, exclude the possibility that the T-cell receptor is an immunoglobulin-related molecule. On the contrary, some evidence is available that both the B-cell and T-cell receptors may share at least their V regions.

As an example of such evidence, we shall mention the experiment reported by Klaus Rajewsky, Klaus Eichmann, and their colleagues. It is a complicated experiment, so, for the sake of clarity, we shall divide it into several steps (Fig. 7.7). In the first step, Rajewsky, Eichmann, and their colleagues immunized A/J-strain mice with group-A streptococcal carbohydrate (A-CHO) and obtained homogeneous antibodies that shared the same A5A idiotype. In the second step, they injected these antibodies into guinea pigs and produced antibodies that reacted with the A5A idiotype carried by the anti-A-CHO immunoglobulin. In the third step, they injected the guinea pig antibodies into another set of A/J mice. In the fourth step, they killed the mice from step two and injected the spleen cells of these mice, together with spleen cells of another group of A/J mice, immunized against a hapten (4-hydroxy-5-iodo-3-nitrophenylacetyl, or NIP) on a carrier protein (chicken gamma globulin), into still another set of X-irradiated A/J mice. In the fifth step, they injected NIP, conjugated to A-CHO, into the irradiated recipients from step four, and measured the antibody response to NIP and to A-CHO. They observed that both NIP and the A-CHO antibodies were produced under these circumstances, and explained this observation by postulating that the antibodies recognizing the A5A idiotype of the anti-A-CHO carbohydrate also reacted with the A5A idiotype of the T-cell receptor (inset in Fig. 7.7), and that this reaction triggered the T-helper cells (a situation analogous to activation of B cells by allotypic antisera; see Chapter 6).

Since the A5A idiotype is characteristic of those V regions capable of reacting with the group-A carbohydrate, the activated T-helper cells must, the investigators argue, have specificity for this carbohydrate. When injected into the irradiated mice, the T cells provide the necessary help to B cells immune to NIP, and NIP antibody production ensues. The simultaneous production of A-CHO antibodies indicates that the A5A antibodies also reacted with the A5A idiotype of the B-cell receptor, and that this reaction activated B cells. Thus, the same idiotypic antibody can react with both B-cell and T-cell receptors, indicating that the two receptors have idiotypes in common. These data can be reconciled with the failure to detect a known immunoglobulin class on T cells by postulating that the T-cell receptor represents a new class of immunoglobulin molecules not expressed on B cells.

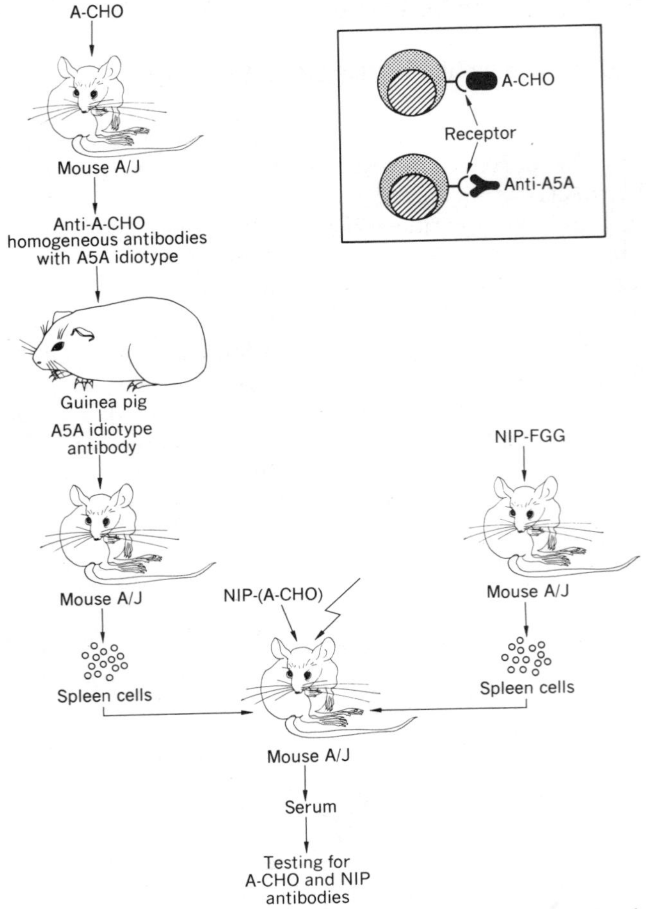

Figure 7.7. Experimental design for T helper-cell activation by idiotypic antibodies. A-CHO, group-A streptococcal carbohydrate; FGG, fowl globulin; NIP, 4-hydroxy-5-iodo-3-nitrophenylacetyl (hapten). Inset shows two modes of T-cell activation: by antigen (A-CHO) and by idiotypic antibody (anti-A5A).

Some immunologists seriously entertain the possibility that the T-cell receptor consists of only one immunoglobulin chain (heavy chain?). The experiments by Rajewsky and Eichmann (and similar studies by Hans Wigzell and Hans Binz), although supporting the immunoglobulin hypothesis of the T-cell receptor, nevertheless do not prove it. Such proof will be possible only when the receptor is isolated and chemically characterized. Until this happens, other interpretations of the T-cell receptor's nature (e.g., that the receptor is controlled, in part, by loci in the MHC) will remain possible.

REFERENCES

General

Bergstrand, H.: Lymphocyte-derived factors affecting cell migration in vitro. *Allergy* **34**:69–96, 1979.

Cohen, S., Pick, E., and Oppenheim, J. J. (Eds.): *Biology of the Lymphokines*. Academic, New York, 1979.

Möller, G. (Ed.): *Acquisition of the T-Cell Repertoire. Immunol. Reviews*, Vol. 42. Munksgaard, Copenhagen, 1978.

Rocklin, R. E., Bendtzen, K., and Greineder, D.: Mediators of immunity: lymphokines and monokines. *Adv. Immunol.* **29**:55–136, 1980.

Rosenau, W. and Tsoukas, C. C.: Lymphotoxin. A review and analysis. *Amer. J. Pathol.* **84**:580–596, 1976.

Zinkernagel, R. M. and Doherty. P. C.: MHC-restricted cytotoxic cells: studies on the biological role of polymorphic major transplantation antigens determining T-cell restriction specificity, function, and responsiveness. *Adv. Immunol.* **27**:51–177, 1979.

Original Articles

Bevan, M. J.: The major histocompatibility complex determines susceptibility to cytotoxic T cells directed against minor histocompatibility antigens. *J. Exp. Med.* **142**:1349–1364, 1975.

Bloom, B. R. and Bennett, B.: Mechanism of a reaction in vitro associated with delayed-type hypersensitivity. *Science* **153**: 80–82, 1966.

David, J. R.: Delayed hypersensitivity in vitro: its mediation by cell-free substances formed by lymphoid cell-antigen interaction. *Proc. Natl. Acad. Sci. U.S.A.* **56**:72–77, 1966.

Eichmann, K. and Rajewsky, K.: Induction of T and B cell immunity by anti-idiotypic antibody. *Eur. J. Immunol.* **5**:661–666, 1975.

Fink, P. J. and Bevan, M. J.: H-2 antigens of the thymus determine lymphocyte specificity. *J. Exp. Med.* **148**:766–775, 1978.

George, M. and Vaughan, J. H.: In vitro cell migration as a model for delayed hypersensitivity. *Proc. Soc. Exp. Biol. Med.* **111**:514–521, 1962.

Gordon, R. D., Simpson, E., and Samelson, L. E.: In vitro cell-mediated immune responses to the male-specific (H-Y) antigen in mice. *J. Exp. Med.* **142**:1108–1120, 1975.

Lawrence, H. S.: The transfer in humans of delayed skin sensitivity to streptococcal M substances and to tuberculin with disrupted leukocytes. *J. Clin. Invest.* **34**:219–230, 1955.

Mackness, G. B.: The immunological basis of acquired cellular resistance. *J. Exp. Med.* **120**:105–120, 1964.

Rich, A. R. and Lewis, M. R.: The nature of allergy in tuberculosis as revealed by tissue culture studies. *Bull. Johns Hopkins Hosp.* **50**:115–131, 1932.

Ruddle, N. H. and Waksman, B. H.: Cytotoxic effect of lymphocyte-antigen interaction in delayed hypersensitivity. *Science* **157**:1060–1061, 1967.

Schimpl, A. and Wecker, E.: Replacement of T-cell function by a T-cell product. *Nature* (*Lond.*) **237**:15–17, 1972.

Shearer, G. M., Rehn, T. G., and Garbarino, C. A.: Cell-mediated lympholysis of trinitrophenyl-modified autologous lymphocytes. Effector cell specificity to modified cell surface components controlled by the H-2K and H-2D serological regions of the murine major histocompatibility complex. *J. Exp. Med.* **141**:1348–1364, 1975.

Takemori, T. and Tada, T.: Properties of antigen-specific suppressive T-cell factor in the regulation of antibody response of the mouse. I. In vivo activity and immunochemical characterizations. *J. Exp. Med.* **142**:1241–1253, 1975.

Taussig, M. J.: T cell factor which can replace T cells in vivo. *Nature* **248**:234–236, 1974.

Zinkernagel, R. M. and Doherty, P. C.: Restriction of in vivo T cell-mediated cytotoxicity in lymphocytic choriomeningitis within a syngeneic or semiallogeneic system. *Nature* (*Lond.*) **248**:701–703, 1974.

Zinkernagel, R. M., Callahan, G. N., Althage, A., Cooper, S., Klein, P. A., and Klein, J.: On the thymus in the differentiation of "H-2 self recognition" by T cells: evidence for dual recognition? *J. Exp. Med.* **147**:882–896, 1978.

Zinkernagel, R. M., Callahan, G. N., Althage, A., Cooper, S., Streilein, D. W., and Klein, J.: The lymphoreticular system in triggering virus plus self-specific cytotoxic T cells: evidence for T help. *J. Exp. Med.* **147**:897–911, 1978.

CHAPTER 8

THE MAJOR HISTOCOMPATIBILITY COMPLEX

We have alluded to the major histocompatibility complex (MHC) many times in the preceding chapters; it is now time to become acquainted with it in detail. The mere fact that we have mentioned it so often testifies to its importance. Yet, the MHC products were the last of the major immunologically important molecules to be discovered, and even after their discovery, it was some time before their significance for immunology was realized.

8.1 DEFINITIONS

The major histocompatibility complex is a group of closely linked loci coding for molecules that restrict the specificity of antigen recognition by T lymphocytes. The loci fall into two classes, which we shall refer to here as class I and class II: class I loci restrict antigen recognition predominantly by cytotoxic T lymphocytes, class II predominantly by regulatory T cells. In addition to these functional differences, the products of the two classes also differ in their serological properties, tissue distribution, and biochemical composition.

The chromosomal segment occupied by class I and class II loci also contains other loci, which may or may not be related to the genuine MHC loci. The most prominent among the accompanying loci are those coding for certain complement components. These loci are considered to be part of the MHC by most immunologists, and are grouped under the heading of class III loci. In this text, we shall discuss the class III loci in the chapter devoted to complement (Chapter 9). All other MHC-associated loci will be referred to as class IV loci.

The word "histocompatibility" in the MHC designation refers to the fact that the recognition of class I or class II MHC molecules by receptors on T lymphocytes determines tissue compatibility or incompatibility. This recognition can be of two kinds: in one, the T cells recognize the MHC molecules alone; in the second, they recognize a non-MHC molecule (a conventional antigen) and an MHC molecule simultaneously. The first kind of recognition normally occurs only in experimental situations, where cells, tissues, or organs are transplanted from one individual to another—provided, of course, that the two individuals differ in their MHC molecules. It was, however, this form of incompatibility that led to the discovery of MHC in the first place (see Chapter 2). The T-cell response to nonself MHC molecules is termed *alloreactivity*. The second kind of recognition occurs whenever a T lymphocyte encounters another cell that expresses nonself matter. The lymphocyte cannot recognize this matter unless it recognizes the MHC molecules on this cell simultaneously.

The term "major" in the MHC designation refers to the fact that there are many tissue compatibility loci, but among these, the MHC loci occupy a special position and are of prime immunological importance. The term "complex" indicates that more than one locus is involved.

MHC is a general term used to refer to this group of loci in any species. The MHCs of individual species have separate names: *histocompatibility*-2, or *H*-2, in the mouse (the use of "2" was explained in Chapter 2), *human leukocyte A*, or *HLA*, in humans, *rat locus* 1, or *RT*1, in the rat, *guinea pig leukocyte antigen locus,* or *GPLA*, in the guinea pig, and the *B* complex in the domestic fowl. (The blood-group antigens of the fowl have been serially designated *A*, *B*, and *C*, and *B* has turned out to be the species' MHC.)

8.2 SEROLOGY

Two individuals often differ in the biochemical composition of their MHC molecules, and this difference is recognized by both T and B lymphocytes when MHC molecules of one individual are introduced into another. The recipient responds to such an introduction by destroying the cells carrying the foreign MHC molecules and by producing antibodies to the foreign antigenic determinants. The analysis of anti-MHC sera is an art (some might say black magic) that one masters only after many years of apprenticeship. Here we shall acquaint ourselves only with the principles of serological analysis and then with the general interpretation of MHC serology; for more detailed treatment of the subject, the reader is referred to one of the specialized manuals listed at the end of this chapter.

8.2.1 Principles

Serological MHC analysis of a species with available inbred strains is performed somewhat differently from that of a species consisting mostly of outbred individuals. In the following, we shall describe the principles of the two types of analysis, using the mouse as an example of the former and the human to illustrate the latter.

The Mouse

Let us consider three inbred mouse strains—X, Y, and Z—and let us assume that we are back in the 1950s, when MHC analysis was just beginning. We have no anti-MHC sera available and we have no idea what kind of MHC molecules the three strains carry. How do we go about defining mouse MHC?

We arrange the three strains into pairs in all possible combinations so that in each pair one strain is the recipient and the other is the donor. We thus have six strain combinations: X anti-Y, X anti-Z, Y anti-X, Y anti-Z, Z anti-X, and Z anti-Y. We then inject tissues of the donor repeatedly into the recipient until antibodies against the donor cells appear in the recipient's serum. Then we obtain as much antiserum as possible by repeated immunization and bleeding, pool the individual bleedings, and use the pools for analysis.

Let us assume that all immunizations were successful, so that we obtained six antisera. When we test these antisera against the three cell types—X, Y, and Z—we may find that each antiserum reacts not only with the immunizing, but also with the third-party strain (Table 8.1). For example, X anti-Y may react not only with Y, but also with Z. The reaction with the third-party strain indicates that this strain shares an antigenic determinant with the immunizing strain. To determine whether the immunizing strain also possesses a determinant lacking in the third-party strain, we must do an *absorption analysis* (Table 8.2). For example, when we incubate the X anti-Y serum with Z cells, the antibodies to the shared determinant will

Table 8.1 Reactivity of Six Hypothetical Antisera Generated by Crossimmunization of Three Hypothetical Inbred Strains

Antiserum	Reactivity with Cells X	Y	Z
X anti-Y	−	+	+
X anti-Z	−	+	+
Y anti-X	+	−	+
Y anti-Z	+	−	+
Z anti-X	+	+	−
Z anti-Y	+	+	−

+, positive reaction; −, negative reaction

bind to these cells and be removed with them from the antiserum when the cells and fluid are subsequently separated by centrifugation. One says that the antibodies are *absorbed out* from the antiserum. If Z cells carry only the shared, but not the Y-specific determinant, antibodies to this determinant should be unaffected by the absorption, and the absorbed antiserum, which no longer reacts with Z cells, should still react with Y cells. If, on the other hand, the X anti-Y serum contains antibodies only against the shared determinant, the absorbed antiserum should react with neither the Z nor the Y cells. In this manner, we take the antisera one by one and determine, by absorption analysis, what antibodies they contain.

Upon completion of this analysis, we have defined a series of antigenic determinants to which we assign numbers. For example, we can designate the shared

Table 8.2 Absorption Analysis of the Six Hypothetical Antisera from Table 8.1

Antiserum	Absorbed by	Reactivity with Cells X	Y	Z
X anti-Y	Z	−	+	−
X anti-Z	Y	−	−	+
Y anti-X	Z	+	−	−
Y anti-Z	X	−	−	+
Z anti-X	Y	+	−	−
Z anti-Y	X	−	+	−

+, positive reaction; −, negative reaction

Table 8.3 Antigenic Determinants Defined by the Six Hypothetical Antisera Analyzed in Tables 8.1 and 8.2

Strain	Antigenic Determinant 1	2	3	4	5	6
X	1	−	3	−	−	6
Y	−	2	3	−	5	−
Z	1	−	−	4	5	−

1, 2, 3, etc., presence of antigenic determinant; −, absence of antigenic determinant

determinant defined by the X anti-Y serum determinant 1, the X-specific determinant 2, the shared determinant defined by the X anti-Z serum determinant 3, and so on. However, some of the determinants defined by different antisera are serologically indistinguishable. For example, X anti-Y and X anti-Z both define determinants shared by Y and Z, and these determinants are regarded as identical until they are proved to be distinct by later inclusion of additional strains into the panel. The maximum number of determinants that can be identified with three strains is thus six (Table 8.3).

If the immunization has been carried out between inbred strains that differ at many genetic loci, we must, as a next step in the analysis, establish by a *linkage test* whether all the determinants belong to the same genetic system. For example, we can produce (X × Y) F_1 × Y backcross progeny and type them for determinants 1 and 6 of the X parent. If the loci coding for the two determinants are on different (nonhomologous) chromosomes, we obtain four types of progeny—1^+6^+, 1^-6^-, 1^+6^-, and 1^-6^+—in approximately equal numbers. If the two determinants are controlled by the same locus, we obtain only two types of progeny—1^+6^+ and 1^-6^-. Finally, if the two determinants are controlled by two linked loci, we obtain four types of progeny, but the parental 1^+6^+ and 1^-6^- types will be in excess of the recombinant types, 1^+6^- and 1^-6^+. A similar test must also be done with the remaining four determinants.

The distinction between determinants controlled by a single locus and those controlled by separate but closely linked loci is a difficult one to make. When one finds rare recombinant types, one can argue that they might have resulted from an intragenic crossingover, and when one does not find such types, one can always say that it is because not enough progeny have been tested. One way of solving this dilemma is to combine the serological analysis with biochemical tests and to determine whether the two determinants controlled by a single chromosome are carried by one or two separate polypeptide chains. In the former case, the two determinants are presumed to be controlled by a single locus, and in the latter case, by two separate loci. Another less convincing way is the cocapping method described in Chapter 6.

Serological analysis of three strains is relatively simple, but as more strains are added, a complete study of the type just described becomes impractical. Modern serological analysis of the MHC, therefore, uses a shortcut approach, carried out as follows. One first prepares a battery of antisera (typing reagents) that define individual antigenic determinants. A typing reagent is usually an antiserum prepared in a strain combination identical or closely related to the one originally used to define a given determinant. But the reagent is conditioned in such a way as to contain, ideally, antibodies to only one determinant. Such an antiserum is referred to as *monospecific*, in contrast to *oligospecific* or *polyspecific* antisera, containing antibodies to several or many antigenic determinants. However, in conventional serological analysis, monospecificity is always defined operationally, which amounts to saying, "I have done everything in my power to eliminate antibodies to all determinants but one; however, the antisera may still contain antibodies to several other determinants I have no way of knowing about." For example, one can make the X anti-Y serum operationally monospecific for determinant 2 by absorption with Z; but it is possible that the X strain carries more than one X strain-specific determinant and that the antiserum may, even after absorption, contain more than one antibody to these determinants. The additional determinants may be distinguished later by the inclusion of new strains in the analyzed sample, or they may never be separated. Operational monospecificity of typing reagents is achieved by extensive absorption and must be ascertained by testing the absorbed sera against a panel of prototype strains carrying known MHC alleles. The battery of typing reagents is then used to test any new strain, and the presence or absence of known antigenic determinants is established. This typing reveals whether the MHC of the new strain resembles any of the MHCs already known. To search for new antigenic determinants, one chooses one or two strains, immunizes them with tissues of the new strain, and analyzes the antisera by testing them against the available panel of inbred strains.

Lately, conventional antisera are being replaced by monoclonal antibodies to MHC determinants. Such antibodies have an advantage in that they are known to be not only operationally, but truly monospecific (or possibly oligospecific, in some instances).

MHC serology is an open-ended system: the more reagents and strains one uses, the more complete the picture becomes. But the system is so complex that to close it completely may not be practical.

The Human

In the outbred human population, no two individuals (with rare exceptions) are genetically the same. Since genetic differences are also reflected in antigenic differences, the chances are low that an antiserum generated by immunization of individual X by cells of individual Y could be reproduced by immunization between two other individuals. Although different antisera may contain antibodies to the same determinant, they will probably also contain antibodies to other determinants, and the composition of these antibodies in different antisera will be different. To analyze such antisera, one must use a strategy different from that used for the analysis of antisera produced in inbred individuals. Instead of concentrating on a few antisera and attempting to identify all the antibodies present by exhaustive absorption analysis with a small number of inbred strains, one obtains a large battery of antisera and tests them against a large panel of cells (Fig. 8.1). The individual results of such a testing are like individual pieces of a jigsaw puzzle that one must assemble in the proper way to obtain a coherent picture. Such an assembly, however, is not an easy task. If one has tested, say, 50 antisera against 100 cells (the usual sample size of a single test in human MHC serology), one is dealing with a jigsaw puzzle consisting of 500 pieces—a challenging proposition even for an experienced puzzle solver. The matter is complicated further by the fact that, in the serological puzzle, one does not know in advance the picture one is assembling. The serologist, however, has certain rules to work by and certain tools to help him get the work done.

The first step in serological puzzle assembly is to group together, on the one hand, antisera with similar reactivity patterns and, on the other hand, antisera with antithetical (opposite) patterns. The former are presumably those that share antibodies to a single determinant or group of determinants; the latter presumably detect determinants controlled by allelic genes. Thus, in contrast to inbred-strain serology, where determinants are defined by individual antisera, outbred serology—at least in its initial phase—is based on the use of blocks of antisera. The antisera within each block are similar to one another in their reactivity pat-

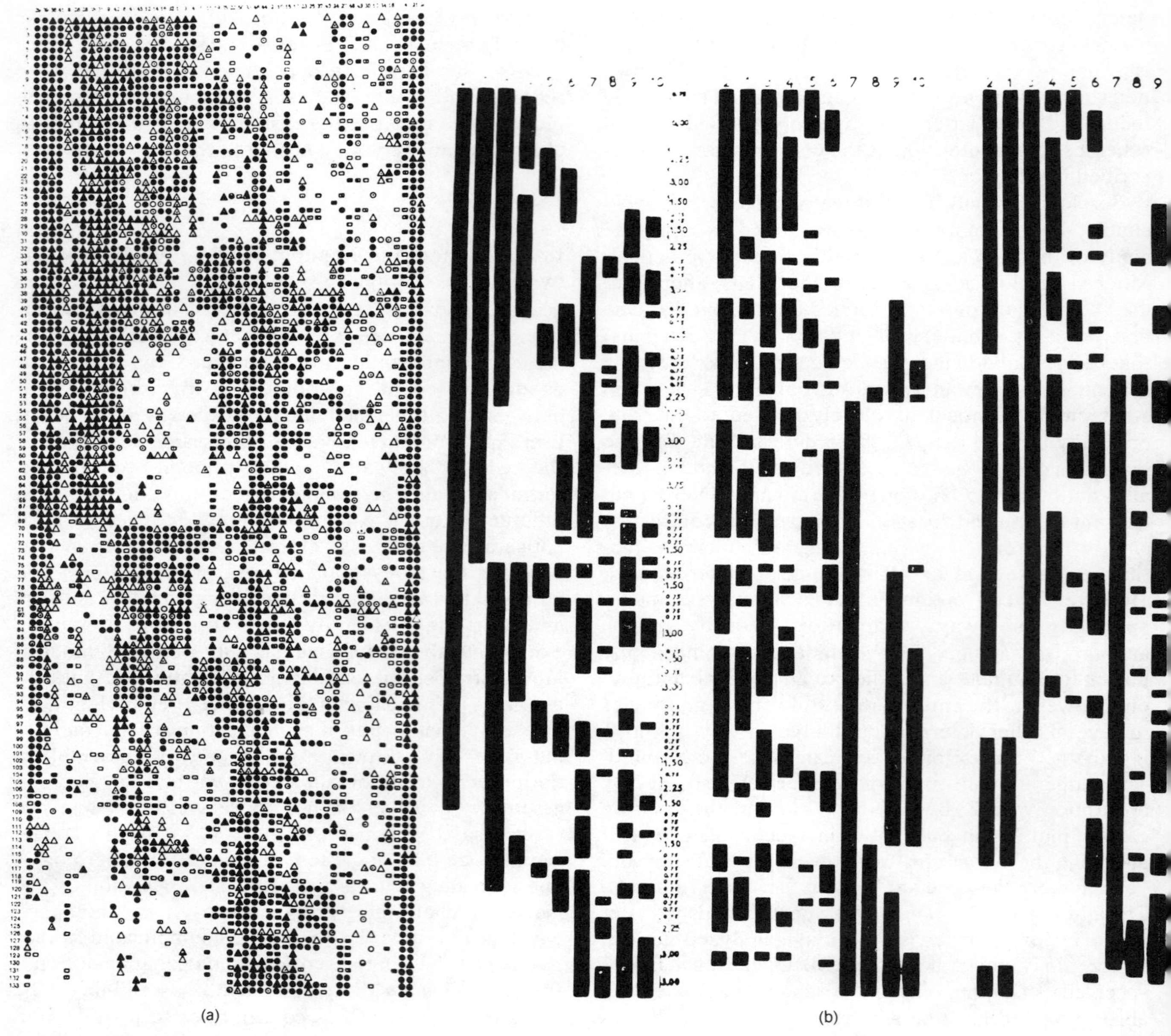

Figure 8.1. Artistic serology (*a, b*) and serological art (*c, d*). (*a*) Results of serological typing of 50 human alloantisera against leukocytes of 133 unrelated donors. Results of cytotoxicity and leukoagglutination (circles), cytotoxicity (triangles), and leukoagglutination (rectangles) tests. Full symbols indicate strong reaction, empty symbols weak reaction, and symbols with a point in the center intermediate reaction. Numbers on the left are code designations of cell donors; numbers on the top are code designations of antisera. (*b*) Typing data organized to show groups of antisera detecting similar or antithetical determinants. Full blocks indicate positive reactions and empty spaces negative reactions. Numbers on the top of the figure are designations of antigens. (*c*) Piet Mondrian: *Broadway Boogie Woogie*. (*d*) Theo van Doesburg: *Rhythm of a Russian Dance*. (*a* and *b* from J. Dausset, P. Ivanyi, and D. Ivanyi; (*In*) *Histocompatibility Testing 1965*, D. B. Amos and J. J. van Rood, eds., pp. 51–62. Williams and Wilkins, Baltimore, 1966.)

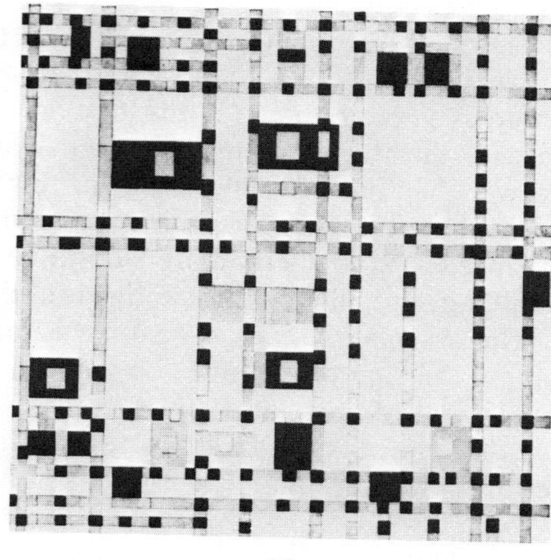

(c)

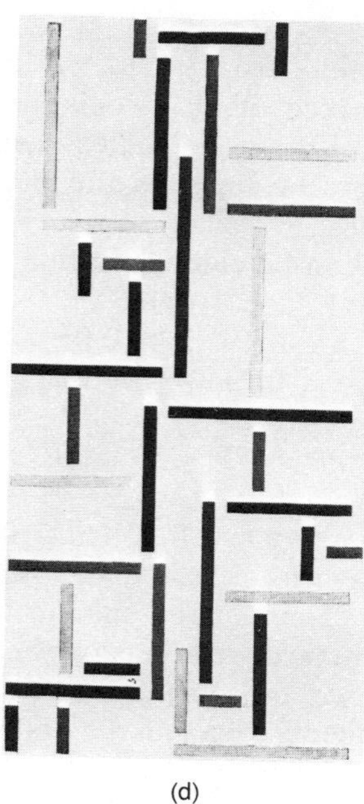

(d)

terns, but only rarely are they identical. To group such antisera into one block, the serologist must learn to ignore certain details of the reactivity pattern and concentrate on the main characteristics. To decide whether the deviation in observed reactivity patterns of an antiserum from that of another antiserum is significant, one must compare the two antisera by a statistical test. The usual way of carrying out such a comparison is first to construct a 2 × 2 contingency table, and then to determine the significance of the associations in this table by one of three statistical tests: Fisher's exact test, the χ^2 test, or the correlation coefficient test. The way a 2 × 2 contingency table is constructed is shown in Table 8.4. The three statistical tests are conducted as follows.

Table 8.4 Construction of a 2 × 2 Contingency Table[a]

		Reactivity with Antiserum 2		
		+	−	
Reactivity with Antiserum 1	+	a	b	a + b
	−	c	d	c + d
		a + c	b + d	n

[a] a, number of individual positive with both antisera; b, number of individuals positive with first antiserum and negative with second; c, number of individuals negative with first antiserum and positive with second; d, number of individuals negative with both antisera; n, total number of individuals tested (a + b + c + d).

The formula used in Fisher's exact test is

$$p = \frac{(a + b)!(c + d)!(a + c)!(b + d)!}{n!a!b!c!d!}$$

$$\text{or} \quad \frac{(a + b)!(c + d)!(a + c)!(b + d)!}{n!} \times \frac{1}{a!b!c!d!}$$

where p is the probability that a given distribution of reactivities has occurred by chance alone. The test can be used only if one of the values for the four observations in the 2 × 2 table (a, b, c, or d) is zero (0). If this is not the case, another 2 × 2 table must be constructed, in which the smallest value of the original table has been reduced by one and the three remaining figures adjusted so that the marginal totals (a + b, c + d, etc.) remain unchanged. If necessary, this is repeated until zero is reached. The p values obtained in each reduction step are then added to the p value calculated from the original 2 × 2 table (Table 8.5).

In cases where a, b, c, and d are relatively large figures, Fisher's exact test becomes inconvenient and must be replaced by another method, usually the χ^2 test. This test cannot be used when observed a, b, c, and d values are smaller than five. With larger numbers, the χ^2 can be calculated using the formula

$$\chi^2 = \frac{(ad - bc)^2 n}{(a + b)(c + d)(a + c)(b + d)}$$

and can reach values of between 0 and n, where n is the number of individuals tested (a + b + c + d). A value

Table 8.5 An Example Illustrating the Use of Fisher's Exact Test for Comparing Reactivity Patterns of Two Antisera

Original 2 × 2 Table

Second Antiserum

		+	−	
First Antiserum	+	5	2	7
	−	3	6	9
		8	8	

$$p_1 = \frac{7!9!8!8!}{16!} \times \frac{1}{5!2!3!6!}$$

$$p_1 = 0.1371$$

First Reduction Step

Second Antiserum

		+	−	
First Antiserum	+	6	1	7
	−	2	7	9
		8	8	16

$$p_2 = \frac{7!9!8!8!}{16!} \times \frac{1}{6!1!2!7}$$

$$p_2 = 0.0196$$

Second Reduction Step

Second Antiserum

		+	−	
First Antiserum	+	7	0	7
	−	1	8	9
		8	8	16

$$p_3 = \frac{7!9!8!8!}{16!} \times \frac{1}{7!0!1!8}$$

$$p_3 = 0.0007$$

(0! = 1 by definition)

Third Step

$$p = p_1 + p_2 + p_3 = 0.1574$$

Conclusion

The probability that the observed reactivity patterns of the two antisera occurred by chance alone is 0.1574.

of $\chi^2 = 0$ (attainable with a = b = c = d) signifies an absence of any association between the two antisera; a value of $\chi^2 = n$ (attainable when a = d and b = c = 0, or when b = c and a = d = 0) signifies an absolute association between the two antisera, meaning that they are either identical (they contain antibodies reacting with the same antigens) or complementary (they contain antibodies reacting with antithetical antigens). Finally, values of χ^2 higher than zero but lower than n can signify either association or lack of association, the decision being made by conversion of a given χ^2 value into a probability value (p), using the χ^2 tables. The tables show that for $\chi^2 > 11$, the corresponding p value with one degree of freedom (if the comparison is made between two antisera) is $p < 0.001$. In other words, if the χ^2 value is greater than 11, the reaction pattern observed with the two antigens can occur by chance alone in fewer than one of 1000 cases. For this reason, two antisera that give $\chi^2 \geqq 11$ when compared by the 2 × 2 contingency table method are said to be associated (containing antibodies against antigens of the same system). The association can be positive or negative, depending on the sign of the ad − bc value.

The coefficient of correlation (r) represents χ^2 corrected for the number of individuals tested. It can be calculated from the formula

$$r = \frac{\text{ad} - \text{bc}}{\sqrt{(\text{a} + \text{b})(\text{c} + \text{d})(\text{a} + \text{c})(\text{b} + \text{d})}} = \pm\sqrt{\frac{\chi^2}{n}}$$

and can reach values from +1 to −1. The value $r = 0$ signifies the absence of an association between two antisera; the value $r = +1$ signifies identity of the two antisera, and $r = -1$ suggests the presence of antithetical antibodies.

If $n \geqq 100$, it can be calculated that for

$$r \geqq 0.19 \quad p \leqq 0.05$$
$$r \geqq 0.23 \quad p \leqq 0.02$$
$$r \geqq 0.25 \quad p \leqq 0.01$$
$$r \geqq 0.32 \quad p \leqq 0.001$$

The value of positive $r \geqq 0.32$ ($p \leqq 0.001$) indicates significant positive association; the value of negative $r \geqq 0.20$ ($p \leqq 0.05$) indicates significant negative association (antithetical relationship between the antibodies of the two antisera).

Thus, the procedure used in the first step of association analysis can be summarized as follows.

Obtain a panel of about 100 different target cell samples from randomly selected individuals.

Prepare a battery of 50 or more antisera.

Test each antiserum against the whole panel.

Compare each antiserum with all other antisera of the battery, one at a time, and arrange the results of this comparison into the 2 × 2 contingency table.

Apply a statistical test (χ^2) to the contingency tables.

Arrange the results of the χ^2 test in descending order so that the highest values, indicating the closest association of two antisera, are at the top of the list and the lowest χ^2 values, indicating no association, are at the bottom.

Select antisera with the highest mutual χ^2 values for further analysis and discard antisera that show no association. Use $\chi^2 = 11$ as a cutoff point for the associated antisera.

Once the antisera are grouped and the antigens defined by the groups, the analysis can proceed to the second step, the definition of the genetic relationship between the antigens. The relationship is determined by using the same statistical methods described above (χ^2 test and the coefficient of correlation test), only this time the methods are applied to the antigens, rather than to the antisera. A significant positive correlation between antigens indicates that they belong to the same system. A significant negative correlation between two antigens indicates that they are controlled by two alleles at the same locus.

The strategy of serological MHC analysis in outbred populations changes once a basic set of antigenic determinants is defined. New determinants are then defined by comparing them to those already recognized and demonstrating that the new determinants are distinct from the existing ones. The comparison is verified by an international body, the *Histocompatibility Workshop*, composed of representatives from individual HLA-typing laboratories. This body, which meets once every two years, also recommends official designations for new determinants and approves typing reagents for individual determinants. These reagents are stored in an antiserum bank at the National Institutes of Health, Bethesda, Maryland, and are distributed, on request, to qualified investigators.

8.2.2 Methods

Preparation of Antisera

To produce anti-MHC sera, inbred animal strains are injected repeatedly at regular intervals with lymphoid tissues (spleen and lymph nodes), which have a high content of MHC antigens. Sometimes as many as 10 injections are needed to produce antibodies to certain MHC determinants. Immunizations on this scale would be unethical in humans, so HLA serologists must obtain their typing reagents in some other way. The sources of HLA antibodies are as follows.

Sera of Patients Who Have Received Multiple Blood Transfusions. The transfused blood is matched for red blood cell antigens (blood groups), but not for white blood cell antigens, and since leukocytes have a relatively high content of MHC molecules, the transfusions, especially when repeated several times, lead to production of MHC antibodies in the patient.

Sera from Women Who Have Had Multiple Pregnancies. During each pregnancy, some fetal white blood cells enter the maternal circulation and immunize the mother against paternal MHC antigens. The concentration of these MHC antibodies increases with repeated exposure to fetal white blood cells in multiple pregnancies following in rapid succession.

Sera from Volunteers Grafted with Small Pieces of Skin or injected with small numbers of white blood cells from selected donors.

Serological Typing

The reaction of MHC antibodies with cell-bound MHC molecules can be visualized in a variety of ways, some based on killing and others on tagging of target cells. The principal method based on cell-killing is the *cytotoxic test*. In this test, antibodies are specifically bound by the MHC molecules of the plasma membrane; the antigen-antibody complexes attract components of the complement system and trigger a cascade reaction, which terminates in perforation of the membrane by multiple lesions, disturbance of the cell's osmotic balance, and cell death (for a description of the complement cascade, see Chapter 9). Dead cells can be distinguished from live ones by a change in the light refraction pattern as observed in a phase-contrast microscope, by their inability to exclude vital dyes such as eosin or trypan blue from their cytoplasm, or by release of radioactive chromium (^{51}Cr) bound in their cytoplasm.

The principal method based on cell tagging is the *fluorescent antibody test*, in which antibodies are labeled by compounds yielding bright light of a characteristic color upon absorption of light of a different color (wavelength). This method is described in Appendix 10.2.5.

In some species (e.g., mouse, rat, domestic fowl), MHC molecules are also present on the surface of red blood cells and can, therefore, be detected by *hemagglutination assays*.

8.2.3 Nomenclature

Individual antigenic determinants are designated by numbers—class I determinants by one series of numbers and class II determinants by another. The numbers are assigned consecutively in the order of determinant discovery. In the mouse *H-2* system (but not, for example, in the human *HLA* system), the determinants and MHC designations are separated by a pe-

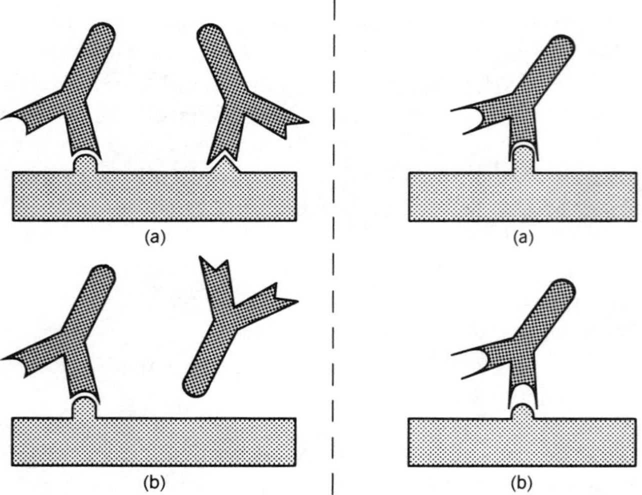

Figure 8.2. Two interpretations of crossreactivity. A and B are antigenic molecules of two inbred strains; the Y-like structures are antibodies. In the left-hand panel, molecule A has two determinants, one of which it shares with molecule B; there are separate antibodies for the two determinants. In the right-hand panel, molecule A has only one determinant; molecule B has a similar, but not identical, determinant, which the antibody fits only imperfectly.

riod (e.g., H-2.1, H-2.2, H-2.3,; but HLA1, HLA2, HLA3). When the locus coding for a given determinant is known, it is indicated by the locus symbol following the generic MHC designation (e.g., H-2K.1, H-2D.2, H-2D.3, or HLA-A1, HLA-A2, HLA-B5). A tentative (Workshop) designation is indicated by a w preceding the determinant designation (e.g., HLA-Bw40, HLA-Bw41).

8.2.4 Crossreactions

The reaction of an antiserum with cells from individuals genetically different from the donor of the immunizing cells is referred to as *crossreaction*. Crossreactions occur for two main reasons (Fig. 8.2). First, the crossreacting individual shares with the immunizing individual *some* antigenic determinants. (When there is complete sharing of determinants, the two individuals are considered genetically identical at the locus concerned and hence, by definition, the reaction with the nonimmunizing individual is not a crossreaction.) Second, the crossreacting individual possesses a determinant that resembles, but is not identical to a determinant of the immunizing strain. In the former situation, crossreactions are caused by the presence of multiple antibody species, each specific for a given determinant, in the antiserum. In the latter situation, the same antibody species reacts with two different determinants but fits the immunizing determinant better than the crossreacting one. To differentiate between these two types of crossreaction is not always easy, and sometimes impossible.

Serologists handle crossreactions of anti-MHC sera differently, depending on the species (inbred versus outbred) they are working with. H-2 serologists deliberately search for crossreactions and register them as if they were always caused by sharing of distinct determinants; HLA serologists, on the other hand, try to avoid crossreactions by selecting for analysis the least crossreactive antisera. Because of this difference in approach, the *H*-2 and *HLA* systems appear to be serologically different. In the *H*-2 system, each allele appears to code for a number of determinants (Tables 8.6 and 7), whereas in the *HLA* system, each allele appears to code for only one (Table 8.8). This difference, however, is illusory: had anti-HLA sera been produced and handled in the same way H-2 sera have been, each *HLA* allele would also appear to control several determinants.

In the *H*-2 system, one can distinguish two kinds of determinant: *private determinants*, characterizing single alleles (or groups of related alleles; see below), and *public determinants*, shared by two or more unrelated alleles. Each allele is thus characterized serologically by one private and several public determinants (Tables 8.6 and 7). The division of determinants into private and public works well for distantly related alleles, but breaks down when, for example, one considers alleles derived from one another by recent mutations: groups of alleles so closely related may share the same private determinants. There is no substantive difference between private and public determinants; the division should be regarded only as an operational means of simplifying the complex picture of H-2 serology. Most of the HLA determinants (Table 8.8) correspond to private H-2 determinants, and one can make the serology of the *H*-2 and *HLA* systems directly comparable by omitting the public determinants from the *H*-2 system.

8.2.5 Classes and Series

When one tests anti-MHC sera against spleen or lymph node lymphocytes, one can, under certain circumstances, distinguish two kinds of antibody: one that reacts with all or almost all cells in the suspension, and another that reacts with only about half of the cells. The former are antibodies detecting class I MHC molecules that are expressed on both T and B lymphocytes, and the latter are antibodies detecting class II molecules that are expressed on B lymphocytes but

Table 8.6 Selected Class I Determinants Controlled by the Mouse *H-2* Complex

H-2 Haplotype	Public K Determinant																Private K Determinant	Public D Determinants												Private D Determinant
	1	3	5	8	11	25	34	35	36	37	38	39	42	45	46	47		1	3	5	6	13	35	36	41	42	43	44	49	
b	—	—	5	—	—	—	—	35	36	—	—	39	—	—	46	—	33	—	—	—	6	—	—	—	—	—	—	—	—	2
d	—	3	—	8	—	—	34	—	—	—	—	—	—	—	46	47	31	—	3	—	6	13	35	36	41	42	43	44	49	4
f	—	—	—	8	—	—	—	—	—	37	—	39	—	—	46	—	26	—	—	—	6	—	—	—	—	—	—	—	—	9
j	1	—	5	—	—	—	—	—	—	—	38	—	—	45	46	47	15	—	—	—	6	—	—	—	—	—	—	45	—	2
k	1	3	5	8	11	25	—	—	—	—	—	—	—	45	—	47	23	1	3	5	—	—	—	—	—	—	—	—	49	32
p	1	—	5	8	—	—	34	—	—	37	38	—	—	45	46	.	16	1	3	5	6	—	35	—	41	—	—	—	49	22
q	1	3	5	—	11	—	34	—	—	—	—	—	—	45	—	—	17	—	3	—	6	13	35	36	—	—	—	—	49	30
r	1	3	5	8	11	25	—	—	—	—	—	—	—	45	—	47	18	1	3	5	6	—	—	—	—	—	—	—	49	10
s	1	—	5	—	—	—	—	—	—	—	—	—	42	45	—	—	19	—	3	—	6	—	35	36	—	42	—	—	49	12
u	1	—	5	8	—	—	—	35	36	—	—	—	—	45	.	.	20	—	3	—	6	13	—	—	41	42	43	44	49	4
v	1	3	5	—	—	—	—	—	—	—	—	—	—	45	—	.	21	—	.	—	.	.	—	—	—	—	43	—	49	14

1, 2, 3, etc., presence of a given determinant; ., no information about this determinant available; —, absence of a given determinant.

considerably less or not at all on T lymphocytes. (In an anti-MHC serum containing both class I and class II antibodies, the latter are obscured by the former; it is primarily for this reason that class II molecules were discovered relatively late.)

In the mouse, the class II determinants are called Ia (from *I* region-associated *a*ntigens, where *I region* is the chromosomal segment occupied by class II loci; see section on immune-response genes). In the human, they are referred to as DR (from *D*-related, where *D* is a locus defined by mixed lymphocyte reaction).

When one considers only the private antigenic determinants in each class, one notices that they can be arranged into series, with determinants in each series being mutually exclusive. In the mouse, there are two class I series (but see below), designated K and D (the origin of these designations will be explained in the section on genetics); in humans, there are three class I

Table 8.7 Selected Class II (Ia) Determinants Controlled by the Mouse *H-2* Complex

H-2 Haplotype	A-Molecule Determinants																				E-Molecule Determinants			
	1	2	3	4	5	6	8	9	10	11	12	13	14	15	16	17	18	19	20	24	7	21	22	23
b	—	—	3	—	—	—	8	9	—	—	—	—	—	15	—	—	—	—	20	—	—	—	—	—
d	—	—	—	—	—	6	8	—	—	11	—	—	—	15	16	—	—	—	—	—	7	—	—	23
f	1	—	—		5	—	—	—	—	—	—	—	14	—	—	17	18	—	—	—	—	—	—	—
j	—		.	—	5	.	—	.	10	—	—	—	—	15	.	—	.	—	—	—	7	.	.	.
k	1		3	—	—	—	—	—	—	—	—	—	—	15	—	17	18	19	—	—	7	—	22	—
p	—	2	—	—	5	6	—	—	—	—	—	13	—	—	—	—	—	—	—	—	7	21	—	—
q	—	—	3	—	5	—	—	9	10	—	—	13	—	—	16	—	—	—	—	—	—	—	—	—
r	1	—	3	—	5	—	—	—	—	—	12	—	—	—	—	17	—	19	—	24	7	—	—	—
s	—	—	—	4	5	—	—	9	—	—	12	—	—	—	—	17	18	—	—	24	—	—	—	—
u	1	—	.	—	5	.	—	.	—	—	—	—	—	—	.	17	.	—	—	24	7	.	.	.
v	—	—	.	—	5	.	8	.	—	—	—	—	—	15	.	—	.	—	—	—	7	.	.	

1, 2, 3, etc., presence of a given determinant; ., no information about this determinant available; —, absence of a given determinant.

Table 8.8 List of HLA Determinants Known in 1980 (According to the Eighth International Histocompatibility Workshop)

HLA-A		*HLA-B*		*HLA-C*		*HLA-D*[a]	
New	Previous	New	Previous	New	Previous	New	Previous
A1	A1	B5	A5	Cw1	T1	Dw1	LD 101
A2	A2	B7	A7	Cw2	T2	Dw2	LD 102
A3	A3	B8	A8	Cw3	T3	Dw3	LD 103
A9	A9	B12	A12	Cw4	T4	Cw4	LD 105
A10	A10	B13	A13	Cw5	T5	Dw5	LD 105
A11	A11	B14	W14	Cw6	T7	Dw6	LD 106
Aw19		B15	W15	Cw7	CVE, TOK	Dw7	LD 107
Aw23	W23	Bw16	W16	Cw8	T8, T9	Dw8	LD 108
Aw24	W24	B17	W17			Dw9	TB9, OH
A25	W25	B18	W18			Dw10	LD 16
A26	W26	Bw21	W21			Dw11	LD 17
A28	W28	Bw22	W22			Dw12	DB4, DHO
A29	W29	27	W27			DRw1	LB1
Aw30	W30	Bw35	W5			DRw2	LB2
Aw31	W31	B37	Bw37, TY			DRw3	LB3
Aw32	W32	Bw38	W16.1			DRw4	LB4
Aw33	W19.6	Bw39	W.16.2			DRw5	LB5
Aw34	MALAY 2	B40	Bw40, W10			DRw6	LB6
Aw36	MO[a]	Bw41	SABELL			DRw7	LB7
Aw43	BK	Bw42	MWA			DRw8	WIA8
		Bw44	B12 non-TT[a]			DRw9	WIA4x7
		Bw45	TT^+			DRw10	ST-1, LTM
		Bw46	HS, SIN 2				
		Bw47	407^+, MO66, CAS, Bw40C				
		Bw48	KSO, JA, Bw40.3				
		Bw49	Bw21.1, SL-ET				
		Bw50	Bw21.2, ET				
		Bw51	B5.1				
		Bw52	B5.2				
		Bw53	HR				
		Bw54	Bw22J, SAP 1, J1				
		Bw55	W55, 22.1				
		Bw56	W56, 22.2, Te92, Da30				
		Bw57	W67, 17.1, 17A, 17 long				
		Bw58	W68, 17.2, 17B, 17 short				
		Bw59	W69, HOK-1, 8.2				
		Bw60	W60, 40.1				
		Bw61	W61, 40.2				
		Bw62	W64, 15.1-TO53, 15B, Te72				
		Bw63	W65, 15.2-TO52, 15A, Te71				
		Bw4	W4, 4a				
		Bw6	W6, 4b				

[a] D determinants, defined by mixed lymphocyte reaction; DR determinants, defined serologically.

series, A, B, and C. Each H-2 private determinant belongs to either the K or the D series but never to both; in humans, each determinant belongs to one, and only one, of the three series. A single mouse cell can have a maximum of two determinants from each series. This behavior suggests that each series is controlled by a separate locus, and this suggestion has been borne out by genetic analysis (see below). Since each cell expresses two alleles at each locus, in an MHC heterozygote, one finds two private determinants from each series, each determinant controlled by one allele. In the mouse, Peter Démant and his coworkers demonstrated that some of the known public class I determinants (in particular, determinant H-2.28) did not fit into the K and D series, and constituted a third series, controlled by a separate locus, *L*.

8.2.6 Determinant Inventory

The serological analysis of the *H-2* and *HLA* systems is far from complete (it may never be complete). New determinants are still being described and existing ones are often split into two or more, as new strains and individuals are typed. In the *H-2* system, there are over 100 class I determinants defined by conventional antibodies, with some molecules carrying at least 30 determinants. Of these, some 30 determinants are private and the rest are public. Among the private determinants, 21 are controlled by the *K* locus and 22 by the *D* locus; the genetic control of the remaining determinants is uncertain. A total of 50 class II determinants have been described, of which 16 are of the private and the rest of the public category. Most of these determinants are controlled by a locus designated *A* and only a few by another locus, referred to as *E*. In addition, several determinants have also been defined by monoclonal antibodies; some of these resemble determinants defined by conventional antisera, but many others are different.

In the *HLA* system, 20 determinants are known to be controlled by the *A* locus, 42 by the *B* locus, and eight by the *C* locus in the class I category (Table 8.8). At the class II *D* locus, two kinds of determinant have been recognized—D determinants, defined by the mixed lymphocyte reaction (see Chapter 12), and DR determinants, defined by serological methods. The interrelationship of the two kinds of determinant is not known; it is not even certain that both kinds are encoded by the same locus. There are 12 D determinants and 10 DR determinants known (Table 8.8).

8.2.7 Topology of Determinants

Little is known about the spatial arrangement of multiple determinants (public and private) on a single class I molecule. Studies of *H-2* mutations have revealed that in some instances, the presumed single amino acid substitution alters some, but not other antigenic determinants. These results may be interpreted as suggesting the existence of multiple *sites* on the same class I molecule, with some sites occupied by one group of determinants and other sites by others. A similar conclusion has also been reached through inhibition studies using monoclonal antibodies. Here, binding of radioactively labeled monoclonal antibodies to a given determinant is inhibited more strongly by the addition of an unlabeled second antibody directed against another determinant, provided the two determinants occupy the same site; binding is inhibited less strongly if the two determinants occupy different, spatially separated sites. The number of sites present on a single class I molecule is not known.

8.3 GENETICS

Although the principles of genetic MHC analysis are the same for inbred and outbred species, to illustrate how the present knowledge has been attained we shall discuss the two most thoroughly studied species (mouse and human) separately.

8.3.1 The Mouse

Present knowledge about the genetic organization of the murine MHC has been obtained by studying the segregation of the individual MHC genes among the progeny of deliberate crosses and the behavior of genes in populations.

Segregation Analysis

History. In 1959, Peter A. Gorer and Z. B. Mikulska tested progeny from the cross (A × C57BL)F_1 × C57BL (A and C57BL are two inbred mouse strains) for class I determinants H-2.4 and H-2.11, carried by the A strain. They observed that, of the 194 animals tested, 192 were of the parental type (95 of the 4^+11^+ type and 97 of the 4^-11^- type); one was of the 4^+11^- type, and one of the 4^-11^+ type. They concluded from these observations that determinants 4 and 11 were encoded by separate but closely linked loci, and that the 4^+11^- and 4^-11^+ animals resulted from genetic recombination between these two loci. At that time, H-2 antigenic determinants were still referred to by capital letters rather than by numbers, so determinant 4 was then called D and determinant 11 was K (the fourth and eleventh letters of the alphabet, respectively).

Gorer and Mikulska therefore designated the loci coding for determinants 4 and 11 as *D* and *K*, respectively, and this designation has been generally accepted. The distance between the two loci was calculated to be 2/194, that is, about one crossover unit (1 cM) (but see below).

Serological typing of the recombinant animals for additional class I determinants at first suggested that there might be more than two class I loci in the *H-2* complex: a separate locus for determinant 3 (*C*), another for determinant 5 (*E*), and still another for determinant 22 (*V*) were thought to exist. But this interpretation quickly ran into difficulties as more *H-2* recombinants were discovered. Different recombinants seemed to require a different order of these hypothetical additional loci—an observation that was without precedent in the history of genetics. In 1971, Donald C. Shreffler and I proposed a solution to these perplexing findings. We suggested that there were only two class I loci, *K* and *D*, and that each allele at any one of these loci coded for one private and several public antigenic determinants. The complications had arisen because many of the public determinants were controlled by both loci, so there were, for example, *K*-encoded 3 and *D*-encoded 3, *K*-encoded 5 and *D*-encoded 5, and so on (Table 8.6). Naturally, these determinants appeared to map now into the *K* end and now into the *D* end of the *H-2* complex, depending on the strain, and so the situation was confused. The two-locus model of the *H-2* complex was confirmed by a variety of serological, biochemical, and functional studies. The finding that the same determinants can be controlled by both the *K* and *D* loci led Shreffler and his associates to the suggestion that the two loci were genetically related by a common origin from a single ancestral locus. This hypothesis, too, was confirmed by amino acid sequence analysis of the K and D molecules (see below).

Other studies, however, demonstrated that there was more to the *H-2* complex than the class I loci. In 1963, Donald C. Shreffler and Ray E. Owen described a serum protein they called *s*erum *s*erological, of Ss, and they proved that the protein was controlled by an *H-2*-linked locus. The *Ss* locus has at least two alleles, one (Ss^h) coding for a high level of the protein and another (Ss^l) coding for protein levels approximately 20 times lower. Ss analysis of recombinants separating the *K* and *D* loci revealed that the *Ss* locus (or *S* locus, for short) resided in the middle of the *H-2* complex. Figure 8.3*a* depicts two such recombinants separating class I determinants 31 (K) and 4 (D) controlled by one chromosome, and 23 (K) and 32 (D) controlled by another. One recombinant inherited determinant 32 *en bloc* with Ss^l and the other inherited determinant 31 *en bloc* with Ss^h. The only arrangement of loci that explains the origin of each of the two recombinants as resulting from a single crossover event is that which places the *Ss* locus between the *K* and *D* loci.

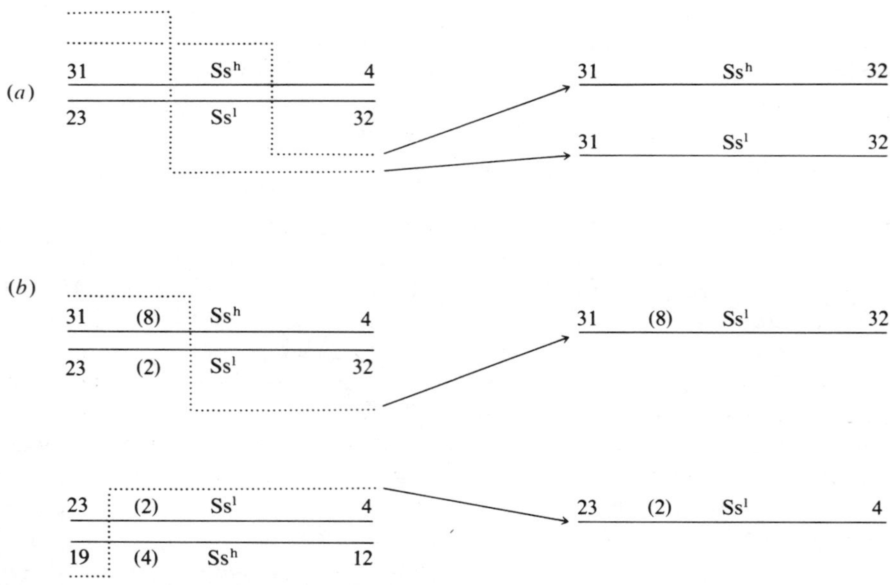

Figure 8.3. Critical *H-2* recombinants that map the *Ss* (*a*) and class II (*b*) loci within the *H-2* complex. Numbers on the left indicate *K* locus-encoded class I determinants, those on the extreme right *D* locus-encoded determinants; class II determinants are in parentheses.

In 1973, two research groups—one headed by Donald C. Shreffler, and the other by myself—discovered a new set of MHC molecules—those controlled by class II loci—and reported that the loci mapped in the region between the *K* and *S* loci. The critical recombinants positioning the class II loci in the indicated region are depicted in Figure 8.3*a*. One of them is the 31 Ss^l 32 recombinant from the *Ss* mapping study; it inherited the class II determinant 8 *en bloc* with K-encoded determinant 31. The other originated from two different chromosomes and inherited the class II determinant 2 *en bloc* with the *S* and *D* loci. Once again, the only order of loci that explains the two recombinants as arising each by a single crossover is that which places class II loci between *K* and *S*. Later studies by Chella S. David and his co-workers demonstrated the existence of at least two class II loci (but see section on biochemistry), and these were designated *A* and *E*. (For these designations, immunogneticists returned to the beginning of the alphabet; see below.)

Nomenclature. The genetic nomenclature of the *H*-2 complex is complicated and confusing. Attempting to improve it, immunogeneticists made it almost incomprehensible to the uninitiated. It will save us considerable difficulty if we completely ignore the official nomenclature and regard the *H*-2 complex as consisting of loci, to which we shall refer by capital letters (i.e., *A*, *B*, *C*, etc.). Each locus has alleles designated by small-letter superscripts (i.e., A^a, A^b, B^a, B^b, etc.). A particular combination of *H*-2 alleles at a single chromosome will be referred to as the *H*-2 *haplotype* and designated by a small-letter superscript in combination with the *H*-2 symbol. In some haplotypes, the superscript designation reflects the allelic designation (e.g., $H\text{-}2^b$ is a combination of alleles K^b, A^b, E^b, S^b, and D^b). In others, the superscript is arbitrary (e.g., $H\text{-}2^a$ is a combination of K^k, A^k, E^k, S^d, and D^d alleles). The allelic combination can also be written *kkkdd* when it is clear to which loci the alleles refer. $H\text{-}2^a$ is an example of a *recombinant haplotype* (Table 8.9), in which one group of alleles (loci *K* through *E*) is known to be derived from one haplotype ($H\text{-}2^k$) and

Table 8.9 The Allelic Composition of Selected *H*-2 Recombinants

Strain	*H*-2 Haplotype	Parental *H*-2 Haplotypes	Alleles at Loci								Originator
			K	A_α	A_β	E_β	J	E_α	S	D	
A	*a*	*k/d*	*k*	*k*	*k*	*k*	*k*	*k* ∣	*d*	*d*	G. D. Snell
A.AL	*a*1	*k/d*	*k*	*k*	*k*	*k*	*k*	*k*	*k* ∣	*d*	D. C. Shreffler
HTG	*g*	*d/b*	*d*	*d*	*d*	*d*	*d*	*d*	*d* ∣	*b*	P. A. Gorer and D. B. Amos
D2.GD	*g*2	*d/b*	*d*	*d*	*d*	*d/b* ∣	*b*	*b*	*b*	*b*	F. Lilly and J. Klein
HTH	*h*	*a/b*	*k*	*k*	*k*	*k*	*k*	*k*	*d* ∣	*b*	P. A. Gorer
B10.A(1R)	*h*1	*a/b*	*k*	*k*	*k*	*k*	*k*	*k*	*d* ∣	*b*	J. H. Stimpfling
B10.A(2R)	*h*2	*a/b*	*k*	*k*	*k*	*k*	*k*	*k*	*d* ∣	*b*	J. H. Stimpfling
B10.A(4R)	*h*4	*a/b*	*k*	*k*	*k*	*k* ∣	*b*	*b*	*b*	*b*	J. H. Stimpfling
HTI	*i*	*b/a*	*b*	*b*	*b*	*b*	*b*	*b*	*b* ∣	*d*	P. A. Gorer
B10.A(3R)	*i*3	*b/a*	*b*	*b*	*b*	*b*	*b* ∣	*k*	*d*	*d*	J. H. Stimpfling
B10.A(5R)	*i*5	*b/a*	*b*	*b*	*b*	*b* ∣	*d*	*d*	*d*	*d*	J. H. Stimpfling
AKR.M	*m*	*k/q*	*k*	*k*	*k*	*k*	*k*	*k*	*k* ∣	*q*	G. D. Snell
C3H.OL	*o*1	*d/k*	*d*	*d*	*d*	*d*	*d*	*d* ∣	*k*	*k*	D. C. Shreffler
C3H.OH	*o*2	*d/k*	*d*	*d*	*d*	*d*	*d*	*d*	*d* ∣	*k*	D. C. Shreffler
A.TL	*t*1	*s/a*l	*s*	*s* ∣	*k*	*k*	*k*	*k*	*k*	*d*	D. C. Shreffler
B10.S(7R)	*t*2	*s/a*	*s*	*s*	*s*	*s*	*s*	*s*	*s* ∣	*d*	J. H. Stimpfling
B10.HTT	*t*3	*s/t*l	*s*	*s*	*s*	*s* ∣	*s*	*k*	*k*	*d*	D. C. Shreffler
B10.S(9R)	*t*4	*s/a*	*s*	*s*	*s*	*s* ∣	*k*	*k*	*d*	*d*	J. H. Stimpfling
B10.AQR	*y*1	*q/a*	*q* ∣	*k*	*k*	*k*	*k*	*k*	*d*	*d*	J. Klein
B10.T(6R)	*y*2	*q/a*	*q*	*q*	*q*	*q*	*q*	*q*	*q* ∣	*d*	J. H. Stimpfling

[a] Vertical line indicates the position of chromosome exchange during crossingover.

Table 8.10 Selected *H*-2 Haplotypes of Independent Origin and Some Strains Carrying Them

H-2 Haplo-type	Strain
b	C57BL/10, C57BL/6, C57L, C3H.SW, LP, 129
d	BALB/c, DBA/2, C57BL/Ks, NZB, SEA, YBR
f	A.CA, B10.M, RFM
j	WB, B10.WB(69NS)
k	AKR, CBA, C3H, B10.BR, C57BR
p	P, B10.P, C3H.NB, F
q	DBA/1, STOLI, B10.Q, BDP
r	RIII, B10.RIII(71NS), LP.RIII
s	A.SW, SJL, B10.S
u	PL, B10.PL(73NS)
v	SM, B10.SM

another group (the *S* and *D* loci) from another haplotype (H-2^d). For certain other haplotypes, no information about the origin of alleles is available, and in these *independent haplotypes* (Table 8.10) all alleles are designated by the same letter—the same one that designates the haplotype (e.g., *bbbbb* in the case of the H-2^b haplotype). Single-letter designations were used for the first 26 haplotypes, and when the alphabet was exhausted it was necessary to use combinations of two letters and numbers. Letters *m* and *v* are reserved for mutations and minor variants, respectively; the letter *w* is reserved for haplotypes derived from wild mice. Different numbers in combination with the same single or double letter refer to related haplotypes. For example, H-2^{bm1} is a mutation of H-2^b observed in the laboratory; H-2^{bv1} is a minor variant of H-2^b that might have arisen by mutation or a series of mutations, but there is no laboratory record of this event; H-2^{g1}, H-2^{g2}, and H-2^{g3} are three recombinant haplotypes that resemble one another in that they share alleles at the *K* and *D* loci but differ at other *H*-2 loci; and finally, H-2^b and H-2^k are two unrelated (as far as one can determine) haplotypes.

The *H*-2 Map. The *H*-2 complex occupies a chromosomal segment that is between 0.3 and 1.5 cM long and contains a minimum of 10 to 15 loci. (The length of the segment and number of loci in it depend on which loci one counts as belonging to the *H*-2 complex.) In the genetic map (the *H*-2 *map*), the loci are arranged in the order indicated by recombination studies, with the locus closest to the centromere (*K*) at the extreme left and the locus closest to the telomere (*D*) at the extreme right (Fig. 8.4). A brief description of the individual loci follows.

Class I Loci. There are three class I loci, *K*, *D*, and *L*. The *K* and *D* loci reside at the opposite ends of the *H*-2 map; the *L* locus maps so closely to *D* that the two have not been separated genetically, and their order with respect to the centromere is not known. The genetic homology of the *K* and *D* loci is firmly established through amino acid sequencing data that demonstrate sharing of some 80 percent of the residues between the K and D molecules (see section on biochemistry). Functionally, the two loci are indistinguishable. The L molecules also share some 80 percent of their amino acids with the K and D molecules, but the functional relationship of the *L* locus to the *K* and *D* loci is not known.

The currently debated question is whether there are more than three class I loci and if so, how their expression is regulated. According to one hypothesis, in at

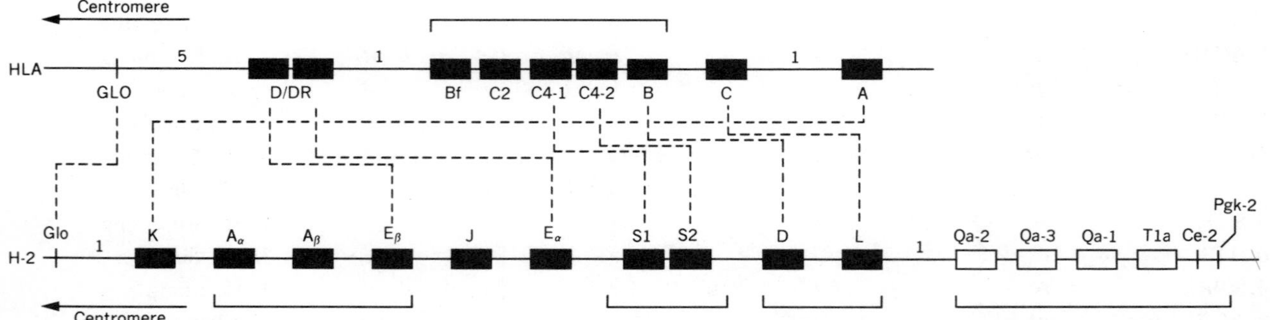

Figure 8.4. Genetic organization of human (*HLA*) and mouse (*H-2*) major histocompatibility complexes. Presumed homology of individual loci is indicated by interconnecting broken lines. Numbers indicate approximate map distance between loci. Order of loci in brackets is not known. *Glo* and *Pgk-2* are two enzyme-encoding loci that are not part of the MHC.

least the K and D regions, there are clusters of structural loci controlled by a regulator locus that allows the expression of only one structural locus in the cluster. Since, according to this hypothesis, all loci but one in each cluster are silent, one gets the erroneous impression that only one locus exists in each of the two regions. There are three reasons for the popularity of this hypothesis. First, the products of the two K or two D alleles differ by some 40 to 50 amino acids, while allelic products at virtually all other known loci differ by only one, or at most a few, amino acids. In this respect, the two K or two D alleles resemble two genes at separate loci, and some investigators believe that, in fact, this is what they are. Second, several investigators have reported the appearance, in tumors, of class I antigenic determinants encoded by alleles that the strain of tumor origin does not possess. The appearance of these "alien determinants" is explained by the activation—during neoplastic transformation—of previously silent H-2 genes. Third, in immunoglobulin systems, certain irregularities in the expression of certain allotypic determinants have been interpreted as evidence for control, through regulator genes, of a family of structural loci (see Chapter 6). These complex allotypes have been used as a precedent in arguing that a similar situation occurs with class I H-2 loci. The three arguments in favor of the gene family hypothesis are either circumstantial or based on controversial data. The final answer to the question of the number of class I loci will probably have to await the results of the DNA cloning analysis.

Class II Loci. The current H-2 map (Fig. 8.4) lists five class II loci—A_β, A_α, E_β, J, and E_α. There is only one piece of circumstantial evidence for grouping these loci into one class—their involvement in regulation (help or suppression) of lymphocyte responses (both B and T; see section on function). Biochemical homologies between individual class II loci have not yet been demonstrated, save for similarities in the size and general organization of some class II molecules (see section on biochemistry). The polypeptides controlled by the A_α and A_β loci combine into $A_\alpha A_\beta$ molecules; similarly, the polypeptides controlled by the E_α and E_β loci combine into $E_\alpha E_\beta$ molecules. No recombinant separating the two A loci has yet been found; the two E loci are separated from each other by the J locus. The order of the A_α, A_β, and E_β loci is yet to be determined.

The J locus was discovered using a functional assay for the suppression of antibody response. The original assay system was as follows. Spleen cells from animals sensitized to a given antigen were mixed with spleen cells from mice preconditioned to suppress antibody formation. Suppressor cells present in the second spleen cell population blocked the antibody response of the first population unless they were killed off by antiserum (and complement) reacting specifically with them. Such an antiserum can be produced by immunization with lymphocytes in certain donor-recipient combinations. Genetic studies have revealed that the antigens with which the antiserum reacts are controlled by a locus that maps in a separate region, J, between E_β and E_α. Thus, antisera reacting with J-locus determinants can be produced, but since the determinants are apparently present only on a small subpopulation of lymphocytes (suppressor T cells), their demonstration using standard serological methods is difficult. Nonetheless, successful detection of J determinants has been reported by several investigators.

Class III Loci. We shall designate MHC or MHC-linked loci controlling the complement system as class III. In the H-2 complex, this class is represented by the S locus, which codes for the C4 component. Biochemical evidence suggests that the S locus may be a composite of two loci, but no recombinants separating the two loci have yet been detected. Class III loci will be discussed in more detail in Chapter 9.

Class IV Loci. In contrast to class I, II, and III loci, for which evidence of intraclass homologies is available, there is virtually no evidence grouping the loci listed below into a single class. For now, they represent miscellaneous loci that have only one feature in common: they all map within a short segment on the telomeric side of the D locus. Whether they belong to the H-2 complex at all can also be debated. It is hoped that future studies will bring some order into this class and allow a more natural grouping of the various loci. The class IV loci are *Tla*, which controls *a*ntigenic determinants expressed on *t*hymocytes and certain *l*eukemias (see Chapter 14), and *Qa*-1 through *Qa*-3, which control the expression of antigenic determinants on different subpopulations of lymphocytes.

Chromosomal Location. The H-2 complex is located in chromosome 17, the third smallest mouse chromosome. Like all other mouse chromosomes, number 17 is acrocentric; the H-2 complex is positioned approximately midway between the centromere and telomere (Fig. 8.5). Located in the same chromosome are loci controlling embryonic differentiation (the t complex), hair growth (*tf* and *thf*), a set of allozymes (*Glo*-1, *Pgk*-2, *Ce*-2, *Apl*, *Map*-2), minor histocompatibility

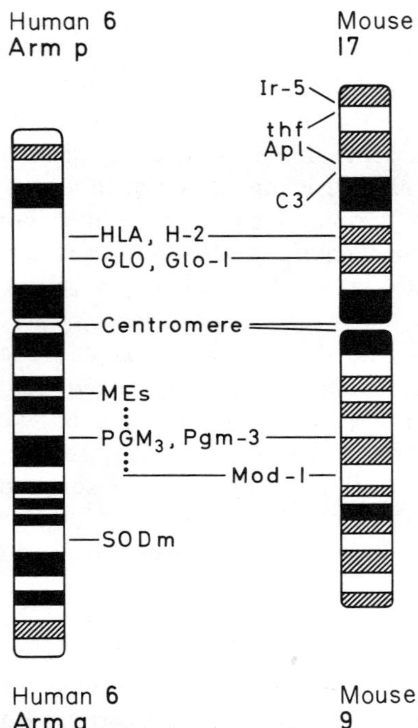

Figure 8.5. Banding patterns and approximate positions of loci of the MHC-bearing chromosomes. Presumed homologies are indicated by interconnecting lines. Mouse chromosome 9 is shown for comparison. *Apl*, acid phosphatase liver; C3, complement component 3; *Glo*, glyoxalase; *Ir-5*, immune response-5; *MEs, Mod-1*, malic enzyme supernatant; *PGM3, Pgm-3*, phosphoglucomutase-3; *SODm*, superoxide dismutate mitochondria; *thf*, thin fur.

antigens (*H*-31, *H*-32, *H*-33), a blood-group antigen (*Ea*-2), and the third component of the complement system (C3).

Population Genetics

Before we can discuss the population genetics of the *H*-2 complex, we must acquaint ourselves with the concept of *genetic polymorphism*. (For the explanation of other terms and concepts used in population genetics, see Appendix 8.1). When one examines a population of individuals for a set of randomly selected loci, one finds that the loci fall into two categories: those carrying the same allele in virtually all individuals typed, and those represented by two or more alleles in the population. The former are referred to as *monomorphic* (Gr. *monos*, single; *morphē*, shape), the latter as *polymorphic* (Gr. *polys*, many). However, the difference between the two types of locus is not so clearcut as it might seem. When one tests enough individuals, one occasionally finds, even at monomorphic loci, a few individuals carrying a different allele than the rest of the population. These are probably individuals in which a recent mutation has occurred. The mutation, however, usually persists in the population only transiently and sooner or later is eliminated by random drift. In contrast, at the polymorphic loci, the alleles generated by mutations persist in the population, so that any time one samples the population, one finds these alleles to be present. The difficulty in classifying loci as polymorphic or monomorphic is in deciding where to draw the line. What frequency must be the mutant alleles achieve in a population for the locus to be considered polymorphic? For lack of a better definition, population geneticists usually stick to an unwritten agreement to consider a frequency greater than 1 percent as an indication of polymorphism. Frequencies below 1 percent are regarded as chance variation. A typical polymorphic locus in the mouse has two or three alleles, of which one is relatively frequent and the other less frequent. Most individuals are homozygous at the given locus and only some 5 to 10 percent are heterozygous. About 60 percent of all loci tested in the mouse show no variation—they are monomorphic.

The *H*-2 loci are in striking contrast to all other loci tested so far. Here, each single class I locus has at least 50 alleles present in a global mouse population, and the number may actually be higher (over 100), since only about half the alleles have been identified. There is no very frequent allele; all are present in similar low frequencies. (In local populations, however, the number of alleles is much smaller and some alleles are more frequent than others, the composition and frequency of alleles being characteristic of a given population.) More than 90 percent of the mice are class I heterozygotes. The polymorphism of A_β and E_β class II loci is probably as high as that of class I loci, although not enough data are yet available to make this statement conclusive. The A_α and E_α loci, on the other hand, are probably not more polymorphic than most non-MHC loci.

This unprecedented high degree of polymorphism is one of the most puzzling characteristics of the *H*-2 complex. Why should the *H*-2 loci differ so much from all other known genetic loci? Why do so many *H*-2 alleles persist in the population? The answer to these questions is probably related in some way to the function of the *H*-2 complex (see section 8.5).

8.3.2 The Human

In the human, as in the mouse, MHC genetics has been approached in two ways—by segregation analysis (family studies) and by population studies.

Family Studies

History. The main events in the study of the *HLA* complex, with the names of investigators who contributed a great deal to these studies, are listed chronologically in Table 8.11. The early history of the *HLA* system was mentioned in Chapter 2.

One of the first *HLA* recombinants was reported in 1969 by Flemming Kissmeyer-Nielsen and his collaborators. They examined several families for segregation of individual HLA determinants and found that determinants encoded by one chromosome were transmitted to the progeny as blocks. In one family, however, they detected an individual that had inher-

Table 8.11 Main Events in the History of HLA Studies

Year	Author	Event
1952	Jean Dausset	Demonstration in patients with certain blood disorders of substances capable of agglutinating leukocytes
1954	Jean Dausset	Observation that patients who received multiple blood transfusions contained leukocyte-agglutinating antibodies in their sera
1958	Jean Dausset	Definition of the first HLA determinant (Mac, now HLA-A2 + A28)
1958	Rose Payne, Jon J. van Rood	Demonstration that pregnancies may induce the formation of leukocyte-agglutinating antibodies in the mother
1962	Jon J. van Rood	Discovery of a diallelic leukocyte antigen system (4a,4b) and introduction of computer analysis to serological studies
1964	Paul I. Terasaki	Introduction of sensitive and rapid microassays for serological leukocyte antigen testing
1964	Bernard D. Amos	The First Histocompatibility Workshop, Durham, North Carolina
1965	Jean Dausset, Pavol Iványi, Dagmar Iványi	Proposal, on the basis of population studies, that most leukocyte antigens are controlled by a single genetic system
1965	Jon J. van Rood	The Second Histocompatibility Workshop, Leiden, The Netherlands
1967	Fritz H. Bach, Bernard D. Amos	Discovery that leukocytes from HLA-identical siblings, when mixed together, fail to give mixed leukocyte reaction, suggesting that the HLA controls MLR antigens
1967	Jean-Louis Amiel	Association between HLA and Hodgkin's disease
1967	Ruggero Ceppellini	The Third Histocompatibility Workshop, Torino, Italy
1967	Ruggero Ceppellini	Suggestion that HLA determinants can be divided into two mutually exclusive series, presumably controlled by two linked loci, *A* and *B*
1968	WHO Nomenclature Committee	Introduction of the term HLA for *H*uman *L*eukocyte *A*ntigen system
1968	Bernard D. Amos, Ruggero Ceppellini	Demonstration that the HLA system is involved in graft rejection (skin grafts transplanted between HLA-identical siblings survive longer than those between HLA-dissimilar siblings)
1969	Flemming Kissmeyer-Nielsen	Discovery of an intra-*HLA* recombinant
1970	Arne Svejgaard, Erik Thorsby, Flemming Kissmeyer-Nielsen	Evidence for the existence of a third series of HLA determinants controlled by a separate locus (*C*)
1970	Paul I. Terasaki	The Fourth Histocompatibility Workshop, Los Angeles, California
1971	Edmond J. Yunis	Demonstration that a locus separate from *A*, *B*, and *C* (locus *D*) controls antigens responsible for mixed lymphocyte reaction
1972	Jean Dausset	The Fifth Histocompatibility Workshop (devoted mainly to anthropological studies), Paris, France
1975	Flemming Kissmeyer-Nielsen	The Sixth Histocompatibility Workshop, Aarhus, Denmark
1977	Walter F. Bodmer	The Seventh Histocompatibility Workshop, Oxford, England
1980	Paul I. Terasaki	The Eighth Histocompatibility Workshop, Los Angeles, California

Table 8.12 Frequency of HLA Genes in Different Races

	Caucasians			Mongolians			Blacks	
Gene	Europe	Middle East	India	Mon-golians	Australia	American Indian	Blacks (average)	Hottentots
A1	17	13	12	2	0	1	4	5
A2	28	20	15	18	11	48	17	12
A3	15	10	7	1	0	1	8	8
Aw23	2	6	2	2	6	0	8	7
Aw24	7	13	12	39	22	25	5	6
Aw25	2	1	1	2	15	0	1	1
Aw26	4	4	6	5	10	0	7	23
A11	6	6	18	13	6	1	1	0
A28	4	6	6	2	0	9	9	10
A29	4	1	1	1	1	0	5	9
Aw30	2	4	1	2	2	1	16	8
Aw31	1	2	1	0	0	9	2	3
Aw32	4	4	3	0	0	0	4	3
A33	2	5	7	7	20	4	7	5
Blank	2	5	8	6	7	1	6	0
B5	6	15	19	9	0	10	8	6
B7	13	3	5	2	0	1	12	13
B8	11	3	8	1	0	0	4	2
B12	16	9	10	3	0	1	12	14
B13	2	3	2	4	11	0	1	1
Bw35	10	13	12	6	0	24	6	8
Bw40	6	4	6	24	32	15	7	7
B14	4	4	0	0	0	1	3	8
Bw15	6	1	8	16	15	14	4	5
Bw16	4	6	1	4	1	12	1	2
Bw17	4	5	8	2	0	1	21	14
B18	5	5	2	1	0	1	3	6
Bw21	2	9	1	0	0	4	1	0
Bw22	3	3	3	13	37	0	1	1
B27	4	2	2	3	0	3	1	3
Blank	4	15	13	12	4	13	15	10

Source. From G. D. Snell, J. Dausset, and S. Nathenson: *Histocompatibility*, p. 214. Academic, New York, 1976.

ited the determinants in a new combination not found in the parents. The family consisted of a father, mother, and six daughters (Fig. 8.6). When one designates the haplotypes of the father *ab* and those of the mother *cd* (a common practice used in HLA family studies), one can designate the haplotypes of three children in this particular family as *bd*, that of one child as *ac*, and that of the fifth child as *ad*. The sixth child carried the *b* haplotype of the father but her second haplotype coded for one determinant inherited from the mother and another determinant inherited from the father. This combination of determinants apparently arose by crossingover between loci controlling these two determinants. Later, other investigators found many other intra-*HLA* recombinants, and by typing these for products of other loci, they were able to arrange these loci into linear order—the genetic map of the *HLA* complex.

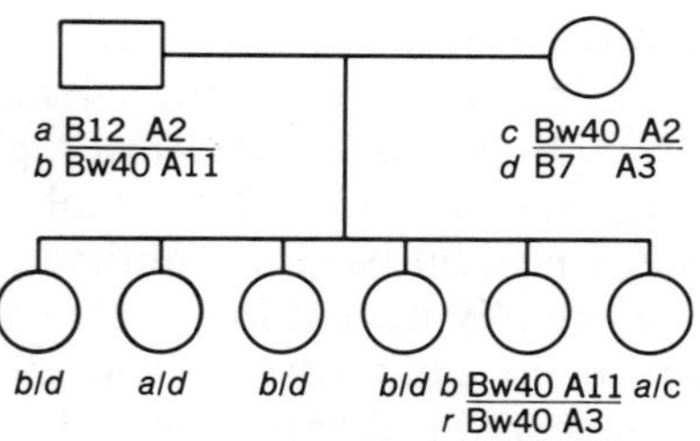

Figure 8.6. Pedigree of a human family with the fifth child carrying intra-*HLA* recombinant chromosome. Squares indicate males (father), circles females (mother or daughters); *a, b, c, d* indicate haplotypes, A and B numbers indicate HLA-A and HLA-B determinants. (Based on data of F. Kissmeyer-Nielsen, A. Svejgaard, and L. S. Nielsen: *Nature* **224**:75–76, 1969.)

The *HLA* Map. The *HLA* complex consists of three class I loci—*A*, *B*, and *C*—and at least one class II locus—*D* (Fig. 8.4). The order of loci from the centromere is *D–B–C–A*. In contrast to the *H*-2 complex, where the class II loci are within the complex between the *K* and *D* class I loci, at least one class II locus in the *HLA* complex lies outside the class I loci. Intercalated between class I and class II loci are the class III loci—*C2*, coding for the second complement component; *C4*, coding for the fourth complement component (and also for the blood-group antigens Chido and Rodgers; see Chapter 9); and *Bf*, coding for the B factor of the alternative complement pathway. The exact location and order of these loci are not known. The recombination frequency between the *A* and *B* loci is approximately 1 percent, and that between *D* and *B* another 1 percent, so that the entire *HLA* complex is about 2 cM long.

Chromosomal Location. The *HLA* complex resides in human chromosome 6, a submetacentric chromosome consisting of one short and one long arm; the complex is located in the long arm (Fig. 8.5). Linked to *HLA* are several enzyme-encoding loci—*SOD*-2, *PGM*-3, *ME*-1, *GLO*, and *Pg*.

Population Genetics

At the population level, the *HLA* system displays many of the same properties as the *H*-2 complex: a

Table 8.13 Frequencies and Δ-Values × 10^3 of Some *HLA*-(*A,B*), (*C,A*), and (*D,B*) Haplotypes in Caucasians

Combination	Haplotype	Frequency	Δ	Combination	Haplotype	Frequency	Δ
A,B	*A1,B8*	98	77	C,A	*C1,A26*	7	6
	A1,B17	15	8		*C2,A2*	33	17
	A2,B12	63	19		*C3,A2*	91	28
	A2,B15	47	16		*C4,A3*	28	15
	A2,B40	50	19		*C4,A11*	15	10
	A3,B7	54	33	C,B	*C1,B22*	16	15
	A3,B35	25	14		*C1,B27*	17	16
	A11,B22	3	2		*C2,B27*	31	29
	A11,B35	25	14		*C2,B40*	14	10
	A25,B18	5	5		*C3,B15*	96	77
	A26,B38	8	7		*C3,B40*	86	68
	A28,B14	5	3		*C4,B35*	69	63
	A28,B15	9	3	D,B	*D1,B35*	33	27
	A28,B18	6	4		*D2,B7*	39	26
	A29,B12	15	11		*D3,B8*	86	72
	A29,B45	2	2		*D4,B15*	43	35
	A32,B41	2	2		*D5,B16*	15	13
					D6,B16	8	7
					D7,B13	9	8
					D8,B40	13	9

Source. Taken from A. Svejgaard, M. Hange, C. Jersild, P. Platz, L. P. Ryder, L. Staub Nielsen, and M. Thomsen: *The HLA System, An Introductory Survey*, 2nd ed., p. 27. Karger, Basel, 1979.

high degree of polymorphism (Table 8.12) and genetic differentiation of individual populations (ethnic groups, races). The latter characteristic is manifested in the presence or absence, in a given population, of certain antigenic determinants (genes), particular gene frequencies, and the occurrence of certain allelic combinations (haplotypes). For example, Caucasians are characterized by the common occurrence of the A1 and B8 determinants, which are infrequent or absent in most other ethnic groups. Furthermore, the A1,B8 combination is a frequent haplotype in European Caucasians. The frequency of A1 and B8 determinants declines from the north to the south of Europe, while the frequency of two other determinants, B5 and B35, displays an opposite trend. Other determinants frequent in Caucasians are A3 and B7, and again, the A3,B7 combination is one of the common haplotypes of this race. Blacks are characterized by the high frequency of A9, A10, A30, and B17, and by three determinants—A36, A43, and B42—that are extremely rare in other races. Mongolians have a high frequency of A9, B40, B15, and B22, and lack determinants A1, A3, B7, and B8. Determinant A9 is particularly frequent in Eskimos, who, in addition, have an Eskimo-specific, *B* locus-encoded determinant. American Indians have only a few determinants, such as A2, A9, A28, A31, A33, B5, B27, B35, B40, B15, and B16. This fact, and the low frequency of blanks (alleles characterized by the absence of all known determinants), suggests a high degree of homozygosity in this race. A2, which is generally the most frequent determinant, reaches a frequency of 80 percent in American Indians. The B15 determinant occurs mainly in South American Indians, whereas B27 is primarily a North American Indian determinant. Australians are characterized by the high frequency of A10 and B22. Polynesians have a high frequency of B22. Similar differences among individual races also exist in terms of haplotypes (Table 8.13).

8.4 BIOCHEMISTRY AND TISSUE DISTRIBUTION

8.4.1 Class I Molecules

Tissue Distribution

Class I molecules are ubiquitous in somatic tissues: there is no tissue known of which one can say with certainty that it completely lacks H-2 or HLA antigens. However, most somatic cells (in particular, muscle cells, fibroblasts, and cells of the nervous system) have only a low content of class I molecules; the only cells with a relatively high concentration are those belonging to the immune system (i.e., lymphocytes of both the T and B categories, and macrophages). But even in the high-content cells, class I molecules constitute less than 1 percent of all membrane proteins.

Embryos generally have a lower content of class I molecules than do adult tissues, and the content is lower the younger the embryos are. Early embryos have very few—or, according to some immunologists, no—class I molecules. Tumors derived from early embryos (teratocarcinomas) are completely devoid of class I molecules. Trophoblastic cells (i.e., embryonic cells that erode the uterus and form a kind of buffer layer between the mother and the fetus) may also be devoid of class I antigens. The presence of class I molecules on germ cells (spermatozoa and eggs) is an open question: some investigators find these cells to react positively with anti-class I sera, while others argue that these reactions are artifacts and that, in actuality, germ cells are devoid of class I molecules.

Biochemistry

All MHC molecules are anchored in the cell membrane; although "free" class I molecules were reported to be present in the plasma and urine, they later proved to be small membrane fragments—remnants of cell destruction. Originally, some biochemists claimed to have found MHC molecules on intracellular membranes as well, but these claims could not be substantiated either. The association with membranes was the main reason it took biochemists more than 10 years to learn how to isolate MHC molecules in a pure form. The pioneering work on MHC biochemistry was done in the laboratories of Stanley G. Nathenson, Jack L. Strominger, and Ralph Reisfeld.

At first, biochemists tried to cleave off the MHC molecules from the membrane by the use of proteolytic enzymes, such as papain, but then they realized that this method left a significant part of the molecule in the membrane. At present, a common method for isolating MHC molecules is dissolving the lipids of the membrane bilayer with detergent and pulling out the molecules from the mixture of proteins thus released with a specific antiserum. One such method, used for purification of both class I and class II molecules, is described below.

Method of MHC Molecule Isolation. The method consists of five main steps: radiolabeling, solubilization, purification, immunoprecipitation, and polyacrylamide gel electrophoresis.

Radiolabeling. There are two principal ways to label MHC molecules: biosynthetic and cell-surface labeling. In the former, lymphocytes from spleen, lymph node, or peripheral blood are incubated in short-term (five to six hours) tissue culture with ^{3}H, ^{14}C-, or ^{35}S-radiolabeled amino acids or carbohydrate precursors. Since there is a relatively rapid turnover of membrane proteins, labeled amino acids are incorporated into the newly synthesized MHC molecules (and of course, into other cellular proteins too), tagging these molecules. In the cell-surface method, radioactive iodine (i.e., ^{125}I) is chemically attached directly to the proteins of the cell membrane. The reaction is catalyzed by the enzyme lactoperoxidase (Fig. 8.7).

Solubilization. After radiolabeling, the cells are harvested and solubilized by a detergent, a substance that provides cleansing properties when dissolved in a liquid. Detergents resemble lipids of the phosphoglyceride type in that they, too, have strong polar head regions and long, nonpolar hydrocarbon tails (see Appendix 5.1). The introduction of a detergent into water results in the formation of *micelles*—small, usually spherical aggregates in which the hydrophobic tails are directed inward and the polar heads are oriented toward the aqueous environment (see Fig. 5.38). When a detergent comes into contact with a lipid, the lipid molecules are incorporated into the micelles by a mechanism, the precise nature of which is dependent on the properties of the lipid. If the lipid is relatively polar, its molecules are simply integrated with those of the detergent; if it is nonpolar, its molecules are engulfed by the micelle and incorporated into the tail portions of the detergent molecules. Because the detergent is dissolved in water (in the form of micelles), the lipid is solubilized by incorporation into the micelles. Solubilization of the cell membrane by the detergent is believed to occur by the same principle—by incorporation of the membrane lipids into the micelles and the release of the membrane proteins into the solution. Detergents can be classified, according to their polar groups, into three major categories: anionic, in which the polar groups carry a negative charge; cationic, with positively charged polar groups; and nonionic, in which the whole molecule carries no charge and produces electrically neutral micelles in solution.

The detergent commonly used for MHC molecule isolation is Nonidet P-40, or NP-40 (a commercial trademark designation by the Shell Oil Company, which developed it). NP-40 detergent preserves the tertiary and the quaternary structure of the MHC molecules and does not interfere with reactions of these molecules with antibodies, lectins, and enzymes. Cell particles insoluble in NP-40 are removed from the mixture by ultracentrifugation.

Partial Purification. The supernatant obtained after ultracentrifugation contains a great variety of proteins, among which the MHC molecules constitute only a small minority. To enrich the mixture for the MHC molecules, the latter are partially purified by the use of lectin obtained from the lentil *Lens culinaris*. Lectins are proteins of plant or animal origin that bind specifically to certain sugars (see Chapter 10 for details). The lentil lectin, for example, binds to glucose and mannose, both of which are present in MHC molecules (see below). Since some other proteins and glycoproteins in the mixture do not contain these two sugars, the MHC molecules (together with other glucose- or mannose-containing glycoproteins) can be separated

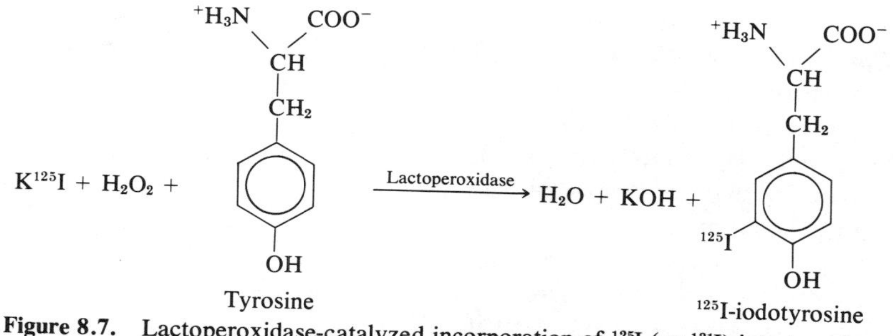

$$K^{125}I + H_2O_2 + \text{Tyrosine} \xrightarrow{\text{Lactoperoxidase}} H_2O + KOH + {}^{125}I\text{-iodotyrosine}$$

Figure 8.7. Lactoperoxidase-catalyzed incorporation of ^{125}I (or ^{131}I) into tyrosine of cell-surface proteins (including those encoded by the major histocompatibility complex). In this reaction, potassium iodide is oxidized to "active iodine," presumably a cationic form of iodine (I^{+}), which then reacts with ionized tyrosine residues of the protein.

from the former by the lentil lectin. The NP-40-solubilized mixture is therefore applied to a column containing lentil lectin bound to Sepharose 4B. The passed (effluent) fraction is collected and the bound fraction is eluted with α-methyl mannoside. (The latter is a glycoside produced by the reaction of mannose with an alcohol; it releases the column-bound MHC molecules by competing with the mannose for their carbohydrate moieties.) The eluted fraction contains less than 10 percent of the applied radioactivity (but most of the MHC activity), indicating a significant purification of the MHC molecules in this step. The α-methyl mannoside does not interfere with antibody binding to the MHC molecules.

Immunoprecipitation. The MHC molecules in the partially purified fraction are reacted with specific anti-MHC sera and the formed immune precipitate is separated from the rest of the molecules in the mixture. However, the antigen-antibody complexes formed by the reaction of MHC and anti-MHC alone do not precipitate; to induce precipitation, a second reagent is needed—either a xenogeneic antibody to the MHC alloantibodies (e.g., rabbit anti-mouse IgG) or the so-called protein A of *Staphylococcus aureus*. Protein A binds to the Fc portion of most mammalian IgG (there are exceptions, however—for example, mouse IgG1), and the complexes of MHC, anti-MHC, and protein A then precipitate from the solution. The precipitate is separated from the rest of the solution by centrifugation.

SDS-PAGE. The MHC molecules are released from the precipitate by boiling in sodium dodecyl sulfate (SDS-nonreducing conditions) or SDS and 2-mercaptoethanol (reducing conditions) and detected by polyacrylamide gel electrophoresis (PAGE; Fig. 8.8).

A modification of this method—the so-called *sequential immunoprecipitation procedure*—can be used for studying whether two antigenic determinants are on the same or different molecules. The preparation containing the two determinants is reacted with an alloantiserum detecting one of the two determinants, the antigen-antibody precipitate is removed by centrifugation, and the supernatant is then tested for the presence of the second determinant. If the second determinant remains in the solution after the removal of the first, it is concluded that the two determinants are carried by different molecules. If the first alloantiserum removes both determinants, one presumes that the determinants are on the same molecule.

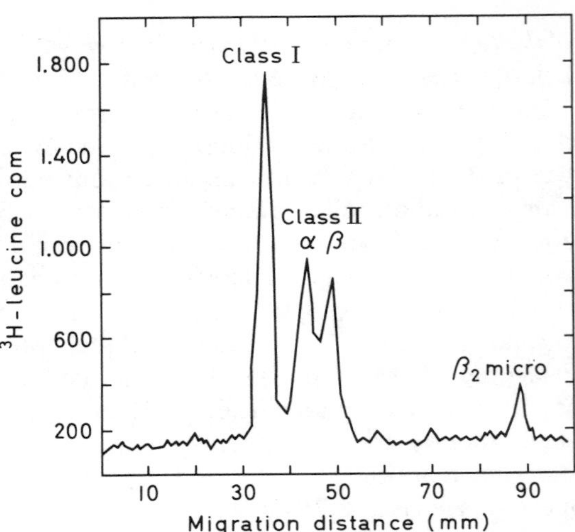

Figure 8.8. The biochemical MHC "signature." SDS-PAGE pattern of H-2 (class I and class II) molecules biosynthetically labelled with ^{3}H-leucine, precipitated with specific antisera, and analyzed using reducing conditions.

General Structure. Each class I MHC molecule consists of one heavy glycoprotein chain and one light protein subunit (Figs. 8.9 and 8.10). Only the protein portion of the heavy subunit is known to be controlled by the MHC region. The light chain is controlled by a locus in a different chromosome (chromosome 2 in the mouse and 15 in humans); the chromosomal position of

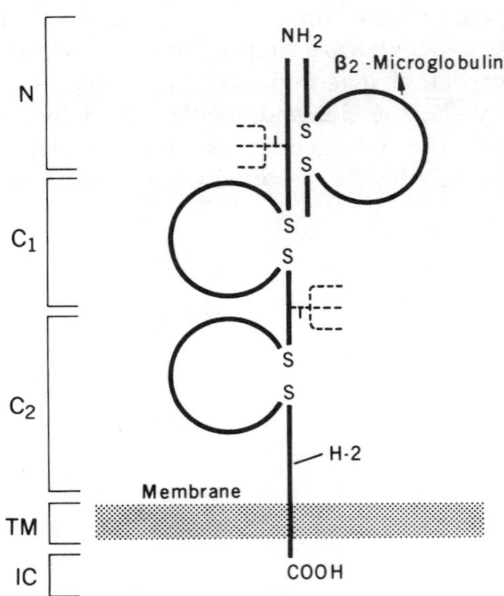

Figure 8.9. Diagrammatic view of a membrane-bound H-2 molecule combined with a molecule of β_2-microglobulin. Broken lines indicate carbohydrate moieties. Regions: N, aminoterminal; C_1, first disulfide loop; C_2, second disulfide loop; TM, transmembrane; IC, intracellular. (From J. Klein: *Science* **203**:516–521, 1979.)

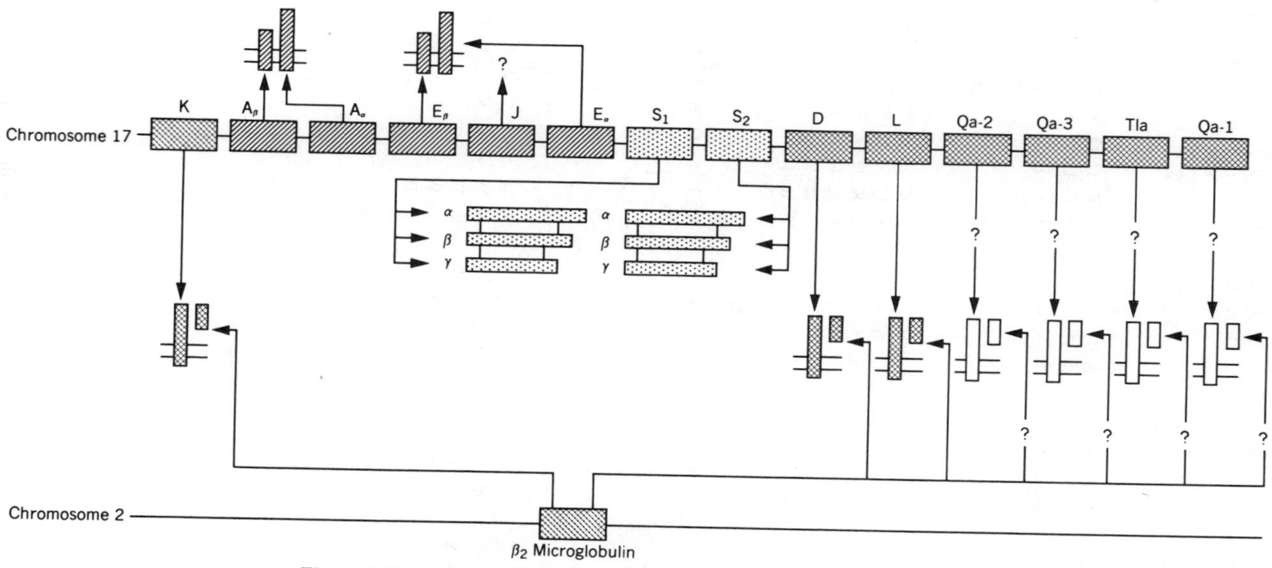

Figure 8.10. The products of the *H-2* loci. ?, product not identified.

the loci controlling the carbohydrate moieties is unknown. The moieties are covalently attached to the heavy chains; the heavy and light chains are both held together by noncovalent bonds. Only the heavy chain is anchored in the cell membrane; the light chain and the carbohydrate moieties are on the outside of the cell. The antigenicity and biological activity of class I molecules reside in the heavy subunit; the function of the light subunit is not known.

The Heavy Chain. The heavy polypeptide chain has a molecular weight of about 39,000 daltons and consists of some 350 amino acids. Covalently attached to each heavy chain are one or two carbohydrate moieties (see below), each weighing about 3000 daltons, so that the entire heavy subunit has a molecular weight of about 44,000 daltons. The polypeptide chain can be divided into three segments, based on the relationship of these segments to the membrane: extracellular, consisting of from 280 to 300 amino acids exposed on the cell surface; transmembrane, consisting of 25 to 30 amino acids and spanning the width of the cell membrane; and intracellular, composed of another 25 to 30 amino acids and extending from the inner membrane surface into the cell's interior. The extracellular segment contains four half-cystines, which pair to form two disulfide bridges. Each bridge forms a loop of some 60 amino acids (Fig. 8.9). The bridges divide the extracellular segment into three regions: amino terminal, first disulfide loop, and second disulfide loop. Complete amino acid sequences have been reported for HLA by Jack L. Strominger and his collaborators, and for H-2 by the laboratories of Stanley G. Nathenson and Thomas J. Kindt (Fig. 8.11). In addition, short N-terminal sequences have been determined for several MHC molecules by the combined efforts of several laboratories (Fig. 8.12). Though incomplete, the data allow one to draw important conclusions about the degree of genetic variation of the class I loci.

Interallelic Variation. The comparison of different *K* and *D* alleles in Figure 8.12 reveals that, in the first 20 residues, two allelic products differ in one amino acid every 10 residues. Deeper into the molecule, this number may increase (see below) so that there may be a difference of some 40 to 50 amino acids between any two heavy chains. This great number of differences is not known for any other two allelic products at any other eukaryotic locus—allelic products normally differ by a single amino acid substitution. But not all class I allelic products differ in this many amino acids; the products of alleles derived from other alleles by recent mutations may differ, like alleles at most other loci, by only one or a few amino acid substitutions.

Interlocus Variation within One Species. The *HLA-A* and *B* loci share some 80 percent of their amino acids (the *C* locus has not been characterized biochemically), and a similar degree of homology also exists between the *H-2K* and *D* loci. This homology supports the hypothesis that the *A* and *B* loci in the human and the *K* and *D* loci in the mouse arose by gene duplication from a common ancestral gene. The degree of homology between class I loci is almost as great as the

```
                          10                  20                  30                  40                  50
HLA-A2   G S H S M R Y F F T S V S R P G R G E P R F I A V G Y V D D T Q F V R F D S D A A S Z R M E P R A P
HLA-B7   G S H S M R Y F Y T S V S R P G R G E P R F I S V G Y V D D T Q F V R F D S D A A S P R E E P R A P
H-2K^b   G P H S L R Y F V T A V S R P G L G E P R Y M E V G Y V D D T E F V R F D S D A E N P R Y E P R A R
H-2K^k   G P H S L R Y F H T A V S R P G L G K P R F I   V G Y       T   F   R F                   Y
H-2D^d   G S H S M R Y F V T A V S R P G F G E P R Y I E V G Y V         F V R F                 R Y
H-2L^d       H   L R Y F V T   V   R     F       R Y M   V   Y V     T   F V R F                 R Y

                          60                  70                  80                  90                 100
HLA-A2     I E Q E Q P E Y W           K V K A H A H T V R V D L G T L R G Y Y N Q S E A G S H T L Q R M Y G
HLA-B7   W I E Q E G P E Y W D R N Y Q I Y K A Q A Q T D R E S L R N L R G Y Y N Q S E A G S H T L Q S M Y G
H-2K^b   W M E Q E G P E Y W E R E T Q K A K G N E Q S F R V D L R T L L G Y Y N Q S K G G S H T I Q V I S G
H-2K^k     M     V       Y       R   T     A K         F R V     R T   L R Y Y                 T       M Y I
H-2D^d     M             Y W                                                                 H         M A
H-2L^d     X             Y W   R I T   I           W F R V     R T                                     M Y

                         110                 120                 130                 140                 150
HLA-A2   C   V G S D W R F L R G Y H Q Y A Y D G K D Y I A L K E D L R S W T A A D T M A Q I T K H K W E A A
HLA-B7   C D V G P D G R L L R G H D Q Y A Y D G K D Y I A L N E D L R S W T A A D T A A Q I T Q R K W E A A
H-2K^b   C E V G S D G R L L R G Y Q Q Y A Y D G C D Y I A L N E D L K T W T A A D M A A L I T K H K W E Q A
H-2K^k                 K L L           Y   Y         Y I           L               M A A L I T K H K W   V
H-2D^d       V         R       R       F                                           M       I T X R W
H-2L^d       V         R       R   Y   F   Y         Y I                 T W       M       I T R R

                         160                 170                 180                 190                 200
HLA-A2   R V A E G R R A Y L E G T C V E W
HLA-B7   R E A E G R R A Y L E G E C V E W L R R Y L E N G K D K L E R A D P P K T H V T H H P I S D H E A T
H-2K^b   G E A E R L R A Y L E G T C V E W L R R Y L K
H-2K^k           R   R   Y L     T   V     L R R
H-2D^d
H-2L^d

                         210                 220                 230                 240                 250
HLA-A2                                                         T E L V E T R P A G D R T F E K W A A V V V P
HLA-B7   L R C W A L G F Y P A E I T L T W Q R D G E D Q T Q D M E L V E T R P A G D G T F Q K W A S V V V P
H-2K^b                                                         M     V   T R           T F   K W
H-2K^k                                                         M     V   T R           T F     W     V V V
H-2D^d                                                         M     V   T R             F     W     V V V
H-2L^d

                         260                 270
HLA-A2
HLA-B7   S G E E Q R Y T C H V Q H E G L P K P L T
H-2K^b   L G K E Q Y Y T C H V Y Q Q G L P
H-2K^k             Y
H-2D^d               Y T       X H
H-2L^d               Y T     V Y H

                         310                 320
HLA-A2             M W R R K S S D R K G G S Y S Q A
HLA-B7             M C R R K S S G G K G G S Y S Q A
H-2K^b
H-2K^k               M R R R         K       Y A L A
H-2D^d
H-2L^d
```

Figure 8.11. Comparison of amino-acid sequence of HLA and H-2 class I polypeptide chains. (Compiled from data produced mainly by the laboratories of Jack L. Strominger, Stanley G. Nathenson, and Thomas J. Kindt.)

	1				5					10					15					20					25			
Human HLA-A2	G	S	H	S	M	R	Y	F	F	T	S	V	S	R	P	G	R	G	E	P	R	F	I	A	V	G	Y	V
B7	G	S	H	S	M	R	Y	F	Y	T	S	V	S	R	P	G	R	G	E	P	R	F	I	S	V	G	Y	V
B12	G	S			M	R	Y	F	Y	T	A	V	S	R	P	G		G	E			F	I	A				
B14	G	S			M	R	Y	F	Y	T	S	V	S	R	P	G		G	E	S	B	F	I					
Mouse H-2K^b	G	P	H	S	L	R	Y	F	V	T	A	V	S	R	P	G	L	G	E	P	R	Y	M	E	V	G	Y	V
K^d	G		H	S	L	R	Y	F	V	T		V	S	R	P	G	L	G		P	R	F	I		V	G	Y	V
K^k	G	P	H	S	L	R	Y	F	H	T	A	V	S	R	P	G	L	G	K	P	R	F	I		V	G	Y	
K^g					L	R	Y	F			A	V		R			L				R	F	I		V		Y	V
K^s					L	R	Y	F	V		A	V		R			F				R	Y					Y	V
D^b	G	P	H		M	R	Y			T	A	V	S	R	P	G	L			P	R	Y	I		V	G	Y	V
D^d	G	S	H	S	M	R	Y	F	V	T	A	V	S	R	P	G	F	G	E	P	R	Y	I	E	V	G	Y	V
D^g		P				R	Y	F			A	V		R	P		L				R	Y			V		Y	V
D^s		R			M	R	Y	F	V		A	V		R			L				R	Y			V		Y	V
L^d			H		L	R	Y	F	V	T		V		R			F				R	Y	M		V		Y	V
Rat RT1-B4					L/I	R	Y	F	Y		A	V										F	I	A	V		Y	V
Guinea pig GPLA-B1			H		L	R	Y	F	Y		A	V			P							F	V				Y	
B2			H		L		Y	V	Y		A	V			P												Y	
B3			H		L		Y	F	Y	I		V													V			
Rabbit RLA-11	G	S	H	S	M	R	Y	F	Y		S	V	S	R	P	G	L	G		P	R	F			V	G	Y	V
Domestic fowl B-2		L	H		L			I	F						P		P		L			F	V		V		Y	V
9		L	H		L	R	Y	I			A				P							Y					Y	
10			H			R	Y	F	R			M																

Figure 8.12. N-terminal amino-acid sequences of molecules encoded by class I MHC loci in different species. (Compiled from different sources.)

homology between alleles at the same locus, so that when one is confronted with an unknown class I sequence, one is unable to tell by which MHC locus this sequence is controlled.

Although the 20 percent of differences between the products of two loci are scattered throughout the polypeptide chain, there are two regions of increased variability—one between residues 60 through 80 in the human HLA-A and B molecules and another between residues 105 through 114. In these regions, the homology between two loci is only about 40 to 50 percent; in the rest of the chain, homology is about 90 percent. Similar distribution of variability is also observed when one compares human and mouse MHC molecules.

Interspecies Variation. Human and mouse class I MHC molecules share about 70 to 75 percent of their amino acids, which is somewhat less than the degree of sharing between two class I loci of a single species. The mouse *K* locus is slightly more similar to the human *A* locus than it is to the *B* locus.

The highly conserved second disulfide loop of HLA shows some degree of homology with the constant-region domains of the immunoglobulin molecule. The significance of this homology is unclear, but some immunologists conclude from this observation that the MHC and immunoglobulin loci are evolutionarily related. However, no MHC-immunoglobulin homology has been found in the other regions of the MHC molecule, and it is possible that the homology of the second disulfide loop is an example of evolutionary convergence—an independent development of similar sequences in two unrelated molecules subjected to similar selective pressures.

The only thing known about the secondary and tertiary structure of the heavy chain is that most of it is arranged into β-pleated sheets.

Like other proteins, the MHC heavy and light chains are synthesized in the cisternae of the rough endoplasmic reticulum (RER) and then transported into the Golgi apparatus. Vesicles containing membrane-integrated MHC molecules are then pinched off from the apparatus and presumably inserted into the cell membrane, by a process resembling that described for cell-surface immunoglobulin (see Chapter 6). The precursor of the heavy chain has a molecular weight of some 39,000 to 40,000 daltons, and contains, at the amino terminal, a signal sequence of about 10 to 20 amino acids (molecular weight of 1000 to 2000 daltons). The signal sequence is needed for the insertion of the precursor into the RER membrane and is cleaved off after the insertion. The membrane-bound 38,000- to 39,000-dalton chain is then glycosylated. However, only a core of oligosaccharide units is attached to the polypeptide chain at this stage; additional glycosylation occurs, apparently in the Golgi apparatus. Insertion into the membrane is not dependent on the concomitant synthesis of the light chain, which is added to the heavy chain after glycosylation in the RER membranes.

The Light Chain. In 1968, Ingemar Berggård and A. G. Bearn isolated, from human urine, a low-molecular-weight component which, on electrophoresis, migrated in the region of β_2-globulins. In reference to these two properties (small size and migration in the electric field), these authors designated the component β_2-microglobulin (abbreviated β_2m or sometimes $\beta_2\mu$). Immunologists became interested in β_2-microglobulin only four years later, when Oliver Smithies and M. David Poulik sequenced the protein and discovered that it was structurally related to immunoglobulins. Still later, several groups of investigators demonstrated almost simultaneously that the β_2-microglobulin is a cell-membrane protein associated with class I MHC molecules.

Human β_2-microglobulin has a molecular weight of 11,800 daltons and contains 100 amino acids (Fig. 8.13). Two half-cysteines, one at position 24 and another at position 81, form a single disulfide bridge spanning a looped-out segment of the polypeptide chain. β_2-microglobulin is a highly conserved protein, as seen from the fact that very little allelic variation has been found at the β_2-m-encoding locus and from the observation that a high degree of homology exists between the corresponding molecules of different species (Fig. 8.14). The protein displays about 28 percent homology with the CH3 domain of human immunoglobulin molecules. The homology is further supported by similar chain length, similar position of the disulfide bridges, and probably similar secondary and tertiary structures. So conspicuous is this homology that the β_2-microglobulin molecule may be regarded as a free single immunoglobulin domain. One can imagine that the β_2m gene originated from the same ancestral gene that gave rise to the immunoglobulin genes and perhaps to at least a portion of the class I heavy chains as well.

No covalent bonds can be demonstrated between the heavy and light chains, and so the two polypeptides must be held together by noncovalent linkages. The precise nature of this association and the spatial arrangement of the two chains are not known.

β_2-microglobulin is synthesized by virtually all somatic cells. Precursors of β_2-microglobulin have a molecular weight of about 15,000 daltons and contain a signal sequence of 19 amino acids, which is cleaved off

	1 ... 10 ... 20
β_2-Microglobulin	I Q R T P K I Q V Y S R H P A — E — — — — N G K S N F L N
EU C_L (residues 109–214)	T V A A P — — S V F I F P P S D E Q — — L K S G T A S V V
EU C_H1(residues 119–220)	S T L G P — — S V F P L A P S S K S — — T S G G T A A L G
EU C_H2(residues 234–341)	L L G G P — — S V F L F P P K P K D T L M I S R T P E V T
EU C_H3(residues 342–446)	Q P R E P — — Q V Y T L P P S R E E — — M T K N Q V S L T

	30 ... 40 ... 50
β_2-Microglobulin	C Y V S G F H P S D I E V — — D L L K D G E R I E K V — E
EU C_L (residues 109–214)	C L L N N F Y P R E A K V — — Q W K V D N — A L Q S G N S
EU C_H1(residues 119–220)	C L V K D Y F P E P V T V — — S W N S — G — A L F S G V
EU C_H2(residues 234–341)	C V V V D V S H E D P Q V K F N W Y V D G — — V Q V H N A
EU C_H3(residues 342–446)	C L V K G F Y P S D I A V — — E W E S N D — — G E P E N Y

	60 ... 70
β_2-Microglobulin	H S D L S F S K N — W S F Y L L Y S Y — T E F T P T — E K
EU C_L (residues 109–214)	Q E S V T E Q D S K D S T Y S L S S T L T L S K A D Y E K
EU C_H1(residues 119–220)	H T F P A V L Q S — S G L Y S L S S V V T V P S S S L G T
EU C_H2(residues 234–341)	K T K P R E Q Q Y — D S T Y R V V S V L T V L H Q N W L D
EU C_H3(residues 342–446)	K T T P P V L D S — D G S F F L Y S K L T V D K S R W Q Q

	80 ... 90 ... 100
β_2-Microglobulin	— D E Y A C R V N H V T L S Q P — — — K I V — K W D R D M
EU C_L (residues 109–214)	H K V Y A C E V T H Q G L S S P V T — K S F — — N R G E C
EU C_H1(residues 119–220)	Q — T Y I C N V N H K P S N T K V — D K R V — — E P K S C
EU C_H2(residues 234–341)	G K E Y K C K V S N K A L P A P I — E K T I S K A K G
EU C_H3(residues 342–446)	G N V F S C S V M H E A L H N H Y F Q K S L S L S P G

Figure 8.13. Comparison of the amino-acid sequence of β_2-microglobulin with that of the constant regions of human γG1 immunoglobulin Eu. Sequences are aligned to maximize homology (indicated by boxes). Numbering is for β_2-microglobulin. (Based on P. A. Peterson et al., *Proc. Natl. Acad. Sci. U.S.A.* **69:**1697, 1972.)

	1				5					10
Human	I	Q	R	T	P	K	I	Q	V	Y
Dog	V	Q	H	P	P	K	I	Q	V	Y
Rabbit	V	Z	R	A	P	B	V	Z	V	Y

	11				15					20
Human	S	R	H	P	A	Z	N	G	K	S
Dog	S	R	H	P	A	Z	B	G	K	P
Rabbit	S	R	H	P	A	Z	B	G	K	P

	21				25					30
Human	N	F	L	N	C	Y	V	S	G	F
Dog	B	F	L	B	C	Y	V	S	G	F
Rabbit	B	F	L	B	C	Y	V	S	G	F

	31				35					40
Human	H	P	S	D	I	E	V	D	L	L
Dog	H	P	?	Z	I	Z	I	B	L	L
Rabbit	H	P	P	Z	I	B	I	Z	L	

Figure 8.14. Comparison of partial amino-acid sequences of β_2-microglobulin from three species of mammal. Homologies are indicated by boxes. (Based on D. Poulik *in Trace Components of Plasma: Isolation and Clinical Significance*, pp. 155–177, Liss, New York 1976.

before the chain combines with the heavy chain. Light chains that fail to combine with heavy chains remain in the precursor form in the cytoplasm.

Attrition of cell surfaces leads to shedding of small amounts of β_2-microglobulin into bodily fluids (i.e., serum, colostrum, seminal fluid, and others). Under normal conditions, serum β_2-microglobulin is filtered through the tufts of the capillary loops (glomeruli) in the kidney and then catabolized in the tubuli. In patients with kidney diseases, damage to the tubuli prevents β_2-microglobulin degradation and results in the increase of this protein's level in the serum and the excretion of β_2-microglobulin into the urine. The latter usually serves as a source of β_2-microglobulin for isolation purposes.

The Carbohydrate Moiety. In the mouse, each K or D heavy chain has two carbohydrate moieties attached to it; in humans, each A and B chain has only one carbohydrate moiety attached, via the asparagine at position 86. A single moiety has a molecular weight of approximately 3300 daltons and consists of 12 to 15 monosaccharides. These include neutral sugars (mannose, galactose, and fucose), the amino sugar galactosamine, and sialic acid. A hypothetical model of the carbohydrate chain is depicted in Figure 8.15. The carbohydrate moiety is apparently invariable and probably functions in biosynthesis and turnover of the glycoproteins or positioning of the molecules in the membrane.

8.4.2 Class II Molecules

Tissue Distribution

Class II molecules are not so ubiquitous as class I molecules. In the mouse, the *A* and *E* locus-encoded molecules are present on B lymphocytes, possibly some T lymphocytes (the possibility that the molecules are acquired passively by T cells has not been excluded), macrophages, some epidermal cells (in particular, the so-called Langerhans cells; see Chapter 5), some epithelial cells, mammary gland cells, and possibly spermatozoa. The *J*-locus molecules have been found on suppressor T cells, a subpopulation of Con-A-responding T cells, T lymphocytes stimulated in mixed lymphocyte cultures, helper T cells, and macrophages.

Biochemistry

In the mouse, the anti-A and anti-E sera precipitate molecules with molecular weights of about 57,000 to 63,000 daltons from detergent-solubilized cell-

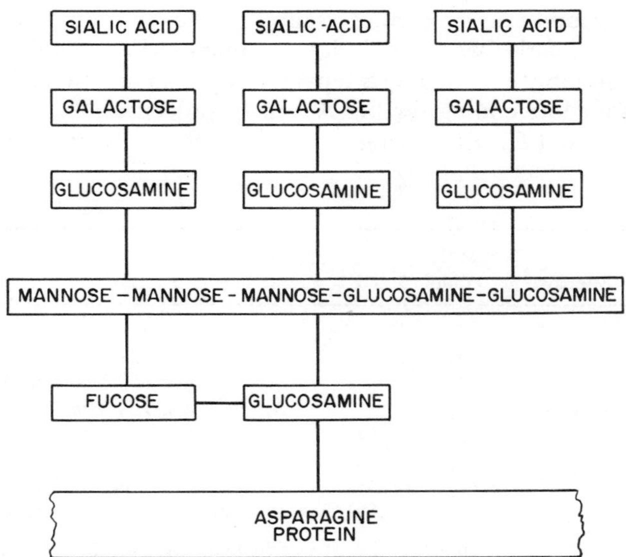

Figure 8.15. Presumed structure of the carbohydrate moiety attached to the heavy chain of the H-2 glycoprotein. (Based on S. G. Nathenson and T. Muramatsu: *in* G. A. Jamieson and T. J. Greenwald (Eds.): *Glycoproteins of Blood Cells and Plasma*, pp. 245–262. Lippincott, Philadelphia, 1971.)

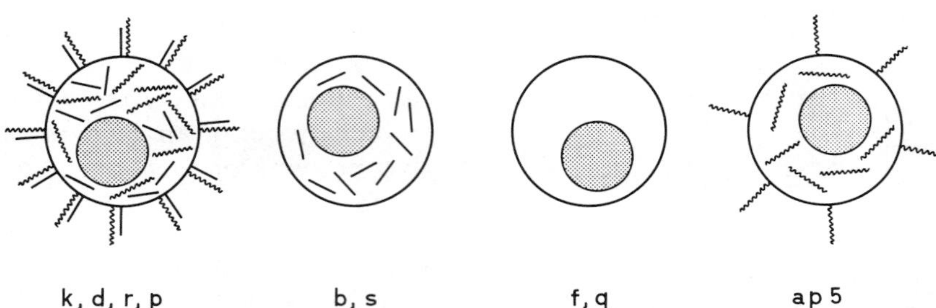

Figure 8.16. Expression of E_{α} and E_{β} chains in the cytoplasm and plasma membrane of mouse cells carrying different *H-2* haplotypes (small letters). Each circle represents a single cell; a straight line indicates the E_{α}, and a wavy line the E_{β} polypeptide.

membrane preparations. After the degradation of noncovalent bonds by treatment with sodium dodecyl sulfate (SDS), the A and E molecules dissociate, each into two chains—the heavier α (molecular weight 31,000 to 34,000 daltons) and the lighter β chain (molecular weight 26,000 to 29,000 daltons). In the human, the D (DR) molecules also consist of two chains, referred to as D_{α}, or p34 (i.e., a protein with a molecular weight of 34,000 daltons), and D_{β}, or p29 (i.e., a protein with a molecular weight of 29,000 daltons). These chains are glycoproteins with the carbohydrate moiety constituting some 10 to 15 percent of the chain's weight (about 3200 daltons). The moieties carried by different chains have similar properties; they also resemble carbohydrate moieties attached to class I molecules but differ from moieties in many other glycoproteins. The antigenic activity resides in the protein component of the glycoprotein molecule; claims to the contrary were apparently based on faulty techniques. Each chain is probably encoded by a separate locus, so that there are four loci coding for the A and E molecules—A_{α}, A_{β}, E_{α}, and E_{β}. Surprisingly, the E_{β}-encoding locus maps in the cluster of *A* loci, so that the E_{α}- and E_{β}-encoding loci are separated by the *J* locus and perhaps some other loci as well (Fig. 8.16).

Peptide mapping and N-terminal amino acid sequencing (Fig. 8.17) have provided the following information concerning chemical homologies and the degree of variation of class II molecules. The four murine chains A_{α}, A_{β}, E_{α}, and E_{β} are not homologous to one another or to class I chains. Murine A_{α} and A_{β} are not homologous to any known human class II molecule; murine E_{α} is homologous to human D_{α} (p34); murine E_{β} is homologous to human D_{β} (p29). The human equivalent of the murine *A* locus has not yet been detected.

The A_{α} is invariable by sequencing (only six residues determined thus far), but shows about 10 percent allelic variation when studied by peptide mapping; A_{β} shows about 35 percent allelic variability as determined by sequencing; E_{α} is invariable by sequencing (11 residues determined thus far), but shows 10 percent or less difference between alleles when tested by peptide mapping; E_{β} shows only about 15 percent allelic

Species	Molecule	1				5					10					15					20			25	
	A_{α}^{b}				Ile		Ala			Val			Tyr				Val	Tyr							Tyr
	A_{α}^{k}				Ile		Ala		Val	Val			Tyr				Val	Tyr							Tyr
	A_{β}^{b}			Ser		Arg	His	Phe	Val	Tyr		Phe					Tyr	Phe							Tyr
Mouse	A_{β}^{k}			Ser		Arg	His	Phe	Val			Phe	Pro	Pro	Phe		Tyr	Phe							Tyr
	E_{α}^{d}	Ile						Ile	Ile		Ala		Phe	Tyr	Leu	Leu						Phe	Phe		Phe
	E_{α}^{k}	Ile	Lys			His		Ile	Ile		Ala		Phe	Tyr	Leu	Leu				Arg		Phe			
	E_{β}^{d}	Val					Pro		Phe	Leu		Tyr	Val			Leu			Phe	Tyr				Val	Tyr
	E_{β}^{k}	Val	Arg		Ser	Arg	Pro		Phe	Leu		Tyr		Lys	Ser				Phe	Tyr					Tyr
	p^{34}	Ile	Lys	Glu	Glu	Arg	Val	Ile	Ile/Leu	Glu	Ala	Glu	Phe	Tyr	Leu	Asn	Tyr	Asp	Phe	Gln	Gly				
Human	p^{29}	Gly	Asp	Thr	Pro	Glu	Arg	Phe	Leu	Glu	Gln	Val													
Guinea pig	4,5	Ile	Tyr		Pro			Phe	Leu	Phe		Phe													

Figure 8.17. N-terminal amino-acid sequences of class II MHC polypeptide chains of the mouse, human and guinea pig. (Compiled from different sources.)

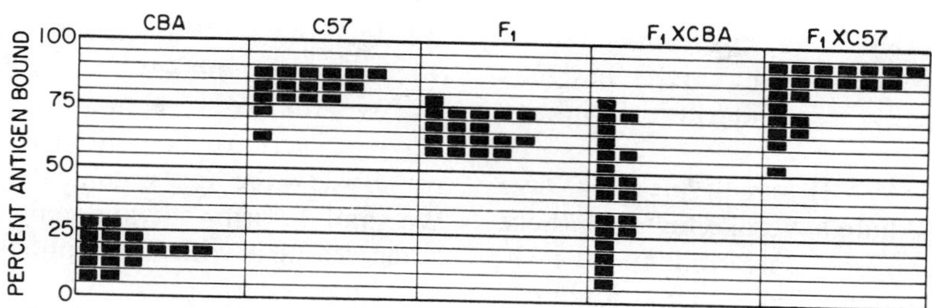

Figure 8.18. Antibody response of CBA and C57 mice and their hybrids to synthetic polypeptide (T,G)-A--L. Each rectangle represents one mouse. (From H. O. McDevitt: *Hospital Practice* **8**:61–74, 1973.)

variation by sequencing (13 residues determined thus far) but 30 to 50 percent variability when studied by peptide mapping. In general, it appears that both β chains are more variable than the two α chains.

Some *H*-2 haplotypes seem to carry mutations affecting the expression of the E molecule. Patricia P. Jones and her co-workers demonstrated that at least four cell types exist, in terms of E-molecule expression (Fig. 8.18). In some cells (i.e., those carrying *H*-2 haplotypes *k*, *d*, *r*, and *p*), both the E_α and E_β chains can be detected in the cytoplasm and on the cell surface. Other cells (i.e., those carrying *H*-2 haplotypes *b* and *s*) lack E_α chains in both the cytoplasm and plasma membrane and have E_β chains in the cytoplasm, but not on the membrane. A third kind of cell (i.e., those carrying *H*-2 haplotypes *f* and *q*) have no detectable E_α and E_β chains in either the membrane or cytoplasm. And finally, a fourth cell type, exemplified by that carrying the $H\text{-}2^{ap5}$ haplotype, expresses the E_α, but not the E_β chain in the cytoplasm and membrane.

These observations indicate that, although the E_α and E_β chains are synthesized independently, the insertion of the β chain into the membrane is dependent upon the simultaneous insertion of the α chain. The opposite, apparently, is not true: the α chain can be inserted into the membrane alone, albeit in a reduced quantity.

These observations also provide a clue to several previously unexplained observations, of which we shall mention only two here. The first concerns serologically detectable class II (Ia) determinants. Typing of some F_1 hybrid mice revealed the presence of certain class II determinants that were lacking in both parents. Since this phenomenon occurs when one parent fails to express the E_α chain in the membrane and the other parent does express it, it can be explained as follows. If one parent is, for example, of the E^b_α E^b_β type, and the other is of the E^k_α E^k_β type, only the latter expresses E_β determinants in the membrane. In the F_1 hybrid, however, the cytoplasmic E^b_β chains combine with the E^k_α chains, the hybrid E^k_α E^b_β molecules are inserted into the membrane, and the previously hidden E^b_β determinants are then expressed.

The second observation concerns the T lymphocyte response in mixed lymphocyte culture (see Chapter 12). Researchers have noted that T lymphocytes of strain A, when stimulated by (A × C57BL/6)F_1 hybrid cells, respond—upon restimulation—more strongly to the F_1 than to the C57BL/6 cells. This observation can be explained as follows. In the A anti-(A × C57BL/6)F_1 combination, two kinds of T cell are activated: those recognizing A^b_β determinants (in combination with A^b_α or A^k_α) and those recognizing E_β determinants on $E^k_\alpha E^b_\beta$ hybrid molecules. When tested against the C57BL/6 parent, which does not express the E molecule in the membrane, only the anti-A^b_β cells can react; the anti-E^b_β cells cannot. For this reason, the response against the F_1 cells is stronger than that against the C57BL/6 cells.

8.5 FUNCTION

More than 60 effects controlled by the MHC have already been described, and new effects are still being discovered and added to this continually growing list. The shape of the mandible, body weight, cyclic adenosine monophosphate levels, rate of DNA synthesis, DNA repair, the number of cells in the spleen, testes' weight, cortisone-induced cleft palate susceptibility, control of mating behavior—these are just a few of the phenomena reported to be controlled by MHC-associated genes. No wonder, then, that so many scientists have been intrigued by the MHC. But none of the above-mentioned effects has actually been mapped to the class I or class II loci, nor is there any reason to believe that any of these, and many other effects, are controlled by these loci. More likely, there are a great many other loci in the MHC chromosome and apart from sharing the same linkage group, they may have nothing to do with the MHC. They may appear to be MHC-associated simply because the MHC antigens are an easy and frequently used marker in linkage studies.

Although class I and class II loci themselves have been demonstrated to mediate several effects, all these effects are immunological in nature and may be reduced to a common denominator—stimulation of T lymphocytes. Most of the apparent versatility of effects results from the fact that the activation of T lymphocytes by MHC molecules can be measured by a variety of assays: mixed lymphocyte reaction, graft-versus-host reaction, cell-mediated lymphocytotoxicity, delayed-type hypersensitivity, and various forms of allograft reaction. These assays, however, all require contact between allogeneic lymphocytes—a situation that almost never occurs naturally in advanced vertebrates. They thus measure responses in human-designed, nonphysiological situations. Although important theoretically (for understanding the mechanisms of T-cell activation and proliferation) and practically (for clinical organ transplantation), the alloreactivity phenomena in advanced vertebrates are not representative of the true MHC function.

The true MHC function is, to the best of our knowledge, to serve as a marker of self in the recognition of nonself by T lymphocytes. The class I molecules as the markers of self for the cytotoxic T lymphocytes, and the class II molecules for the regulatory T cells. We discussed the evidence leading to this conclusion in the preceding chapter. This evidence indicates that T lymphocytes always recognize an antigen along with the individual's MHC molecules. T-cell recognition of an antigen alone is not possible, unless the antigen is an MHC molecule itself. What, exactly, the significance of this linked recognition is and how it is actually accomplished are not known.

Nor is exactly what happens in the allogeneic situation clear. Perhaps the responding T lymphocytes recognize part of the allogeneic MHC molecule as self and the other part as nonself, so that the stimulation occurs on the same principle as in the physiological situation. The allogeneic class I molecules, like the syngeneic ones, are predominantly (but not exclusively) recognized by T lymphocytes that have the ability to develop into cytotoxic cells, whereas allogeneic class II molecules stimulate predominantly (but again, not exclusively) T lymphocytes programmed to become regulatory cells. The former are measured, in the allogeneic situation, by their ability to kill target cells in vitro (in the cell-mediated lymphocytotoxicity assay) or in vivo (in the allograft reaction assay). The latter are detected by their proliferation in the cell culture (the mixed lymphocyte reaction) or in the host (the graft-versus-host reaction or delayed-type hypersensitivity reaction). The allogeneic phenomena thus mirror closely the physiological T-lymphocyte reaction. We shall describe the allogenic reaction in Chapter 12, when we deal with T lymphocyte-mediated effects in more detail.

There is, however, one MHC-related phenomenon that does not seem to fit into the scheme just described—the phenomenon of *immune response regulation* by MHC lymphocytes. Already, at the turn of the century, investigators had observed that in experimental animals, as well as in the human, certain diseases ran in families, suggesting that disease susceptibility or resistance could be controlled genetically. Similar hints of genetic control of antibody response to disease-related and innocuous antigens were reported sporadically throughout the first half of this century. However, the phenomenon did not come under thorough scrutiny until the 1960s, first by Baruj Benacerraf and his colleagues and then by groups headed by Hugh O. McDevitt and Paul H. Maurer. All three groups used antigens prepared synthetically by linking together selected amino acids. These synthetic polypeptides (see Chapter 10) have the advantage that, in contrast to natural antigens, they carry only a limited assortment of antigenic determinants, simplifying the genetic analysis of the otherwise complicated immune-response control. An example of an immune response to a synthetic polypeptide is depicted in Figure 8.19. In this experiment, Hugh O. McDevitt and Michael Sela immunized two inbred strains, C57 and CBA, with (T,G)-A--L, a multichain polypeptide, consisting of a poly-L-*l*ysine backbone with poly-D,L-alanine sidechains and L-*t*yrosine and L-*g*lutamic acid peptides attached to the amino-terminal groups of the poly*a*lanine (see Chapter 10). Both strains produced antibodies to (T,G)-A--L, but the CBA strain produced low, and the C57 strain high, antibody levels. The F_1 hybrids gave intermediate responses, compared to the two parental strains. The $F_1 \times$ CBA backcross animals could be divided into two groups, low and intermediate responders, whereas the $F_1 =$ C57 backcross animals were all high responders. These results suggest that the response to (T,G)-A--L is controlled by a single, codominant *immune response*-1, or *Ir*-1, *gene*. Later, McDevitt and his colleagues mapped the *Ir*-1 gene in the *H*-2 complex in the same region in which loci controlling class II molecules map.

Following these studies, Benacerraf, McDevitt, Maurer, and others discovered many other *Ir* genes

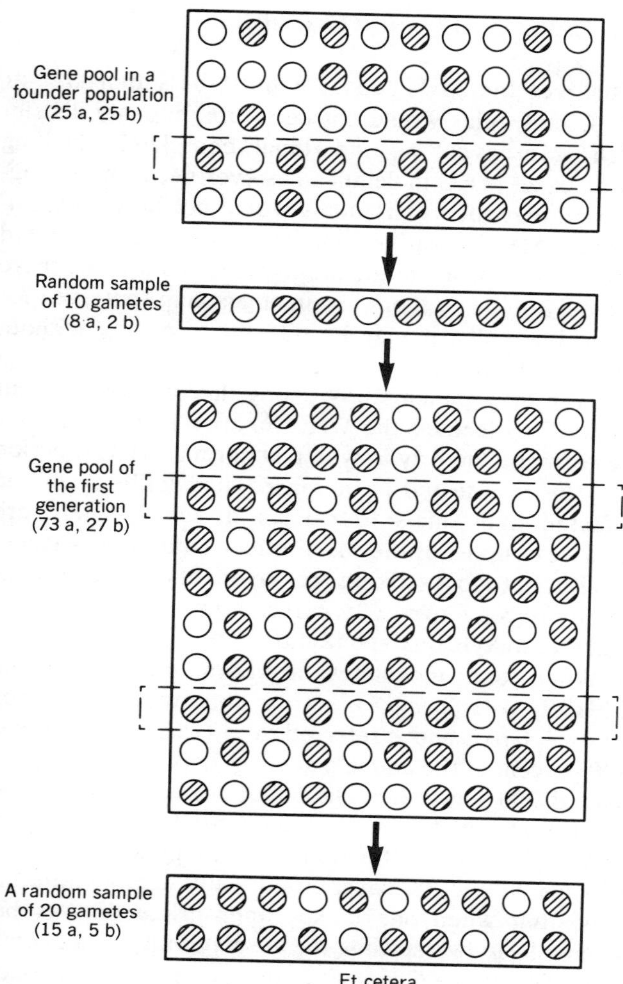

Figure 8.19. Simulation of random genetic drift in a small population. Circles represent individual genes; shaded circles represent the *a* allele, open circles the *b* allele.

controlling responsiveness to other antigens and mapped them, one after another, all in the same region of the *H-2* complex. In addition, similar *Ir* genes were described in other species, and there too they were mapped within the species' MHC. The major conclusions from these studies can be summarized as follows.

Certain alleles of class II loci confer high responsiveness to a given antigen, while other alleles confer low responsiveness, or, in rare instances, complete unresponsiveness. Thus, in most cases, the effect of class II genes is a quantitative one, and low responder animals can often be converted into high responders by increasing the dose of the immunizing antigen. In fact, the genetic control of the immune response can usually be observed only when the challenging antigen is of restricted heterogeneity.

Originally, the control of the immune response was described using synthetic polypeptides as the immunizing antigen, but later, numerous studies demonstrated similar control by many other antigens. Now the prevailing belief among immunologists is that class II loci control the response to antigens that can stimulate thymus-derived lymphocytes—that is, the so-called T-dependent antigens; no instance of *Ir* gene-controlled immune response to T-independent antigens has been reported.

The usual way of measuring the control of immune response is by determining the level of humoral antibodies. However, *Ir* genes also affect the response in delayed-type hypersensitivity, in vitro stimulation of T lymphocytes by conventional antigens, and production of the soluble regulatory (helper or suppressor) factor.

Regulation of immune response occurs in two ways—through helper and suppressor effects. A genetic low responder or nonresponder can, therefore, be the result either of lack of help or of active suppression. Genes controlling helper effects are referred to as *immune response* or *Ir* genes, whereas those affecting suppressive phenomena have been designated *immune suppression* or *Is genes*. The relationship between the two types of gene is not known. Genetically, however, they are quite similar and may represent two sides of the same coin.

Ir genes are concerned with the recognition of the carrier portion of the hapten-carrier complex (see Chapter 13), so that by attaching a hapten to a different carrier, one can turn a nonresponder to this hapten into a responder. In some instances, *Ir* genes have a preferential effect on IgG antibody production, but in other instances they affect both the IgG and IgM classes. Outwardly, the *Ir*-gene effect is highly specific: often the same *H-2* haplotype affects high responsiveness to some antigen but unresponsiveness to other closely related antigens. In most instances, *Ir* genes do not influence the specificity of the antibodies the production of which they control. Antibodies to a given antigen often crossreact with antigens the response to which is controlled by different *Ir* genes. However, instances have been described in which certain *Ir* genes preferentially affect response to certain antigenic determinants of a given multideterminant molecule.

There has been a long, protracted debate concerning the cell type in which *Ir* genes are expressed. The debate has ended in a kind of limbo. It may have been the wrong question to ask in the first place. *Ir* genes now appear to immunologists as light does to physicists, showing different sides of its nature depending on how one looks at it. When studied in a certain way, *Ir* genes appear to be expressed in T lymphocytes; when studied in a different way, they seem to affect B lymphocytes primarily, or macrophages.

The formal genetics of the *Ir* phenomenon, which at first seemed so simple (single MHC-linked, Mendelian *Ir* gene controlling response to a given antigen, with responsiveness dominant over nonresponsiveness), has become muddled by later studies. Not only have other *Ir* loci not linked to the MHC been described, but the control by the complex itself has turned out to be quite involved. Not only do multiple *Ir* loci affect responsiveness to the same antigen, but they also interact with one another in a complicated way. These interactions sometimes occur between different genes; at other times they seem to concern alleles at the same locus. They may sometimes occur in *cis* and other times in *trans* configuration of the genes involved; and often certain genes may interact only with certain other genes (see below).

Two principal hypotheses have been proposed to explain the MHC-controlled immune-response reaction. According to one hypothesis, the *Ir* genes are distinct and separate from the class I and class II genes. The *Ir* genes may function, for example, by controlling the T-cell receptor. Animals genetically lacking the receptor for a given antigen behave as low responders; animals possessing the right *Ir* gene (i.e., gene that codes for the receptor capable of recognizing this antigen) behave as high responders. There are many possible variants of this basic hypothesis, but all presuppose a large number of genes in the MHC, distinct from the already known loci. However, to this day, no evidence for the existence of these hypothetical genes has turned up. On the contrary, the perfect correlation between *Ir* and class II genes in the MHC suggests that the two might be identical.

Identity of the *Ir* and class II genes is the basic tenet of the second, and more likely, hypothesis. According to this hypothesis, the difference between the high and low responder arises from the ability or inability of the T-cell receptor to recognize certain combinations of class II molecules and antigens. An animal incapable of recognizing a given combination will appear to be a low responder, while an animal recognizing this combination seems to be a high responder. The nonrecognition could be the consequence either of the lack of the appropriate receptor or the inability of a given antigen to be seen in the company of a given class II molecule. The immune response appears to be MHC-controlled because of this involvement of the class II molecules in the recognition of the antigen.

8.6 DEFECTS OF MHC FUNCTION

Whatever the MHC does, it must be important, or MHC molecules would not be so ubiquitously distributed. Moreover, no individual completely lacking some or all MHC molecules has ever been found, suggesting that such individuals would not be viable. Although MHC-negative cell lines have been isolated from adult tissues (e.g., the human Daudi line), there are only a few of them, again suggesting that even for individual cells, it may be difficult to get by without MHC molecules.

Even in organisms possessing the full complement of MHC molecules, the MHC function may not always be normal. One way in which abnormal MHC function may be manifested is increased susceptibility of the affected individuals to certain diseases. There are many examples of the MHC effect on disease susceptibility, but most striking are the effects on the susceptibility of mice to virally induced leukemia and of humans to ankylosing spondylitis.

When one inoculates newborn mice of strain C3Hf/Bi with a *leukemia virus* that was isolated by Ludwik Gross and is referred to as Gross virus, almost 100 percent of the animals develop leukemia before the age of 200 days. Inoculation of the same virus into newborn mice of another strain, C57BL, results in only about 25 percent of the animals coming down with the disease within 200 days. Frank Lilly demonstrated in 1966 that when one makes appropriate crosses between these two strains, the susceptibility to leukemia induction by the Gross virus segregates as if controlled by two loci, one of which is closely linked to the *H-2* complex. Hence, the *H-2* complex has a strong influence on the development of a disease—in this instance, neoplasms of the lymphoid system.

Ankylosing spondylitis is a rare human disease causing inflammation and stiffening of vertebrae and thus deformities of the spine (Gr. *ankylōsis*, stiffening of a joint; *spondylos*, vertebra; suffix *-itis*, inflammation). Approximately 90 percent of Caucasians with this disease carry the HLA-B27 determinant. Since this determinant is present in only about 7 percent of the control population, its frequency in patients with ankylosing spondylitis is increased 15 times, suggesting that individuals with B27 are significantly more susceptible to the disease than individuals carrying other HLA determinants. There is also an obvious correlation between the incidence of B27 and ankylosing spondylitis in non-Caucasian races. The Pima American Indians have a high frequency of both B27 (10 percent) and the disease (5 percent), while in African blacks, both B27 and the disease are rare (B27 occurring in less than 1 percent of the population). Furthermore, a higher than normal incidence of B27 was also found among patients with diseases related to or associated with ankylosing spondylitis, notably acute anterior uveitis (inflammation of the uvea—the iris, cilliary body, and choroid coat of the eye), psoriasis (a skin disease characterized by circumscribed red patches covered with white scales), and Reiter's disease (inflammation of the urethra, eye, and joints, appearing in that order).

Ankylosing spondylitis is not the only example of an association between a particular disease and a particular HLA determinant, but it is the most striking one. Other associations are much weaker and can be demonstrated only by the use of statistical methods. The significance of the association is established using the χ^2 test described earlier in this chapter, and comparing a group of patients suffering from a particular disease with a control group of healthy individuals:

	HLA Determinant		
	Positive	Negative	Total
Patients	a	b	a + b
Controls	c	d	c + d
Total	a + c	b + d	a + b + c + d = n

The actual values are then used to compute the χ^2, according to the formula given in the section on serology. The significance of the association is strongly influenced by the sample size: the larger the sample, the weaker the associations that can be detected. The strength of the association can be expressed in terms of relative risk, ad/bc, which indicates how many times more frequently the disease occurs in a group of individuals carrying the determinant relative to the group lacking it. A relative risk of >1 indicates that the frequency of the determinant is increased in the patients, while a risk <1 indicates decreased frequency. Because of the weakness and variability of many HLA-disease associations, contradictory findings are abundant: some investigators find a particular disease associated with a particular determinant, others do not. Some of the reported associations are listed in Table 8.14.

The following hypotheses have been proposed to explain the MHC-disease associations.

The Receptor Hypothesis. MHC molecules may serve as receptors for the adsorption of pathogens, particularly viruses, to the cell surface. According to this hypothesis, the presence of a particular MHC molecule (determinant) allows the penetration of a particular virus into the cell; absence of these molecules precludes virus penetration and makes the individual resistant. However, despite considerable efforts by several laboratories, no correlation has been found between adsorption of viruses to cells and the presence of particular MHC molecules. In only one instance was a virus found with affinity for MHC molecules. This so-called Semliki Forest virus (lipid-containing, RNA virus belonging to arboviruses of group A), however, associates with all HLA molecules, regardless of their polymorphic variation. Indications are that the virus does not even distinguish between MHCs of different species. Such affinity cannot, therefore, explain the association of different diseases with specific MHC molecules. There is, thus, no evidence for the receptor hypothesis of HLA-disease association.

Mimicry Hypothesis. An accidental sharing of determinants between a pathogen and its host (a kind of molecular mimicry) could result in failure of the host to mount an immune response to the infectious agent and in susceptibility to a given disease. Experiments on mice suggest that such sharing does occasionally occur, for example, between pneumococcal and streptococcal polysaccharides and histocompatibility antigens. In one experiment, for example, mice pretreated with membranes of heat-killed streptococci rejected allografts more rapidly than did untreated mice, suggesting that streptococcal antigens induced immunity to antigens present in the allografted tissue. But it is unlikely that such immunity has any bearing on immunity to MHC molecules, for in these molecules, as we already know, antigenicity resides in the protein, rather than in the carbohydrate portion. Furthermore, sharing of one or two determinants would not suffice to make the host tolerant of a pathogen, and the probability of complete sharing of determinants is low.

Ir Gene Hypothesis. We already know that antigens, including viral and bacterial antigens, are recognized in the context of host MHC molecules. We also know that, in some individuals, some combinations of antigen and MHC molecules, for unknown reasons, fail to stimulate immune response. Hence, the most probable explanation of MHC-disease association is that pathogens responsible for a given disease control antigens which, in combination with a particular MHC determinant, form blind spots in the host's immune response system. Supporting this hypothesis is the finding that many MHC-associated diseases are proved to have or suspected of having an immunological component. The association with the disease of a particular

Table 8.14 Examples of Association Between Particular Diseases and the MHC in Humans

Disease	HLA Determinant (Locus)	Relative Risk[a]	Symptoms of Disease
Inflammatory diseases			
Ankylosing spondylitis	B27 (*HLA-B*)	100–200	Inflammation of the spine, leading to stiffening of vertebral joints
Reiter's syndrome	B27 (*HLA-B*)	40	Inflammation of spine, prostate, and parts of the eye (the uvea, which is the iris, the ciliary body and the choroid)
Acute anterior uveitis	B27 (*HLA-B*)	30	Inflammation of iris and ciliary body
Juvenile rheumatoid arthritis (Type III)	B27 (*HLA-B*)	10–12	A multisystem inflammatory disease of children characterized by joint disease, fever, and rapid onset
Psoriasis	B13 (*HLA-B*)	4–5	An acute, recurrent, localized inflammatory disease of the skin (usually scalp, elbows, knees), often associated with arthritis
Celiac disease	Dw3 (*HLA-D*)	9–10	A chronic inflammatory disease of the small intestine; probably a food allergy to gluten, a protein in grains
Multiple sclerosis	Dw2 (*HLA-D*)	5	A progressive chronic inflammatory disease of brain and spinal cord that causes hardening (sclerosis) and loss of function in affected foci
Allergic diseases			
Ragweed hay fever	Many loci; direct linkage shown in family studies	Difficult to calculate	An IgE-mediated allergic response to ragweed extracts
Endocrine diseases			
Addison's disease	B8 (*HLA-B*)	4	A deficiency in production of adrenal gland cortical hormones
Diabetes mellitus (juvenile)	Dw2, Dw3, Dw4, (*HLA-D*)	2–5	A deficiency of insulin production; pancreatic islet cells usually absent or damaged
Graves' disease	Dw3 (*HLA-D*)	10–12	A hyperactivity of the thyroid; patients often produce an IgG antibody that stimulates thyroid function (LATS: long-acting thyroid stimulator)
Malignant diseases			
Acute lymphocytic leukemia	A2 (*HLA-A*)	1.2–1.4	A cancer of lymphocytes, usually in children, and usually of the T-lymphocyte series
Hodgkin's disease	A1 (*HLA-A*)	1.5–1.8	A cancer of lymph node cells; local inflammation is prominent, as well as selective deficiency in cellular immunity and T-cell functions

Source. Modified from L. D. Hood, I. L. Weissman, and W. B. Wood: *Immunology*, p. 147. Benjamin/Cummings, Menlo Park, 1978.
[a] Disease risk of persons who bear the determinant, relative to that of a control population.

class of MHC molecules and a particular MHC allele may depend on the nature of the inducing pathogen and the type of immune response this pathogen normally stimulates.

Linked-Locus Hypothesis. Among the MHC-associated diseases are some in which involvement of the immune system cannot be demonstrated. In such instances, it is quite possible that, in fact, it is not the MHC, but a locus linked to the MHC, which is responsible for the association. The function of this locus may be MHC-linked by chance. It may code, for example, for an enzyme of a metabolic pathway, and it may be the interruption of this pathway that causes a disease. The illness then appears to be associated with a particular MHC allele because of a linkage disequilibrium (see Appendix 8.1) in the population between the metabolic locus and the MHC. Some diseases may also be affected by defects in the MHC-linked complement-encoding genes (see Chapter 9).

The interpretation of the MHC-disease association is complicated by the fact that in almost none of the diseases is the causative agent known. Most of the diseases appear to have an immunological component, probably of an autoimmune character (see Chapter 14), and many of them are suspected to be of viral etiology. But the nature of the disturbance is not known.

Most of the known associations are with determinants controlled by the *B* locus, but this fact too may be the consequence of linkage disequilibrium with another locus—perhaps the *D* locus, which is closer to *B* than to *A* or *C*, and which may be the human immune response locus.

The weakness of most of the associations is not surprising. The development of a disease is a complex process, influenced by many factors, both genetic and environmental. The MHC-associated genes represent only one of these factors and their effect may be overridden by other components of the system.

The practical value of the HLA-disease association studies is in the identification of individuals at risk of developing a given disease, in more precise diagnosis of certain disorders, and in predicting the course of the disease.

8.7 EVOLUTION

The MHC has been identified in every mammalian species that has been studied, so it is probably safe to assume that all mammals possess an MHC. In birds, the MHC has been demonstrated so far only in the domestic fowl, but there is every reason to believe that all other species of this vertebrate class possess this complex. Information about the presence of the MHC in vertebrates other than mammals and birds is sketchy. It is based exclusively on functional tests, such as rapid allograft rejection and mixed lymphocyte reaction. On this basis, predictions have been made about the presence of the MHC in amphibians, at least some reptiles, and some fish. In fact, there is no evidence that would argue against the presence of the MHC in *all* vertebrates. Nothing is known about the presence of the MHC in invertebrates, although the experiments in earthworms described in Chapter 1 and other experiments on tunicates have been interpreted by some immunologists as suggestive of the presence of MHC-like systems in these taxons. Thus, the MHC may be an old genetic system, the elements of which existed in invertebrates and which has been vastly improved and exploited by the vertebrates, particularly mammals. In this sense, the evolution of the MHC parallels that of the immunoglobulin system, so much so that several immunologists have been impelled to speculate about common evolutionary origins of these two systems. According to this speculation, the first few rounds of duplication of the primordial immunoglobulin gene described in Chapter 6 founded three evolutionary branches—one leading to immunoglobulins, another to the MHC, and the third to the β_2-microglobulin. Cited in favor of this hypothesis is the finding of homologies in primary and tertiary structure of immunoglobulins, the MHC, and the β_2-microglobulin. However, these homologies are extremely weak and could have arisen, as already discussed by evolutionary convergence rather than by common origin. The whole problem of MHC origin thus remains largely open.

In the thoroughly studied mammalian and avian species, the MHC displays a remarkable degree of evolutionary conservation in that it always occupies a chromosomal region of less than 1 cM and consists of the same classes of loci. The homologous loci are not always in the same order, indicating that chromosomal rearrangements within the MHC do occur. Possibly, there are different numbers of loci in different species, but this point is not firmly established. In at least some species, the evolutionary conservation concerns not only the MHC itself, but also some of the linked loci. For example, the locus coding for the enzyme glyoxalase is closely linked to the MHC in both the human and the mouse. It could be, therefore, that, at least in mammals, a relatively large segment of the MHC chromosome has been retained during speciation, despite possible rearrangement within this segment (see Fig. 8.5). This conservation could be a chance effect (there are other chromosomal segments in which the gene constellation has been retained from species to species) or it could mean that for some reason it is important for an organism to keep all the MHC loci together.

8.8 APPENDIX 8.1: BASIC TERMS AND CONCEPTS IN POPULATION GENETICS

A population geneticist views a population not as a group of individuals occupying a certain geographical or otherwise defined region, but as a group of genes in

Table 8.15 Computation of Gene Frequencies by Gene Counting

	Genotype				
	aa	*ab*	*bb*	Total	Gene Frequency
Number of individuals	80	18	2	100	
Number of *a* genes	160	18	0	178	178/200 = 0.89 = 89%
Number of *b* genes	0	18	4	22	22/200 = 0.11 = 11%
Total number of genes	160	36	4	200	

this region—a *gene pool*. The first thing he wants to know about a population is the numerical relationships among the genes in the pool. To obtain such information, he samples the population, counts the genes, and extrapolates from these the counts for the population as a whole. As an example, let us assume that we have obtained, from a given population, a sample of 100 randomly chosen individuals (i.e., 200 genes, since each individual has two genes at a given locus), determined whether they are of the *a* or the *b* type, and found 80 a^+b^-, 18 a^+b^+, and two a^-b^+ individuals in the sample (Table 8.15). From this finding we can calculate the *gene frequency* (the proportion of the *a* or *b* genes in the pool) as follows: the 80 a^+b^- individuals are apparently *aa* homozygotes, and, as such, they carry 168 genes altogether (each individual carries two *a* genes); the 18 a^+b^+ individuals are presumably *ab* heterozygotes and so they carry 18 *a* genes; the a^-b^+ individuals can be regarded as *bb* homozygotes that carry no *a* genes. Hence, the total number of *a* genes in the sample is 160 + 18 = 178, and the frequency of the *a* genes in the population is 178/200 = 0.89 = 89 percent. Similarly, we can calculate the frequency of the *b* gene to be 22/200 = 0.11 or 11 percent (Table 8.15).

The calculation of gene frequencies is this simple only when one can detect both alleles, even when they occur together in one individual (i.e., when they are in the heterozygous condition). Often, however, the heterozygote expresses just one of the two alleles phenotypically—one allele is dominant, the other recessive. In such a situation, one determines the *phenotypic frequency* of the products controlled by the two alleles by dividing the number of individuals expressing a given allele by the total number of individuals tested—100 in our sample. Then one corrects this calculation by taking into account, as best one can, the fact that some alleles have remained undetected. There are several ways of making this correction, the most simple of which is to calculate gene frequencies by using the formula $g = 1 - \sqrt{1 - f}$, where g is the gene and f the phenotype frequency. (For the derivation of this formula, the reader is referred to a population genetics textbook.)

Once population geneticists know the gene frequencies, they calculate the frequencies of homozygotes and heterozygotes for each of the two alleles and compare the calculated frequencies with those expected on the basis of population genetics theory. The expected frequencies are given by the formula $p^2 + 2pq + q^2$, known as the *Hardy-Weinberg Law*. In this formula, p

Table 8.16 Comparison of Expected and Observed Gene Frequencies From Table 8.5

		Number of Individuals in Population of 100	
Genotype	Expected Genotype Frequency	Expected[a]	Observed
aa	$p^2 = (0.89)^2 = 0.7921$	79	80
ab	$2pq = 2(0.89)(0.11) = 0.1958$	19	18
bb	$q^2 = (0.11)^2 = 0.0121$	1	2

[a] The expected number of individuals is computed by multiplying the expected genotype frequency by the population size ($N = 100$).

is the frequency of *a* and q the frequency of the *b* gene. The formula predicts that, in the population, the frequency of *a* homozygotes will be p^2, the frequency of *ab* heterozygotes $2pq$, and the frequency of *b* homozygotes q^2. A comparison of the expected and observed gene frequencies in our example is given in Table 8.16. The Hardy-Weinberg Law can be derived simply by considering the chance with which genes carried by gametes meet in the zygote. The chance is obviously dependent upon gene frequencies and one can determine it by considering all the theoretical possibilities.

	Eggs	
	p	q
Sperm p	p^2	pq
q	pq	q^2

The Hardy-Weinberg Law is a probability law and probability provides accurate predictions only when the numbers are large. Hence, the law applies only to large (theoretically infinite) populations. The law also requires that the gene frequency not be disturbed by external or internal factors. For example, if there were a sudden immigration of a large number of new individuals into the population from outside, the validity of the Hardy-Weinberg Law would be suspended temporarily until the population had stabilized again and reached an equilibrium. Other factors affecting *Hardy-Weinberg equilibrium* are mutation and selection. (In the latter case, if one allele is preferred over the other, the randomness of one gene's meeting another gene is changed.) Hence, by determining whether a population is in equilibrium, the geneticist obtains valuable information about the population itself.

A population in equilibrium is usually stable over a long period of time—more precisely, it changes so slowly that one is unable to notice it. In the example that we used, if we were to come to the population, say, in 10 years' time and sample another 100 individuals, we would again find the *a* and *b* alleles in the same frequencies (i.e., 89 percent for the *a* and 11 percent for the *b* allele). The stability of the population follows from what we said about the population earlier. If the population is not disturbed by migration, mutation, and selection and if it is sufficiently large, the probabilities governing the meeting of genes at fertilization remain the same and the gene pool itself does not change.

One may ask, however, why the gene frequencies are not equal in the first place. Why does gene *a* occur with the frequency of 89 percent and gene *b* with the frequency of 11 percent? There is no simple answer to this question. One possibility is that the genetic constitution of a given population reflects its history—the way the population evolved to its present form from a few founding individuals. When the population was small, the behavior of genes in it was governed by laws different from those governing a large population. A major force affecting gene behavior in a small population is *random genetic drift*—a chance fluctuation in gene frequencies.

As an example, consider a founding population containing a total of 50 genes at locus 1 (i.e., consisting of 25 individuals; see Fig. 8.19). Suppose further that the two alleles *a* and *b* are equally represented in this population so that there are 25 *a* and 25 *b* alleles present. Only a small fraction of these genes—say, 10—is passed into the next generation. The selection of these genes is completely random and so it can happen, as is shown in Figure 8.19, that the sample, instead of containing five *a* and five *b* genes, by chance contains eight *a* and two *b* genes. When these founding genes multiply in the next generation, they remain in the same proportion, so that now the population contains 80 percent *a* and 20 percent *b* genes. So drastic a change in gene frequency from generation to generation could never happen in a large population because there, the sample of genes drawn for the next generation would be large and would probably contain the *a* and *b* alleles in the same proportion as in the parental population (in an infinitely large sample, the effect of random fluctuation is nonexistent). Let us assume, however, that the conditions for the expansion of the small founding population are so favorable that the number of individuals in the next generation doubles. We then have 100 genes, of which 80 are of the *a* and 20 of the *b* type. Now the effect of random fluctuation is not so drastic as in the previous generation, and in the third generation the gene frequencies may depart from those in the previous generations by only a few percent. As the population continues to expand and the sample from which the genes are drawn for the next generation continues to grow, there is less and less variation in gene frequencies from one generation to another, until—at a certain large size—the frequencies no longer vary at all. The gene frequencies thus freeze at a certain value—the value detected in present-day, large populations.

Another explanation for the differences in gene frequencies is that the frequencies are determined by *natural selection*. For example, a situation may arise wherein the *ab* heterozygote is at an advantage over both *aa* and *bb* homozygotes. To produce heterozygotes continually, both alleles must be maintained in the population in substantial frequencies. So a compromise is worked out, balancing out the heterozygous advantage against a particular frequency of *a* and a particular frequency of *b*—a situation referred to as *balanced polymorphism*.

Until now, we have considered only the behavior of a single locus in a population. But the MHC is a cluster of loci and so we have to ask questions about the behavior of linked loci. Let us assume that there are two linked loci, 1 and 2, each with two alleles, *a* and *b*. Let us assume further that the population was founded by animals carrying only two haplotypes, 1^a2^a and 1^b2^b. In each generation that the population passes through, there is a certain probability that the two loci will be separated by crossingover, and generally, this chance is the greater the further apart in the chromosome the two loci are. No matter how closely linked the loci are, sooner or later recombination between them will occur and animals with haplotypes 1^a2^b and 1^b2^a will appear, in addition to animals carrying the original 1^a2^a and 1^b2^b haplotypes. Given enough time, an equilibrium among the four possible haplotypes will be established, so that the haplotypes will occur with certain frequencies determined by the gene frequencies. If the frequencies of the four genes 1^a,1^b, 2^a,2^b are p_1, p_2, q_1, q_2, respectively, then the frequencies of the four possible haplotypes are p_1q_1 for 1^a2^a, p_1q_2 for 1^a2^b, and p_2q_2 for 1^b2^b. Hence, when one knows the gene frequencies, one can calculate the expected haplotype frequencies by simply multiplying the former. When one finds that the observed haplotype frequencies do not match the expected frequencies, one says that the relevant genes show *linkage disequilibrium*. The strength of linkage disequilibrium is expressed by the so-called Δ value (read "delta"), defined as Δ = expected haplotype frequency less observed haplotype frequency. [If there is no association between genes at two loci (i.e., the two genes are in equilibrium), the frequency of their cooccurrence in the same chomosome is the product of their gene frequencies, *pq*, which is also the expected frequency of the haplotype formed by these two genes.] Positively associated genes show positive Δ values, while negative association gives negative Δ. Genes display linkage disequilibrium for two main reasons: either they have not had enough time to reach equilibrium (for closely linked loci, it takes many generations before equilibrium is attained), or there is a force in the population acting against the attainment of equilibrium. The latter situation may arise when certain gene combinations are favored by natural selection over other combinations.

REFERENCES

General

Bodmer, W. F. and Cavalli-Sforza, L. L.: *Genetics, Evolution, and Man*. Freeman, San Francisco, 1976.

Braun, W. E.: *HLA and Disease. A Comprehensive Review*. CRC Press, Boca Raton, Florida, 1979.

Götze, D. (Ed.): *The Major Histocompatibility System in Man and Animals*. Springer-Verlag, New York, 1977.

Klein, J.: *Biology of the Mouse Histocompatibility-2 Complex. Principles of Immunogenetics Applied to a Single System*. Springer-Verlag, New York, 1975.

Möller, G. (Ed.): Ir genes and T lymphocytes. *Immunol. Rev.*, Vol. 38. Munksgaard, Copenhagen, 1978.

Poulik, M. D. and Reisfeld, R. A.: β_2-microglobulins. *Contemp. Top. Molec. Immunol.* **4**:157–204, 1975.

Schwartz, B. D. and Cullen, S. E.: Chemical characteristics of Ia antigens. *Springer Sem. Immunopathol.* **1**:85–109, 1978.

Selwood, N. and Hedges, A.: *Transplantation Antigens—A Study in Serological Data Analysis*. Wiley, Chichester, 1978.

Snell, G. D., Dausset, J., and Nathenson, S.: *Histocompatibility*. Academic, New York, 1976.

Svejgaard, A., Hauge, M., Jersild, C., Platz, P., Ryder, L. P., Nielsen, L. S., and Thomsen, M.: *The HLA System. An Introductory Survey*, 2nd ed. Karger, Basel, 1979.

Original Articles

Amiel, J. L.: Study of the leucocyte phenotypes in Hodgkin's disease. *Histcompatibility Testing 1967*, pp. 79–81. Munksgaard, Copenhagen, 1967.

Amos, D. B., Seigler, H. F., Southworth, J. G., and Ward, F. E.: Skin graft rejection between subjects genotyped for HLA. *Transplant. Proc.* **1**:342–346, 1969.

Bach, F. H. and Amos, D. B.: Hu-1: major histocompatibility locus in man. *Science* **156**:1506–1508, 1967.

Berggård, I. and Bearn, A. G.: Isolation and properties of a low molecular weight β_2-microglobulin occurring in human biological fluids. *J. Biol. Chem.* **243**:4095–4103, 1968.

Ceppellini, R., Curtoni, E. S., Mattiuz, P. L., Miggiano, V., Scudeller, G., and Serra, A.: Genetics of leukocyte antigens. A family study of segregation and linkage. *Histocompatibility Testing 1967*, pp. 149–185. Munksgaard, Copenhagen, 1967.

Ceppellini, R., Mattiuz, P. L., Scudeller, G., and Visetti, M.: Experimental allotransplantation in man. I. The role of the HLA system in different genetic combinations. *Transplant. Proc.* **1**:385–389, 1969.

Dausset, J.: Leuco-agglutinins. IV. Leucoagglutinins and blood transfusion. *Vox Sang.* **4**:190–198, 1954.

Dausset, J. and Nenna, A.: Présence d'une leuco-agglutinine dans le sérum d'un cas d'agranulocytose chronique. *Compt. Rend. Soc. Biol. (Paris)* **146**:1539–1541, 1972.

Dausset, J., Iványi, P., and Iványi, D.: Tissue alloantigens in humans. Identification of a complex system (Hu-1). *Histcompatibility Testing 1965*, pp. 51–62. Munksgaard, Copenhagen, 1965.

David, D. S., Shreffler, D. C., and Frelinger, J. A.: New lymphocyte antigen system (Lna) controlled by the Ir region of the mouse

H-2 complex. *Proc. Natl. Acad. Sci. U.S.A.* **70**:2509–2514, 1973.

Démant, P., Snell, G. D., Hess, M., Lemonnier, F., Neauport-Sautes, C., and Kourilsky, F.: Separate and polymorphic loci controlling two types of polypeptide chains bearing the H-2 private and public specificities. *J. Immunogenetics* **2**:263–271, 1975.

Gorer, P. A. and Mikulska, Z. B.: Some further data on the H-2 system of antigens. *Proc. Roy. Soc. (London)* **B151**:57–69, 1959.

Hauptfeld, V., Klein, D., and Klein, J.: Serological identification of an Ir-region product. *Science* **181**:167–169, 1973.

Jones, P. P., Murphy, D. B., and McDevitt, H. O.: Two-gene control of the expression of a murine Ia antigen. *J. Exp. Med.* **148**:925–939, 1978.

Kissmeyer-Nielsen, F., Svejgaard, A., and Nielsen, L. S.: Crossing over within the HLA-system. *Nature, Lond.* **224**:75–76, 1969.

Klein, J. and Shreffler, D. C.: The H-2 model for major histocompatibility systems. *Transplant. Rev.* **6**:3–29, 1971.

Levine, B. B., Ojeda, A., and Benacerraf, B.: Studies on artificial antigens. III. The genetic control of the immune response to hapten poly-L-lysine conjugates in guinea pigs. *J. Exp. Med.* **118**:953–975, 1963.

Lilly, F.: The inheritance of susceptibility to the Gross leukemia virus in mice. *Genetics* **53**:529–539, 1966.

McDevitt, H. O. and Chinitz, A.: Genetic control of the antibody response: relationship between immune response and histocompatibility (H-2) type. *Science* **163**:1207–1208, 1969.

McDevitt, H. O. and Sela, M.: Genetic control of the antibody response. I. Demonstration of determinant-specific differences in response to synthetic polypeptide antigens in two strains of inbred mice. *J. Exp. Med.* **122**:517–531, 1965.

McDevitt, H. O., Deak, B. D., Shreffler, D. C., Klein, J., Stimpfling, J. H., and Snell, G. D.: Genetic control of the immune response. Mapping of the *Ir*-1 locus. *J. Exp. Med.* **135**:1259–1278, 1972.

Payne, R. and Rolfs, M. R.: Fetomaternal leucocyte incompatibility. *J. Clin. Invest.* **37**:1756–1763, 1958.

Rood, J. J., van: *Leucocyte Grouping. A Method and Its Application.* Pasmans, Haag, 1962.

Rood, J. J., van, Leeuwen, A., van, and Eernisse, J. G.: Leucocyte antibodies in sera from pregnant women. *Nature, Lond.* **181**:1735–1736, 1958.

Rood, J. J., van, Leeuwen, A., van, Schippers, A., Vooys, W. H., Frederiks, H., Balner, H., and Eernisse, J. G.: Leucocyte groups, the normal lymphocyte transfer test and homograft sensitivity. *Histocompatibility Testing 1965,* pp. 37–50. Munskgaard, Copenhagen, 1965.

Sandberg, L., Thorsby, E., Kissmeyer-Nielsen, F., and Lindholm, A.: Evidence of a third sublocus within the HLA chromosomal region. *Histocompatibility Testing 1970*, pp. 165–169. Munksgaard, Copenhagen, 1970.

Shreffler, D. C. and Owen, R. D.: A serologically detected variant in mouse serum: inheritance and association with the histocompatibility-2 locus. *Genetics* **48**:9–25, 1963.

Shreffler, D. C., David, C. S., Passmore, H. C., and Klein, J.: Genetic organization and evolution of the mouse *H*-2 region: a duplication model. *Transplant. Proc.* **3**:176–179, 1971.

Smithies, O. and Poulik, M. D.: Initiation of protein synthesis at an unusual position in an immunoglobulin gene? *Science* **175**:187–189, 1972.

Svejgaard, A., Nielsen, L. S., Ryder, L. P., Kissmeyer-Nielsen, F., Sandberg, L., Lindholm, A., and Thorsby, E.: Evidence of a "new" segregant series. *Histocompatibility Testing 1972*, pp. 465–473. Munksgaard, Copenhagen, 1972.

Terasaki, P. I. and McClelland, J. D.: Microdroplet assay of human serum cytotoxins. *Nature, Lond.* **204**:998–1000, 1964.

WHO IUIS Terminology Committee: Nomenclature for factors of the HLA system. *Histocompatibility Testing 1975,* pp. 5–20. Munksgaard, Copenhagen, 1975.

Yunis, E. J., Plate, M., Ward, F. E., Seigler, H. F., and Amos, D. B.: Anomalous MLR responsiveness among siblings. *Transplant. Proc.* **3**:118–126, 1971.

(See also references 19, 34, 60, 75, 83, and 88 in Chapter 2.)

CHAPTER 9

COMPLEMENT AND OTHER ACTIVATION SYSTEMS

9.1 INTRODUCTION TO ACTIVATION SYSTEMS

Vertebrate blood plasma contains several activation systems, each consisting of a series of proteins coordinated in their functions like members of a relay-race team. Normally, the proteins are in an inactive form, but on a specific signal, the first protein of the team is activated (it receives the baton and starts the race), it activates the second protein of the team (passes the baton), the second activated protein activates a third protein, and so on. The last members of the team then perform a certain function (they cross the finish line): they form a clot that stops the blood flow in damaged tissues (the *clotting system*), they decompose (lyse) the clot when it is no longer needed (the *fibrinolytic system*), they widen the lumen of blood vessels and increase capillary permeability (the *bradykinin system*), or they destroy pathogens and pathogen-infected cells (the *complement system*).

The inactive proteins represent zymogens (*proenzymes*)—precursors of enzymes in which the active site is masked by an inhibitory fragment. Activation of

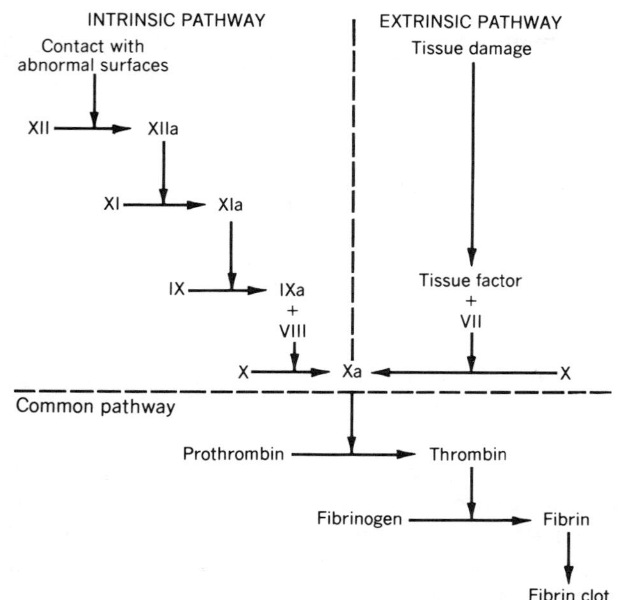

Figure 9.1. The clotting (coagulation) cascade.

the zymogen involves removal of the masking fragment and exposing of the enzymatically active site. Although the main function of the system is carried out by the last members of the relay team, the intermediate members have their tasks to perform as well. Once activated, they (and the freed inhibiting fragments) may become involved in other reactions, some of which interconnect with individual systems in a complicated manner. Furthermore, the race is often regulated by additional proteins that either speed up or slow down the activity of some of the competitors. This complexity is apparently necessary for keeping the systems under tight control, for a malfunction could easily turn beneficial effects into harmful ones.

The activation systems have three properties in common.

Sequentiality. Individual members of each system are activated in a certain sequence, so that a protein cannot be activated unless the protein preceding it in the sequence is activated first. The graphic depiction of the system thus resembles a series of small waterfalls—a cascade (Fig. 9.1).

Rapid Inactivation. Activated components are short-lived: they are either quickly cleared from the circulation or are inactivated by inhibitors present in the plasma, so they have only a short time in which to act.

Amplification. A single activated molecule can activate a number of components rapidly. These second-generation components activate an even greater number of third-generation components, producing a shower effect and greatly amplifying the original action.

The *clotting* (*coagulation*) *system* (Fig. 9.1) consists of more than 10 proteins (factors), referred to either by Roman numerals in the order of discovery (rather than in the order of their participation in the cascade), or by

Table 9.1 Blood-Clotting Factors

Factor	Synonyms	Function of Active Form	Pathway[a]
I	Fibrinogen	Forms fibrin clot	C
II	Prothrombin	Activates fibrinogen (I)	C
III	Thromboplastin, tissue factor	Required to activate X	E
IV	Calcium ions	Required for the interaction of all clotting factors except II, XI, and XII	E, I, C
V	Labile factor, accelerator globulin	Stimulates activation of II	C
VI	Unidentified		E
VII	Serum prothrombin, stable factor, proconvertin		
VIII	Antihemophilic factor A	Required to activate X	I
IX	Christmas factor		
X	Stuart-Power factor	Activates II	C
XI	Plasma thromboplastin antecedent (PTA)	Activates IX	I
XII	Hageman factor, contact factor	Activates XI	I
XIII	Fibrin-stabilizing factor, fibrinase	Stabilizes clot by crosslinking fibrin	C

[a] C, common; E, extrinsic; I, intrinsic

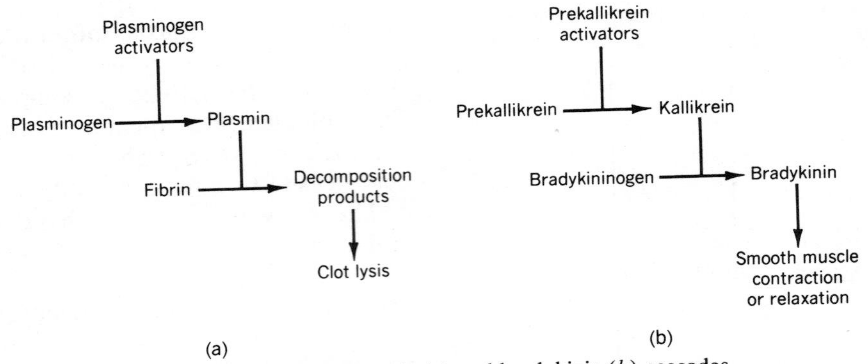

Figure 9.2. The fibrinolytic (*a*) and bradykinin (*b*) cascades.

names—either those of the discoverers (e.g., *Hageman* factor, *Stuart-Power* factor) or those of the patients with defects in the particular factor (e.g., *Christmas* factor; see Table 9.1). The active form of a factor is indicated by a small letter *a* added to the Roman numeral.

The system can be activated in two principal ways and can run along two different tracks—the intrinsic and extrinsic pathways. The two tracks meet at the level of factor X and then continue as a single, common pathway. The *intrinsic pathway* is activated by contact of plasma with abnormal surfaces, a fact first recognized in 1863 by Joseph Lister, the English surgeon who introduced antiseptic methods into operating rooms. Lister observed that blood remained fluid when maintained in the excised vein of an ox, but clotted

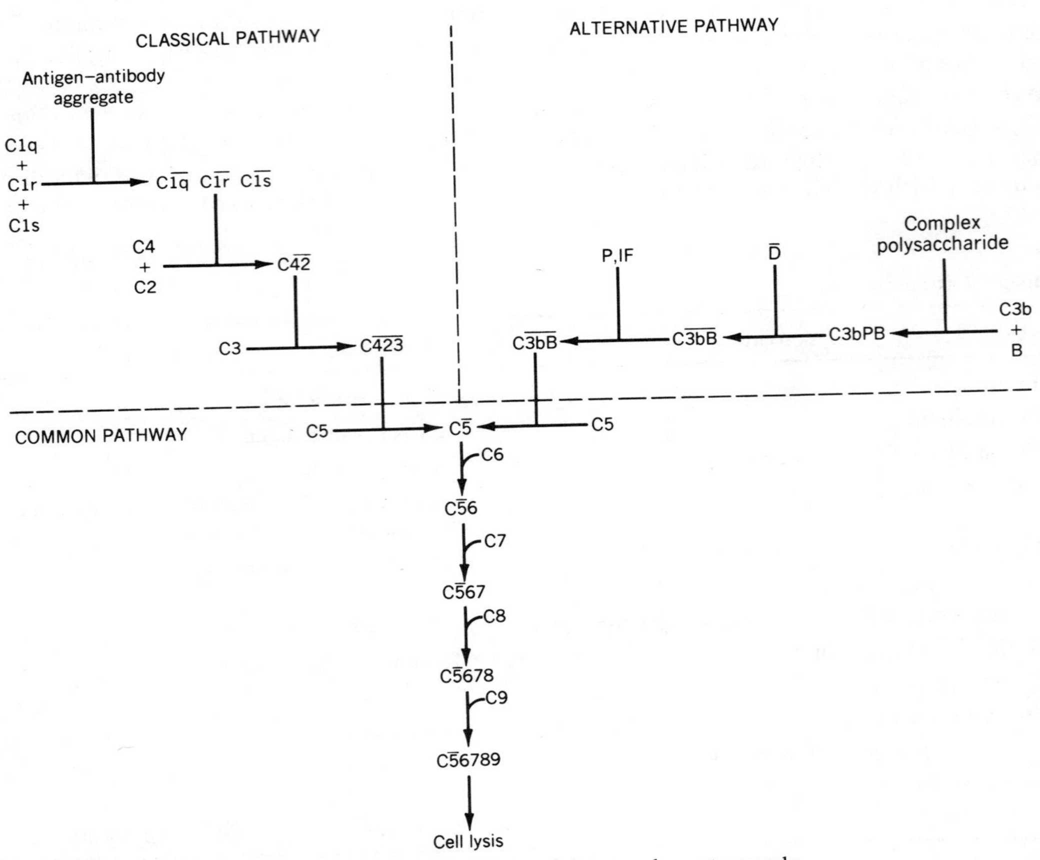

Figure 9.3. General scheme of the complement cascade.

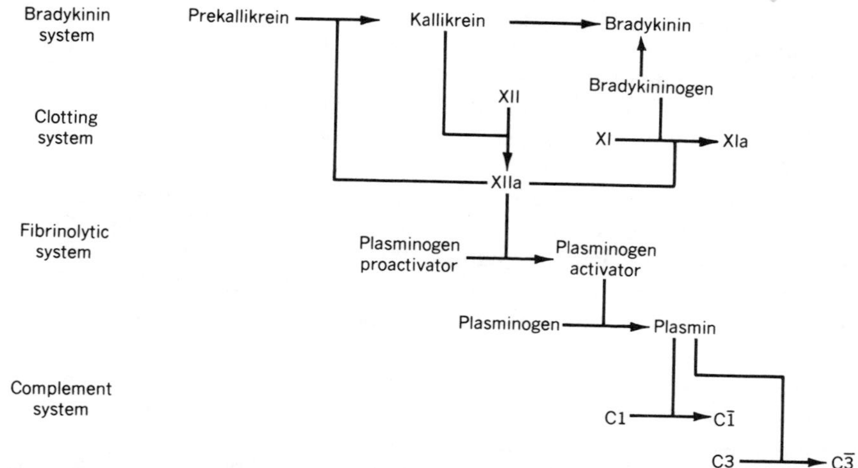

Figure 9.4. A simplified scheme of interaction among the four major activation systems.

rapidly when transferred to a glass vessel. The first protein known to be activated by changes in the surface properties of the damaged blood-vessel walls is the Hageman factor (XII), but there may be other, so far undetected proteins, the activation of which may precede the activation of factor XII. The precise mechanism of activation is not known. The *extrinsic pathway* is activated by a tissue factor, a lipoprotein released by damaged blood vessels. The final step of the *common pathway* is the conversion of the highly soluble fibrinogen into insoluble fibrin. Molecules of fibrin associate to form long fibers, which are staggered one upon another and then crosslinked. The network of fibrin fibers traps blood cells, so that a damlike barrier is formed, preventing blood seepage from the damaged vessel. Hereditary absence of some of the clotting factors results in hemophilia (Gr. *haima*, blood; *philos*, fond), a disease marked by a tendency toward spontaneous bleeding.

Clots usually disappear after lengthy standing. The disappearance is caused by the activation of the *fibrinolytic system* (Fig. 9.2*a*), the main component of which is plasminogen. This substance can be activated by a number of factors (e.g., organic solvents and the enzymes streptokinase, trypsin, and urokinase) and converted into active plasmin (fibrinolysin), which solubilizes fibrin and thus dissolves the clot.

In the *bradykinin system* (Fig. 9.2*b*), activators convert inactive prekallikrein into active kallikrein (Gr. *kallikreas*, pancreas—the organ from which kallikrein was first isolated), an enzyme that then converts bradykininogen into bradykinin (Gr. *bradys*, slow; *kinesis*, movement), a peptide consisting of only nine amino acids. Bradykinin affects smooth muscle contraction and blood vessel permeability.

In the *complement system* (Fig. 9.3), the initial activation occurs either by antigen-antibody complexes or by other activators (e.g., complex polysaccharides in bacterial or yeast cell walls). Each of these two types of activation initiates a separate activation pathway, but as in the case of the clotting system, the two pathways eventually meet and follow a common track. The end result of the activation is killing (lysis) of cells on which the components of the complement system have assembled.

The clotting, fibrinolytic, bradykinin, and complement systems interact in a complex way and so form one supersystem. Some of the interactions are summarized in Figure 9.4. Although all four activation systems participate in one way or another in immunological phenomena, the complement system is the most important of the four for the defense of the organism.

9.2. INTRODUCTION TO THE COMPLEMENT SYSTEM

9.2.1 History

As we already know from Chapter 2, the notion of a serum substance distinct from antibodies and involved in the killing of bacteria crystallized in the last two decades of the nineteenth century. In 1895, Jules Bordet formally demonstrated the existence of the new substance by proving that it lost activity upon heating of serum to 56°C, whereas antibodies did not. Different investigators suggested different names for the substance that completed the action of antibodies; the term eventually accepted—complement—was introduced by Paul Ehrlich and Julius Morgenroth. Following the realization that complement combines with antibodies to kill not only bacteria but also eukaryotic cells, Bordet simplified the study of complement by designing a model system consisting of sheep erythrocytes (E) as target cells, rabbit antibodies to sheep red blood cells, and guinea pig serum as the source of complement. The system is used to this day; its main advantage is that complement activity can be measured easily through the release of hemoglobin from the lysed erythrocytes. Because of their preoccupation with the hemolytic system, immunologists sometimes speak of *hemolytic complement*. Not until half a century after Bordet's discovery did immunologists realize that to learn about the bactericidal effects of complement, they had to go back to studying bacteria.

The first indication that complement might be a complex consisting of several components was obtained in 1907 by A. Ferrata. He dialyzed fresh guinea pig serum against water and observed, as other researchers had before him, the formation of a precipitate in the serum. He then separated the precipitate from the supernatant fluid and redissolved it in an NaCl solution. When tested separately, the supernatant and the redissolved precipitate lacked hemolytic activity, but when mixed together, they lysed erythrocytes.

In the same year, E. Brand discovered that the factor in the supernatant reacted with antibody-coated cells only after the factor in the precipitate had attached to them. He postulated that complement consisted of two "pieces" and that the complement-mediated reaction proceeded in three steps: in the first step, antibody attached to the cell; in the second step, the precipitin component, which he named "midpiece" (because it acted in the middle section of the reaction), attached to the antibody; in the third step, the supernatant component ("endpiece") attached to the midpiece. Later the names were changed to numerical designations: the midpiece became component C1 and the endpiece component C2.

In 1912, H. Ritz observed that treatment of whole serum with cobra venom destroyed the serum's hemolytic activity. But when fresh serum in which the activity of both the midpiece (C2) and endpiece (C1) had been destroyed by heating to 56°C was added to the cobra venom-treated serum, the hemolytic activity of the latter reappeared. Ritz concluded from this observation that normal serum contained a third, relatively heat-stable component—C3.

Fourteen years elapsed before the discovery of the fourth complement component. In 1926, J. Gordon and his collaborators observed that there were at least two heat-stable complement factors—one (C3) that could be removed by mixing the serum with yeast cells (a fact then known for 12 years), and another, the activity of which was not affected by yeasts. The latter component (C4) could be inactivated by treating the serum with ammonia or hydrazine.

For the next 32 years, immunologists lived under the impression that there were only four complement components—C1, C2, C3, and C4. (The procedures for isolation of these four components are summarized in Figure 9.5.) Around 1958, however, evidence for additional components began to accumulate. The isolation and characterization of the complement components was the work of several laboratories, in particular those headed by Hans J. Müller-Eberhard, Manfred M. Mayer, and Irwin H. Lepow. The work resulted in the identification of five more components (C5 through C9) and the splitting of C1 into three subcomponents (C1q, C1r, and C1s). All these components belonged to a single activation pathway. The realization that there was an alternative to this classical pathway dawned slowly on immunologists.

The discovery of the alternative pathway came about from studies designed to isolate the C3 component by binding it to yeast cells or to *zymosan*, the insoluble residue obtained from yeast cells following their digestion with trypsin and extraction with water and alcohol. Zymosan is composed mainly of carbohydrate derived from the yeast cell wall. Treatment of human serum with zymosan at 37°C inactivates C3 selectively. Originally, immunologists thought that the inactivation occurred by the adsorption of C3 to zymosan, but all attempts to elute C3 from zymosan were unsuccessful. When zymosan was added to human

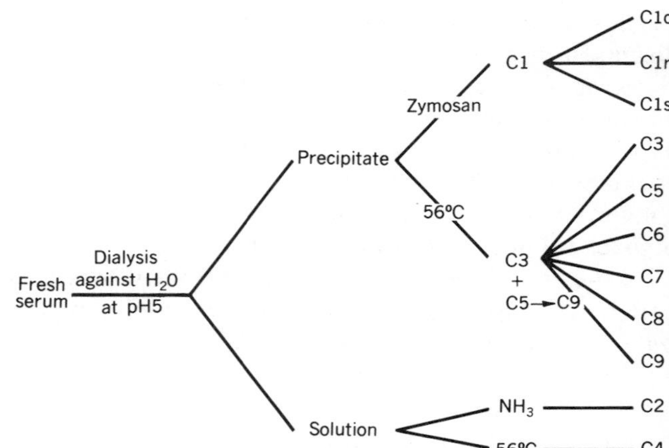

Figure 9.5. Diagrammatic representation of how the first four complement components were distinguished from one another.

serum at 17°C, neither C3 nor any other complement component was inactivated, although some change in the complement did occur since, when zymosan was removed and the serum warmed to 37°C, the addition of fresh zymosan to the warm serum failed to inactivate C3. (When zymosan was not removed from the serum after the original incubation at 17°C and the temperature was raised to 37°C, inactivation of C3 did take place.) These observations, largely the work of Louis Pillemer and his co-workers, were interpreted as follows: at 17°C zymosan, Z, combines with a substance, P, in the serum to form an insoluble complex, PZ, capable of inactivating C3 at 37°C, but not at 17°C. By removing zymosan, one also removes P, and when fresh zymosan is added and the temperature raised to 37°C, no P is present and zymosan can react with neither P nor C3. Pillemer and his co-workers called the hypothetical serum substance *properdin* (L. *perdere*, to destroy) and suggested, in 1954, that the properdin system represented a new complement pathway activated by sugars in yeast or bacterial cell walls, rather than by antibodies. This hypothesis was viciously attacked by other immunologists, properdin was proclaimed to be an artifact, and the entire set of experiments was dismissed as fabrication. So emotional and fierce was the attack that Pillemer took his own life and immunologists forgot about the alternative pathway for 10 years. Only in the 1970s did several investigators begin to realize that Pillemer and his collaborators had been right after all, and that properdin and the properdin pathway of complement activation did exist. By then it was too late for Pillemer to find consolation in La Rochefoucauld's maxim: "The biggest disadvantage of a penetrating intellect is not failure to reach the goal but going beyond it." Later studies proved the existence of other components of the alternative pathway, in addition to properdin, and also demonstrated that the pathway joined the classical pathway at the level of C5.

9.2.2. Definitions and Nomenclature

Complement (originally abbreviated as C′ and now as C) is a multimolecular, self-assembling activation system that irreversibly alters biological membranes, causing cell death, and that also carries out a series of specialized functions related to body defense. The complement system can be divided into three compartments, concerned with *activation*, *effector function*, and *regulation* (Fig. 9.6). Two pathways, the classical and the alternative, constitute the activation compartment.

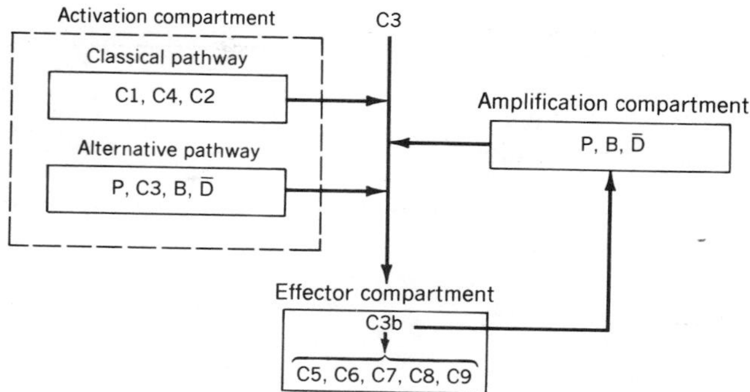

Figure 9.6. The three compartments of the complement system. (Based on D. F. Fearon and K. F. Austen: *in* L. E. Glynn and M. W. Steward (Eds.): *Immunochemistry: An Advanced Textbook*. Wiley, Chichester, 1977.)

The *classical pathway* consists of six proteins (Table 9.2), referred to by Arabic numerals (C2, C3, and C4) or by numbers and letters (C1q, C1r, and C1s). The numbers reflect the sequence in which the components are activated, with the exception of C4, which is activated after C1 and before C2 (the numbers were assigned before the reaction sequence was fully known).

The *alternative pathway* consists of at least five components not used by the classical pathway (Table 9.2); these are referred to either by names (initiation factor, properdin, C3b proactivator, C3 activator, and C3 proactivator convertase) or by symbols (I, F, P, C3PA or B, C3A or B̄, and C3PAse or D̄). The alternative pathway shares with the classical pathway the component C3.

The *effector function* is carried by the *common pathway* shared by the classical and alternative pathways. The common pathway consists of five components, referred to, as in the case of the components of the classical pathway, by Arabic numerals (C5, C6, C7, C8, and C9).

The *regulatory compartment* is only now being discovered. It consists of at least four components, referred to by an assortment of names and symbols (C1 inhibitor, C3̄b inactivator, B1H globulin, and anaphylatoxin inactivator).

Polypeptide chains of a given component are designated by Greek letters (e.g., $C4_{\alpha}$, $C4_{\beta}$, $C4_{\gamma}$). Physiological fragments resulting from enzymatic cleavage of components by other complement components are distinguished by small letters in combination with the component designation (e.g., C4a, C4b, C4e, C4d).[1] A

[1] The suffix "a" is sometimes used for the activated form of a given component (e.g., C1a is the activated form of C1). This usage, however, confuses the situation.

Table 9.2 Properties of Complement Components

Component	Serum Concentration (μg/ml)	Activation Products	Molecular Weight	Polypeptide Chains
Classical pathway				
C1q	180		410,000	6 × 24,000
				6 × 23,000
				6 × 22,000
C1r	50		170,000	2 × 85,000
		C$\bar{1}$r	170,000	2 × 58,000
				2 × 27,000
C1s	100		85,000	
		C$\bar{1}$s	85,000	58,000
				27,000
C4	500		210,000	
			90,000	
			78,000	
			33,000	
		C4a	10,000	
		C4b	200,000	85,000
				78,000
				33,000
C2	30		115,000	
		C2a	80,000	
		C2b	35,000	
C3	1300		195,000	
			110,000	
			85,000	
		C3a	9000	
		C3b	186,000	110,000
				75,000
Alternative pathway				
B	200		93,000	
		Ba	30,000	
		Bb	63,000	
D	1–5		25,000	
		$\bar{\text{D}}$	25,000	
P	25		184,000	4 × 46,000
I	20–50	NF (?)	170,000	2 × 85,000
N			170,000	2 × 85,000
Common pathway				
C5	75		205,000	
			120,000	
			85,000	
		C5a	11,000	
		C5b	195,000	110,000
				85,000
C6	60		128,000	
C7	55		121,000	
C8	80		155,000	77,000
				63,000
				14,000
C9	200		75,000	
Regulatory proteins				
C$\bar{1}$-INH	180		100,000	
C$\bar{3}$b-INA	25		100,000	55,000
C4b-binding protein	?		540,000	n × 70,000
β1H globulin	670		150,000	

Source. Modified from R. R. Porter and K. B. M. Reid: *Adv. Prot. Chem.* **33**:1–71, 1979.

transiently activated site of a fragment is indicated by an asterisk (C3b*), the inactivated form of the fragment by a subscript "i" (C3b_i). A bar over the number (C$\bar{1}$, C$\bar{2}$, C$\bar{3}$, etc.) indicates that this component possesses enzymatic activity. Complexes formed by the joining of two or more components are indicated by the corresponding combination of symbols (C$\overline{42}$).

9.2.3 Methods of Study

To study complement activation, an investigator uses one of the following three experimental methods: bacteriolysis, hemolysis, or complement fixation. In the *bacteriolysis method*, the investigator coats bacteria with antibodies directed against surface antigens and, upon addition of complement, observes, with the aid of a microscope, cell breakage and disintegration (lysis). However, complement kills only some Gram-negative bacteria, such as *Vibrio*, *Salmonella*, or *Treponema*, and has no effect on Gram-positive bacteria with thick cell walls and large quantities of surface mucopolysaccharides (see Chapter 10). Because of the small size of most bacteria, direct observation of their lysis is often difficult, so this method of complement testing is used only infrequently.

In the *hemolysis method*, the investigator produces antibodies (hemolysins) to antigens on the surface of red blood cells, coats the erythrocytes with these antibodies, and upon addition of complement, observes the release of hemoglobin from the damaged cells. The released hemoglobin changes the color and optical density of the solution. The color change can be measured colorimetrically by comparing the solution's color with that of a standard solution; the change in optical density is measured spectrophotometrically by the decrease in intensity of monochromatic light passing through the solution. The advantage of hemolysis is that erythrocytes are easy to obtain in large quantities and easy to store and count, and that the release of hemoglobin can be measured quantitatively. The most commonly used erythrocytes are those of sheep; a frequently used antibody is that of a rabbit to the Forssman antigen—a cell-surface antigen shared by many different vertebrate species. When all other conditions (erythrocyte concentration, dilution and quality of hemolysins) are constant, the extent of erythrocyte lysis is a function of complement concentration. When one makes serial dilutions of complement and then plots the degree of lysis at the different dilutions, one obtains a sigmoid (S-shaped) curve (Fig. 9.7) that is nearly linear in its central portion (between 30 and 70 percent lysis). The initial leg of the curve (less than 30 percent lysis) can be attributed to, among other things, the fact that, at lower complement concentration, one or more complement components are not available in quantities sufficient for the completion of the lytic sequence. The departure from linearity in the range above 70 percent lysis can be explained by the inefficiency of the hemolytic reaction at high complement concentrations. Hemolysis is a one-hit phenomenon, which means that a single puncture of the membrane suffices to kill the cell; binding of complement at additional sites of the membrane is therefore superfluous. Since multiple binding is more frequent the higher the complement concentration is, the reaction loses its efficiency beyond the point needed to produce 70 percent lysis.

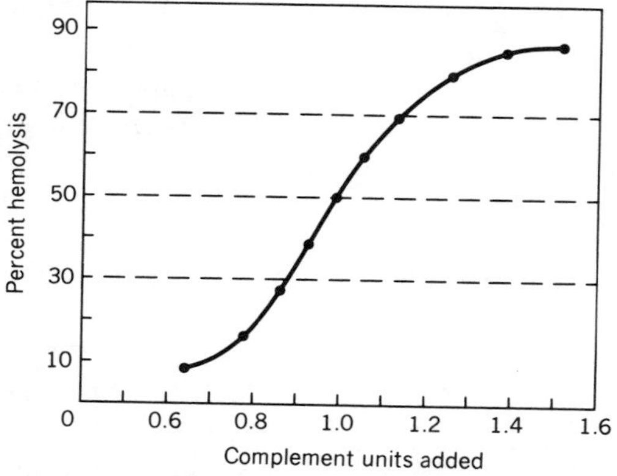

Figure 9.7. The relationship between the degree of hemolysis and the amount of complement added.

Rather than measuring the actual amount of complement in the serum, one can express the complement concentration in arbitrary units, where one unit is the amount necessary for 50 or 100 percent lysis. The former (CH_{50} or 50 percent hemolytic unit) is the preferred way of expressing complement concentration, since it corresponds to the steeper and thus more precisely defined region of the lytic curve.

The hemolytic reactions are sometimes expressed by a kind of immunological shorthand, in which E stands for erythrocyte, A for antibody, and EA for erythrocytes coated with antibody. Components already bound are designated by adding their numbers to the EAC symbol (e.g., EAC142 is a complex of erythrocytes, antibodies, and complement components C1, C4, and C2). Addition of another component can be written as a chemical equation:

$$\text{EAC142} + \text{C3} \rightarrow \text{EAC1423}$$

In the bacteriolysis and hemolysis methods, the binding of complement to antibody produces a visible effect (cell lysis). Such an effect does not occur when soluble antigen reacts with an antibody: the antigen-antibody complex binds complement, but outwardly this binding cannot be seen. To study complement in such a situation, one uses the *complement-fixation test*, originally described by Jules Bordet and Octave Gengou. The basis for complement fixation is the observation that the complex resulting from the combination of antigen (e.g., egg albumin) with antibody (e.g., rabbit antibody to egg albumin) takes up (fixes) complement, and that after this fixation, complement is no longer available to lyse red blood cells. Since the absence of erythrocyte lysis indicates, first, that antibody-antigen reaction has taken place, and second, that complement has been fixed, the test can be used for the detection of the antibody, the antigen, or complement.

The reagents necessary for the complement fixation test can be divided into the hemolytic (indicator) system, the test system, and complement. The *hemolytic system* consists of sheep red blood cells and an amboceptor—a term introduced by Paul Ehrlich (L. *ambo*, both; *capio*, to take) for antibodies to sheep erythrocytes. The most frequently used amboceptor is rabbit antibody to Forssman antigen. The *test system* consists of the test antigen and antibodies; the usual source of *complement* is normal guinea pig serum.

The test for the presence of antibodies to a particular antigen is carried out as follows. First, serum suspected of containing the antibody is heated to inactivate its own complement and is serially diluted. Second, the same (predetermined) amounts of antigen and complement are added to each dilution and the mixture is incubated to allow reaction of antibodies with the antigen and the attachment of complement to the antigen-antibody complexes. Third, simultaneously, the hemolytic indicator system is prepared, by adding a suspension of sheep red blood cells to heated rabbit anti-sheep erythrocyte serum. (The heating is necessary to prevent lysis of the sheep red blood cells by complement in the rabbit serum.) The antiserum is diluted so that it contains an insufficient amount of antibody to cause hemagglutination. The attachment of antibody to sheep red blood cells is referred to as *sensitization*, and the antibody-coated erythrocytes are described as *sensitized*. Fourth, the sensitized erythrocytes are added to the antigen-antibody-complement mixture and the degree of hemolysis is measured. Principally, two situations can occur (Fig. 9.8*a*,*b*). Antibody may be present in the test system, all the added complement may be adsorbed to the antigen-antibody complexes, and no free complement would remain to lyse the sensitized sheep red blood cells. Absence of hemolysis, therefore, would indicate presence of antibody. Alternatively, antibody may be absent in the test system, in which case complement would not be fixed, but would remain free to attach to the antibody on the sensitized sheep red blood cells and to lyse those cells. Occurrence of hemolysis would thus indicate absence of antibody in the test serum.

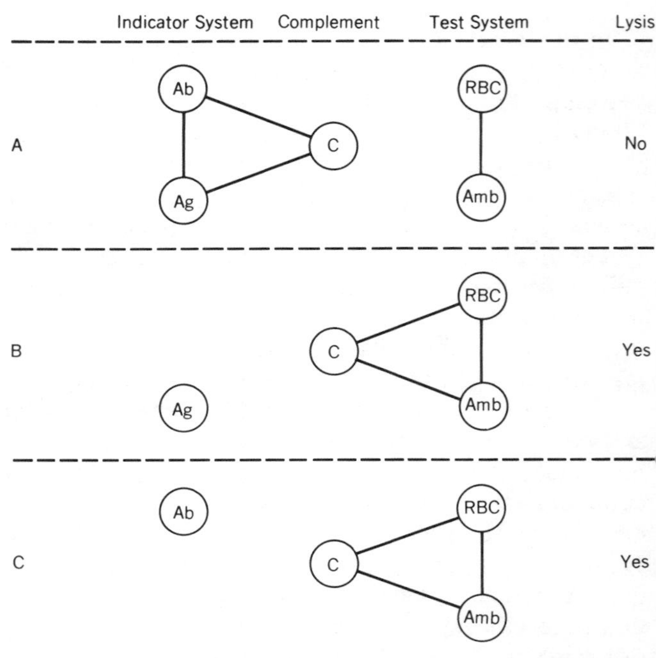

Figure 9.8. Diagrammatic representation of the three principal situations in the complement fixation test. (*a*) All components are present, complement is bound (fixed) by the antigen-antibody complex, no free complement is left to attack the sensitized erythrocytes, and hence no lysis occurs. (*b*) No antibody is present for a given antigen, free complement binds to sensitized erythrocytes and lyses them. (*c*) No antigen with which the antibody is capable of reacting is present, free complement binds to sensitized erythrocytes and lyses them. Ab, antibody; Ag, antigen; Amb, sensitizing antibody (amboceptor); C, complement; RBC, red blood cells. (Modified from W. C. Boyd: *Fundamentals of Immunology*, 4th ed. Interscience, New York, 1966.)

The assay must always be checked by a system of four controls: *antibody control*, in which the antigen has been omitted; *antigen control*, in which the antiserum has been omitted; *erythrocyte control*, in which unsensitized sheep red blood cells are used; and *hemolytic control*, in which both the antigen and antibody have been omitted. The first two controls are necessary because sometimes the antibody or antigen preparation may contain anticomplementary substances—substances that inhibit the action of complement. The third control is necessary because occasionally the sheep red blood cells may be damaged and lyse spontaneously. And the fourth control is needed to prove that the complement and sensitized antibodies are active at the dosages used. The test is meaningful only when total lysis occurs in the antigen, antibody, and hemolytic controls, and no lysis occurs in the erythrocyte control.

The system can also be modified to test an unknown preparation for the presence of an antigen (rather than the presence of antibody; see Fig. 9.8*a*). In this modification, it is the antigen that is serially diluted, while the other components of the system are kept constant.

The assay works only when properly standardized by using the individual reagents in predetermined amounts. The sheep red blood cells are normally used in concentrations between 2 and 5 percent; the dilution of the sensitizing antibody and of the antigen are determined by trial and error. The dose of complement is selected by setting up the guinea pig serum in a series of dilutions against a standard dose of coated sheep red blood cells. The commonly used doses are those corresponding to two CH_{100} or five CH_{50} units.

The complement fixation test is useful not only for the study of complement, but also for the analysis of antibody structure and function, for the detection of cell-bound macromolecules, for the detection and quantitation of antigens in bodily fluids, and for establishing immunochemical relationships among antigens. The test has also been widely used in medicine, in the diagnosis of infectious diseases. The best example of the clinical application of the complement fixation test is the *Wassermann reaction* for syphilis. August P. von Wassermann observed, in 1906, that sera from patients infected with *Treponema pallidum*—the causative bacterium of syphilis—contained a substance that reacted with alcoholic liver extracts from the fetuses of syphilitic mothers. (The disease is transmitted from the mother to the fetus in the uterus.) The reaction fixed complement—in other words, it prevented lysis of sensitized sheep red blood cells added to the reaction mixture. Wassermann thought that the extract contained *Treponema*-specific antigens, but later research revealed that the same antigen could also be obtained from liver, heart, and other tissues of nonsyphilitic persons or animals; nowadays the usual source of antigen is ox heart. The antigen has been designated *cardiolipin*, and it has been demonstrated to consist of three glycerol residues joined by two phosphate groups, with four fatty acid chains attached to the hydroxyl groups of the terminal glycerol molecules (Fig. 9.9). Cardiolipin alone does not stimulate antibody production, although it binds antibodies produced by other means; to activate antibody-synthesizing cells, cardiolipin must be attached to a carrier molecule. Researchers believe that the *Treponema* infection leads to the release of normally cytoplasmic cardiolipin into bodily fluids and to immunization of the patient. The substance in the serum of syphilitic persons is thus an autoantibody directed against cardiolipin; the antibody is, however, not totally specific for syphilis, since a similar substance also occurs in a variety of infectious and noninfectious conditions. Originally, when the

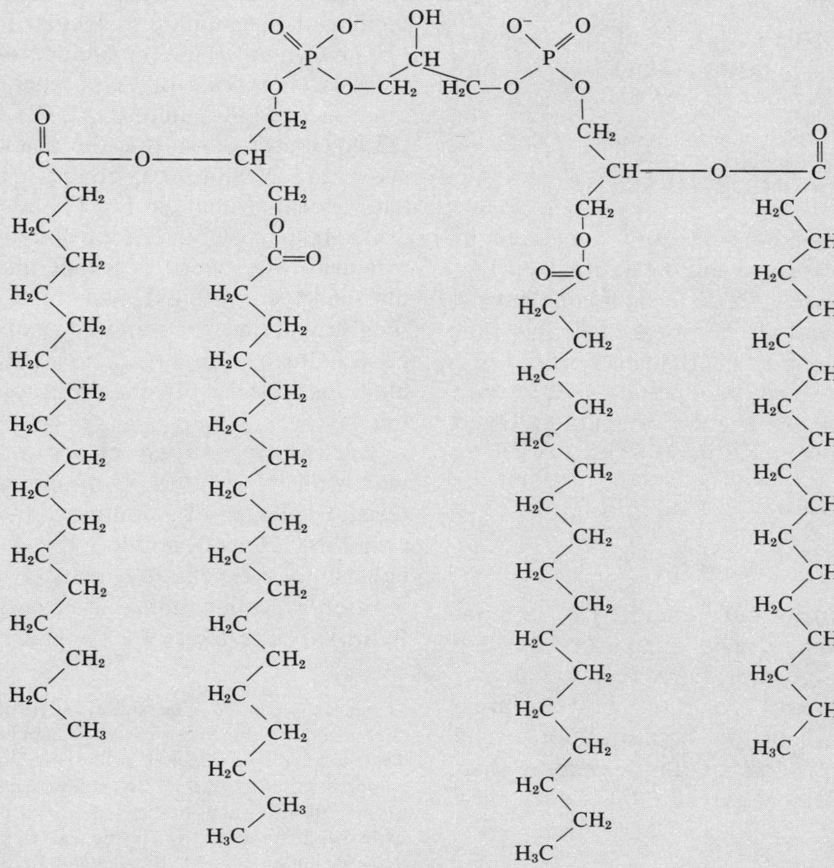

Figure 9.9. Cardiolipin.

immunoglobulin nature of the serum substance was doubted, the antibody was referred to as *reagin* (not to be confused with reaginic antibodies of the IgE type).

To isolate individual complement components from the serum, biochemists use standard techniques of protein fractionation, such as euglobulin precipitation, ammonium sulfate fractionation, and column chromatography on ion-exchange and molecular-sieve supports. Purification is not an easy task because most complement components are present in plasma at relatively low concentrations and because some of them are highly labile. Once the individual complement components are isolated and purified, antibodies can be produced against them and the complement system studied, using standard serological assays.

To study the alternative complement pathway, one must inactivate the classical pathway. Such inactivation can be achieved in two ways—genetically or by chemical treatment of the serum. In the former instance, one uses serum of animals genetically deficient in C1, C2, or C4 (see section 9.9). In the latter case, one incubates the serum with compounds, such as ethylene glycoltetraacetic acid (EGTA), which bind Ca^{2+} ions necessary for the activation of the classical, but not of the alternative pathway. (The latter requires Mg^{++} ions, which EGTA binds far less than Ca^{++} ions.)

9.3 THE ACTIVATION COMPARTMENT

Activation of the complement cascade can occur in one of two ways—the classical and the alternative. (As has already been discussed, these designations have a historical connotation and are not meant to imply that one pathway is more important than the other.) We shall discuss the two pathways separately and, in each case, we shall first describe the components involved and then the activation process itself.

9.3.1 The Classical Pathway

Components

Almost all the complement components (i.e., components of all three complement compartments) are high-molecular-weight glycoproteins, containing between 5 and 10 percent carbohydrate. Most are present in plasma at relatively low concentrations. The classical pathway components are (in the order of their activation in the complement cascade) C1, C4, C2, and C3 (Table 9.2).

The C1 Component. The C1 component consists of three subcomponents—C1q, C1r, and C1s—which

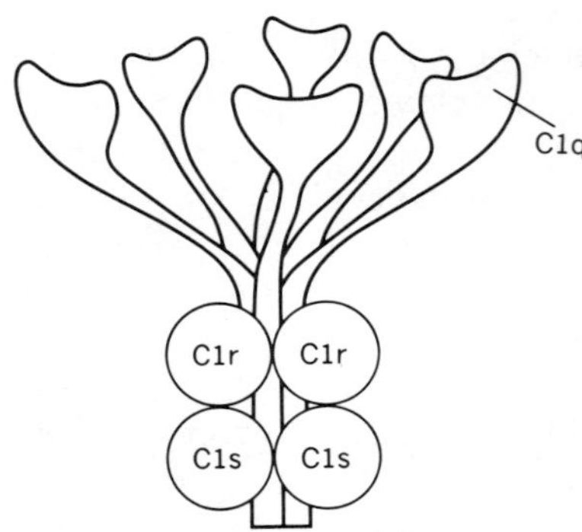

Figure 9.10. Complex of one C1q, two C1r, and two C1s molecules.

interact with one another in a way not yet entirely clear to us. The following combinations of the subcomponents have been found in the serum: $C1q–C1r_2–C1s_2$ (Fig. 9.10), $C1r_2–C1s_2$, $C1q–C1r_2$, C1q–C1s, and free C1q, $C1r_2$, C1s molecules. Of these, the $C1q–C1r_2$ and $C1r_2–C1s_2$ complexes are relatively stable, provided Ca^{2+} ions are available: removal of Ca^{2+} ions by the addition of EDTA breaks the complexes and the $C1r_2$ dimers; the remaining molecular forms are unstable.

The C1q molecule (molecular weight of 410,000 daltons) is comprised of 18 polypeptide chains of three kinds—A (24,000 daltons), B (23,000 daltons), and C (22,000 daltons)—so that the whole molecule contains six A, six B, and six C chains (Fig. 9.11). The A, B, and C chains contain 12, 8, and 4 percent carbohydrate, respectively. The carbohydrates are composed primarily of glucose (a rather unusual component of plasma glycoproteins), galactose, and small amounts of glucosamine, neuraminic acid, mannose, and fucose. Glucose and galactose are linked as disaccharides to the hydroxyl group of hydroxylysine (see below).

Each chain consists of about 200 amino acids, of which the N-terminal 89 amino acids have a characteristic collagen-like composition: starting with position 3 in C, 6 in B, and 9 in the A chain, the sequence consists of a repeating triplet, glycine–X–Y, where X is often a proline and Y is usually hydroxyproline or hydroxylysine (Fig. 9.12).[2] The regularity of the se-

[2] Collagen (Gr. *koilla*, glue; suffix *-gen*, producing) is a major protein of connective tissue fibers, cartillage, and bone (see Appendix 4.1.2). The amino acid sequence of collagen is highly regular, with glycine comprising nearly every third residue, and the most frequent sequence being glycine–proline–hydroxyproline. Hydroxylysine and hydroxyproline differ from lysine and proline, respectively, only by the substitution of one hydrogen with the hydroxyl group OH; these two amino acids occur in only a few proteins other than collagen and C1q.

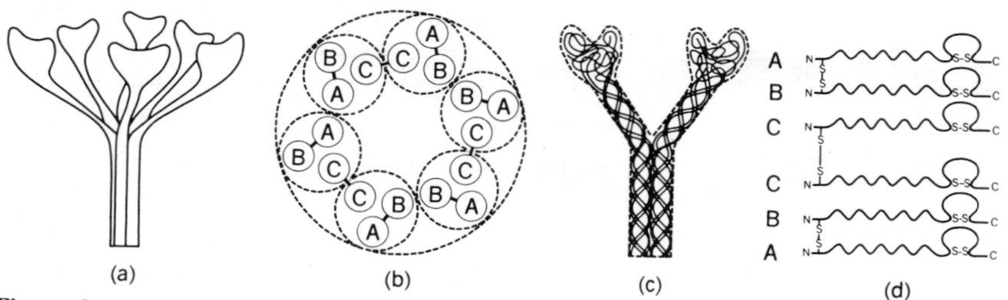

Figure 9.11. The structure of the C1q molecule. (*a*) The "bouquet of tulips," each "tulip" consisting of three polypeptide chains. (*b*) Cross section through the "stalk" region of the bouquet. Each solid circle represents one polypeptide chain, the broken circle represents chain grouping, and the connecting lines indicate disulfide bridges. (*c*) One double "tulip." (*d*) Arrangement of polypeptide chains, helical and globular regions, and disulfide bridges.

quence is disturbed only by alanine's replacing glycine at position 9 in the B chain, threonine inserted between positions 38 and 39 in chain A, and alanine's replacing glycine at position 36 in chain C.

Starting with position 90 and continuing toward the C terminal, the regularity of the sequence is lost. This region in each of the three polypeptide chains contains one intrachain disulfide bridge. There is a high degree of sequence homology among the three chains throughout their entire length, suggesting common evolutionary origin of the encoding genes (Fig. 9.12). Intrachain disulfide bridges form at the N terminal between the A and B and between the C and D chains (Fig. 9.11*d*). The 18 chains are arranged into six triplets, each triplet consisting of one A, one B, and one C chain; the triplets are then joined into pairs by the disulfide bridges between their C chains (Fig. 9.11*b*). In each triplet, the three chains form a triple helix in the N-terminal region of the molecule (up to residue 89), while the rest of the molecule is globular (Fig. 9.11*c*). The entire complex resembles a bouquet of six tulips (with the helical regions representing the stalks and the globular regions the flowers) or a six-headed dragon. This resemblance is enhanced by the bending

	1									10										20										30		
A chain	E	D	L	C	R	A	P	D	G	K	L^+	G	E	A	G	R	P^+	G	R	R	G	R	P^+	G	L	L^+	G	E	Q	G	E	P^+
B chain	E	L	S	C	T	G	P	P^+	A	I	P^+	G	I	P^+	G	I	P	G	T	P	G	P	N	G	Q	P^+	G	T	P^+	G	I	L^+
C chain	N	T	G	C	Y	G	I	P^+	G	M	P^+	G	L	P^+	G	A	P^+	G	K	D	G	Y	D	G	L	P^+	G	P	P^+	G	E	P

									40										50										60				
A chain	G	A	P^+	G	I	R	T	G	I	Q				G	L	P^+	G	D	Q	G	Q	L^+	G	P	S	G	N	P^+	G	K	V	G	Y
B chain	G	E	L^+	G	L	P^+		G	L	A	G	D	H	G	E	F	G	E	L^+	G	D	P	G	I	P^+	G	D	P^+	G	K	V	G	P
C chain	G	I	P^+	A	I	L^+		G	I	R				G	P	P^+	G	Q	L^+	G	E	P	G	L	P^+	G	K	H	G	L^+	D	G	P

						70										80										90							97
A chain	P^+	G	P	S	G	P	L	G	A	R	G	I	L^+	G	I	L^+	G	T	P^+	G	S	P	G	N	I	K	D	Q	P	R	P	A	F.....
B chain	L^+	G	P	M	G	P	L^+	G	P	P^+	G	A	P^+	G	A	P^+	G	P	L^+	G	E	S	G	D	Y	K	A	T	Q	K	I	A	F.....
C chain	N	G	P		G	M	P^+	G	V	P^+	G	P	M	G	I	P^+	G	E	P	G	E	E	G	R	Y	K	Q	K	F	Q	S	V	F.....

	130									140					145
A chain	...F	V	C	T	V	P	G	Y	Y	Y	F	T	F	Q	V	L
B chain	...F	T	C	K	V	P	G	L	Y	Y	F	T	F	Q	V	L
C chain	...F	T	C	K	V	P	G	L	Y	Y	F	Y	V	Q	A	S

Figure 9.12. Partial amino-acid sequence of the A, B, and C chains of human C1q. The numbering is based on the B-chain sequence. Gaps in the sequence had been introduced to give the optimal alignment for maximum homology. Each chain is about 200 residues long. L^+ stands for hydroxylysine, P^+ for hydroxyproline. (From R. R. Porter and K. B. M. Reid, *Adv. Prot. Chem.* **33**:1–71, 1979.)

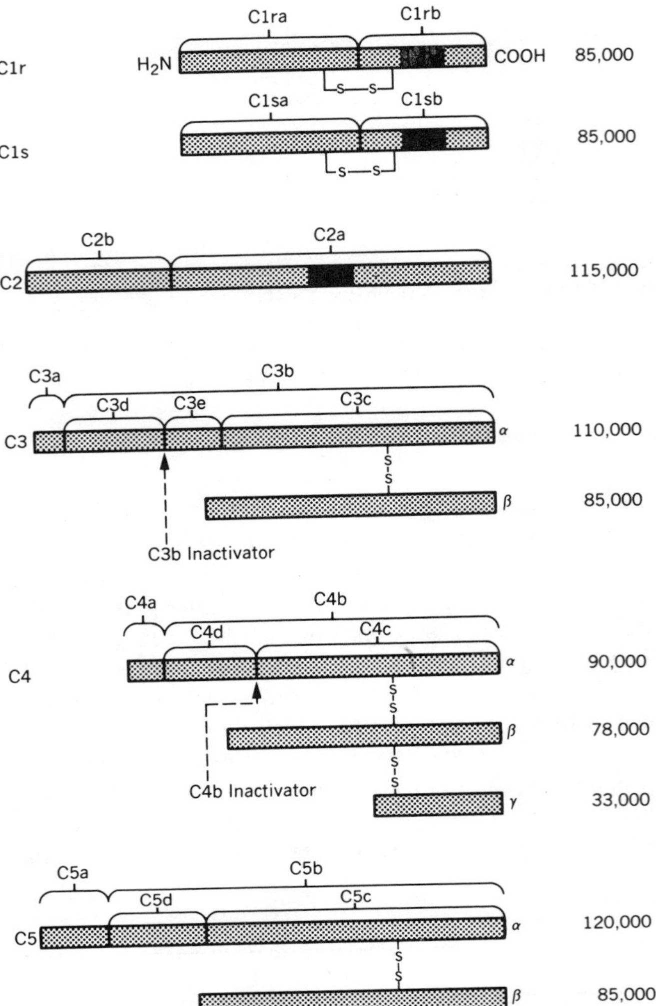

Figure 9.13. Diagrammatic representation of the early components of the classical complement pathway. Sites of proteolytic cleavage are indicated by vertical bars, approximate positions of enzymatically active sites by black areas. The number and position of disulfide bridges linking the individual chains are not known. The numbers at the right-hand side of the figures indicate the molecular weights of the chains.

of the stalk, probably at positions 39 and 36 in the A and C chains, respectively, in the area where the sequence regularity is interrupted.

C1r and C1s have similar molecular weights (83,000 daltons), structure (each consisting of a single polypeptide chain; Fig. 9.13), and amino acid sequence (Fig. 9.14), suggesting that they are products of duplicated genes. When not associated with C1q, the C1r molecules occur as dimers (molecular weight of 170,000 daltons) in which the two chains are held together by Ca^{++} ions. The C1q molecules, on the other hand, are usually monomers. In the C1q–C1r$_2$–C1s$_2$ complex, both C1r and C1s are probably attached to the collagenous stalks of C1q, so that all three subcomponents are in physical contact with one another (see Fig. 9.10). Reports describing a fourth C1 subcomponent, referred to as C1t, have not been substantiated.

The C4 Component. In terms of serum concentration, C4 is one of the major complement components (500 μg/ml). It has a molecular weight of 210,000 daltons and consists of three disulfide bridge-linked chains—α (90,000 daltons), β (78,000 daltons), and γ (33,000 daltons; cf. Fig. 9.13). Only short stretches of the three chain N terminals have been sequenced (Fig. 9.15) and the sequences do not show any obvious homology with other sequenced proteins, including the large chain of C3, often considered homologous in function to C4.

The C2 Component. C2 is difficult to isolate because it is present in serum only in trace amounts (30 μg/ml) and because it is highly susceptible to proteolysis. The C2 molecule consists of a single polypeptide chain with a molecular weight of some 115,000 daltons and with two free SH groups positioned in close proximity to each other. Upon oxidation with iodine, the groups form intramolecular disulfide bridges and this modification increases the hemolytic activity of the molecules from 10 to 20 times.

	1 10 20	
Human C$\overline{1s}$ A chain	E P T M Y G E I L S P N Y P Q A Y P X E	
Human C$\overline{1r}$ B chain	I I G G Q K A K M G N F P W Q V F T N Z	
Human C$\overline{1s}$ B chain	I I G G S D A D I K N F P W Q V F F D N	A C G L D S G E X R
Bovine chymotrypsin	I V N G E E A V P G S W P W Q V S L Q D	
Bovine trypsin	I V G G Y T C G A N T V P Y Q V S L N S	S C Q G D S G G P V
Bovine thrombin B chain	I V E G Q D A E V G L S P W Q V M L F R	A C E G D S G G P F
Human plasmin B chain	V V G G C V A H P H S W P W Q V V L L R	S C Q G D S G G P L

Figure 9.14. Comparison of N-terminal and active site amino-acid sequences of C$\overline{1r}$ and C$\overline{1s}$ with the corresponding polypeptide chains of other serine proteinases. (Based on R. R. Porter and K. B. M. Reid, *Adv. Prot. Chem.* **33**:1–71, 1979.)

	1				5					10					15							20					25	
α chains																												
Human C5a			T	L	Q	K	K	I	E	E	I	A	A	K	Y	K		H	S	V	V	K	K	C	C	Y	D	G
Human C4	N	V	N	F	Q	K	A	I	N	E	K	L	G	E	Y	A		S	P	T	A	K						
Human C3a	S	V	Q	L	T	E	K	R	M	N	K	V	G	K	Y	P		K	E	L		R	K	C	C	E	D	G
Pig C3a	S	V	Q	L	M	E	R	K	M	N	K	L	G	Q	Y	S		K	E	L		R	R	C	C	E	H	G
Rat C3a	S	V	Q	L	M	E	R	R	M	D	K	A	G	Q	Y	T	D	K	E	L		R	K	C	C	E	D	G
β chains																												
Human C4		K	P	R G	L Y	L	L I	F L T	F P V	P C D	V																	
Human C3		S	P	M	Y	S	I	G	T	P	B																	
γ chain																												
Human C4		E	A	P	K	V	V	E H	E	Q	E	S	R	V A	H	Y	T	V	C	I C	W	G						

				30					35					40					45					50				
α chains																												
Human C5a	A	C	V	N	N	D	E		T	C	E	Q	R	A	A	R	I	S	L	G	P	R	C	I	K	A	F	T
Human C4	M	R	Q	N	P	M	R	F	S	C	Q	R	R	T	R	F	I	S	L	G	E	A	C	K	K	V	F	L
Human C3a	M	R	N	N	P	M	K	F	S	C	Q	R	R	A	Q	F	I	H	Q	G	N	A	C	V	K	A	F	L
Pig C3a	M	R	D	I	P	M	D	Y	S	C	Q	R	A	T	R	L	I	T	Q	G	E	S	C	K	L	A	F	M

	55						60					65					70							75		
α chains																										
Human C5a	E	C	C	V	V	A	S	Q	L	R					A	N	I	S	H	K	C	M	Q	L	G	R
																								L	Q	R
Human C4	N	C	C	N	Y		I	T	E	L	R	R	Q	H	A	R	A	S	H			L	G	L	A	R
Human C3a	N	C	C	E	Y		I	A	K	L	R	Q	Q	H	S	R	N	K	P			L	G	L	A	R
Pig C3a	D	C	C	N	Y		I	T	K	L	R	E	Q	H	R	R	D	H	V			L	G	L	A	R

Figure 9.15. Comparison of amino-acid sequences of C3, C4, and C5 components of different species. (Based on R. R. Porter and K. B. M. Reid, *Adv. Prot. Chem.* **33**:1–71, 1979.)

The C3 Component. The serum concentration of C3 is 10 times greater than that of most other components (1300 μg/ml). The C3 molecule consists of two disulfide-bridged chains of about 105,000 and 75,000 daltons, so that the intact C3 molecule weighs about 195,000 daltons.

The Activation Sequence

The complement cascade of the classical pathway begins with the activation of C1q, although other initiation points are also possible (see below). The C1q thus acts as the starter, who fires the shot that begins the complement relay race. The activated C1q converts C1r from its inactive proenzyme form to an enzymatically active molecule that then activates C1s. The latter cleaves away small fragments from C4 and C2, exposing sites that permit the two molecules to fuse and the C4 molecule to attach to the cell surface. The enzymatically active C4–C2 complex acts on C3, cleaving it into two fragments, and associates with one of the fragments (C3b) to form a C4–C2–C3b complex, which then acts on C5, the first component of the effector compartment (Fig. 9.16).

All components of the activation compartment, with the exception of C1q, are enzymes—proteins capable of catalyzing chemical reactions. In the native (proenzyme, zymogen) form, the active site of the component (i.e., the region of the enzyme that binds the substrate and makes or breaks bonds) is concealed in the interior of the molecule. The proenzyme is activated by the cleavage of a single peptide bond (effected by the enzyme preceding a given component in the activation cascade); the cleavage results in the clipping off of a low-molecular-weight fragment and exposure of the active site. The activated enzyme then acts on the subsequent component of the cascade, cleaving its apolypeptide chains. In addition to this proteolytic activity (i.e., ability to break peptide bonds), many of the complement enzymes also act as esterases, catalyzing

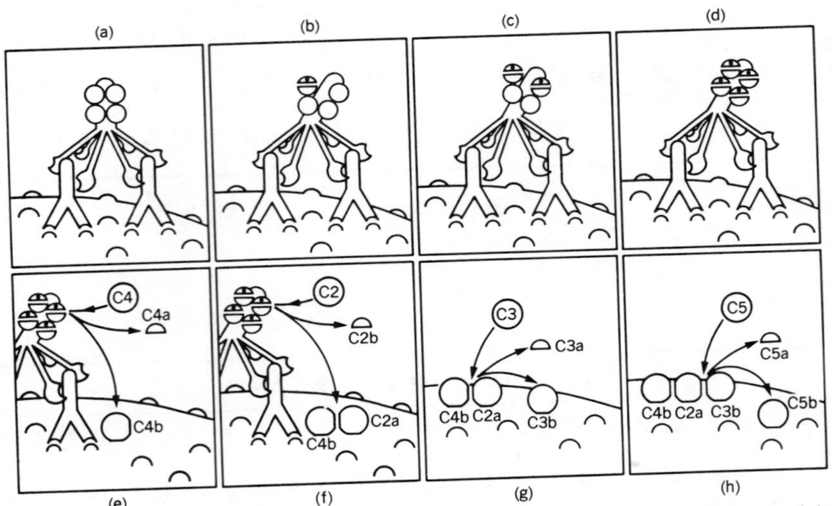

Figure 9.16. The activation compartment of the classical complement pathway. (*a*) Two IgG molecules bind to adjacent antigenic sites on the cell's surface and are bridged by a $C1q–C1r_1–Ca^{++}–C1s_2$ complex. (*b*) Conformational changes in C1q expose an active site in one of the two C1r molecules; the activated enzyme breaks one peptide bond in the second C1r molecule of the complex, activating this molecule. (*c*) The activated second molecule breaks a peptide bond in the first C1r monomer. (*d*) The activated $\overline{C1r}$ molecules break peptide bonds in the two C1s monomers, activating the latter. (*e*) Activated $\overline{C1s}$ chips off, from a C4 molecule, a small fragment (C4a), which moves out from the complement cascade; the remainder of the molecule (C4b) attaches to the cell membrane. (*f*) Activated $\overline{C1s}$ acts on C2, chipping off a C2b fragment; the remainder of the C2 molecule (the C2a fragment) fuses with C4b on the cell surface. (*g*) The C4bC2a complex cleaves a C3 molecule into C3a, which moves out of the complement cascade, and C3b, which binds to the membrane in the vicinity of the C4bC2a complex, forming the C5 convertase, which splits the C5 component into C5a and C5b. The C5b fragment attaches to yet another membrane site—that at which, eventually, the membrane lesion occurs.

the hydrolysis of esters according to the equation:

$$\underset{\text{Ester}}{R_1\text{—}\overset{\overset{\displaystyle O}{\|}}{C}\text{—}O\text{—}R_2} + H_2O \rightarrow \underset{\text{Acid}}{R_1\text{—}C\begin{smallmatrix} \diagup O^- \\ \diagdown\!\!\diagdown O \end{smallmatrix}} + \underset{\text{Alcohol}}{HO\text{—}R_2} + H^+.$$

The activated forms of the complement components are usually unstable and are often rapidly inactivated, either spontaneously or by a system of regulatory molecules.

After this brief introduction to the activation process, let us now examine in detail the individual steps of this process.

Initiation of the Complement Cascade (C1 Activation). To initiate the cascade, C1q must be activated by interaction with an immunoglobulin molecule or some other agent. However, since complement components coexist with immunoglobulins in the serum without undergoing significant activation, it seems that the antibody molecule itself must first change somehow in order to be recognized by C1q. This change occurs either when the antibody binds to an antigen, or when immunoglobulin molecules aggregate, following heating, ultrasonication, or chemical coupling. The nature of the change in the immunoglobulin molecule is not known. According to some immunologists, antigen binding or aggregation results in a conformational change of the immunoglobulin molecules and exposure of the C1q binding site. According to others, it is the proximity of several antigen-bound or aggregated antibody molecules that counts. The problem with the first hypothesis is that antigen binds to the Fab region, whereas C1q, as we shall see shortly, binds to the Fc region, which means that a change at one end of the molecule must somehow be transmitted to the other end. Conformational changes in the Fc region following antibody binding have, indeed, been recorded, but this observation does not satisfy the critics of the conformation hypothesis. They argue that such changes may have nothing to do with C1q activation, particularly since monovalent antigens do not cause complement binding. Furthermore, some antigens induce conformational changes without conferring the ability to bind complement on the Fc region. It is possible, however, that there are different kinds of conformational changes, only some of which expose the C1q binding site. Arguments, counterarguments—obviously, it is best to wait until the experts resolve the issue.

Not all immunoglobulins are capable of binding C1q: of the known classes, only IgM and IgG can activate the classical complement pathway; IgA, IgE, and IgD cannot. But IgA and IgE can activate complement via the alternative pathway (see below). Of the known human IgG subclasses, IgG3 and IgG1 bind and activate C1q readily, IgG2 does so poorly, and IgG4 almost does not at all. However, there is some evidence indicating that even the immunoglobulin molecules that do not bind and activate C1q do possess the C1q binding site in a concealed form not available for binding. It is possible that, in complement-fixing antibodies, the binding with an antigen results in a quarternary rearrangement of the domains and thus in exposure of the C1q binding site, and that the nonfixing immunoglobulins have lost their rearrangement ability. IgM molecules display, by far, the strongest C1q-binding ability, possibly because they possess five interaction sites and so can bind several complement molecules simultaneously. Binding of a single C1q molecule to a single, erythrocyte-bound IgM molecule suffices for lysis by complement to occur, whereas binding of a single C1q molecule to two IgG molecules simultaneously is necessary to achieve this same effect. Simultaneous attachment of C1q on two IgG molecules can occur only when the two antibody molecules bind to two antigenic sites that are very close to each other on the cell surface. The probability of such an attachment varies, depending on the density of the antigenic sites, but for an average antigen, about 800 IgG molecules must coat the erythrocyte to generate conditions for C1q binding and cell lysis. Since, under the same conditions, cell lysis can occur following the binding of a single IgM molecule, IgM is obviously a far more efficient hemolytic antibody than is IgG.

The C1q binding site resides in the CH2 domain of the IgG molecule (Fig. 9.17) and probably in the CH4 domain of the IgM molecule. Although each IgG molecule has two CH2 domains, apparently only one is necessary for C1q binding. Amino acid sequence comparisons of Fc regions that fix complement and those that do not have failed to identify a stretch in the primary structure responsible for the binding, but several lines of evidence indicate that tryptophan and tyrosine may play an important role. Furthermore, synthetic hexapeptides containing these two amino acids have been demonstrated to be involved in complement activation.

In addition to antibodies, C1q can also be activated by the following agents.

Protein A. As has already been discussed, protein A from the cell wall of *Staphylococcus aureus* binds to the

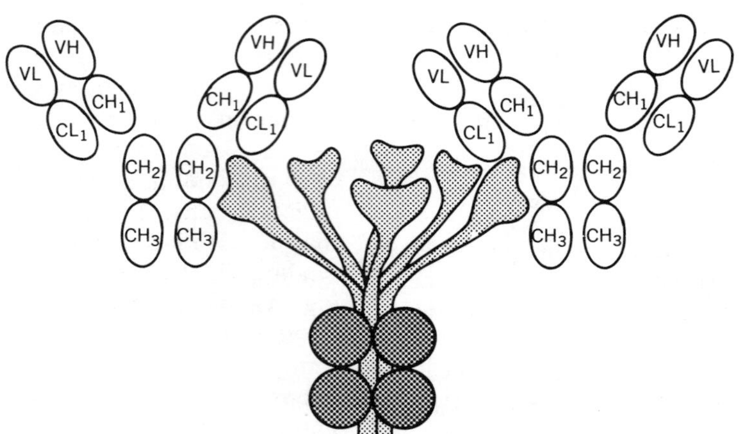

Figure 9.17. Binding of C1 components to CH2 domains of two IgG molecules.

Fc portion of Ig molecules and thus precipitates the antibodies. The precipitate binds C1q in the same way as do antigen–antibody complexes or aggregated immunoglobulins. Erythrocytes passively coated with protein A lyse upon addition of fresh normal serum.

Polyanions. Polyinosinic acid, deoxyribonucleic acid, dextran sulfate, polyvinylsulfonate, polyethanol sulfate, carrageenin, cellulose sulfate, and other negatively charged compounds consisting of repeated subunits often bind C1q more strongly than do aggregated immunoglobulins.

Polyanion-Polycation Interaction. Marked depletion of C1q and other complement components occurs following the interaction of strongly positively charged compounds with strongly negatively charged compounds. For example, heparin (polyanion) and protamine (polycation), when added to serum at the same time, deplete complement activity in amounts far below those required when either agent is added alone.

Viruses. Certain RNA-containing viruses (e.g., Moloney leukemia virus or vesicular stomatitis virus) bind C1q directly, without the participation of immunoglobulins. The binding leads to activation of the classical pathway, depositing of complement components on the viral surface, and destruction of viral particles.

C-Reactive Protein. Normal serum contains trace amounts of a protein that, in the presence of Ca^{2+}, precipitates pneumococcal polysaccharide C. This *C-reactive protein* has a molecular weight of from 120,000 to 140,000 daltons and consists of six (according to some authors, five) identical, noncovalently associated subunits. Species as widely separated as the rabbit and human show considerable amino acid sequence homology of their C-reactive proteins. A weak homology has been reported to exist between the C-reactive protein and the CH3 domain of the immunoglobulin molecule and possibly also between the C-reactive protein and murine and human MHC molecules, suggesting that all these proteins may have a common evolutionary origin. The C-reactive protein also resembles immunoglobulins in that it can bind C1q, and in its ability to initiate precipitation, agglutination, and enhancement of phagocytosis. Furthermore, C-reactive protein binds selectively to T (but not B) lymphocytes and platelets and has the ability to inhibit certain of their functions. The protein is synthesized by hepatocytes in the liver, and this synthesis is accelerated a thousandfold by inflammatory stimuli, suggesting that the protein's function may somehow be related to the inflammatory response (see Chapter 14).

In some instances, activation of the complement cascade can occur through later components of the system without the involvement of the earlier components. For example, evidence has been presented to suggest that C1r may also attach to immunoglobulin (to a site in the Fc region distinct from the C1q attachment site), and that it may be activated directly by antigen-antibody complexes; C1s can be activated directly by plasmin or kallikrein; certain snake and insect venoms may activate C4 and C2; plasmin, trypsin, tissue proteases, and thrombin can activate C3; trypsin and lysosomal enzymes derived from peripheral leukocytes may activate C5; and finally, a variety of complement components can be induced, in the presence of substances such as silinic acid, tannic acid, or polyethylene glycol, to attach directly to unsensitized erythrocytes and thus initiate a reaction leading to hemolysis.

What exactly happens during C1q activation is not clear, but since no breakage of covalent bonds, no formation of new bonds, and no appearance of catalytic activity can be demonstrated, the process probably involves a mere conformational change of the molecule. The change in shape of the C1q molecule is believed to induce, in turn, conformational alteration in one of the monomers of the C1r dimer. This alteration probably exposes an enzymatic site, which then cleaves the second monomer of the dimer in such a way that two disulfide-bonded fragments, one larger (a, molecular weight of 58,000 daltons) and one smaller (b, molecular weight of 27,000 daltons), result. The breakage exposes an enzymatically active site in the smaller fragment, which then cleaves the first monomer that was previously only distorted by C1q. The cleavage also splits the first monomer into the same disulfide-bonded fragments (a and b) as those of the second monomer. The two active sites in the two smaller fragments then attack the two monomers of the C1s dimer, cleave these chains in a similar fashion, each into 58,000-dalton (a) and 27,000-dalton (b) fragments, and so expose the enzymatically active sites in the two smaller fragments of C1s (see Fig. 9.13).

Activation of C4. Activated C1s acts first on C4 and then on C2, activating these two components in turn (Fig. 9.16). The activation of C4 consists of clipping off a low molecular-weight fragment (10,000 daltons) from the N terminal of the α chain. The fragment, referred to as C4a, moves out of the complement sequence and into the fluid phase (we shall describe its fate in section 9.6 of this chapter). The remainder of the molecule, now referred to as C4b (molecular weight of 200,000 daltons), has no enzymatic activity but possesses two interaction sites, probably both located in the α chain and both exposed by the removal of C4a. One site is hydrophobic and has an affinity for membranes and thus a capacity to transfer C4b from the fluid phase (serum) to the solid phase (cell or immune complex). However, this site is active only for a fraction of a second; if, during this time, the C4b molecule does not collide with a membrane, it is inactivated and the molecule converted into C4i. The latter can no longer attach to the membrane, although it can perform all other functions of C4b. Because of the short half-life of the binding site, only about 10 percent of activated C4b attaches to the membrane, while the remaining 90 percent remains in the fluid phase, where it is converted to C4i. This relative inefficiency of membrane binding is compensated by the high concentration of C4 in the serum and the fact that one C1s molecule can activate more than 200 C4 molecules around a single hemolytic site. The membrane-bound C4b has the ability to bind firmly to receptors on the surface of a variety of mammalian cells, and thus to enhance phagocytosis of complement-coated granulocytes, monocytes, and macrophages (see section 9.7). The second interaction site exposed after the C4a fragment has been clipped off has affinity for activated C2.

Activation of C2. The interaction of C1s with C4 apparently modifies the former so that it can activate the next component in the cascade, C2. How C4b or C4i changes the specificity of C1s to include C2 as its substrate is not known, but one possibility is that the interaction with C4 alters the conformation of C1s and fully uncovers the active site for C2. The action of C1s on C2 results in fission of the molecule into two fragments—larger C2a (molecular weight, 80,000 daltons), which leaves the complement cascade (see section 9.6), and smaller C2b (molecular weight, 35,000 daltons; see Figs. 9.13 and 16); note that the designation of fragments relative to their size is illogically inverted in the case of C2. The activation exposes two sites in the C2a fragment: one interacts with the corresponding region on the C4b fragment and the two fragments unite (how is not clear) to form a bimolecular complex, C4bC2a, which has a sedimentation constant of 11S and a molecular weight of 300,000 daltons. The second site is enzymatically active and has specificity for the next complement component in the sequence, C3 (for this reason, the C4bC2a complex is referred to as *C3 convertase*), and for certain esterases. This site is active only so long as C2a is united with C4b; if the former dissociates from the latter, the site loses its C3-cleaving activity, while retaining its esterase activity. To initiate the process leading to cell lysis, C3 convertase must bind to a membrane via its C4b portion; C4b thus serves as a bridge between the membrane and the C2a molecule. When the membrane-binding site is lost, the soluble enzyme can still act on C3, but cannot attach to the cells. The C3 convertase undergoes temperature-dependent and time-dependent decay with a half-life of from five to 10 minutes at 37°C. The decay process is mediated by factors in serum that convert the C2a into an inactive C2d. The latter is then released from the C4b molecule into the fluid phase, but the activity of the enzyme can be restored when another active C2a unites with C4b.

Activation of C3. The C3 convertase cleaves off, from the N terminal of the C3 α chain, a 77-residue peptide (molecular weight, 9000 daltons), thus splitting the C3 molecules into the smaller C3a and larger C3b fragments (Figs. 9.13 and 16). Like the other small products of complement activation so far described, the C3a fragment leaves the complement cascade to become active elsewhere (see section 9.6). And, as in the case of C4 and C2, the removal of the small fragment exposes two regions on the large fragment—one for binding to cell membrane and another for interaction with the cleaving enzyme, the C3 convertase. Current evidence suggests that the surface-binding site involves an intramolecular thioester bond and that the activation occurs in the following manner.

O=C
S
Activation by proteolytic enzymes
(−C3a)
Native C3

O=C
S
Unstable C3b
Receptive surface
(+ROH)
O=C—OR
SH
Surface-bound C3b

$(+H_2O)$
O=C—OH
SH
Fluid-phase C3b

The binding to the membrane occurs in the vicinity of the C4bC2a attachment site, and C3b molecules often arrange themselves radially around this site.

The second exposed region of the activated C3 molecule serves to attach the C4bC2a complex (the C3 convertase) to the C3b fragment and to form a trimolecular complex, C4bC2aC3b, referred to as *C5 convertase*. (C5 convertase can also assemble in the fluid phase, but then it is far less efficient than the membrane-bound convertase.) The substrate of C5 convertase is the next component to be activated, C5. For this activation, the C5 convertase probably uses the same active site as the C3 convertase —that in the α chain of the C2a fragment (thus, the C3 component, like the C4, does not display any enzymatic activity), and the actual cleaving process is probably similar in both instances (hydrolysis of a peptide bond, which involves the carboxyl group of arginine). Presumably, the addition of the C3b molecule to the complex changes the configuration of the enzyme, unmasks a C5-binding site, and thus makes attack on C5 possible.

9.3.2. The Alternative Pathway

Although the existence of the alternative pathway is now generally accepted and although this pathway is the subject of intensive research by many immunologists, it is still far from being understood, even in principle. Contradictory data and different interpretations abound, and it may take a few years before a general consensus is reached.

Components

The following components have been identified in the alternative pathway: C3 and cobra venom factor, initiation factor, properdin, factor B, and factor D.

C3 and Cobra Venom Factor. C3, as we shall learn shortly, plays a central role in the alternative pathway. Referred to also as *hydrazine-sensitive factor*, or HSF, and *factor A*, it is the same component that participates in an important way in the classical pathway, described in the preceding paragraphs.

Immunologists have known for some time that the addition of cobra venom to human serum depletes this serum of C3 and of all components in the classical pathway following C3 in the sequence. They attributed this depletion to a hypothetical *cobra venom factor*, and since this factor also activated the alternative complement pathway, they considered it to be a component of this pathway. However, recent studies have demonstrated that the cobra venom factor is, in fact, cobra C3b. Why it depletes serum of most of the classical pathway components and activates the alternative pathway will become clear shortly.

Initiation Factor. The discovery of this factor is tied to the so-called *nephritic factor*, present in the sera of patients suffering from chronic glomerulonephritis (a kidney disease characterized by protracted inflammation of the glomeruli—the tufts of capillary loops), partial lipodystrophy (a defect in fat metabolism), and systemic lupus erythematosus (an inflammatory connective tissue disease resembling rheumatoid arthritis;

see Chapter 14). The one thing these three diseases have in common is that they all affect the kidneys and are accompanied by the reduction of complement levels. The addition of sera from these patients to normal human sera causes a depletion of C3 similar to that observed upon addition of the cobra venom factor. This depletion has been ascribed to a pathological serum protein—the nephritic factor. Antiserum made against the nephritic factor crossreacts with a component in normal serum, and this component is referred to as the *initiation factor* because it is believed by some immunologists to initiate the alternative complement pathway. Nephritic and initiation factors have very similar structures, so much so that the former may be a pathological form of the latter. The initiation factor (factor I) has a molecular weight of 170,000 daltons and consists of two presumably identical disulfide-bridged chains, each weighing 85,000 daltons. The protein has no enzymatic activity and is stable when heated at 56°C for 30 minutes. It shows some similarities to IgG.

Properdin. Originally believed to play a pivotal role in the alternative complement pathway, properdin has been dethroned from this eminent position by later studies. However, its function in the alternative pathway is still far from being fully elucidated. The properdin molecule is a glycoprotein containing about 10 percent carbohydrate and present in serum at a concentration of from 20 to 25 μg/ml. It has a molecular weight of 184,000 daltons and consists of four similar or identical chains, associated by noncovalent bonds. Each chain has a molecular weight of 46,000 daltons. Like the initiation factor, properdin has no enzymatic activity.

Factor B. Other names for this key factor of the alternative pathway are *C3 proactivator* (*C3PA*) and *glycine-rich β-glycoprotein* (*GBG*). Its role in the alternative pathway is analogous to that of C2 in the classical pathway, and the two components may be evolutionarily related. It has a molecular weight of 93,000 daltons and consists of a single polypeptide chain. Its concentration in serum is approximately 200 μg/ml. It is inactivated when serum is heated at from 50 to 52°C for 30 minutes.

Factor D. Also referred to as *C3 proactivator convertase*, or *C3PA convertase*, it is the smallest of all known complement components, with a molecular weight of only 25,000 daltons. It is present only in trace amounts in serum, where its role may be analogous to that of C1s, or possibly of the $\overline{C1s}$ fragment.

The Activation Sequence

The alternative pathway can be initiated by a variety of agents: complex microbial polysaccharides such as zymosan, plant polysaccharides such as inulin (from a composite plant, *Inula*), bacterial products such as dextrans and levans, rabbit erythrocytes, human erythrocyte stroma, aggregated human IgA and aggregated $F(ab')_2$ fragments of guinea pig IgG1 (but not human IgG or IgM), cobra venom factor, and the nephritic factor. It is difficult to find any common denominator among all these substances, and it is possible that none exists and that the initiation occurs in a different way with different substances. It is important to realize, however, that antibodies are, under certain circumstances, capable of activating the alternative pathway, but they are not obligatory for this activation.

An activation scheme favored by immunologists at the time of this writing is this (Fig. 9.18). In normal plasma, the α chain of the C3 molecule spontaneously incorporates one molecule of water, thus breaking the intramolecular thioester bond:

O=C–S (Native C3) $\xrightarrow{+H_2O}$ O=C—OH, SH ($C3(H_2O)$)

A similar change can also occur, for example, by methylamine modification:

O=C–S (Native C3) $\xrightarrow{+CH_3NH_2}$ O=C—$NHCH_3$, SH ($C3(CH_3NH_2)$)

The $C3(H_2O)$ and $C3(CH_3NH_2)$ molecules behave functionally as does C3b, but unlike C3b, they fail to release the C3a fragment. The activated C3b-like molecules associate reversibly with factor B into loose C3B complexes, and the B molecule in the complex is enzymatically activated by the D factor, as described below. Alternatively, the C3 molecule in C3B induces a conformational change in B, unmasking an active site with specificity for intact C3 molecules. The activated C3B complex, referred to as the *initiating C3 convertase*, acts on C3 (thus, a C3-containing enzyme uses another C3 molecule as its substrate) and cleaves it into C3a and C3b, just as the C3 convertase (composed

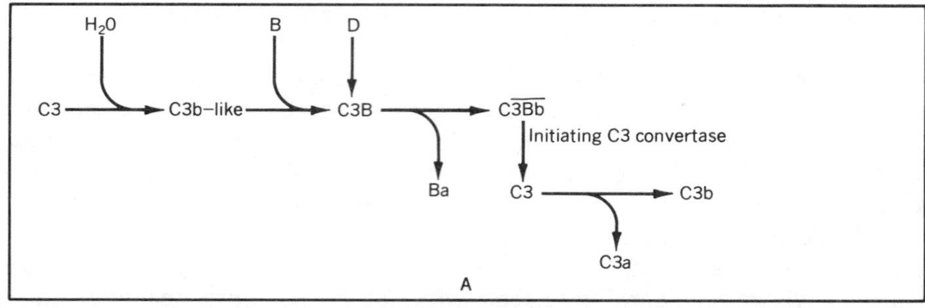

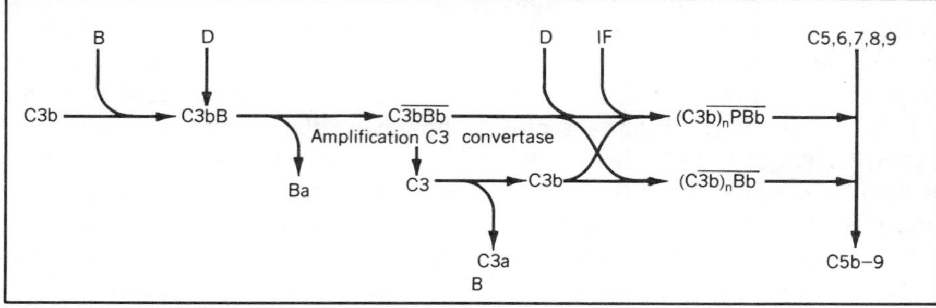

Figure 9.18. Activation compartment of the alternative complement pathway. (*a*) In the absence of activating substances. (*b*) In the presence of activating substances. Explanation in text.

of activated C3bC2a components) does in the classical pathway. However, the C3b fragment in the plasma is acted upon immediately by a powerful inhibitor, C3bINA (see Section 9.5), which cleaves C3b into inactive fragments, removing the activated C3 from the complement cascade. Hence, in normal plasma, C3 activation and inactivation constantly occur at a low rate through the interplay between the spontaneously formed initiating C3b convertase and C3bINA, and the concentration of the unstable C3b never rises above a certain low level.

But the situation changes in the presence of alternative pathway-activating substances such as zymosan. These substances apparently bind C3b generated by the initiating C3 convertase, and this binding protects C3b against immediate degradation by C3bINA. (Whether the binding of C3b to activators is direct or mediated by other factors, particularly the initiation factor, is still a matter of controversy.) The C3b molecule attached to an activator particle binds an intact B molecule with the help of Mg^{2+} ions, generating a labile C3bB complex with weak C3 cleaving activity. The C3b in this complex induces a conformational change in the B molecule and makes the latter susceptible to the action of the D factor. This enzyme is unique among the plasma proteins in that it does not need to be activated and is present all the time in an active form (although some immunologists might dispute this statement). The action of D (or $\overline{D}$) consists of cleaving the B molecule in the C3bB complex into two fragments—a larger $\overline{Bb}$ (molecular weight of 63,000 daltons; also referred to as β_2-glycoprotein II, or β_2II, and *g*lycine-rich γ-*g*lobulin, or GGG) and a smaller Ba (molecular weight of 30,000 daltons). The cleavage exposes an active site in the Bb fragment that remains associated with C3b in a complex now referred to as *amplification C3 convertase*.

The substrate of the highly active $\overline{C3bBb}$ convertase is the intact C3 molecule. However, this convertase is extremely labile and decays rapidly by the release of Bb from the complex unless it is stabilized by other factors. It is here that properdin comes into play. In a manner not yet fully understood, properdin is incorporated into the $\overline{C3bBb}$ convertase, forming a trimolecular complex, $\overline{C3bPBb}$. (The controversy centers on the question of whether properdin needs to be activated to enter into the complex, and if it does, whether the activation is of an enzymatic nature.) The $\overline{C3bPBb}$ complex, in which properdin is bound to C3b, has a half-life of 30 minutes at 30°C, which is 10 times longer than that of the bimolecular $\overline{C3bBb}$ complex. Further stabilization of the C3 convertase is thought to be achieved by the interaction with the initiation (or nephritic) factor, although the manner in which this interaction occurs is not clear.

Thus, because of the interaction with an activator, the equilibrium in the spontaneous formation of C3b swings in favor of C3b via stabilization of the C3 convertase. Once stable $\overline{C3bPBb}$ enzyme is formed, it cleaves more C3b, more stable $\overline{C3bPBb}$ is formed, which produces still more C3b, and so on (hence the name, *amplification* C3 convertase). So, in contrast to the classical pathway, which is based on specific recognition between two molecules (antibodies and C1q), activation in the alternative pathway can be achieved by much more diverse substances—all those to which C3b is attracted and by which it can be at least temporarily stabilized. This interpretation also explains the activation of the alternative pathway by the cobra venom factor. Cobra venom floods the system with excess C3, which escapes the normal control mechanisms (cobra C3b is resistant to the action of human C3bINA) and quickly amplifies the cascade.

The next step in the activation process is the deposit of additional C3b molecules at the site at which the $\overline{\text{C3bPBb}}$ complex is located and the formation of a $\overline{(\text{C3b})_n\text{PBb}}$ complex, where n is a multiple of C3b. The addition of the second C3b molecule to the $\overline{\text{C3bPBb}}$ complex induces further conformational modification of the $\overline{\text{Bb}}$ molecule in this complex, exposing the enzymatic site for the cleavage of the C5 molecule and turning the complex into *C5 convertase*. Hence both enzymatic sites, the one with specificity for C3 and the other with specificity for C5, are located on the same Bb fragment. C5 convertase can form only when the initial C3b molecule attaches to a particulate substance (activator); it cannot form in the fluid phase. This arrangement represents a further control mechanism in the alternative pathway process.

At the stage of C5 activation, the alternative pathway converges with the classical complement cascade and the two pathways then use a common lytic sequence, described in the next section.

9.4 THE EFFECTOR COMPARTMENT

The terminal components of the complement cascade assemble into a *membrane attack complex* (MAC) capable of disrupting cell-surface structures. The molecular interactions of these components are of a different character than those in the activation compartment: none of the final components has any enzymatic activity, and there is just one enzymatic cleavage in the entire attack system—that of the first component in the effector sequence; all the other components assemble spontaneously.

9.4.1 Components

The membrane attack complex consists of five components—C5, C6, C7, C8, and C9—which assemble into a complex in this order.

The C5 Component. The C5 component resembles, in many ways, the C3 component of the activation compartment. It has a molecular weight of 205,000 daltons and consists of two disulfide-bridged chains—α (120,000 daltons) and β (85,000 daltons). Its concentration in serum, however, is considerably lower than that of C3 (about 75 μg/ml, compared to 1,300 μg/ml of C3).

The C6 and C7 Components. These are very similar to each other. Each consists of a single polypeptide chain, weighing 128,000 daltons (C6) and 121,000 daltons (C7) and containing some 20 to 30 percent ordered structure (α helix or β-pleated sheets). The amino acid composition of the two components is almost indistinguishable, but the extent of this homology at the primary structure level has not yet been determined.

The C8 Component. The C8 component has a molecular weight of 155,000 daltons and is a rather peculiar molecule, consisting of three polypeptide chains—α (77,000 daltons), β (63,000 daltons), and γ (14,000 daltons). The α and γ chains are covalently linked through disulfide bridges, whereas the third chain is noncovalently associated with the other two. The α chain, which is highly hydrophobic in character, is probably located in the interior of the molecule.

The C9 Component. The C9 component has a molecular weight of 75,000 daltons and consists of a single polypeptide chain. It has the mobility of an α globulin and is present in plasma at a higher concentration than those of the other components of the membrane attack system (approximately 200 μg/ml).

9.4.2 The Assembly

The assembly of the membrane attack complex (Fig. 9.19) starts with the activation of C5 by C5 convertase. This enzyme [which, in the classical pathway, is a trimolecular complex of C4bC2a and C3b, and, in the alternative pathway, consists of $(\text{C3b})_n$, P, and Bb] liberates a small polypeptide from the N terminal of the C5 α chain, splitting the molecule into the smaller C5a and larger C5b fragments (molecular weights, 11,000 and 195,000 daltons, respectively; see Fig. 9.13). The C5a fragment drifts off into the fluid phase and out of the complement sequence to become involved in other cellular activities (see section 9.6). The C5b fragment is unstable and short-lived. It can bind immediately to the membrane at the site where the C5 convertase is attached, combine with C6 in the fluid phase to form the C5bC6 complex, or become irreversibly inacti-

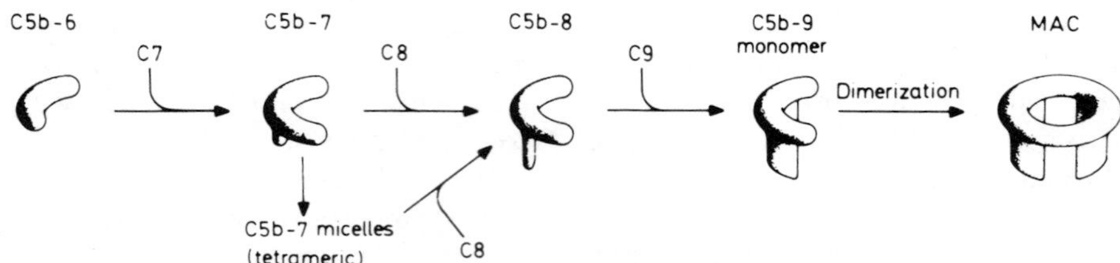

Figure 9.19. The effector compartment of the complement cascade: the formation of the membrane attack complex. (From E. R. Podack, A. F. Biesecker, and J. H. Müller-Eberhard: *J. Exp. Med.* **151**:301–313, 1980.)

vated and converted, in the fluid phase, into C5i. The membrane-bound C5b combines with C6 and then with other proteins of the membrane attack complex. There are, then, three topologically distinct sites on the target cell at which the components of the classical pathway interact with the membrane (Fig. 9.20): site I, where C1 binds to the antibody; site II, where C4bC2a (site IIA) and C3b (site IIB) attach to the membrane and form C3 and C5 convertases; and site III, where C5b settles down. It is at this last site that membrane lesions eventually occur. The fluid-phase C5b can also bind C6 and then C7, and the C5bC6C7 complex is deposited at the same cell or one different from that carrying the C5 convertase. If it deposits the complex at a different cell, cells are lysed without the deposit of early complement components—a phenomenon known as *reactive lysis*. The main route of the attack process, however, depends on the deposit of C5b at membrane site III in the vicinity of site II, where C5 convertase is attached. The site III-bound C5bC6 complex combines spontaneously with C7 and then with C8. In the latter step, the complex induces a conformational change in C8 that leads to the unmasking of a hydrophobic polypeptide from the interior of the molecule (possibly the α chain). The polypeptide interacts with the lipid bilayer of the membrane and begins to wedge the complex into the membrane. The membrane-penetration process is greatly speeded up by the addition of C9 to the complex. When isolated from lysed cells, the membrane attack complex has a molecular weight of 1,700,000 daltons, so it must contain more than one molecule of each of the five terminal complement components. According to some immunologists, it may, in fact, contain 14 molecules, arranged according to the formula $(C5b,C6,C7,C8,C9_3)_2$. The entire process of MAC formation can be summarized as follows (see also Fig. 9.19):

$$C5 \xrightarrow{\text{C5 convertase}} C5a + C5b^*$$

$$C5b^* + C6 \longrightarrow C5b - 6$$

$$C5b - 6 + C7 \longrightarrow C5b - 7^*$$

$$4C5b - 7^* \longrightarrow (C5b - 7)_4$$

$$(C5b - 7)_4 + 4C8 \longrightarrow 4\ C5b - 8$$

$$2C5b - 8 + 6C9 \longrightarrow 2C5b - 9$$

$$2C5b - 9 \longrightarrow (C5b - 9)_2$$

where the asterisks denote unstable intermediate forms.

The process of cell lysis by the membrane attack complex is not yet fully elucidated. According to the *doughnut hypothesis*, proposed by Manfred M. Mayer in 1972, the complex forms a hollow cylinder that pos-

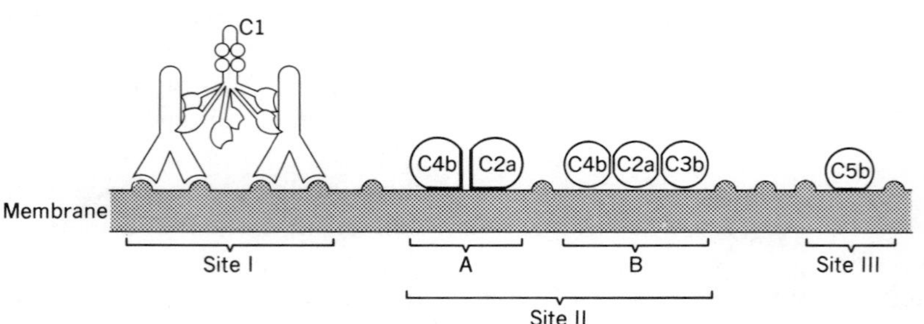

Figure 9.20. The three membrane sites to which the complement components of the classical pathway attach.

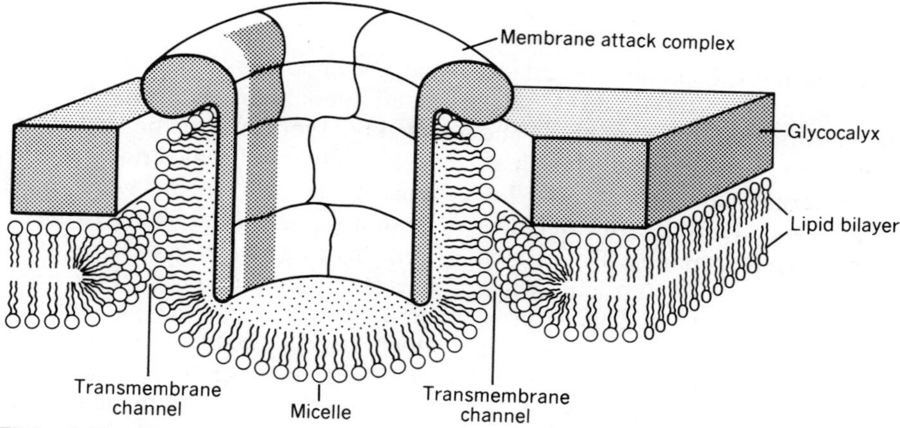

Figure 9.21. The presumed structure of the membrane attack complex of the complement system.

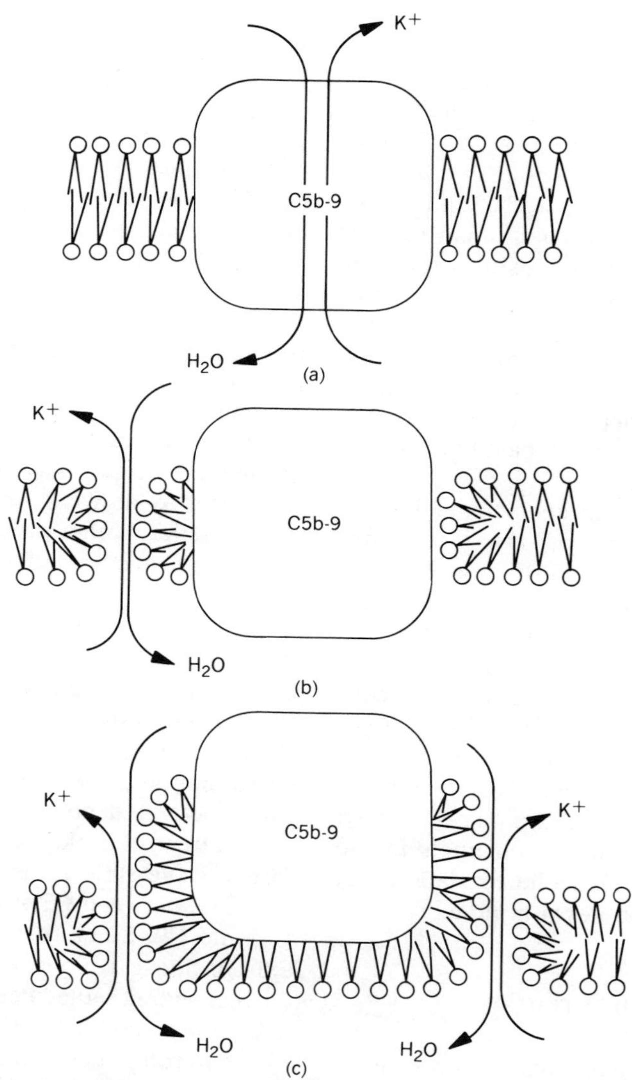

Figure 9.22. Three models of membrane damage by the membrane attack complex. (*a*) Protein-channel model. (*b*) Lipid-channel model. (*c*) Mixed micelle model. (From E. R. Podack, G. Biesecker, and H. J. Müller-Eberhard: *Proc. Natl. Acad. Sci. U.S.A.* **76**:897–901, 1979.)

sesses lipid binding regions at one end and so is able to penetrate into the lipid bilayer (Fig. 9.21). The cylinder projects above the outer surface of the membrane and widens at the noninserted end into an annulus (a thick rim). The internal and external diameters of the cylinder are 100 Å and 200 Å, respectively; its total height is 150 Å, of which 30 Å make up the annulus. The portion embedded in the bilayer is only about 40 Å long, while the rest of the cylinder is external to it. This external part, however, is embedded in the glycocalyx—the cell's outer coating of carbohydrate-rich molecules; only the annulus projects above the cell surface. (On electronmicrographs of lysed cells, only the electrondense rims can be seen, so that the membrane attack complexes look like craters or doughnuts; hence the designation.)

The inserted cylinders open up transmembrane channels (pores) that connect the cell interior with the external environment. Since the concentration of proteins inside a normal cell is higher than that in the extracellular fluid, water will begin to pour through the channels into the cell. Similarly, since the concentration of potassium is higher on the inside than on the outside of the cell—while just the opposite is true for sodium—potassium will move out of and sodium into the cell. The result of this movement will be swelling of the cell, which will make the cell membrane permeable for macromolecules. Proteins, nucleic acids, and other high-molecular-weight substances will begin to leave the cell until it is reduced to an empty bag: the cell has lysed.

Exactly how the transmembrane channels are formed has not yet been decided. The three possibilities that exist are depicted in Figure 9.22. In model *a*, the membrane attack complex traverses the entire membrane and the channel is formed by the hollow space inside the cylinder. In model *b*, the membrane attack complex also traverses the membrane, but here the channels are formed either in the lipid bilayer adjacent to the complex or in the lipid *and* in the cylinder. In model *c*, the displaced lipid binds to the membrane attack complex, forming a mixed protein-lipid micelle and opening up channels in the lipid bilayer as a result of the micelle formation. All experimental data are compatible with model *c*.

9.5 THE REGULATORY COMPARTMENT

For organisms, the complement system must have been a hard nut to crack. Some of the problems they had to solve were these. First, because potentially dangerous to the organism's own cells, the complement components could be made available only in small amounts; yet, since the system had to act quickly, there had to be a way of amplifying small effects into a full-scale attack within a short time. Second, if the components were to be present in small quantities, and if they were to act in a concerted fashion, there had to be a way of ensuring that they were present at the right place at the right time, so that they could find one another and interact physically. And third, once activated, the system had to be kept from derailing; in other words, there had to be a way of stopping the system after it had fulfilled its function. Accordingly, there are at least three aspects to complement system regulation: amplification, coordination, and inactivation.

9.5.1 Amplification

As was mentioned earlier, one of the reasons plasma activation systems have many components is probably the necessity of providing opportunities for rapid amplification. The most striking example of amplification in the complement system is the handling of C3b by the alternative pathway. Here, as was discussed in section 9.3, once the rate of C3 convertase formation becomes, via the stabilizing effect of one of the activators, greater than that of its degradation, increasing quantities of C3b are rapidly produced by this enzyme. Furthermore, since C3b is shared by both activation pathways, production of C3b following the activation of the classical pathway probably activates the alternative pathway as well. Amplification probably also occurs at several other points in both pathways, producing a chain-reaction effect.

9.5.2 Coordination

Coordination in time is achieved by the strict orderliness of the system, in which component Y cannot be activated unless component X has been activated first. Coordination in space is assured in at least two ways. First, activated components that interact with each other already display mutual affinity in their inactive forms. Reversible associations exist among C1q, C1r, and C1s, between C2 and C4, and among C5, C6, C7, C8, and C9. Since these groups of components often exist in loose complexes even in normal plasma, the corresponding molecules do not have to "search" for each other upon activation. Second, although all complement components are present in a soluble form in the plasma, fixation on solid or semisolid surfaces (e.g., cell membranes) often occurs upon activation. This transfer from a fluid to a solid phase, which occurs in very few other molecular systems, speeds up the assembly of molecules through the formation of activation foci. However, even with the help of these two "tricks," there are a great many misses. Immunologists have calculated that about 400 C4 molecules are needed to place one molecule into the right position on the cell surface, and for C2 the number is probably even higher.

9.5.3 Inactivation

An activated complement component can be inactivated by one of three mechanisms—spontaneous decay, stoichiometric inhibition, and enzymatic degradation. *Spontaneous decay* plays an important role in the control of binding ability of C4, C3, and C5 components. The binding site apparently consists of relatively hydrophobic amino acid residues that are not in a thermodynamically stable configuration. As a result, spontaneous rearrangement and loss of binding ability occurs after activation unless stabilization of the binding site has occurred through the attachment to a membrane. *Stoichiometric inhibition* (i.e., inhibition by interaction of two molecules in molar proportions without enzymatic cleavage, but with consumption of the inhibitor by the reaction) and *enzymatic degradation* are mediated by special regulatory proteins. Of these, only four have been characterized: $C\bar{1}$ inhibitor, β1H globulin, C4b-binding protein, and C3b inactivator; the first three are stoichiometric inhibitors, the third is an enzyme.

$C\bar{1}$ inhibitor ($C\bar{1}$-INH) is a α-globulin with a molecular weight of 100,000 daltons. Its molecule probably consists of a single polypeptide chain and a carbohydrate moiety that comprises about 40 percent of the molecular weight and includes significant amounts of sialic acid. $C\bar{1}$-INH combines and forms stable complexes with C1r and $C\bar{1}$r, inhibiting these enzymes and consequently preventing $C\bar{1}$s from cleaving C4 and C2 in the classical complement pathway.

Factor I (*C3b inactivator*, *C3b-INA*, sometimes also referred to as conglutinogen-activating factor, or KAF, because it reacts with fixed C3 and makes it reactive with conglutinin) is a β-globulin with a molecular weight of 100,000 daltons and with molecules composed of two chains (55,000 and 41,000 daltons). It acts enzymatically on C3b, thereby degrading this molecule; the degradation proceeds in two steps (Fig. 9.23). In the relatively rapid first step, C3bINA cleaves a single peptide bond in the α chain of the C3b molecule and produces an intermediary C3bi (C3b′) molecule. The only difference between C3b and C3bi is apparently the one break in the α chain of C3bi; but this break fully inactivates the molecule. When the broken α chain is separated from the β chain, it splits into two fragments of 40,000 and 60,000 daltons; the two fragments do not separate because both are connected to the β chain by disulfide bridges. In the slower second step, the C3bINA, aided by so far unidentified plasma proteases (the effect of which can be simulated by trypsin), scisses the α chain at another position and breaks the C3bi molecule into two fragments—C3d (molecular weight of 30,000 daltons, representing a clipped-off N-terminal portion of the α chain) and C3c (molecular weight of 157,000 daltons, representing the rest of the molecule); it should be noted, however, that the terms "C3c" and "C3d" were originally used for C3 fragments found in aged sera, and that the identity of these fragments with those produced by controlled enzymatic degradation has not been established. The degradation of C3b by C3bINA proceeds in the same way, regardless of whether C3b is in the fluid phase or bound to a membrane. In the latter case, however, after completion of the reaction, the C3d fragment remains membrane-bound, whereas C3 is released into the medium. Apparently, the membrane-binding site of C3b is located in the C3d portion of the α chain. There are conflicting data about the requirement for proteins other than C3bINA in the first step of the reaction. According to some authors, the reaction proceeds only when β1H globulin is also present (see below). According to other immunologists, plasma contains a high-molecular-weight protein that binds C4 (*C4b-binding protein*; see below) and also serves as a cofactor in the enzymatic degradation of C3b. Molecules of C4b and C5b are also cleaved into c and d fragments by an enzyme that is probably identical to C3bINA.

C4b-binding protein (C4b-BP) has been isolated

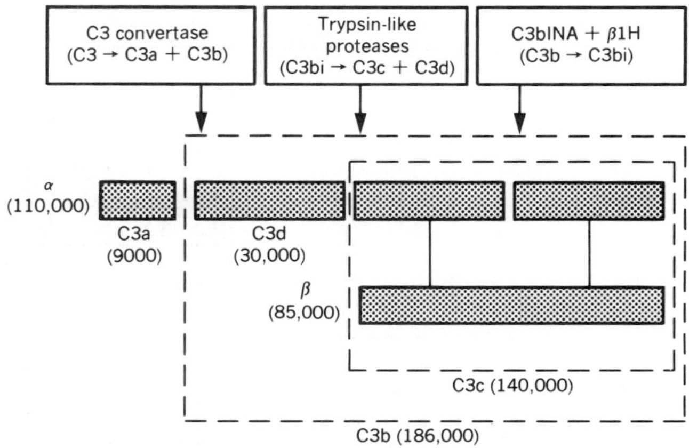

Figure 9.23. Fragmentation of the C3 molecule by C3 convertase, C3bINA, and trypsin-like proteases.

from human and mouse sera. Human C4b-BP has a molecular weight of from 540,000 to 590,000 daltons and consists of several disulfide-bridged subunits, each with a molecular weight of about 70,000 daltons. It participates as a cofactor in the cleavage of the C4b α chain by the C3b (C4b) inactivator. Furthermore, C4b-BP also interferes with the assembly of the membrane-bound, classical pathway C3 convertase and accelerates the decay of C42.

Factor H (*β1H globulin*, *C3b inactivator accelerator*) has a molecular weight of 150,000 daltons and consists of a single polypeptide chain. It binds to C3b and thereby increases the susceptibility of this molecule to proteolysis by C3bINA. In addition, it probably dissociates Bb from the $\overline{\text{C3bBb}}$ complexes and thereby abolishes the activity of the amplification C3 convertase. Like $C\bar{1}$ inhibitor, β1H globulin displays no enzymatic activity itself and exerts its inhibitory effect by complexing with the target molecule.

9.6 SECONDARY PRODUCTS OF COMPLEMENT ACTIVATION

Cleavage of some complement components produces two fragments—a larger (primary) one that participates directly in the reactions of the complement cascade, and a smaller (secondary) one that leaves the cascade and plays a role in other defense reactions. The first indication of the existence of secondary complement products was obtained as early as the first decade of this century. In 1909, in an attempt to determine whether anaphylaxis (see Chapters 2 and 13) was mediated by cellular or humoral factors, E. Friedberger added antigen-antibody precipitate to a fresh guinea pig serum and, after a short incubation, reinjected the treated serum into the donor animals. When some of the animals went into a state of shock resembling anaphylaxis as it had been described earlier by Portier and Richet (see Chapter 2), Friedberger postulated that the treatment produced a toxic substance, which he termed *anaphylatoxin*. Although the suspicion that anaphylatoxin had something to do with complement arose shortly after the discovery of this substance, it was not until 1959 that the first direct experimental evidence for the derivation of anaphylatoxin from complement was presented. And its true nature was revealed only in the late 1960s, when several immunologists demonstrated anaphylatoxins to be identical with the small fragments released from C3 and C5 after the attack by C3 convertase and C5 convertase, respectively. Only recently have immunologists dem-

	1				5					10					15						20
Porcine C3a	S	V	Q	L	M	E	K	R	M	N	K	L	G	Q	Y	S	K	E	L	—	R
Human C3a	S	V	Q	L	T	E	K	R	M	N	K	V	G	K	Y	P	K	E	L	—	R
Human C5a			T	L	Q	K	K	I	E	E	I	A	A	K	Y	K	H	S	V	V	K

					25					30					35					40
Porcine C3a	R	C	C	E	H	G	M	R	N	N	P	M	K	F	S	C	Q	R	R	A
Human C3a	K	C	C	E	D	G	M	R	Q	N	P	M	R	F	S	C	Q	R	R	T
Human C5a	K	C	C	Y	D	G	A	C	V	N	N	D	E		T	C	E	Q	R	A

					45					50					55					60	
Porcine C3a	Q	F	I	H	Q	G	N	A	C	V	K	A	F	L	N	C	C	E	Y	I	A
Human C3a	R	F	I	S	L	G	E	A	C	K	K	V	F	L	D	C	C	N	Y	I	T
Human C5a	A	R	I	S	L	G	P	R	C	I	K	A	F	T	E	C	C	V	V	A	S

				65					70							75		
Porcine C3a	K	L	R	Q	Q	H	S	R	N	K	P			L	G	L	A	R
Human C3a	E	L	R	R	Q	H	A	R	A	S	H			L	G	L	A	R
Human C5a	Q	L	R				A	N	I	S	H	K	D	M	Q	L	G	R

Figure 9.24. Amino acid sequence of human C3a, porcine C3a, and human C5a. Gaps (indicated by boxes) were introduced to maximize sequence homology. (Based on T. E. Hugli and H. J. Müller-Eberhard: *Adv. Immunol.* **26**:1–53, 1978.)

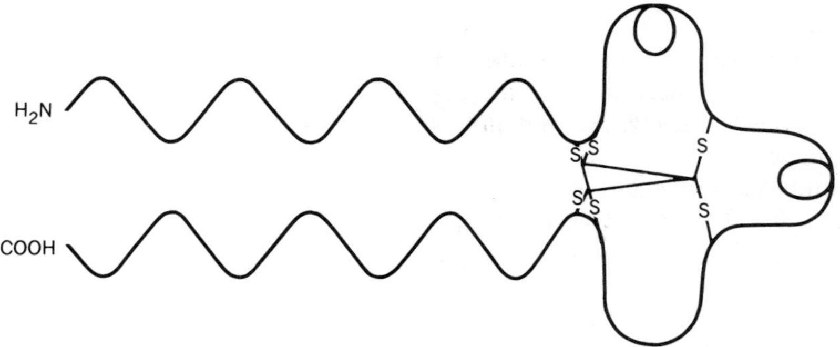

Figure 9.25. Presumed structure of the human C3a molecule. (Modified from T. E. Hugli: *Contemp. Top. Mol. Immunol.* **7**:181–214, 1978.)

onstrated that the small fragment of C4, released by the action of the $\overline{C1}$s enzyme, also possesses anaphylatoxic activity. There are thus three known anaphylatoxins: C3a, C5a, and C4a. Because of the late discovery of the third anaphylatoxin, most of the work has been done on C3a and C5a, and far less is known about C4a.

Complete amino acid sequence has been determined for human C3a, porcine C3a, and human C5a (Fig. 9.24). All three molecules have a molecular weight of about 9000 daltons, the C3a fragments consisting of 77 amino acids and the C5a fragments of 74 amino acids. When properly aligned, human and porcine C3a show about 70 percent homology, and C3a and C5a show about 40 percent. (In the latter case, to maximize the homology, some deletions had to be introduced.) Each molecule contains six half-cystines, located at positions 22, 23, 36, 49, 56, and 57 in the C3a molecule and at positions 21, 22, 34, 47, 54, and 55 in the C5a molecule. The half-cystines form three disulfide bridges, apparently all located in one knot in the same region of the molecules (Fig. 9.25). About 40 percent of the molecule is arranged into an α helix. The functionally active site of C3a and C5a resides at the C terminal, particularly in the terminal arginine residue: removal of this residue abrogates anaphylatoxic activity. A synthetic octapeptide with a sequence identical to residues 70 to 77 of human C3a exhibits all the biological activities of intact C3a, but with much lower efficiency (about 1 to 2 percent of the natural C3a). C5a differs from C3a in that it has a high content of carbohydrate (about 25 percent; in contrast, C3a contains none).

The C4a fragment has a molecular weight of 8600 daltons and shows a limited structural homology with C3a and C5a. As in the other two anaphylatoxins, in C4a, the C-terminal amino acid is arginine and the removal of this residue abolishes the fragment's biological activity. The C4a molecule possesses activities similar to those of C3a and C5a but is considerably less efficient.

C3a, C5a, and C4a induce histamine release from mast cells and release of hydrolytic enzymes from neutrophils, cause smooth muscle contraction, and increase blood vessel permeability. In addition, C5a effects directed migration (chemotaxis) of granulocytes and monocytes. These functions will be dealt with in detail in Chapters 11 and 13.

A secondary product is also released by the activation of the C2 component. The C2b fragment, however, is not an anaphylatoxin; rather, it displays kinin-like activity.

9.7 COMPLEMENT RECEPTORS

The system of complement components and regulatory proteins is supplemented by a system of complement receptors—a group of cell-membrane structures capable of reacting specifically and reversibly with certain complement molecules or their fragments. Complement receptors are distinct from the nonspecific attachment sites to which complement components may bind via their unstable binding regions, exposed for a fraction of a second immediately after activation. The attachment sites are not specialized structures, since the activated component can attach through the binding region almost anywhere on the membrane.

9.7.1 Discovery

Early in this century, several immunologists noticed that parasites or microorganisms adhered to host cells (e.g., leukocytes or platelets) in the presence of specific antibody. Further analysis of the phenomenon revealed that four ingredients were necessary for the adherence to occur: antigen-bearing cells or particles (parasites, bacteria, viruses, and particulate or soluble antigens), antibodies to these antigens, complement, and indicator cells (i.e., cells adhering to the antigen-bearing cells or particles). Later, immunologists learned the mechanism of this *immune adherence* phenomenon: the interaction of antibodies with antigens activates the complement cascade and produces activated complement components, which are then deposited on the cell surface of antigen-bearing cells; some of these components bind to complement receptors on the surface of the indicator cells and thus form a bridge connecting the two cells so that they adhere to each other (Fig. 9.26*b*).

9.7.2 Methods of Study

One can observe immune adherence of cells directly, through the microscope, or one can use erythrocytes as indicator cells and detect adherence by hemagglutination. (Since each antigen-bearing cell may be covered by complement components at many sites and each erythrocyte possesses many complement receptors, immune adherence leads to clumping of cells.) However, the most common way of detecting immune adherence is by the rosetting technique, in which conditions are set such that multiple indicator cells (erythrocytes) encircle a single antigen-bearing cell. To avoid reaction with receptors for the Fc region of the IgG molecule, IgM antibodies are used. Mouse serum is particularly suitable for the immune adherence test because it is poorly lytic.

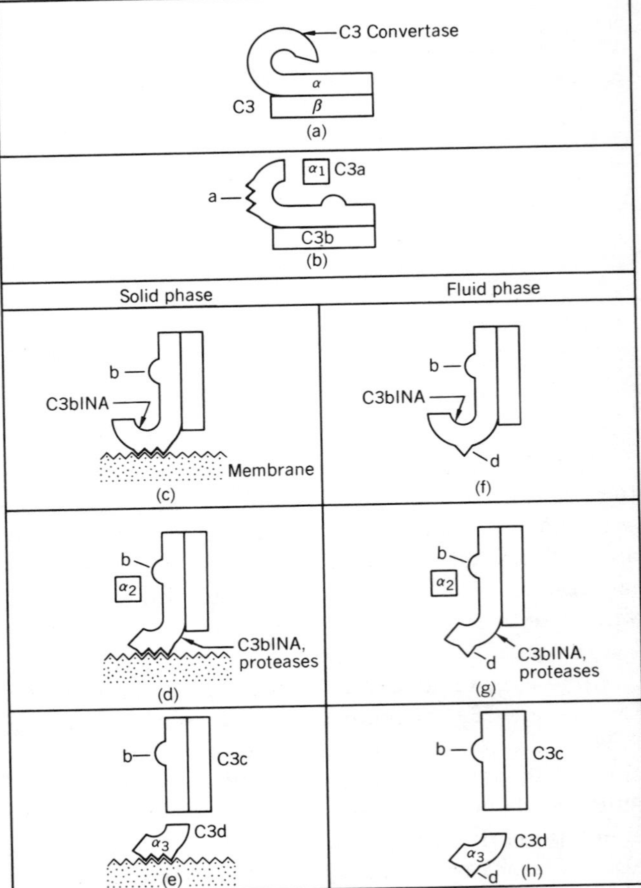

Figure 9.26. Fragmentation of the C3 molecule and appearance of membrane-binding sites in solid and fluid phase. a, short-lived, unstable binding site through which the nascent C3b molecule can attach to any cell surface; b, stable binding site through which the molecule attaches to the C3b receptor on the surface of some cells; d, stable binding site through which the fragment attaches to the C3d receptor carried by some cells. The binding abilities at the different stages of fragmentation: (*a*) Uncleaved, inactive molecule cannot attach to cell surfaces. (*b*) Nascent C3b molecule can attach to any cell surface. (*c*) and (*d*) C3b receptor-binding site exposed, but since the molecule is already cell-bound, its further binding abilities are restricted; whether the molecule expresses the binding site for the C3d receptor is not clear: the receptor may be masked by the already existing attachment to the membrane. (*e*) The C3c fragment can bind to the C3b, but not to the C3d receptor, and perhaps also to both simultaneously. (*f*) and (*g*) Corresponding changes in the fluid phase. (*h*) The C3c fragment in the fluid phase can bind to the C3b, but not the C3d receptor, and the C3d fragment can bind to the C3d, but not to the C3b receptor.

9.7.3 Survey of Receptors

The three complement receptors described so far react with the C3b, C3d, and C1q components.

The C3b receptor (complement receptor I, or CRI) binds to the larger fragment of C3 produced by the action of C3 convertase (see Figs. 9.13 and 23). The binding of C3b to the C3b receptor should not be confused with the interaction between the unstable, hydrophobic binding site and the membrane (any membrane, even a liposome) that occurs immediately after the activation of C3; a C3b molecule that has lost this unstable site binds perfectly well to the C3b receptor (Fig. 9.26). The binding of C3b to its receptor requires an intact C3b molecule; fragmentation of C3b by C3bINA abrogates the binding activity. However, C3c can partially inhibit the adherence of C3b-coated erythrocytes to complement receptor I, indicating that the binding site in C3b resides in the portion of the molecule that becomes C3c. The same receptor also binds C4b molecules.

C3b-coated cells adhere to receptors on epithelial cells of the kidney glomerulus and on monocytes, but not to those on human erythrocytes, suggesting that the *glomerulus complement receptor* (GCR) recognizes portions of the C3 molecule different from those recognized by either erythrocyte or monocyte receptors.

The *C3d receptor* (complement receptor II, or CRII) binds one of the fragments (C3d) generated by the action of C3bINA on C3b. The site interacting with the receptor is available only on soluble C3b; on membrane-bound C3b, the interaction site is not normally accessible and is revealed only after proteolytic breakdown of C3b, and possibly also following the interaction between C3b and β1H. The C3d receptors apparently also bind C4d fragments.

The *C1q receptor* binds C1q in the absence of antibodies. The distinctiveness of this receptor is evidenced by the fact that cells lacking other receptors still bind C1q.

9.7.4 Distribution

The C1q receptor is present on both T and B lymphocytes and on certain lymphoblastoid cells. The distribution of the C3b and C3d receptors is given in Table 9.3. Only a few cells have the C3d, but not the C3b receptors (e.g., chronic lymphocyte leukemia cells, lymphoid cell lines, and immature neutrophils of the mouse). In B lymphocytes, the expression of the C3b and C3d receptors occurs only at certain differentiation stages, since both immature B cells and plasma cells lack these structures.

Table 9.3 Tissue Distribution of C4b (C3b) and C3d Complement Receptors

Cell Type	Species	Receptor Type b (C4b, C3b)	Receptor Type d (C3d)
Erythrocytes	Human and primates	+	−
	Other mammals	−	−
Platelets	Human and primates	−	−
	Other mammals	+	−
B lymphocytes	Mammals	+	+
T lymphocytes	Mammals	−	−
Granulocytes	Mammals	+	−
Monocytes	Mammals	+	−
Macrophages (lung)	Human	+	−
Macrophages (resident/ peritoneal cavity)	Mouse, guinea pig	+	−
Activated macrophage (peritoneal cavity)	Mouse, guinea pig	+	−

Source. From C. Bianco: *in* N. K. Day and R. A. Good (Eds.): *Biological Amplification System in Immunology*, p. 70. Plenum, New York, 1977.

9.7.5 Physicochemical Properties

None of the receptors has been isolated in a pure form. The difficulties encountered during attempts to purify the C3 receptors may stem from their being protein-lipid complexes. The proteinaceous nature of the receptors is indicated by the observation that trypsin and papain destroy the activity of these structures. The fact that the receptors become nonfunctional after treatment with reducing agents suggests that disulfide bridges may be required for activity. The interaction between complement components and their receptors is temperature-dependent: it is minimal at 0°C and maximal at 37°C. The interaction may, therefore, be influenced by membrane fluidity.

9.7.6 Genetic Control

The genes coding for complement receptors have not been identified. In the mouse, the percentage of complement-receptor–bearing splenocytes at two weeks of age is influenced by the *H*-2 complex. This influence, however, may be indirect, since *H*-2 is known to control the absolute number of cells in the spleen. For example, at 15 days of age, the spleens of DBA/2 mice contain five times more cells than the spleens of AKR mice. And while the proportion of complement-receptor–bearing lymphocytes in AKR spleens is much higher than in DBA/2 spleens, in absolute numbers, DBA/2 spleens contain more complement-receptor–bearing lymphocytes than do AKR spleens.

9.7.7 Biological Function

Adherence of antibodies and complement-coated bacteria to host cells, particularly macrophages and monocytes, facilitates phagocytosis. Adherence of complement-coated particles or cells to platelets promotes the release of substances affecting the tone and diameter of blood vessels. And interaction between complement and complement receptors on lymphocytes may stimulate the release of chemotactic factors and facilitate antibody response to antigen, either by promoting bridging between antigen-bearing macrophages and lymphocytes or by enhancing antigen binding to B-cell surfaces.

9.8 BIOSYNTHESIS

To learn where complement components are synthesized, an immunologist can explant different tissues and cells, grow them in tissue culture, and look for the protein in the culture medium, using an appropriate antiserum or a functional assay for complement activity. Alternatively, he can transplant different tissues into animals genetically deficient for a given component and determine which tissue restores the full complement activity of the recipient. To describe the molecular mechanisms involved in complement biosynthesis, an immunologist isolates messenger RNA carrying the information for the particular component and translates it in a cell-free system capable of sustaining protein synthesis.

The information so far obtained about complement biosynthesis is still rather sketchy. The only components we know something about are C1, C2, C3, C4, C5, C6, C9, and $C\bar{1}INH$; the remaining components either have not been studied at all or the data obtained were inconclusive. The C1, C2, C3, C4, and C5 components are known to be synthesized by macrophages—from the peritoneum, blood (monocytes), or liver; C5, C6, C9, and C1INH are synthesized in the liver, probably by macrophages too. The C1q subcomponent is perhaps also synthesized by epithelial cells of the small and large intestines.

The C3, C4, and C5 components are synthesized as single polypeptide chains that are post-translationally cleaved into the corresponding number of chains (Fig. 9.27). The human 197,000-dalton, pro-C3 molecule is cleaved into the α and β chains; the 200,000-dalton, pro-C4 molecule is cleaved into α, β, and γ chains; and the 175,000-dalton, pro-C5 molecule is cleaved into α and β. (The increase in molecular weight of the processed C5 is probably caused by the addition of carbohydrate to the polypeptide chains.) The three subcomponents of C1 are known to be synthesized separately, from different mRNA molecules. In some instances (e.g., C3), the precursor form is probably also present, in a small amount, in plasma.

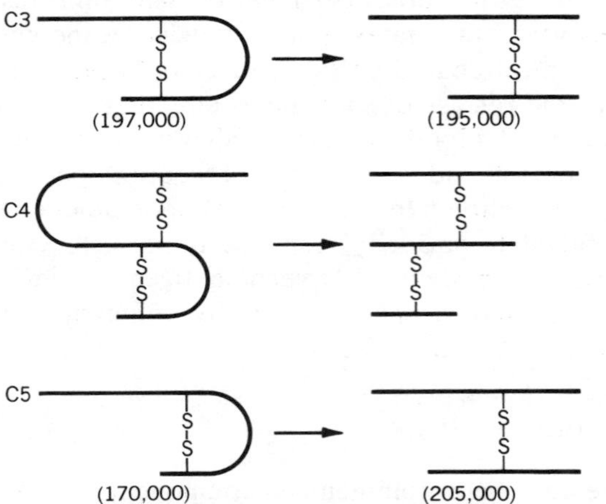

Figure 9.27. Precursor forms of C3, C4, and C5 components.

The human fetus begins to synthesize complement components in the first three months of gestation. Placental transfer of complement does not occur in either direction (from mother to fetus, or the other way around). At birth, the plasma concentration of complement components is approximately half the level of the maternal levels. The concentrations reach adult levels at six months of age. Although colostrum contains significant amounts of C3, C4, and factor B, there is no evidence that any of these components reach the plasma of breast-fed infants.

9.9 GENETIC CONTROL

9.9.1 Complement Loci

There is at least one locus for each of the complement components, but for some components, there may be more (e.g., the C4 locus may be duplicated in some human chromosomes; see below). The individual chains in a multichain molecule such as C3, C4, or C5 are apparently encoded by the same locus, transcribed into a single messenger RNA, and translated into a single polypeptide chain; the scission into chains comprising the final product occurs only after translation. Whether this observation also applies to the three chains of the C1q molecule is not known, but the three C1 subcomponents (C1q, C1r, and C1s) are probably controlled by separate loci. Consequently, the genome of a given species must contain at least 18 loci coding for complement components and regulatory proteins.

9.9.2 Linkage Groups

In the human, the complement-encoding loci are distributed in at least four linkage groups: the MHC group, the C6-C7 group, the C3 group, and the C5 group. The most interesting of these is the MHC linkage group. The human MHC group consists of loci coding for the B, C2, and C4 components. *HLA* linkage of loci coding for C6 and C8 has also been reported, but later studies have proved that C6 is definitely not controlled by chromosome 6; the location of C8 is still uncertain. The B-, C2-, and C4-encoding loci are relatively close to the *HLA* complex (see Fig. 8.4), but their exact positions are still being investigated. It is interesting to note that the three components encoded by the MHC linkage group are all involved in the activation of C3, and that the C3 locus, although not linked to the human *HLA*, is linked to the mouse *H-2* complex. In the mouse, linkage to *H-2* has been demonstrated for C3- and C4-encoding loci. The C4 locus is identical to the *S* locus, which codes for the Ss protein (see below) and is located between the E_α and *D* loci within the *H-2* complex. The C3-encoding locus is some 10 map units away from *H-2* on the *D*-end side (see Fig. 8.5). The C4-encoding locus is also linked to the MHC in the guinea pig, and the B-encoding locus is linked to the MHC of the rhesus monkey. Furthermore, an unidentified complement locus is linked to the MHC of the domestic fowl. Thus the C-encoding loci constitute a habitual companion to the MHC and are often considered as part of it (class III loci; see also section 9.7).

The chromosomal location of the other three complement linkage groups is not known in any species. The human C6- and C7-encoding loci are closely linked to each other, as is evidenced by the fact that no recombinants have been found between them and that the deficiency of C6 is sometimes associated with a deficiency of C7.

9.9.3 Polymorphism

Genetic variation in complement components can be detected in three ways: immunologically, by using specific antibodies to complement allotypes; by electrophoresis; and as a deficiency of the particular protein.

Allotypic Variation

We shall mention three examples of allotypic variation in complement components: the human Chido and Rodgers systems, the mouse Ss-Slp-H-2.7 complex, and the mouse MuB system.

Chido-Rodgers Antigens. Human blood group serologists have a special category of antibodies they call ''unsolved,'' ''difficult,'' or ''nebulous,'' because, for one reason or another, these antibodies are difficult to analyze. One such antibody, called anti-Chido because it was found in the serum of a patient named Chido, reacted with almost all red blood cells in a panel (99 percent, to be precise), gave many weak reactions that were difficult to distinguish from negative ones, and could not be absorbed out, even by strongly reactive cells. Serotyping and genetic studies with such an antibody were obviously almost impossible to carry out. But the situation improved dramatically when serologists discovered that a substance reacting with Chido antibodies was present in the plasma of all Chido-positive individuals but not in the plasma of Chido-negative individuals. At once, a reliable method for detecting Chido-negative individuals became available, since the Chido substance could be used to inhibit agglutination of Chido-positive red blood cells by Chido antibodies. Using this improved typing method, close linkage of the Chido-encoding gene (Ch^a) with *HLA* could be demonstrated. (The absence of Ch^a is associated with antigens HLA-B12 and Bw35.)

Another ''difficult'' antibody was detected in the serum of a Mr. Rodgers and the corresponding antigen was, therefore, designated by his name. Like Chido, the Rodgers antigen could be detected not only on red blood cells, but also in the sera of the positive individuals, and this fact greatly facilitated the typing for this blood group. Again like Chido, the Rodgers antigen is also found at a high frequency (97 percent) in the population and the Rodgers-encoding gene (Rg^a) is closely linked to *HLA*. (The absence of Rg^a is associated with antigen HLA-B8.) Most individuals are $Ch(a^+)Rg(a^+)$; $Ch(a^-)Rg(a^-)$ individuals are extremely rare.

When electrophoretic variants of C4 were discovered, a remarkable correlation between C4 types and the Chido and Rodgers blood groups was found. Three main electrophoretic patterns of C4 were observed: F, consisting of four fast-moving anodal bands; S, consisting of four slow-moving cathodal bands; and FS, consisting of a combination of the F and S bands (Fig. 9.28). The correlation was as follows: all F individ-

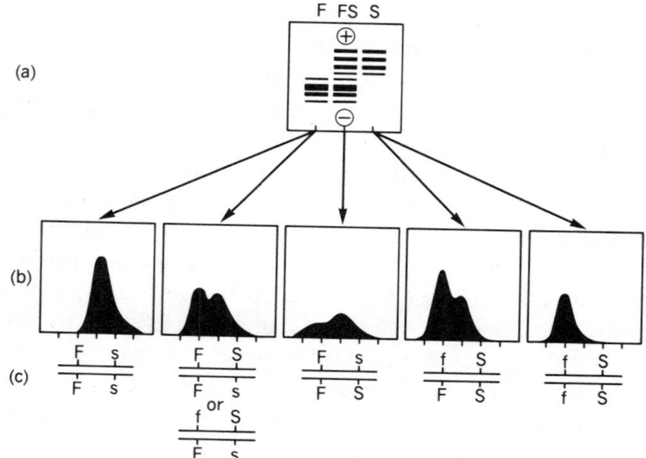

Figure 9.28. Polymorphism of the human C4 component. (*a*) Three main agarose electrophoresis patterns of C4: C4S, four cathodal bands; C4FS, eight bands; and C4F, four anodal bands. (*b*) Crossed immunoelectrophoresis patterns of the five detected phenotypes of C4. (*c*) Genetic interpretation of the patterns based on the assumption of two closely linked loci, *F* and *S*. (Based on the data of G. J. O'Neill, S. Y. Yang, J. Tegoli, R. Berger, and B. Dupont: *Nature* **273**:668–670, 1978, and Z. L. Awdeh, D. Raum, and C. A. Alper: *Nature* **282**:205–207, 1979.)

uals were $Ch(a^-)Rg(a^+)$; all S individuals were $Ch(a^+)Rg(a^-)$; all FS individuals were $Ch(a^+)Rg(a^+)$; and rare C4-deficient individuals were $Ch(a^-)Rg(a^-)$. Furthermore, purified C4FS was shown to inhibit both anti-Ch^a and anti-Rg^a; purified C4F inhibited anti-Rg^a, but not anti-Ch^a; and purified C4S inhibited anti-Ch^a, but not anti-Rg^a. The removal of C4 from serum containing Ch^a and Rg^a antigens resulted in the removal of these two blood-group substances. These findings probably mean that the substance carrying the Chido and Rodgers antigens is a fragment of the C4 molecule (recent evidence suggests that the antigens are located in the C4d portion of the molecule), and that the antigenicity of erythrocytes arises by passive adsorption of C4 fragments to these cells. The electrophoretic patterns and the correlation of the Ch^a and Rg^a antigens suggests that there are two loci coding for C4—one for the C4F pattern and the Rg^a allotype, and another for the C4S pattern and the Ch^a allotype.

The Ss-Slp-H-2.7 Antigens. Immunization of rabbits with mouse serum produces a plethora of antibodies, among which is one that reacts with all mice—but with some more strongly than others. (The strength of the reaction can be determined, for instance, from the position of the precipitin band formed when the antibodies are allowed to diffuse in agar against the serum carrying the antigen.) The *S* locus coding for this *serum serological,* or Ss, substance maps within the *H*-2 complex, between the E_α and *D* loci (see Chapter 8). Most inbred strains and wild mice carry the Ss^h allele, which determines a high level of the Ss substance, and a few carry the Ss^l allele, controlling concentrations of Ss in the serum that are 20 times lower.

Immunization of Ss^l mice with serum of Ss^h donors induces alloantibodies reacting with an antigen that can be detected easily in the male serum of some strains, but not in the female serum of most strains, nor in the male or female serum of certain other strains. This *sex-limited protein*, or Slp (the designation is probably not quite correct because even females of the Slp^+ strains do have this antigen, though only in small amounts), is encoded by an *Slp* gene that maps in the same region as the *Ss* gene (the two genes have not been separated genetically). The variation in the Slp level is influenced by male hormones—by testosterone, in particular.

The function of Ss and Slp remained unknown until Peter Démant and his co-workers demonstrated that these substances were related to complement. This was the first demonstration of the MHC's involvement in the control of complement proteins. Later studies by several laboratories identified the Ss protein as the murine C4 component.

The relationship between the Ss and Slp substances is not yet completely clear. They are probably distinct, because Slp, in contrast to Ss, does not have complement activity, and because there are small structural differences between the two, suggesting that the proteins are controlled by separate loci. If so, this situation would be similar to that in the human, where the C4 locus is also duplicated. The similarity between the human and the mouse may go even further. The mouse possesses a blood-group antigen originally considered to be a class I H-2 antigen and therefore designated H-2.7. Recent studies, however, indicate that the H-2.7 antigen differs in many respects from class I H-2 antigens, is not controlled by either the *K* or *D* locus, is present in the serum, and can be passively adsorbed to red blood cells, turning H-2.7^- cells into H-2.7^+ ones. This antigen may thus be the homologue of either the Chido or the Rodgers antigen in humans.

The MuB1 Antigen. In the search for immunoglobulin allotypes in the mouse, an antibody was produced against a serum substance designated murine B1 antigen, or MuB1. The substance later was found to be the mouse C5 component.

Electrophoretic Variations

A mutation in a complement-encoding gene results in the replacement of one amino acid by another that may have an electric charge different from the original one. The component controlled by the mutated gene may still carry out its function normally, but it may have a changed mobility in an electric field and when subjected to electrophoresis, it may end up in a region of the supporting gel (e.g., starch gel or agarose) different from that of the original protein. Hence, electrophoresis is a simple way of identifying polymorphic variants, but since it is carried out with the whole serum, which contains many other proteins in addition to complement components, it must be supplemented by a method of identifying the studied proteins. For complement components this method is referred to as *immunofixation* and consists of fixing the proteins after electrophoresis by precipitating them with a specific antiserum. Unfixed proteins are then washed out and the precipitate is stained with a protein dye. The variants are designated according to their relative migration distances toward either cathode or anode: the migration of the most common variant is taken as unity, and all other mobilities are expressed as decimals (e.g., 1.1 or 0.9) with respect to this distance.

Table 9.4 **Hereditary Complement Deficiencies in the Human**

Affected Component	Frequency[a]	Manifestations
C1q	F	Associated with hypogammaglobulinemia and severe combined immunodeficiency
C1r	I	Kidney and skin lesions, glomerulonephritis, recurrent infections, lupus-like syndrome
C1s	I	Found in one patient with systemic lupus erythematosus (SLE)
C2	F[b]	Often no sign, sometimes increased incidence of SLE and other autoimmune disorders
C3	I	Frequent infections
C4	I	Lupus-like syndrome
C5	I	Recurrent infections, lupus-like syndrome
C6	I	No disease
C7	I	No disease
C8	I	Found in a patient with *N. gonorrhoeae* infection
$C\bar{1}INH$	F	Hereditary angioneurotic edema
C3bINA	I	Frequent infections

[a] F, relatively, frequent (several cases reported; I, relatively infrequent
[b] Most frequently observed deficiency

In humans, electrophoretic variants have been detected in all complement components studied. Usually, a population contains one common, one or two less common, and several rare variants. Different variants often occur in different populations and races in different frequencies.

Complement-Component Deficiencies

Individuals that completely lack a certain complement component or that possess it at a drastically reduced level are rarely found. Such variants can result from a deletion or inactivation of the corresponding gene or from a block in the expression of this gene. In humans, deficiencies have been reported for most of the complement components (Table 9.4). Some of the deficiencies have no apparent deleterious effect on the bearer; others cause various degrees of disturbance in the individual's normal physiology (see section 9.11). Complement deficiencies have also been described in animals (Table 9.5): C5 deficiency in the mouse (in fact, almost 40 percent of inbred mouse strains are C5-deficient, probably because of a defect in C5 secretion), C4 deficiency in the guinea pig, and C6 deficiency in the rabbit and Syrian hamster.

9.10 FUNCTION

Body defense is a tricky business, for parasites use all kinds of maneuvers to overcome defense lines and invade the host. To counteract these ploys, defense systems must be manifold and equipped to meet all possibilities of attack. The complement system is a telling example of this multiplicity. Originally regarded as basically a system for direct killing of bacteria, it has since been proved to participate in many diverse defense reactions. Some of the functions in which complement components are known to participate are these.

Cytolysis. Because of its attack compartment, the complement system is capable of lysing a variety of cells marked for destruction—microorganisms of all kinds, erythrocytes, leukocytes, platelets, and others.

Neutralization. Complement components, with the help of specific antibodies, can bind and incapacitate viruses. Some viruses can also be lysed via the

Table 9.5 **Hereditary Complement Deficiencies in Animals**

Species	Affected Component	Frequency	Manifestations
Guinea pig	C4	One strain	No abnormality
Mouse	C5	Several strains	No abnormality
Rabbit	C6	Numerous cases	Blood-clotting defect
Syrian hamster	C6	Several strains	Inflammation of the intestine

classical pathway in combination with the attack mechanism.

Enhancement of Phagocytosis. Binding of complement components to cells via receptors facilitates phagocytosis of these cells.

Pharmacological Effects. Secondary products of complement activation affect smooth muscle contraction, increase in blood vessel permeability, histamine release, and leukocyte chemotaxis. All these effects constitute important features of the inflammatory reaction (see Chapter 14).

Enhancement of Antibody Response. In a way not yet fully understood, certain complement components enhance the production of antibodies to antigens. Mechanisms of complement involvement in these functions will be discussed in Chapters 11 and 12.

In addition, the complement system is also connected, through some of its components, to other plasma-activation systems.

9.11 DISTURBANCES OF COMPLEMENT FUNCTION

Although vigorously regulated, the complement system is nonetheless subject to disturbances that can result either in an elevation to above-normal levels of one or more components (*hypercomplementemia*), or, in contrast, a decrease in complement levels to below normal (*hypocomplementemia*). The former condition is frequently associated with inflammatory reactions; the latter can result from increased consumption, increased catabolism, or decreased production of complement components.

Increased consumption and *increased catabolism* of complement are the most frequent causes of hypocomplementemia accompanying certain diseases (e.g., membranoproliferative glomerulonephritis, autoimmune hemolytic anemia, leukopenia, and thrombocytopenia; see Chapter 14). The decrease in complement level is presumably caused by excessive activation of the cascade or abnormally rapid degradation of complement components.

The *decreased production* of complement components can result either from environmental effects, such as malnutrition or hepatitis (both affecting the organ of complement synthesis—the liver), or hereditary deficiencies.

Hereditary complement deficiencies usually affect one (rarely two) complement component, and are presumably caused by defects in the genes controlling complement synthesis. Some of the known deficiencies, their frequencies, and effects on the carriers are listed in Table 9.4. At least one of the deficiencies has such characteristic manifestations that it is considered a distinct disease. This condition, known to clinicians by the name *hereditary angioneurotic edema*, is caused by defective C$\bar{1}$ inhibitor. In about 85 percent of the patients, C$\bar{1}$INH is lacking almost completely; in the remaining 15 percent, C$\bar{1}$INH is present, but inactive. The absence of C$\bar{1}$INH results in uncontrolled activation of C1. The interaction of the activated C$\bar{1}$ with C4 and C2 generates vasodilators—factors increasing blood vessel permeability (Gr. *angeion*, vessel). The escaped fluid causes swelling of tissues (Gr. *oidema*, a swelling), mainly in the limbs, trunk, and neck. When swelling occurs in the upper airways, the patient is in danger of suffocating; swelling in the intestinal wall causes severe abdominal pain, diarrhea, and vomitting. After all the available C$\bar{1}$ has been consumed, the level of the vasodilators returns to normal, and the swelling subsides; but as soon as new C$\bar{1}$ is generated, the patient suffers another attack of the disease. Although the attacks are unpredictable, they often occur subsequent to excessive fatigue and mental stress (hence the *neurotic* in the name).

9.12 EVOLUTION

The two main approaches to the study of complement evolution are the functional and the biochemical. In the *functional approach*, an immunologist tests sera or other bodily fluids of a given species for their capability to perform a certain function attributed to complement (usually hemolysis). The test is done either by using all ingredients (i.e., fluids, antibodies, and cells) of the tested species, or by using cells and antibodies of one species and attempting to replace this species' complement with the addition of serum from the tested species. Both tests have their disadvantages: in the former, one cannot be sure that the observed effect (i.e., hemolysis) is caused by complement and not by some other substance mimicking its effect; in the latter, absence of the effect could simply mean that the two species are phylogenetically too far apart for the mixed ingredients to interact functionally. The value of the functional approach is thus rather limited, and any conclusions based on this approach must be taken with reservations.

In the *biochemical approach*, one draws conclusions about the phylogenetic relationships from the structure of the presumably homologous molecules. The disadvantage of this approach is its laboriousness: a great deal of work goes into sequencing a single molecule! However, even limited biochemical data are often more informative than an exhaustive series of functional tests, since one does not need to sequence the entire molecule to learn whether it is homologous to another.

The functional studies suggest that, in vertebrate phylogeny, the components of the classical complement pathway first appear at the level of fishes—more precisely, the *Elasmobranchii* (sharks). The components seem to be absent in the most primitive vertebrates—the cyclostomes exemplified by the hagfish and the lamprey—and in all invertebrates. Thus, the evolution of the classical pathway parallels, to a certain degree, that of immunoglobulins. The alternative pathway appears to be older than the classical, with its origins extending as far back as the more advanced invertebrates. Hemolymph of several invertebrate species contains substances capable of interacting with cobra venom factor and activating a lytic system analogous to the alternative complement pathway in humans.

The evolutionary advantage of the classical complement pathway is obvious: any antigen can activate this pathway by reacting with specific antibodies, while only certain structures can activate the alternative complement pathway. The classical pathway, in combination with the immunoglobulin system, thus introduces into the defense mechanisms a high degree of specificity and refinement of the recognition process. Recognition of nonself in the alternative pathway is possible because the cell membrane of pathogens contains certain structures that the host cell membrane does not have. This recognition, however, is crude, and it fails when the parasite adapts to the host and the differences between their membranes become more refined. The classical pathway, in combination with the immunoglobulin system, might be a response to this adaptation, for it provides a way of recognizing the invader even if its cell surface differs only minutely from that of the host. The reason vertebrates kept the alternative pathway even after the emergence of the classical might be the usefulness of the former in rapid antibody-independent identification of those parasites that have retained crudely different cell surfaces. In addition, the interplay of the two pathways is an important amplification mechanism that greatly increases the effects of the complement system.

The origins of the classical pathway are not clear. In part, it probably used and modified some of the proteins of the alternative pathway (e.g., the factor B), but it probably also called upon other proteins (e.g., the ancestors of C1) and modified them to function in specific steps of the cascade. However, once they had evolved, both pathways remained evolutionarily conservative, as is evidenced by the fact that components of one species can functionally replace components of another, unrelated species. A case in point is the activation of the human alternative pathway by cobra C3b (the cobra venom factor), although in this case, cobra C3b is sufficiently different structurally from its human counterpart to be insensitive to the normal control by human C3bINA.

Some indication as to where the individual complement components came from has been provided by limited biochemical studies. Based on structural homologies, the components can be divided into several groups, with proteins within each group presumably related by common origin. The relatedness of proteins in each group is often underscored by the linkage of their encoding loci. The following groups can be distinguished at present: C1q (if the A, B, and C chains are encoded by separate loci, these three loci probably have originated by duplication from a single ancestral locus); C1r and C1s; C2 and B; C3, C4, and C5; and C6 and C7. The origin and interrelationship of these groups is not clear. As was discussed earlier, part of the C1q molecule bears a striking resemblance to collagen, so that the two might have a common ancestor. (One should remember, however, that "collagen" is a generic name for a group of proteins with common, as well as different, properties). The C1r and C1s components belong to a group of enzymes referred to as *serine proteases*, because they all have serine at a certain position in the active site (see Fig. 9.14). Other members of this group are chymotrypsin, trypsin, thrombin, plasmin, and factor X of the coagulation cascade. The enzymes display striking amino acid sequence homologies, not only in the active site, but also at the N terminal (see Fig. 9.14), suggesting that they share a common ancestry. The presence of coagulation factors in this group formally ties the complement cascade to this activation system. The superficial similarities between the different activation systems were discussed at the beginning of this chapter.

The linkage of loci coding for the C2, B, C3, and C4 components with the MHC remains unexplained. Several possibilities can be considered. First, the linkage might have arisen by chance: a single chromosome carries thousands of genes and it is improbable that all are related. Second, the function of the complement components might somehow be tied to that of the MHC loci, and it might be advantageous for the organism to keep these functionally related loci together (for example, to simplify the regulation and synchronization of the expression of these loci). But so far nobody has been able to come up with a reasonable proposal as to what this functional relationship might be. Third, the loci might be related in their origin and the linkage relationships might be a relic of this circumstance. However, no biochemical evidence for genetic homology between complement and MHC loci has been provided. Thus, the relationship between complement and MHC loci remains one more unresolved immunological puzzle.

Taken together, the biochemical data suggest that the complement cascade might have been assembled from various sources, by taking proteins from other systems and adjusting their function to fit this or that complement compartment. A system as complex as the complement cascade perhaps could not have been assembled in any other way.

REFERENCES

General

Alper, C. A. and Rosen, F. S.: Genetics of the complement system. *Adv. Hum. Genet.* **7**:141–188, 1976.

Bianco, C. and Nussenzweig, V.: Complement receptors. *Contemp. Top. Mol. Immunol.* **6**:145–176, 1977.

Day, N. K. and Good, R. A.: *Biological Amplification Systems in Immunology*. Plenum, New York, 1977.

Fothergill, J. E. and Anderson, W. H. K.: A molecular approach to the complement system. *Curr. Top. Cell. Regul.* **13**:259–311, 1978.

Hugli, T. E. and Müller-Eberhard, H. J.: Anaphylatoxins: C3a and C5a. *Adv. Immunol.* **26**:1–53, 1978.

Mayer, M. M.: The complement system. *Sci. Am.* **229**:54–66, 1973.

Möller, G. (Ed.).: *Biology of Complement and Complement Receptors. Transplant. Rev.*, vol. 32, 1976.

Müller-Eberhard, H. J.: Complement. *Annu. Rev. Biochem.* **44**:697–724, 1975.

Porter, R. R. and Reid, K. B. M.: Activation of the complement system by antibody-antigen complexes: the classical pathway. *Adv. Prot. Chem.* **33**:1–71, 1979.

Original Articles

Bordet, J.: Les leucocytes et les propriétés actives du sérum chez les vaccinés. *Ann. Inst. Pasteur* **9**:462–509, 1895.

Bordet, J. and Gengou, O.: Sur l'existance de substances sensibilisatrices dans la plupart des sérums antimicrobiens. *Ann. Inst. Pasteur* **15**:289–302, 1901.

Ferrata, A.: Die Unwirksamkeit der komplexen Hämolysine in salzfreien Lösungen und ihre Ursache. *Berlin Klin. Wochenschr.* **44**:366–368, 1907.

Friedberger, E.: Kritik der Theorien über die Anaphylaxie. *Z. Immunitätsforsch. Exp. Ther.* **2**:208–224, 1909.

Gordon, J., Whitehead, H. R., and Wormall, A.: The action of ammonia on complement. The fourth component. *Biochem. J.* **20**:1028–1035, 1926.

Pillemer, L., Blu, L., Lepow, J. H., Ross, O. A., Todd, E. W., and Wardlaw, A. C.: The properdin system and immunity. I. Demonstration and isolation of a new serum protein, properdin, and its role in immune phenomena. *Science* **120**:279–285, 1954.

Ritz, H.: Über die Wirkung des Cobragiftes auf die Komplemente. *Z. Immunitätsforsch. Exp. Ther.* **13**:62–83, 1912.

Wassermann, A., Neisser, A., and Bruck, C.: Eine serodiagnostische Reaktion bei Syphilis. *Dtsch. Med. Wochenschr.* **32**:745–746, 1906.

CHAPTER 10

LYMPHOCYTE-ACTIVATING SUBSTANCES

In the preceding chapters, we described the elements of defense; in this chapter we shall discuss the substances that incite defense reactions. And since the central event in vertebrate immune reactions is lymphocyte activation—the transformation of small, quiescent cells into large blasts and their differentiation into immunologically active cells—we shall concentrate on substances that bring this event about.

Lymphocyte-activating substances can be divided into two broad categories—substances that activate lymphocytes by interacting specifically with the combining site of the T- or B-cell receptors, and substances that activate lymphocytes by some other mechanism. We shall devote most of this chapter to the former category of substances, which we shall call antigens; of the latter category we shall discuss lectins and lipopolysaccharides in detail and mention the other substances only in passing.

10.1 ANTIGENS

10.1.1 What Is an Antigen?

To ask an immunologist what an antigen is is like asking a physicist what matter is, or a biologist what life is. You may name one thing after another and the immunologist, the physicist, and the biologist will tell you—most of the time without hesitation—whether the thing is or is not an antigen, is or is not matter, or is or is not alive. But you will put them at a loss if you ask them for a definition of the broadest category dealt with in their disciplines. In Paul Ehrlich's era, *antigen* was defined as a substance that generated antibody production (Gr. *anti,* against; suffix *-gen,* producing), but we now know that there are at least three things wrong with this definition. First, it covers only one arm (the humoral) of immunity and completely ignores cell-mediated reactions. Second, it covers only one aspect of the immune process (responsiveness) and ignores the other aspect (unresponsiveness). And third, it is tautological, which means that it uses one term to explain another, and then this second term to explain the first ("Antigens are substances that produce antibodies; antibodies are substances induced by antigens").

Modern immunologists distinguish three not very precisely defined terms—antigen, immunogen, and hapten. By *antigen* they usually mean the substance recognized by T- and B-cell receptors (antibodies); as an *immunogen* they designate a substance capable of eliciting immune response; and by *hapten* they mean substances of low molecular weight (less than 4000 daltons) that can bind antibodies (and presumably T-cell receptors as well), but induce immune response only if covalently attached to a large *carrier* molecule. Some immunologists use a fourth term, *ligand*[1], as a designation for molecules (haptens and antigens) that interact with antibodies.

In this text, we shall define *antigen* as *the substance that activates lymphocytes (positively or negatively) by interacting with the combining sites of T- or B-cell receptors. Positive activation leads to responsiveness, negative activation to unresponsiveness (tolerance)*. This definition makes the use of the term *immunogen* superfluous, and we shall use it only when we want to emphasize the role of a given substance in the induction phase of lymphocyte activation. We shall use the terms *hapten*, *carrier*, and *ligand* as defined above. Substances that enhance immune response nonspecifically will be designated *adjuvants*.

10.1.2 What Makes Antigens Antigenic?

Not everything in the world activates lymphocytes by interacting with T- and B-cell receptors, but neither is there any single property the possession of which would make a substance an antigen. In fact, so diverse are the substances called antigens that there is no simple answer to the question posed as the title of this section. The most we can do in attempting to answer it is to enumerate some of the properties that seem to be required, at least in certain circumstances, to make a substance antigenic.

Chemical Nature

No inorganic substance has ever been found to activate lymphocytes by binding specifically with their T- or B-cell receptors (though lymphocytes can be activated by the attachment of certain inorganic molecules at sites other than the immune receptors; see Chapter 12), and no one has ever produced antibodies to inorganic matter. This unresponsiveness to the inorganic world can be accounted for, at least partially, by the generally low molecular weight of inorganic substances. But there must be other reasons, since even large crystals, such as kidney stones, do not induce immune response. Probably, the T- and B-cell receptors are simply not constructed in such a way as to interact with inorganic substances. This specialization

[1] The term—derived from the Latin *ligo*, to bind—is used by chemists for organic molecules or ions grouped around a center, such as an iron ion, and attached to this center by multiple coordinate bonds.

of receptors for the recognition of organic molecules undoubtedly has evolutionary justifications, for it is organic, and not inorganic matter that poses the greatest danger to the integrity of an organism.

Many organic substances do not behave as antigens simply because they are too small. However, when attached to larger molecules (carriers), they can interact with immune receptors and activate lymphocytes. These organic substances thus behave as haptens that, alone, do not activate lymphocytes, but react with activated (immune) lymphocytes or immune molecules.

Proteins. Among organic macromolecules, by far the most efficient antigens are proteins. Some immunologists believe that all proteins are antigenic, but such a statement is difficult to prove or disprove when one realizes how many proteins there are and how few have been tested. It is true, however, that all proteins that *have* been tested have eventually proved to be antigenic. (Some proteins, such as collagen, were long thought to be nonantigenic, but eventually conditions were found in which even they behaved as antigens.) The antigenicity of proteins is not restricted to naturally occurring molecules; synthetic polypeptides produced by biochemists in the laboratory can often be as effective antigenically as are peptides or polypeptides extracted from living matter. Furthermore, peptides composed of D amino acids that normally do not occur in living matter produce antibodies as well as (if not better than) L amino acids. (D and L forms of a given amino acid are identical except that one is a mirror image of the other.) However, antibodies made against polypeptides composed of D amino acids usually do not react with polypeptides composed of L amino acids, and vice versa. The variation among proteins in the degree of antigenicity depends, to a certain extent, on their amino acid composition, particularly on the ratio of aromatic and nonaromatic acids. Proteins containing a large proportion of aromatic amino acids—in particular, tyrosine—are often better antigens than proteins composed largely of nonaromatic amino acids. In addition, weak antigens, such as collagen, can be turned into strong ones by attaching tyrosine residues to them.

Polysaccharides. In comparison to proteins, everything else is less antigenic, including polysaccharides. Furthermore, it may be that only proteins are able to initiate T-cell responses in any significant way, while all other antigens activate predominantly B lymphocytes (we shall return to this point later in this chapter). Polysaccharides induce strong antibody response in some species (e.g., human, mouse) and poor or no response in others (e.g., rabbit, guinea pig). The reason for this difference is not known. It is extremely difficult to raise antibodies to some polysaccharides in any species.

Lipids. Pure lipids are unable to activate lymphocytes; however, when mixed with proteins, they often function as haptens, which bind antibodies produced with the help of the carrier molecule. An example of such a hapten is cardiolipin, the molecule detected by the Wassermann test for syphilis (see Chapter 9).

Nucleic Acids. Pure nucleic acids, like pure lipids, are probably incapable of inducing any form of specific immune response. However, antibodies to nucleic acids can be produced by immunization with nucleoproteins (complexes in which the proteins apparently function as carriers and the nucleic acids as haptens). Antibodies to nucleic acids also appear in the serum of patients with systemic lupus erythematosus, a connective tissue disease of autoimmune character (see Chapter 14). Some of the antibodies react best with denatured DNA, others with native DNA, and still others with both native and denatured molecules. Antibodies to double-stranded RNA or even to isolated nucleotide triplets (e.g., AAA, AAC, or AUC) have also been obtained.

Chemical Complexity

In general, the more complex a molecule is, the better it functions as an antigen. A molecule composed of subunits of a single kind (such as amino acids in a synthetic polypeptide) either does not function as an antigen at all or activates lymphocytes poorly. The introduction into a molecule of another kind of subunit usually improves antigenicity, but a good antigen is, as a rule, composed of several different subunits.

Molecular Size

Unless coupled to large carriers, small molecules, such as amino acids or monosaccharides, usually do not activate lymphocytes at all. To serve as antigen, a substance must have a molecular weight of at least 4000 daltons; to become a good antigen, a substance must weigh more than 10,000 daltons: the most potent antigens have molecular weights greater than 100,000 daltons. However, there are exceptions to this rule, the most striking of which is a molecule consisting of three tyrosines coupled to *p*-azobenzene arsonate (see Fig. 10.1). Although it has a molecular weight of only about 400 daltons, it does elicit antibody production.

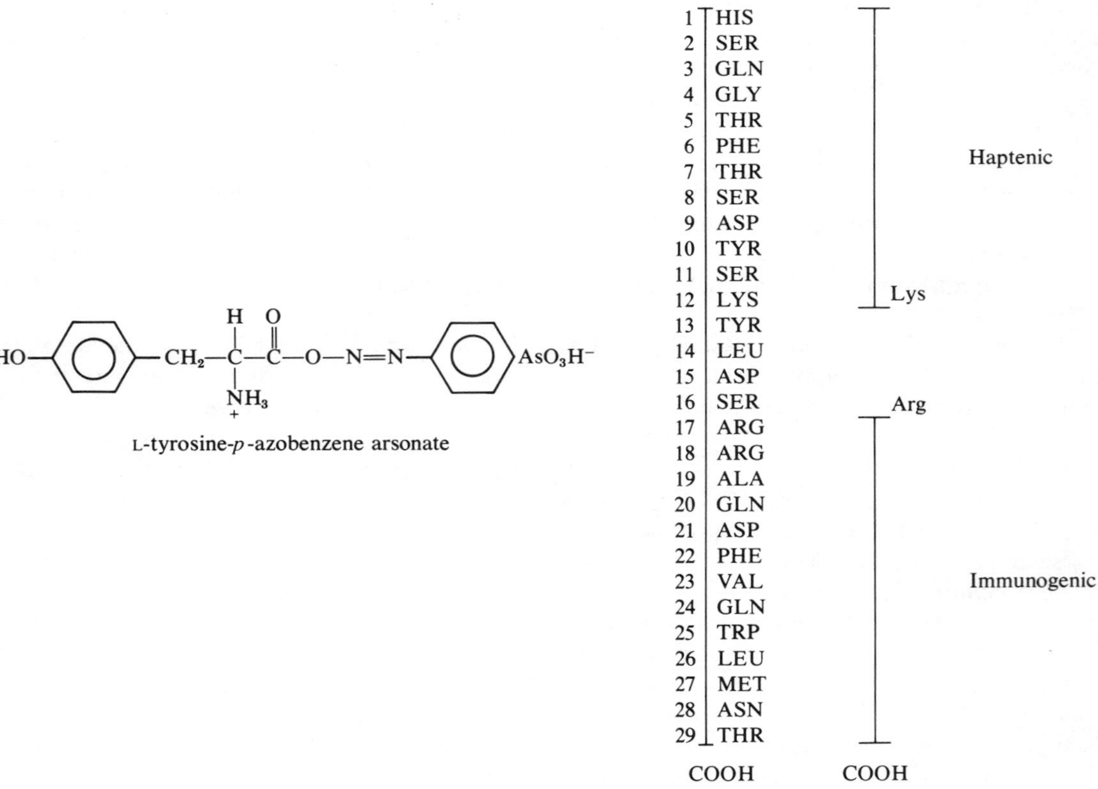

Figure 10.1. Two examples of small molecules functioning as antigens: L-tyrosine-azobenzene-*p*-arsonate (ABA-Tyr) and bovine glucagone. (Based on J. W. Goodman *in* M. Sela (ed.): *The Antigens*, vol. 3, pp. 127–187, Academic Press, New York, 1975.)

Conformation

Change of conformation by denaturation, or unfolding of the molecule, results in a change in the antigenic properties of the compound, at least as far as B-cell responses are concerned. The denatured molecule does not cease to function as an antigen, but its antigenic properties are often different from those of the original molecule (some antigenic determinants are lost and new ones appear). The way a molecule is folded and assembled thus determines what kind of antigen it is—again, at least as far as B cells go.

Charge

Molecules need not be charged to function as antigens, and over a wide range, charge does not influence the amount of antibody elicited. However, an excessively high charge depresses the antibody response. Nonspecific electrostatic interactions between the antigenic molecule and the cell surface may contribute to the selection of lymphocytes by antigens. These interactions may, at least in part, occur outside the combining site of the lymphocyte receptor, and may be one of the reasons for the observed inverse relationship between the net charge of the antigen and that of the antibody without any apparent change in antibody specificity.

Foreignness

Normally, an organism responds immunologically only to nonself substances, and the recognition of nonself is generally easier the more distinct nonself is from self. When a substance from one organism is introduced into another organism, the recipient's response often depends on the foreignness of the introduced matter and thus on the phylogenetic relationship between the two organisms. If the recipient possesses a substance similar to that introduced, the latter will act as a poor antigen; but if the introduced substance is unlike anything the host possesses, the response to this antigen will be vigorous. To give an example: collagens are poor antigens because they vary little from species to species; on the other hand, class I molecules controlled by the major histocompatibility complex are generally good antigens, because even individuals of the same species differ in these molecules.

Antigens can be divided into two broad categories, according to the genetic distance between the donor and the recipient—*alloantigens*, differentiating members of the same species, and *xenoantigens*, differentiating individuals of two different species. There is also a third category—the so-called *autoantigens*—the response to which is observed only in abnormal situations. The recognition of self is not an inherent, but a learned property; to recognize a substance as self, lymphocytes must, in some critical phase of their own development, somehow be made aware of the substance's existence. There are, however, substances in every organism that are normally hidden from lymphocytes, either in the cell's interior or in organs, such as the brain or testes, to which lymphocytes do not have access. Since, during maturation, lymphocytes do not encounter these substances, when mature, they identify them as foreign if they are accidentally exposed to them (e.g., testis extract can act as an autoantigen when injected into the animal from which it originated).

Mode of Administration

Immunologists are able to predict the outcome of an experimental immunization with about the same accuracy with which meterologists predict weather. The same substance may provoke a vigorous response when introduced in one way and no response when administered in another. The main variables are the route of antigen administration, antigen dose, immunization schedule, and time of testing the response. Normally, antigens are administered *parenterally*—that is, by some means other than through the digestive tract (Gr. *para*, alongside; *enteron*, intestine); *peroral* administration (L. *per*, through; *os*, mouth) is used only rarely, because the digestive enzymes of the stomach normally destroy potential antigens before they can be absorbed into the blood. (For this reason, food, which contains many antigens, normally does not immunize an animal.) Parenteral administration can be carried out by injecting a substance into the skin (*intradermally*; Gr. *derma*, skin), beneath the skin (*subcutaneously*; L. *cutis*, skin), into the muscle (*intramuscularly*), in the vein (*intravenously*), or into the peritoneal cavity (*intraperitoneally*). When administered by one of the first three of these routes, the antigen usually ends up in the regional lymph node; when administered intravenously or intraperitoneally, it accumulates predominantly in the spleen. The difference in the site at which the antigen is processed probably influences the type of ensuing response.

Each antigen has a certain optimal dose at which it produces the highest response: too low a dose fails to activate lymphocytes altogether; too high a dose may induce unresponsiveness. Some antigens induce immune response after a single injection, but most must be administered repeatedly, over prolonged periods, before a response can be recorded. The number and distribution in time of the individual injections must be determined empirically for each antigen. The time of assaying should coincide with the peak of the response, which also must be determined by trial and error.

Genetic Constitution of the Immunized Animal

The course of the immune response—from antigen entrance into the body to the appearance of immune lymphocytes or secretion of immune molecules—is a long one. Since several steps in this course are controlled by the recipient's genes, the recipient's genetic constitution influences not only the type of response, but sometimes whether the animal will respond at all. The best-characterized of these *immune response genes* are those constituting the major histocompatibility complex (see Chapter 8), but there are also others that are not part of the MHC. The cause of unresponsiveness may lie in the hereditary absence of lymphocyte receptors recognizing a particular antigen, or in the failure of an antigen to be recognized in the context of a given MHC molecule.

10.1.3 Antigens Activating T and B Cells

The fact that there are two kinds of lymphocyte, T and B, also reflects on antigens. Although both T and B lymphocytes are activated via antigen-specific receptors, there are two main differences in the way this activation transpires. First, with some exceptions (see below), activation of B cells is dependent on T cells, but T-cell activation is independent of B cells. And second, T cells recognize antigens and MHC molecules simultaneously (although they can recognize MHC molecules alone, at least the allogeneic ones, they cannot, again with some exceptions, recognize antigens alone); there is no evidence that MHC molecules are required for antigen recognition by B cells.

These asymmetries in antigen recognition by T and B cells explain a puzzling phenomenon long known to immunologists—the *hapten-carrier relationship*. As was mentioned earlier, certain small molecules (haptens) induce antibody formation only when attached to larger carriers. Haptens alone, without carriers, bind antibodies, but do not induce them. Modern immunology explains this observation as follows. When haptens, attached to their carriers, are presented to the immune system, they bind to the B-cell receptors and the carriers bind to the T-cell receptors, so that a functional connection is established between the two kinds of lymphocyte. This connection need not necessarily be an actual physical bridge, although such a link between the two cells would certainly be the simplest one could imagine (see Chapter 13 for details). At any rate, the establishment of the functional connection generates conditions that lead to the activation of B cells and secretion of antibodies with the same specificity as the receptors carried by these cells (i.e., antibodies against the hapten). When the hapten is presented to the immune system alone, without the carrier, it binds to the B cell; but there is nothing that would also stimulate the T cells necessary for B-cell activation, so no antibodies are produced. Carrier alone, on the other hand, can activate T cells (and, in at least some instances, B cells) because no connection to B cells is necessary for this activation. Where exactly the MHC enters this picture is not clear. The simplest possibility is that T cells recognize the carrier portion of the antigen bound to the B cell via the hapten in the context of the B cell's abundant class II MHC molecules. In situations in which the T cells are stimulated in the absence of B cells, the contextual MHC molecules may be provided by macrophages; but this explanation may be too simplistic, and cooperation may occur in some other, more sophisticated way (see Chapter 13 for discussion).

Whatever the correct interpretation of T–B cooperation, it is clear that there is no magical difference between haptens and carriers. What counts is the number of antigenic determinants: molecules that carry only one determinant (monovalent antigens) cannot activate B lymphocytes, because a second determinant—to activate the B cell-stimulating T cells—is needed. At least some monovalent molecules, however, can activate T cells that do not depend on B cells for activation. An example of such a monovalent antigen is L-tyrosine-*p*-azobenzene arsonate (ABA-Tyr; Fig 10.1), which, despite its small size (molecular weight of only 409 daltons), induces cellular (T-cell), but not humoral (B-cell) immunity. Molecules carrying two determinants (bivalent antigens) can activate both T and B cells, because one of these two determinants (hapten) can interact with the B and the other (carrier) with the T cell.

Haptens, as has already been discussed in Chapter 7, do not often activate T cells, but this is hardly surprising since few small molecules bring about lymphocyte activation. Large size, as we recall, is one of the conditions of antigenicity, and for the B cells, this condition is fulfilled by the conjugation of the hapten to the carrier. However, many haptens, even when they are part of a larger molecule, fail to activate T cells; again, this is not unexpected. In addition to size, many other conditions, some of which we mentioned in the preceding section, must be fulfilled for a molecule to be immunogenic. Since the activation of a B cell probably has a mechanism different from that of the activation of a T cell (after all, T cells are needed for B-cell activation, but not vice-versa), there are probably different requirements for T-cell and B-cell antigenicity. Hence, a portion of a molecule that fulfills one set of requirements may not fulfill the other set, and consequently, one molecular region may act as a T-cell and another as a B-cell determinant.

A good example of this differentiation of determinants has been provided by Joel W. Goodman and his co-workers, who have contributed greatly to our understanding of the requirements for T- and B-cell triggering. This example is *glucagon*, a glycogenolysis-controlling hormone produced by the pancreas. The hormone, which consists of only 29 amino acids, carries two determinants—a B cell-binding determinant in the N-terminal region and a T cell-activating determinant in the C-terminal region (Fig. 10.1). The intact molecule, therefore, activates both B and T cells. However, the molecule can be broken up by trypsin into two fragments—the N-terminal fragment, which combines with antibodies produced against the intact glucagon but is no longer able to stimulate antibody production, and the C-terminal fragment, which continues to activate T cells. The N-terminal portion of the molecule does not activate T cells, apparently because it does not fulfill some of the conditions necessary for T-cell activation.

We mentioned at the beginning of this section that there are exceptions to the requirements for T–B cooperation in B-cell activation: certain molecules can trigger antibody synthesis even in animals completely lacking in T lymphocytes. Such molecules are referred to as *T-independent antigens*, in contrast to *T-dependent antigens*, which stimulate antibody synthesis only when T cells are present. T-independent antigens are usually large molecules (polymers), such as some bacterial polysaccharides or some polymerized proteins that consist of repeated units (monomers; see next section). However, since not all polymers act as T-independent antigens, there must be more than mere repetition of a unit structure that makes these antigens behave as they do. How T-independent antigens bypass the requirements for T cooperation is not known (see also Chapter 13), but we know that the bypass is not complete since few IgG antibodies are elicited by these antigens; the antibodies produced are largely or exclusively of the IgM class.

10.1.4 Some Favorite Antigens Used in Immunological Research

From the large universe of antigens, immunologists use only a few. How these "pet antigens" have been selected is not always immediately apparent, although the choice has probably been empirical, for the most part. A brief description of some of these favorite antigens follows (Fig. 10.2).

Bovine Serum Albumin (*BSA*). Albumins are heat-coagulable glycoproteins of the eggwhite ("eggwhite" is the literal meaning of "albumin" in Latin) and of the serum. In contrast to water-insoluble globulins, albumins are water-soluble (see Chapter 2). Serum albumin is a major serum protein, constituting about half of the total protein content. Its functions include regulation of plasma volume, storage of amino acids, and acceptance of fatty acids in lipid metabolism. Bovine serum albumin (BSA) has a molecular weight of about 66,000 daltons and consists of a single, long polypeptide chain that can, however, be divided into three compact regions (domains) having a high degree of homology with one another. Each region consists of about 190 amino acids and the entire chain contains 585 residues. Seventeen disulfide bridges arrange the molecule into 18 loops, each domain containing six loops. The albumin-encoding gene was one of the first genes to be cloned in a bacterial plasmid. The advantage of BSA as an antigen is, in addition to its potent immunogenicity, its easy isolation and availability in large quantities—cattle, after all, are among the largest nonexotic animals to which immunologists have access.

Ovalbumin (*OA*). OA is the major protein of the eggwhite. It functions as a source of nutrient amino acid for the developing hen embryo. Structurally, it resembles serum albumin, to which it is evolutionarily related. The main source of OA is the egg of the domestic fowl. Crystallized ovalbumin has a molecular weight of some 40,000 daltons.

Bovine γ-Globulin (*BGG*). This is the immunoglobulin fraction (predominantly IgG) of normal cattle serum.

Keyhole Limpet Hemocyanin (*KLH*). Limpets are molluscs with low conical shells; they are particularly abundant on rocks of the seashore. Keyhole limpets are so named because of a characteristically shaped opening in the shell's apex. There are several species of keyhole limpet, but the one usually used by immunologists is the giant keyhole limpet, *Megathura*

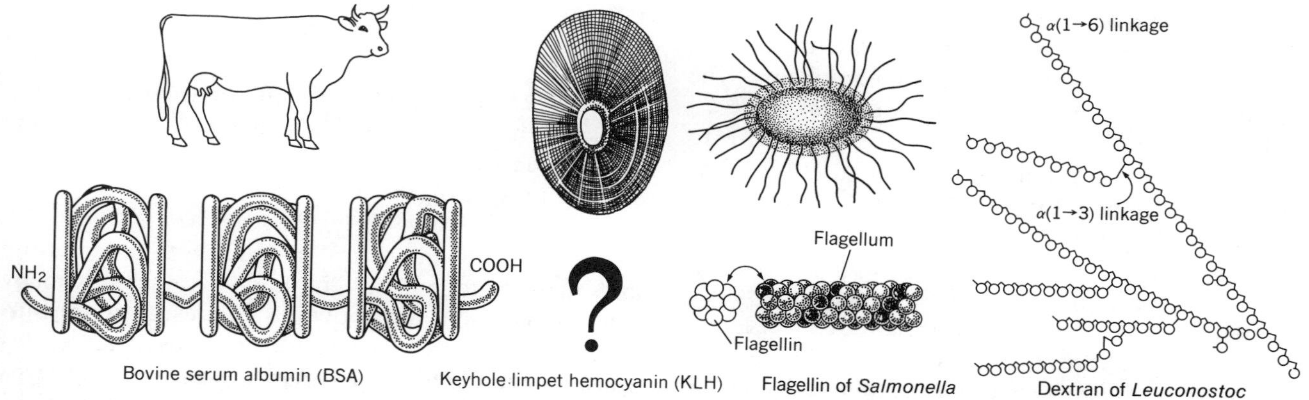

Figure 10.2. Four commonly used antigens. Bovine serum albumin, together with hen ovalbumin (which has a structure similar to BSA) and bovine gamma globulin (which has the structure of a typical IgG molecule) are typical T-dependent protein antigens. Keyhole limpet hemocyanin, the structure of which is not known, is a frequently used protein carrier. Flagellin is an example of a T-independent antigen. Dextran from yeasts and Gram-positive bacteria is an example of a polysaccharide antigen. (From various sources.)

crenulata (Fig. 10.2), found in relative abundance along the Pacific coast. By making an incision in the mollusc's soft body and then placing the animal on a screen wire overnight, one can "bleed" it and collect the hemolymph (the bloodlike fluid of animals with open circulatory systems) in a Petri dish placed beneath the wire. From the hemolymph one can isolate hemocyanin (Gr. *haima*, blood; *kyanos*, dark blue), the oxygen-carrying substance that performs the function of hemoglobin in molluscs and some arthropods. Hemocyanin contains copper as an essential element and it is this that gives the hemolymph a bluish tint. Hemocyanin, which has a molecular weight of several million daltons, is among the most immunogenic proteins known.

Flagellin. Flagellin is the main protein of the flagella, the long, thin filaments attached at one end to the body of some highly motile bacteria such as *Salmonella* (Fig. 10.2). The wall of the filament is made of flagellin molecules arranged into several helical fibrils. Treatment with heat, extreme pH, or concentrated urea solution dissociates flagella into individual flagellin molecules. The addition of salt to the flagellin solution results in repolymerization of flagellin and formation of flagellalike structures. The flagellin molecules, then, can exist in three physical states: as subunits of native flagellin, as dissociated monomers, and as reaggregated polymers. The monomers, which have a molecular weight of 40,000 daltons, are weak, T-independent antigens; polymerized flagellin (POL) is a highly immunogenic T-independent antigen.

Dextran. A storage polysaccharide of some yeasts and Gram-positive bacteria, such as *Leuconostoc mesenteroides*, dextran is a polymer consisting of glucose subunits joined into long, branched chains. The predominant bond joining the individual links is α(1–6)—that is, a bond from carbon 1 of one glucose to carbon 6 of the adjacent glucose (Fig. 10.2). The branches are joined by α(1–2), α(1–3), or α(1–4) bonds, depending on the particular dextran type. (The letter α means that the hydroxyl group attached to carbon 1 is below the plane of the ring.) Dextran of microbial origin has a molecular weight of several million daltons; the hydrolyzed dextrans used in the laboratory have a molecular weight of about 75,000 ± 25,000 daltons.

Sheep Red Blood Cells. In contrast to all previously mentioned antigens, which were either single molecular species or groups of closely related molecules, sheep erythrocytes are a heterogeneous mosaic of several molecules, most of them residing in the cell's stroma. The antigens can be divided into two groups—heat-stable (remaining antigenic even after boiling of erythrocyte stromata) and heat-labile. The predominant antigen in the former group is the one first described by the Swedish pathologist John Forssman in 1931. The original source of the antigen, however, was not sheep erythrocytes, but ground-up guinea pig organs (liver, kidney, adrenals, testicles, and brain). When injected into rabbits, the homogenate produced antibodies that reacted not only with guinea pig tissues, but also with sheep red blood cells. Because of its presence in tissues other than those used for immunization, the antigen—together with other antigens displaying similar properties—is referred to as *heterogenetic* (Gr. *heteros*, other, *genesis*, production), or *heterophilic* (Gr. *philē*, to love); sometimes it is simply called *Forssman antigen* and the corresponding antibodies *Forssman antibodies*. The antigen is widely distributed in the animal, and even in the plant kingdom. It occurs either in organs or in erythrocytes, but usually not in both. Red blood cells of guinea pigs, humans, sheep, goats, and mice are Forssman antigen-positive; those of the rabbit, rat, pig, and cattle are Forssman antigen-negative.

Blood-Group Antigens. This designation encompasses a variety of antigens in many different species; the one thing they all have in common is their presence on red blood cells. Some of the antigens, particularly those present on human red blood cells, are among the serologically best-characterized substances. A well-known representative of this group is the human ABO antigens. Because of their practical and theoretical importance, we shall describe them in detail in Appendix 10.3.

Major Histocompatibility Complex Antigens. MHC antigens have been studied extensively in many species, particularly in the human and mouse. We described these antigens in Chapter 8.

Cell-Surface Alloantigens. In addition to blood-group and major histocompatibility complex antigens, many other alloantigens are known to be present on the surfaces of a variety of cells. Most are used merely as markers for different cell populations (e.g., antigens controlled by the *Thy-1* or *Lyt* loci in the mouse), while serologically and chemically they remain poorly characterized (see Chapter 5).

Synthetic Polypeptides. These antigens are made in the laboratory by polymerization of activated amino acids. The usual method of activation is phosphogenation, which turns an amino acid into *N*-carboxy-α-amino acid anhydride:

$$H_2N\text{—}\overset{\displaystyle R}{\underset{\displaystyle H}{C}}\text{—}COOH \xrightarrow[\text{Inert solvent}]{COCl_2} \begin{array}{c} HN\text{——}\overset{\displaystyle H}{C}\text{—}R \\ | \qquad\quad | \\ C \qquad\quad C \\ O\diagup\;\; \diagdown O \diagup \;\;\diagdown O \end{array} + 2\ HCl.$$

The polymerization of anhydrides takes place as follows:

$$\begin{array}{c} HN\text{——}\overset{\displaystyle H}{C}\text{—}R \\ | \qquad\quad | \\ C \qquad\quad C \\ O\diagup\;\; \diagdown O \diagup \;\;\diagdown O \end{array} + NH_2\text{—peptide} \rightarrow$$

$$H_2N\text{—}\overset{\displaystyle R}{\underset{\displaystyle H}{C}}\text{—}\overset{\displaystyle O}{\overset{\|}{C}}\text{—}\overset{\displaystyle H}{N}\text{—}\overset{\displaystyle R}{\underset{\displaystyle H}{C}}\text{—}\overset{\displaystyle O}{\overset{\|}{C}}\text{—}\overset{\displaystyle H}{N}\text{—peptide} + CO_2.$$

Peptides composed of a single repeating amino acid are referred to as *homopolymers*; peptides composed of two or more different kinds of amino acid are called *copolymers*. In the latter, the amino acids can be put together in a sequence determined purely by chance (*random copolymers*), or they can be arranged in a specific order (*ordered copolymers*); short peptides of known sequence can be linked into *block polymers*. Random, ordered, and block polymers can be either *linear* or *branched* (Fig. 10.3). Copolymers are designated by abbreviations of the constituting amino acids and superscripts that indicate their percentage composition. For example, poly($Ala^{60}Glu^{40}$) is a copolymer containing 60 percent alanine and 40 percent glutamic acid. Homopolymers are usually poorly immunogenic; copolymers are far better antigens and their immunogenicity increases with increasing complexity. Pioneering work on the synthesis and characterization of synthetic polypeptides was carried out by Michael Sela, Paul H. Maurer, Thomas J. Gill III, and others.

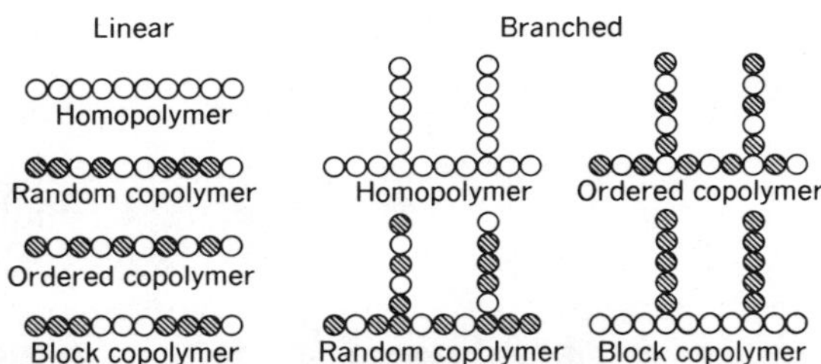

Figure 10.3. Types of synthetic polypeptide. Each circle represents one amino acid residue. Open circles, one type of amino acid; shaded circles, a different type.

10.1.5 Determinant Analysis

We shall define an *antigenic determinant* (*epitope*) as the region of a molecule that fits into the combining site of a T-cell receptor, B-cell receptor, or antibody. Isolated antigenic determinants are, therefore, relatively small molecules and as such, usually do not induce antibody formation—they act as haptens. In fact, the terms ''antigenic determinant'' and ''hapten'' overlap to a great extent.

The size of an antigenic determinant corresponds roughly to that of the combining site: in proteins, they consist of six or seven amino acids, in polysaccharides of six sugar residues, and in nucleic acids of four to six nucleotides. Although all residues composing a determinant participate in defining its specificity, usually one residue plays a crucial role in this definition. The small portion of the antigenic determinant that is of prime importance in establishing the determinant's specificity is termed *immunodominant*.

Complex molecules often carry more than one determinant.[2] The identification of these determinants, elucidation of their composition, and determination of their topographical distribution can be a long and arduous task: it may take one laboratory more than 10 years to elucidate the entire antigenic structure of a single protein.

The four main methods serving as a source of information about the determinant composition of a protein molecule are these. First, the molecule is degraded enzymatically or chemically into fragments carrying single, intact antigenic determinants; the fragments are isolated and their structure is determined. Second, conformational changes are induced in the molecule and the effect of these changes on antigenicity is determined. Third, the molecule is modified by the attachment of certain simple compounds to specific amino acids, and changes in antigenicity introduced by such modification are delineated. Fourth, once the antigenic regions of the molecule are identified, peptides that overlap to different degrees with the individual

[2] If one of the determinants induces more rigorous response than other determinants, it is sometimes referred to as *immunopotent*; under certain circumstances, some determinants may remain *immunosilent*.

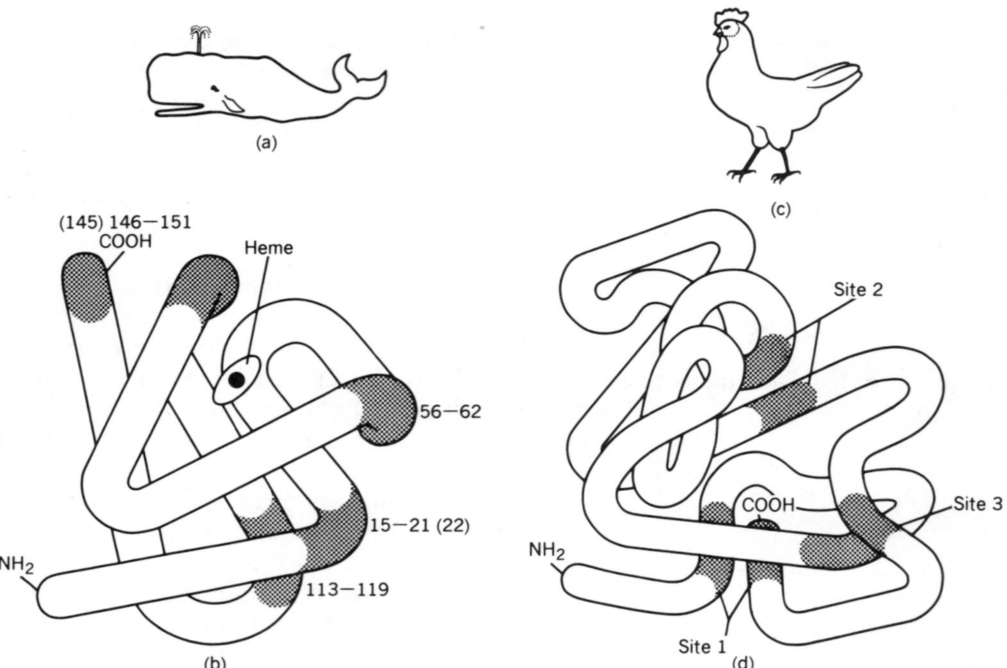

Figure 10.4. Distribution of antigenic determinants on protein molecules. (*a*) Sperm whale. (*b*) Sperm whale myoglobin. (*c*) A hen. (*d*) Hen eggwhite lysozyme. Shading indicates position of antigenic sites (reactive regions); numbers show positions of amino acid residues constituting antigenic determinants. (Based on data of M. Z. Atassi and A. L. Kazim: *Adv. Exp. Med. Biol.* **98**:9–40, 1978.)

regions are synthesized, and antibody reactivity of these peptides is determined.

So far, only a few proteins—of which we shall mention two, myoglobin and lysozyme—have been completely elucidated antigenically. What we know about these proteins is due mainly to the efforts of M. Zouhair Atassi, Emanuel Margoliash, Eli Benjamini, Morris Reichlin, and others.

Myoglobin is the oxygen-transporting protein of the muscle, resembling one-fourth of the hemoglobin molecule. (It contains only one heme, rather than the four that hemoglobin has.) A rich source of myoglobin is the skeletal muscles of the sperm whale (Fig. 10.4*a*), which the animal uses to store oxygen for diving. Myoglobin consists of a single polypeptide chain with a molecular weight of 17,600 daltons. When immunized with sperm whale myoglobin, rabbits or goats produce antisera that recognize five sharply delineated antigenic determinants. All five are located in the "corners," bends, or rod-shaped endings on the molecule's surface (Fig. 10.4*b*). The determinants are formed by short, continuous sequences, each six to seven amino acid residues long. The sequences are rich in basic amino acids, so binding of the determinants with the combining site of the antibody is thought to occur mainly through polar interactions; the nonpolar amino acids probably just stabilize the binding through hydrophobic interactions. Antigenicity is conferred by both the primary sequence and conformational structural features. Amino acid comparisons of sperm whale and rabbit myoglobins revealed that two of five determinants in the two myoglobins had identical sequences, and yet the rabbit produced antibodies to these two determinants. (The other determinants in the two molecules differed in one or two amino acid residues.) One could argue that perhaps sperm whale and rabbit myoglobins differ conformationally in the two determinants because of an effect of other molecular regions, but no conformational differences could be found. Furthermore, rabbits immunized with rabbit myoglobin made antibodies that reacted with the same five determinants defined by antibodies to sperm whale myoglobin. (Since myoglobin is an intramuscular protein, and thus normally inaccessible to the body's immune system, animals are not tolerant of it.) The important conclusion to be drawn from these studies is that antigenic determinants need not always be in regions in which homologous proteins differ.

Lysozyme is an enzyme present in tears and other bodily fluids, eggwhite, and some plant tissues (see

Chapter 11). Rabbit or goat antisera to hen eggwhite lysozyme recognize three antigen determinants (Fig. 10.4*c*,*d*). Each is made up of amino acids that are adjacent to one another on the surface of the molecule, but—in contrast to myoglobin—some are not directly peptide bonded: determinant 1 is composed of residues 5, 7, 13, 14, and 125; determinant 2 of residues 62, 87, 89, 93, 96, and 97; determinant 3 of residues 33, 34, 113, 114, and 116. These amino acids, although noncontiguous, come together into three small, circumscribed regions on the surface of the lysozyme molecules—the three determinants. The three regions are examples of *conformational determinants*, which depend on the tertiary structure of a molecule.

Detailed knowledge is also available about the composition and distribution of antigenic determinants on several polysaccharide molecules. We shall give an example of polysaccharide determinant analysis in section 10.3.

Thus far we have discussed only antigenic determinants defined by antibodies; however, there is also evidence for the existence of discrete, T cell-defined determinants, particularly on some of the molecules controlled by the major histocompatibility complex. Analysis of these determinants has been facilitated by the availability of mouse strains carrying mutations in *H*-2 genes; molecules controlled by these genes differ from the standard molecules only in determinants altered by the mutation.

10.1.6 Haptens

Discovery

In 1921, Karl Landsteiner observed that an alcoholic extract of horse kidney failed to induce antibody formation when injected into rabbits, but this same extract combined with antibodies from rabbits immunized to a kidney tissue homogenate. Subsequently, he also demonstrated that the extract induced antibody production after covalent attachment to a carrier. Landsteiner designated the small molecules that induced antibody formation only when fastened to a larger molecule as *haptens* (Gr. *hapto*, to fasten, to bind). The formulas of some of the commonly used haptens are given in Figure 10.5.

Carrier Coupling

To produce antibodies with antihaptenic activity, one must couple the hapten to a carrier—a protein such as albumin or γ-globulin, a red blood cell, a bacteriophage, a synthetic macromolecule, or an insoluble particle such as an agarose bead. Some of the chemical reactions used in this coupling are described below.

Diazotization. The prefix *diazo-* denotes a compound containing the –N=N– or –N≡N$^+$ group (Gr. *di-*, two; Fr. *azote*, nitrogen). The diazo group can be added to any aromatic or heterocyclic compound by treatment of this compound with nitrous acid at low temperatures. This treatment converts the compound into a diazonium salt,

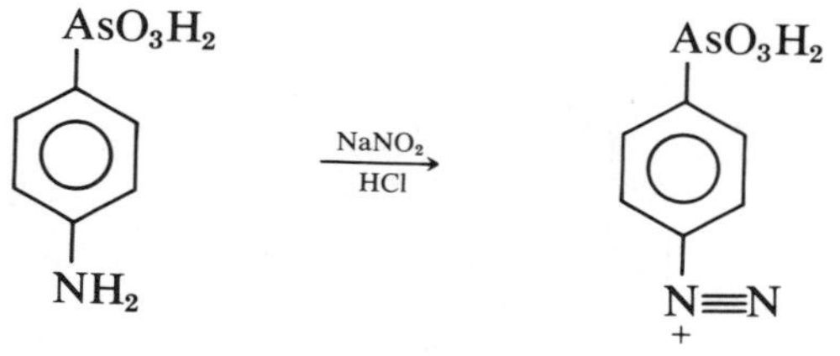

AsO_3H_2 / NH_2 $\xrightarrow[HCl]{NaNO_2}$ AsO_3H_2 / $\overset{+}{N}\equiv N$

p-Aminobenzenearsonate *p*-Benzenearsonate diazonium salt

which can then bind to amino acids, such as tyrosine or histidine. The coupling of a diazonium salt to a tyrosine occurs as follows:

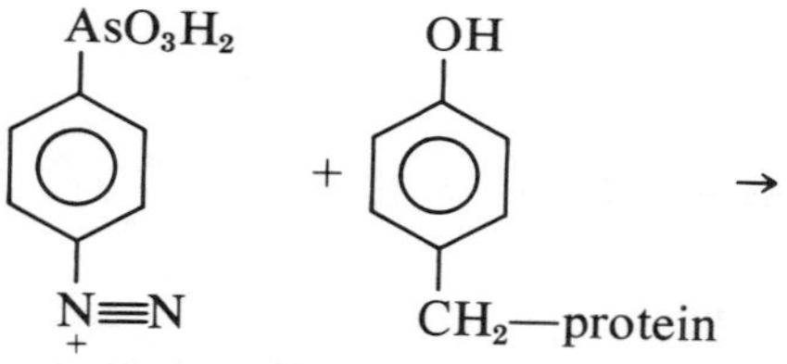

AsO_3H_2 / $\overset{+}{N}\equiv N$ + OH / CH_2—protein →

p-Benzenearsonate diazonium salt Tyrosine residue

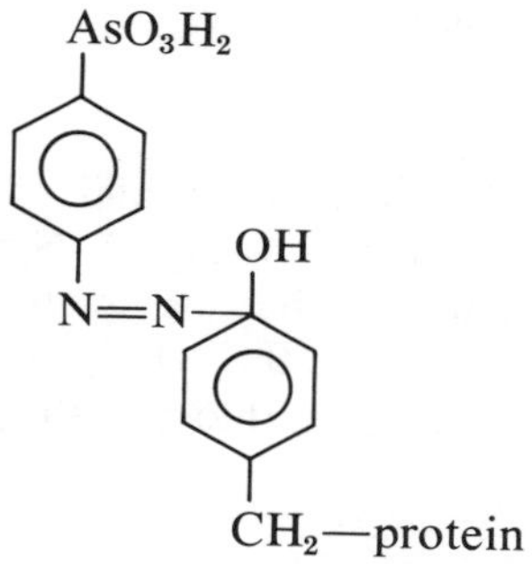

AsO_3H_2 / N=N— / OH / CH_2—protein

Conjugated protein

Conjugation of Isocyanates and Isothiocyanates. The prefix *cyano-* (Gr. *kyanos*, a dark blue mineral) indicates compounds containing the cyanide group, CN; *iso-* (Gr. *isos*, equal) refers to an isomer (i.e., isocyanate is an isomer of cyanate—the two compounds have identical compositions but differ in the arrangement of atoms within the molecule); *thio-* indicates that sulfur has replaced oxygen in the particular compound. Thus,

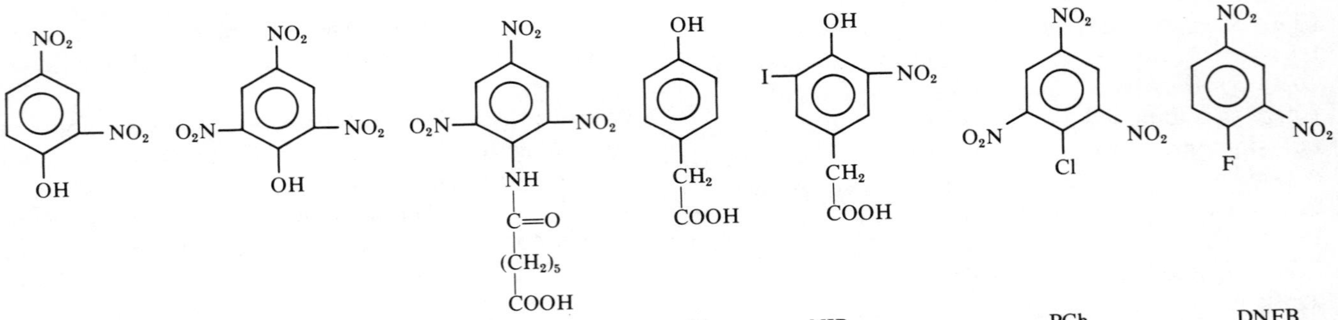

DNP TNP TNP-CAP P NIP PCh DNFB

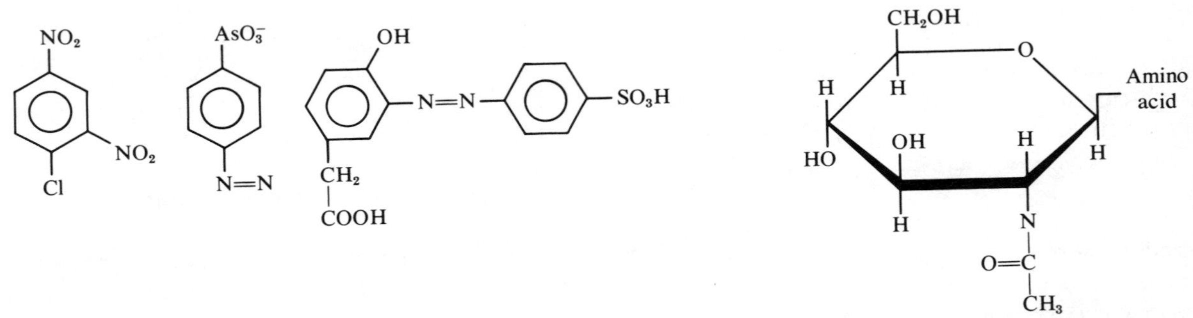

DNCB PABArs SP NAcGlu

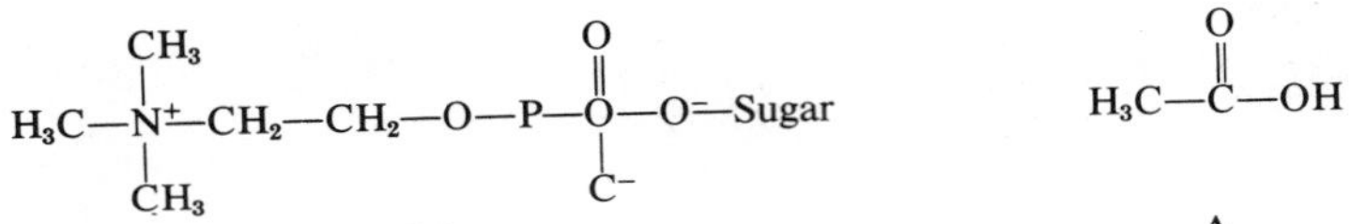

PC A

Figure 10.5. Examples of some commonly used haptens. A, acetic acid; DNCB, dinitrochlorobenzene; DNFB, dinitrofluorobenzene; DNP, dinitrophenol; NAcGlu, N-acetyl-glucosamine; NIP, 3-iodo-4-hydroxyl-5-nitrophenylacetic acid; P, *p*-hydroxyphenylacetic acid; PABArs, *p*-azobenzenearsonate; PC, phosphorylcholine; PCh, picrylchloride; SP, *p*-sulfanilic acid; TNP, trinitrophenol; TNP-CAP, trinitrobenzene-ε-aminocaproic acid.

the isocyanate and the isothiocyanate groups are R–N=C=O and R–N=C=S, respectively. A hapten carrying the isocyanate or isothiocyanate groups is attached to the NH_2 group of a protein by amide (CO–NH) or isothiocyanate (CS–NH) bonds:

R–N=C=O + NH_2—protein
Isocyanate

→ R-NH-CO-NH-protein
Conjugated protein

or

R–N=C=S + NH_2—protein
Isothiocyanate

→ R-NH-CS-NH-protein
Conjugated protein

The two haptens frequently used with isocyanate and isothiocyanate groups are toluene 2,4-diisocyanate (TDIC) and fluorescein isothiocyanate (FITC):

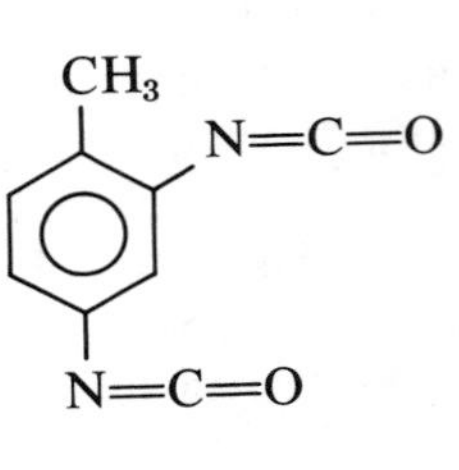

2,4-Diisocyanate 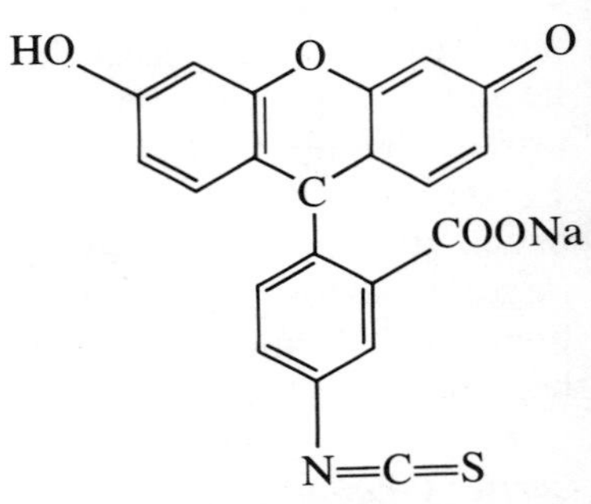 Fluorescein isothiocyanate

TDIC has two isocyanate groups and can, therefore, bind to one protein (e.g., immunoglobulin) with one group, and to another protein (e.g., ferritin) with the other.

Conjugation of Nitrophenyl Derivatives. Nitrophenyl derivatives are compounds with nitro groups (NO_2) attached to benzene. Examples are dinitrophenol (DNP), trinitrophenol (TNP), picrylchloride, and dinitrofluorobenzene (see Fig. 10.5). Nitrophenyls bind to proteins by interacting with the ϵ-NH_2 group of lysine, the α-NH_2 group of the terminal amino acids, or the SH group of cysteines. For example:

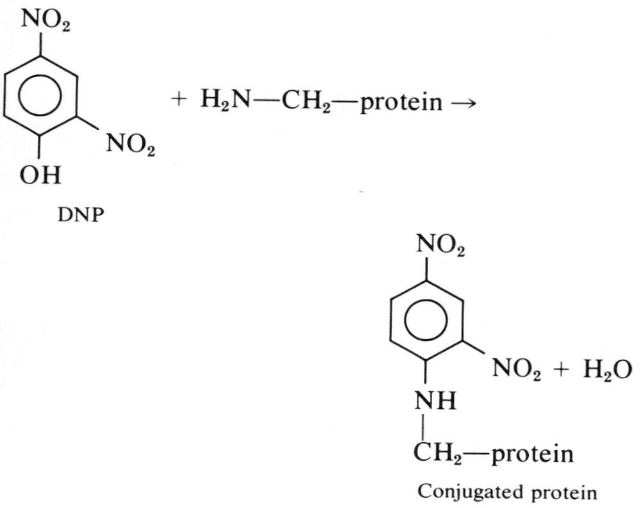

DNP $+ H_2N—CH_2—\text{protein} \rightarrow$

NO_2, NO_2, NH, CH_2—protein $+ H_2O$

Conjugated protein

Conjugation of Mixed Anhydrides. Anhydride is an oxygen-containing compound that can combine with water to form an acid, or is derived from an acid by the removal of water. If the anhydride contains a carboxyl (–COOH) group, it can be attached to proteins directly; if not, a carboxyl group must first be added to the hapten:

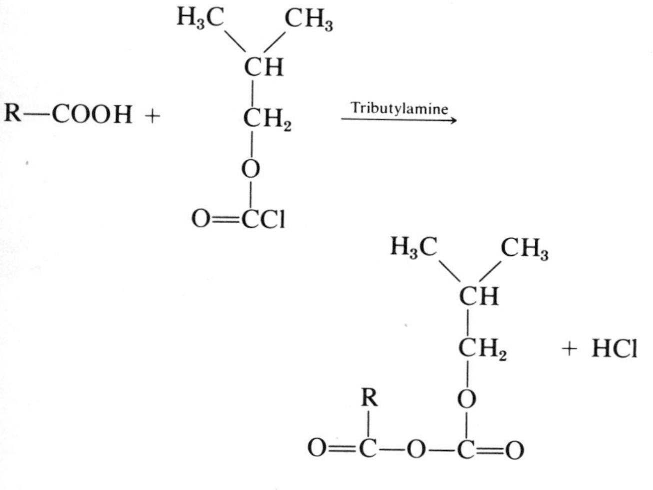

$$R—COOH + (H_3C)(CH_3)CH—CH_2—O—C(=O)Cl \xrightarrow{\text{Tributylamine}} (H_3C)(CH_3)CH—CH_2—O—C(=O)—O—C(=O)—R + HCl$$

Through the carboxyl group, the anhydride can then attach to any free amino (NH_2) group of a protein:

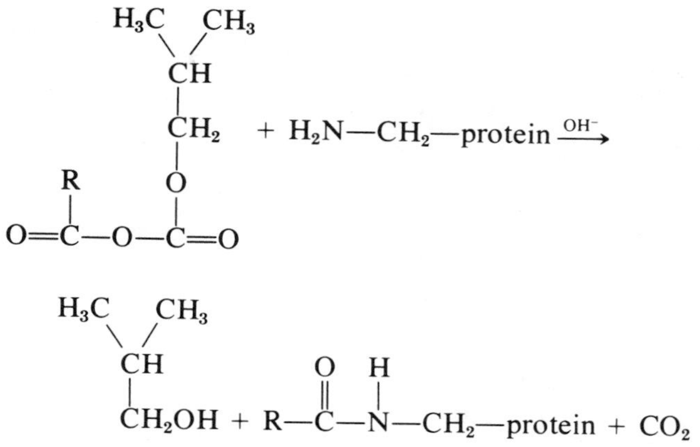

$$(H_3C)(CH_3)CH—CH_2—O—C(=O)—O—C(=O)—R + H_2N—CH_2—\text{protein} \xrightarrow{OH^-}$$

$$(H_3C)(CH_3)CH—CH_2OH + R—C(=O)—N(H)—CH_2—\text{protein} + CO_2$$

Conjugation Using Carbodiimides. Carbodiimides have a general formula, RN═C═NR′, where R and R′ are aryl and alkyl groups, respectively. (Aryl derives from an aromatic compound by the removal of a hydrogen atom; alkyl is a radical of the general formula C_nH_{2n+1}.) The carboxyl group containing hapten is first combined with the carbodiimide:

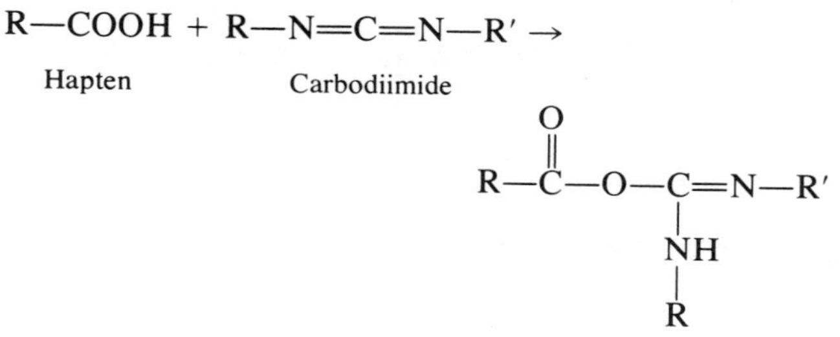

$$\underset{\text{Hapten}}{R—COOH} + \underset{\text{Carbodiimide}}{R—N═C═N—R'} \rightarrow$$

$$R—C(=O)—O—C(—NH—R)═N—R'$$

and then conjugated to a protein carrier:

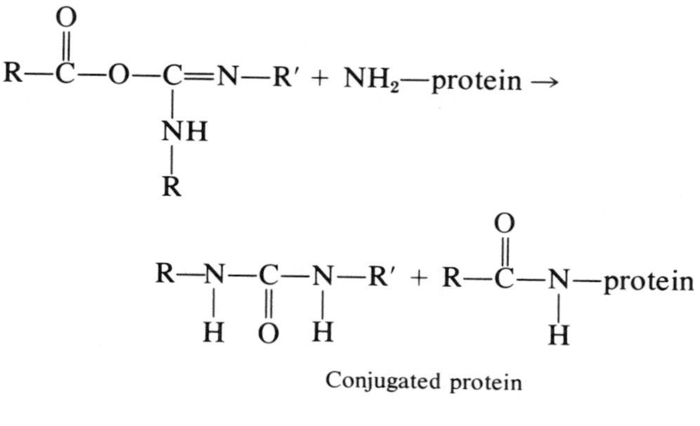

$$R—C(=O)—O—C(—NH—R)═N—R' + NH_2—\text{protein} \rightarrow$$

$$R—N(H)—C(=O)—N(H)—R' + R—C(=O)—N(H)—\text{protein}$$

Conjugated protein

Conjugation of Penicillin. Penicillin may combine directly with the NH_2 and SH groups of proteins by forming amide bonds (penicilloyl-protein conjugation):

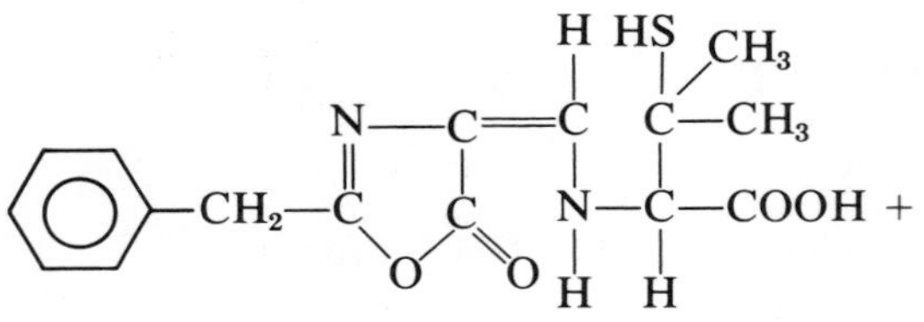

$$\text{Benzylpenicillenic acid} + \text{Lysine-containing protein} \longrightarrow \text{Benzylpenicilloyl protein}$$

Benzylpenicillenic acid

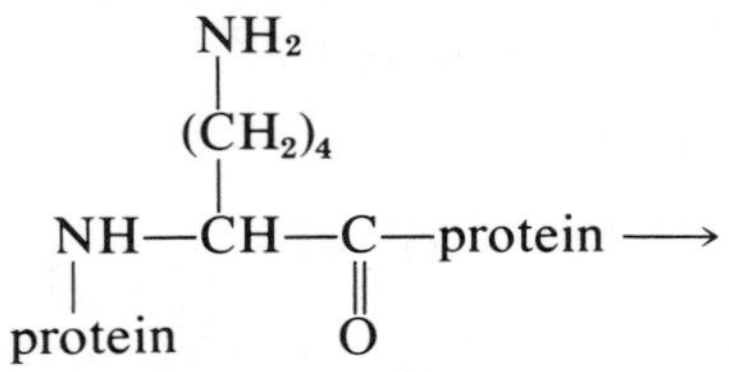

Lysine-containing protein

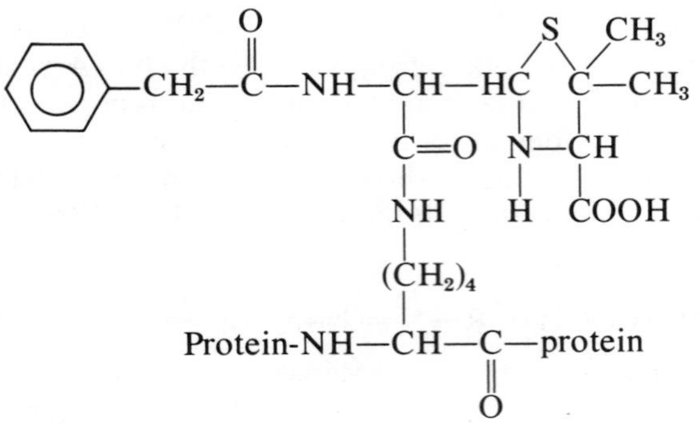

Benzylpenicilloyl protein

or disulfide bridges (penicillenic acid-protein conjugation):

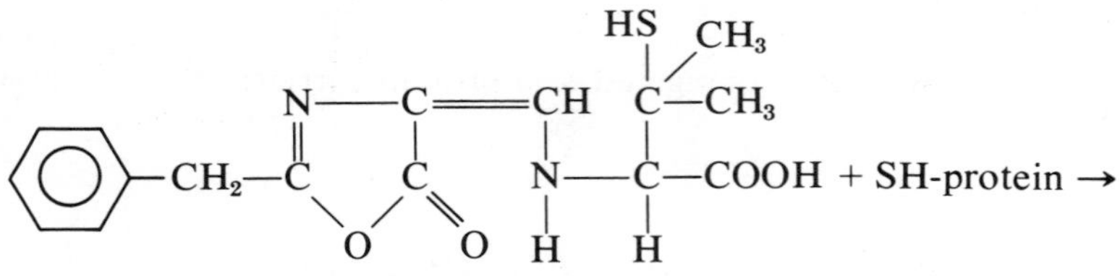

$$\text{Benzylpenicillenic acid} + \text{SH-protein} \rightarrow \text{Benzylpenicilloyl protein}$$

Benzylpenicillenic acid

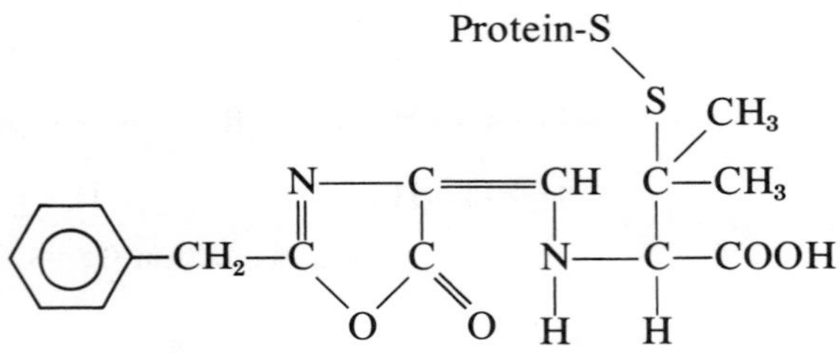

Benzylpenicilloyl protein

Coupling of Ribonucleosides and Nucleotides. The ribose ring of a nucleoside or nucleotide can be opened by oxidation with periodic acid, and the resulting dialdehyde can be coupled to a free amino group of a protein and stabilized by reduction with sodium borohydride:

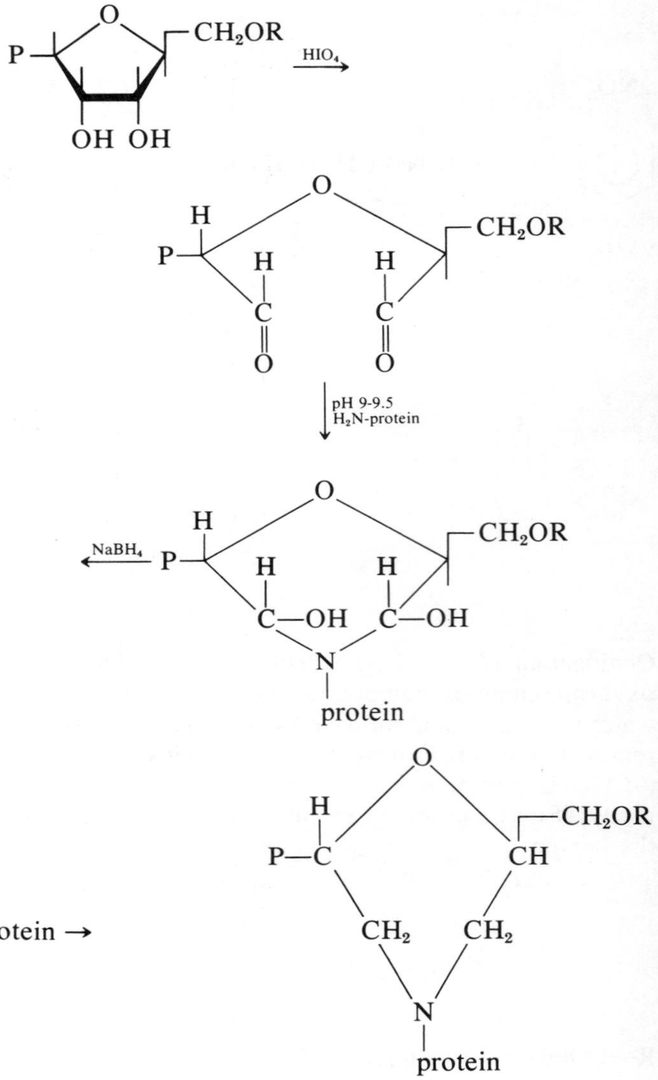

$$\xrightarrow{HIO_4} \quad \xrightarrow[H_2N\text{-protein}]{pH\ 9\text{-}9.5} \quad \xrightarrow{NaBH_4}$$

where P is purine, or pyrimidine, and R is H, or

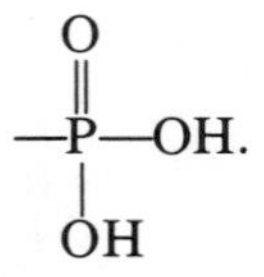

$$-\overset{\overset{\displaystyle O}{\|}}{\underset{\underset{\displaystyle OH}{|}}{P}}-OH.$$

10.1.7 Adjuvants and Immunostimulants

Discovery

That mixing additional substances with antigen intensifies immune response was observed by Louis Pasteur and G. Joubert as early as 1877. But the discovery of the adjuvant effect is usually credited to G. Ramon, who, during repeated immunizations of horses with diphtheria toxoid (protein exotoxin of the diphtheria bacillus rendered nontoxic by formalin treatment) some 50 years later, noticed that particularly good antibody titers resulted when a collection of pus developed at the injection site. To verify this observation, he isolated some pus, added it to the toxoid, and then immunized the animal with the mixture: the response was indeed far better, in comparison to immunization with the antigen alone. In 1930, L. Dienes and E. W. Schoenheit observed that the injection of antigen into the tuberculous foci of animals infected with *Mycobacterium tuberculosis* gave a better response than injection of the same antigen into noninfected animals. This observation inspired Jules Freund and Katharine McDermot in 1942 to the development of the popular Freund's adjuvant. To disperse the tuberculi bacilli, which they suspected were responsible for the augmentation of the immune response, Freund and McDermot used a lanolinlike substance, which later proved to have an adjuvant effect itself.

Definitions

Adjuvants (L. *adjuvere*, to help) are substances that nonspecifically augment specific immune response to an antigen when mixed with the antigen prior to injection, or when injected separately but into the same site. Substances that cause transient general increase in immune response without having to be mixed with the antigen are referred to as *immunostimulants*. These differ from adjuvants in that they boost overall response (rather than the response to a single antigen) and in that they can be administered separately from the antigen. However, the dividing line between the two groups of immunopotentiating substances is not a sharp one.

Classification

The diverse and heterogeneous substances included in the adjuvant category can be divided loosely into five groups: oil adjuvants, mineral salts, polynucleotides, natural substances, and others.

Oil Adjuvants. The best-known representative of this category is Freund's adjuvant, which is used in one of two forms—complete or incomplete. *Complete Freund's adjuvant* is prepared by mixing mineral oil, heat-killed *Mycobacterium tuberculosis*, and an emulsifying agent, such as lanolin or Arlacel A (a mannide monooleate, which acts as a detergent, dispersing the oil into small droplets), adding a saline solution of the antigen to the above, and emulsifying the mixture. The adjuvant is then a creamy emulsion, consisting of tiny drops of antigen surrounded by mineral oil; the bacilli stick to these droplets because of their lipophilic properties. *Incomplete Freund's adjuvant* is prepared in the same way but the bacilli are left out. Of the two, complete Freund's adjuvant is the more potent stimulator of immune response. For maximum effect, the adjuvant must be injected subcutaneously or intradermally. Another oil used as adjuvant is Bayol F, composed of paraffin (42.5 percent), monocyclic naphthalene (31.4 percent), and polycyclic naphthalene (26.1 percent).

Mineral Salts. Aluminum sulfate with K^+, Na^+, or NH_4^+ ions is another frequently used adjuvant. Its formula is $AlK(SO_4)_2.12H_2O$, $AlNa(SO_4)_2.12H_2O$, or $AlNH_4(SO_4).12H_2O$. When added to a solution, the salt precipitates the antigen and the precipitate is then injected into the animal. Other mineral substances with adjuvant effect are silica, kaolin, and carbon.

Polynucleotides. This group includes synthetic polyribonucleotides such as polyinosinic-polycytidilic (poly IC) and polyadenylic polyuridylic (poly AU) acids.

Natural Substances. These are produced by fungi, parasites, and especially by bacteria. The best-known representative of this group is wax D, the active principle extracted by chloroform from *Mycobacterium tuberculosis*. It is composed of glycolipids and peptidoglycolipids; the minimal structure required for activity is *N*-acetyl-muramyl-L-alanyl-D-isoglutamine (muramyldipeptide, or MDP). Other active substances are present in *Corynebacterium parvum*, *Bordetella pertussis*, and in bacteria of the *Brucellae* group.

Others. This group includes all adjuvant substances that do not fit into any of the previous groups. Examples are vitamin A and tapioca (starch from the root of a tropical American plant, *Janipha manihot*).

Mechanism of Action

The augmentation of the immune response by adjuvants is the result of the combined effect of several factors, some of which are enumerated below.

Adjuvants trap the antigen and cause the formation of depots from which the antigen is released slowly over a prolonged period. The destruction of the antigen is thus delayed and the organism's exposure to the antigen lengthened.

Adjuvants stimulate nonspecific migration of cells to the site of antigen injection and thus increase the probability of interaction of the antigen with these cells. Often a dense, granular mass of cells—a granuloma—develops at the site of adjuvant injection.

Adjuvants increase antigen dispersion in the recipient's body by continually delivering the antigen in small droplets from the injection site to the regional lymph nodes or spleen.

Some adjuvants have a mitogenic effect and so stimulate the proliferation of lymphocytes nonspecifically.

Some adjuvants (e.g., synthetic polyribonucleotides) help to stimulate lymphocytes by activating adenylate cyclase and other chemical messengers.

Adjuvants may increase the number of T-helper cells in relation to the number of T-suppressor cells.

Adjuvants may increase the probability of contact among T and B cells, macrophages, and antigen through the activation of lymphocyte-trapping mechanisms.

Adjuvants may tip the balance between tolerance and immunity in favor of the latter.

Some adjuvants act predominantly on T cells, others on B cells, and still others on both T and B cells.

Immunostimulants

Only two examples of these substances will be mentioned here, BCG and *C. parvum*. BCG is an abbreviation for *bacille bilié de Calmette-Guérin*—an attenuated strain of tuberculi bacilli (*Mycobacterium tuberculosis*) named after its originators. BCG vaccination results in generalized enhancement of immune response, characterized by increased antigen clearance and phagocytosis, enhanced humoral immunity, accelerated graft rejection, increased resistance to infection, and augmented tumor immunity (see Chapter 14). *Corynebacterium parvum* is a Gram-negative bacterium which, when given in a nonviable form, stimulates macrophage functions primarily and acts as an antitumor agent.

10.2 LECTINS

10.2.1 Discovery

In 1888, H. Stillmark observed that the press cake formed during the extraction of castor oil from the seeds of castor beans, *Ricinus communis*, contained a highly toxic substance, ricin, which also had a remarkable capability to agglutinate erythrocytes from human and animal blood. A few years later, other investigators isolated another toxic and hemagglutinating substance, abrin, from the seeds of the jequirity beans, *Abrus precatorius*. Immunologists, particularly Paul Ehrlich, became interested in ricin and abrin because of the toxicity of these compounds, which reminded them of bacterial toxins. Although Karl Landsteiner and H. Raubitschek established as early as 1908 that various seed extracts agglutinated erythrocytes of different animals differently, immunologists of that time generally believed that the plant hemagglutinins were nonspecific. It was not until the end of the 1940s that K. O. Renkonen and William C. Boyd, together with Rose M. Reguera, discovered almost simultaneously (though independently) that certain seed extracts contained agglutinins specific for some human blood-group antigens. Thus, for example, extracts of the kidney bean, *Phaseolus vulgaris*, reacted specifically with the A antigen, and only when highly concentrated did they display weak activity with the B antigen. Soon, a whole series of plant agglutinins more or less specific for different blood-group substances was discovered. The usefulness of the agglutinins in blood-group typing and in the investigation of the chemical basis of blood-group antigenicity stimulated a search for more of these substances and the list soon grew into the hundreds. In 1954, Boyd and his co-worker, Elizabeth Shapleigh, proposed to name the various agglutinins *lectins* (L. *legere*, to select or choose—in reference to these substances' ability to choose between different blood groups), and we shall use this designation here.

The most exciting development in lectin research, however, did not take place until 1960, when Peter C. Nowell discovered the mitogenic properties of phytohemagglutinin. Nowell's was a chance discovery, made during an attempt to culture blood leukocytes. At that time, leukocytes and lymphocytes were generally regarded as dead-end cells that had reached the terminal stage of their development and could neither divide nor differentiate further. However, to his great surprise, Nowell found a number of lymphoblasts that seemed to be on a proliferation course in some of his cultures. It seemed as if something in the culture medium turned the lymphocytes on and transformed them from quiescent to differentiating cells; but a systematic search for the mysterious mitogenic substance failed. Only then did it occur to Nowell that the mitogenic stimulus might have come, not from the culture, but from the solution used for the separation of leukocytes from other blood cells. Because many lectins agglutinate erythrocytes better than they do leukocytes, they can be used to prepare relatively pure leukocyte suspensions. In this particular case, Nowell used phytohemagglutinin (PHA), a lectin extracted from the kidney bean, to obtain a pure leukocyte suspension, and apparently it was this PHA treatment that provided the differentiation stimulus. Surprisingly, however, it was not immunologists, but cytogeneticists who immediately took advantage of Nowell's discovery. To them, PHA stimulation of leukocytes represented an easy and inexpensive method of obtaining mitoses for chromosome analysis. Only later, when other lectins also proved to be mitogenic and some lectins were demonstrated to act specifically on certain lymphocyte subpopulations, did immunologists become interested.

10.2.2 Isolation

To separate lectins from other proteins in an extract, biochemists can either use conventional methods of protein fractionation, or take advantage of the lectins' ability to bind sugars specifically and reversibly. In the latter case, they couple the sugar to a column of beads and then pass the extract through the beads. The lectin specifically binds to the sugar and is retained by the column, while the rest of the extract passes through, unhindered. The retained lectin is then eluted from the beads in a virtually pure form.

10.2.3 Properties

Definition

Lectins are a heterogeneous group of compounds that have no structural features in common except that they are all proteins. They are characterized by the following three properties, of which only the first is mandatory for a protein to be considered a lectin: specific binding to sugars, agglutination of cells, and stimulation of lymphocytes. In these properties, lectins resemble antibodies, from which they differ in that they are not produced in response to a specific stimulus, in that they are restricted in their specificity to carbohydrates, and in that they are not immunoglobulins, but a rather diverse group of proteins.

Distribution

Extracts with hemagglutinating activity have been obtained from over 800 species of plant, numerous invertebrates (snails and horseshoe crabs), some microorganisms (e.g., *Pseudomonas*), and a few vertebrates (e.g., the rabbit). Among plants, the main lectin source is the legumes, the family characterized by butterflylike flowers; but legumes are not the only lectin-producing plants, for agglutinins have also been isolated from pokeweed, castor beans, wheat, potatoes, and many other species. Most lectins are found in the seeds, but some are also present in other parts of plants, such as roots, leaves, and bark. Plant lectins are sometimes referred to as *plant hemagglutinins*, *phytohemagglutinins* (Gr. *phyton*, a plant), or *phytomitogens*. Of the large number of lectins, only about 50 have been isolated in a pure form; some of these are available commercially.

Specificity

All lectins bind sugars, but different lectins display varying degrees of specificity. Most lectins interact preferentially with a single sugar, such as galactose or fucose, but some have a broader specificity, reacting with a number of closely related sugars (e.g., mannose, glucose, and arabinose); still others interact only with complex carbohydrates, such as those present in glycoproteins and on the cell surface. The carbohydrate specificity of the more common lectins is given in Table 10.1.

Binding to Cells

The interaction between lectins and cells occurs via a binding site of the former and a receptor of the latter. The binding site is specific for the carbohydrate carried by the receptor. A single lectin molecule contains at least one, but often more than one, binding site; a single cell may carry up to 10^7 lectin-binding receptors. At the onset, the receptors are evenly distributed on the cell surface, but shortly after binding, they begin to form patches and caps, just as other molecules do when crosslinked by antibodies. Normal cells, with the exception of erythrocytes, bind lectins only at high lectin concentrations. An initial observation that malignant cells and cells transformed in culture often bind lectins better than do corresponding normal cells raised hopes for using lectin binding as a marker for malignancy and transformation; however, subsequent studies have blurred the originally sharp dividing line between malignant and normal cells in this situation.

In some instances, lectin binding leads to cell agglutination; in other instances, agglutination does not occur, even though lectin attachment to the cell surface can be demonstrated. The mechanism of lectin-mediated cell agglutination is not yet fully understood, but the process apparently involves complex interactions leading to the formation of multiple cross-bridges between adjacent cells.

Table 10.1 Lectins Used in Immunological Research.

Name of Lectin	Source	Specificity: Sugar	Specificity: Human Erythrocytes Agglutinated
Concanavalin A	*Canavalia ensiformis* (Jack bean)	α-D-Man α-D-Glc D-Fru	A,B,O,AB (weakly)
Ricin RCA I	*Ricinus communis*	β-D-Gal; L-Rha	A,B,O,AB
RCA II		D-Gal; D-GalNAc	A,B,O,AB
Soy bean	*Glycine max*	α-D-GalNAc; α-D-Gal	A,B,O,AB
Wheat germ	*Triticum vulgaris*	D-GlcNAC	A,B,O,AB (weakly)
Pokeweed	*Phytolacca americana*		A,B,O,AB
Fructosan specific protein (FSP) shark	Nurse shark	β-D-Fructofuranose	None
Phytohemagglutinin E-PHA	*Phaseolus vulgaris* (Kidney bean)	D-GalNAC	A,B,O,AB
L-PHA		D-GalNAC	None
Sponge agglutinin	*Axinella polypoides*	D-Gal	A,B,O,AB
Sponge agglutinin	*Aaptos papillata*		A,B,O,AB
Limulus hemagglutinin	*Limulus polyphemus*	*N*-acetylneuraminic acid	A,B,O,AB
Lotus I II III	*Lotus tetragonolobus*	α-L-Fuc α-L-Fuc α-L-Fuc	O(H), A_2
Ulex I II	*Ulex europeus*	L-Fuc D-GlcNAc	O(H), A_2
Eel	*Anguilla rostrata*	α-L-Fuc	O(H), A_2
Hepatic binding protein (HBP)	Rabbit liver		A,B,O,AB
Snail	*Helix pomatia*	α-D-GalNAc; α-D-GalNAc; α-D-Gal, weak	A
Dolichos	*Dolichos biflorus*	α-D-GalNAc	A
Lima bean I II	*Phaseolus lunatus*	α-D-GalNAc	A
Sophora japonica	*Sophora japonica*	α-D-GalNAc; α-D-Gal	A,B
Bandeiraea simplicifolia	*Bandeiraea simplicifolia*	α-D-Gal	B,AB (A weak)

Source. From E. A. Kabat: *Structural Concepts in Immunology and Immunochemistry*, 2nd ed., Holt, Rinehart & Winston, New York, 1976.

Mitogenic Effect on Lymphocytes

Following the addition of a lectin, nondividing lymphocytes grow, differentiate, and proliferate; in other words, the lectin acts as a mitosis-stimulating substance, or *mitogen*. The mitogenic effect can be measured by counting enlarged lymphocytes (blasts) or by determining the increase in the incorporation rate of labeled thymidine, uridine, or leucine into DNA, RNA, or protein, respectively.

Molecular Weight	Number of Subunits	Association Constant (Number of Binding Sites)	Metallo-Protein	Biological Properties
102,000	4(α_4)	1.4×10^4 (4)	Mn^{2+} Ca^{2+}	Mitogen for T cells; B cells if aggregated
118,000–120,000	4($\alpha_2\beta_2$)			Low toxicity
60,000–65,000	2($\alpha\beta'$)			Toxic
120,000	4(α_4)	3×10^4 (2)		
23,000	1			
32,000	1			
280,500	4	9×10^3		Mitogenic for T and B cells
140,000	4($\alpha_2\beta_2$)			Mitogenic for T cells (α subunit)
140,000	4(α_4)			Mitogenic for T cells (α subunit)
400,000	18		Ca^{2+}	
120,000	4	6×10^3	Zn^{2+}	
		3.7×10^3	Zn^{2+}	
120,000	4	1.2×10^3	Zn^{2+}	
170,000			Ca^{2+}	
			Zn^{2+} or Mn^{2+}	
123,000	3			Precipitates directly with L-Fuc, not with methyl α-L-Fuc
				Binds asialoglycoproteins; agglutinates neuraminidase-treated rat, mouse, and guinea pig erythrocytes
100,000	6	5×10^3 (6)		
113,000; 109,000	4			
269,000	8	1×10^3	Mn^{2+}, Ca^{2+}	
138,000	4	0.9×10^3	Mn^{2+}, Ca^{2+}	
135,000				
	4			
114,000	4			

Lectin-stimulated lymphocytes display the same spectrum of functional characteristics as do lymphocytes stimulated by antigens: stimulated B lymphocytes secrete immunoglobulins, whereas stimulated T lymphocytes produce lymphokines and act as cytotoxic cells. The difference between antigen activation and lectin activation is in the number of activated lymphocyte clones: while an antigen activates only those T- or B-cell clones bearing the corresponding receptors (usually only about 0.02 to 0.1 percent of the cells), lectins activate many clones that carry receptors with different antigen-binding specificity, often as many as from 30 to 60 percent of the cells. (For this reason, lectins are sometimes referred to as *polyclonal activators*.) Lectins, however, never activate all lymphocytes; most activate only certain lymphocyte subpopulations (T or B cells), and even in each subpopulation, they activate only about one-third of the cells. The reason for this restricted activation is not clear, but it is certain that the restriction is not caused by the absence of lectin receptors, since, when crosslinked or bound to sepharose beads, even lectins normally specific for T cells will activate B cells. The mitogenic effect is not common to all lectins; some do not stimulate lymphocytes at all.

Toxicity

Several lectins (e.g., ricin and abrin) are highly toxic to mammalian cells. Once taken up by these cells, they inhibit protein synthesis by interfering with polypeptide-chain elongation on polyribosomes. Many other lectins (for example, those commonly used in immunological studies) are also toxic, but at least 1000 times less so than ricin and abrin. The cytotoxic effect can be inhibited by the addition of the sugar for which the lectin is specific. Some lectins preferentially kill cells that have undergone malignant transformation.

10.2.4 Function

The exact role that lectins play in the life of a plant is not known, but several possibilities have been suggested: defense against soil bacteria, phytopathogens, and insect predators; transport and storage of sugars; mediation of enzyme attachment in multienzyme systems; regulation of development, cell differentiation, and cell cohesion; binding of nitrogen-fixing bacteria; and regulation of plant cell wall extension. However, none of these suggestions has been proved or disproved.

10.2.5 Use in the Laboratory

Immunologists, cell biologists, and biochemists have found a variety of uses for lectins: generation of dividing lymphocytes for chromosome analysis; separation and differentiation of cell subsets; isolation of glycoproteins (see Chapter 8); study of lymphocyte activation; membrane fluidity studies; and others.

10.2.6 Immunologically Important Lectins

The three lectins most frequently used in immunology laboratories are concanavalin A, phytohemagglutinin, and pokeweed mitogen.

Concanavalin A

In 1911, F. Assman demonstrated hemagglutinating activity of extracts from jack beans, *Canavalia ensiformis* (Fig. 10.6). In an attempt to identify the active compound of these extracts, D. B. and C. O. Jones, five years later, distinguished two fractions based on

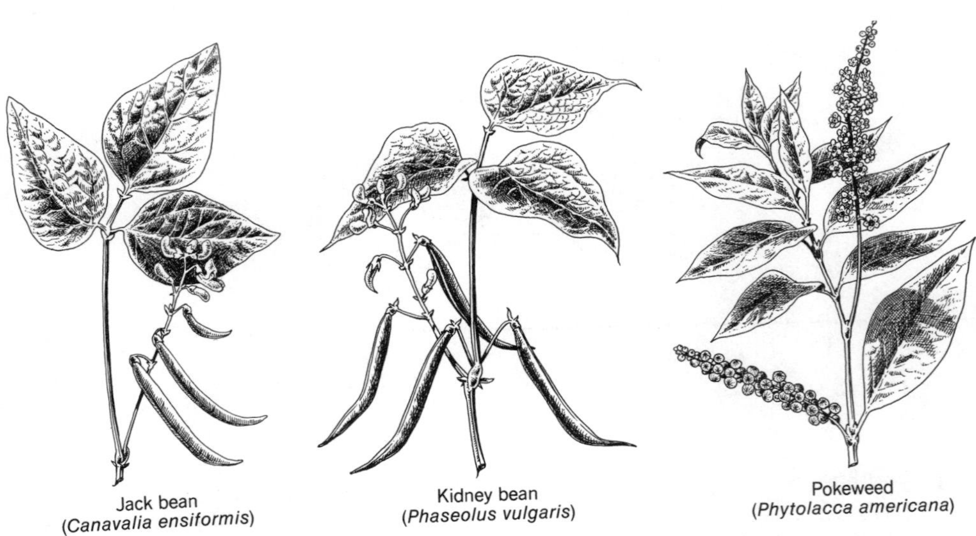

Figure 10.6. Plants from which the three commonly used lectins are extracted: jack bean, *Canavalia ensiformis*, the source of Con A; kidney bean, *Phaseolus vulgaris*, the source of PHA; and pokeweed, *Phytolacca americana*, the source of pokeweed mitogen.

their solubility in ammonium sulfate—*canavalin*, precipitable by saturation with ammonium sulfate, and *concanavalin*, precipitable with 0.6 saturated ammonium sulfate. In 1919, J. G. Sumner succeeded in separating the concanavalin fraction further into two subfractions—A, soluble only in concentrated sodium chloride solution, and B, soluble in 10 percent sodium chloride solution. Of the two, only fraction A agglutinated red blood cells of various animal species; it is the present-day *concanavalin A*, or *Con A*.

Con A is the most extensively studied lectin—the subject of several books and conferences. It is a pure protein (contains no carbohydrate) that constitutes about 3 percent of the total jack bean protein content. It binds to saccharides containing α-D-mannose or α-D-glucose residues in either terminal or internal positions. The Con A molecule (molecular weight of 102,000 daltons) consists of four identical subunits (monomeres), each composed of one polypeptide chain that is 237 amino acid residues long (molecular weight of 25,500 daltons). However, isolated Con A spontaneously forms dimers or higher molecular-weight aggregates, depending on pH. The helmet-shaped monomers are paired, base to base, into dimers, and the dimers are then paired at right angles into tetramers (Fig. 10.7). Part of the polypeptide chain in the monomer is arranged into two antiparallel, β-pleated sheets, while the rest forms a random coil. Each monomer has one carbohydrate-binding site, and one binding site each for the Ca^{++} and Mn^{++} ions needed for carbohydrate attachment. Con A is a T cell-specific mitogen.

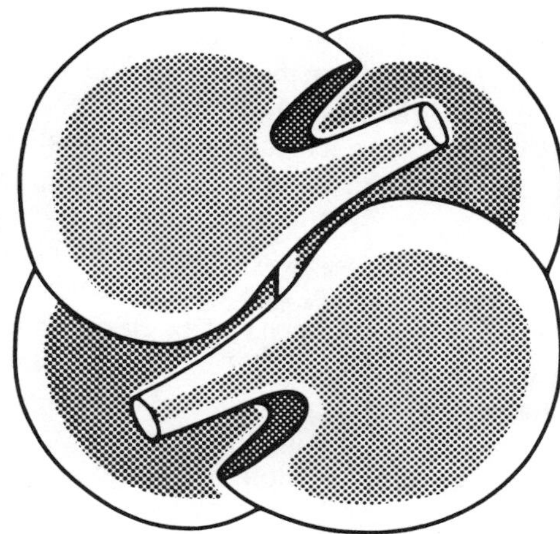

Figure 10.7. The arrangement of monomers in the tetrameric molecule of concanavalin A.

Phytohemagglutinin

Phytohemagglutinin (PHA), the crude extract from the kidney bean (Fig. 10.6; however, the designation is sometimes used as a generic name for hemagglutinins of plant origin), was the first lectin shown to be mitogenic. Like Con A, PHA (molecular weight of 140,000 daltons) is a tetramer, but unlike Con A, it is composed of two kinds of subunit, L and R. The L form agglutinates leukocytes (hence the designation), but not erythrocytes, and is mitogenic; the R form agglutinates red blood cells but has no mitogenic activity. The tetramers can be composed of one of five possible monomeric combinations: L_4, L_3R, L_2R_2, LR_3, and R_4. Mixtures of L_4 and L_3R molecules agglutinate leukocytes and are therefore referred to as L-PHA; mixtures of L_2R_2 and LR_3 (H-PHA) agglutinate both leukocytes and erythrocytes; and R_4 molecules agglutinate erythrocytes but, in contrast to the other two PHA preparations, do not possess mitogenic activity. Commercially available PHA is a mixture of these various forms. The R and L monomers are homologous in structure and probably related in their origin. PHA is a T-cell mitogen, specific for N-acetylgalactosamine.

Pokeweed Mitogen

Pokeweed mitogen (PWM), found in the roots of pokeweed, *Phytolacca americana* (Fig. 10.6), is a mixture of at least five mitogenic proteins. One of these is a polymer, mitogenic for both T and B lymphocytes, while the other four are T-cell mitogens. The carbohydrate specificity of PWM is not known.

10.3 BACTERIAL LIPOPOLYSACCHARIDES

The bacterial cell surface abounds with lymphocyte-stimulating substances. Some of these stimulate lymphocytes specifically via immune receptors (i.e., they function as antigens), while others function as nonspecific activators. The best-known example of the latter group is the lipopolysaccharide (LPS), to which we now turn our attention. We shall first review briefly the natural setting of these complex molecules—the bacterial cell wall—and then describe the properties of the LPS itself.

10.3.1 The Structure of the Bacterial Cell Wall

With the exception of *Mycoplasma* and a few other genera, all bacteria are enveloped in a *cell wall*, in addition to the plasma membrane. The main reason that most bacterial cells have cell walls and most animal cells do not is the fact that bacteria live in an environment that exerts less osmotic pressure on the cell membrane from the outside than the cytoplasm (because of a higher concentration of metabolites) does from the inside. The cell wall thus protects bacterial cells from bursting. Other functions of the bacterial cell wall involve mechanical support, maintenance of distinctive shape, and interactions with host cells.

There are two main types of bacterial cell, distinguished by a stain discovered in 1884 by the Danish bacteriologist Hans C. J. Gram. The *Gram staining* procedure is carried out in three steps: staining with the basic dye, crystal violet; fixation with diluted iodine (I_2-KI); and washing with organic solvents (acetone or alcohol). All bacteria stain with the dyes, but the so-called Gram-positive bacteria maintain the dark purple-black color even after washing, whereas the stain is washed out of the Gram-negative bacteria. The reason for this difference is that the cell wall of Gram-positive bacteria prevents the crystal violet–iodine complex from getting out of the cell, whereas the wall of Gram-negative bacteria is permeable to this complex. All bacteria fall into one or the other category: they are either Gram-positive or Gram-negative. Examples of Gram-positive bacteria are the various staphylococci and streptococci; representatives of Gram-negative bacteria are *Pseudomonas*, *Azotobacter*, *Nitrosomonas*, and *Enterobacteriaceae* (e.g., *Escherichia coli*, *Salmonella*, *Shigella*, *Klebsiella*, *Serratia*, *Proteus*, and *Enterobacter*). The cell walls of the two bacterial groups differ morphologically and biochemically.

The cell wall of *Gram-positive bacteria* consists of a single uniform layer, about 20 to 80 nm in width (Fig. 10.8*a, b*). Its two major constituents are peptidoglycan and teichoic acid. *Peptidoglycan* is a heteropolymer consisting of two acetylated amino sugars (N-acetylglucosamine, abbreviated G, and N-acetyl muramic

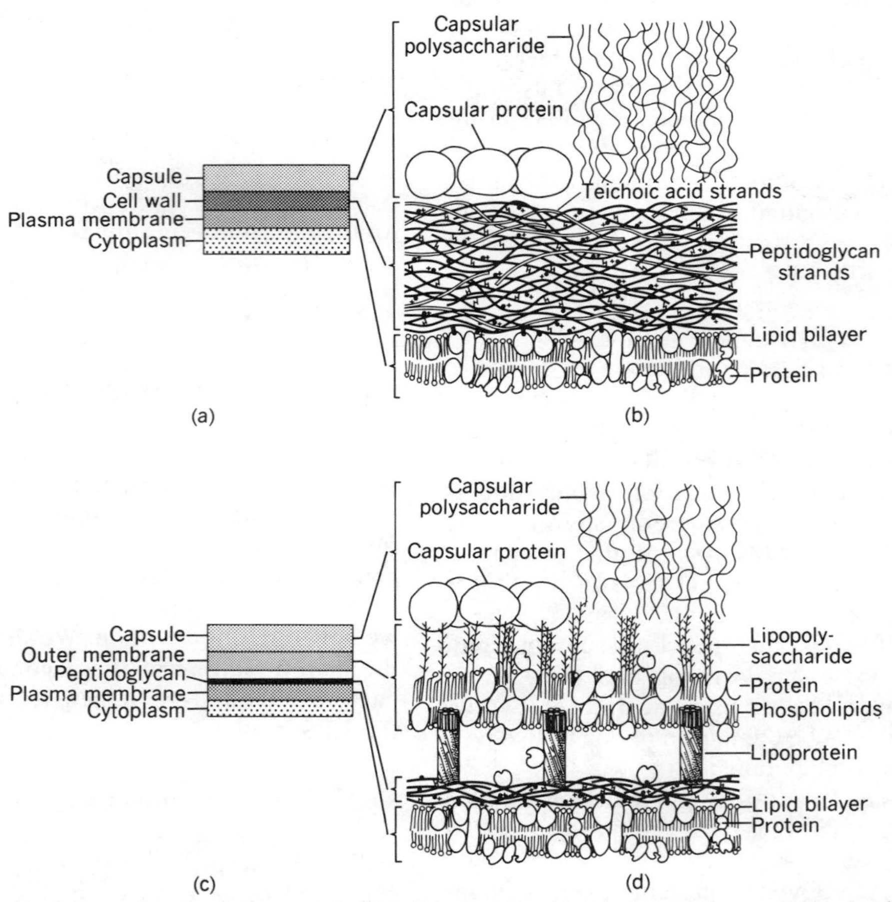

Figure 10.8. Structure of bacterial cell wall in Gram-positive (*a, b*) and Gram-negative (*c, d*) bacteria. (Based in part on J. W. Costerton *in* (Ed.): *Microbiology*.

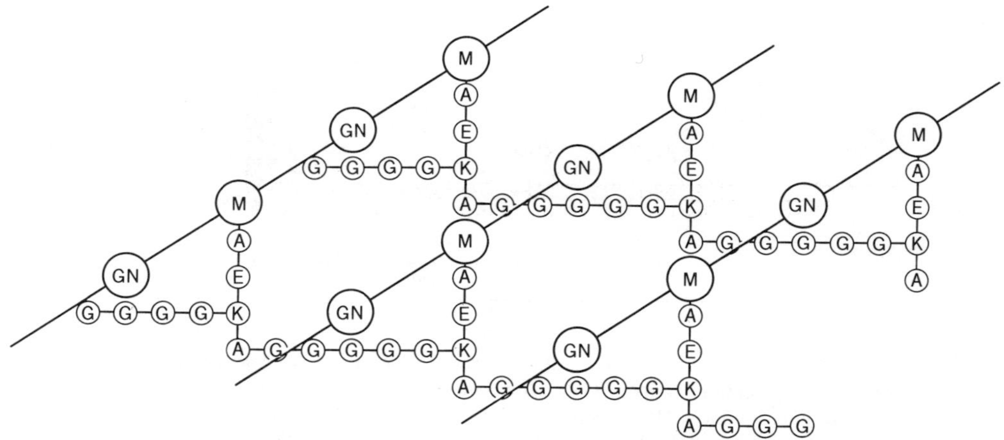

Figure 10.9. Composition and organization of the bacterial cell-wall peptidoglycan. Glycan strands (heavy lines), are composed of alternating N-acetylglucosamine (G) and *N*-acetylmuramic acid (M) residues. Circles vertical from M represent the amino acid residue of the tetrapeptide subunit: A, alanine, E, glutamic acid, K, lysine, and A, alanine. Circles on the horizontal represent the peptide crosslinking bridges consisting of five repeated glycine (G) residues.

acid, abbreviated M) and a small number of amino acids, some of which are "unnatural" in that they never occur in proteins (they have the D, rather than the usual L configuration). The amino sugars are arranged into glycan strands of alternating G and M units, each strand consisting of from 10 to 65 disaccharide units. The strands are crosslinked by tetrapeptides in the manner shown in Figure 10.9. *Teichoic acid* (Gr. *teichos,* wall), a linear polymer derived from either glycerol phosphate or ribitol phosphate (Fig. 10.10), occurs as a wall constituent only in Gram-positive bacteria. Some of the teichoic acid polymers are covalently linked to the glycan strands of the peptidoglycan net; others are anchored in the plasma membrane (Fig. 10.8*b*).

The cell wall of *Gram-negative bacteria* consists of at least two layers, a thin (2 to 3 nm wide) inner (*rigid*) layer of peptidoglycan (with some protein attached to it) and a thicker (8 to 10 nm wide) outer membrane (Fig. 10.8*c*, *d*). Some bacteria have a third, loose layer on top of the outer membrane. The peptidoglycan of the inner layer forms a sac enveloping the cell. The outer membrane bears a superficial morphological resemblance to the plasma ("unit") membrane, but the two are structurally and chemically distinct. The major

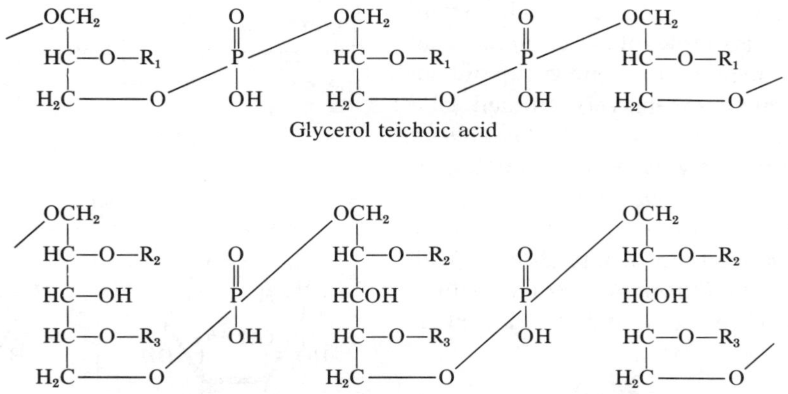

OCH_2 — $HC—O—R_1$ — $H_2C—O$ — $P(=O)(OH)$ — OCH_2 — $HC—O—R_1$ — $H_2C—O$ — $P(=O)(OH)$ — OCH_2 — $HC—O—R_1$ — $H_2C—O$

Glycerol teichoic acid

OCH_2 — $HC—O—R_2$ — $HC—OH$ — $HC—O—R_3$ — $H_2C—O$ — $P(=O)(OH)$ — OCH_2 — $HC—O—R_2$ — $HCOH$ — $HC—O—R_3$ — $H_2C—O$ — $P(=O)(OH)$ — OCH_2 — $HC—O—R_2$ — $HCOH$ — $HC—O—R_3$ — $H_2C—O$

Ribitol teichoic acid

Figure 10.10. Structure of typical teichoic acids. R_1, hydrogen, glycosyl, or D-alanyl (in about half of the glycerol residues the R_1 is H); R_2, D-alanyl; R_3, glycosyl, Ala-D-alanyl.

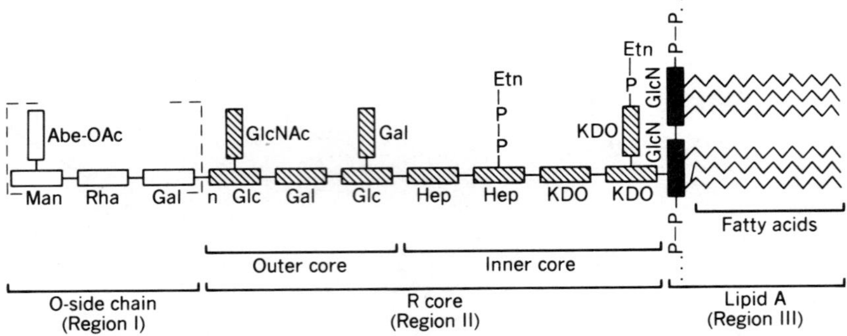

Figure 10.11. The basic unit of the lipopolysaccharide molecule. Abe, abequose; Ac, acetyl; Etn, ethanolamine; Gal, D-galactose; Glc, D-glucose; GlcNAc, *N*-acetyl-D-glucosamine; Hep, heptose; KDO, 2-keto-3-deoxyoctonic acid; Man, D-mannose; P, phosphate; Rha, L-rhamnose.

components of the outer membrane are phospholipids, proteins, lipoproteins, and lipopolysaccharides. The phospholipids are similar in composition and arrangement to those found in the plasma membrane. The proteins—structural and enzymatic—are irregularly distributed through the phospholipid bilayer. The lipoproteins form columns interconnecting the inner and outer layers, with the bases of the columns attached to the peptidoglycan and the lipid heads buried in the phospholipid layer, so that the wall resembles an ancient Greek temple. The space between the inner and outer layers is only loosely filled with the protein molecules usually associated with the lipoprotein columns. Dispersed in the outer membrane are groups of lipopolysaccharide molecules.

10.3.2 Properties of the Lipopolysaccharide

The lipopolysaccharide (LPS) constitutes a major component of the outer wall in most, if not all, Gram-negative bacteria. The LPS molecule is complex, and its chemical composition varies from one group of bacteria to another. The most extensively studied LPS molecules are those extracted from the *Salmonella* group; the LPS most frequently used in immunology is that isolated from *Escherichia coli*. The chemical and antigenic structure of LPS has been elucidated by a number of scientists, among them André Boivin, Walter T. J. Morgan, Fritz Kaufmann, Bruce White, Anne-Marie Staub, Otto Westphal, and Otto Lüderitz.

Isolation

LPS can be extracted from the cell wall after treating the bacteria with a hot (65 to 68°C) phenol-water mixture. On cooling, the homogeneous mixture separates into an upper (water) and a lower (phenol) phase. LPS, in the form of large aggregates, remains in the water phase, together with nucleic acids, and can be recovered for further purification by ultracentrifugation.

Structure

The basic structural unit of the LPS molecule consists of three regions, designated I (O-side chain), II (R core), and III (lipid A). The first two regions consist of saccharides, the third of a saccharide and a lipid (Fig. 10.11). The *lipid-A region* consists of two sugars (glucosamines), to which are attached long-chain fatty acids (lauric, palmitic, and 3-D-meristoxymyristic acid). The lipids impose hydrophobicity on this region of the LPS molecule. The *core region* (in *Salmonella*) consists of 10 sugar residues, including, in the inner portion, two unusual substances—2-keto-3-deoxyoctonic acid (KDO) and heptose (Fig. 10.12); the outer portion of the core contains conventional sugars—glucose, galactose, and *N*-acetyl-glucosamine. The composition and structure of the core region is the same in all *Salmonella* species; in other bacterial

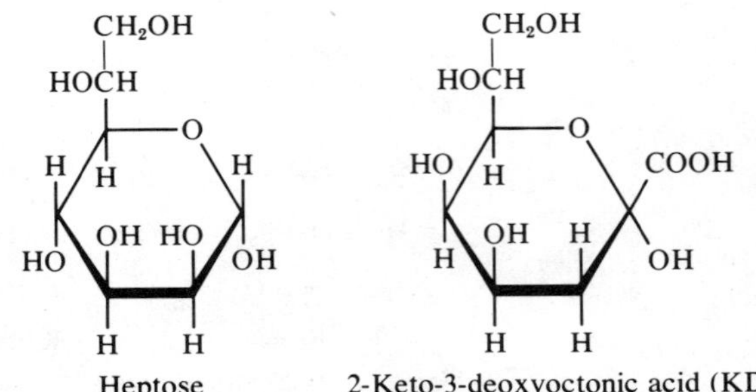

Figure 10.12. The C_7 and C_8 constituents of the lipopolysaccharide inner-core region.

genera, the region may have a different structure. The O-side chain region of *Salmonella typhimurium* contains four or five monosaccharide residues (abequose, mannose, rhamnose, galactose, and glucose) arranged into a branched unit, which is repeated in the chain several times (the number of repeats depending on the particular bacterial strain). In the cell wall, region III is buried in the outer membrane, whereas the long chains of regions I and II protrude to the outside (the regions are arranged in the order I–II–III). In *Salmonella*, the basic units just described form aggregates of three, and the aggregates associate with cell-wall proteins. The complexes of multiple LPS chains and proteins are referred to as *endotoxins*.

Biosynthesis

The mechanism of lipid-A biosynthesis is unknown. Presumably, the first step involves the formation of the disaccharide skeleton, to which specific enzymes then attach the individual fatty acids.

The core is synthesized by sequential addition of monosaccharides to the growing chain, starting with the attachment of the KDO residue to the disaccharide backbone of lipid A. The synthesis is catalyzed by two series of enzymes—synthetases, involved in the actual formation of monosaccharide residues, and transferases, involved in the transfer of these residues to the growing chain.

The O-side chain is assembled from prefabricated tetra- or pentasaccharide units, manufactured separately. In each unit, the four or five monosaccharides are assembled sequentially, with the aid of specific synthetases and transferases, and once the first unit is assembled, it is attached by another enzyme (ligase) to the core. Individual units are then added, one by one, to the growing chain.

Serology

Rabbits immunized with different species and strains of a given Gram-negative bacterium (e.g., *Salmonella*) form antibodies that specifically recognize antigens on the bacterium's cell surface. The antigens fall into one of three categories, designated K, H, and O. The K antigens are located in the bacterium's capsule (the designation derives from the German *Kapsel*), a loose slime layer present on top of the cell wall in some bacteria. The H antigens were first identified in motile bacteria capable (because of their motility) of forming a continuous film (the German word for film is *Hauch*); they are located in the bacterium's flagella. The O antigens were first identified in nonmotile bacteria that colonize the substrate without forming a film (the German *ohne Hauch* means "without film"); they are located in the bacterial body (soma), in region I of the lipopolysaccharide.

The anti-O sera can be subjected to a standard serological analysis: they can be tested against a large panel of strains and made monospecific by absorption, and the monospecific antisera can be used to identify individual determinants. Over 70 such determinants have been described in *Salmonella* and designated by serial numbers 1, 2, 3, 4, and so on. Some strains of *Salmonella* possess only one determinant, others have two or three, and a few may have up to four. When multiple determinants are present, their combination—*serotype*—is characteristic of a given strain. Serotypes sharing at least one determinant form a *serogroup,* designated by capital letters (A, B, C, etc.) or letters and numbers (C1, C2, C3, etc.). The classification of *Salmonella* strains according to serogroups and serotypes is called—in reference to its originators—the *Kauffmann-White scheme* (Table 10.2). Serotyping is an important tool for identification of bacteria in the diagnosis of infectious diseases.

Immunochemistry

Based on the chemical composition of their polysaccharide chains (regions I and II), the different species and strains of *Salmonella* can be divided into 16 *chemotypes*, designated I through XVI. Species and strains within each chemotype have identical sugar compositions, whereas *Salmonella* species belonging to different chemotypes differ in one or more sugars. For example, *Salmonella* species of chemotype I contain D-glucosamine, KDO, heptose, D-glucose, and D-galactose; *Salmonella* strains of chemotype II contain these same four monosaccharides and, in addition, D-galactosamine; *Salmonella* strains of chemotype III contain the four sugars and D-mannose, and so on (see Table 10.3). Comparison of the serological and chemical classification reveals that all bacteria belonging to the same serogroup also belong to the same chemotype (but a given chemotype may encompass several serogroups; for example, chemotype I includes serogroups J, B, X, Y, and 58).

A complete chemical analysis of the LPS polysaccharide portions has revealed the structural basis of the serotype grouping and of the individual antigenic determinants. The serotypes are determined by the order of sugar residues and the type of linkage between neighboring sugars in the repeating region-I units of the LPS molecule. Examples of serotypes and corresponding tetra- or pentasaccharide sequences are given

Table 10.2 Established Serogroups and Serotypes of *Salmonella* O-Antigen

Serogroup	Serotype	Serogroup	Serotype
A	1,2,123	L	21
B	1,4,5,12	M	$28_1,28_2$
	1,4,12,27		$28_1,28_3$
	4,12,27	N	$30_1,30_3$
	4,12		30_1
	4,5,12	O	35
	1,4,12	P	38
C1	6,7	Q	39
	6,7,Vi	R	$40_1,40_2$
C2	6,8		$40_1,40_3,1$
C3	8	S	41
	8,20	T	42_1
C4	6,7,14		$42_1,42_2,1$
D1	1,9,12	U	$43_1,43_2,43_3$
	9,12		$43_1,43_2,43_4$
	9,12,Vi	V	44
D2	9,46	W	$45_1,45_2$
	9,12,46		$45_1,45_3$
E1	3,10	X	$47_1,47_2$
E2	3,15		$47_1,47_3$
E3	3,15,34	Y	$48_1,48_2$
E4	1,3,19		$48_1,48_2,48_3$
	1,3,10,19		$48_1,48_3,48_4$
	1,3,15,19	Z	$50_1,50_2,50_3$
F	11		$50_1,50_2,50_4$
G1	13,22		$50_1,50_3$
	1,13,22	51	51
G2	1,13,23	52	52
	13,23	53	53
H	1,6,14,25	54	54
	6,14,24	55	55
	1,6,14,24	56	56
	6,14	57	57
I	16	58	58
J	17	59	59
K	18	60	60
	6,14,18		

in Table 10.4. Single determinants usually encompass more than one sugar residue (or one intersaccharide linkage), but among the multiple residues, one—the so-called *immunodominant sugar*—is usually more important than the others (Fig. 10.13). The immunodominant sugar is the one that inhibits the reaction of an antibody with a given antigenic determinant most strongly (in other words, the antibody has the highest affinity for this particular sugar).

The structure and antigenicity of region-I LPS chains may change following the infection of *Salmonella* by certain lysogenic phages. For example, infection with bacteriophage Φ27 converts *Salmonella* of serogroup B with determinants 1, 4, and 12 into bacteria carrying determinants (4), 12, and 27. At the chemical level, this *lysogenic conversion* is accompanied by a change of the Gal-1,4-Man linkage in the parental strain to a Gal-1,6-Man linkage in the converted strain:

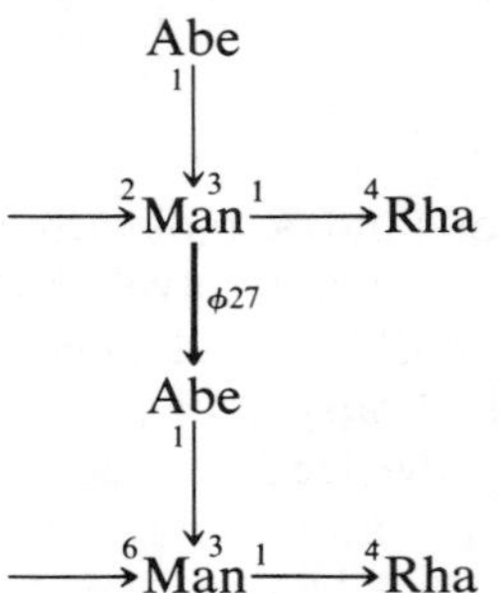

The change can be explained as follows: the infection is followed by the incorporation of the phage nucleic acid into the bacterial chromosome; the integrated phage genes change one or more enzymes involved in

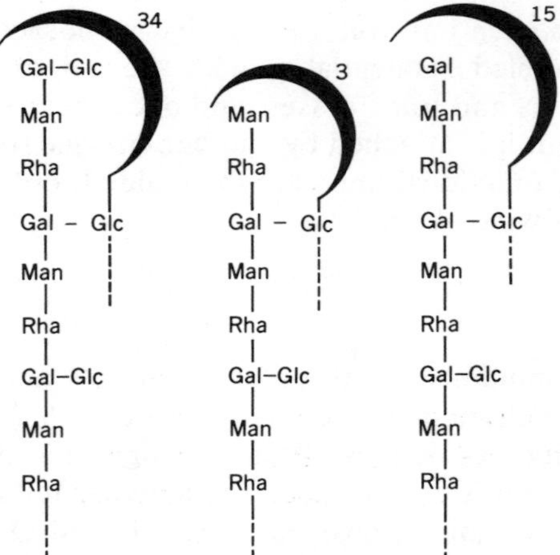

Figure 10.13. Location of antigenic determinants 3, 15, and 34 on O-side chains of *Salmonella* group E_3 polysaccharides. The lines around the chains symbolize the strength of interaction (affinity) between the antibody combining site and the corresponding sugars of the polysaccharide (the thicker the line, the greater the affinity). The antibody has the strongest affinity for the immunodominant sugar. Abbreviations are the same as in Figure 10.11. (From O. Lüderitz, A. M. Staub, and O. Westphal: *Bacteriol. Rev*. **30:**192–255, 1966.)

Table 10.3 Chemotypes of *Salmonella*. (The first four sugars are in the R core region, the remaining sugars in the O side chain.)

Chemotype	Presence (X) of Sugar														Found in Serogroups
	D-Glucosamine	2-Keto-3-Deoxyoctonic Acid	L-Glycero-D-Mannose	D-Galactose	D-Glucose	D-Galactosamine	D-Mannose	L-Fucose	L-Rhamnose	Ribose	Colitose	Abequose	Paratose	Tyvelose	
I	X	X	X	X	X										J,V,X,Y,58
II	X	X	X	X	X	X									L,P,51,55
III	X	X	X	X	X		X								C_1,C_4,H,S
IV	X	X	X	X	X	X	X								K,R
V	X	X	X	X	X			X							W
VI	X	X	X	X	X	X		X							G,N,U
VII	X	X	X	X	X				X						T,59
VIII	X	X	X	X	X	X			X						M,(28_1,28_3)53,57
XXV	X	X	X	X	X					X					52
IX	X	X	X	X	X	X				X					M,(28_1,28_2),56
X	X	X	X	X	X						X				O
XI	X	X	X	X	X	X					X				Z
XII	X	X	X	X	X	X	X	X							I,Q
XIII	X	X	X	X	X		X		X						E,F,54
XIV	X	X	X	X	X		X		X			X			B,C2,C3
XV	X	X	X	X	X		X		X				X		A
XVI	X	X	X	X	X		X		X					X	D1,D2

Source. From O. Lüderitz, A. M. Staub, and O. Westphal: *Bacteriol. Rev.* **30:**192–255, 1966.

the biosynthesis of the repeating units; and the altered enzyme then changes the linkage (or, in some instances, the sugars themselves too) in these units. The altered linkage of sugar residues is then responsible for the altered antigenic properties of the converted bacteria. In the example mentioned, part of determinant 4 changed into determinant 27, but other phages acting on the same or different bacteria can cause other types of conversion (Table 10.5).

R Antigens

Most Gram-negative bacteria isolated from nature form colonies with a smooth surface. However, from time to time, these S-type bacteria mutate to "rough" types, characterized by an irregular, coarsely granular colony surface. When analyzed chemically, the R-type bacteria can be demonstrated to lack region-I side chains in their LPS molecules. The basis for the S → R change is a mutation in one of the synthetase or transferase genes coding for the enzymes involved in biosynthesis of region-I repeating units. Functional failure of one of these enzymes means that one of the sugars is not incorporated into the repeating unit, and hence, that the latter is not attached to the terminal sugar of region II. Consequently, in R mutants, region II remains bare, without the O-side chains.

By immunization of rabbits with different R mutants, one can produce antisera specific for region-II determinants (i.e., for R antigens). Analysis of such antisera has revealed an additional series of R mutations (designated R_a through R_e), responsible for shortening of the region-II chain. These mutations affect genes controlling the sequential addition of sugar residues to the growing oligosaccharide chain of region II. The addition of residues beyond a particular position is blocked whenever an enzyme responsible for the placement of a sugar in this position is inactivated

Table 10.4 Repeating Sugar Units of Some *Salmonella* Lipopolysaccharides.

Serogroup	*Salmonella* Species (O factors)	Antigenic Determinants	Repeating Units
A	*S. paratyphi* A	1,2,12	Par $\downarrow$ 1,3 α (to Man); Glc $\downarrow$ 1,4/1,6 α (to Gal) $\xrightarrow{2}$ Man $\xrightarrow[\alpha]{1,4}$ Rha $\xrightarrow[\alpha]{1,3}$ Gal $\xrightarrow[\alpha]{1}$ OAc (on Rha)
B	*S. bredeney*	1,4,12	Abe $\downarrow$ 1,3 α (to Man); Glc $\downarrow$ 1,4/1,6 α (to Gal) $\xrightarrow{2}$ Man $\xrightarrow[\alpha]{1,4}$ Rha $\xrightarrow[\beta]{1,3}$ Gal $\xrightarrow[\alpha]{1}$
	S. typhimurium	4,5,12	2-OAc-Abe $\downarrow$ 1,3 α (to Man); Glc $\downarrow$ 1,4 α (to Gal) $\xrightarrow{2}$ Man $\xrightarrow[\alpha]{1,4}$ Rha $\xrightarrow[\beta]{1,3}$ Gal $\xrightarrow[\alpha]{1}$
D_1	*S. typhi*	9,12	Tyv $\downarrow$ 1,3 α (to Man); (2-OAc-)Glc $\downarrow$ 1,4 α (to Gal) $\xrightarrow{2}$ Man $\xrightarrow[\alpha]{1,4}$ Rha $\xrightarrow[\alpha]{1,3}$ Gal $\xrightarrow[\alpha]{1}$
D_2	*S. strassbourg*	(9),46	Tyv $\downarrow$ 1,3 α (to Man); Glc $\downarrow$ 1,4 α (to Gal) $\xrightarrow{6}$ Man $\xrightarrow[\alpha]{1,4}$ Rha $\xrightarrow[\alpha]{1,3}$ Gal $\xrightarrow[\alpha]{1}$
E_1	*S. anatum*	3,10	$\xrightarrow{6}$ Man $\xrightarrow[\beta]{1,4}$ Rha $\xrightarrow[\alpha]{1,3}$ Gal $\xrightarrow[\alpha]{1}$ (OAc) (on Gal)
E_2	*S. newington*	3,15	$\xrightarrow{6}$ Man $\xrightarrow[\beta]{1,4}$ Rha $\xrightarrow[\alpha]{1,3}$ Gal $\xrightarrow[\beta]{1}$
E_3	*S. illinois*	(3),(15),46	Glc $\downarrow$ 1,4 α (to Gal) $\xrightarrow{6}$ Man $\xrightarrow[\beta]{1,4}$ Rha $\xrightarrow[\alpha]{1,3}$ Gal $\xrightarrow[\beta]{1}$
E_4	*S. senftenberg*	1,3,19	Glc $\downarrow$ 1,6 α (to Gal) $\xrightarrow{6}$ Man $\xrightarrow[\beta]{1,4}$ Rha $\xrightarrow[\alpha]{1,3}$ Gal $\xrightarrow[\alpha]{1}$

Source. From K. Jann and O. Westphal *in* M. Sela (Ed.): *The Antigens,* Vol. 3, pp. 1–125. Academic, New York, 1975.

Abe, abequose; OAc, O-acetyl; Gal, D-galactose; Glc, D-glucose; Man, D-mannose; Par, paratose; Rha, L-rhamnose; Tyv, tyvelose.

by a mutation. A series of mutant strains with progressively longer region-II chains can thus be produced (Fig. 10.14).

10.3.3 Endotoxin

The aggregate of several LPS chains (the number depends on the particular bacterial genus, species, and strain) and the associated protein is called the *endotoxin* (Gr. *endon,* within; Fig. 10.15). The name refers to the fact that the aggregate acts as a poison but, in contrast to exotoxins, is normally not freely liberated into the surrounding medium; it is released only when the integrity of the cell wall is disturbed. When injected into an animal, endotoxin acts as a *pyrogen*—that is, as a substance causing a rise in temperature (Gr. *pyr,* fire; *-gen,* producing). The high pyrogenic activity of this substance (10^{-6} g of endotoxin produces fever in a horse weighing 700 kg) complicated the production of pure bacterial vaccines for a long time. It was so difficult to get rid of contaminating trace amounts of endotoxin in the vaccines that some bacteriologists began to refer to these ghostlike substances as "the little blue devils." The pyrogenic ac-

Table 10.5 Examples of Phage Conversion.

Phage	Alteration	Bacteria	Antigen Structure: Before	Antigen Structure: After Conversion
P22	Glucosylation	*Salmonella* A, B, D	↓ (on Man) →Man→Rha→Gal—	↓ (on Man), α-Glc ↓ (on Gal) →Man→Rha→Gal—
ϵ34	Glucosylation	*Salmonella* E	→Man→Rha→Gal—	α-Glc ↓ (on Gal) →Man→Rha→Gal—
ϵ15	Deacetylation	*Salmonella* E	O.Ac | (on Gal) →Man→Rha→Gal—	→Man→Rha→Gal—
ϵ15	Polymer configuration	*Salmonella* E	O.Ac | (on Gal) →Man→Rha$\xrightarrow{\alpha}$Gal—	→Man→Rha$\xrightarrow{\beta}$Gal—
ϕ27	Polymer configuration	*Salmonella* A, B, D	↓ (on Man) →2Man→Rha→Gal—	→6Man→Rha→Gal—

Source. From I. W. Sutherland *in* L. E. Glynn and M. W. Steward (Eds.): *Immunochemistry. An Advanced Textbook*, pp. 399–443. Wiley, Chichester, 1977.

Abe, abequose; OAc, O-acetyl; Gal, D-galactose; Glc, D-glucose; Man, D-mannose; Rha, L-rhamnose.

tivity of endotoxin is indirect: it acts on granulocytes, causing them to release a pyrogenic substance, which then acts on thermoregulatory centers in the brain and produces fever (see also Chapter 14).

Other effects of endotoxin include toxicity (it induces symptoms characteristic of inflammatory diseases), killing of certain tumor cells (but the strong side effects make the substance unsuitable for tumor therapy), activation of the fibrinolytic and complement systems, adjuvanticity, and induction of interferon

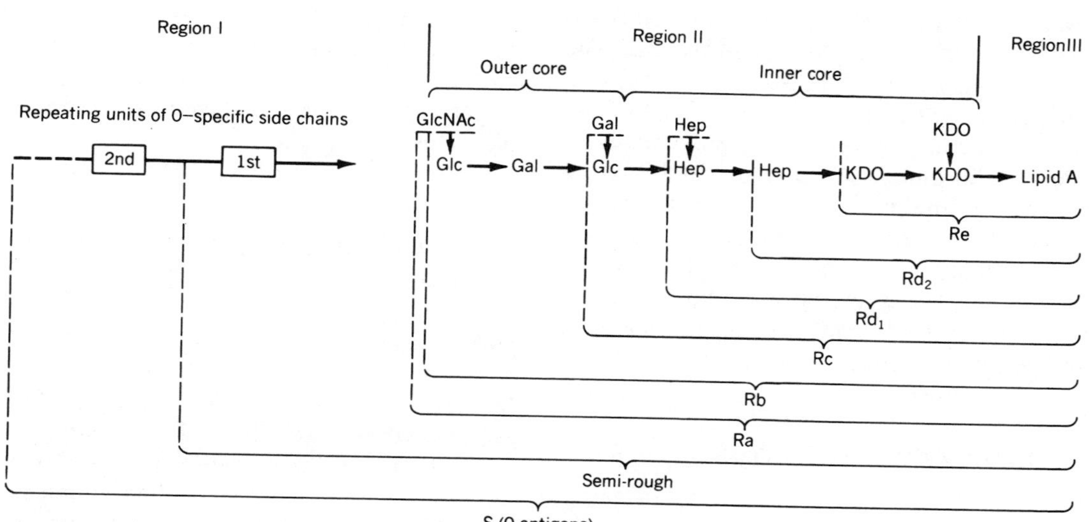

Figure 10.14. Structure of the various rough mutants of *Salmonella*. Each R mutant synthesizes only the portion of the R core indicated by the brace. (Based on O. Lüderitz, A. M. Staub, and O. Westphal: *Bacteriol. Rev.* **30:**192–255, 1966.)

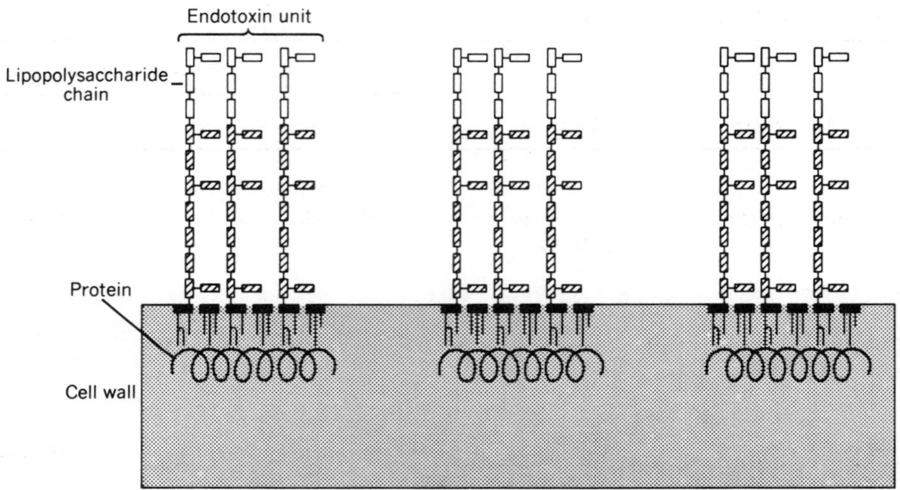

Figure 10.15. Endotoxin aggregates (three are shown) in bacterial cell wall.

production. However, the main reason that we discuss endotoxin and LPS in such detail here is their mitogenic effect.

10.3.4 Mitogenic Action of LPS

In 1972, Göran Möller and his colleagues reported that *Escherichia coli*-derived LPS causes proliferation when added to lymphocyte culture. The effect of LPS on lymphocytes is similar to that of lectins: the LPS acts as a polyclonal activator, nonspecifically stimulating lymphocyte clones with different lymphocyte-receptor specificity. The LPS is specific for B lymphocytes, although the presence of helper T cells in the culture enhances LPS stimulation. However, even under optimal conditions, only about 20 percent of B lymphocytes in a given population are activated. The activated lymphocytes undergo blastogenesis, mitosis, and maturation into antibody-secreting cells, but the produced antibodies are extremely heterogeneous in their specificity. The mitogenic activity of LPS molecules resides in their lipid moieties; the polysaccharide portions are nonmitogenic. How LPS activates B cells is not clear; probably the lipid A interacts with the lipid bilayer of the plasma membrane and induces a conformational change of some of its components, which then triggers the activation process.

10.4 OTHER LYMPHOCYTE-ACTIVATING SUBSTANCES

Lymphocytes can be activated by a variety of other substances in addition to antigens, lectins, and lipopolysaccharides. The most important of these are antibodies to immunoglobulin receptors. Class- or allotype-specific antibodies activate B lymphocytes, but not T lymphocytes; idiotype-specific antibodies and xenogeneic antibodies to certain other cell-surface molecules may activate both B and T lymphocytes.

Other lymphocyte-activating substances are certain lymphokines, periodate, zinc ions, mercury, proteolytic enzymes (trypsin, chymotrypsin), walnut extracts, granulocyte extracts, polyanions (dextran sulfate, polynucleotides), and agents that cause the formation of aldehyde groups on the lymphocyte surface. Mild activation can also be accomplished by physical agents, such as heat, cold, and ultrasonication. The mechanism of activation by these substances and agents is not understood; in at least some instances, the agents might act indirectly by changing the surface properties of lymphocytes in such a way that the change is then recognized as foreign by other lymphocytes.

10.5 APPENDIX 10.1: ANTIGEN-ANTIBODY INTERACTIONS

10.5.1 Binding Forces

Molecules of liquids are in constant motion: they bump into each other like billiard balls, bounce apart, collide with other molecules, rebound, collide again, and so on, and so on—a never-ending, aimless *perpetuum mobile*. However, if one of the colliding molecules is an antigen (hapten) and the other is the corresponding antibody, the molecules may not rebound after the collision; rather, the antigenic determinant may slip into the antibody's combining site and the two may stick together. The reason that the two molecules do not recoil from the collision is that, at the moment when their complementary surfaces come into contact, weak binding forces glue them together. These forces are the same as those governing protein-to-protein interactions in general: hydrogen bonds, ionic bonds, van der Waals bonds, and hydrophobic interactions—all described in Appendix 6.1. The bond holding the molecules together may be stronger in some cases and weaker in others, depending on how well the antigenic determinants fit into the combining sites and how strong the forces are that develop between the molecules.

10.5.2 The Law of Mass Action

However, the binding of antigen to antibody is not irreversible; no matter how good the fit between the two is, they will sooner or later come apart again. The reasons for this dissociation are the slight conformational changes induced by the interactions and thermal motion of molecules: other molecules collide with the antigen-antibody complexes, and during each collision, some energy is passed on to the complexes, making them less stable. The dissociated molecules can then associate again or associate with other molecules, and so it may go on and on—constant coming together and parting. This situation can be expressed by an equation:

$$\mathrm{Ag} + \mathrm{Ab} \leftrightarrows \mathrm{AgAb} \qquad (1)$$

where Ag represents the antigen, Ab the antibody, and AgAb the antigen-antibody complex. (For clarity, individual equations in this section will be numbered.)

According to the physicochemical law known as the *law of mass action*, the association rate (i.e., the rate at which antigen-antibody complexes form) is proportional to the concentration of antigen and antibody, and can thus be expressed as $k_1[\mathrm{Ag}][\mathrm{Ab}]$, where k_1 is the *association rate constant* and the brackets indicate concentrations. Similarly, the dissociation rate of the antigen-antibody complexes is equal to $k_2[\mathrm{AgAb}]$, where k_2 is the *dissociation rate constant*. After mixing of the antigens with the antibodies, the solution eventually reaches *equilibrium*, in which the association rate equals the dissociation rate:

$$k_1[\mathrm{Ag}][\mathrm{Ab}] = k_2[\mathrm{AgAb}] \qquad (2)$$

The k_1/k_2 quotient, the ratio of complexed to free reactants at equilibrium, is known as the *equilibrium constant*, K:

$$K = \frac{k_1}{k_2} = \frac{[\mathrm{AgAb}]}{[\mathrm{Ag}][\mathrm{Ab}]} \qquad (3)$$

This equation can also be written

$$K[\mathrm{Ag}][\mathrm{Ab}] = [\mathrm{AgAb}] \qquad (4)$$

Let us first consider a situation wherein each antibody possesses only one combining site and each antigen molecule only one antigenic determinant. The total concentration of antibody molecules $[\mathrm{Ab}_t]$ equals the sum of concentrations of free antibodies $[\mathrm{Ab}_f]$ and those bound to the antigen $[\mathrm{Ab}_b]$:

$$[\mathrm{Ab}_t] = [\mathrm{Ab}_f] + [\mathrm{Ab}_b] \qquad (5)$$

The concentration of free antibodies is thus:

$$[\mathrm{Ab}_f] = [\mathrm{Ab}_t] - [\mathrm{Ab}_b]. \qquad (6)$$

If we now introduce the Ab value from equation (6) into equation (4), we obtain

$$K[\mathrm{Ag}]([\mathrm{Ab}_t] - [\mathrm{Ab}_b]) = [\mathrm{AgAb}] \qquad (7)$$

After multiplying out the left-hand side of equation (7) and rearranging, we obtain

$$K[\mathrm{Ag}][\mathrm{Ab}_t] = [\mathrm{AgAb}](1 + K[\mathrm{Ag}]) \qquad (8)$$

and after dividing both sides of equation (8) by $[\mathrm{Ab}_b](1 + K[\mathrm{Ag}])$, we obtain

$$\frac{[\mathrm{AgAb}]}{[\mathrm{Ab}_t]} = \frac{K[\mathrm{Ag}]}{1 + K[\mathrm{Ag}]} \qquad (9)$$

The ratio $[\mathrm{AgAb}]/[\mathrm{Ab}_t]$, which we shall designate as r, is the fraction of antibody molecules bound to the antigen (number of molecules of bound antigen per antibody molecule). Equation (9) thus becomes:

$$r = \frac{K[\mathrm{Ag}]}{1 + K[\mathrm{Ag}]} \qquad (10)$$

If we now consider, instead of monovalent antibodies, identical (homogeneous) antibodies with n number of combining sites (n is the valency of the antibody), we can write equation (10) as

$$r = \frac{nK[\text{Ag}]}{1 + K[\text{Ag}]} \tag{11}$$

By multiplying both sides of this equation by $(1 + K[\text{Ag}])$, and rearranging, we obtain

$$r = nK[\text{Ag}] - rK[\text{Ag}] \tag{12}$$

and after dividing by [Ag], we obtain

$$\frac{r}{[\text{Ag}]} = nK - rK \tag{13}$$

or, if we designate [Ag] as c (the concentration of free antigen),

$$\frac{r}{c} = nK - rK \tag{14}$$

When one has a set of values for r and c over a range of antigen concentrations available, one can plot r/c versus r. This so-called *Scatchard plot* (developed by G. Scatchard in 1949; see Fig. 10.16) should, theoretically, give a straight line of slope K (provided all antibody-combining sites are identical and independent). The x (abscissa) intercept of this line gives the n, and the y (ordinate) intercept gives the nK value.

To calculate K and n from equation (14), one must know $[\text{Ab}_t]$, or the total concentration of antibody molecules, [AgAb], or the concentration of antigen bound by the antibody, and [Ag], or the concentration of free antigen. However, the determination of total antibody concentration is possible only when one works with a pure antibody preparation. To bypass the pure-antibody requirement, one can use an alternative method for calculating K, a method in which one needs to know only the concentration of the free and bound antigen. In this method, one derives K for the antibody-combining site, rather than for the antibody molecule, and thus eliminates the n from consideration. Up to equation (9), the derivation proceeds the same way as in the preceding method, with the exception that the symbol Ab now means antibody-combining site. If we take the reciprocal of equation (9), we get

$$\frac{[\text{Ab}_t]}{[\text{AgAb}]} = \frac{1 + K[\text{Ag}]}{K[\text{Ag}]} \tag{15}$$

Dividing both sides of equation (15) by $[\text{Ab}_t]$ produces

$$\frac{1}{[\text{AgAb}]} = \frac{1 + K[\text{Ag}]}{[\text{Ab}_t]K[\text{Ag}]} \tag{16}$$

Expanding the right-hand portion of equation (16), we obtain

$$\frac{1}{[\text{AgAb}]} = \frac{1}{[\text{Ab}_t]K[\text{Ag}]} + \frac{1}{[\text{Ab}_t]} \tag{17}$$

By plotting 1/[AgAb] against 1/[Ag], we obtain a straight line, with a slope $1/K[\text{Ab}_t]$ and y intercept $1/[\text{Ab}_t]$.

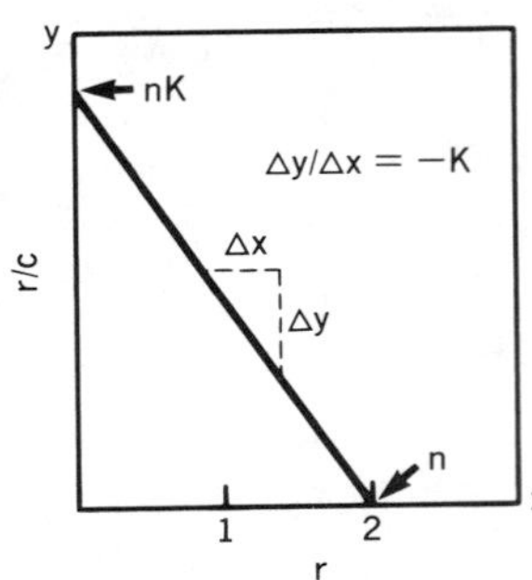

Figure 10.16. Scatchard plot of antigen binding to a homogeneous antibody. Explanation in the text. (From R. N. Pinckard and D. M. Weir *in* D. M. Weir (Ed.): *Handbook of Experimental Immunology*, 2nd ed., pp. 16.1–16.21. Blackwell, Oxford, 1973.)

10.5.3 The Average Association Constant

One of the conditions in the preceding considerations was monovalency of antibodies: we assumed that each antibody had only one combining site, but we know that antibodies normally have at least two. To take this fact into account, we can calculate K from a point on the straight line where, on the average, each antibody reacts with only one, instead of two antigenic determinants (haptens)—in other words, a concentration at which antibody molecules behave as if monovalent. Since, for bivalent antibodies, r is equal to 2, it should be equal to 1 for monovalent antibodies, so that if $r = 1$, and $n = 2$, then equation (14) becomes

$$\frac{1}{c} = 2K - 1K \tag{18}$$

or

$$\frac{1}{c} = K \tag{19}$$

When defined in this way, K is referred to as the *average association constant* and designated K_o. The average association constant is thus the reciprocal of free-antigen concentration. It is obtained by reading the r/c value from the straight line at $r = 1$. Concentration, c, is expressed in moles per liter, and r/c (K_o) in liter moles.

10.5.4 Correction for Antibody Heterogeneity

Another assumption we made in the derivation of the association constants was homogeneity of antibodies: we presumed that all antibodies in a given preparation had the same association constant. In practice, however, antibodies are often a heterogeneous mixture of molecules with different association constants. It is, therefore, desirable to express in some way the range and distribution of association constants in a given antibody preparation. Since individual association constants are randomly distributed around K_o, their spread may be expressed by an error function, such as *Gaussian (normal) distribution*, used in statistics. However, a more common way of evaluating antibody heterogeneity is by the so-called *Sips distribution* (described by R. Sips in 1949), which is similar to the normal distribution, and is expressed by an equation,

$$\frac{r}{n} = \frac{(K_o c)^a}{1 + (K_o c)^a} \tag{20}$$

in which a is the index of heterogeneity (dispersion index of association constants about the average constant, K_o, corresponding to the standard deviation in the normal distribution). Values of a range from 0 to 1; the value $a = 1$ means that all antibodies have the same K (they are homogeneous), and in this case, equation (20) becomes the Scatchard equation. Equation (20) can also be written

$$\log(r/n - r) = a \log c + a \log K_o. \tag{21}$$

A plot of $\log(r/n - r)$ versus $\log c$ gives a straight line, the slope of which is a; the x intercept in this plot gives K_o. For the derivation of equations (20) and (21), the reader should consult the original Sips paper.

10.5.5 Thermodynamics of Antigen-Antibody Interactions

Thermodynamics, in case you have forgotten, is the branch of physics dealing with energy and its transformation. (The literal translation of this term is "heat movement," a designation referring to the fact that heat is used to measure energy.) Energy, or the ability to produce a change (to accomplish work), is measured in calories, where one calorie (kilogram calorie, or kilocalorie) is the amount of heat required to raise the temperature of one kilogram of water from 14.5°C to 15.5°C.

The passage of a system (matter within a defined region) from one state to another is accompanied by a change of energy; indeed, energy is revealed only by change. Consider again the motion of antigen and antibody molecules in a solution. The motion itself is a form of energy (so-called *kinetic energy*). When two molecules collide, the kinetic energy of one molecule can be transferred to the other molecule. As a result, the molecule that gained energy increases its velocity and the one that passed it slows down until it is hit by another molecule with higher kinetic energy. When an antigen molecule collides with an antibody molecule and the two combine, part of the kinetic energy is transferred into the bonds that glue the molecules together. The bonds thus become a storage place of *potential energy*; when the bonds break, the potential energy may be released as heat. The energy changes associated with a reaction such as

$$\text{Ag} + \text{Ab} \leftrightarrows \text{AgAb}$$

can therefore be determined by measuring the amount of heat released (or taken up) during the reaction. However, not all the molecule's energy is used for its movement or for the generation of bonds; some of it is "wasted," for example, on overcoming frictional forces. The usable ("nonwasted") energy is referred to as *free*, and denoted by the symbol G (or F, in the older literature), in honor of the nineteenth-century physicist J. Willard Gibbs. Free energy can be measured only in terms of change (indicated by the Δ sign), either positive or negative, depending on whether energy is consumed or released during a reaction. Hence, ΔG stands for a *change of free energy* that occurs when a system passes from one state to another. In a given system, under given conditions, the change in usable (free) energy equals the change in total energy minus the change in unusable energy: expressed mathematically,

$$\Delta G = \Delta H - T\Delta S \tag{22}$$

where ΔH denotes change in total energy (so-called *enthalpy*, from Gr. *enthalpein*, to warm up), T is the absolute temperature, and ΔS is the change of unusable energy (so-called *entropy*, from Gr. *entropia*, a turning towards). ΔH is positive when energy is absorbed and negative when it is given off. T is obtained by adding the temperature in degrees centigrade to 273.15.

The equilibrium constant, K, is related to free energy change, G, by the expression

$$\Delta G = -RT \ln K \quad (23)$$

where R is the gas constant (1.987 calories/mole) and $\ln K$ the natural logarithm of K, equal to 2.303 log K. Hence,

$$\Delta G = -4.576\ T \log K \quad (24)$$

which means that ΔG can be calculated when K is known. In the antigen-antibody reaction, ΔG is the gain or loss of free energy in calories as one mole of antigen (hapten) and one mole of antibody (combining site) combine to form one mole of AgAb complex. When K is high, ΔG is negative, and the reaction proceeds with a decrease in free energy; when $K = 1$, then $\Delta G = 0$, and the system is at equilibrium, neither liberating nor consuming energy. The values for ΔG for various antigen-antibody combinations range from -6000 to $-11{,}000$ calories (per mole antigen bound), which corresponds to equilibrium constants of 10^5 to 10^9 liters mole^{-1} at 30°C.

10.5.6 Affinity and Avidity

The strength of a reaction between monovalent antigen (hapten) and monovalent antibody (combining site) is referred to as *affinity*. Antibodies that combine loosely with antigens and dissociate readily are said to have low affinity, while those that bind tightly are said to have high affinity. Antibody affinity is influenced by many factors, among which are the closeness of the stereochemical fit between the combining site and the antigenic determinant, and the size of the region over which attractive or repulsive forces act. A measure of affinity is either the equilibrium constant, K, or the free energy change, ΔG. The binding strength of a heterogeneous mixture of antibodies with diverse equilibrium constants is referred to as *average affinity*; the measure of average affinity is the average equilibrium constant, K_o.

Affinity must be distinguished from *avidity*, a term introduced by Rudolf Kraus to explain the observation that the antitoxin content did not always correlate with the protective ability of an antiserum. Kraus postulated that the protective ability of antibodies depended on their binding power, or avidity. Contemporary immunologists use "avidity" as a designation for the overall tendency of antibodies to combine with antigens, particularly antibodies with multiple combining sites and antigens with multiple determinants. Hence, affinity is a more precise, and avidity a more nebulous, designation for the rate of antigen-antibody reaction.

But just to complicate things, some immunologists use avidity synonymously with affinity, and others define affinity and avidity in a manner exactly the opposite of that described above. Had there been no Biblical Tower of Babel, scientists would have built one.

Avidity is expressed in terms of *titer*—that is, the last serial dilution of antibodies that still gives a visible reaction with the antigen. Avidity is influenced by affinity, valency of antigens and antibodies, and composition of antibodies.

10.5.7 Factors Influencing Antigen-Antibody Reactions

Temperature

Theoretically, raising the temperature should increase the thermal motion of molecules, the number of molecular collisions, and consequently, the speed of specific antigen-antibody reactions. By the same token, nonspecific reactions should be slowed by raising the temperature, since increased motion prevents molecules from forming weak bonds. In actuality, however, many antigen-antibody interactions are conspicuously unaffected by temperature changes in the range between 4° and 40°C. An exception is the reaction mediated by the so-called *cold agglutinins*, which, for reasons unknown, react better at 4°C than at 37°C (see Chapter 14). Increasing the temperature above 55°C usually slows antigen-antibody reactions, mainly because of protein denaturation and an increased dissociation rate.

Ionic Strength and pH

All antigen-antibody bonds involve charge interactions; it is therefore not surprising that the concentration of ions in the solution affects these interactions. A decrease in ionic strength increases antigen-antibody reaction, not only by affecting charge interactions at the combining site, but perhaps also by minimizing perturbations of antibody structure caused by ionic attractions. An increase in ionic strength decreases antibody uptake, and high salt concentrations are sometimes used to elute antibodies from antigen-antibody complexes. Similarly, lowering pH usually results in decreasing antigen-antibody interaction, and this fact,

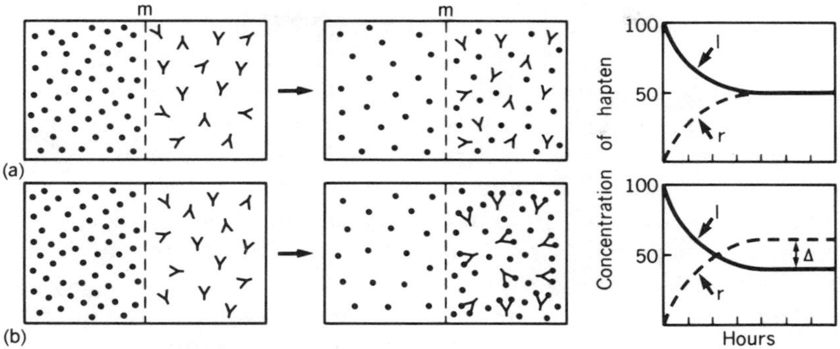

Figure 10.17. Principle of equilibrium dialysis. (*a*) Antibody separated by a semipermeable membrane (m) does not react with hapten in the solution. (*b*) Antibody does react with the hapten. Explanation in the text; l, hapten concentration in left chamber; r, hapten concentration in right chamber; Δ, difference between l and r at equilibrium.

too, is used for the elution of antibodies from immunoadsorbent columns.

10.5.8 Kinetics

A chemical reaction cannot proceed faster than the speed with which molecules meet by diffusion; since the antigen-antibody reactions approach this limit, the majority of collisions between antigens and antibody molecules result in bond formation. The antigen-antibody interaction is thus one of the fastest chemical reactions known. In comparison, interactions leading to covalent bond formation have an association rate a million times lower. Such fast reactions are difficult to study, and it has been necessary to devise special techniques to measure them.

10.5.9 Methods of Measuring Equilibrium Constants

Several methods are available for determining the value of the equilibrium constant, K, for a given antigen (hapten)-antibody reaction: equilibrium dialysis, fluorescent quenching, hapten-inhibition of precipitation, and ultracentrifuge measurement. (In actuality, however, all the methods are calibrated against the determinations by equilibrium analysis.)

Equilibrium Dialysis

To calculate K, one needs to know the concentrations of free and bound hapten (antigen) after the hapten-antibody equilibrium has been established. To determine these two values, one uses a dialysis cell, consisting of two compartments separated by a semipermeable membrane. One places a known amount of the low-molecular-weight, radioactively labeled hapten in one compartment and the high-molecular-weight antibody in the other, and then samples the solution in the antibody compartment periodically. The pores in the separating membrane are too small for the antibodies to move out of the compartment but large enough for the hapten molecules to move into it, so the hapten will diffuse into the antibody compartment until its concentration in both compartments is the same. However, some of the diffusing hapten will react with the antibody, so that at equilibrium, the amount of *free* hapten will be the same in both compartments. But since the bound hapten does not "count," the concentration of *total* hapten will be greater in the antibody compartment than in the hapten compartment (Fig. 10.17). The difference in the total hapten concentration between the two compartments indicates the amount of hapten bound to the antibody.

Fluorescence Quenching

Tryptophan residues in a protein such as the antibody absorb ultraviolet (UV) light with a wave length of 280 nm and emit fluorescent light with a wave length of from 330 to 350 nm. When an antibody reacts with an antigen, some of the energy that would ordinarily be emitted is transferred to the bound molecules and dissipated. Binding of antigens to antibodies thus extinguishes, or quenches, the fluorescence of UV-irradiated molecules. Since the degree of fluorescence quenching is proportional to the number of antibody-combining sites interacting with the antigen, by measuring fluorescence of an antibody solution during gradual addition of small amounts of antigen, one can determine the amount of bound antigen.

Inhibition of Precipitation by a Hapten

After a univalent hapten has bound to an antibody combining site, this site is no longer available for subsequent binding of bivalent antigens; since bivalent antigens are needed for precipitation of antigen-antibody complexes to occur (see Appendix 10.2), the addition of a hapten inhibits antigen precipitation. Furthermore, since the more hapten added, the greater the inhibition, using this assay, one can determine the amount of free hapten.

Ultracentrifuge Measurements

In this assay, the hapten is reacted with antibody and the mixture spun down in an ultracentrifuge. Since free hapten sediments at a rate slower than that of hapten-antibody complexes, the two components can be separated and the concentration of free hapten determined.

10.5.10 Specificity of Antigen-Antibody Reactions

The most striking characteristic of antigen-antibody reactions is their *specificity*: an antibody produced against a given antigen will react with this antigen and perhaps a few other, related antigens, but will not react with the rest of the antigen universe. The question, then, is what determines whether an antibody reacts not only with the inducing (*homologous*) antigen, but also with some other (*heterologous*) antigen. A partial answer to this question was provided by Karl Landsteiner and his colleagues, who, in the years between 1917 and 1943, systematically analyzed the conditions affecting the specificity of antigen-antibody reactions. Landsteiner summarized these studies in the now-classic treatise, *The Specificity of Serologic Reactions* (see *References*). Many aspects of serological specificity have also been elucidated by Michael Heidelberger, Elvin A. Kabat, Herman N. Eisen, Fred Karush, and David Pressman. The general approach used in these studies is based on the observation by F. Obermayer and E. P. Pick that the specificity of proteins can be modified by the attachment of simple chemicals. The idea is to immunize an animal (say, a rabbit) with a hapten, X, attached to a protein derived from another animal (say, a horse) and to test the antibodies against a series of haptens—X, Y, and Z—where Y and Z differ from X only slightly, but in a precisely defined manner. The testing can be either direct (with the haptens attached to a protein of still another species—say, a fowl—so that reactivity of antibodies to the immunizing protein itself is excluded), or indirect (haptens Y and Z are used for inhibition of anti-hapten-X reaction). Landsteiner and his colleagues evaluated the reactions on a plus-minus basis; other investigators made quantitative determinations and used the equilibrium constant, K, as a measure of the reaction.

Some of the factors influencing serological specificity are discussed below; for other factors, the interested reader should consult Landsteiner's book and the monograph by Pressman and Grossberg (see *References*).

Table 10.6 The Effect of Different Ionic (Acidic) Groups on the Specificity of Hapten Antibody Reactions

	Reactivity with			
Antiserum Against	NH_2 (benzene ring) Aminobenzene (Aniline)	NH_2 (benzene ring) $COOH$ *p*-Amino-Benzoic Acid	NH_2 (benzene ring) SO_3H *p*-Aminobenzene Sulfonic Acid	NH_2 (benzene ring) AsO_3H_2 *p*-Aminobenzene Arsenic Acid
Aminobenzene	+++	0	0	0
p-Aminobenzoic acid	0	+++±	0	0
p-Aminobenzene sulfonic acid	0	0	+++±	0
p-Aminobenzene arsenic acid	0	0	0	+++±

Source. Based on K. Landsteiner: *The Specificity of Serologic Reactions*. Dover Press, New York, 1962.
0, no reactivity; +++, strong reactivity

Table 10.7 The Effect of Different Nonionic Groups on the Specificity of Hapten-Antibody Reactions

	Reactivity with			
Antiserum Against	Aminobenzene (Aniline) [NH_2–C$_6$H$_5$]	*p*-Chloro-amino Benzene [NH_2, Cl]	*p*-Toluidine [NH_2, CH_3]	*p*-Nitroamino Benzene [NH_2, NO_2]
Aminobenzene	+++±	+	+±	+
p-Chloroaminobenzene	±++±	++	++	+±
p-Toluidine	+±	++	++	+
p-Nitroaminobenzene	+	++	+±	+

Source. Based on K. Landsteiner: *The Specificity of Serologic Reactions.* Dover Press, New York, 1962.
+, +±, ++, different degrees of reactivity

The Effect of Ionic Groups. Table 10.6 compares the reactivity of four antisera made against aminobenzene derivatives with different ionic (acidic) groups in the para position. In every instance, the antiserum reacts only with the immunizing hapten, not with any of the three related haptens. This finding indicates that ionic groups play a dominant role in determining specificity of antigen-antibody reactions.

The Effect of Nonionic Groups. In sharp contrast to ionic groups, nonionic groups have a much less striking effect on the specificity of antigen-antibody reactions. In Table 10.7, antibodies to aminobenzene derivatives with different nonionic groups in the para position react not only with the immunizing hapten, but also with the other three haptens. Some of the reactions with the nonhomologous haptens are as strong as those with the homologous haptens; others are weaker.

The Effect of Spatial Arrangement. In Table 10.8, antisera were produced against aminobenzene deriva-

Table 10.8 The Effect of Position of a Chemical Group (–COOH) on the Specificity of Hapten-Antibody Reactions

	Reactivity with			
Antiserum Against	Aminobenzene [NH_2]	*o*-Aminobenzoic Acid [NH_2, COOH]	*m*-Aminobenzoic Acid [NH_2, COOH]	*p*-Aminobenzoic Acid [NH_2, COOH]
Aminobenzene	+++	0	0	0
o-Aminobenzoic acid	0	+++	0	0
m-Aminobenzoic acid	0	0	++++	0
p-Aminobenzoic acid	0	0	0	+++±

Source. Based on K. Landsteiner: *The Specificity of Serologic Reactions.* Dover Press, New York, 1962.
0, no reactivity; +++ and ++++ strong reactivity

tives differing only in the respective positioning of the amino and carboxyl groups (ortho-, meta-, and para-arrangement). Yet, in each case, the antisera are absolutely specific for the immunizing hapten and fail to react with any of the other isomers. Thus, even when the overall composition of a molecule is the same, the spatial distribution of the chemical groups matters very much in determining whether the molecule will react with a given antibody.

The Effect of Stereoisomerism. In some instances, antibodies even distinguish between haptens carrying the same, but somewhat differently oriented, groups at the same position. In Table 10.9, *p*-aminophenyl-α-glucoside differs from *p*-aminophenyl-β-glucoside only in that, in the former, the aminobenzene is located above and, in the latter, below the plane of the glucose ring; yet this difference is enough to lower the reactivity of antibodies with the heterologous hapten significantly. An even more drastic effect of orientation is seen with *p*-aminophenyl-β-galactoside, which differs from the β-glucoside in the arrangement of one of the hydroxyl (OH) groups in relation to the sugar ring. Here, antibodies to one molecule do not react at all with the other molecule. Similarly, as is shown in Table 10.10, the arrangement of the hydroxyl groups in tartaric acid is decisive in determining the cross-reactivity of anti-sera produced against this hapten. Only antisera against the meso form, which may be regarded as half dextro and half levo, also react weakly with the other two forms (D and L).

The Effect of Terminal Groups. In haptens consisting of two amino acids (dipeptides) attached to a protein carrier, it is often the free-terminal group that determines the specificity of the antigen-antibody reaction. Thus, for example, an antibody to glycyl-leucyl-protein does not react with a leucyl-glycyl-protein, and vice versa (Table 10.11), despite the fact that both haptens contain the same two amino acids: it is the free amino acid (i.e., the amino acid not conjugated directly to the protein) that matters.

The Effect of Chain Length. By attaching aliphatic chains to aminobenzene and then coupling the entire molecule to a protein, Landsteiner demonstrated that chain length also plays a role in determining specificity of antigen-antibody reaction. Antisera against short-chain (oxanilic and succinanilic) acids reacted only with the immunizing hapten, but antisera against the longer-chain acids also reacted with some heterologous haptens (Table 10.12). A difference of one or two

Table 10.9 The Effect of the Glycoside Bond on the Specificity of Hapten-Antibody Reactions

	Reactivity with		
Antiserum Against	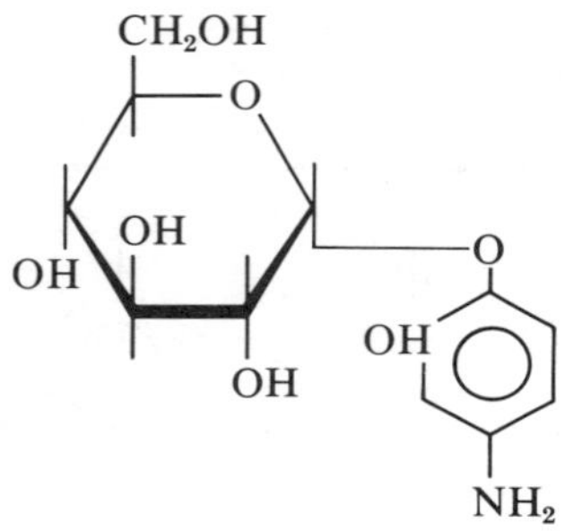 *p*-Aminophenyl-α-Glucoside	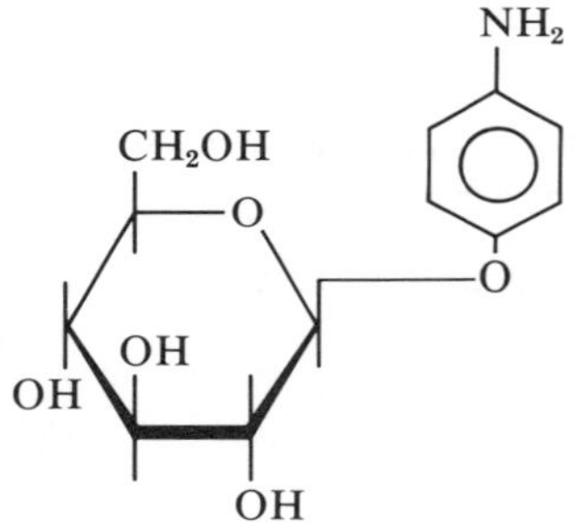 *p*-Aminophenyl-β-Glucoside	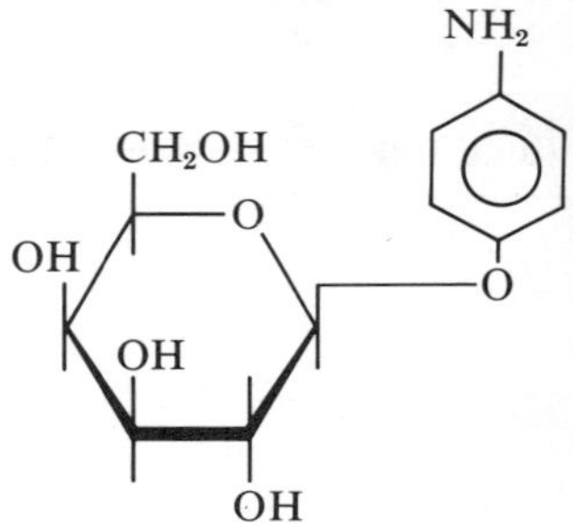 *p*-Aminophenyl-β-Galactoside
p-Aminophenyl-α-glucoside	+++	+	0
p-Aminophenyl-β-glucoside	++	++++	0
p-Aminophenyl-β-galactoside	0	0	+++

Source. Based on K. Landsteiner: *The Specificity of Serologic Reactions*. Dover Press, New York, 1962.
0, no reactivity; + through ++++, different degrees of reactivity

Table 10.10 The Effect of Stereoisomerism on the Specificity of Hapten-Antibody Reactions

Antiserum Against	Reactivity with		
	COOH HO—CH HC—OH COOH D-Tartaric Acid	COOH HC—OH HO—CH COOH L-Tartaric Acid	COOH HC—OH HC—OH COOH M-Tartaric Acid
D-tartaric acid	++±	0	±
L-tartaric acid	0	++±	±
M-tartaric acid	±	0	+++

Source. Based on K. Landsteiner: *The Specificity of Serologic Reactions*. Dover Press, New York, 1962. 0, no reactivity; ±, weak reactivity; ++± and +++, strong reactivity

carbon atoms completely changed the reactivity of a short chain; much more extensive changes were needed to alter the reactivity of a long chain.

10.5.11 Crossreactivity

The reactivity of an antibody with nonhomologous antigens is referred to as *crossreactivity*. In Chapter 6, we considered crossreactivity from the standpoint of antibodies; here, we shall briefly discuss crossreactivity in relation to antigens. At the antigen level, crossreactivity can occur because of antigen heterogeneity, determinant sharing, or determinant similarity (see Fig. 8.2).

Antigen Heterogeneity

An immunizing preparation containing several different antigenic molecules will produce a mixture of antibodies, each antibody specific for different molecules. Any preparation containing one or more of these molecules, but differing from the immunizing preparation in other molecules, will crossreact with the polyspecific antiserum.

Determinant Sharing.

An antigenic molecule carrying several antigenic determinants may produce a mixture of determinant-specific antibodies. A molecule distinct from the immunizing antigen but sharing at least one of the determinants with it will crossreact with the polyspecific antiserum.

Determinant Similarity.

An antibody produced to a given determinant is often not absolutely specific; it may also crossreact with determinants different from, but resembling the immunizing determinant. Examples of this type of crossreactivity were described in the preceding section. One way of distinguishing between these three types of crossreactivity is by absorption, as described in Chapter 8.

10.5.12 Main Forms of Antigen-Antibody Reaction: Precipitation and Agglutination

Precipitation

A Historical Note. When a small molecule, such as a hapten, combines with an antibody, the resulting antigen-antibody complex remains soluble, and is thus invisible to the immunologist's eye; but when a macromolecule enters such a reaction, the insoluble antigen-antibody complex falls out (precipitates) of the solution in a visible form. The discovery of this *precipitin reaction*[2] by Rudolf Kraus in 1897 (see Chapter 2) provided a means of quantitating antigen-antibody interactions and thus set the stage for understanding the chemistry and mechanism of these interactions. Before Kraus, all immunologists could do was make serial dilutions of an antiserum and demonstrate that, at a certain concentration, the antibodies ceased to agglutinate bacteria or ceased to protect an animal in whose blood deadly toxins were circulating. Since

[2] Precipitating antibodies, or *precipitins*, were originally thought to be a special class of antibodies induced by a special class of antigens—*precipitinogens*.

Table 10.11 The Effect of Terminal Groups on the Specificity of Hapten-Antibody Reactions

	Reactivity with			
	$^{+}H_3N-CH_2-CO-NH-CH_2-COO^-$	$^{+}H_3N-CH_2-CO-NH-CH(CH_2CH(CH_3)_2)-COO^-$	$^{+}H_3N-CH(CH_2CH(CH_3)_2)-CO-NH-CH_2-COO^-$	$^{+}H_3N-CH(CH_2CH(CH_3)_2)-CO-NH-CH(CH_2CH(CH_3)_2)-COO^-$
Antiserum Against	Glycyl Glycine	Glycyl Leucine	Leucyl Glycine	Leucyl Leucine
Glycyl glycine	++±	0	0	0
Glycyl leucine	0	++±	0	±
Leucyl glycine	+	0	+++	0
Leucyl leucine	0	+	0	++

Source. Based on K. Landsteiner: *The Specificity of Serologic Reactions*. Dover Press, New York, 1962.
0, no reactivity; ± through +++, different degrees of reactivity

Table 10.12 The Effect of Chain Length on the Specificity of Hapten-Antibody Reactions

	Reactivity with						
Antiserum Against	$NH_2-C_6H_4-NH-CO-COOH$ *p*-Amino Oxanilic Acid	$NH_2-C_6H_4-NH-CO-CH_2-COOH$ *p*-Amino Malonanilic Acid	$NH_2-C_6H_4-NH-CO-(CH_2)_2-COOH$ *p*-Amino Succinanilic Acid	$NH_2-C_6H_4-NH-CO-(CH_2)_3-COOH$ *p*-Amino Glutaranilic Acid	$NH_2-C_6H_4-NH-CO-(CH_2)_4-COOH$ *p*-Amino Adipanilic Acid	$NH_2-C_6H_4-NH-CO-(CH_2)_5-COOH$ *p*-Amino Pimelanilic Acid	$NH_2-C_6H_4-NH-CO-(CH_2)_6-COOH$ *p*-Amino Suberanilic Acid
p-Aminooxanilic acid	++	0	0	0	0	0	0
p-Aminosuccinilic acid	0	0	+++	+	0	0	0
p-Aminoadipanilic acid	0	0	±	+	++	+±	+±
p-Aminosuberanilic acid	0	0	±	+±	++±	+++±	++++

Source. Based on K. Landsteiner: *The Specificity of Serologic Reactions*. Dover Press, New York, 1962.
0, no reactivity; ± through ++++, different degrees of reactivity

Table 10.13 Reaction of Rabbit Antiovalbumin Serum with Increasing Amounts of Ovalbumin

Antigen Added (μg)	Precipitated Antigen (μg)	Total Precipitated Protein (μg)	Precipitated Antibody (μg)	Antibody: Antigen Ratio	Precipitated Antibody Calculated from Equation (μg)	Tests on Supernatant
9.1	Total	156	147	16.2	137	Excess Ab
15.5	Total	236	220	14.2	225	Excess Ab
25	Total	374	349	14.0	343	Excess Ab
40	Total	526	468	12.2	499	Excess Ab
50	Total	632	582	11.6	582	Excess Ab
65	Total	740	675	10.4	677	Excess Ab
74	Total	794	720	9.7	714	No Ab or Ag
82	Total	830	748	9.1	738	No Ab, 1 μg Ag
90	87	826	739	8.5	746	Excess Ag
98	89	820	731	8.2		Excess Ag
124	87	730	643	7.4		Excess Ag
135	(72)[a]	610	(538)	7.5		Excess Ag
195	(48)	414	(366)	(7.6)		Excess Ag
307	(4)	106				Excess Ag
490		42				Excess Ag

Source. Data from M. Heidelberger and F. E. Kendall: *J. Exp. Med.* **62:**617, 1935.
Ab, antibody; Ag, antigen (ovalbumin)
[a] Values in parentheses are considered uncertain.

some antisera could be diluted more than others before they ceased to be active, researchers assumed that the former were "stronger" than the latter. But immunologists had no means of elucidating the cause of these differences until the precipitin reaction was discovered. Here, pure antigen-antibody complexes separated from the rest of the molecules in the solution and made themselves available from chemical analysis. Still, it took more than 40 years before the first such analysis was actually carried out, by Michael Heidelberger and Forrest M. Kendall.

The Assay. To measure the precipitin reaction, one sets up a series of tubes and adds to each tube a constant amount of antibody and an amount of antigen that increases progressively from the first tube to the last. (One can also do the test the other way around, keeping the concentration of antigen constant and increasing the antibody concentration, but this variant is rarely used.) After incubation in the refrigerator for at least 24 hours (to allow completion of the reaction), one centrifuges the tubes, separates the sediment (precipitate) from the supernatant, and determines the following values: the amount of precipitate (antigen-antibody complexes); the amount of antigen and antibody in the precipitate; the presence or absence of antigen and antibody in the supernatant.

To measure the amount of precipitate formed following the interaction of a protein antigen and antibody, Heidelberger and Kendall used the so-called micro-Kjeldahl technique of nitrogen determination.[3] They reasoned that since most proteins contain nitrogen, and since the antigen-antibody complexes were proteins, the determination should give the amount of precipitin after the values obtained had been multiplied by a factor corresponding to the nitrogen content of the proteins (about 16 percent). In modern immunological laboratories, the protein is measured in a less laborious way—for example, by determining the absorption of ultraviolet light, by using the color reaction of ninhydrin with amino groups, or by using the so-

[3] In this technique, named after the nineteenth-century chemist Johan G. C. Kjeldahl, the organic substance is digested with concentrated sulfuric acid in the presence of an appropriate catalyst and distilled, and ammonia is determined in the ammonium sulfate thus formed.

called Folin-Ciocalteu reagent. (Sometimes it suffices to know only the amount of the precipitated antigen or of the precipitated antibody. To determine these values, one can use radioactively labeled reagents—either antigens or antibodies).

The determination of antigen and antibody content in the precipitate is tied in with the determination of antigen and antibodies in the supernatant (see below). In tubes in which the supernatant does not contain any demonstrable antigen after the reaction has taken place, it is assumed that all of the antigen has entered into the precipitate. In this case, the amount of antigen in the precipitate equals the amount of antigen added to the tube, and the amount of antibody equals the total amount of precipitated protein minus the amount of antigen. In tubes in which some antigen remains in the supernatant even after the completion of the reaction, one must determine how much of the antigen is left behind and subtract this value from the total amount of antigen added, to obtain the amount of antigen in the precipitate.

The data thus obtained are arranged in a table (Table 10.13) and plotted (Fig. 10.18), with the total protein (or antibody) precipitated on the ordinate and the amount of antigen added on the abscissa.

The Precipitin Curve. Figure 10.18 depicts a typical plot of a quantitative precipitin reaction, based on the data Heidelberger and Kendall obtained with rabbit antiserum to fowl ovalbumin. One can see that, with the addition of increasing amounts of antigen, the amount of precipitate rises until it reaches a maximum (*point of maximum precipitation*) and then declines. This precipitation curve starts at the 0 value on the abscissa; other curves, however, may start at some positive value and instead of having the parabolic shape shown, may be bell-shaped (Fig. 10.19). This latter type of curve is often obtained with horse antisera, so it is sometimes referred to as *horse-type*, in contrast to the *rabbit-type* shown in Figure 10.18. Another name for the horse-type curve is the *flocculation curve*, derived from *flocculation* (L. *floccus*, tuft of

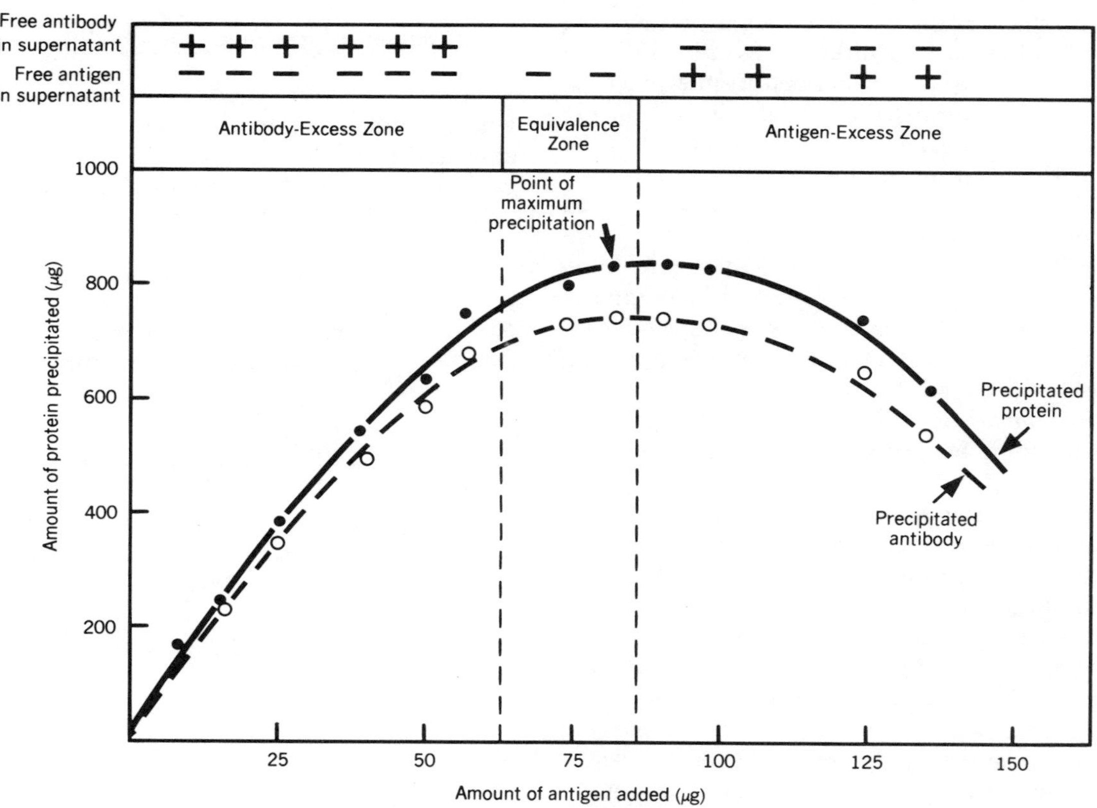

Figure 10.18. The precipitin curve. Quantitative precipitin reaction between ovalbumin and rabbit antibody to ovalbumin. (Based on the data of M. Heidelberger and F. E. Kendall: *J. Exp. Med.* **62:**697–000, 1935.)

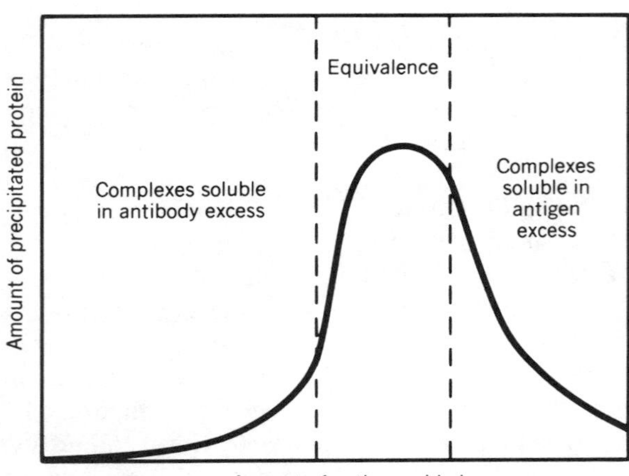

Figure 10.19. The flocculation curve.

wool), a term used for a precipitin reaction inhibited by extreme antibody, as well as antigen excesses. The shape of the curve probably depends, to a large degree, on the predominant class of the antibody in the antiserum, and on the solubility of antigen-antibody complexes in the antibody excess.

Based on the results of supernatant testing, the curve can be divided into three zones: the *antibody-excess zone* (*prozone*), characterized by the presence of free antibody and absence of free antigen in the supernatant; the *equivalence zone*, characterized by the absence in the supernatant of both the antigen and antibody; and the *antigen-excess zone*, characterized by the presence of antigen and absence of free antibody (Fig. 10.18). The point of maximum precipitation usually lies in the equivalence zone or in the zone of slight antigen excess. The portion of the antigen-excess zone in which the quantity of antigen-antibody precipitate decreases is called the *inhibition zone*. In Figure 10.18, the antigen-excess and -inhibition zones overlap, but with some horse antisera, the curve levels in the antigen-excess zone before it starts to decline, and in such instances, the inhibition zone constitutes only part of the antigen-excess zone; some immunologists even divide this zone further into zones of complete and partial inhibition.

With monospecific antisera, the supernatants in individual test tubes are Ag^-Ab^+, Ag^-Ab^-, or Ag^+Ab^-, but never Ag^+Ab^+. With polyspecific antisera, on the other hand, Ag^+Ab^+ supernatants may occur, and can be explained by different equivalence zones of the two or more antibodies involved: the doubly positive supernatants probably represent an $Ag_1^+Ag_2^-Ab_1^-Ab_2^+$ situation, where Ag_1 and Ag_2, and Ab_1 and Ab_2 are two different kinds of antigen and antibody, respectively (the antigen-excess zone of one antigen overlaps the antibody-excess zone of the other antigen). The occurrence of doubly positive supernatants thus represents a simple means of detecting polyspecificity of antisera in the precipitation test.

Composition of the Precipitate. The ratio of antibody and antigen in the precipitate varies, depending on the amount of antigen added and on other factors, such as the molecular weight of the antigen. In most instances, nearly all of the precipitate is made up of the antibody (Fig. 10.18); only in the case of a few high-molecular-weight antigens does the antigen dominate quantitatively over the antibody. When one plots the ratio

$$\frac{\text{amount of precipitated antibody}}{\text{amount of antigen added}}$$

against the amount of antigen added, one obtains a straight line, extending over the antibody-excess zone and leveling in the antigen-excess zone (Fig. 10.20). The straight segment of the line can be expressed by an equation,

$$\frac{\text{amount of precipitated antibody}}{x} = a - bx \quad (25)$$

where x is the amount of antigen added and a and b are constants (a is the intercept of the line on the ordinate and b is the slope of the curve). After multiplying both sides of equation (25) by x, one obtains

$$\text{amount of precipitated antibody} = ax - bx^2 \quad (26)$$

By substituting x for the actual values of antigen, one can then calculate the expected amount of precipitated

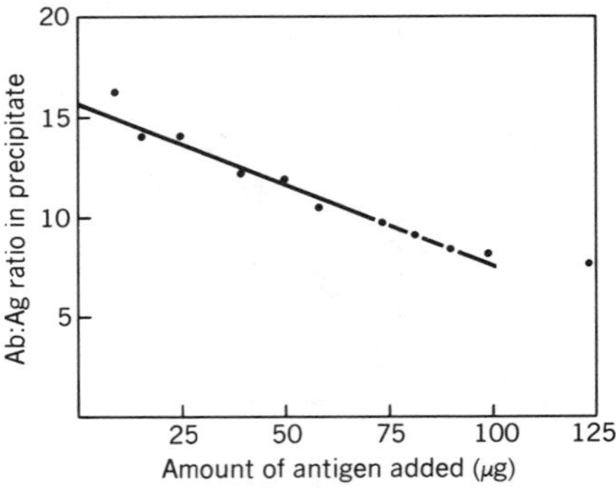

Figure 10.20. The plot of [amount of precipitated antibody/amount of added antigen] against the added antigen. Plotted values obtained from the antibody-excess zone in Figure 10.18.

antibody. For the experiment in Table 10.13, the calculated values are given in column 6; one can see that there is a good agreement between the expected (column 6) and obtained (column 4) values. Equation (25) was originally derived empirically, but it can also be derived theoretically from the law of mass action.

Conversion of Ab : Ag Ratios into Molecular Ratios. Once one knows the amount of precipitated antibody, one can calculate the molecular ratio in which antigens and antibodies combine in the precipitate. For this calculation, one uses the formula:

$$\frac{\text{amount of precipitated antibody}}{\text{molecular weight of antibody}} : \frac{\text{amount of added antigen}}{\text{molecular weight of antigen}}$$

In the example used, ovalbumin has a molecular weight of 42,000 daltons, and the predominant antibody in the hyperimmune rabbit anti-ovalbumin serum is IgG, with a molecular weight of 165,000 daltons. The ratios for three of the 15 tubes in Table 10.13 are:

$$\text{Antibody-excess zone:}\quad \frac{147/165{,}000}{9.1/42{,}000} = 4.1$$

$$\text{Equivalence zone:}\quad \frac{748/165{,}000}{82/42{,}000} = 2.3$$

$$\text{Antigen-excess zone:}\quad \frac{643/165{,}000}{124/42{,}000} = 1.3$$

The values corroborate the statement made above that the Ab : Ag ratios in the precipitate depend on the amount of added antigen: when 9.1 μg of antigen were added, four antibody molecules combined with one antigen molecule; the addition of 82 μg of antigen resulted in the binding of two antibody molecules with one antigen molecule; and the addition of 124 μg of antigen resulted in a one-antibody-to-one-antigen ratio. Examples of ratios for other antigens are given in Table 10.14. These calculations can also be used to obtain the valency of the antigen—the ratio of antibody to antigen molecules at the extreme antibody excess where every antigenic determinant binds a separate antibody molecule. The valency is equal to the a value, the intercept of the line in Figure 10.20 with the ordinate. It correlates reasonably well with the molecular weight (Table 10.15), which is not surprising since, the larger a molecule is, the more antigenic determinants it can carry.

The Lattice Theory. The molecular composition of the antigen-antibody complexes in the different zones of the precipitin curve influences the size, and thus the solubility (or precipitability), of these complexes. In the antibody-excess zone, virtually every antigenic molecule is complexed with an antibody, but since there is not enough antigen to bind to all antibody molecules, some of these remain free. And because of the relatively small number of antigenic molecules, there is only a low probability of a single antibody molecule's binding two antigenic molecules simultaneously, so that the predominant type of complex consists of one antigen molecule surrounded by several antibody molecules. (The number of the latter depends on, among other things, the valency of the particular molecule; see Fig. 10.21.) Since small complexes are soluble and since large, insoluble complexes form only with low

Table 10.14 Molecular Composition of Antigen (Ag)–Antibody (Ab) Precipitates in Different Zones of the Precipitin Curve

		Composition of Precipitate at				
Antigen	Antibody	Extreme Antibody Excess	Antibody Excess, End of Equivalence Zone	Antigen Excess, End of Equivalence Zone	Zone of Partial Inhibition	Composition of Soluble Compound in Zone of Partial Inhibition
Ovalbumin	Rabbit	Ab_5Ag	Ab_3Ag	Ab_5Ag_2	Ab_2Ag	(Ab Ag)
Ovalbumin	Horse	(Ab_4Ag)	Ab_2Ag		Ab Ag	$(Ab\ Ag_2)$
Serum albumin	Rabbit	Ab_6Ag	Ab_4Ag	Ab_3Ag	Ab_2Ag	(Ab Ag)
Thyroglobulin	Rabbit	$Ab_{10}Ag$	$Ab_{14}Ag$	$Ab_{10}Ag$	Ab_2Ag	(Ab Ag)
Tobacco mosaic virus	Rabbit	$Ab_{900}Ag$	$Ab_{450}Ag$	—	—	—
Diphtheria toxin	Horse	Ab_8Ag	Ab_4Ag	Ab_3Ag_2	Ab Ag	$(Ab\ Ag_2)$

Source. From W. C. Boyd: *Fundamentals of Immunology*, 4th ed., Wiley, New York, 1966.

Table 10.15 Correlation Between Molecular Weight and Valence of Antigens

Antigen	Molecular Weight	Approximate Mole Ratio Ab/Ag of Precipitates in Extreme Antibody Excess
Bovine pancreatic ribonuclease	13,600	3
Chicken ovalbumin	42,000	5
Horse serum albumin	69,000	6
Human γ-globulin	160,000	7
Horse apoferritin	465,000	26
Thyroglobulin	700,000	40
Tomato bushy stunt virus	8,000,000	90
Tobacco mosaic virus	40,000,000	650

Source. Based on E. A. Kabat *in* Kabat and Mayer: *Experimental Immunochemistry*, 2nd ed. Thomas, Springfield, Illinois, 1961.

probability, only a small amount of precipitate falls out of the solution. However, as the amount of added antigen increases, more antibody molecules crosslink individual antigen molecules and form a reasonably stable network, or lattice, of alternating antigen and antibody molecules (Fig. 10.21*b*). This lattice is most developed in the equivalence zone, when almost all antigen and antibody molecules participate in the formation of relatively large complexes that precipitate easily out of solution. Then, as the concentration of antigen continues to increase, many antigen molecules surround each antibody molecule, separating it from other antibody molecules and thus preventing lattice formation (Fig. 10.21*c*). The size and precipitability of the antigen-antibody complexes gradually decline and the antigen excess begins to inhibit lattice formation. This *lattice theory*, originally proposed by John R. Marrack in 1934, explains why antigen-antibody complexing, unlike other biochemical reactions, goes through a maximum and then declines.

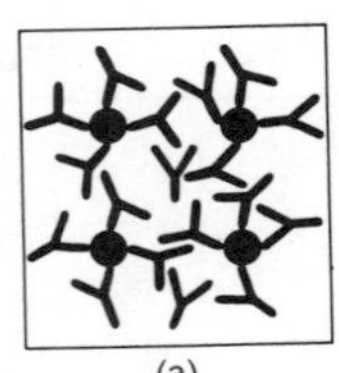
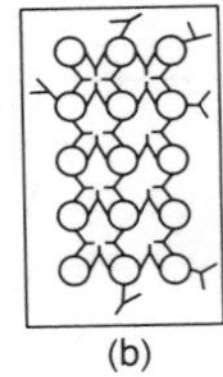
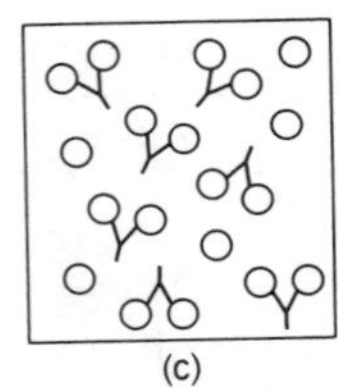
(a) (b) (c)

Figure 10.21. Schematic representation of the predominant type of antigen-antibody complexes present in (*a*) the zone of extreme antibody excess, (*b*) the equivalence zone, and (*c*) the zone of extreme antigen excess.

Reversibility of Precipitation. Originally, immunologists believed that precipitates, once formed, could not dissolve spontaneously into free antigens and antibodies. The one observation that seemed to support this belief was the *Danysz phenomenon*. In 1902, J. Danysz reported that, when one adds to a given amount of diphtheria toxin an equivalent amount of antitoxin, the residual toxicity of the mixture varies, depending on how the two reagents are mixed. If antigen is added to the antibody all at once, the antibody is nontoxic when injected into animals. If, on the other hand, one mixes, say, only half the antigen with the antibody, waits 15 to 30 minutes, and then adds the second half, the mixture is toxic. Danysz interpreted this result to mean that the first half of the antigen engages all the antibody in the formation of irreversible complexes, so that no free antibody remains to neutralize the second half of the toxin added half an hour later. This observation and its interpretation seem to be contradictory to what we know about the antigen-antibody reaction. Since the reaction obeys the law of mass action, the binding of the first half of the toxin should be reversible, so that free antibody for the binding of the second half should be available. However, it is only a *seeming* contradiction, and can be explained by the slowness of the dissociation rates of certain antigen-antibody complexes, of which the toxin-antitoxin system is an example. The release of the free antitoxin from the initial complex is simply so slow that the reaction appears irreversible and the complex insoluble. It should be added, however, that some immunologists consider the Danysz phenomenon to be an artifact.

Another striking example of antigen-antibody reaction with a slow dissociation rate is the binding of antibodies to viruses, in which the establishment of equilibrium often requires days, or even months. It is apparently the antibody, rather than the antigen, that is responsible for the stability of some antigen-antibody complexes. In contrast to these systems, in many other systems the addition of fresh antigen to already formed complexes results in dissolution of the precipitate as expected: the additional antigen pushes the system into the antigen-excess zone in which the antibody, freed by the dissociation, forms small, soluble complexes.

Nonprecipitating Antibodies. In some instances, no visible precipitation occurs, although one can prove, by other means, that antigen-antibody reaction is taking place and although the same antigen tested with other antibodies precipitates normally. It must, therefore, be the antibodies that are responsible for the absence of precipitation in systems containing precipitable antigens. What it is that makes antibodies nonprecipitable is not known. Originally, immunologists thought such antibodies to be univalent, and hence incapable of antigen crosslinking, which is needed for lattice formation; but we now know that all antibodies are at least bivalent. A more likely explanation is that nonprecipitating antibodies are of low affinity, so that antigen must be added in relatively high concentration to sway the reaction in favor of the antigen-antibody complex formations; however, since in the antigen-excess zone, only small, soluble complexes form, no precipitate is discernible. Another interpretation of the nonprecipitating systems assumes that the antibodies bind preferentially with both their combining sites to determinants on the same antigenic molecule, rather than on different molecules. This type of *monogamous binding* precludes crosslinking of the antigen, and so prevents lattice formation.

To detect nonprecipitating antibody, one uses a trick introduced by R. S. Farr. The *Farr assay* is based on the observation that 50 percent saturation of a serum with ammonium sulfate results in the precipitation of immunoglobulins, but not, for example, of albumin. One can therefore add radioactively labeled antigen to a constant amount of serially diluted antiserum and, after incubation, precipitate the globulin in each tube with ammonium sulfate. The radioactivity of the precipitate indicates the amount of antigen bound—in other words, the antigen-binding capacity of the antiserum. (For this reason, the assay is sometimes also called the *ABC test*.)

Application of the Precipitin Reaction. In addition to the study of the mechanism of antigen-antibody interaction, the precipitin reaction can also be used to measure the amount of antibody and antigen in a solution. The amount of antibody can be determined from the precipitin curve. As has already been discussed, in the equivalence zone, this amount is equal to the amount of total precipitate minus the amount of added antigen. To determine the amount of antigen in an unknown sample, one first plots a precipitin curve for a known antigen-antibody combination and then uses the same antibody in the antibody-excess zone to test the unknown antigen. In this zone, all the added antigen is precipitated, so that the concentration of the tested antigen equals the amount of total precipitated protein minus the amount of precipitated antibody (predetermined in the test with the known antigen).

The precipitin reaction is also the basis for several other methods of antibody quantitation—in particular, the radioimmunoassay that will be described later in this chapter.

Agglutination

The only principal difference between precipitation and agglutination is the size of the antigen: in the former, the antigen is a soluble macromolecule, in the latter, a microscopic particle (a bacterial cell or an erythrocyte). And since the general principles described for the precipitin reaction also apply to agglutination, we shall discuss the latter only briefly.

Mechanism. Agglutination (clumping) results from the crosslinking of particles (cells) by antibodies (agglutinins) specific for antigens (agglutinogens) on the particle's surface. For agglutination to occur, the multivalent antibody must bind to an antigen on one particle with one combining site, and to an antigen on another particle with the other combining site, and thus form a lattice similar to that in the equivalence zone of the precipitin reaction. In the zone of antibody or antigen excess, antibodies bind to particles but do not crosslink with (and hence do not agglutinate) them. For this reason, agglutinins often display a *prozone*—absence of agglutination at highest antibody concentrations. This fact must be kept in mind when testing agglutinating antisera, for not diluting an antiserum enough may produce false negative results. Agglutination is strongly influenced by the ionic strength of the medium in which the clumping takes place. Apparently, at neutral pH, bacterial cells and erythrocytes have a strong negative electric charge that normally

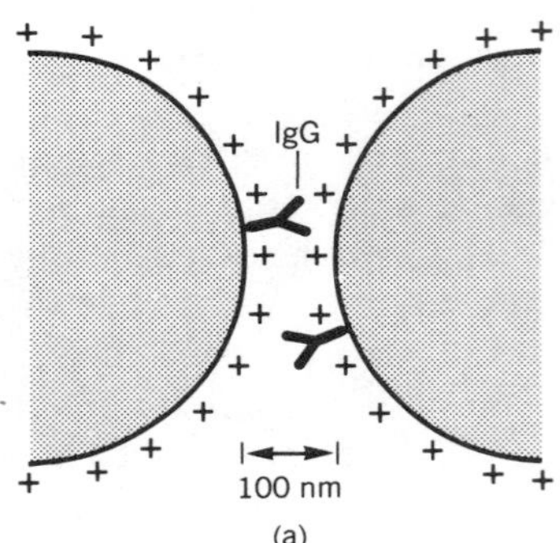

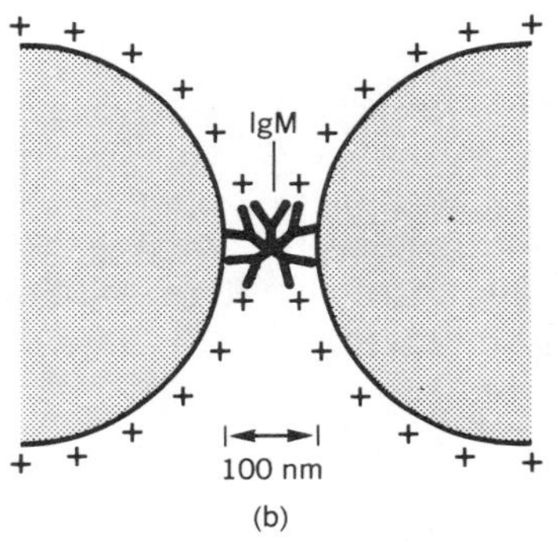

Figure 10.22. The zeta potential of red blood cells. (*a*) The ion cloud surrounding the negatively charged erythrocyte in physiological salt solution prevents IgG molecules from agglutinating the corpuscles. (*b*) The larger IgM molecule can bridge the gap between the two corpuscles and agglutinate them.

keeps them at a distance and prevents their bridging by antibodies (Fig. 10.22). One can observe the effect of the repulsive forces on a diluted erythrocyte suspension: in a light microscope, one sees that the cells are regularly distributed in the field, as if something were keeping them from coming too close to one another. The repulsive forces can be expressed in terms of a zeta potential (ζ):

$$\zeta = \frac{1}{\mu D}$$

where μ is the ionic strength of the solution and D the dielectric constant. An increase in ionic strength or in the dielectric constant results in a decrease in zeta potential and thus in closer packing of cells.

In a heterogeneous mixture of particles, the antibodies to the different particles are independent of one another (provided the particles do not share antigens), so that each antibody-particle system agglutinates separately.

Assay. To detect agglutination, an antiserum is serially diluted in a row of test tubes or wells, a constant number of particles is added to each tube, and after incubation of the mixture, the presence of clumps is determined macro- or microscopically. The usual diluent is physiological salt solution (0.15 M NaCl), but for some antibodies, special macromolecular diluents—such as dextran, polyvinyl pyrrolidone (PVP), or serum albumin—are necessary. The mechanism of the enhancement of agglutination by macromolecular substances is not fully understood; one possibility is that the molecules reduce the strong negative charge surrounding the particles (Fig. 10.22); another explanation presupposes that the macromolecular diluents increase the probability of particle contact more or less mechanically.

Blocking (Incomplete) Antibodies. As in the precipitin reaction, in the agglutination reaction, too, some antibodies combine with antigens without producing a visible effect. And like the nonprecipitating antibodies, the nonagglutinating antibodies were believed to be univalent ("*incomplete*") until it became clear that no univalent antibodies exist naturally. Current explanations as to why nonagglutinating antibodies do not agglutinate are the same as those proposed for nonprecipitating antibodies.

The usual way of demonstrating nonagglutinating antibodies is by a *blocking assay* (hence the designation *blocking antibodies*): cells are incubated with a test antiserum, washed, and then exposed to an antiserum known to contain agglutinating antibodies. If the treated cells are no longer agglutinated in the presence of agglutinating antibodies, one concludes that the test antiserum contains incomplete antibodies that have blocked the reaction by coating the antigenic sites on the cell surfaces. Other ways of demonstrating nonagglutinating antibodies involve replacing physiological salt solution with macromolecular diluents, or treatment of red cells with proteolytic enzymes such as trypsin, papain, bromelin, or ficin. The latter technique is an empirical one: just how it works it not clear.

10.6 APPENDIX 10.2: METHODS FOR THE DETECTION OF ANTIGEN-ANTIBODY REACTIONS

To complete the discussion of antigen-antibody reactions, we shall now give a few specific examples of how these reactions are used. We shall limit the description to a mere outline of each method; for a more detailed description, the reader is referred to one of the method books listed in the References.

10.6.1 Methods Based on the Precipitin Reaction

Precipitation in Liquid Medium (Ring Test).

Antiserum is dispensed into small tubes and carefully overlaid with an antigen-containing solution so that the two do not mix. Usually the amount of antiserum per tube is constant, whereas the antigen concentration increases from tube to tube. The precipitate produced at the interface of the antigen-antibody solution forms an opaque, clearly visible band or ring (hence the designation *ring test*).

Precipitation in Semisolid Media

In these methods, one (*simple* or *single diffusion method*) or both (*double diffusion method*) of the two immune reagents (antigens and antibodies) diffuse through a gel (usually agar) and the precipitin forms at the site where the two reagents meet (*immunodiffusion methods*). The agar gel can form either a thin column (*one-dimensional methods*) or a plate (*two-dimensional methods*).

Simple (Single) Diffusion in One Dimension (Oudin Tube Technique; Fig. 10.23*a*). The antiserum is incorporated in the melted agar, and the antigen-agar mixture is poured into tubes and allowed to gel. The antigen solution is then added to the top of the vertical gel column and the tube is sealed to prevent evaporation. The antigen diffuses downward into the gel, creating a concentration gradient that decreases from top to bottom. The diffusing antigen reacts with the antibody present in the gel, forming antigen-antibody complexes. In the region of the gradient where the concentration of the diffusing antigen is equivalent to that of the antibody, the complexes connect and form a lattice of visible precipitate. Behind the moving front, the antigen concentration becomes too high relative to the concentration of the antibody, and the formed precipitate dissolves again—just as in the antigen-excess zone of the precipitin curve. The precipitate thus forms a narrow band that moves down the tube with the front of the antigen concentration gradient. The speed of the downward movement depends on the speed of the antigen diffusion, which, in turn, depends on the size and shape of the antigen molecules, and on the antiserum concentration in the upper reservoir. If the reservoir contains several antigens, each with a different molecular weight, the antigens diffuse with different speeds and each forms a distinct precipitin band.

Simple Diffusion in Two Dimensions (Mancini Radial Technique; Fig. 10.23*b*). The flat bottom of a glass dish or slide is covered with antibody-containing agar. Holes are then punched out of the agar and the wells

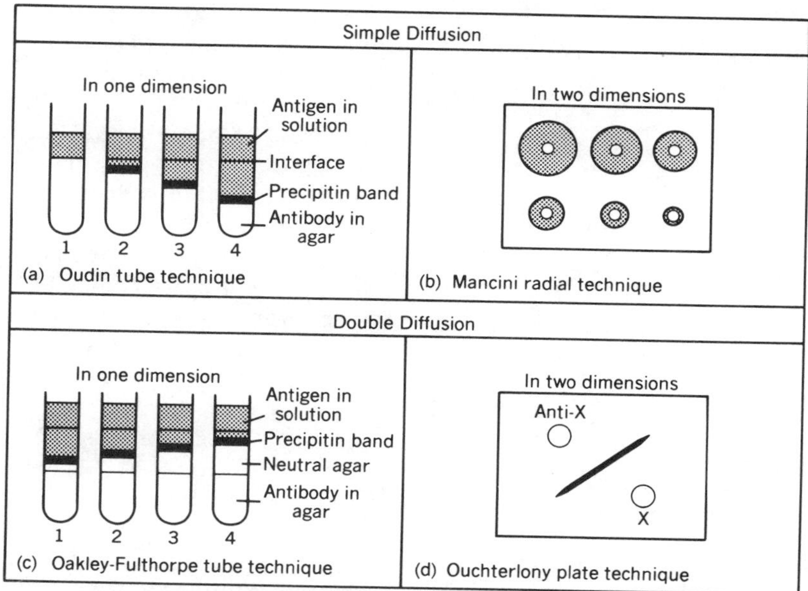

Figure 10.23. Types of precipitin (immunodiffusion) assay in agar.

are filled with the antigen solution. As the antigen diffuses through the agar radially from each well, it reacts with the antibodies, and a growing circle of precipitate forms, most of it accumulating at the circle's periphery. The diameter of the circle for a given antigen depends on antigen concentration in the well: the higher the concentration, the larger the circle.

Double Diffusion in One Dimension (Oakley-Fulthrope Tube Technique; Fig. 10.23*c*). The antibody is incorporated into the agar and the agar is allowed to gel in a tube. Fresh agar is poured on top of the agar-antibody column—fresh, but this time with no antibody in it ("neutral agar"). When the second agar column gells, an antigen solution is placed on top of it. Hence, in this setup, the antibody diffuses upward and the antigen downward, and where the two meet in the neutral gel, they form a precipitin band.

Double Diffusion in Two Dimensions (Ouchterlony Plate Technique; Fig. 10.23*d*). In the simplest setup using this method, one prepares an agar plate, punches out two wells in it, and fills one with the antigen solution and the other with antibodies. The two reagents then diffuse radially and meet at some point between the two wells, forming a precipitin line (Fig. 10.24). The position of the line will depend on the factors influencing the two reagents' speed of diffusion, above all on the relative reagent concentration: if the concentration of the antigen is higher than that of the antibody, the line will form closer to the antibody well; in the reverse situation, the line will develop close to the antigen well. Neither the antigen nor the antibody can diffuse past the line: on the antibody side of the line, there is always enough free antibody to bind the diffusing antigen and deposit it onto the line in the form of antigen-antibody complexes; similarly, there is always enough free antigen on the antigen side of the line to stop any migration of antibodies. However, antigens that do not react with a given antibody pass freely through the line, only to be stopped at another line formed by the corresponding antibody. Thus, in general, as many precipitin lines develop as there are antigen-antibody systems in the two wells.

The test is useful for establishing the identity of antigens. Consider, as an example, a situation where an antiserum gives a single precipitin line when tested separately with two antigens: are the two antigens identical, or does the antiserum contain two antibodies, one reacting with one and the other with the other antigen? To answer this question, one makes three triangularly arranged holes in an agar plate (Fig. 10.24) and places the antiserum in one well and one antigen in each of the two other wells. Lines now form between the antiserum well and the two antigen wells; if the two antigens share determinants, the two lines fuse smoothly (*line of identity*; Fig. 10.24*a*); if the antigens carry different determinants, the two lines cross each other (*lines of nonidentity*; Fig. 10.24*b*); and finally, if the antiserum contains antibodies to two different determinants, both of which are present on one antigen and only one of which is present on the second, one of the two lines fuses with the other line, but the other line spurs over the first (*lines of partial identity*; Fig. 10.24*c*). How these three types of line pattern arise during the diffusion of the immune reagents is apparent from Figure 10.25. More complex line patterns arise when one of the two antigenic preparations contains two distinct types of antigen molecules. In such a case, one of the two antigens might be shared by both preparations, while the other may occur only in one preparation (depending on the speed of migration of the two, one obtains either the pattern shown in Fig. 10.24*d* or that in Fig. 10.24*e*); or one of the two molecules may share antigenic determinants with the second preparation, while the other molecule may again be present only in the first preparation (Fig. 10.24*f*). Even more complex patterns arise when more than two antibodies are present in the antiserum and several antigenic molecules occur in the antigenic preparations. Furthermore, one can change the number and arrangement of the wells and again obtain different line patterns.

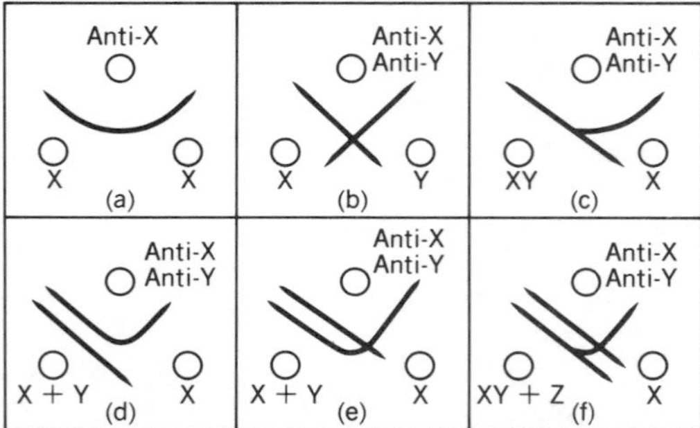

Figure 10.24. Precipitin lines formed by diffusion of antibodies and antigens from wells (circles) in agar gel. (*a*) Line of identity. (*b*) Line of nonidentity. (*c*) Line of partial identity. (*d*), (*e*), (*f*) More complicated patterns arise when one of the two antigen wells contains two sorts of molecule differing in their antigenic determinants.

Immunoelectrophoresis

As the name suggests, this technique is a combination of gel electrophoresis and immunodiffusion. There are

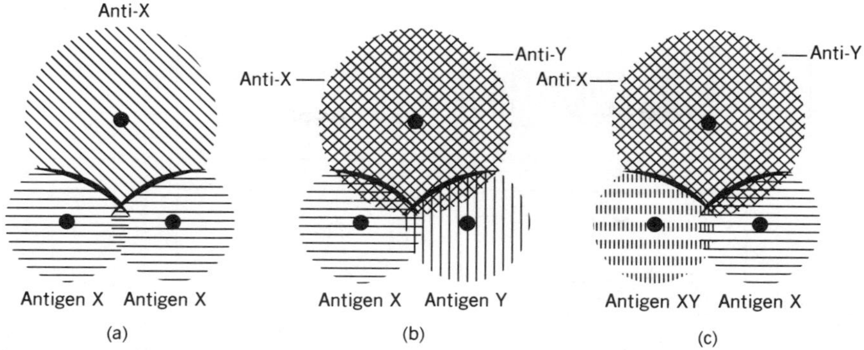

Figure 10.25. Diagrammatic representation of how (*a*) the precipitin line of identity, (*b*) line of nonidentity, and (*c*) line of partial identity form through the diffusion of anti-X + anti-Y antibodies from one well, X (or XY) antigen from another well, and Y antigen from yet another well. The basic premise is that neither anti-X nor X can pass beyond the anti-X + X precipitin line, while anti-Y and Y can. (Based on C. J. van Oss *in* N. R. Rose, F. Milgrom, and C. J. van Oss (Eds.): *Principles of Immunology*, pp. 30–55. MacMillan, New York, 1973.)

many variants of the immunoelectrophoretic method, of which we shall describe only three.

Standard Immunoelectrophoresis (Grabar-Williams Technique). Melted agar is poured onto a glass plate and allowed to gel. A hole is then punched out of the agar and filled with the antigen solution. The plate is placed as a bridge between electrolyte-containing anode and cathode compartments, the agar is connected with the fluid in these compartments by electrolyte-soaked filter paper strips (Fig. 10.26), and an electric current is introduced. The substances in the sample separate, according to their net electric charge, into different regions along the cathode-anode axis (Fig. 10.27*a*). Following this separation, the plate is removed from the electrophoresis apparatus, a longitudinal trough is cut in the gel, the trough is filled with antiserum, and the plate is incubated to allow diffusion to take place. Where the diffusing antigens meet the corresponding diffusing antibodies, characteristic arcs of precipitate form—one arc for each antigen-antibody system (Figs. 10.27 and 28).

Crossed Electrophoresis (First Laurell Technique; Fig. 10.27*b*). A transverse slit cut in a gel on a plate is filled with the antigen sample, and the individual antigens are separated by electrophoresis in one direction. A longitudinal strip containing the separated bands is then cut out from the middle of the gel and laid on another plate, covered with antibody-containing gel. Electrophoresis is repeated, but perpendicular to the original direction. The individual antigens diffuse from the strip into the underlying gel and migrate in the second direction. The precipitin zones for the individual antigen-antibody systems form in areas of antigen excess and appear as a series of peaks, the height of which is proportional to antigen concentration (the antibody concentration being constant).

Rocket Immunoelectrophoresis (Second Laurell Technique; Fig. 10.27*c*). A series of holes cut out along the edge of the agar-coated plate is filled with antigen at increasing dilutions. Since the agar, as in the first Laurell technique, is soaked with antibodies, a series of rocket-shaped peaks of precipitate develops when electric current is introduced perpendicular to the row of holes. And since the distance travelled by the precipitate is again directly proportional to antigen concentration, the technique can be used for antigen quantitation (by comparison with samples containing known amounts of antigen).

Counter Immunoelectrophoresis (Lang and Haan Technique; Fig. 10.27*d*). Two rows of wells are cut out in the gel, wells of one row are filled, each with the same amount of antibody, and wells of the second row with different dilutions of the antigen. A current is then

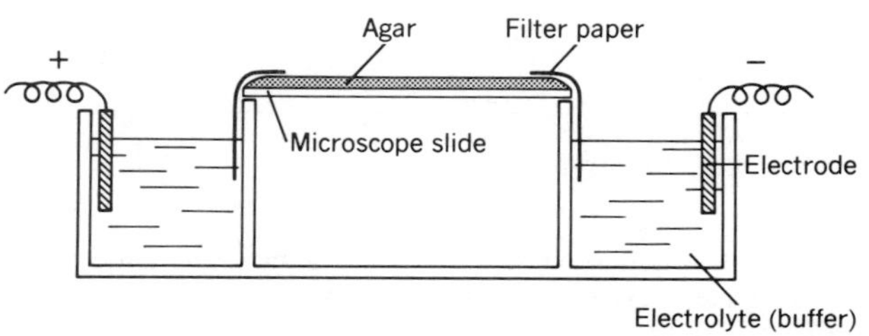

Figure 10.26. Diagram of an apparatus for immunoelectrophoresis.

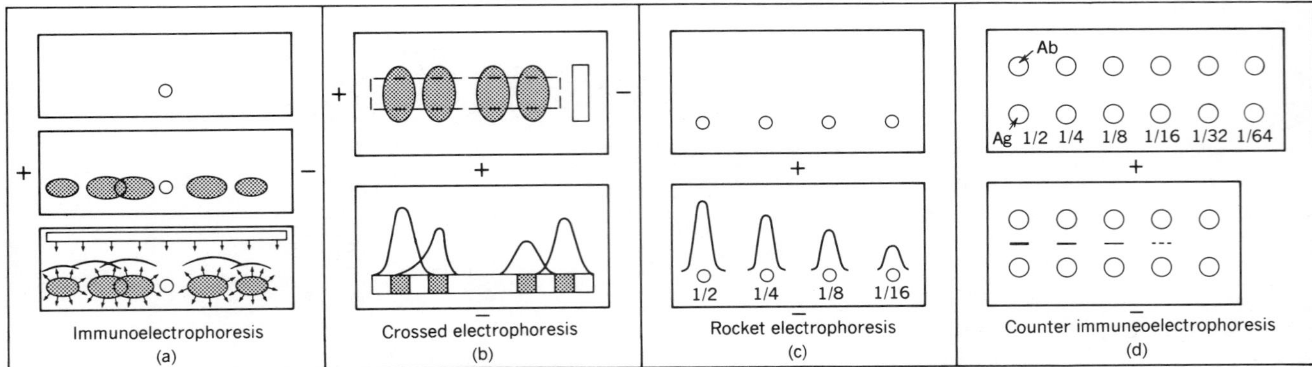

Figure 10.27. Various forms of immunoelectrophoresis. Explanation in the text.

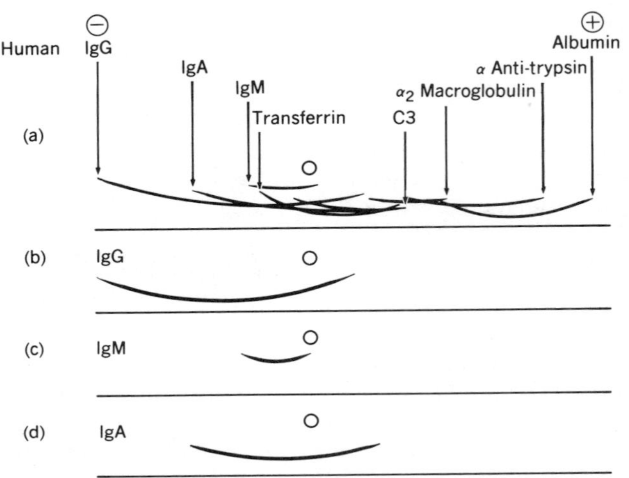

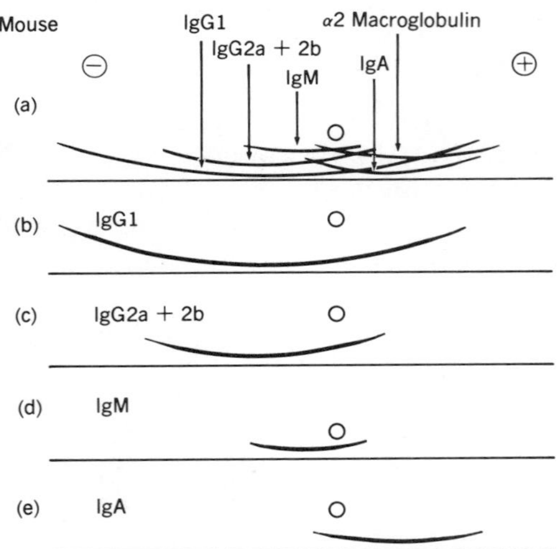

Figure 10.28. Immunoelectrophoresis of human and mouse normal sera. (*a*) Plates developed with antiserum made against the whole serum. (*b*), (*c*), (*d*), (*e*) Plates developed with antiserum specific for individual immunoglobulin classes.

passed in such a way that the antigen migrates toward the antibody well (the mobility of the antigen must be greater than that of the antibody at a given pH). Because of a backward flow of the electrolyte (electro-osmosis[4]), the antibodies travel in the opposite direction, and precipitin lines form where the antigen and antibody meet between the two rows of wells. Since all the antigens and antibodies are brought into contact, the technique is about 10 times more sensitive than the double immunodiffusion method.

10.6.2 Methods Based on Agglutination

Agglutination assays are extremely versatile. One can agglutinate bacteria, erythrocytes, spermatozoa, or even polystyrene particles; one can carry out the assay on a microscope slide, in a test tube, or in wells of a plastic tray; the diluent can be physiological salt solution, normal serum, albumin, dextran, or polyvinyl pyrrolidone; and one can score the result from the shape of the sediment, from shaking the tubes and observing into how many pieces the clump breaks, from flushing the sediment with fluid, or from observing, with the aid of a microscope, clustering of cells. The scores are usually expressed semiquantitatively in numbers of plus signs (4+ indicating the strongest reaction and − standing for the absence of agglutination) and the overall result in titer (or the reciprocal thereof). The assay is thus rather imprecise, but this disadvantage is offset by the high sensitivity of the agglutination reaction.

There are two principal forms of the agglutination

[4] In alkaline pH, agar molecules assume a negative charge, but since they themselves cannot move, the electrolyte present in the gel assumes a positive charge and moves toward the cathode, carrying some protein molecules with it and slowing others down.

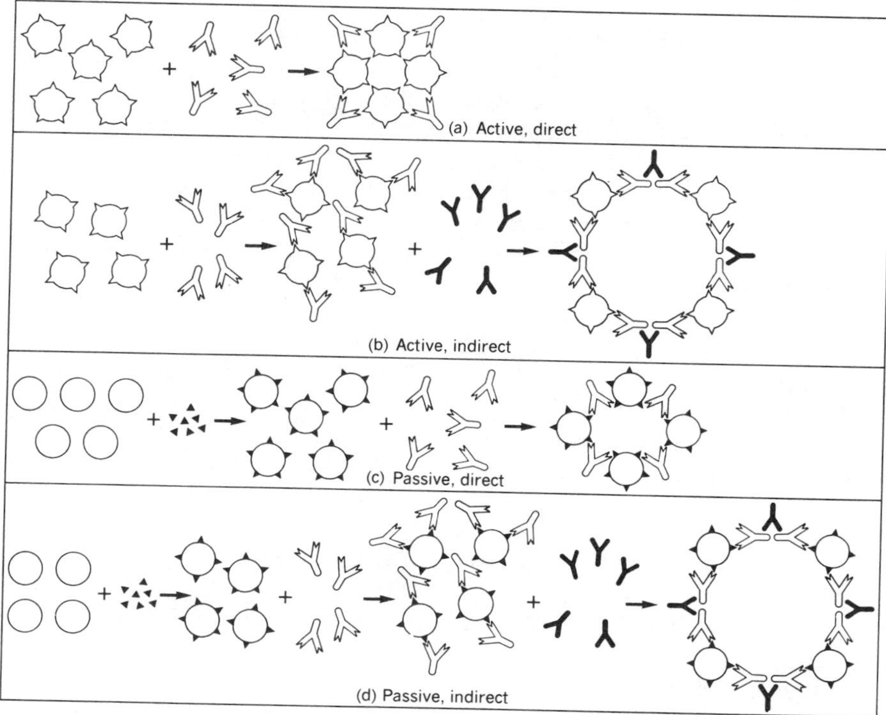

Figure 10.29. Principal forms of the agglutination assay.

assay—active and passive (Fig. 10.29). In the *active agglutination assay*, the antigen is indigenous to the particles and one can therefore achieve agglutination by simply mixing the particles with the antiserum. The active test can be either direct or indirect. In the *direct agglutination test* (Fig. 10.29*a*), particles are agglutinated by antibodies directed against antigens on the particles' surface. In the *indirect agglutination assay* (Fig. 10.29*b*), particles carrying antigen X are first allowed to react with anti-X (which alone is unable to agglutinate the particles) and then xenogeneic antiserum against anti-X immunoglobulins is added to the mixture. The xenogeneic antibodies combine with the coating antibodies and bridge the particles. Because of the use of anti-immunoglobulin reagents, the system is also referred to as the *antiglobulin test* or, after its discoverer, the *Coombs test*.

In the *passive agglutination assay*, the antigen is passively attached to the particles' surface. The attachment occurs in one of two ways. It can occur spontaneously via noncovalent bonds (e.g., erythrocytes spontaneously adsorb certain lipopolysaccharides of Gram-negative bacteria, and this phenomenon can sometimes be enhanced—for unknown reasons—by treatment of erythrocytes with tannic acid or chromic chloride); it can also occur via special linkers and covalent bonding. Commonly used linkers are *bis*-diazotized benzidine and glutaraldehyde. The conjugation of an antigen to an erythrocyte via the former linker takes place as follows:

$$H_2N\text{—}C_6H_4\text{—}C_6H_4\text{—}NH_2 \xrightarrow{\text{HONO}} {}^{+}NN\text{—}C_6H_4\text{—}C_6H_4\text{—}NN^{+}$$

Benzidine → *Bis*-diazotized benzidine

$${}^{+}NN\text{—}C_6H_4\text{—}C_6H_4\text{—}NN^{+} \xrightarrow[\text{Antigen}]{\text{Erythrocyte}} \text{Erythrocyte-NN—}C_6H_4\text{—}C_6H_4\text{—NN-antigen}$$

Bis-diazotized benzidine → Antigen conjugated to erythrocyte

Like the active agglutination, the passive reaction too can be either direct (mediated solely by antibodies to the antigen; Fig. 10.29*c*) or indirect (mediated by anti-immunoglobulin serum directed against the coating antibody; Fig. 10.29*d*).

The principle of competitive inhibition, which will be described in the section on the radioimmunoassay later in this chapter, forms the basis of the *agglutination inhibition assays*. Here, soluble antigens are added to the agglutination system and as their concentration increases, they occupy more and more of the antibody combining sites, making them unavailable for particle agglutination. A special case of agglutination inhibition occurs with certain viruses, which bind directly to erythrocytes via special cell-surface receptors. The resulting erythrocyte clumping can be inhibited by the addition of antibodies that react with the viruses, rendering them incapable of attaching to the red-cell receptors.

10.6.3 Methods Requiring Complement Participation

Since we discussed the complement assays in the preceding chapter, there is no need to dwell on them here. We can summarize by saying that these assays can be either direct or indirect. In the *direct assays*, activation of the complement cascade results in the lysis of cells—be they bacteria (*bacteriolytic tests*), erythrocytes (*hemolytic tests*), or nucleated cells (*cytotoxic tests*). The dead cells can be identified by their changed morphology, altered light transmission properties, release of hemoglobin, uptake of vital stains such as trypan blue or eosin, or release of ^{51}Cr previously fixed to cytoplasmic components. In the *indirect* (*complement fixation*) *tests*, the sign that antigen-antibody reaction has taken place is the disappearance of complement (its fixation to the antigen-antibody complexes) from the mixture, as measured by a special indicator system. A variant of the complement fixation test is the *conglutination complement adsorption test*. *Conglutinin* (L. *conglutino*, to glue together[5]) is a protein in the serum of cattle and other ruminants that adsorbs to erythrocyte-antibody-complement complexes and agglutinates them (in systems in which the antibody alone is unable to effect agglutination). The protein is not an immunoglobulin and its level does not increase after immunization; it has specificity for certain sugars of the C3 complement component (the binding requires Ca^{++}). In the conglutination complement adsorption test, conglutinin is used in an indicator system to test whether complement has been fixed: if an antigen-antibody reaction has consumed all free C3, antibody-coated erythrocytes are not agglutinated by the addition of conglutinin.

10.6.4 Methods Based on Neutralization of Biological Activities

Many biologically active agents are inactivated when they combine with antibodies; so a loss of biological activity in these situations is an indication that antigen-antibody reaction has taken place. The commonly used agents are toxins, viruses, bacteriophages, and enzymes.

Toxin Neutralization

Toxins (Gr. *toxicos*, poison) are noxious substances produced by microorganisms, plants, or animals that, in a high dose, are often lethal for higher forms of life (see Chapter 14). They are a highly heterogeneous group of substances and they exert a variety of biological effects. But these effects are often abrogated (neutralized) when toxins combine with corresponding antibodies (*antitoxins*). This neutralization can be measured by injecting the antibody directly into the toxin-containing animal, or by combining toxins and antitoxins in vitro and demonstrating the innocuousness of the mixture following animal inoculation.

Phage Neutralization

Bacteriophages, or phages, are viruses that attack and often destroy (lyse) bacteria. The spraying of a suspension of bacteriophages over a confluent bacterial culture produces clear areas (plaques) at the deposit sites of individual phage particles (in these areas, the phages multiply and lyse the bacteria). The plaque formation can be reduced or totally inhibited by preincubation of phages with specific antibodies.

Virus Neutralization

Inactivation of viruses by antibodies can be measured in several ways. One can inoculate the mixture of antibody and virus into a susceptible animal and demonstrate absence of virally induced disease (in comparison to a control group of animals). One can inoculate the virus-antibody mixture into chicken eggs that contain embryos and demonstrate the absence of the visible lesions (pocks) normally formed on the egg mem-

[5] Conglutinin must not be confused with *immune conglutinin*, or *immunoconglutinin*, which is an IgM autoantibody specific for activated C3 or C4 components; it is present at low levels in most normal sera but its concentration increases after various infections and after immunization with many antigens; animals are not tolerant of the determinants detected by immunoconglutinins because these determinants are normally hidden in the molecule and become exposed only after C3 or C4 activation.

brane when virus alone is inoculated and caused by cell death (cytopathogenic effect). Or one can spray a tissue culture with the virus-antibody mixture and demonstrate the absence of the clear areas (plaques) that normally result from cell lysis caused by the virus alone.

Enzyme Neutralization

Incubation of enzymes with specific antibodies often blocks the enzymatic activity (many toxins are, in fact, enzymes). However, this blocking occurs only when the antibody recognizes a determinant close to the active site of the enzyme and thus sterically prevents the enzyme from acting on its substrate. Antibodies to determinants at a distance from the active site do not exert a neutralizing effect. A third category of antibodies reacts with determinants that are close enough to the active site to prevent other (neutralizing) antibodies from attaching to the site but, at the same time, are far enough away that they themselves do not prevent combination of the enzyme with the substrate. Antibodies in this last category block the action of the neutralizing antibodies but do not neutralize the enzymes.

10.6.5 Methods Based on the Use of Tagged Antibodies

One can make the antigen-antibody reaction visible by attaching a tag to the antibody (or the antigen). The tag is a molecule demonstrable through some special property: emission of light (fluorescent antibody techniques), enzymatic activity (enzyme immunoassays), high electron-scanning capacity (the immunoferritin method), or radioactivity (radioimmunoassays). The branch of science based on the use of tagged antibodies is called *immunocytochemistry*, or *immunohistochemistry*.

Fluorescent Antibody Techniques

When a photon (a quantum of light) strikes an atom, some of the electrons absorb energy and the atom enters an energy-rich, excited state. Excited atoms are unstable and quickly return to their original low-energy ground state. This return is accompanied by the release of energy in the form of a chemical reaction, heat, or visible light. In which of these three forms the energy is released depends, to a large degree, on the structure of the molecule of which the atom is a part. For example, molecules with freely rotating bonds, such as those in the aliphatic-saturated compounds, dissipate the absorbed energy in the rotational movement; structurally rigid molecules release energy in the form of light. The emission of absorbed light is called *fluorescence* and the structurally rigid molecules capable of fluorescence are *fluorochromes*. The emitted light has a lower energy (different color) than the absorbed light and fluorescence is noticeable when the former is in the visible and the latter in the invisible, ultraviolet range.

A fluorochrome attached to an antibody molecule makes the latter—as demonstrated first by Albert H. Coons in 1941—easily identifiable through its fluorescence. The two fluorochromes commonly used in immunology are *fluorescein* and *rhodamine disulfonic acid* (lissamine rhodamine B200; Fig. 10.30). Before they can be conjugated to proteins (antibodies), fluorescein and rhodamine must first be converted into isothiocyanates, using the reaction described earlier in this chapter. The fluoresceinated (or rhodaminated) antibodies are then combined with cellular antigens, the unbound proteins are removed by washing, and the cell preparation is observed in a fluorescence microscope. This instrument contains a source of high-intensity UV light and two sets of special filters: the *excitation filters* let through only light with a wave-

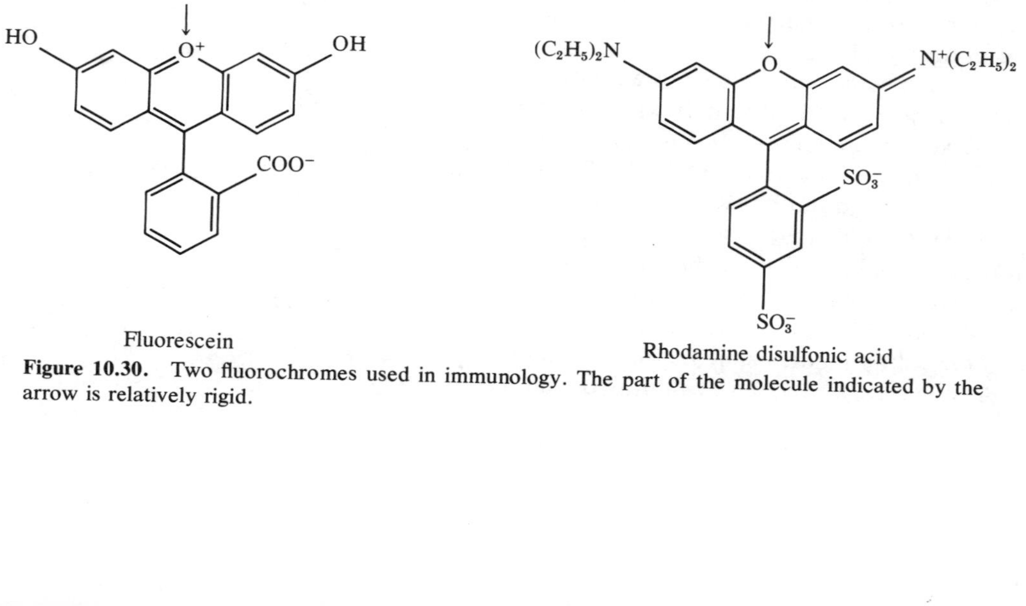

HO O+ OH COO−

Fluorescein

$(C_2H_5)_2N$ O $N^+(C_2H_5)_2$ SO_3^- SO_3^-

Rhodamine disulfonic acid

Figure 10.30. Two fluorochromes used in immunology. The part of the molecule indicated by the arrow is relatively rigid.

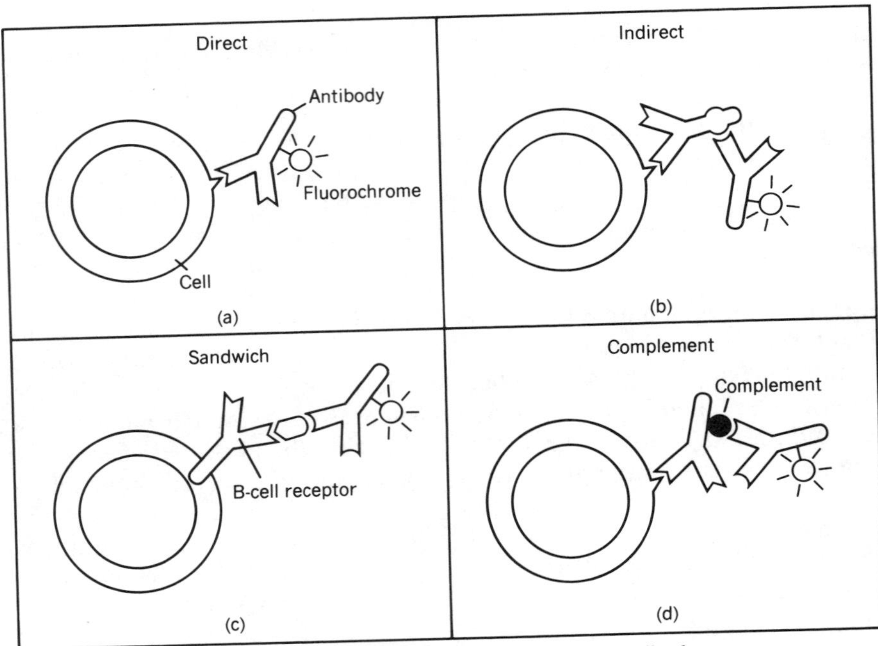

Figure 10.31. Principal forms of the fluorescent antibody assay.

length capable of fluorescent activation (490 to 495 nm in the case of fluorescein isothiocyanate, and 550 nm in the case of tetramethylrhodamine isothiocyanate); the *barrier filters* let through only light emitted by the fluorochrome (green light with a wavelength of 517 nm in the case of fluorescein, and red light with a wavelength of 580 nm in the case of rhodamine). This arrangement cuts down on light dispersion and enhances the intensity of the fluorescence. In the original design of fluorescent microscopes, the light came from below and passed through the preparation; most modern microscopes use the epi-illumination system (light coming from above), introduced by J. S. Ploem.

The actual test can be carried out in one of four ways (Fig. 10.31*a* through *d*): in the *direct test* the cell is coated with fluorochrome-tagged antibodies specific for cell-surface antigens; in the *indirect test*, the cell is first coated with the specific, unconjugated antibody, which is then reacted with fluorochrome-tagged xenogeneic anti-Ig serum; in the *sandwich test*, an antigen is reacted with cell-surface immunoglobulin (B-cell receptor) and then a tagged antibody is reacted with the bound antigen (the antigen is thus sandwiched between two antibodies); and finally, in the *complement technique*, cells are coated by specific antibodies, complement is allowed to bind to the antigen-antibody complexes, and tagged antibodies specific for complement components are then reacted with the bound complement.

Enzyme Immunoassays

In these tests, one attaches enzymes (instead of fluorochromes) to antibodies and takes any sign of enzymatic activity in a given tissue or cell as an indication that the tissue or cell possesses antigens to which the antibodies bind. There are only a few enzymes suitable for this kind of antibody tagging; the most frequently used among these is the *horseradish peroxidase*. This enzyme can be attached to a protein via bifunctional agents, such as 4,4′-difluoro-3,3′-dinitro-phenylsulfone:

F–C₆H₃(NO₂)–SO₂–C₆H₃(NO₂)–F $\xrightarrow{\text{protein—NH}_2}$

4,4′-difluoro-3,3′-dinitro-phenylsulfone
or glutaraldehyde:

Protein-NH–C₆H₃(NO₂)–SO₂–C₆H₃(NO₂)–NH-protein

protein conjugate

or glutaraldehyde:

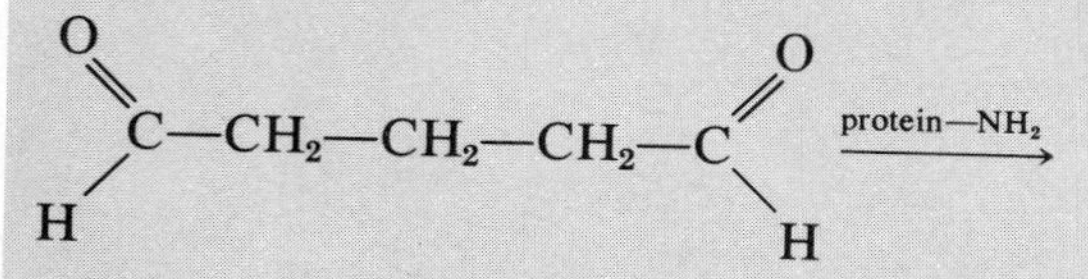

$$\mathrm{OHC{-}CH_2{-}CH_2{-}CH_2{-}CHO} \xrightarrow{\text{protein—NH}_2}$$

$$\text{protein-N}{=}\mathrm{CH{-}CH_2{-}CH_2{-}CH_2{-}CH}{=}\text{N-protein.}$$

The conjugated antibodies are then reacted with cellular antigens, unbound antibodies are removed by washing, and the enzyme is allowed to convert its substrate, hydrogen peroxide (H_2O_2) to water:

$$2H_2O_2 \xrightarrow{4H} 4H_2O$$

The reaction can take place only when electron donors, such as diamino benzidine, are provided. The electron donors are oxidized by this reaction and the oxidation products rapidly polymerize into an amorphous, insoluble, brown substance deposited at the site of antibody binding and visible in a light microscope:

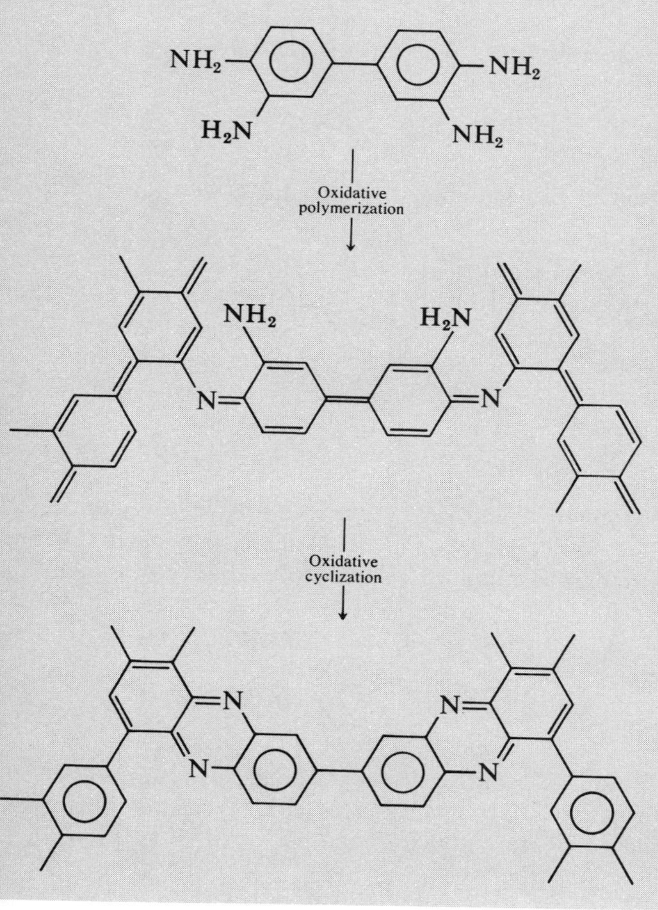

NH₂, H₂N, NH₂, NH₂ (diaminobenzidine)

Oxidative polymerization

NH₂, H₂N, N=, =N

Oxidative cyclization

=N, N=, N, N

The polymers combine with osmium tetroxide, OsO_4, to form a highly electron-opaque chelate, visible in the electron microscope.

Immunoferritin Techniques

In ferritin-labeling methods, the antibodies are tagged by ferritin molecules, visible in the electron microscope. Ferritin is a protein containing about 20 percent iron in the form of a ferric hydroxyphosphate complex. Each ferritin molecule has a protein shell enveloping an inner core of four iron micelles, with high electron-scattering capacity. Ferritin molecules can be attached to antibodies either chemically or immunologically. The chemical attachment in the *direct ferritin-labeling technique* proceeds in two steps (Fig. 10.32*a*). In the first, ferritin molecules are treated with a coupling agent, such as toluene-2,4-diazocyanate, and in the second step, the resulting complex is conjugated with antibody molecules. The ferritin-labeled antibodies are then applied directly to cells and the specimens are prepared for electron microscopy. In the *indirect ferritin-labeling technique*, ferritin is coupled to xenogeneic antibodies reacting with alloantibodies that are specific for a given antigen on the cell surface. An example of this technique is the *hybrid-antibody method* in which one uses ferritin-specific antibodies (Fig. 10.32*b*), produced, for instance, in rabbits. The antibody molecules are split enzymatically into Fab fragments and then reconstituted with Fab fragments obtained from rabbit antibodies to immunoglobulins of another species—say, a mouse. Hybrid $F(ab)_2$ molecules are thus produced whereby each molecule consists of one rabbit anti-ferritin and one rabbit anti-mouse Ig fragment. The cells to be examined are first exposed to an alloantibody, then to the hybrid $F(ab)_2$ reagent, and finally to ferritin. Each hybrid $F(ab)_2$ molecule binds, via its first combining site, with the alloantibody on the cell surface, and, via its second combining site, with the ferritin molecule (Fig. 10.32*b*). The hybrid antibody method obviates the loss of antibody activity caused by the chemical coupling and permits the use of markers other than ferritin—for example, plant viruses or bacteriophages.

In the *hybrid antibody bridge method*, a hapten (e.g., benzylpenicilloyl) is coupled chemically to an alloantibody, which is then allowed to bind to cells. The cell-bound antibodies are then bridged to the marker (ferritin or virus) by a hybrid $F(ab)_2$ antibody containing one combining site for the hapten and another for the marker. In the *untreated anti-hapten antibody bridge method*, the hapten is coupled chemically to both the alloantibody and the marker (ferritin, virus), cells are

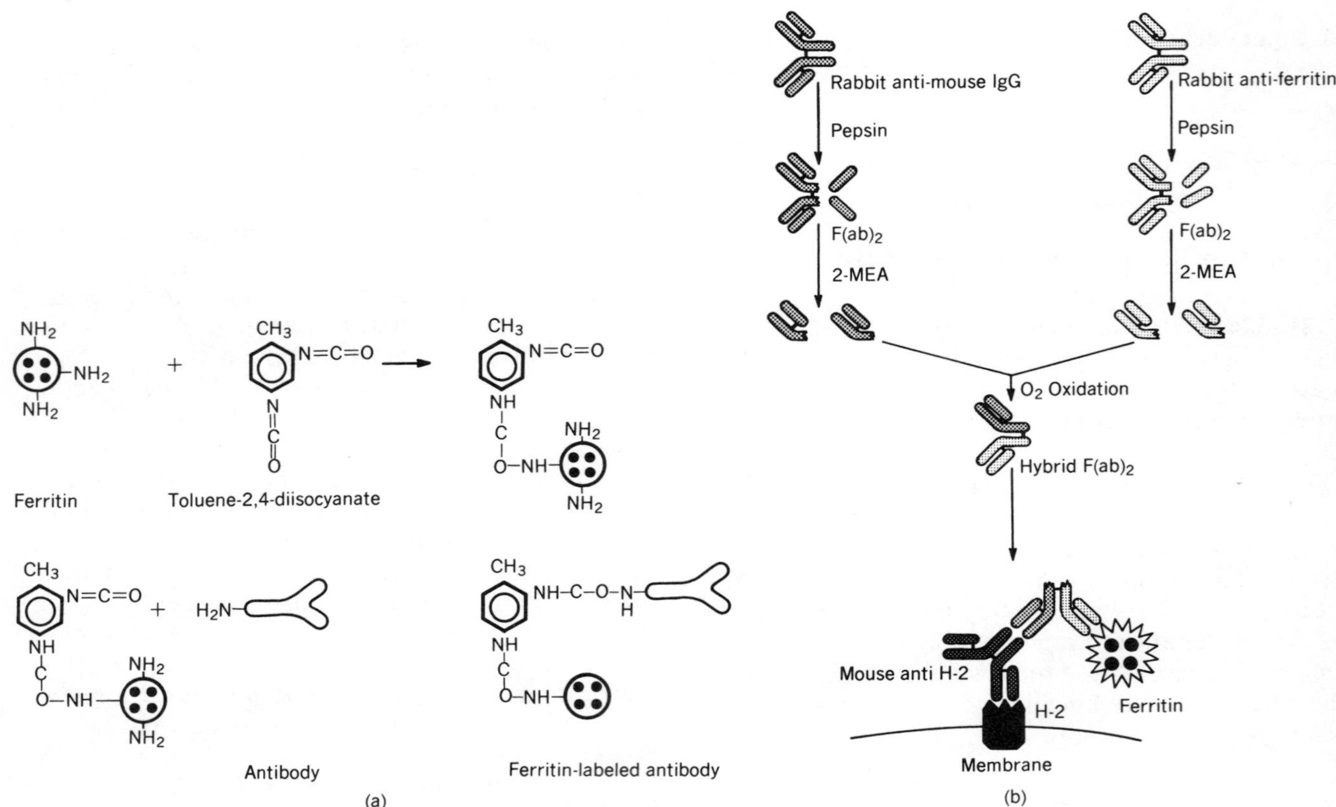

Figure 10.32. Principle of (*a*) the direct and (*b*) indirect ferritin-labeling techniques. 2-MEA, 2-mercaptoethanol. (From J. Klein: *Biology of the Mouse Histocompatibility-2 Complex*. Springer-Verlag, New York, 1975.)

then coated with the hapten-coupled alloantibodies, and the latter are bridged to the hapten-coupled marker by the rabbit anti-hapten immunoglobulins.

Radioimmunoassay

This assay was developed in 1960 by Solmon A. Berson and Rosalyn S. Yalow for the quantitation of plasma insulin, but has since been used for the detection of many other hormones. In fact, the method can be used for the detection of any substance that can be isolated in a sufficiently pure form for labeling. The main steps of this method are as follows.

Step One. An antiserum to substance X is produced. If the substance is of small molecular weight and, as such, is nonantigenic, it can be attached, before immunization, to a macromolecular carrier, and used as a hapten.

Step Two. Substance X is labeled with a radioactive isotope. If the substance is a tyrosine-containing protein, it can be labeled with radioactive iodine, ^{125}I or ^{131}I:

$$\text{O}^-\text{-C}_6\text{H}_4\text{-CH}_2\text{-} + I_2^* \rightleftharpoons \text{O-C}_6\text{H}_3(\text{I}^*)\text{-CH}_2\text{-} + \text{HI}.$$

(Asterisks indicate radioactivity.) The attachment of the iodine to tyrosine is facilitated by an oxidizing agent, chloramine T (*N*-chloro-*p*-toluene sulfonamide)

$$\text{Na}^+\left[\text{H}_3\text{C}-\text{C}_6\text{H}_4-\text{SO}_2-\text{N}\!-\!\text{Cl}\right]^-$$

a nontoxic antiseptic, occasionally used for wound irrigation. If the substance lacks tyrosine, it can be labeled internally, for example, with ^3H.

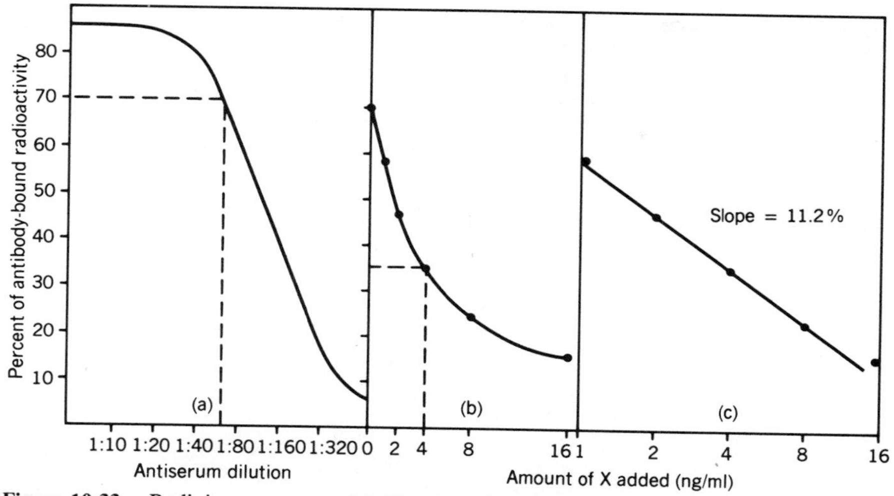

Figure 10.33. Radioimmunoassay. (*a*) Titration of anti-X against X*. (*b*) Standard curve for substance X (linear scale). (*c*) The same as (*b*), but plotted on a semilogarithmic scale.

Step Three. A constant amount of the labeled antigen (X*) is mixed and incubated with different dilutions of the anti-X serum, and the antigen-antibody complexes are precipitated with a xenogeneic serum against immunoglobulins contained in the anti-X serum. (The amount of X* for the test is chosen empirically so that the antigen-antibody reaction occurs in a large antibody excess in which only soluble antigen-antibody complexes form.) The precipitate is separated, the radioactivity of the precipitate and of the remaining free X* determined, the ratio of the two values (the percent of X* bound by the antibody) calculated, and the percentage plotted against the antiserum dilution (Fig. 10.33). For further experimentation, an antiserum dilution is chosen that binds 70 percent of the radioactive substance X* (a point on the titration curve where the straight region of the curve begins and where the assay is most sensitive).

Step Four. The diluted anti-X serum is distributed in constant amounts into several tubes containing a constant amount of X*. Known, increasing amounts of X (unlabeled substance) are then added to the individual tubes, the antigen-antibody complexes are precipitated

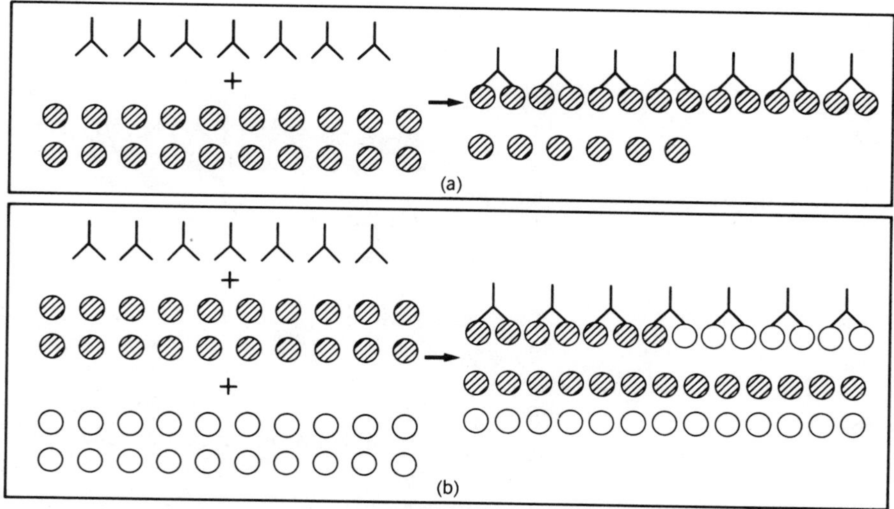

Figure 10.34. Principle of competitive inhibition. Explanation in the text. ⅄ , antibody; ⊘, labeled antigen (X*); ○, unlabeled antigen (X).

Table 10.16 Sensitivity of Methods for Detecting Antibody

Method	Minimal Amount of Antibody Detected
Precipitation	
Micro-Kjedahl	125μg
Colorimetry (absorbance at 280 nm, Lowry, Nessler)	6–25 μg/ml
Optimal proportions	50 μg/ml
Ring test	20–30 μg/ml
Nephelometry	
Molecular	0.5 μg/ml
Bacterial	0.005–0.01 μg/ml
Gel Diffusion	
Preer method (double diffusion tube)	20–50 μg/ml
Oudin method (single diffusion tube)	12–110 μg/ml
Ouchterlony method (double diffusion plate)	<40 μg/ml
Mancini method (radial diffusion plate)	10 μg/ml
Immunoelectrophoresis	
Standard microtechnique	100 μg/ml
Crossed (Laurell technique)	>100 μg/ml
Radio technique (with anti-globulin)	0.02 μg/ml
Agglutination	
Bacteria	
Salmonella typhi	0.12 μg/ml
Pneumococcus	60–120 μg/ml
Red blood cell alloaglutinins	0.6–1.2 μg/ml
Rh-positive blood cells-anti-globulin test	0.03 μg/ml
Passive hemagglutination with protein-sensitized cells	0.03 μg/ml
Complement fixation (micro method) with rabbit antibody	1–0.1 μg
Anaphylaxis	
Passive cutaneous, with rabbit antibody	0.02 μg
Schultz-Dale test with rabbit antibody	6 μg/ml
Fluorescence polarization	3–10 μg/ml
Fluorescence quenching	<40 μg/ml
Radioimmunoassay	μg–ng/ml range
Specific immunoadsorbent	20 μg/ml
Specific immunoadsorbent-inhibition technique	0.01–0.02 μg/ml
Farr binding technique (ABC-33)	0.05–0.1 μg/ml
P_{80}-binding technique	<1 μg/ml
Antiglobulin technique	μg–ng/ml range
Nonprecipitating antibody by copre-cipitation	50–100 μg/ml
Diphtheria toxin neutralization (rabbit skin test)	0.01 μg/ml
Specific bioassay	μg–ng̃/ml range
Enzyme activity	
Count of viable bacteria	
Syphilis flocculation test	
Neutralization tests	1 molecule of antibody[a]
Phage (φX174)	
Viruses (polio, etc.)	
Fluorescent dye uptake	1 molecule of antibody[a,b]
Cytoxic antibody technique	1 cell coated with antibody[a]
Jerne plaque technique	1 antibody-producing cell[a]
Immunocytoadherence	1 cell coated with antibody[a]
Red cells (rosette formation)	
Bacterial adherence	
Coons tissue fluorescence technique	1 antibody-producing cell[a]
Ethidium bromide uptake	1 molecule of antibody[a]
Cunningham monolayer technique	1 antibody-producing cell[a]

Source. From T. J. Gill III: *Immunochemistry* 7:997–1000, 1970.
[a] This is a theoretical limit of detection. Technical problems, such as sampling, greatly reduce the sensitivity of the method.
[b] Applicable only with β-galactosidase as the antigen.

with an antiglobulin serum, and the radioactivity of these complexes is plotted against the amount of X added (Fig. 10.33*b*).

Step Five. A standard curve (Fig. 10.33*b*) is then used to evaluate substance X (or a substance related to X) in an unknown sample. To this end, one mixes the unknown sample with the same amount of antiserum and X* as was used in the preceding step, then determines radioactivity of the precipitate and of the remaining free X*, calculates the percentage of X* bound by anti-X, and reads off, from the standard curve, the corresponding concentration of X in the unknown sample. In Figure 10.33*b*, an example is given of an unknown sample that reduced the percent of antibody-bound radioactivity from 70 percent (absence of unlabeled X) to 35 percent; this value corresponds to 5 ng of X per 1 ml.

The radioimmunoassay is based on the principle of *competitive inhibition*, which can be explained in simplified form as follows. Consider a mixture of seven bivalent antibody molecules and 20 molecules of labeled antigen (Fig. 10.34*a*). If all the antibody-combining sites react with the antigen, 14/20, or 70 percent, of the antigen molecules become antibody-bound and will be brought down with the precipitate. Consider another mixture, again consisting of seven antibody molecules and 20 labeled antigen molecules, and, in addition, 20 unlabeled antigen molecules (Fig. 10.34*b*). Both the labeled and unlabeled antigens have an equal chance of combining with antibodies, so that probably half the bound molecules will be labeled. In this case, only 7/20, or 35 percent, of the labeled antigen molecules will be precipitated out of the solution; the rest of the combining site will be occupied by unlabeled antigen molecules. Thus, the competition of unlabeled molecules inhibits the binding of the labeled ones, and this inhibition is the greater the more unlabeled molecules one adds to the mixture. If one knows that 35 percent reduction of antibody-bound radioactivity is brought about by 20 unlabeled antigen molecules, one can conclude that any unknown sample causing this much reduction must contain 20 antigen molecules. This consideration applies only to situations where the standard and test antigens are identical. If, on the other hand, the test antigen is only similar to, but not identical with, the standard antigen, the antibody may react with the two antigens with different affinities and the quantitative relationships may change. However, if such a situation were to occur, one would become aware of it because of a change in the slope of the inhibition curve in comparison to the slope of the curve given by the standard antigen.

In the assay as we described it, the soluble antigen-antibody complexes were separated from the free antigen by an antiglobulin serum. However, one can also separate the two by other means—chromatography, gel diffusion, electrophoresis, and so on. Or one can attach the antibodies to a solid surface, wash off the free antigen, and determine the radioactivity of this surface. Radioimmunoassays can detect extremely small amounts of antigen and are thus among the most sensitive methods at the immunologist's disposal.

10.6.6 Conclusions

Just as there is no unicorn among experimental animals, there is no ideal technique for the detection of antigen-antibody reaction. Some techniques are more suitable under a given set of conditions, others give better results under other conditions, but there is no single technique tailored for all conditions. Although there are immunologists who use the same technique all their lives and manage to remain productive, most scientists do not like doing assembly-line work. The more intellectually ambitious immunologist will therefore want to choose a technique on the basis of the particular question being asked. Among the many factors one must consider when selecting a technique (amount of reagents available, the type of antigen, quantitative versus qualitative character of the test, and so on), the sensitivity of the test—the minimum detectable concentration of antibodies—often stands in first place. How much the individual tests differ in their sensitivity is shown in Table 10.16.

10.7 APPENDIX 10.3: HUMAN ABO AND OTHER BLOOD-GROUP ANTIGENS

We shall conclude this chapter on lymphocyte-activating substances with a description of antigenic systems that have fascinated immunologists, geneticists, and biochemists for more than half a century. Since this is the only section of the text that will deal with blood groups, the description will be more detailed than a chapter on lymphocyte-stimulating substances would otherwise call for.

10.7.1 Discovery

In 1901, Karl Landsteiner collected blood from five of his colleagues, as well as from himself, separated erythrocytes from the sera, mixed each serum with each of the five erythrocyte suspensions, and after incubation, scored the mixtures for red-cell agglutination. A summary of the results he obtained is shown in Table 10.17. (Only those individuals whose sera and cells reacted differently from sera and cells of other individuals are listed; see also Chapter 2.) Landsteiner interpreted these results as indicating the presence in normal sera of antibodies against antigens on red blood cells. Thus, Dr. Sturli's serum contained an antibody (β) that agglutinated only Dr. Pletschnig's erythrocytes, indicating that Dr. Pletschnig's erythrocytes carried a unique antigen (B). Dr. Pletschnig's serum contained an antibody (α) that detected an antigen (A) present only on Dr. Sturli's erythrocytes. And finally, Dr. Landsteiner's serum contained both α and β antibodies because it agglutinated both Dr. Pletschnig's and Dr. Sturli's erythrocytes; but Dr. Landsteiner's erythrocytes lacked both the A and B antigens because

Table 10.17 Landsteiner's Experiment Revealing the Existence of ABO Blood-Group Antigens

Serum Donor	Agglutination of Erythrocytes from			Antibody in Serum
	Dr. Sturli	Dr. Pletschnig	Dr. Landsteiner	
Dr. Sturli	−	+	−	β
Dr. Pletschnig	+	−	−	α
Dr. Landsteiner	+	+	−	α,β
Antigen on erythrocytes	A	B	C(O)	

Source. Based on K. Landsteiner: *Wien. Klin. Wochenschr.* **14:**1132–1134, 1901.
+, erythrocytes agglutinated; −, erythrocytes not agglutinated

they failed to be agglutinated by either Dr. Sturli's or Dr. Pletschnig's serum. Landsteiner could thus distinguish three blood groups—A (Dr. Sturli), B (Dr. Pletschnig), and C (Dr. Landsteiner; the "C" symbol was later changed to "O"). A fourth blood group, AB (erythrocytes agglutinated by both α- and β-containing sera), was discovered a few years later by W. L. Moss, Jan Janský, and Alfred Decastello and by Adriano Sturli. The agglutination pattern observed with the four ABO blood group-defining sera is depicted in Figure 10.35.

In 1910, Emil von Dungern and Jan Hirszfeld discovered an additional complexity in the A antigen. They observed that some anti-A sera absorbed by erythrocytes from certain A-positive individuals ceased to react with these individuals, but still reacted with erythrocytes of other A-positive individuals. They interpreted these results to mean that there were two subgroups of A—A_1 and A_2.

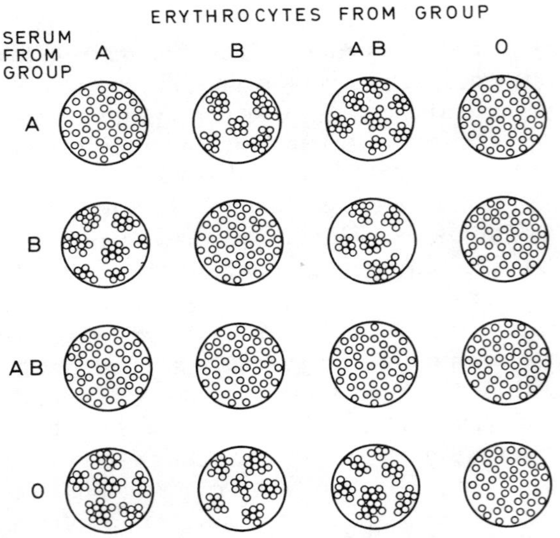

Clues about the mechanism of gene action in the ABO system were provided by several observations, some of which were originally thought to be unrelated to the ABO system. In 1930, Michael Eisler reported that goat antisera made against *Shigella dysenteriae* agglutinated not only bacteria, but also human red blood cells. Apparently, human erythrocytes and bacteria shared a "heterogenetic," or H, antigen. The only indication that the H antigen might be part of the ABO system was the finding that anti-H sera agglutinated erythrocytes of type O more strongly than they did other human red blood cells.

In 1926, K. Yamakami, as well as Karl Landsteiner and Philip Levine, observed that mixing of seminal fluid or spermatozoa with anti-AB sera removed the anti-AB activity, and he suggested that bodily fluids contain AB antigens. This observation was later confirmed by many other investigators, and AB substances were found in a variety of bodily fluids—urine, saliva, milk, and amniotic fluid.

In 1932, F. Schiff and H. Sasaki discovered that AB substances occurred in secretions of some, but not of other individuals, and thus divided humankind into secretors (about 75 to 80 percent of all individuals) and nonsecretors.

In 1946, A. E. Mourant observed that the serum of a Mrs. Lewis agglutinated about 25 percent of unselected blood samples from the British population, and he attributed this activity to an antibody he designated anti-Le^a. Two years later, P. H. Andresen obtained a

Figure 10.35. Reactions of four human sera with four human erythrocyte suspensions. The distribution of positive (clumping) and negative (nonagglutination) reactions defines four basic blood groups: A, B, AB, and O. Large circles represent the field of vision of a microscope, small circles, erythrocytes.

serum that agglutinated most Le^a-negative and failed to agglutinate any Le^a-positive red blood cells. He attributed the activity to an antibody that reacted with an Le^b antigen. Population studies revealed that about 20 percent of individuals were Le^a-positive, 70 percent were Le^b-positive, and 10 percent were Le-negative (i.e., reactive neither with anti-Le^a nor anti-Le^b sera). The relationship of the Lewis system to the ABO-secretor system was suggested by the observation that all Le^a-positive individuals were nonsecretors. These observations set the stage for the correct interpretation of how the ABO system operates. It took many years, however, before such an interpretation of the AB-H-Le system was reached.

10.7.2 Genetics

We now know that the ABO antigens are controlled by at least four loci: *ABO*, which control the AB substances and are located at the distal end of the long arm of chromosome 9; *H*(*h*), which controls the hetrogenetic substances (individuals carrying the *H* alleles possess the H antigen; *hh* individuals lack the antigen); *Se* (*se*), which controls the secretor status of an individual (*Se*/*Se* and *Se*/*se* individuals are secretors, whereas *se*/*se* individuals are nonsecretors); and *Le* (*le*), which controls the Lewis substance (but the presence or absence of the Lewis substance and the type of the substance when present are determined by an interaction with other genes of the ABO system—namely, *Se* and *H*). The ABH-secretor-Lewis phenotype of a red blood cell depends on a particular combination of alleles at these four loci. The various phenotypes determined by the different gene combinations are listed in Table 10.18. How these phenotypes arise will become clear only after we have discussed the chemical nature of the ABO and related antigens.

10.7.3 Chemistry

Studies by Walter T. J. Morgan, Winifred M. Watkins, K. O. Loyd, Elvin A. Kabat, and other investigators have established that the ABHLe antigenicity resides in oligosaccharide chains of varying length: some chains are only a few sugar residues long, while others contain up to 60 residues. The chains can exist in three forms—free, attached to proteins, or attached to lipids. *Free oligosaccharides* have been isolated from milk, colostrum, and urine. Protein-bound ABHLe antigens (*glycoproteins*) are secreted by goblet cells (mucus-producing epithelial cells, columnar in shape but extended at the free end) and by mucus glands of the gastrointestinal tract (producing saliva, gastric juice, bile, and meconium—the first intestinal discharge of the newborn infant), genitourinary tract (producing spermatic fluid, vaginal secretions, ovarian cyst fluid, urine), and respiratory tract; they are also present in amniotic fluid, milk, sweat, and tears. The oligosaccharide side chains are attached, through *N*-acetyl-D-galactosamine, to a serine or threonine of the protein backbone. The lipid-bound ABHLe antigens (*glycolipids*) are incorporated into the plasma membrane of red blood cells and of cells of other tissues such as liver, spleen, kidney, pancreas, and stomach. Here, the oligosaccharide is attached by a glucose to a sphingolipid (consisting of *N*-acetyl-sphingosine or ceramide and fatty acids; see Fig. 5.37). Thus, in contrast to ABHLe-active glycoproteins, which always contain *N*-acetyl-D-galactosamine, glycolipid may—but need not—contain this sugar.

Most of the work on chemical characterization of blood-group substances has been done on *water-soluble glycoproteins*, which can be isolated relatively easily in large quantities from bodily fluids (especially the ovarian cyst mucins). The water-insoluble, membrane-bound glycolipids have only recently been extracted from cells in quantities sufficient for chemical analysis, so our knowledge of the glycoproteins is far more complete than that of the glycolipids.

The basic structural unit of all *oligosaccharide chains* with ABHLe activity is a disaccharide composed of D-galactose (Gal) and *N*-acetyl-glucosamine (GlcNAc; Fig. 10.36). The variation in length of the chains depends on how many times this basic unit is repeated. Further variation is achieved by chain

Table 10.18 The Relationship between Genotype and Phenotype in the Human ABO System

Gene Combination	Antigens on RBC					Antigens in Secretion				
	A	B	H	Le^a	Le^b	A	B	H	Le^a	Le^b
AB H Se, *Le*	+	+	+	−	+	+	+	+	+	+
AB H sese, *Le*	+	+	+	+	−	−	−	−	+	−
AB H Se, *lele*	+	+	+	−	−	+	+	+	−	−
AB hh, *Se* or *sese*, *Le*	−	−	−	+	−[a]	−	−	−	+	−[a]
AB hh, *Se* or *sese*, *lele*	−	−	−	−	−[a]	−	−	−	−	−[a]

[a] The Bombay phenotype

+, presence of antigen; −, absence of antigen

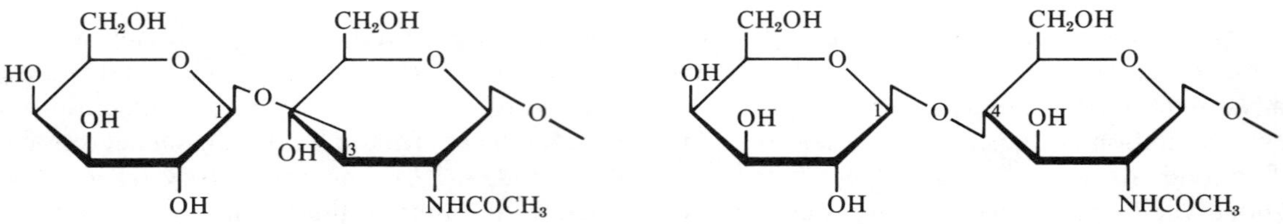

βGal(1 → 3) βGlcNAc
Type 1

βGal(1 → 4) βGlcNAc
Type 2

Figure 10.36. Two types of carbohydrate chain ending found in ABHLe-active oligosaccharides.

branching, for example, in the following manner:

```
Gal-GlcNAc
           >Gal-GlcNAc-Gal-GlcNAc—
Gal-GlcNAc
```

The chains attached to lipids contain glucose at one end; the attachment to proteins occurs via *N*-acetyl-D-galactosamine. The free end of the chain can terminate with the basic disaccharide unit or can have an L-fucose (Fuc) and *N*-acetyl-D-galactosamine (GalNAc) attached to one of the terminal residues. It is this composition and arrangement of the terminal sugar residues that determines the blood-group activity of the oligosaccharide chain. Chains lacking L-fucose at their free termini do not have any ABH activity. (Since it was first found in a person from Bombay, this characteristic is referred to as the *Bombay phenotype*.) Chains carrying L-fucose attached to the terminal D-galactose

```
Fuc
 |
Gal—GlcNAc—
```

have H, but no AB or Le activity. Chains ending with *N*-acetyl-D-galactosamine and with the L-fucose attached to the penultimate D-galactose

```
          Fuc
           |
GalNAc—Gal—GlcNAc—
```

have H and A activity. Chains ending with D-galactose and with L-fucose attached to the adjacent galactose

```
       Fuc
        |
Gal—Gal—GlcNAc
```

have H and B activity.

To explain the origin of the Le activity, we must first consider the types of linkage joining the D-galactose with the *N*-acetylglucosamine in the basic disaccharide unit. Two types of linkage are possible (Fig. 10.36): in *Type 1*, carbon 1 of D-galactose is linked with carbon 3 of *N*-acetylglucosamine; in *Type 2*, carbon 1 of D-galactose is linked with carbon 4 of *N*-acetylglucosamine. In a single chain the linkage is always *either* of Type 1 *or* Type 2, although in Type 2 chains, the disaccharide units are joined by a 1 → 3 linkage from GlcNAc of one unit to the D-galactose of the adjacent unit:

```
[Gal(1 → 4)GlcNAc] (1 → 3) [Gal(1 → 4)GlcNAc]
          (1 → 3) [Gal(1 → 4)GlcNAc] (1 → 3)
```

In a branched chain, one prong of the fork may be based on Type 1 and the other on Type 2 linkages:

```
Fuc
↓1,2
Gal(1 → 3)GlcNAc 1,3
                    >Gal—
Gal(1 → 4)GlcNAc 1,6
↑1,2
Fuc
```

However, the "hybrid" branched chains have so far been found only in glycoproteins; branched chains of glycolipids are either of Type 1 or Type 2, but never of the hybrid type. The H, A, and B antigens can be present on both Type 1 and Type 2 chains, but Le antigens can occur only on Type 1 chains.

The reason for this restriction is as follows. The appearance of Le antigens requires the attachment of L-fucose to the *N*-acetyl-D-glucosamine of the terminal disaccharide. But since the Fuc → GlcNAc linkage is of the 1 → 4 type, this attachment is not possible in Type 2 chains, where carbon 4 of the GlcNAc is involved in the 1 → 4 linkage with the D-galactose. The Le^a phenotype arises when H antigen-determining L-fucose is present, and Le^b arises when it is not. Chains lacking the terminal D-galactose-linked

L-fucose

Fuc
↓1,4
Gal(1 → 3)GlcNAc—

display Le^a activity (and lack H activity). Chains carrying both L-fucose and residues at the terminus

Fuc ↓1,2   Fuc ↓1,4
Gal(1 → 3)GlcNAc

display Le^b activity (and also H activity). The relationship between structure and antigenicity of oligosaccharide chains is summarized in Table 10.19.

The structural basis for the A_1 and A_2 antigens remains unclarified. Some investigators believe that the A-encoded enzyme (see below) exists in two forms (controlled by two alleles), one less effective than the other. The less effective enzyme adds fewer galactose residues to oligosaccharide chains than the more effective enzyme and the resulting quantitative difference is then the basis for the distinction between A_1 and A_2 subgroups. Other investigators believe that there is some as yet unidentified qualitative difference between the A_1 and A_2 antigens.

10.7.4 Mechanism of Gene Action

Loci controlling the attachment of the first *N*-acetylgalactosamine to the protein backbone and D-glucose to the lipid backbone, and genes controlling the joining of D-galactose with *N*-acetylglucosamine in the basic disaccharide unit and the joining of the disaccharide units have not yet been identified. The four known loci (*H, Se, ABO,* and *Le*) are all concerned with the synthesis of the oligosaccharide free ends.

The *H* gene codes for an enzyme, *fucosyltransferase*, which attaches L-fucose to the terminal or subterminal D-galactose, producing the H antigen. Whether the *h* allele produces a protein is not known, but if it does, the product must be enzymatically inactive. In *hh* individuals, L-fucose fails to attach to the oligosaccharide endings and since the ABO gene cannot act on these endings unless the L-fucose is attached first, the chains bear neither H nor AB antigens (i.e., the individuals have the Bombay phenotype). The *Le* gene acts independently of the *H* and *ABO* genes (individuals with the Bombay phenotype can be Le-positive).

The expression of the *H* gene is somehow controlled by the *Se* locus, but only in the secretory cells; in hemopoietic cells (and erythrocytes), the *H* gene acts independently of *Se*. In secretory cells, the *se* allele, when present in a homozygous state, shuts off the

Table 10.19 Relationship between ABHLe Antigenicity and Oligosaccharide Structure

Antigen	Structure of Oligosaccharide Free End: Type 1	Type 2
H	Fuc ↓1,2 Gal(1 → 3)GlcNAc—	Fuc ↓1,2 Gal(1 → 4)GlcNAc—
A	Fuc ↓1,2 (on Gal) GalNAc(1 → 3)Gal(1 → 3)GlcNAc—	Fuc ↓1,2 (on Gal) GalNAc(1 → 3)Gal(1 → 4)GlcNAc—
B	Fuc ↓1,2 (on Gal) Gal(1 → 3)Gal(1 → 3)GlcNAc—	Fuc ↓1,2 (on Gal) Gal(1 → 3)Gal(1 → 4)GlcNAc—
Le^a	Fuc ↓1,4 Gal(1 → 3)GlcNAc—	
Le^b	Fuc ↓1,4 Gal(1 → 3)GlcNAc—	

H gene, so that no L-fucose is added to the terminal D-galactose and no H activity (and consequently, no AB activity) appears in secretions. The *se/se* individuals thus appear as nonsecretors, although this designation is a misnomer since they secrete glycoproteins, which lack ABH activity. The presence of glycoproteins in secretions of nonsecretors is evident, for example, from their reaction with anti-Le^a sera. (The expression of the Le^a gene is independent of both the *H* and the *se* gene, and hence the Le^a antigen appears even in the absence of H and AB antigens; however, as is discussed below, the expression of the Le antigen depends on the presence of the H antigen.) The *Se* allele permits normal expression of the *H* gene. On hemopoietic cells and erythrocytes, the *Se* locus is either not expressed at all or has no control over the *H* gene or its products. Consequently, nonsecretors who lack ABH antigens in their secretions have a normal amount of these antigens on red blood cells.

The *ABO* locus codes for two *glycosyltransferases*, an *N-acetyl-D-galactosaminyltransferase* controlled by the *A* gene, and a *galactosyltransferase* controlled by the *B* gene. The former links up *N*-acetyl-D-galactosamine to the terminal D-galactose, while the latter places a D-galactose in this position instead. Both transferases can act only on oligosaccharides that already have the *H* gene-determined L-fucose attached to the terminal. The *O* gene codes for functionally inactive proteins.

The *Le* gene codes for an enzyme, *fucosyltransferase*, which attaches additional L-fucose to an *N*-acetyl-D-glucosamine at the chain's end. If the chain also bears the L-fucose specified by the *H* gene, it will appear as Le^b-positive (the Le^b antigenic determinant thus involves both L-fucoses, one controlled by the *H* and the other by the *Le* gene); if the chain bears no other L-fucose (in *hh* individuals), it will possess Le^a activity. The *le* gene is inactive, producing neither the Le^a nor the Le^b antigen (no L-fucose attached to *N*-acetyl-D-glucosamine). Erythrocytes do not express the *Le* gene; although they may carry Le antigens, these are not an integral part of the red cell membrane, but are acquired secondarily from the plasma in which the erythrocytes circulate. The acquired antigens are glycolipids, rather than glycoproteins; they are not derived from secretions. The Le-positive glycolipids are synthesized at an as yet unidentified site and carried in the plasma by high- and low-density lipoproteins. In secretions, Le^a and Le^b antigens are carried by the same glycoprotein molecules as are the ABH antigens.

We stated earlier that the appearance of the Le^b antigen requires the addition of L-fucose to the oligosaccharide end by the *H* gene-determined fucosyltransferase. We also said that the *H* gene (or its product) is turned off in *se/se* individuals (nonsecretors). It follows from these two observations that nonsecretors can never produce Le^b-positive secretions—a conclusion reached empirically many years ago by blood group serologists.

10.7.5 Function

Like the characters who search for an author in Pirandello's famous play, most cell-surface antigens are searching for a function. The ABO blood-group antigens are no exception in this respect. For, despite three-quarters of a century of research, the function of ABO antigens remains unknown. The fact that persons with the Bombay phenotype lead a normal life, combined with the finding that some 45 percent of all individuals in a human population have blood group O, indicates that the AB antigens are not essential for normal bodily functioning. The significance of the ABO variation is more likely at the population, not the individual level; it may somehow be advantageous for the *species* to have the different red blood cell variants in store. Scientists have put an enormous effort into finding out what the selective advantage of the individual antigens might be, but they have failed to come up with any clues. A number of diseases have been claimed to be associated with one or the other of the ABO antigens but, in each case, closer scrutiny revealed this association to be due to a sampling error or some other technical flaw. Now, as in 1901, when they were discovered, ABO blood groups remain a mystery.

10.7.6 Other Blood-Group Antigens

In addition to the ABHLe system, some 200 other antigens belonging to more than 20 different systems are known in humans. Many other antigenic systems are known in other mammals. The chemical structure of most of these antigens has not been elucidated. Of great clinical importance is the human *Rh system*, so named because it was discovered with the aid of rabbit antibodies to rhesus monkey erythrocytes. The system is quite complex, consisting of many antigens for which three different notations systems have been proposed—one by Ronald A. Fisher and R. R. Race, another by Alexander S. Wiener, and still another by Richard E. Rosenfield (Table 10.20). All three systems are in use and there seems to be no willingness to compromise. As someone once remarked, scientists would rather share their toothbrushes than their nomenclatures.

The first two notations are based on two different genetic interpretations of the Rh system. According to Fischer and Race, the system consists of three closely linked loci—*D* (*d*), *C* (*c*), and *e*—and each allele (with the exception of *d*, which is serologically silent) codes for a single antigen (D, C, c, or e). The recombination frequency among these loci is so low that the human population carries only a limited number of gene combinations (one could say haplotypes, the main haplotypes being *Dce*, *DCe*, *DcE*, *DCE*, *dce*, *dCe*, *dcE*, and *dCE*). According to Wiener's interpretation, there is only one *Rh* locus with many alleles, each allele coding for several antigens designated by a rather baroque array of symbols. Rosenfield's nomenclature tries to avoid taking a stand on the genetic interpretation of the Rh system by assigning neutral numbers to individual determinants. Rosenfield's is clearly the best solution to the Rh jungle and one would hope that, eventually, human serologists will unite and accept his notation.

Table 10.20. Rh Antigens and Their Frequencies

Name of Determinant According to			
Rosenfield et al.	Fisher and Race	Wiener	Frequency in Caucasians (percent)[a]
Rh1	D	Rh_0	85
Rh2	C	rh′	70
Rh3	E	rh″	30
Rh4	c	hr′	80
Rh5	e	hr″	98
Rh6	ce or f	hr	64
Rh7	Ce	rh_i	70
Rh8	C^w	rh^{w1}	1
Rh9	C^x	rh^x	<1
Rh10	V or ce^s	hr^v	<1
Rh11	E^w	rh^{w2}	<1
Rh12	G	rh^G	85
Rh13		Rh^A	85
Rh14		Rh^B	85
Rh15		Rh^C	85
Rh16		Rh^D	85
Rh17		Hr	100
Rh18		Hr^0	100
Rh19		hr^s	98
Rh20	VS or e^s		<1
Rh21	C^G		70
Rh22	CE		<1
Rh23	D^w		<1
Rh24	E^T		30
Rh25	LW		100
Rh26	c-like		80
Rh27	cE		30
Rh28		hr^H	<1
Rh29	RH		100
Rh30	D^{Cor}		<1
Rh31		hr^B	98
Rh32			<1
Rh33			<1
Rh34			<1
Rh35			100

[a] Since a single individual may possess more than one antigenic determinant, the frequencies do not add up to 100 percent.

REFERENCES

General

Atassi, M. Z. (Ed.): *Immunochemistry of Proteins*, Vols. 1 and 2. Plenum, New York, 1977.

Bittiger, H. and Schnebli, H. P. (Eds.): *Concanavalin A as a Tool*. Wiley, London, 1976.

Borek, F. (Ed.): *Immunogenicity*. North-Holland, Amsterdam, 1972.

Campbell, D. H., Garvey, J. S., Cremer, N. E., and Sussdorf, D. H.: *Methods in Immunology*, 2nd ed. Benjamin, New York, 1970.

Hudson, L. and Hay, F. C.: *Practical Immunology*. Blackwell, Oxford, 1976.

Jollès, P. and Paraf, A.: *Chemical and Biological Basis of Adjuvants*. Springer-Verlag, Berlin, 1973.

Landsteiner, K.: *The Specificity of Serologic Reactions*. Dover, New York, 1962.

Lefkovits, I. and Pernis, B. (Eds.): *Immunological Methods*. Academic, New York, 1979.

Ling, N. R. and Kay, J. E.: *Lymphocyte Stimulation*. North-Holland, Amsterdam, 1975.

Pressman, D. and Grossberg, A. L.: *The Structural Basis of Antibody Specificity*. Benjamin, New York, 1968.

Sela, M.: *The Antigens*, Vols. I-V. Academic, New York, 1973–1979.

Sharon, N. and Lis, H.: Lectins: cell-agglutinating and sugar-specific proteins. *Science* **177**:949–959, 1972.

Weir, D. M. (Ed.): *Handbook of Experimental Immunology*, Vols. 1–3, 2nd ed. Blackwell, Oxford, 1973.

Williams, C. A. and Chase, M. W. (Eds.): *Methods in Immunology and Immunochemistry*, Vols. I–V. Academic, New York, 1967–1976.

Original Articles

Andresen, P. H.: The blood group system L. A new blood group, L_2. *Acta Path. Microbiol. Scand.* **25**:728–731, 1948.

Assmann, F.: Beitrage zur Kenntnis pflanzlicher Agglutinine. *Arch. Ger. Physiol.* **134**:489–510, 1911.

Boyd, W. C. and Reguera, R. M.: Hemagglutinating substances for human cells in various plants. *J. Immunol.* **62**:333–339, 1949.

Boyd, W. C. and Shapleigh, E.: Specific precipitating activity of plant agglutinins (lectins). *Science* **119**:419, 1954.

Danysz, J.: Contribution à l'étude des proprietés et de la nature des mélanges des toxines avec leurs antitoxines. *Ann. Inst. Pasteur* **16**:331–345, 1902.

DeCastello, A. and Sturli, A.: Über die Isoagglutinine im Serum gesunder und kranker Menschen. *Münch. Med. Wochenschr.* 1090–1095, 1902.

Dienes, L. and Schoenheit, E. W.: Certain characteristics of the infectious process in connection with the influence exerted on the immunity response. *J. Immunol.* **19**:41–61, 1930.

Eisler, M.: Über ein gemeinsames Antigen in den Zellen des Menschen und in Shigabazillen. *Zschr. Immunitätsforsch.* **67**:38–48, 1930.

Farr, R. S.: A quantitative immunochemical measure of the primary interaction between I*BSA and antibody. *J. Infect. Dis.* **103**:239–262, 1958.

Forssman, J.: Die Herstellung hochwertiger spezifischer Schafhämolysine ohne Verwendung von Schafblut. *Biochem. Z.* **37**:78–115, 1911.

Janský, J.: Hematologické studie u psychotiků. *Klinický Sborník* **8**:85–139, 1907.

Jones, D. B. and Jones, C. D.: Some proteins from the jack bean, *Canavalia ensiformis*. *J. Biol. Chem.* **28**:67–75, 1916.

Landsteiner, K.: Über heterogenetisches Antigen und Hapten. XV. Mitteilung über Antigene. *Biochem. Z.* **119**:294–306, 1921.

Landsteiner, K. and Levine, P.: On group specific substances in human spermatozoa. *J. Immunol.* **12**:441–460, 1926.

Landsteiner, K. and Raubitschek, H.: Über die Adsorption von Immunstoffen. V. Mitteilung. *Biochem. Z.* **115**:33–51, 1908.

Möller, G., Andersson, J., and Sjöberg, O.: Lipopolysaccharides can convert heterologous red cells into thymus-independent antigens. *Cell. Immunol.* **4**:416–424, 1972.

Moss, W. L.: Studies on isoagglutinins and isohemolysins. *Bull. Johns Hopkins Hosp.* **21**:63–70, 1910.

Mourant, A. E.: A "new" human blood group antigen of frequent occurrence. *Nature (Lond.)* **158**:237, 1946.

Nowell, P. C.: Phytohaemagglutinin: an initiator of mitosis in cultures of normal human leukocytes. *Cancer Res.* **20**:462–466, 1960.

Pasteur, L. and Joubert, G.: Charbon et scepticémie. *C.R. Acad. Sci. (Paris)* **85**:101–115, 1877.

Ramon, G.: Sur la concentration du sérum antidiphtérique et l'isolement de l'antitoxine. *C.R. Soc. Biol. (Paris)* **88**:167–168, 1923.

Ramon, G.: Pouvoir floculant et pouvoir toxique de la toxine diphtérique. *C.R. Soc. Biol. (Paris)* **89**:2–4, 1923.

Renkonen, K. O.: Studies in hemagglutinins present in seeds of some representatives of the family of *Leguminosae*. *Ann. Med. Exp. Biol. Fenniae* **26**:66–72, 1948.

Scatchard, G.: The attractions of proteins for small molecules and ions. *Ann. N.Y. Acad. Sci.* **51**:660–672, 1949.

Schiff, F. and Sasaki, H.: Der Ausscheidungstypus, ein auf serologischen Wege nachweisbares mendelndes Merkmal. *Klin. Wochenschr.* **11**:1426–1429, 1932.

Sips, R.: On the structure of a catalyst surface. *J. Chem. Phys.* **16**:490–495, 1948.

Stillmark, H.: Über Rizin, ein giftiges Ferment aus dem Samen von *Ricinus communis* L. und einigen anderen Euphorbiaceen. *Inaug. Diss.*, Dorpat, 1888.

Sumner, J. B.: The globulins of the jack bean, *Canavalia ensiformis*. *J. Biol. Chem.* **37**:137–144, 1919.

Yamakami, K.: The individuality of semen, with reference to its property of inhibiting specifically isohemagglutination. *J. Immunol.* **12**:185–189, 1926.

(See also references 17, 22, 31, 36, 42, 50, 52, 53, 54, 59, 67, 68, 69, and 95 in Chapter 2.)

THE THIRD MOVEMENT
Mechanisms

CHAPTER 11

IMMUNE RESPONSES DOMINATED BY CELLS OF THE MONOCYTIC SERIES

Now that we have described the instruments of the immunological orchestra, we shall analyze the music they play. We shall proceed like a conductor who has just received the score of a new composition. Instead of trying to follow all the instruments at once, we shall first study the music played by individual *groups* of instruments—the woodwinds, brass, and strings—and only then shall we try to perceive the composition in its entirety. In other words, we shall first describe the activities of the individual cell groups (cells of the monocytic and granulocytic series in this chapter, T lymphocytes in Chapter 12, and B lymphocytes in

Chapter 13), and then, in Chapter 14, we shall put all this knowledge together to attain an understanding of how the different activities intertwine in securing the integrity of an organism.

In this chapter, we shall first learn about the functional activity (phagocytosis) shared by neutrophils and macrophages (section 11.1), and then have a look at some other activities of macrophages (sections 11.2 through 11.5). It might seem logical to include the discussion of responses mediated by mast cells and granulocytes here, but for reasons that will become apparent later, we shall postpone this discussion until Chapters 13 and 14.

11.1 PHAGOCYTOSIS AND RELATED PHENOMENA

The plasma membrane of a cell is in constant motion, even if the cell itself is stationary. The membrane ruffles, folds, and sends out fingerlike protrusions and invaginations. From time to time, some of the protrusions close over a small volume of the external milieu and form a vesicle, which is then internalized by pinching off from the membranes (Fig. 11.1*a*). Exogenous material is thus constantly taken up by the cell and the plasma membrane is continually internalized. This uptake of material by cells is called *endocytosis* (Gr. *endon*, within; *kytos*, cell; suffix *-osis*, condition). Although most, if not all, eukaryotic cells take up material by endocytosis, some cells (e.g., neutrophils, macrophages, monocytes, capillary endothelial and thyroid epithelial cells, yolk sac cells, and oocytes) do so at a much faster rate than other cells. Macrophages, for example, interiorize 180 percent of their surface area as endocytic vesicles in an hour. Most of the interiorized membrane is exteriorized again by *exocytosis* (Gr. *exo*, outside), which is the reverse of endocytosis: the vesicle attaches to the plasma membrane from the cell's inside, opens up at the attachment site, integrates into the membrane, and, at the same time, discharges its contents into the extracellular environment (Fig. 11.1*b*). The endo-exocytosis cycle thus provides the means of getting things into and out of a cell or transporting them across it.

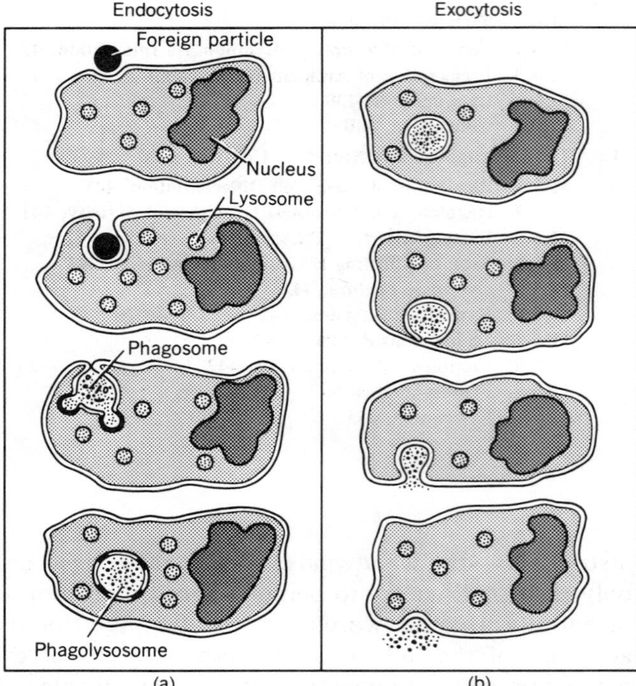

Figure 11.1. Endocytosis and exocytosis.

Endocytosis can be of two kinds, depending on the consistency and size of the material taken up. If this material is fluid, or in a macromolecular form, or if there are small particles dissolved in the fluid, one speaks of *pinocytosis* (Gr. *pineo*, to drink), if the material is a large particle, one refers to the take-up process as *phagocytosis* (Gr. *phagein*, to eat). A pinocytic vesicle is always filled with fluid; a phagocytic vesicle, on the other hand, is almost completely occupied by the particle and contains very little, if any, fluid. Pinocytosis is carried out by most cells most of the time; phagocytosis, on the other hand, is carried out by specialized cells—mainly neutrophils, monocytes, and macrophages. In pinocytosis, the interiorized material need not attach to or interact with the membrane, although when it does, its uptake may be speeded several thousandfold. But to be phagocytosed, most particles must first interact with the membrane. Uptake by pinocytosis is therefore directly related to the concentration of the substance in the environment; uptake by phagocytosis depends on the number and affinity of membrane-binding sites capable of interacting with the particle.

Phagocytosis, the ingestion and digestion of a particulate substance by cells (*phagocytes*), can be divided conveniently into five stages: recognition and attachment, engulfment, lysozyme and granule fusion (degranulation), killing and digestion of microorganisms, and exocytosis. It is preceded, at least in vivo, by a chemically guided movement (chemotaxis) of phagocytic cells toward the target particle. The ingested particle can be many things—a microorganism, a fragment thereof, the body's own cell whose usefulness has been exhausted by attrition or a structural defect, a cell fragment, a grain of inorganic matter introduced into the body by an experimenter (e.g., colloidal iron) or through breathing (e.g., a speck of dust), or a protozoal parasite. The two major types of cell capable of phagocytosis are macrophages (monocytes) and neutrophils. The former is a mononuclear cell—that is, a cell with a single nonsegmented nucleus, and the latter is a polymorphonuclear cell, with a segmented nucleus that gives the appearance of being several nuclei.

Before we describe the five stages of phagocytosis, let us first discuss how phagocytes and phagocytosed particles are brought together.

11.1.1 Chemotaxis

Neutrophils and macrophages move constantly. Most of the time the movement is random: it may occur in any direction with equal probability. But occasionally the behavior of these cells changes. As if called by an invisible signal, they stop their random browsing, take a direction, and head straight to the apparent signal. The directed movement of cells in response to a signal is called *chemotaxis* (Gr. *chemos*, juice, liquid; *taxis*, an arrangement, also movement). Chemotaxis is not limited to neutrophils and macrophages: it is also exerted by lymphocytes, fibroblasts, melanoblasts, plant spermatozoa, or bacteria. (To distinguish the directed movement of leukocytes from that of other cells, the former is sometimes referred to as *leukotaxis*.) Chemotaxis can be either positive, when cells are heading toward the signal, or negative, when they are moving away from it. Leukotaxis is almost always positive; negative chemotaxis is exerted, for example, by certain bacteria.

Methods of Study

Of the many different methods available for the study of chemotaxis only two will be mentioned here—an in vivo and an in vitro method.

Skin Window Technique (Fig. 11.2*a*). In this technique, an area of an animal's skin (e.g., the surface of the forearm) is shaved and cleaned with alcohol, and the epidermis is carefully scraped with a sterile scalpel over a region of from three to four millimeters in diameter until very fine bleeding points are seen, indicating that the capillary layer of the corium has been reached. The abraded area is covered with a sterile glass cover slip, held in place by adhesive tape. Leukocytes migrate to the injured site and adhere to the undersurface of the cover slip. At intervals, the cover slip is replaced with another, the removed slip is air-dried and stained, and the number of adhering leukocytes is determined microscopically. To determine a substance's chemotactic activity, one applies this substance over the abraded area before attaching the cover slip, then determines the number of adhering leukocytes, and compares this number with that in a skin window to which no substance has been applied.

The Boyden Chamber Technique (Fig. 11.2*b*). In 1962, S. Boyden devised a simple, quantitative technique for studying leukotaxis in vitro in a specially designed chamber. The *Boyden chamber* has two compartments, separated by a filter with pores small enough to prevent cells from simply falling through them, but at the same time, large enough that cells can squeeze their way through. A leukocyte suspension is placed in the upper compartment and the material to be tested for chemotactic activity in the lower compartment. Responding to chemotactic stimuli, cells migrate through the filter, and the response can be quantitated by counting those cells that have accumulated on the lower surface of the filter after a certain incubation period.

Chemotactic Factors

Substances capable of causing directional movement of cells are called *chemotactic factors*. Their action can be either direct, in which case they are referred to as *cytotaxins*, or indirect, in which case they are called *cytotaxigens* (i.e., substances that generate chemotactically active compounds). The bewildering array of chemotactic factors can be divided into four groups: factors of bacterial and viral origin, components of plasma activation systems (complement components and components of the clotting and fibrinolytic systems), factors elaborated by cells of the immune system, and miscellaneous other factors.

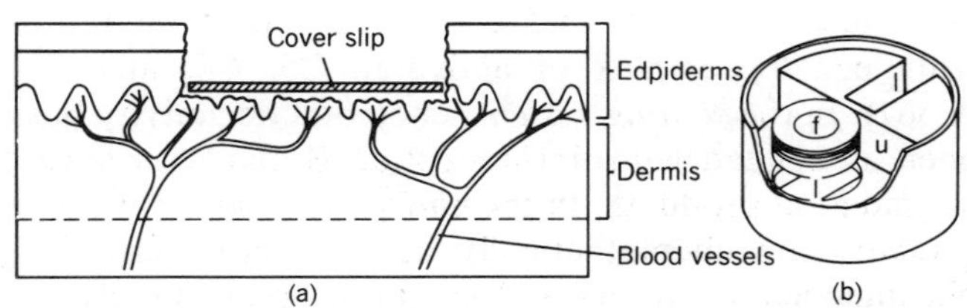

Figure 11.2. Two methods used in the study of chemotaxis. (*a*) The skin window technique. (*b*) The Boyden chamber technique. The chamber consists of two compartments—upper (u) and lower (l)—separated from each other by a filter (f). The filter is fixed in place by a cap, which fits into the aperture between the two compartments. (*b* from S. Boyden: *J. Exp. Med.* **115**:453–466, 1962.)

Chemotactic Factors Produced by Microorganisms. Most bacteria produce chemotactic factors, and often a single bacterium makes several, usually during its growth phase. The relationships among factors manufactured by different bacteria and the nature of the individual factors are not known. Some have a molecular weight as low as 150 daltons, while others are much larger. Chemically, they can be peptides (proteins) or lipids.

Bacteria may also induce chemotaxis indirectly: they may stimulate production of specific antibodies, the antibody-bacterial antigen complexes may activate the complement cascade, and some of the complement components may induce chemotaxis; protein A of the *Staphylococcus* cell wall may bind IgG and thus activate the complement pathway; endotoxins of Gram-negative bacteria may activate the alternative complement pathway; some bacteria may produce proteolytic enzymes capable of activating certain complement components; bacterial endotoxins may activate the Hageman factor of the coagulation cascade, and the activated components of this cascade may act as chemotactic factors; and finally, the clotting cascade can also be activated by other events accompanying bacterial infection (tissue damage, local platelet aggregation, and accumulation of leukocytes).

Similar mechanisms also operate in viral infections. Viral replication may release chemotaxins from infected cells, or it may lead to cell destruction and the release of proteolytic enzymes capable of activating complement components. Alternatively, virus-encoded cell-surface antigens may bind specific antibodies and the antigen-antibody complexes may activate the complement cascade, or they may bind sensitized lymphocytes and induce them to secrete chemotactically active lymphokines.

Components of the Plasma Activation Systems. Components of all four activation systems described in Chapter 9 have been implicated in chemotaxis. In the *complement system*, four chemotactic factors have been identified: C3a, C5a, C3 convertase, and the trimolecular complex of activated C5, C6, and C7 ($C\overline{567}$). In the *clotting system*, chemotactic activity has been associated with fibrinopeptide B and with fibrin degradation products. In the *fibrinolytic* and *bradykinin systems*, the chemotactically active factors are the plasminogen activators and kallikrein, respectively.

Mediators Produced by Cells of the Immune System. Chemotactic factors are produced by neutrophils, lymphocytes, and macrophages. The neutrophil-derived factors are probably not actively secreted by these cells but rather released upon cell death. The adaptive value of such a phenomenon could be to amplify the chemotactic reaction: when the first neutrophils arrive at the site of bacterial invasion, attracted either directly by bacterial products or indirectly through activation of plasma proteins, they immediately begin to phagocytose the invaders; during this process, however, some of the cells die, releasing a variety of cytotaxins and cytotaxigens, which then attract more neutrophils to the site.

Lymphocytes, on the other hand, are active secretors of chemotactic factors. The secretion commences following the stimulation of lymphocytes either by antigen or by one of the many polyclonal activators. The lymphocyte-derived chemotactic factors act mainly on monocytes and macrophages and less on neutrophils. But chemotactic activity is also associated with the transfer factor (see Chapter 7), the main target of which seems to be the polymorphonuclear cells.

Little is known about the macrophage-derived chemotactic factors. They seem to be produced by active secretion too and appear to be active on polymorphonuclear cells.

Miscellaneous Chemotactic Factors. This group contains factors that do not fit into any of the three previous groups and are not numerous enough or important enough to form groups of their own. They are leukogresin (probably modified IgG); synthetic formylated peptides, such as N-formyl methionine or N-formylmethionyl-leucine; lipids, such as arachidonic acid or eicosapentaenoic acid; collagen and collagenase; cyclic adenosine monophosphate; prostaglandins; cassein; IgM fragments; and purified bee venom (mellitin). The only thing most of these factors have in common is the presence of nonpolar groups. In native proteins, these groups are hidden away from the aqueous environment in the molecule's interior, but upon activation and unfolding of the molecule, they become exposed. The exteriorization of the nonpolar groups increases the molecule's hydrophobicity and thus the ability to form hydrophobic bonds with similar groups on the cell surface. However, hydrophobicity alone is probably not sufficient to make a molecule chemotactic; other characteristics we do not yet know might also be required.

Mechanism of Chemotactic Activation

The chemotactic signals are probably received by defined regions of the target-cell surface. One might call these regions "receptors," but there is no good evidence for a high degree of specificity in the interaction between them and the chemotactic molecules. If hydrophobic bond formation were indeed the basis for this interaction, one could envision the receptor simply as a patch of the membrane in which the constellation of building blocks favors formation of multiple bonds in a small area. This postulate would explain why only some molecules carrying nonpolar groups act as chemotactic factors; in these molecules, the groups may be arranged in such a way that they match the arrangement of groups on the corresponding membrane patch. It would also explain the observed diversity of chemotactic factors, since any molecule with this arrangement of polar groups, no matter what its nature otherwise, would be able to interact with the corresponding membrane patch. (I use the word "patch" to emphasize that the receptor site on the membrane may not be a single molecule and may not always be the *same* molecule.)

After receiving the chemotactic signal, the cell translates it into motion. The translation involves a series of events, such as serine esterase activation; fluxes of calcium, sodium, and potassium; changes in transmembrane electropotential; reduced surface charges; metabolic activation; and release of enzymes from granules. The last two of these events resemble those occurring during phagocytosis; they will be described in detail later in this chapter. The sequence of these events and their interrelationships are unknown.

The energy necessary for movement is supplied largely through adenosine triphosphate, generated by anaerobic glycolysis. The movement itself involves the extension of pseudopods and the formation of a broad, thin veil (*lamellipodium*) at the advancing front of the cell and a knoblike tail with trailing retraction fibers at the rear (see also Chapter 5). In the moving cell, the cytoplasm streams into the lamellipodia in the direction of the movement and away from the tail. Pseudopods, lamellipodia, and cytoplasmic streaming are probably produced through the polarized formation of the contractile system, which is composed of microtubules and microfilaments, with the former determining the direction of the movement and the latter supplying the work. Polarized microtubule polymerization may occur because of a localized alteration in cytoplasmic calcium. The speed of polymerization, and thus of the movement as well, may be controlled by cyclic nucleotides.

The directed movement of a cell toward the source of the chemotactic factor is based on the cell's ability to recognize the concentration gradient formed by this factor as it diffuses from its source. Apparently, the cell is somehow able to distinguish differences in concentration between two points in space. How does it do it? There are two principal possibilities: either the evenly distributed surface receptors inform the cell that fewer chemotactic molecules have been bound at one end of the cell than at the other, or there is a special concentration-determining region on the cell that must be moved around constantly during the cell's random migration to sense where the concentration is highest. The difference between these two possibilities is not unlike that between our ability to determine a source of heat or sound. Since we have heat receptors all over the body, we can tell, even when we are completely still, where the warmth comes from because one side of the body is warmer than the other; but to determine the source of a sound, we must often turn our heads so that the ear is better aligned with it. The available evidence suggests that cells determine the direction of a concentration gradient the way we determine the source of heat. Apparently, sensors of chemotactic molecules are distributed all over the cell surface and the cell selects the direction of movement based on which of its regions is bombarded most heavily by these molecules. The cell reacts to changes of a gradient direction almost instantly; it does not stop to "feel its way" as one would expect it to do if it had to align itself to determine the gradient direction before making a directed move.

Inhibitors of Chemotaxis

Like many other biological processes, chemotaxis, if not stopped when it is no longer needed, may cease to be beneficial and begin to harm the body. To prevent such a rampage of chemotaxis, the body has developed a series of control mechanisms that operate on one of two principles: inactivation of the chemotactic factors, or shutting off their production. A number of agents that inhibit chemotaxis by one or the other control mechanism have been identified. Representative of the factor-inactivating inhibitors are the various regulatory proteins associated with the complement cascade and with other activation systems in plasma. Among the agents that decrease neutrophil chemotactic responses are cyclic nucleotides; a neutrophil-immobilizing factor extracted from human polymorphonuclear cells and mononuclear leukocytes; a number of pharmacological substances, such as hydrocortisone, cyclophosphamide, or aspirin; certain bacterial products (e.g., staphylococcus cell-wall mucopeptide and streptolysin O); plasma esterase inhibitors; tuftsin (a phagocytosis-enhancing tetrapeptide, Thr-Lys-Pro-Arg); and altered physicochemical environment (changes in pH, osmolarity, and temperature).

11.1.2 Adherence

Once the phagocyte and the foreign particle have come into contact, either by chance encounter or as a result of chemotaxis, the first step of phagocytosis commences: the particle interacts with the plasma membrane of the phagocyte. But before we discuss the attachment (adherence) of a particle to a phagocyte, we must first answer one question: how does the phagocyte know which particle to ingest?

There are two principal ways to select particles for phagocytosis—immunological and nonimmunological. In the *nonimmunological way*, the particle is so obviously out of place in the body that the phagocyte has no difficulty in identifying it as foreign. Some inert materials (e.g., carbon, silica, berylium, or asbestos)—but some bacteria too—interact with phagocytes nonspecifically, perhaps via the formation of electrostatic and hydrophobic bonds in a manner that sets them apart from the body's own substances (Fig. 11.3*a*). This form of recognition plays a major role, for example, in the alveolar macrophages' clearing of dust particles from miners' lungs. The *immunological way* of recognition requires that the particle first be coated by certain serum proteins. This covering process, referred to as *opsonization* (the covering proteins are *opsonins*), serves two purposes: it identifies a particle as foreign, and it facilitates its engulfment by phagocytes. Particles that are not opsonized and that cannot be recognized in the nonimmunological way are not engulfed by phagocytes. One type of such a particle is an encapsulated bacterium, for which the capsule serves as an armor coat, protecting it from phagocytosis. These bacteria, however, can be engulfed by phagocytes after they have been opsonized.

Immunologists have known for some time that the opsonizing substances in the serum fall into two categories—thermostable and thermolabile (the latter being inactivated by heating to 56°C). Thermostable opsonins were later identified as immunoglobulins, and thermolabile opsonins as complement components. The most important, if not the sole, opsonizing immunoglobulin is IgG. Although IgM-associated opsonizing activity has also been reported, the evidence is not conclusive; other Ig classes do not seem to participate in opsonization to any measurable degree. Of the four human IgG subclasses, IgG1 and IgG3 are the most efficient opsonins, the order of effectiveness being IgG1 > IgG3 > IgG2 > IgG4. The most important opsonizing complement component is C3b; less important complement opsonins are C4b and C5b.

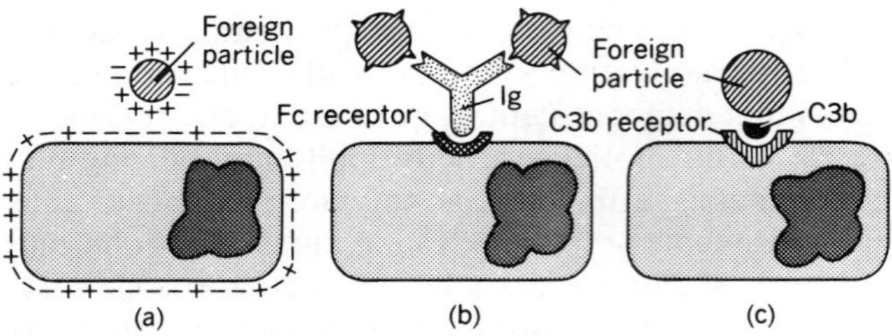

Figure 11.3. Three modes of adherence of a macrophage to a foreign particle. (*a*) Nonimmunological adherence mediated, perhaps, by electrostatic attraction. (*b*) Immunological adherence mediated by antibodies and Fc receptors. (*c*) Immunological adherence mediated by C3b fragments and C3b receptors.

Opsonization by IgG is immunologically specific, which means that only IgG molecules with combining sites complementary to antigens carried by a given particle bind to these particles. The binding exposes a site in the Fc region of the IgG molecule that is then recognized by a corresponding receptor, the *Fc receptor*, on the phagocyte. In this manner, the IgG molecule forms a bridge between antigens on the particle to which it binds via its combining sites and the Fc receptor of the phagocyte to which it attaches via its Fc region (Fig. 11.3*b*).

The C3b molecules are generated by clipping off the small C3a fragment from C3. The C3 cleavage occurs either by sequential complement activation (in either the classical or alternative pathway), or when C3 is acted upon by proteases derived from host tissues, host phagocytes, or bacteria. After the cleavage, C3b is deposited at the nearest membrane—for example, that of an invading bacterium. The attached C3b molecule is then recognized by the *C3b receptor* of the phagocyte and a bridge is formed between the particle and the phagocyte—but this time the bridging element is the C3b molecule (Fig. 11.3*c*).

Opsonization by IgG cannot take place before antibodies specific for the bacterial particles are produced. It is therefore likely that, in the first stage of infection, the invading bacteria are opsonized by C3b, which is generated by tissue phagocytes or bacterial proteases. Only later, when specific antibodies begin to appear, do IgG molecules join in; so at the height of the infection, opsonization by both C3b and IgG occurs concurrently, often on the same particle. The outcome of an infection often depends on whether the mobilization of opsonizing mechanisms manages to outrun the proliferation of the invaders.

In sum, then, there are three principal forces that bind a foreign particle to a phagocyte: nonspecific surface interaction, bridging via IgG molecules, and bridging via C3b molecules (Fig. 11.3). As will be discussed in section 11.4, nonparticulate antigens can apparently be taken up by phagocytes through pinocytosis.

11.1.3 Engulfment (Phagocytosis *Per Se*)

The period that runs from the attachment of a particle to a phagocyte until the complete disappearance of the particle inside the cell represents the third stage of phagocytosis—the engulfment, or phagocytosis in the strict sense of the word.

Methods of Study

Several procedures exist by which one can ascertain the phagocytic ingestion of particles; some of these are enumerated below.

Microscopic Methods. Particles (bacteria) are added to a suspension of phagocytes and the mixture is incubated and spread on a slide. The smears are fixed, stained, and examined with a light microscope. The results are expressed either as a *phagocytic index* (mean number of particles ingested per phagocyte) or the *percent of phagocytes* containing ingested particles. Although this method is the oldest, it is also the least accurate.

Isotopic Methods. There are two principal ways in which one can employ isotopes for the measurement of phagocytosis. In the first, one labels the particles themselves, either by attaching radioactive substances to them chemically, or by growing them in media containing radioactive metabolites. The other method is based on the observation that a small amount of the fluid surrounding the particle is taken up by the phagocyte during engulfment (a phenomenon sometimes referred to as *"piggy-back" phagocytosis*). One can therefore measure phagocytosis by adding a radioactive compound (e.g., ^{125}I-labeled human serum albumin) to the medium and determining the radioactivity of the washed cells.

Extraction Methods. When one uses particles that are normally not found in cells, one can measure the degree of phagocytosis by simply extracting the particles from the cells after engulfment. For example, one can incubate phagocytes with paraffin oil droplets containing a dye, Oil Red O, then separate the cells by gentle centrifugation and determine the amount of cell-associated dye spectrophotometrically. Or one can use polystyrene latex particles, extract the polystyrene from the phagocytes with dioxane, and again, determine its amount spectrophotometrically.

Indirect Methods. Engulfment of a particle is followed by a series of intracellular changes that can be used indirectly as indicators of phagocytosis. For example, one can measure the increase in the oxygen consumption that accompanies phagocytosis, the reduction of nitroblue tetrazolium dye, or an increased chemiluminescence. These changes will be discussed later in this chapter.

In Vivo Methods. In these procedures, one injects the particles into an animal and periodically samples the animal's blood to determine the particles' clearance rate.

Mechanism of Engulfment

The contact of the particle with the plasma membrane of the phagocyte initiates a series of events, the nature and sequence of which are still poorly understood. According to the hypothesis proposed in 1976 by T. P. Stossel and J. H. Hartwig (Fig. 11.4), a central role in the event is played by the so-called *actin-binding protein*. When added to a solution of actin (see Appendix 5.1), this high-molecular-weight protein isolated from macrophages and neutrophils causes assembly of the actin molecules into filaments, and gelation of the solution. In the cell, actin-binding protein is thought to be located either in the plasma membrane or close to it. The perturbation of the membrane caused by the adherence of the ingestible particle activates—in a manner not yet known—the actin-binding protein, which begins to polymerize actin molecules in the cytoplasm underlying the attachment site. The assembled actin filaments are acted upon by *myosin* in the presence of an actin-myosin co-factor, which accelerates the reaction. The actin-myosin interaction results in the myosin's contraction in the region of cell–particle contact, causing the formation of narrow pseudopods. As the pseudopods move around the particle, additional cell–particle contacts are made, and the actin-binding protein activation and regional formation of contractile microfilaments spreads. The pseudopod thus circumnavigates the entire particle and gradually engulfs it. The extent of circumnavigation depends on the degree of coating of the particles by opsonin molecules. If opsonins cover only half the

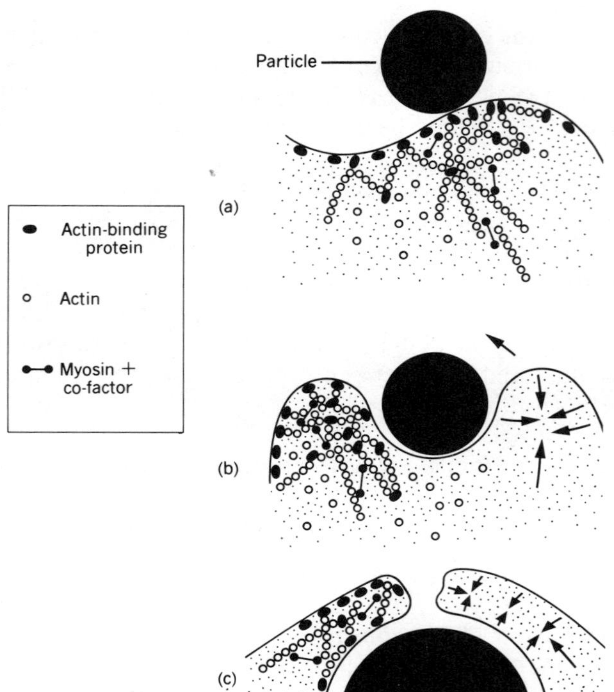

Figure 11.4. Proposed mechanism for pseudopod formation. (*a*) Contact between particle and phagocyte leads to the activation or release of actin-binding protein from the plasma membrane. (*b*) The released protein initiates an interaction among actin, myosin, and actin-myosin co-factor, the result of which is gelation of the cytoplasm. (*c*) The contraction of the cytoplasmic gel causes the formation of a narrow, translucent pseudopod. (From T. P. Stossel and J. H. Hartwig: *J. Cell Biol.* **68:**602–619, 1976.)

particle, only the coated half is engulfed by the phagocyte: it seems that the opsonin molecules lead the pseudopods by juxtaposing themselves to the corresponding receptor molecules on the phagocyte. Because the opsonins and receptors interact in a zipper-like fashion, this explanation is known as the *zipper model of phagocytosis* (Fig. 11.5). The activation signal passes from the opsonin via the receptor to the actin-binding protein by an unknown number of intermediates.

Once all the circumnavigating pseudopodia meet, the particle disappears from the phagocyte surface—it is ingested. The particle is now in the phagocyte cytoplasm as a vacuole, surrounded by a thin rim of the external medium and by what used to be the cell's plasma membrane. At first this *phagocytic vacuole* (*phagosome*) is connected with the cell surface by a stalk formed by the fusing of the pseudopodia, but later the stalk dissolves and the vacuole floats free in the cytoplasm.

Metabolic Burst

Mature phagocytes, particularly neutrophils, are in a quiescent, metabolically dormant state. The attachment of an ingestible particle to the cell surface changes this situation within seconds: the cell enters a stage of increased metabolic activity, the so-called *metabolic* (*respiratory*) *burst*. The transition is associated with a series of characteristic changes, of which the most important are increase in oxygen consumption, activation of the hexose monophosphate shunt (HMPS), and activation of the nicotinamide adenine dinucleotide phosphate (NADP) system. The initial event of the metabolic burst is apparently activation of an oxidative enzyme (oxidase) capable of capturing

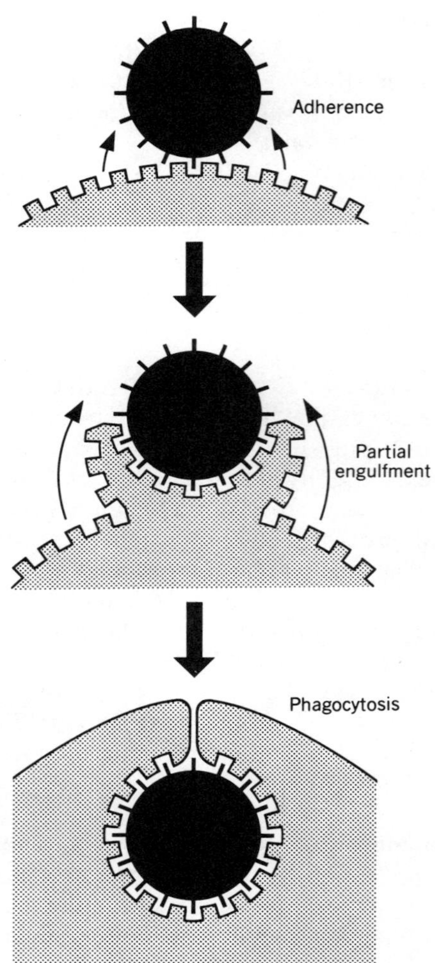

Figure 11.5. The zipper model of phagocytosis. (From S. J. Klebanoff and R. A. Clark: *The Neutrophil: Functional and Clinical Disorders*. North-Holland, Amsterdam, 1978.)

Table 11.1 Composition of the Electron Cloud Surrounding the Nucleus of the Oxygen Atom

Shell	Subshell	Orbital	Number of Electrons
K	1*s*	1*s*	2
L	2*s*	2*s*	2
	2*p*	$2p_x$	2
		$2p_y$	1
		$2p_z$	1

free molecules of oxygen and converting them into hydrogen peroxide, H_2O_2. The identity of this oxidase is controversial; several enzymes have been proposed, but the two most likely candidates are NADPH oxidase and NADH oxidase. We will discuss these two enzymes after we have reviewed briefly the basic chemistry of oxygen, the atom that plays a crucial role in the metabolic burst.

The oxygen atom has eight electrons, two in the inner K and six in the outer L shell (Table 11.1). The K shell consists of only one orbital, the 1*s* orbital, occupied by two electrons with opposed spins (the electrons form an electron pair). The L shell consists of two subshells, 2*s* (inner) and 2*p* (outer), containing two and four electrons, respectively. The 2*s* shell, like the 1*s* shell, consists of only one orbital occupied by a single electron pair. The 2*p* subshell consists of three orbitals—*x*, occupied by an electron pair, and *y* and *z*, occupied each by a single electron. The unpaired electrons impose instability on the oxygen atom, as a result of which two atoms combine to form an O_2 molecule

$$:\ddot{\underset{\cdot}{O}}\cdot + \cdot\ddot{\underset{\cdot\cdot}{O}}: \rightarrow :\ddot{\underset{\cdot}{O}}:\ddot{\underset{\cdot\cdot}{O}}:$$

where dots represent electrons in the L shell. However, this interaction still leaves two unpaired electrons in the outer orbitals of molecular oxygen, O_2. The electrons occupy separate orbitals and have their spins in the same direction. The addition of one electron to molecular oxygen produces the *superoxide anion*, $:\ddot{\underset{\cdot}{O}}:\ddot{\underset{\cdot\cdot}{O}}:$, written variously as $\cdot O_2^-$, $O_2^{-\cdot}$, or simply O_2^-; the addition of two electrons produces the *peroxy anion*, $:\ddot{\underset{\cdot\cdot}{O}}:\ddot{\underset{\cdot\cdot}{O}}:$ or O_2^{2-}.

Upon absorption of energy, the outer electrons of oxygen change their spin and the molecule enters an excited state termed *singlet oxygen*, or $^1O_2$. Two such excited states exist: in one, the two unpaired electrons occupy the same orbital, leaving the previously occupied orbital empty; in the other, the two electrons remain in their separate orbitals, but they are now of opposite spin. The excited, high-energy singlet oxygen exists for only a fraction of a second, until the excess energy dissipates into heat, light, or chemical energy.

The interaction of the superoxide anion with hydrogen peroxide, H_2O_2, leads to the production of a *hydroxyl radical*, $\cdot OH$:

$$\cdot O_2^- + H_2O_2 \rightarrow \cdot OH + OH^- + O_2$$

A hydroxyl radical is also produced when ionizing irradiation passes through water. The radical is highly unstable and reacts almost instantaneously with most organic molecules it encounters.

Let us now return to our discussion of the two oxidases, both of which use O_2 as their substrate and act only when another molecule, a coenzyme, is present. They differ in the coenzyme they use: the *NADH oxidase* uses nicotinamide adenine dinucleotide (NAD) as coenzyme, and the *NADPH oxidase* uses nicotinamide adenine dinucleotide phosphate (NADP). These two coenzymes are very similar, differing only by a single phosphate (PO_3^{2-}) group (Fig. 11.6). Each can exist in two interconvertible forms: oxidized (NAD^+ or $NADP^+$, a form in which the nicotinamide ring has donated one H^+ ion and two electrons), and reduced (NADH or NADPH, a form in which the nicotinamide has accepted one H^+ ion and two electrons; Fig. 11.6). The NADH oxidase converts O_2 directly into H_2O_2, according to the reaction

$$NADH + H^+ + O_2 \xrightarrow[\text{oxidase}]{\text{NADH}} NAD + H_2O_2$$

The H_2O_2 can then be converted into water and oxygen according to the reaction

$$2\ H_2O_2 \xrightarrow{\text{catalase}} 2\ H_2O + O_2$$

or, according to another reaction

$$H_2O_2 + 2\ GSH \xrightarrow[\text{peroxidase}]{\text{GSH}} 2\ H_2O + GSSG$$

where GSH is the reduced, and GSSG the oxidized form of glutathione (the latter is Glu–Cys–Gly tripeptide, with SH on Cys; see Fig. 11.7). GSSG can then be converted by GSSG reductase back into GSH:

$$GSSG + 2\ NADPH \xrightarrow[\text{reductase}]{\text{GSSG}} 2\ GSH + 2\ NADP$$

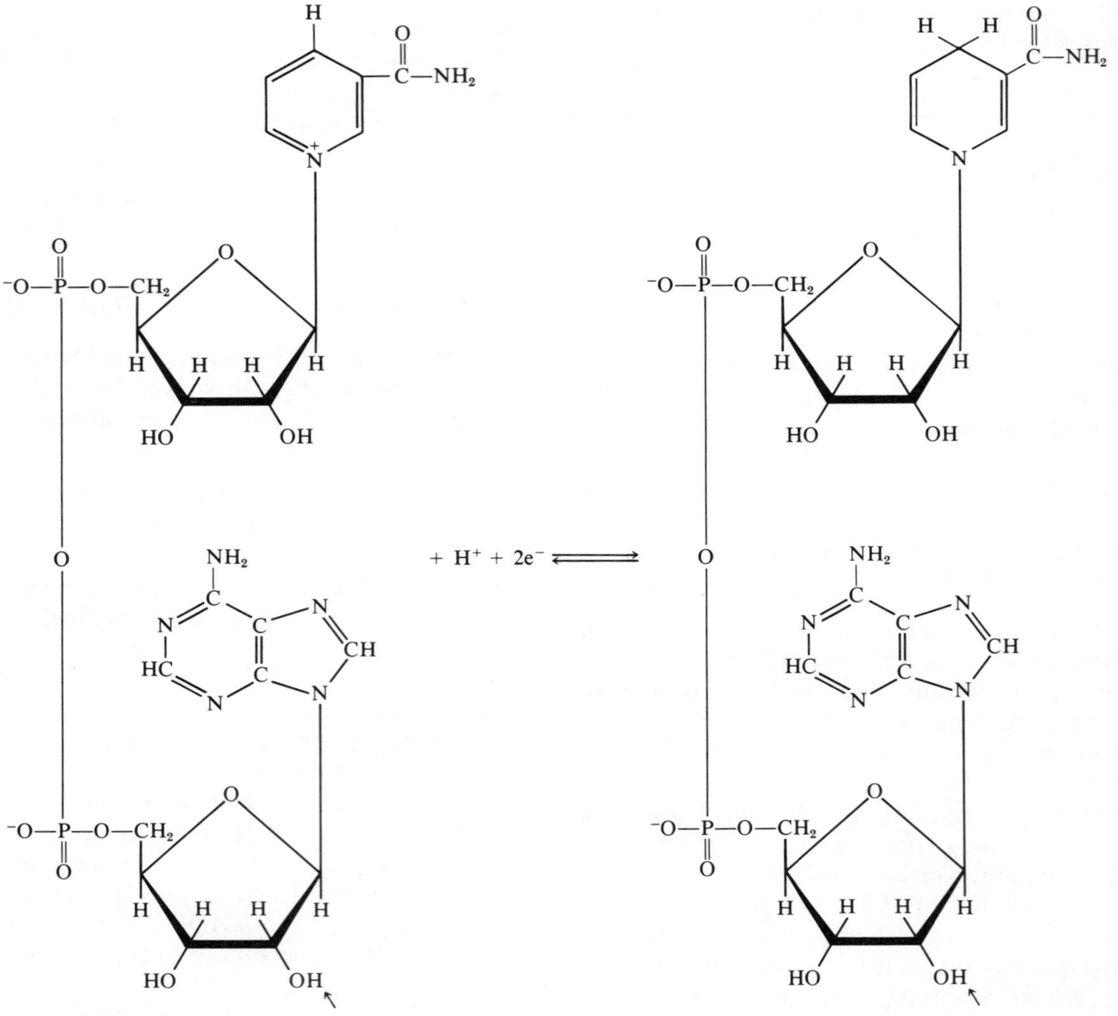

$$+\ H^+ + 2e^- \rightleftharpoons$$

NAD$^+$ NADH

Figure 11.6. The oxidized (NAD$^+$) and reduced (NADH) form of nicotin amide adenine dinucleotide. When the hydrogen atom, indicated by an arrow, is replaced by a PO_3^{2-} group, the compounds turn into nicotinamide adenine dinucleotide phosphate (NADP$^+$ or NADPH).

The NADP generated by this reaction enters the so-called *hexose monophosphate shunt*, a series of chemical reactions degrading cytoplasmic glucose into six molecules of CO_2, and releasing 24 hydrogen atoms in the process. In this pathway, glucose is first converted into glucose 6-phosphate (G6P), which is then converted into ribose 5-phosphate (R5P, a five-carbon sugar) in the second step of the reaction. From here on the pathway becomes a pentose phosphate shunt:

$$\text{G6P} + 2\ \text{NADPH} + H_2O \xrightarrow{\text{G6P dehydrogenase}} \text{R5P} + 2\ \text{NADPH} + 2\ H^+ + CO_2$$

The NADPH generated by this reaction is then used by the second of the two oxidases, NADPH oxidase, for the conversion of oxygen into the superoxide anion:

$$\text{NADPH} + O_2 \xrightarrow[\text{oxidase}]{\text{NADPH}} \text{NADP} + \cdot O_2^-$$

The superoxide anion can be converted into hydrogen peroxide by several reactions; here we shall describe only the two most important ones. In the first reaction,

$$\cdot O_2^- + \cdot O_2^- + 2\ H^+ \xrightarrow[\text{dismutase}]{\text{superoxide}} O_2 + H_2O_2$$

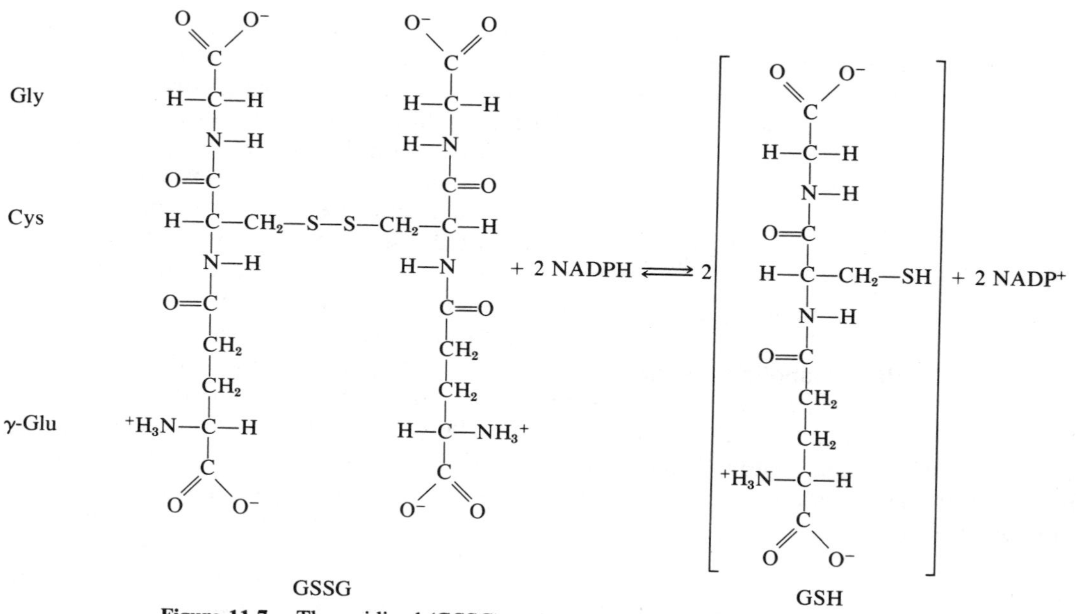

Gly

Cys

γ-Glu

$$\mathrm{GSSG} + 2\,\mathrm{NADPH} \rightleftharpoons 2\,\mathrm{GSH} + 2\,\mathrm{NADP^+}$$

GSSG

GSH

Figure 11.7. The oxidized (GSSG) and reduced (GSH) form of glutathione.

one $\cdot O_2^-$ anion donates its extra electron to another $\cdot O_2^-$ anion and is thus converted into O_2. So one $\cdot O_2^-$ anion serves as an electron donor (reductant), and the other as an electron acceptor (oxidant). A reaction in which oxidation and reduction occur by interaction of two molecules of the same kind is known as *dismutation* (Gr. *dis*, two; L. *muto*, to change), and an enzyme catalyzing such a reaction is called a *dismutase*. The enzyme catalyzing the decomposition of the superoxide anion to O_2 and H_2O_2 is referred to as *superoxide dismutase*.

The second reaction occurs spontaneously and produces, in addition to H_2O_2 singlet oxygen:

$$\cdot O_2^- + \cdot O_2^- + 2\,H^+ \rightarrow {}^1O_2 + H_2O_2$$

Singlet oxygen can, however, also be generated by other reactions involving superoxide anions. It can then react with any oxidizable molecule of the ingested particle—for example, any hydrocarbon (olefin) possessing one or more double bond in the carbon chain, breaking the chain as follows:

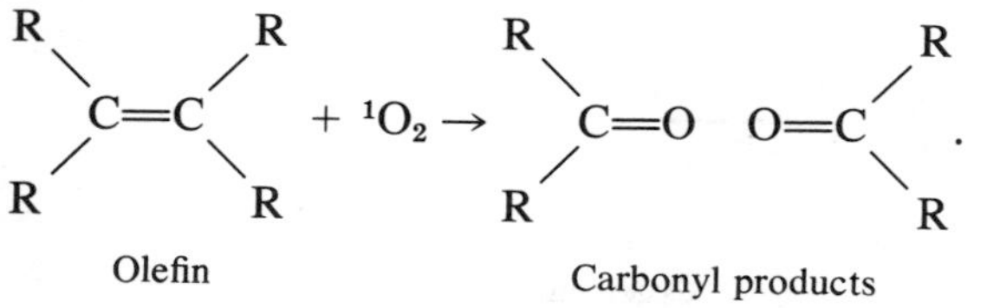

$$R_2C{=}CR_2 + {}^1O_2 \rightarrow R_2C{=}O \quad O{=}CR_2 .$$

Olefin — Carbonyl products

During this reaction, the singlet oxygen atoms return from the excited to the ground state, releasing some of their energy in the form of light. This light production by chemical action, or *chemiluminescence* is one of the characteristics associated with the metabolic burst. However, chemiluminescence also results from several other chemical reactions of the burst. Light production by neutrophils is maximal about 15 minutes after the ingestion of microorganisms. The flashes of light are too weak to see, but they can be recorded in a standard liquid scintillation counter.

The hydrogen peroxide produced by interaction of superoxide anions can react with chloride, iodide, bromide, or fluoride anions to produce water:

$$H_2O_2 + Cl^- + H^+ \xrightarrow{\text{myeloperoxidase}} HOCl + H_2O$$

The reaction is catalyzed by *myeloperoxidase*, an enzyme contained in phagocytic granules. The hypocholorous acid (HOCl) can react with amino acids of the ingested microorganism to form chloramines:

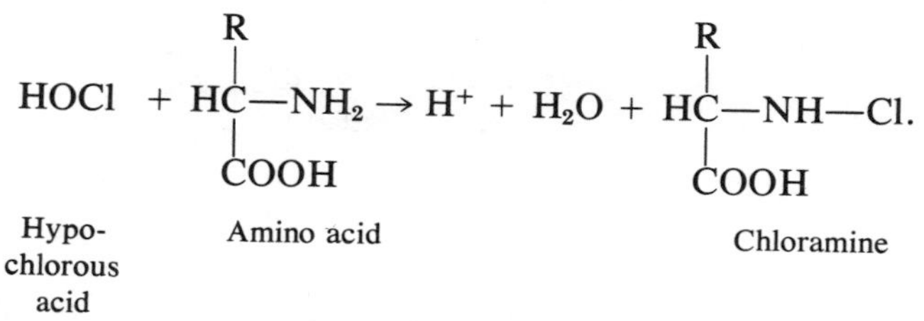

$$HOCl + HC(R)(COOH){-}NH_2 \rightarrow H^+ + H_2O + HC(R)(COOH){-}NH{-}Cl.$$

Hypochlorous acid — Amino acid — Chloramine

Chloramines decompose spontaneously into NH_3, CO_2, chloride, and aldehyde (RCHO):

$$\begin{array}{l} R \\ | \\ CH{-}NH{-}Cl + H_2O \rightarrow \\ | \\ COOH \end{array}$$

$$RCHO + NH_4^+ + CO_2 + Cl^-$$

The decomposition is part of the phagocyte's attack on the ingested particle.

The main reactions of the metabolic burst are summarized in Figure 11.8. Its occurrence can be determined by the addition of *nitroblue tetrazolium* (NBT) to the phagocyte suspension. The yellow NBT reacts with the superoxide anions generated by the burst and turns into blue-black formazan:

$$NBT + \cdot O_2^- \rightarrow formazan + O_2$$

Precipitation of formazan in cells can be visualized microscopically; alternatively, the dye can be extracted from the cells and measured spectrophotometrically.

11.1.4 Degranulation

The cytoplasm of a neutrophil or a macrophage is full of small, membrane-enclosed bags filled with an assortment of enzymes. In the neutrophil, these bags are called *granules*; in the macrophage they are referred to as *lysosomes*, the difference between the two being primarily in their enzyme content. However, the classification of granules as neutrophil organelles and lysosomes as macrophage organelles is not absolute: macrophages and monocytes do contain some granules, and lysosomes are a standard cell organelle (for a discussion of granule morphology, see Chapter 5). In a quiescent cell, the bags remain closed and meticulously separated from the cytoplasm, but as soon as the phagocytic vacuole begins to form, the bags empty their contents into it, one by one. This emptying process is most striking in the neutrophil, where the cytoplasm gradually becomes (and remains) granule-free, or *degranulated*, as a result.

The commencement of degranulation can be imagined as follows. Granules and lysosomes float freely and randomly in the cytoplasm, pushed around by the forces of the Brownian motion, until they bump into the phagosome. Whether there is directed movement of granules toward the vacuole in addition to the random movement has not yet been demonstrated, but the swiftness of the degranulation process suggests that this might be so. One can imagine, for example, a granule sliding along microtubules toward the phagosome. At collision, the membrane of the phagocytic vacuole adheres to that of the granule. The membranes fuse and dissolve in the contact region, forming an opening through which the content of the granule passes into the vacuole. The undissolved portion of the granule's membrane becomes an integral part of the vacuole membrane, so that by each fusion, the vacuole (now referred to as a *phagocytic lysosome*, or

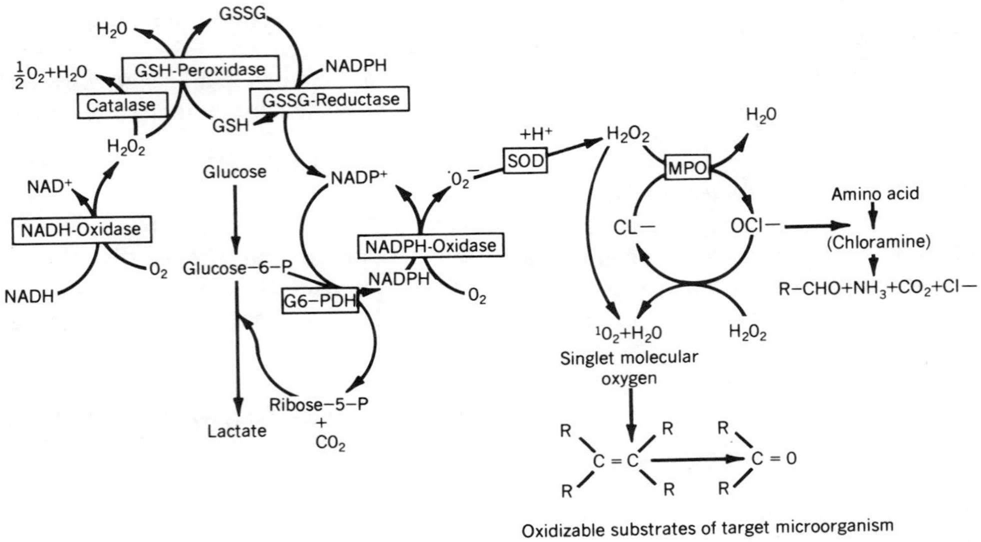

Figure 11.8. Reactions constituting the "metabolic burst." (From A. Cruchand: *Schweiz. Med. Wochenschr.* **107**:1721–1728, 1977.)

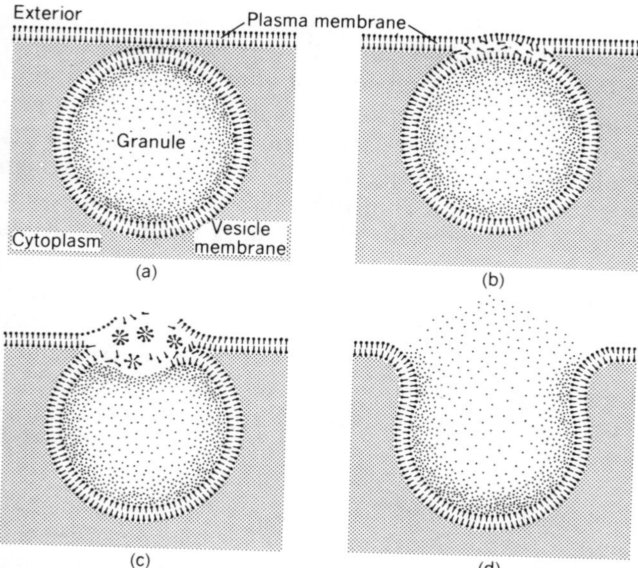

Figure 11.9. Postulated mechanism of granule fusion with the plasma membrane. (*a*) The granule approaches the plasma membrane. (*b*) The granule membrane contacts the plasma membrane. (*c*) The contacting membrane begins to dissolve. (*d*) The granule opens up and discharges its contents into the cell exterior.

phagolysosome) grows a bit larger. At no time during degranulation do the membranes open into the cytoplasm: the cell handles granules as if each were a bag of poisonous snakes. A possible mechanism of membrane fusion and dissolution is depicted in Figure 11.9.

Because the emptying of granules into the phagocytic vacuole has already begun when the vacuole is still open through a membrane channel to the cell exterior, some of the granule's contents may be discharged to the outside. Extracellular enzyme release may also occur under many other circumstances, most notably when the cell dies—before, during, or after phagocytosis. The enzymes and other active substances released by extracellular degranulation are probably responsible for the tissue injury associated with a variety of immunological reactions (e.g., Arthus phenomenon, serum sickness, anaphylaxis, some forms of arthritis and nephritis, antibody-mediated graft rejection, and others; these will be discussed in Chapters 12 and 13). In many instances, the effect of these enzymes is probably similar to that which occurs during intracellular degranulation (described below), but there may also be some important differences.

11.1.5 Killing, Digestion, and Exocytosis

Once inside a vacuole, the ingested particle is immediately attacked in a variety of ways, all aimed at killing and digesting the foreign body. If the particles are live bacteria, the progress of the killing process can be monitored by removing cell aliquots at various time intervals, lysing the cells, plating the diluted lysate on agar, and counting the number of bacterial colonies formed. The count is proportional to the number of surviving bacteria.

The multiplicity of the attack systems is probably the result of host-parasite coevolution. A microorganism with a novel kind of protective coating may survive phagocytosis and kill most of the hosts. The hosts that survive will be those that have evolved a new attack system capable of destroying the resistant microorganisms. The new hosts will thrive until another parasite comes up with yet another trick to escape the defense mechanism. And so the hosts will accumulate a series of attack systems tailored to different parasites.

The known or proposed attack mechanisms are listed in Table 11.2. They fall into two categories, oxygen-dependent and oxygen-independent. *Oxygen-dependent mechanisms* have already been described in the discussion of phagocytosis-associated metabolic burst. The two most significant effectors of this form of attack are hydrogen peroxide and oxygen radicals. Peroxide-mediated reactions lead to iodination of

Table 11.2 Postulated Bactericidal Mechanisms

Oxygen-dependent mechanisms
H_2O_2 production
Peroxidase-mediated
Iodination
Aldehyde formation
Peptide cleavage
Peroxidase-independent
Interaction with ascorbate
Lipid peroxidation
Oxygen-free radicals
Superoxide anion ($\cdot O_2^-$)
Singlet oxygen ($^1O_2$)
Hydroxyl radical ($\cdot OH$)
Oxygen-independent mechanisms
Peroxidase
Lysozyme
Lactoferrin
Hydrolytic enzymes
Permeability factor
Cationic proteins

bacterial proteins, aldehyde formation, and cleavage of polypeptide chains. However, peroxide can also interact with ascorbic acid (vitamin C) and form so far unidentified compounds that are toxic for many bacterial species. Finally, peroxide may produce bactericidal effects by removing certain lipids—for example, arachidonic acid—from the bacterial membrane. The action of the three free radicals of oxygen (O_2^-, the superoxide anion; $^1O_2$, the singlet oxygen; and $OH\cdot$, the hydroxyl radical) was described in the section dealing with the metabolic burst. The end effect of this action is degradation of bacterial cell constituents.

Another oxygen-dependent attack mechanism is mediated by lactic acid and hydrogen ions that accumulate in the cell during the metabolic burst, as a result of glycolysis. The acid and excess hydrogen ions are probably largely responsible for the rapid drop in pH in the phagocytic vacuole. The normal physiological pH is around seven; but within three minutes of particle uptake, the pH in the vacuole drops to six, and within seven minutes, it reaches the value of four or lower. Few bacteria can live at such a low pH, and those that survive cannot multiply. In addition, the low pH probably facilitates the action of many enzymes emptied into the vacuoles, since their pH optima are between 4.5 and 5.0.

The best-characterized of the *oxygen-independent mechanisms* are peroxidases, lysozymes, lactoferrin, hydrolytic enzymes, permeability factors, and cationic proteins.

Peroxidases. The enzymes catalyzing the oxidation of various substrates in the presence of H_2O_2 are called peroxidases. They act by removing a hydrogen atom from the substrate (hydrogen or electron donor) and transferring it to another substance (hydrogen or electron acceptor). The substrate is thus oxidized and the hydrogen acceptor reduced. The substrate could be an iodide (which is thus converted by the reaction into iodine); the hydrogen acceptor is the H_2O_2, which is converted into H_2O. Most peroxidases are iron-containing proteins (hemeproteins) functionally related to hemoglobin; in fact, hemoglobin itself exhibits some peroxidase activity but with a low reaction rate. Peroxidases alone have not been demonstrated to have antimicrobial activity, but they may catalyze the conversion of other substances from weak to strong microbicidal agents. The enzymes are present in milk, saliva, and leukocytes. In the preceding sections we mentioned two peroxidases, myeloperoxidase and catalase. *Myeloperoxidase* has been so named because of its presence in cells of myeloid origin (it occurs in granulocytes, but also in monocytes). Its concentration is exceptionally high: it constitutes from 1 to 5 percent
of the dry weight of the cell. It is this enzyme that is
responsible for the green color of pus (the purified protein is intense green in color). Myeloperoxidase is a
basic protein with an isoelectric point of about 10. Its
molecular weight ranges in the different mammalian
species from 130,000 to 160,000 daltons. The molecule
consists of several subunits arranged around two heme
groups, each containing one iron atom. The iron forms
complexes with cyanide, azide, and hydroxylamine
leading to the inactivation of the enzyme. The enzymatic activity is highest in the presence of co-factors.
Catalase is particularly effective in reactions in which
H_2O_2 is both oxidant and hydrogen donor (*catalytic
reactions*).

Lysozyme (*Muraminidase*). Lysozyme was discovered in 1922 by Alexander Fleming, who observed that
an addition of nasal mucus to a culture of growing
bacteria resulted in rapid clearing of the areas where
drops of mucus fell. Because the lysis of bacteria resembled the action of an enzyme, Fleming called the
bactericidal substance in the mucus *lysozyme*. Later
the substance indeed proved to be an enzyme.
Lysozyme is present in eggwhite (the usual source fo
its isolation) and many mammalian tissues, in additio
to bodily secretions. In birds, there are two types c
lysozyme—a smaller "chicken type" (molecula
weight of about 14,000 daltons) and a larger "goos
type" (molecular weight of about 20,000 daltons), th
names referring to the origin of the enzyme. The tw
types also differ in amino acid composition, im
munological properties, and catalytic activity. Th
mammalian lysozyme is evolutionarily derived fror
the chicken type, with the different mammalian specie
differing slightly in the primary structure of this er
zyme. Structurally, the lysozyme is one of the bes
characterized enzymes. It consists of a single polyper
tide chain of 129 amino acids. Both the amino aci
sequence and the tertiary structure of the lysozym
molecule are known (see Chapter 10). The enzyme act
by breaking the bond between acetyl muramic acid an
N-acetyl-glucosamine in the peptidoglycan layer of th
bacterial cell wall (Fig. 11.10). In a few bacteria (e.g
Micrococcus lysodeikticus or *Bacillus megaterium*) th
peptidoglycan layer is directly accessible to the en
zyme, and these species are then killed directly by th
lysozyme. In other bacteria, the peptidoglycan laye
becomes accessible only after the cell wall has bee
damaged by other agents (e.g., antibody and comple
ment, ascorbic acid and H_2O_2, proteases, or chelatin
agents), and in these species the lysozyme kills only i
conjunction with these agents. Lysozyme is not abs

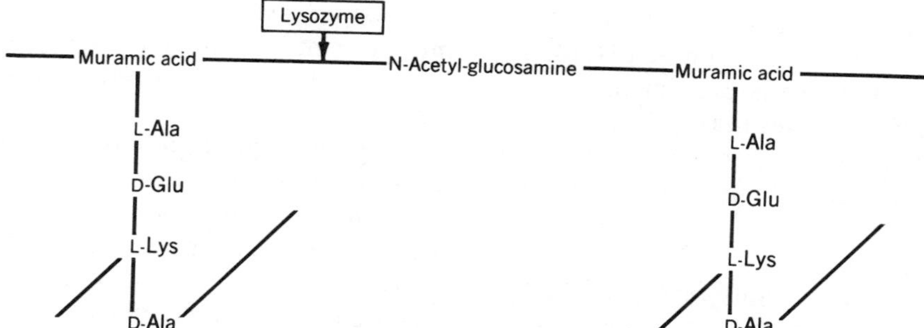

Figure 11.10. The site of lysozyme action.

lutely necessary for the survival of the species, as is evidenced by the fact that several mammals (e.g., cattle, goats, sheep, cats, hamsters, rhesus monkeys, and a mutant rabbit strain) completely lack this enzyme.

Lactoferrin (*Lactotransferin*, *Lactosiderophilin*). So named because it is an iron-binding protein first discovered in milk, lactoferrin is related to serum transferin, has a molecular weight of from 77,000 to 93,000 daltons, and has no known enzymatic activity. It occurs in a variety of bodily secretions, in addition to milk (i.e., tears, saliva, nasal and bronchial secretions, bile, and urine) and in leukocyte granules (where it may constitute up to 10 percent of the total cell protein). Lactoferrin acts as a potent chelating agent.[1] It binds iron, depriving bacteria of this essential nutrient, required for their normal growth. However, it may also have some more direct bactericidal effect, and furthermore, it may potentiate the effect of lysozyme.

Hydrolytic Enzymes. Hydrolytic enzymes cleave the substrate by adding H_2O_2 to the cleavage points. They serve as digestive, rather than bactericidal agents, although they may be toxic to some bacteria. They are divided arbitrarily into three groups, according to the pH at which they function best. *Acid hydrolases* act at acidic pH and cleave phosphate esters according to the following general scheme:

$$\underset{\text{Ester}}{R_1{-}\overset{\overset{\displaystyle O}{\|}}{C}{-}O{-}R_2} + H_2O \rightleftarrows \underset{\text{Acid}}{R_1{-}C\genfrac{}{}{0pt}{}{\nearrow O}{\searrow O^-}} + \underset{\text{Alcohol}}{HO{-}R_2} + H^+.$$

The ester bond can occur in a protein, polysaccharide, lipid, or nucleic acid, so that the enzymes have the capability to lyse all the biologically important compounds. They form a heterogeneous group with individual enzymes distinguished by their electrophoretic mobility and substrate specificity. Some have special names, usually referring to the substrate on which they act (e.g., acid β-glycerophosphatase, β-glucuronidase, α-mannosidase, β-galactosidase, 5-nucleosidase, etc.). Others are included in a group of *cathepsins*—enzymes responsible for protein hydrolysis in dead animals (Gr. *kathepsis*, boiling down). They are designated by letters A, B, C, and so on. Acid hydrolases are present in granules and lysosomes. Their activity is strongly inhibited by heparin and chondroitin sulfate, presumably because of ionic interaction between the anionic groups of these two compounds and the cationic groups of the enzymes. Chondroitin sulfate may be involved in the control of acid hydrolase activity in situ.

Neutral hydrolases are maximally active at neutral pH. They too have esterolytic activity and, like acid hydrolases, are a heterogeneous group of enzymes. The three best-characterized representatives are chymotrypsin-like protease, elastase, and collagenase. *Chymotrypsin-like protease* (cathepsin G) is a highly cationic protein that acts, like chymotrypsin, on tyrosine residues. Its natural substrates are cartilage, proteoglycans, fibrinogen, and cassein. *Elastase* has the ability to hydrolyse long chains consisting of aliphatic amino acids, such as alanine and glycine; such chains are common in elastin. But the enzyme also acts on many other substrates. Elastase is not microbicidal itself, but it makes possible the activity of myeloperoxidase and chymotrypsin-like protease. *Collagenase* splits collagen molecules into two pieces and thus unwinds the normal triple helical configuration of these molecules, changing them into the random coils found in gelatin. The fragments then become the target of attack by other enzymes.

[1] Chelation is the bond formation between a metal ion and two or more polar groups of a single molecule.

Alkaline hydrolases are exemplified by *alkaline phosphatase*, which has a reaction optimum at pH 10. In the rabbit, alkaline phosphatase is present in neutrophil granules; in humans, it resides in the plasma membrane. Its activity is changed by various hematological disorders (e.g., it is absent in certain forms of chronic granulocytic leukemia).

Cationic Proteins. A heterogeneous family of highly basic compounds extracted from tissues by diluted acid, cationic proteins can be separated into a number of fractions by electrophoretic techniques. These positively charged molecules probably act by sticking to the negatively charged bacterial surfaces, thus interfering with the growth of the microorganisms and killing bacteria without lysing them (*bacteriostatic effect*). Two of these proteins, *phagocytin* and *leukin*, have been characterized to the degree that they have been given identifying names.

Permeability-Increasing Factors. Certain cationic proteins act by increasing the permeability of the bacterial membrane, thereby opening the cell to many deleterious agents. The precise identity of these proteins and the mechanisms of their actions are unknown.

Killed microorganisms are digested enzymatically in the phagolysome and their components degraded into individual building blocks. The contents of the phagolysosome are then discharged into the extracellular space. This discharge, or *exocytosis*, is the reverse of phagocytosis: the vacuole fuses with the plasma membrane at one point, then ruptures, integrates into the plasma membrane, and releases its contents (see Fig. 11.1*b*).

11.2 ACQUIRED CELLULAR RESISTANCE TO INFECTION

11.2.1 Definitions

Acquired resistance is an ill-defined term that immunologists keep using—perhaps because it is so vague and noncomittal. To explain what it means, we must make sure we understand the meaning of the term's three components—"infection," "resistance," and "acquired." *Infection* is defined as the presence, in an animal, of microorganisms capable of damaging the animal's cells and tissues. *Resistance* is a word of Latin origin with a general meaning of "to stand back" or "withstand." In connection with infection, a resistant animal is one that never becomes sick when infected, that becomes sick but recovers, that develops milder forms of a disease in comparison to another animal, or that becomes sick only when exposed to a large dose of microorganisms. Since the early days of immunology, scientists have recognized two forms of resistance, natural and acquired. *Natural resistance* (also referred to as native, innate, inherent, genetic, or nonspecific) is usually defined as resistance manifested by animals that have not previously been exposed to an infecting organism or its constituents. *Acquired resistance*, on the other hand, is that of animals that have previously mounted a response against a given microorganism or its constituents (*actively acquired resistance*), or that have received serum or cells from a previously exposed animal (*passively acquired resistance*). Acquired resistance can be mediated either by antibodies (*humoral resistance*) or by cells (*cellular resistance*). In practice, it is often difficult to draw the line between natural and acquired resistance. There are, for example, so-called *natural antibodies* that are present in an animal for most of its life, and no one really knows when they are formed or what induces their formation. Should they be considered part of natural or acquired resistance? Or another example: natural resistance is usually regarded as something laid down in one's heredity (hence the synonyms "genetic" and "constitutional"); but we now know that many of the typical *acquired* responses are genetically controlled. These and many other paradoxes make the perpetuation of the terms "natural" and "acquired" untenable, except for distinguishing between constitutive and inducible forms of response. According to this definition, *natural* would be all forms of resistance not influenced by an infecting agent, while *acquired* would be those forms that are either augmented or diminished by exposure to a microorganism. An example of a natural resistance mechanism is the action of lysozyme in bodily fluids on microorganisms; an example of acquired resistance is the production of antibodies after bacterial infection. The term "resistance" is partly or completely included in the term "immunity" (partly when one uses "immunity" in its usual narrow sense, and completely when one defines immunity more broadly, as in this book; see Chapter 1).

In this section we shall deal with one particular form of acquired resistance, characterized by the following attributes.

First, it functions in the absence of antibodies and cannot be transferred by serum; but it is transferable by cells, and thus qualifies for the category of cellular responses.

Second, it involves organisms that can survive and multiply within normal macrophages and monocytes; most of these organisms are bacteria (e.g., *Listeria monocytogenes, Salmonella enteritidis, S. typhimurium, Mycobacterium tuberculosis, Corynebac-*

terium parvum, *C. granulosum*, *Brucella abortus*), but the list includes viruses (e.g., vaccinia, psittacosis, and meningo pneumonitis viruses), yeastlike fungi (e.g., *Histoplasma*, *Candida*), parasitic protozoa (e.g., *Toxoplasma*, *Plasmodium*, *Trypanosoma*, *Leishmania*, *Besnoitia*), and small metazoal parasites (e.g., *Nippostrongulus brasiliensis*). Many of these agents cause characteristic diseases, referred to by names derived from the names of the organism (i.e., listeriosis, salmonellosis, tuberculosis, brucellosis, histoplasmosis, candidiasis, leishmaniasis, etc.).

Third, with few exceptions, the resistance can be induced only by live, avirulent organisms, or it follows recovery from the disease; it cannot be induced by killed organisms.

Fourth, the resistance is usually accompanied by delayed-type hypersensitivity (see Chapter 12).

The mechanism of this form of acquired cellular resistance has been studied extensively by George B. Mackaness and his colleagues, using infection of mice with *Listeria monocytogenes* as a model. On the following pages, we shall first describe the model, then discuss what is known about the mechanism of resistance to *Listeria*, and finally mention one special case of this form of resistance that concerns a disease of great medical import—tuberculosis.

11.2.2 Model System

Listeria monocytogenes is a small, motile, aerobic, rod-shaped, Gram-positive bacterium with a ubiquitous distribution worldwide. Its generic name honors Joseph Lister, the English surgeon noted for his introduction of antiseptic methods into operating rooms; its specific name refers to the fact that large numbers of monocytes (up to 6000 times higher than normal) are often found in the peripheral blood of *Listeria*-infected animals. The bacterium has a remarkably broad host range, which involves at least 37 mammals, including the mouse and human, 17 birds, ticks, flies, fish, and crustaceans. However, most of the naturally occuring *Listeria* forms are avirulent, so that cases of *listeriosis*, particularly in humans, are relatively rare. When the disease does occur, it can be fatal. In ruminants (e.g., sheep or cattle), the infection involves the central nervous system and causes encephalitis, meningitis, and various other neurological disorders. In nonruminant mammals and in birds, the main causes of death are liver necrosis and septicemia (poisoning by flooding the blood with bacteria—a word derived from Gr. *sepsis*, putrefaction, and *haima*, blood).

In mice, *L. monocytogenes* is highly virulent only when injected intravenously and thus given the opportunity to seed the liver and spleen, the two crucial organs for its multiplication, directly. The bacteria grow in macrophages residing in the liver and spleen and in monocytes recruited to these organs from blood; they kill these cells and cause extensive organ damage. If not contained, the infection eventually spreads into the blood, leading to overproduction of blood monocytes, blood poisoning, and eventually, death of the host. When injected in a sublethal dose, the bacteria multiply for three or four days in the liver and spleen, but thereafter their number begins to decline and the mice stay healthy. The host will then survive even when challenged with a high dose of bacteria—the host has acquired resistance to the infection.

Mouse macrophages can also be infected with *Listeria* in tissue culture. When derived from untreated animals, most of the infected macrophages die, whereas those coming from resistant animals withstand the attack.

11.2.3 Mechanism

Resistance to *Listeria* infection involves two cell types—macrophages (monocytes) and lymphocytes. Since the macrophage is the target of the infection, it is probably this cell that encounters the pathogen first. Many of the infected macrophages die, killed by the bacteria, but some may survive, kill and degrade the pathogen, and display its components on the cell surface (see section 11.4). The displayed antigens activate T lymphocytes, which then secrete soluble mediators; these in turn activate macrophages. Activated macrophages differ from normal ones in their morphological, biochemical, and functional characteristics: they are larger; they attach more rapidly to glass and plastic and spread more extensively on the substrate; they display a characteristic undulating (ruffled) plasma membrane; they contain a greater number of mitochondria, lysosomes, and ribosomes and more extensive Golgi apparatus; they manifest an increased rate and speed of phagocytosis; and they display increased total protein synthesis, increased ATP, increased lysosomal enzyme and hexose monophosphate shunt activity, and increased oxygen consumption. The functional change in activated macrophages manifests itself in their increased ability to destroy pathogens. So conspicuous is the change that immunologists, who are not profuse with hyperbole, refer to these cells as "angry" or even "blood-thirsty."

Exactly how activated macrophages kill and eliminate bacteria is not known. Most of the killing probably occurs intracellularly, after the pathogen has been enclosed in the phagocytic vacuole, the vacuole has fused with lysosomes, and the lysosomal content has been discharged on the particle. A major part of the killing is carried out by lysosomal acid hydrolases, but these enzymes are not the sole bactericidal factors of activated macrophages. What the other factors are is not known; several substances that inhibit growth of bacteria or fungi have been isolated from macrophages and monocytes and given names such as "mycosuppressin" or "monocytin," but they remain poorly characterized. In contrast to its function in neutrophils, the peroxidase-halide system does not seem to play a role in bacterial killing by macrophages and monocytes. It is likely that activated macrophages possess several killing systems and use different ones on different pathogens.

In addition to intracellular killing, activated macrophages may also attack target cells extracellularly. What role this extracellular killing plays in resistance to infection, particularly infection by protozoal parasites, remains to be determined; cell lysis by macrophages is, however, a dominant form of attack in certain other forms of defense reaction (for example, tumor immunity or allograft reactions; see Chapters 12 and 14).

The question of whether activated macrophages are qualitatively (rather than quantitatively) different from normal macrophages is unresolved. Clearly most of the activities displayed by activated macrophages are also present in unactivated macrophages, but at much lower levels; what is not known is whether activated macrophages also possess certain properties that unactivated macrophages lack. The emergence of acquired resistance is accompanied by widespread macrophage proliferation, but the significance of this event is not clear.

Macrophages can be activated by pathogens, their products (e.g., endotoxin of Gram-negative bacteria and peptidoglycan), lymphokines, and many other agents that have nothing to do with infection (e.g., double-stranded DNA and polyinosinic-polycytidilic acid). Lymphokines seem to shorten the activation process, making activated macrophages available sooner than they would be normally. Hence, the interaction between macrophages and lymphocytes in the development of acquired resistance is a true coöperative endeavor.

The major difference between macrophage and lymphocyte responses to infection is their specificity. The macrophage response is totally nonspecific: for example, mice infected with *Brucella abortus* or with *Salmonella typhimurium* are also resistant to *Listeria*, and vice versa. This nonspecificity extends even to different types of organisms, as is evidenced by the observation that, for example, mice infected with the protozoa *Toxoplasma* or *Besnoitia* are resistant to bacteria such as *Salmonella* and *Listeria*. But the lymphocyte response is specific. For instance, spleen cells of animals immunized with *Mycobacterium tuberculosis* can confer tuberculin sensitivity (see Chapter 12) upon normal recipients, but they do not make the secondary host resistant to *Listeria* infection (although the original host is resistant to both *Mycobacterium* and *Listeria*). In other words, transfer of activated macrophages makes the new host resistant not only to the original infecting pathogens, but also to many unrelated pathogens. Transfer of activated lymphocytes makes the new host hypersensitive to the stimulating pathogens, but not to others.

11.2.4 Resistance to Tubercle Bacilli

The tubercle bacilli *Mycobacterium tuberculosis* get into the body by being inhaled, settle in the lungs, and attack alveolar macrophages. Once within the macrophage, the avirulent forms of *M. tuberculosis* are quickly destroyed by one of the intracellular killing mechanisms noted above. The virulent forms, on the other hand, escape destruction, perhaps by producing substances that prevent fusion of lysosomes with the phagosomes they inhabit. The infected macrophage assumes a characteristic elongated shape that is called epitheloid because it resembles the shape of an epithelial cell, and the *epitheloid cells* arrange themselves concentrically, forming a little nodule—the *tubercle* (Fig. 11.11). As the tubercle grows, the cells in its center fuse to form *giant cells* with dozens of nuclei at their periphery and viable bacilli in the cytoplasm. The surface of the nodule becomes coated with a mantle of lymphocytes and proliferating fibroblasts. Isolated from the outside by this fibrous wall, the cells in the core of the tubercle die, perhaps because of a lack of oxygen, and the core may become calcified and give rise to the characteristic shadow visible in X-ray pictures of tuberculous lungs. Some of the tubercles may rupture, discharging infectious bacilli to neighboring areas of the lung and leaving a cavity in the lung parenchyma. As the disease progresses, more and more of the parenchyma is destroyed, until a stage is reached at which the lung is no longer capable of supplying the body with sufficient oxygen. Expectorated sputum and droplets spread the bacilli to other individuals.

The virulent tubercle bacilli, like the *Listeria* bacteria, activate macrophages, but the activated macrophages are not capable of ridding the body of the infection. The bacilli also activate lymphocytes, which

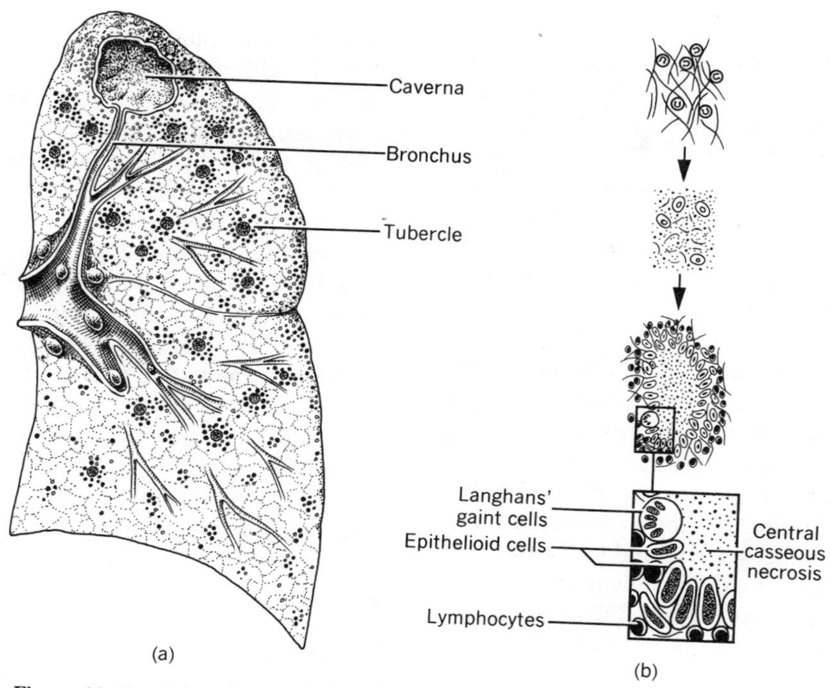

Figure 11.11. Tubercle formation in the lungs of a patient infected with *Mycobacterium tuberculosis*. (*a*) Infected lung. (*b*) Structure of a tubercle.

are then responsible for the delayed-type hypersensitivity (tuberculin) reaction (see Chapter 12). In contrast to *Listeria*, however, tubercle bacilli need not be alive to activate macrophages. This peculiarity probably constitutes the basis for the adjuvant action of tubercle bacilli (see Chapter 10).

11.3 TARGET-CELL LYSIS BY MACROPHAGES

11.3.1 Discovery

In the 1950s, circumstantial evidence accumulated to indicate that macrophages can also kill target cells by nonphagocytic mechanisms. Most of the evidence was provided by tumor biologists who observed that, for example, transplanted tumors were usually full of macrophages, and that on histological preparations, tumor cells were often surrounded by macrophages. Some histologists even reported noting direct contact between plasma membranes of tumor cells and those of macrophages. The first direct evidence for the killer function of macrophages was not provided until 1964, in an in vitro study by Gale A. Granger and R. S. Weiser. They inoculated tumor cells of strain-X origin intraperitoneally into Y mice, harvested peritoneal macrophages from the immunized animal after 10 days, cultured the macrophages for 12 hours in vitro, and then added them in small drops to a culture of strain-X embryonic fibroblasts. They observed that within 60 hours each added drop caused a dissolution of cells, visible as a clear plaque, in the area where it landed. Before this experiment, lymphocytes were the only cells known to cause immunological destruction of target cells by nonphagocytic mechanisms. Now Granger and Weiser added immune macrophages to the killer cell category (macrophages from unimmunized animals are incapable of killing target cells). Later, many other investigators confirmed the Granger-Weiser observation and demonstrated, moreover, that macrophages killed not only allogeneic, but also syngeneic tumor cells, and hence that macrophages probably played an important role in tumor immunity.

11.3.2 Methods of Study

Macrophages can exert three kinds of effect on target cells: cytostatic, cytolytic, and cytotoxic. The *cytostatic effect* results in an inhibition of target cell proliferation (cessation of tumor growth) without overt signs of cell damage; it can be measured by ^{3}H-thymidine incorporation into replicating DNA. The *cytolytic effect* results in cell death, leading to an extensive leakage of cell content as assessed by isotope release or dye uptake. The *cytotoxic effect* leads to impairment of cell function as a result of cell damage that varies in degree from detachment from a glass or plastic substrate to cell death. The cytotoxic effect, which is usually less severe than that caused by cytolysis, can be measured by the release of ^{125}I-iododeoxyuridine from labeled cells. However, the terms "cytolytic" and "cytotoxic" are often used indiscriminately.

Although cytostatic, cytolytic, or cytotoxic effects of activated macrophages can be measured in vivo (by determining a slowdown in tumor growth following macrophage inoculation), in vitro is usually the method of choice. The principle of the in vitro method is the same as that of the original Granger-Weiser experiment: activated macrophages are added to a culture of target cells and target cell death is measured by one of many available assays (dye exclusion, ^{51}Cr-release, inhibition of colony formation, inhibition of DNA synthesis, etc.).

11.3.3 Mechanism

As was noted above, macrophages become killer cells only when appropriately activated by one of many activating stimuli. The same agents that turn macrophages into angry cells also turn them into killers. In fact, the process of macrophage activation in these two situations is probably the same: intracellular and extracellular killing are just two different ways in which activated macrophages carry out the same function.

In cases where the activating agent is a tumor cell, the activating signal is probably provided by cell-surface antigens—histocompatibility antigens in allogeneic-tumor systems and tumor-specific transplantation antigens in systems involving syngeneic tumors (see Chapters 12 and 14). After fortuitously digesting and processing some debris of the tumor cells, macrophages display the foreign antigens in a form that activates T lymphocytes, which then secrete macrophage-activating factors. The latter attract monocytes, immobilize them in the tumor, and transform them into macrophages, and the activated macrophages then kill the tumor cells. The similarity of macrophage activation in bacterial infection and in tumor immunity is underscored by the fact that macrophages activated by bacteria exert a cytotoxic effect on tumors.

Most of the killing is nonspecific: activated macrophages destroy any cell that happens to be in their vicinity. Since the activation occurs directly in the tumor, the malignant cells are the natural targets of the killers. In addition, however, tumor cells seem to possess some property by which the macrophage distinguishes them from normal cells (see below). As a consequence, normal cells are only rarely killed (at a high effector-to-target-cell ratio). But as long as the cell is malignant, it makes no difference to the activated macrophage what its source is: macrophages activated by one tumor not only kill it but also tumors derived from unrelated individuals or strains.

In some situations, however, at least part of the macrophage-mediated killing of target cells can be specific: the activated macrophages kill the activating target cells and not genetically unrelated cells. The mechanism of this specific killing is still largely undiscovered. As far as is known, macrophages lack receptors capable of distinguishing antigens, so the discriminatory power must be conferred upon them by exogenous factors with cytophilic properties. Two groups of such factors have been identified—immunoglobulins (cytophilic antibodies) and T cell-derived factors. *Cytophilic antibodies* can be detected by a variety of methods: a commonly used one is the rosetting technique. Cultured macrophages are allowed to form a monolayer, which is then incubated with serum containing cytophilic antibodies specific for a particular antigen—say, sheep red blood cells. The sensitized macrophages are washed to remove free serum components and incubated with antigen (sheep red blood cells). After washing to remove the unbound antigen, the presence of rosettes is established by microscopic examination. Cytophilic antibodies can belong to either the IgG or IgM class. They bind via their Fc regions to the Fc receptors on the macrophages and the attached antibodies then bind to antigens via their Fab regions.

In the case of tumor cells, B cells produce antibodies to tumor antigens, and the antibodies then bind to unstimulated macrophages, arming them with an antigen-specific receptor. The *armed macrophages* recognize the antigen on the tumor cell and kill it upon activation. In this situation, only the antigen recognition by armed macrophages is specific—the killing is not. But since the arming and killing follow in close sequence, the first target of the macrophage attack is the cell to which the macrophage is bound through its arming factor—the tumor cell. But the mechanism does not exclude innocent bystanders from being attacked too, as is evidenced by the following observation. After the removal of the activating agent, arming persists longer than activation (and hence cytotoxicity), so that macrophages that are no longer activated still remain armed. When such macrophages are injected, together with tumor cells, into a host, they rapidly destroy the transplant. But when the armed macrophages are injected at one site in the host and the tumor cells at another, rapid killing does not occur.

The nature of the *T cell-derived specific macrophage-activating factor* (SMAF) is unknown. Some immunologists believe it to be related to the T-cell receptor; another possibility is that the activating factor is a cytophilic molecule that recognizes some widely distributed determinant common to most dividing cells. The factor is functionally distinct from the macrophage-inhibiting factor (MIF) and from lymphotoxins (see Chapter 7). Its relation to other lymphokines remains to be determined.

The actual mechanism of target cell killing by activated macrophages is unclear. The killing seems to require direct contact between the killer and its target and may involve transfer (by "exocytosis") of lysosomes from the former to the latter—a kind of Kamikaze mission, since the interaction destroys not only the target but usually the activated macrophage as well. An alternative mechanism—the release of soluble cytotoxic factors—seems less likely. Although macrophage-derived cytotoxic factors apparently do exist, they probably play no more than an accessory role in the killing, which may involve temporary, focal, fusion-favoring destabilization of the target cell and macrophage membranes (manifested by increased membrane fluidity). In fact, one of the reasons that activated macrophages attack tumor cells preferentially might be that tumor cells are already destabilized by neoplastic transformation.

11.4 ANTIGEN HANDLING AND MACROPHAGE-LYMPHOCYTE INTERACTIONS DURING IMMUNE RESPONSE

11.4.1 Technical Problems

Immunologists generally agree that most, if not all, specific immune responses—be they humoral or cellular—require *accessory cells*—macrophages or macrophage-like cells[2], in addition to lymphocytes. But the agreement ends when one begins to discuss the *form* of macrophage involvement in the individual responses. And it is not difficult to see why immunologists still argue about how macrophages contribute to lymphocyte-mediated responses. Three important variables contribute to the controversy.

First, the almost absolute requirement for a good experiment—the standardization of experimental conditions—is often not fulfilled in experiments involving macrophages. For instance, no one has yet succeeded in producing a macrophage-free animal. This basic difficulty means that whenever one transfers accessory cells into a recipient, one must reckon with an unknown number of unidentified macrophages already present in the animal. The situation is somewhat better in in vitro experiments, but even there, an immunologist is never certain that he has removed all macrophages from a given cell population.

Second, macrophages, like lymphocytes, are probably heterogeneous cells, but since one knows next to nothing about this heterogeneity, one is unable to control it. Consequently, two inocula prepared under what seem to be identical conditions may not have the same composition of macrophage types, and this fact can greatly influence the outcome of an experiment.

And third, there is probably not one, but a variety of ways in which macrophages participate in an immune response, but an immunologist is often unable to distinguish these from one another. So the same result may be accomplished—without the immunologist's being aware of it—by different means, involving different macrophage functions.

Because of these difficulties, there is a great deal of controversy, ambiguity, and irreproducibility in macrophage studies, and the studies themselves do not always enjoy the reputation they should have.

11.4.2 Forms of Macrophage-Lymphocyte Interaction

Macrophages are known to interact with lymphocytes in at least three ways. First, they provide factors necessary for lymphocyte growth. This function can best be studied in a tissue culture where lymphocytes often live in nonphysiological and strenuous conditions. Here macrophage-derived factors become an absolute requirement for lymphocyte survival. The factors are totally nonspecific, as indicated by the fact that they can be replaced by simple compounds, such as mercaptoethanol. When cultured in the presence of mercaptoethanol, lymphocytes can often do without macrophages.

Second, macrophages provide factors participating in lymphocyte activation. Turning on a lymphocyte is a

[2] Until recently immunologists believed that almost any macrophage could perform the antigen-handling function described in this section. In the last few years, however, evidence has been accumulating indicating that this function may be limited to a relatively small subpopulation of macrophages, usually referred to as *dendritic cells*. In this text we shall not differentiate between the various subpopulations of macrophages; however, the reader should keep in mind that the statements made in this section may apply only to a small percentage of macrophages.

complex process (see Chapter 12), and at a certain stage, the lymphocyte must receive a signal from the macrophage if the activation is to proceed further. The signal is apparently a soluble molecule secreted by the macrophage and received by a special site on the lymphocyte membrane. Whether receiving a signal is an absolute requirement for the completion of the activation process or whether lymphocytes can bypass this requirement by some other means is not yet known. The question of what makes the macrophage produce the activating signal and whether all lymphocytes, or only some types, depend on this signal remains unresolved too. Specific examples of macrophage-lymphocyte cooperation will be given in Chapter 12.

Third, macrophages prepare antigens for recognition by specific lymphocyte receptors; it is this macrophage function to which we shall devote the rest of this section.

11.4.3 Preparation of Antigens for Recognition by Lymphocytes

The protracted debate over whether lymphocytes or macrophages recognize the antigen first is drawing to an end: it is becoming clear that it is the macrophage that handles the antigens first. The two possible, and still unconfirmed, exceptions to this rule are the recognition of cell-bound antigens (e.g., those controlled by the major histocompatibility complex) and that of T-independent antigens by B lymphocytes. In both these cases, some evidence exists to implicate macrophages in lymphocyte recognition, but other evidence contradicts such involvement. In all other physiological situations, the lymphocyte is probably not able to recognize antigen directly; the antigen must be presented to the lymphocyte by the macrophage. In T-dependent antigen recognition by B cells, the involvement of macrophages might be indirect: the macrophage may present the antigen to the T cell, which may then present it to the B cell; but evidence suggesting that macrophages may interact directly with B cells in some situations has also been reported. Nevertheless, the possibility remains open that, under unusual circumstances or in certain specialized responses, the lymphocyte might be able to bypass the macrophage-interaction requirement and recognize the antigen directly. Antigen presentation by macrophages can be divided arbitrarily into three stages: uptake, processing, and presentation.

Antigen Uptake

Particulate antigens are taken up via phagocytosis, soluble antigens via pinocytosis. In the latter process, the antigen need not be recognized by the macrophage as foreign; it is ingested merely because it is present in the extracellular fluid. However, if a macrophage happens to be coated by cytophilic antibodies capable of recognizing the antigen, the antigen uptake is greatly accelerated. The uptake rate is influenced by the form in which the antigen is present in the fluid. Aggregated albumin, for example, is taken up much more rapidly than nonaggregated, and peroxidase-antibody complexes are taken up more rapidly than are peroxidase molecules alone. In the absence of cytophilic antibodies, the uptake is completely nonspecific since, for example, autologous and heterologous albumin or autologous and heterologous immunoglobulin are taken up by macrophages at comparable rates. To ingest the antigen, a macrophage does not need to be in any kind of activated state: drinking comes as naturally to macrophages as it does to people.

Antigen Processing

Some 90 percent of the taken-up antigen is completely degraded within two to six hours, presumably by lysosomal enzymes. The remaining 10 percent is only partially degraded and persists in the cell in a macromolecular form for several days. It can be found associated with the plasma membrane, segregated into a special compartment and inaccessible to lysosomal enzymes. How it gets to the membrane and what form the membrane association takes is not known, but at least part of the antigen must be located on the outside of the cell, since it can be released from the membrane by treatment with trypsin and since it is accessible to antibodies. Activated macrophages seem to possess greater quantities of the membrane-associated antigen than do nonactivated cells. The persistence of a macromolecular antigen in cells with intense phagocytosis, pinocytosis, and catabolism is a paradox no one has solved yet. A small amount of the ingested antigen is released back—probably by exocytosis—into the surrounding fluids. The released antigen is probably independent of the membrane-associated antigen, since trypsin treatment has no effect on the release. Particulate antigens are released in higher quantities than soluble antigens. The released antigen is apparently still in a macromolecular form, although its molecular weight is lower than that of the native molecule, presumably because of partial degradation inside the cell. The physiological significance of antigen release is not understood. Of the three forms of processed antigen (lysosome-associated, plasma membrane-associated, and released), the one presumably used for presentation is the membrane-associated antigen; however, there is some evidence that the other two may occasionally be used as well.

It is unclear whether antigen *must* be processed for presentation. Some antigens can attach to the macrophage membrane without going through the interiorization stage. The attachment, mediated by cytophilic antibodies, may play a role when the antigen is present at low concentrations; at high concentrations, the preferred route is via interiorization. However, even the passively adsorbed antigen appears to be altered somehow by the macrophage, since it is protected from degradation. Uptake of a first dose of antigen has no effect on processing a second dose of the same or different antigens. Once it was thought that processing of the antigen involved its complexing with RNA, but the evidence for antigen-RNA association has remained unconvincing.

Antigen Presentation

Theoretically, antigen can be presented by the macrophage in two ways—by direct macrophage-lymphocyte contact and by way of soluble factors. Some evidence suggests that both modes of antigen presentation might operate. Direct macrophage-lymphocyte contact has been amply documented by both light and electron microscopic observations. Lymphocytes have been seen clustering around macrophages, each cluster consisting of one macrophage and several lymphocytes. Both T and B lymphocytes can take part in the clustering but there is some controversy over which lymphocyte attaches directly and which attaches indirectly, via the other lymphocyte, to the macrophage. The macrophage-lymphocyte clusters can be of two kinds, antigen-independent and -dependent. *Antigen-independent clusters* form even in the absence of antigen, but the binding is reversible and the clusters are short-lived. If no antigen becomes available, the clusters dissociate without any consequences for the participating cells. However, if antigen is present, more stable bonds form between the macrophage and lymphocytes, the cells remain in contact, and the cluster turns into the *antigen-dependent type*. In a culture of macrophages, lymphocytes, and antigen, one observes a progressive shift from antigen-independent to antigen-dependent clusters. The former arise even between histoincompatible macrophages and lymphocytes, while antigen-dependent cluster formation requires histocompatibility between the participating cells.

The main objective of antigen presentation by macrophages, at least as far as T cells are concerned, is to provide the lymphocytes with the opportunity of recognizing the antigen in the context of class I or class II major histocompatibility complex molecules. Part of the processing might be the placement of the antigen in the vicinity of the MHC molecules, and part of the

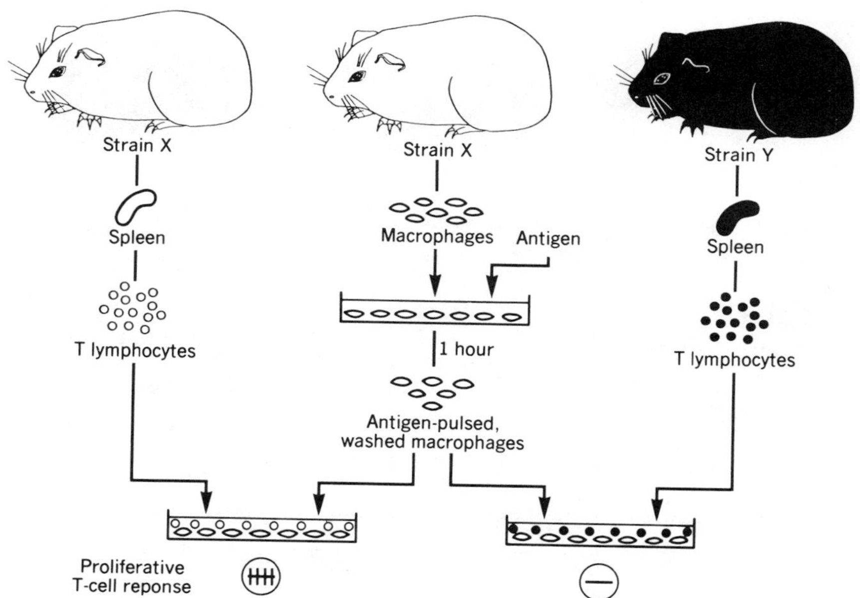

Figure 11.12. An experiment demonstrating that antigen-pulsed macrophages can activate MHC-compatible, but not MHC-incompatible, T lymphocytes. Explanation in the text.

presentation might involve the display of the antigen in conjunction with these molecules. The most convincing experiments supporting this interpretation were performed in 1973 by Alan S. Rosenthal and Ethan M. Shevach (Fig. 11.12). These investigators exposed macrophages to an antigen in culture but only for a short time—say, one hour (the macrophages are said to be "pulsed" by the antigen). They then washed the macrophages (to remove any free uningested antigen) and mixed them with T lymphocytes from guinea pigs immunized against the same antigen. When cultured together, the lymphocytes in the mixture became activated by the antigen presented to them by the macrophages and the activation could be measured by ^{3}H-thymidine incorporation into the DNA-synthesizing cells (see Chapter 12). Rosenthal and Shevach observed that significant lymphocyte activation occurred only when the macrophage carried the same class II molecules as the donor of the T lymphocytes. In other words, the activation of lymphocytes by the antigen-presenting macrophages was restricted by class II MHC molecules. Moreover, these investigators were able to demonstrate that the in vitro T-cell response to macrophage-presented antigen correlated well with antibody response to this antigen (Fig. 11.13). In this experiment, they selected two guinea pig strains, one of which was a high responder (HR) and the other a low responder (LR) to a given antigen in terms of antibody formation (the response being controlled by the class II MHC loci). They produced (HR × LR)F_1 hybrids, immunized the animals to the antigen, isolated T cells from the immunized animals, and mixed the T cells in cell culture with antigen-pulsed HR- or LR-strain macrophages. They observed that HR macrophages, but not LR, were able to activate lymphocytes. This experiment further strengthened the conclusion that interaction between lymphocytes and antigen-presenting macrophages involves class II MHC molecules.

Not much is known about the form of macrophage-lymphocyte interaction mediated by soluble factors, except that the factors are of two kinds—specific, carrying information for lymphocyte activation via antigen-specific receptors, and nonspecific. The specific factors seem to contain class II MHC molecules and they may represent complexes of these molecules with the antigen. The nonspecific factors might, in fact, be regulatory signals necessary for lymphocyte activation.

11.4.4 Conclusion

The gist of the preceding discussion is that only lymphocytes are capable of specific immune response to a given antigen, but that to respond, the lymphocyte

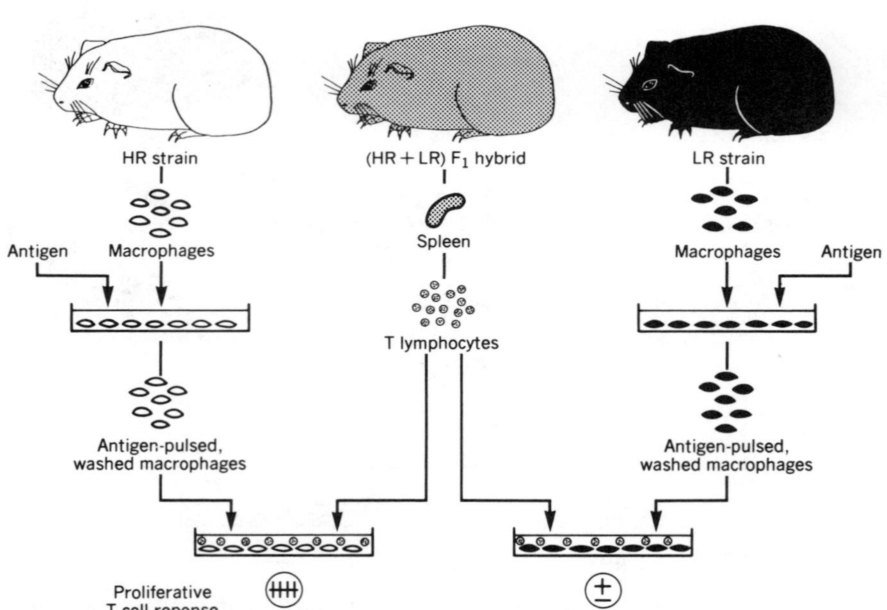

Figure 11.13. An experiment demonstrating that antigen-pulsed macrophages can activate T lymphocytes from a high (HR)-, but not from a low (LR)-responder strain, where responsiveness is controlled by *Ir* genes of the major histocompatibility complex.

must first interact directly or indirectly with a macrophage. The main purpose of this interaction is to present the antigen to the lymphocyte in the context of the macrophage's MHC molecules. The macrophage thus determines whether an animal is going to mount a specific lymphocyte response. Macrophages may also determine whether the response will be predominantly of the T-cell or B-cell type, whether the lymphocytes will secrete antibodies or turn into memory cells, and whether lymphocytes will respond positively (and so induce immunity) or negatively (and so induce tolerance), or remain indifferent. All these decisions are apparently made *before* any involvement of lymphocytes. But once lymphocytes are activated, they, in turn, influence macrophage behavior by secreting a variety of soluble mediators (see Chapter 7). Although many gaps still remain in our knowledge of macrophage-lymphocyte interaction, it is clear that hardly any form of immune response is unaffected by macrophages.

11.5 THE MACROPHAGE AS A SECRETORY CELL

In the preceding sections we described two ways in which macrophages participate in defense reactions—intracellular killing of ingested particles and killing of target cells by cell-to-cell contact. In this section, we shall discuss a third way, consisting of secretion by the macrophage of soluble substances that play a role in defense. The macrophage synthesizes and secretes a great many substances, some of which are listed below.

11.5.1 Regulators of Stem-Cell Differentiation

Mice injected with endotoxin display an increased stem-cell proliferation in bone marrow, and serum from such mice supports the growth and differentiation of bone marrow cells in vitro. Since endotoxin is known to activate macrophages and monocytes, the effect on bone marrow cells could be the result of this activation. Supporting this conclusion is the observation that the medium from cultured monocytes, or the monocytes themselves, when used as feeder cells, support the establishment of granulocytic or mononuclear colonies from bone marrow stem cells. The factor responsible for this *colony-stimulating activity* (CSA) is produced at a low rate by unactivated macrophages; endotoxin activation of macrophages greatly increases this production. The adaptive significance of the factor is in that it regulates the differentiation of stem cells into monocytes and granulocytes, according to the needs of the organism. The factor is a glycoprotein; upon electrophoresis it migrates between α_1 globulins and albumins; and it has a molecular weight of between 45,000 and 60,000 daltons.

11.5.2 Regulators of Fibroblast Growth and Activity

When one cultures macrophages in the presence of silica (silicon dioxide, SiO_2, here used as a macrophage activator), harvests the medium, and then adds it to a culture of fibroblasts, one observes an increased conversion of radiolabeled proline into hydroxyproline, and incorporation of the latter into collagen of the fibroblasts. Apparently, activated macrophages (unactivated macrophages less so) produce a soluble factor that speeds fibroblast growth. In vivo, the factor probably plays a role in wound healing: wounds attract large numbers of monocytes, which speed the migration of fibroblasts into the wound and induce increased collagen production by the fibroblasts. Researchers have repeatedly observed that, when immigration of monocytes is prevented or reduced, fibroblasts immigration is delayed. The interaction between monocytes and fibroblasts might be a two-way street, for the fibroblasts seem to secrete a factor that stimulates macrophage proliferation. As was discussed in Chapter 5, macrophages normally do not divide in culture, but when incubated with medium from a fibroblast culture, they begin to synthesize DNA within 24 to 48 hours following the exposure, and prepare themselves for proliferation.

11.5.3 Factors Affecting T Lymphocyte Activity

Macrophages cultured in the presence of endotoxin or some other macrophage activator secrete a substance into the medium, which when added to the culture of T lymphocytes, stimulates the incorporation of ^{3}H-thymidine into the T cells. The substance, usually referred to as *lymphocyte-activating factor* (LAF) (see Chapter 7), is most actively produced within the first 48 hours of challenge by the activator. As with the preceding factor, unstimulated macrophages produce some LAF and the activation merely increases the production. The factor production is regulated by a feedback mechanism: the LAF-stimulated lymphocytes produce lymphokine, which increases LAF production by macrophages. The factor probably plays a role in the expansion of T-lymphocyte clones (see Chapter 12); it has no effect on B cells.

11.5.4 Factors Affecting B Lymphocyte Activity

B lymphocytes seem to be acted upon by another macrophage-produced factor, the *B lymphocyte-acti-*

vating factor (BAF). In some unknown manner, this factor enhances the production of antibodies by B lymphocytes. It can act in the absence of T cells and its production is enhanced by some macrophage-activating stimuli (e.g., endotoxin) but apparently not by others (e.g., latex particles). Its molecular weight is between 15,000 and 21,000 daltons.

11.5.5 Cytotoxic Factors

As was already mentioned in section 11.3, activated macrophages secrete soluble factors that can kill various target cells. Different laboratories have given different names to these factors (e.g., specific macrophage cytotoxin or SMC, growth-inhibiting factor or GIF, and macrophage cytotoxic factor or MCF), but whether there really are several cytotoxic factors has not been established. Of the three factors mentioned, SMC and GIF are probably the same, and the two are probably different from MFC. The *specific macrophage cytotoxin* is produced by macrophages activated by allogeneic cells; it kills the activating target cells specifically in vitro, and its molecular weight is around 100,000 daltons. The *macrophage cytotoxic factor* is produced by macrophages incubated overnight on glass or plastic surfaces. In contrast to SMC, MCF is completely nonspecific and kills allogeneic and syngeneic target cells equally well. Because of its extreme lability, MCF is not detected under normal culture conditions.

11.5.6 Hydrolytic Enzymes

The same enzymes that are involved in intracellular killing of microorganisms are also found in extracellular fluids and the medium of cultured macrophages. Some are passively released into the medium when macrophages and monocytes die, but most are actively secreted. The evidence for this conclusion is provided by the observation that the level of hydrolytic enzymes in the medium increases by the addition of almost any macrophage-activating agent to the culture. The secreted enzymes derive in part from a preformed store contained in lysosomes, and in part from *de novo* synthesis. The enzymes play a major role in defense reactions stimulated by tissue injury: they degrade connective tissue substances, activate the inactive forms of several humoral mediators—including the components of the complement, coagulation, and kinin systems, and modify cell function by limited hydrolysis of certain plasma membrane constituents.

11.5.7 Endogenous Pyrogen

You may recall from Chapter 10 that bacterial endotoxin stimulates macrophages and monocytes to release a protein, which induces fever by stimulating the thermoregulation center of the hypothalamus. Endotoxin is therefore sometimes referred to as exogenous pyrogen, and the monocyte-produced protein as *endogenous pyrogen*. In addition to monocytes and macrophages, endogenous pyrogen is also produced by neutrophils, but the two pyrogens differ in their molecular weights: the monocyte-derived pyrogen has a molecular weight of 38,000 daltons; the neutrophil-derived pyrogen is smaller (molecular weight of 15,000 daltons). The release of pyrogen by unactivated macrophages is quite slow (one must culture these cells for at least five days before one detects the protein in the medium); activated macrophages, on the other hand, secrete enough pyrogen within four hours to induce fever in rabbits injected with the culture supernatant. The adaptive role and significance of fever for bodily defense are still unclear.

11.5.8 Complement Components

We described these macrophage products in Chapter 9; here it suffices to say that a complement component not secreted by macrophages is yet to be discovered.

11.5.9 Prostaglandins

Prostaglandins are a family of biologically highly active fatty acids, derived from *prostanoic acid* (Fig. 11.14). Their designation refers to the fact that they were originally discovered in secretions of the prostate gland, discharged at the time of semen emission. Prostanoic acid consists of a five-carbon ring, to which are attached two carbon tails (both chains together contain 20 carbon atoms). It is synthesized from phospholipids of the plasma membrane. The first step in this synthesis is the amputation of the fatty acid chains from the phospholipid—a reaction catalyzed by the enzyme phospholipase A_2. The amputated fatty acid then becomes the precursor of prostanoic acid, provided, of course, that it is of the right composition (its chain must contain 20 carbon atoms). A common precursor of prostanoic acid is *arachidonic acid* (Fig. 11.14), also called 5,8,11,14-eicosatetraenoic acid (the numbers indicate the positions of double bonds), present in abundance in *Arachis*, the common soybean. After its release from the plasma membrane, the arachidonic acid bends in the middle and assumes the hairpin shape shown in Figure 11.14. The addition of oxygen to the atoms in the bend (atoms C_8 and C_{12}) results in closing (cyclization) of the five-carbon ring of the prostanoic acid. Cyclization of the arachidonic acid is catalyzed by the enzyme *cyclooxygenase*; the requirement for molecular oxygen ties the arachidonic cascade to the

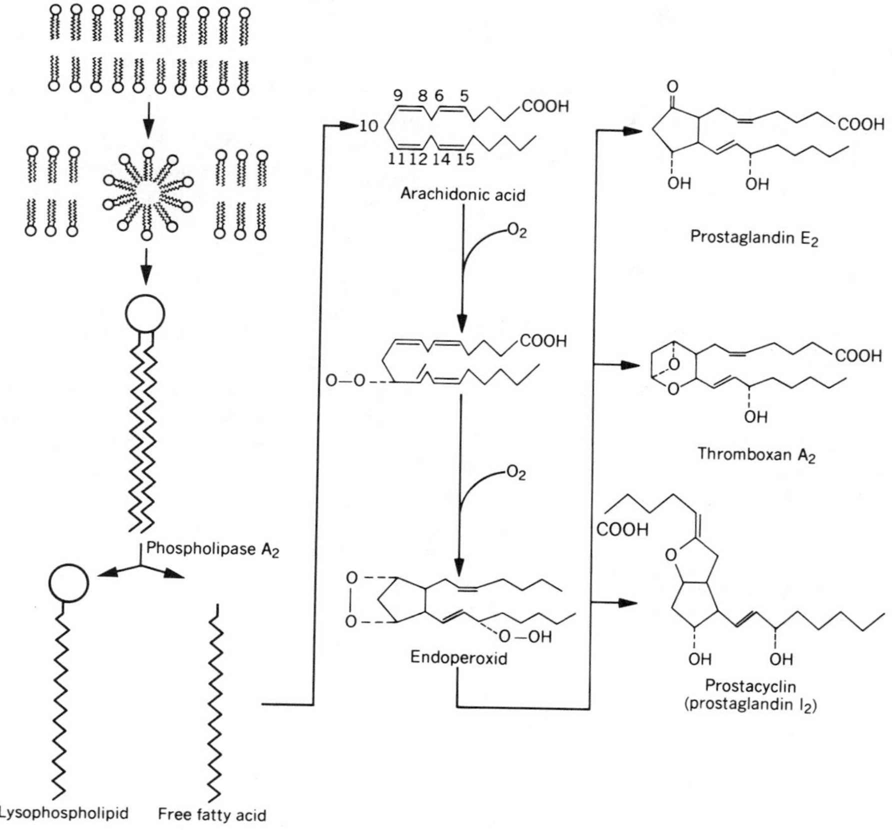

Figure 11.14. Derivation of the prostaglandins thromboxan and prostacyclin from plasma-membrane phospholipids.

metabolic burst system that occurs during phagocytosis. The cyclization product, the so-called *endoperoxid,* is then converted into one of the prostaglandins—thromboxan or prostacyclin (Fig. 11.14). The different *prostaglandins* differ mainly in the position of the double bond in the carbon tail; *thromboxan* contains an additional oxan ring; *prostacyclin* contains two joined five-carbon rings. The main classes of prostaglandin are designated PGA, PGE, and PGF, followed by a subscript that denotes the number of double bonds outside the ring.

Prostaglandins are synthesized by many other cells (e.g., lymphocytes, fibroblasts, and granulocytes) in addition to macrophages and monocytes. In the body, they are ubiquitous, present in virtually all major tissues. Since they are biologically highly active (and in that they resemble hormones), but are not secreted by specialized glands, they are sometimes referred to as *local* or *cellular hormones*. They are important messengers in intercellular communications and have a broad range of biological activity: they regulate blood flow to particular organs by narrowing or widening blood vessels; they stimulate intestinal and uterine smooth muscles (infusion of PGE_2 induces uterine contractions within a few hours); they act as antagonists of hormones regulating lipid metabolism; they control transport of ions across the plasma membrane; they modulate synaptic transmission (see Chapter 14); and they are involved in bone resorption. Thromboxan and prostacyclin are involved in platelet (thrombocyte)-mediated blood clotting. For us, the most important function of prostaglandins is their involvement in the so-called inflammatory reactions accompanying tissue injury and wound healing, which will be discussed in Chapter 14.

Prostaglandin synthesis is inhibited by aspirin, which interferes with the enzymatic cyclization of the linear fatty acids. This interference is one of the mechanisms of aspirin action: prostaglandins enhance inflammatory reactions; aspirin diminishes them.

REFERENCES

General

Badwey, J. A. and Karnovsky, M. L.: Active oxygen species and the functions of phagocytic leukocytes. *Annu. Rev. Biochem.* **49:**695–726, 1980.

Carr, I.: *The Macrophage. A Review of Ultrastructure and Function*. Academic, London, 1973.

Klebanoff, S. J. and Clark, R. A.: *The Neutrophil: Function and Clinical Disorders*. North-Holland, Amsterdam, 1978.

Murphy, P.: *The Neutrophil*. Plenum Medical Press, New York, 1976.

Nelson, D. S.: *Macrophages and Immunity*. North-Holland, Amsterdam, 1969.

Pearsall, N. N. and Weiser, R. S.: *The Macrophage*. Lea and Febiger, Philadelphia, 1970.

Silverstein, S. C., Steinman, R. M., and Cohn, Z. A.: Endocytosis. *Annu. Rev. Biochem*. **46**:669–722, 1977.

Vernon-Roberts, B.: *The Macrophage*. Cambridge University Press, 1972.

Wilkinson, P. C.: *Chemotaxis and Inflammation*. Churchill Livingstone, Edinburgh, 1974.

Original Articles

Boyden, S.: The chemotactic effect of mixtures of antibody and antigen on polymorphonuclear leukocytes. *J. Exp. Med*. **115**: 453–466, 1962.

Granger, G. A. and Weiser, R. S.: Homograft target cells: specific destruction *in vitro* by contact interaction with immune macrophages. *Science* **145**:1427–1429, 1964.

MacKaness, G. B.: Resistance to intracellular infection. *J. Infect. Dis*. **123**:439–445, 1971.

Rosenthal, A. S. and Shevach, E. M.: Function of macrophages in antigen recognition by guinea pig T lymphocytes. I. Requirement for histocompatible macrophages and lymphocytes. *J. Exp. Med*. **138**:1194–1212, 1973.

Shevach, E. M. and Rosenthal, A. S.: Function of macrophages in antigen recognition by guinea pig T lymphocytes. II. Role of the macrophage in the regulation of genetic control of the immune system. *J. Exp. Med*. **138**:1213–1229, 1973.

Stossel, T. P. and Hartwig, J. H.: Interaction of actin, myosin, and a new actin-binding protein of rabbit pulmonary macrophages. *J. Cell. Biol*. **68**:602–619, 1976.

CHAPTER 12

RESPONSES DOMINATED BY T LYMPHOCYTES

12.1 INTRODUCTION

The ancient Romans had a special god of doorways, departures and returns, and of all means of communication. He was Janus, the two-faced god, with one face to watch the exterior and the other the interior of a house. Janus was also the god of beginnings (the first month of the year still bears his name), promoter of all initiative, the god of gods. The gates of his temple were closed only in times of peace and so they were almost always open.

In immunological mythology, the macrophage is Proteus and the T lymphocyte is Janus. Like Janus, the T cell has two faces, one for the outside world (nonself) and the other for the body's interior (self), and like Janus, T cells are at the beginning of all things, for there is hardly an event in the specific immune response that occurs without their participation. T cells are the prime movers of the immunological universe.

The T lymphocyte that has just left the thymus is a small cell that does little but cruise the body and perform the usual housekeeping functions. This state changes, however, when the lymphocyte is shown an antigen—probably by a macrophagelike cell. The encounter with the antigen initiates a chain of events that transforms the small, quiescent lymphocyte into a large, highly active *blast cell*—a phenomenon called *blast transformation*. The blast then divides mitotically (*proliferates*) and during these divisions gradually returns to the size of the original small lymphocyte (Fig. 12.1). However, the new small lymphocyte is a changed cell, for it is now capable of performing functions the original cell probably was not—it has become an *effector cell*. The function of the effector cell is twofold: some specialize in killing target cells carrying the same antigen that activated the lymphocyte in the first place (*cytotoxic T cells*), while others turn into regulatory cells that either enhance or suppress the activity of target cells (*helper* and *suppressor T cells*).

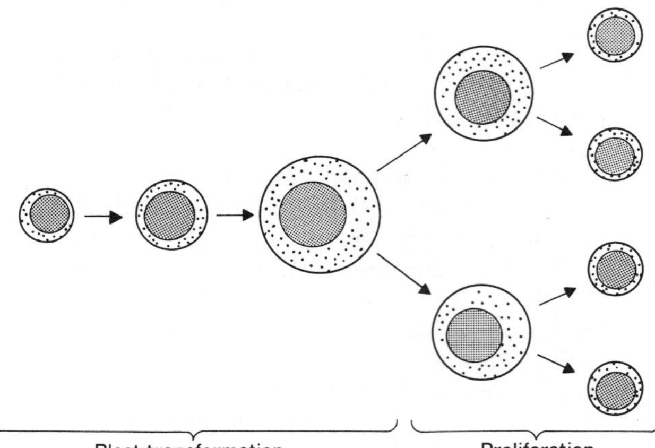

Figure 12.1. Morphological changes following lymphocyte activation.

To be activated by an antigen, a T lymphocyte must recognize not only the antigen itself (a nonself component) *but also the individual's own major histocompatibility complex (MHC) molecules* (a self component). This requirement for the simultaneous interaction of the T-cell receptor with self and nonself components is a *sine qua non*, an essential condition, of T-cell recognition. There is only one highly artificial situation in which T cells might possibly bypass this requirement, and that is when they interact with MHC molecules of another, genetically disparate individual (i.e., allogeneic MHC molecules), but even here it is not at all certain that some form of self recognition does not take place. In all other situations, T cells are unable to use their antigen-specific receptors unless nonself is presented to them in the context of self. And since MHC molecules are normally present on cell surfaces, it follows that, to be recognized, the antigen must be presented to T lymphocytes on the surface of another cell, a cell that expresses the appropriate MHC genes (usually a macrophage). In this respect—as we shall learn in the next chapter—T cells differ from B cells, which can recognize an antigen alone, without MHC, and do not require that it be presented to them on the cell surface.

In this chapter, we shall deal first with changes occurring during lymphocyte activation in general (with changes common to both T *and* B cells), then describe several forms of T-lymphocyte responsiveness as well as one form of unresponsiveness, and finally consider what the forms tell us about the natural functions of T lymphocytes in a body undisturbed by an experimenter. (The individual forms are all artificial situations set up by the experimenter to measure each particular facet of the T-cell response; they reflect the natural T-lymphocyte function only indirectly.)

12.2 LYMPHOCYTE ACTIVATION

As you will recall from Chapter 5, the life of a cell (the cell cycle) can be divided into four phases: mitotic (M), first growth phase (G_1), synthetic (S), and second growth phase (G_2). Unstimulated lymphocytes are all in the G_1 phase—they are quiescent, or resting. Upon receiving a proper activating signal, the lymphocytes leave the G_1 phase and enter the S phase, in which they synthesize DNA and prepare for cell division. What happens between the receiving of the signal and the start of DNA synthesis is largely unknown. It is as if the signal disappeared in, as one immunologist put it, "a dark, if not altogether black box." Immunologists assume that the signal initiates a train of events that culminates in cell division, but the elucidation of these events is proving to be a formidable problem. To solve this problem, immunologists divide their work into three stages: in the first stage, they compare stimulated and unstimulated lymphocytes and search for differences between the two; in the second, they try to decide which of the differences found pertain in a critical way to lymphocyte activation rather than being nonessential side effects of the process; and in the third stage, they try to arrange the events into a causally linked chain. So far the work on lymphocyte activation has not progressed far beyond the first stage: a few wagons of the train have been identified, but how they link up is not at all clear. To simplify the discussion we shall divide the process of lymphocyte activation more or less arbitrarily into five phases: signal receiving, membrane alteration, transmission of the signal into the cell interior, changes in the nucleus, and attainment of the effector status.

12.2.1 Signal-Receiving Phase

The activation signal is received by a cell-surface receptor probably represented by membrane-spanning glycoprotein molecules. The signal-receptor interaction raises a number of questions, some of which are discussed below.

Does Activation Require Not Only Binding But Also the Entry of the Stimulating Molecule into the Lymphocyte? There has been a long controversy among immunologists as to the correct answer to this question. It is still not fully resolved, but most immunologists would probably agree that, although in some instances the stimulating molecules do indeed enter lymphocytes, this entry is probably irrelevant to lymphocyte activation.

Are Crosslinking and Capping of Receptors Necessary for Lymphocyte Activation? Although initially, stimulating molecules bind to many receptors diffusely distributed on the cell surface, eventually they are found concentrated in a cap at one pole of the cell in the area of the uropod. The cap is then either shed or internalized. But is this receptor rearrangement from a diffused to a concentrated state an essential part of activation, or merely the result of receptor crosslinking by the stimulating molecules—an event of no functional significance? Since lymphocyte activation also occurs with lectins, which often do not cap receptors, it would seem that capping is not necessary to initiate the activation process. Other experiments also demonstrate that capping is not sufficient for lymphocyte activation.

How Long Does the Signal Need To Act on Lymphocytes to Activate Them? There are two apparent possibilities: either the activation is like pressing a button, in which all the signal does is provide the initial impulse, or it is like starting a car engine, where the key must remain in the ignition to keep the car running. The actual answer seems to lie somewhere between the two possibilities. The presence of the stimulating molecule is required even after the initial binding to the receptor, but the molecule can be removed several hours before the cell begins to synthesize DNA. Apparently, as soon as the cell becomes committed to DNA synthesis, the stimulating molecule is no longer needed—the car runs by itself.

Is the Stimulating Molecule Alone Sufficient for Lymphocyte Activation? Another controversial issue is whether a lymphocyte is activated by one or two signals (the one signal being the activating molecule and the other a nonspecific inducer, like a lymphokine, provided by another cell). It is clear that a second signal increases the probability of activation, but whether a lymphocyte can also be activated by the mere binding of a stimulating molecule still remains an open question. The second signal might merely be a way of amplifying the response so that the lymphocyte might be turned on by either the first or second signal, rather than by both signals simultaneously. We shall return to this question in Chapter 13, where we shall discuss B-lymphocyte activation.

Need Other Cells Be Present To Activate a Lymphocyte? This question is difficult to answer for purely technical reasons: lymphocytes grow very poorly in culture when their density drops below a certain (relatively high) number and nobody has yet designed a method for culturing single lymphocytes. The observation that lymphocytes at certain low densities no longer respond to activating stimuli could therefore reflect some basic metabolic deficiency of lymphocytes in tissue culture, or it could signify that the activation depends on inducing stimuli from other cells: the question remains open. Whether the presence of lymphocytes alone is sufficient for activation to occur or whether some other cell types are needed has not been decided either. Many lymphocyte responses either do not occur at all or are inferior in the absence of macrophages; the addition of no more than 1 percent of macrophages (of the total lymphocyte number) often suffices to improve the responses conspicuously. But the question of whether macrophages are an essential ingredient of T-cell responses or merely amplify these responses remains unanswered.

12.2.2 Plasma-Membrane Changes Following the Binding of Stimulating Molecules

Changes in Entry Rate of Compounds into the Cell

Very shortly (within minutes) after the binding of the stimulating molecule to cell-surface receptors, one observes an increase in the entry rate of nucleosides, sugars, amino acids, phosphate, choline, K^+, Na^+, and Ca^{2+} into lymphocytes. Some of these increases are clearly irrelevant to lymphocyte activation as is evidenced, for example, by the fact that when one cultures lymphocytes, one can leave uridine or phosphate out of the medium without any effect; others seem to be essential for activation. The most thoroughly studied of the latter category of changes is the increase in transport of K^+ and Na^+ ions.

Not only lymphocytes, but virtually all cells are low in sodium (average concentration of about 10 μM/ml) and high in potassium (100 μM/ml). Just the opposite is true for extracellular fluids (e.g., plasma), where the concentration of Na^+ is about 140 μM/ml and that of K^+ about 5 μM/ml, which is close to the concentration of these ions in sea water. The ionic imbalance between the cell interior and exterior is maintained by an *ion pump*, which, through the expenditure of about 25 percent of the cell's basal energy, pumps K^+ in and Na^+ out of the cell. An essential part of the pump is an enzyme, Na^+,K^+-dependent adenosine triphosphatase (Na^+, K^+ATPase)—a membrane-spanning protein that picks up K^+ on the cell's outside and transports it across the membrane into the cell; simultaneously, this protein picks up Na^+ on the inside and transports it to the cell's outside (Fig. 12.2).

Within 30 seconds after the addition of mitogen to lymphocyte culture, the K^+ and Na^+ transport rate increases to approximately double that observed in unstimulated lymphocytes. Evidence indicating that this increase is essential for lymphocyte activation comes from studies with quabain, a steroid used by African tribesmen as an arrow poison and by cardiologists for heart failures caused by clogging of blood vessels. Quabain is specific for Na^+,K^+ATPase and its action inhibits lymphocyte transformation: no DNA synthesis occurs in lymphocytes upon the addition of this drug.

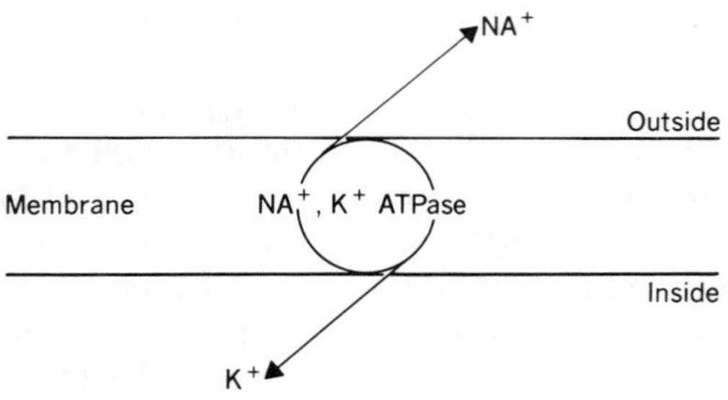

Figure 12.2. The ion pump.

The role of the increased ion pump flux in stimulated lymphocytes is not known. The increase might represent a preparatory adjustment for the cell volume increase characteristic of blast transformation (the rate returns to normal before the cell actually begins to increase in size), or it might somehow be tied to changes in cyclic adenosine monophosphate (cAMP) concentration in the stimulated lymphocyte. Some biochemists believe that lymphocyte triggering requires a drop in cAMP concentration, and since adenylate cyclase, the enzyme that converts adenosine triphosphate (ATP) into cAMP (see below), and N^+,K^+ATPase compete for a common ATP pool, the increased function of the ion pump rapidly exhausts this pool. However, several other explanations are also possible.

Changes in Membrane Lipids

Lipids, you might recall, are prominently represented in the cell membrane, forming the lipid bilayer and providing conditions for membrane fluidity. The degree of membrane fluidity varies under the influence of two main factors: cholesterol content and the extent of unsaturation of the phospholipid's fatty acid side chains (see Appendix 5.1). Lymphocyte stimulation leads to changes in phospholipid metabolism—among other things, to enrichment in the content of polyunsaturated fatty acids. As a consequence of these changes, the phospholipid become more loosely packed and the membrane more fluid. The change in membrane fluidity may, in turn, affect transport and other membrane functions.

Interpretation of Membrane Changes Preceding Activation

One view of what might be happening in the lymphocyte membrane before the lymphocyte begins to synthesize DNA is depicted in Figure 12.3. Here, the binding of a ligand (an antigen or a mitogen) to a membrane receptor is thought to activate two membrane-bound enzymes, phospholipid methyltransferases I and II (PMT I and PMT II). The two enzymes are positioned

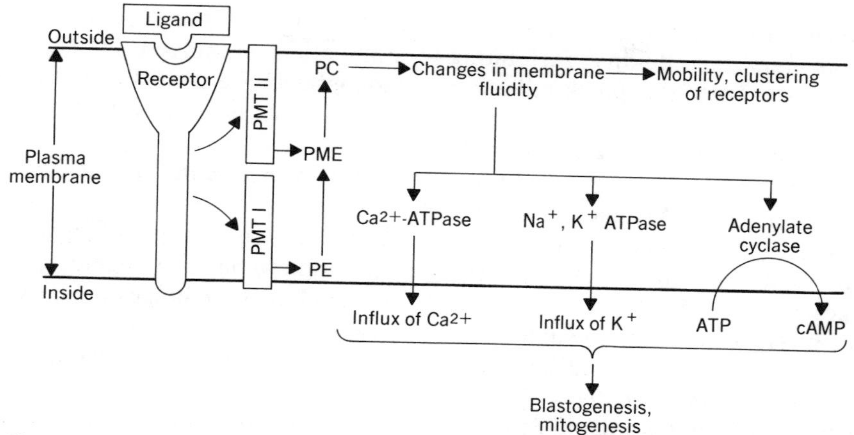

Figure 12.3. Membrane changes following the binding of a ligand (antigen, lectin) to a lymphocyte receptor. PC, phosphatidylcholine; PE, phosphatidylethanolamine; PME, phosphatidyl-*N*-mono-methylethanolamine; PMT I and II, phospholipid methyltransferase I and II.

on opposite sides of the membrane: PMTI faces the cytoplasmic side, PMTII the outside. This location matches the distribution of the phospholipids that are the substrates of the two enzymes: phosphatidylethanolamines (PE), the substrate of PMTI, are mostly on the cytoplasmic side, whereas phosphatidvlcholines (PC), the substrate of PMTII, are mostly oriented toward the outside.

The activated PMTI methylates (adds methyl group $-CH_3$ to) PE and thus converts it into phosphatidyl-*N*-monomethylethanolamine (PME; Fig. 12.4). PME is then acted upon by PMT II and converted, by the addition of two methyl groups, into phosphatidylcholine (Fig. 12.4). The methylated phospholipid molecules are then translocated from the cytoplasmic side of the membrane to the exterior surface (they are said

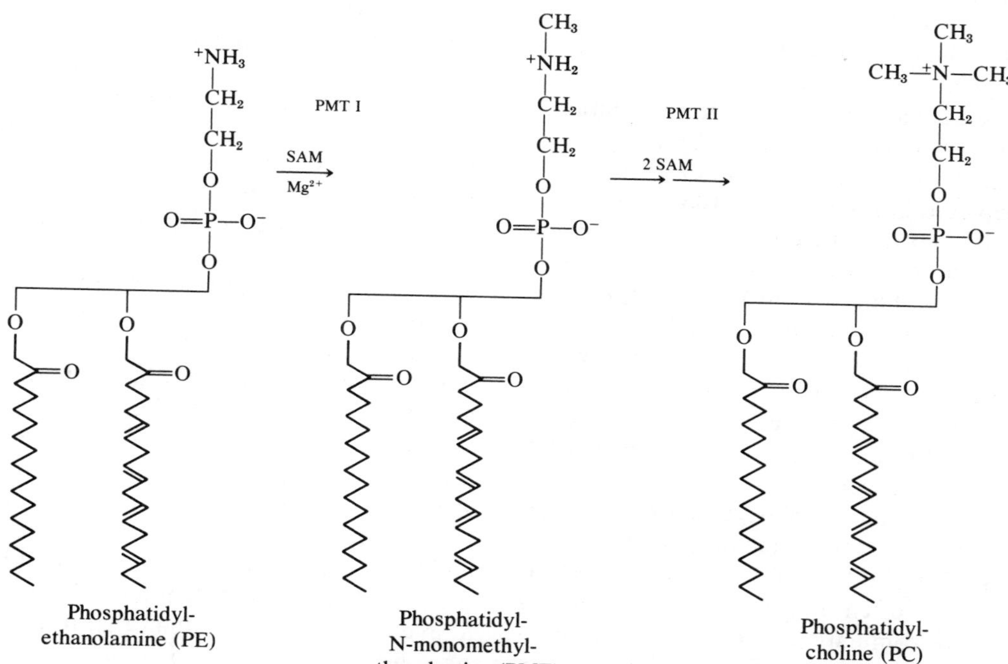

Figure 12.4. The enzymatic conversion of phosphatidylethanolamine to phosphatidylcholine. PMTI and II, phospholipid methyltransferase I and II; SAM, S-adenosyl-L-methionine. (From H. Hirata and J. Axelrod, *Science* **209**:1082–1090, 1980.)

to flip-flop). This translocation decreases lipid viscosity and hence increases membrane fluidity, facilitating lateral movement and clustering of receptors and other membrane molecules.

The increased fluidity is thought to be responsible for at least three major changes in the membrane. First, it affects the Ca^{2+}-dependent ATPase, an enzyme regulating the efflux of Ca^{2+} from cells. The enzyme is surrounded in the membrane by an annulus of phospholipids; the changes in the viscosity of the membrane lipids somehow alter this enzyme in such a way that it opens the calcium ion channels and allows an influx of Ca^{2+} into the cell. Second, the decreased viscosity of membrane lipids affects Na^+,K^+ATPase and so the ion pump. And third, the lipid changes affect adenylate cyclase by an unknown factor and so influence the level of cAMP in the cytoplasm.

12.2.3 Signal Transfer from Membrane to Nucleus

This phase is the least understood of the entire lymphocyte activation process. The signal transfer is thought to be mediated by a hypothetical "second messenger" (the first messenger being the lymphocyte-stimulating molecule), but its nature remains totally obscure. Two candidates have been considered for the messenger function—Ca^{2+} ions and cAMP—but evidence implicating one or the other in signal transmission is lacking.

An increase in the Ca^{2+}-uptake rate of stimulating lymphocytes has been observed, but the possibility that changes in Ca^{2+} concentration affect the nucleus and lead to gene activation remains idle speculation.

Cyclic adenosine monophosphate (cAMP) is a substance synthesized from adenosine triphosphate (ATP) in a manner depicted in Figure 12.5. (Biochemists use the word "cyclic" to designate compounds in which the constituting atoms form a ring.) The reaction occurs primarily in muscles and is catalyzed by a membrane-associated enzyme, *adenylate cyclase*. Since cyclic AMP plays the role of a second messenger in many biological processes (for example, it mediates the action of some polypeptide hormones on their target cells), immunologists thought that it might also mediate information transfer from the membrane to the nucleus in stimulated lymphocytes. However, no clear evidence has yet been marshalled in support of this hypothesis. The addition of exogenous cAMP to lymphocyte culture often inhibits, rather than enhances lymphocyte stimulation, and attempts to measure changes of endogenous cAMP during lymphocyte stimulation have provided contradictory results: different investigators found increased, decreased, or unchanged cAMP levels. Now some immunologists think that the role of the second messenger in lymphocyte stimulation is played instead by cyclic guanosine monophosphate (cGMP, see Fig. 12.5), but here, too, the evidence is equally controversial.

12.2.4 Changes in the Nucleus

Originally, some immunologists believed lymphocyte activation to be accompanied by widespread gene activation. Indeed, changes in acetylation and phosphorylation of histones and other chromosomal proteins have been reported to occur after the interaction of lymphocyte-activating molecules with corresponding receptors; but some of these changes are probably artifacts, while others may be unrelated to lymphocyte activation. In fact, widespread gene activation now appears extremely unlikely and a few genes that might be activated would be difficult to detect with available methods. Lymphocyte activation, however, does lead to changes in the nucleus that result in the synthesis of DNA, RNA, and protein.

DNA synthesis begins 24 hours after mitogen addition to lymphocyte culture, reaches a maximum at 72 hours, and then gradually declines unless lymphocytes are restimulated. The synthesis can be measured by the incorporation of radioactively labeled nucleic acid building blocks added to the culture medium. The cell, which normally synthesizes these precursors itself, takes up the prefabricated building blocks and uses them to construct new DNA molecules. The radioactivity of DNA extracted from activated lymphocytes then provides evidence that DNA synthesis has occurred. The most frequently used precursor is thymidine, a nucleoside composed of a sugar (deoxyribose), a phosphate, and a nitrogenous base (thymine, which is one of the four bases found in DNA, the others being adenine, guanine, and cytosine; see Fig. 12.5). The frequently used isotopes are ^3H (tritium) and ^{14}C (the former is preferred because it is cheaper and is available with high specific activity).

The increase in *RNA synthesis* concerns the ribosomal and transfer RNA. No definite difference in messenger RNA synthesis between stimulated and unstimulated lymphocytes has yet been demonstrated. Stimulated lymphocytes also use pre-existing ribosomes for protein synthesis at an increased rate.

The rate of *protein synthesis* increases soon after the addition of mitogen to lymphocyte culture and prior to the induction of DNA synthesis. Eventually it reaches a level 10 times higher than that in unstimulated lymphocytes. The increase is caused by the removal of inhibitors in activated lymphocytes; in normal lymphocytes, these inhibitors inactivate the initiation factors that are necessary to begin the synthesis.

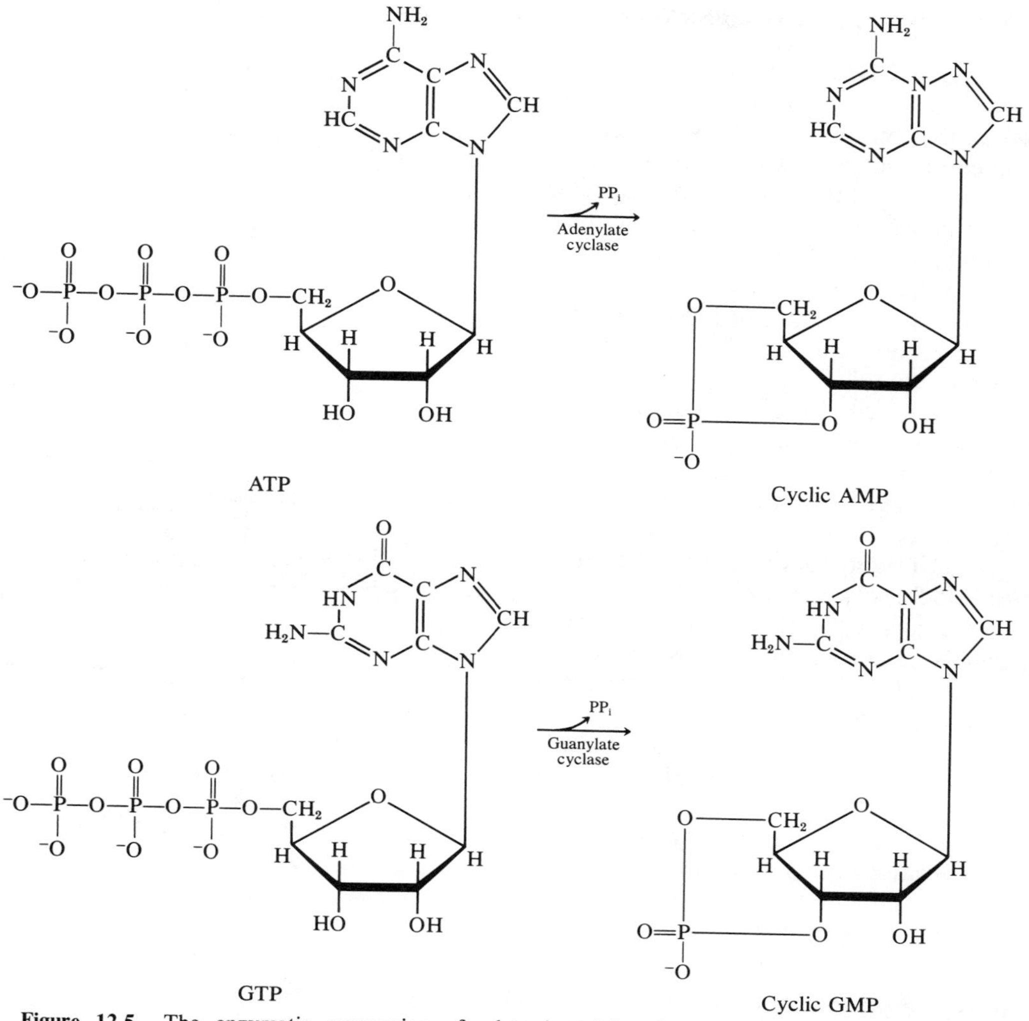

Figure 12.5. The enzymatic conversion of adenosine-triphosphate (ATP) to cyclic adenosine monophosphate (cAMP) and of guanosine triphosphate (GMP) to cyclic guanosine monophosphate (cGMP).

12.2.5 Induction of Effector Functions

The activated lymphocytes perform acts—such as the secretion of lymphokines and other factors, or killing of target cells—that the unstimulated lymphocytes cannot do. Unfortunately, we know nothing about the manner in which this functional lymphocyte maturation occurs. The functions are already expressed in the blast cell stage but are most pronounced after the reversal of the lymphocyte to the small-cell stage.

Lymphocyte activation is accompanied by pronounced morphological changes: increase in cell diameter (within 24 hours after mitogen stimulation, the cell diameter more than doubles, corresponding to an increase in cell volume of more than one order of magnitude), the appearance of the nucleolus, an increase in the number of mitochondria and lysosomes, and the decondensation of nuclear heterochromatin. However, the stimulated effector cells are morphologically indistinguishable from unstimulated small lymphocytes.

After this general description of lymphocyte activation, we shall now discuss specific forms of T-lymphocyte activation. The individual forms differ from one another in the manner in which they are induced (by a lectin, an alloantigen, or a conventional antigen), carried out (in vitro or in vivo), and measured (cell proliferation, killing of target cells, generation of regulatory factors, or a combination of all three effects). Although all these forms are artificial in one way or another, they are important tools for learning about the natural functions of T lymphocytes.

12.3 LECTIN-INDUCED T-CELL PROLIFERATION

Certain lectins activate T lymphocytes in culture (see also Chapter 10). This activation differs from other T-cell responses in that the first signal is not received by the T-cell receptor, but by a lectin-binding molecule. In contrast to the receptor, the binding molecule is not clonally distributed and probably has some function other than binding lectins but happens to contain the sugars for which the lectin has specificity. A given lectin activates a considerable proportion of lymphocytes that carry the lectin-binding molecule—namely, all members of a particular subset of lymphocytes in a particular stage of differentiation, regardless of the T-cell receptors these cells carry. In a given T-cell population, about one-third of the cells at any given time are usually at a stage in which they can be activated by a particular lectin. As a result, lectins stimulate many clones of T lymphocytes with different T cell-receptor specificities—they are *polyclonal activators*. What role, if any, lectin stimulation might play in bodily defense is not known. Since certain bacteria and certain parasites carry lectin molecules, it is conceivable that these molecules might, under certain circumstances, contribute to the amplification of T-cell responses; but it is unlikely that lectins play a major role in vertebrate defense.

To activate lymphocytes, one simply adds a lectin in appropriate concentrations to a lymphocyte culture and then measures stimulation by the incorporation of ^{3}H-thymidine into the DNA-synthesizing cells.

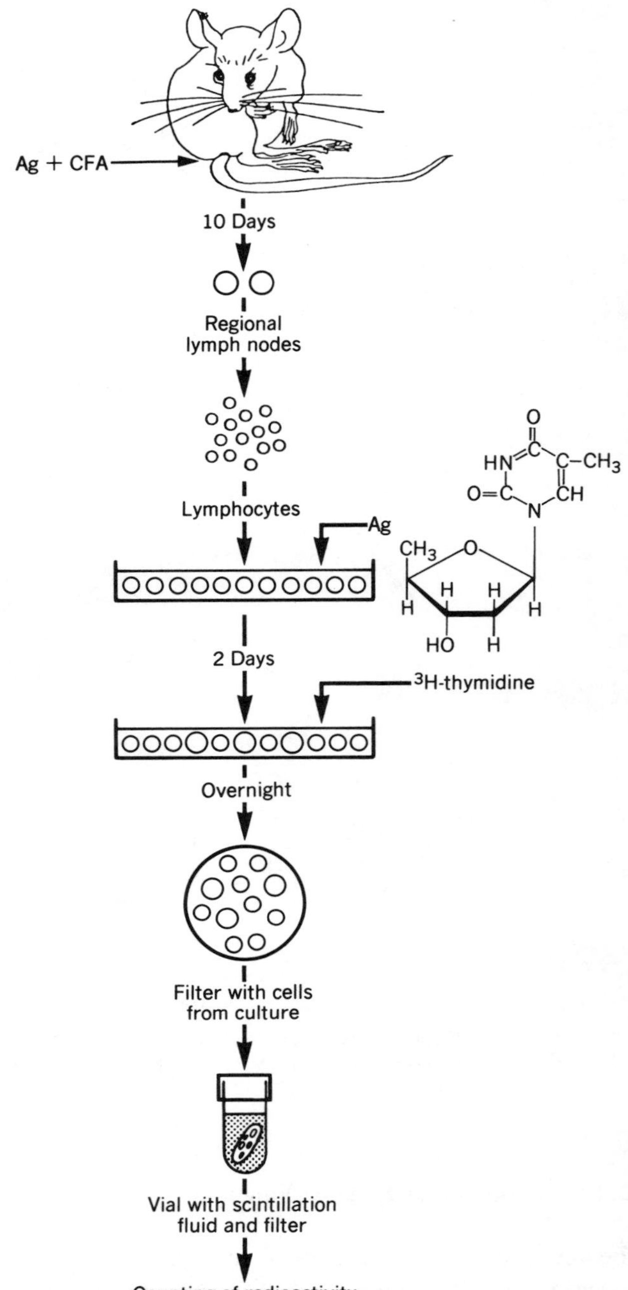

Figure 12.6. An assay for antigen-stimulated proliferation of T lymphocytes in vitro. Ag, antigen; CFA, complete Freund's adjuvant.

12.4 T-CELL PROLIFERATION INDUCED BY SOLUBLE ANTIGENS

In 1963, G. Pearmain and his colleagues reported that lymphocytes of tuberculine-positive individuals transformed in vitro in the presence of purified protein derivative (PPD); no such transformation occurred in cultures of lymphocytes from normal (tuberculine-negative) individuals. Later, other investigators demonstrated that cultured lymphocytes, human or otherwise, can be activated by a variety of antigens, provided the lymphocyte donors have been immunized to these antigens.

The usual protocol used to demonstrate antigen-induced lymphocyte activation in vitro is as follows (Fig. 12.6). The antigen in complete Freund's adjuvant is injected into the animals, and from one to four weeks later, the animals are killed and peritoneal exudate cells or lymph node T lymphocytes are obtained. The cells are cultured together with the antigen for from two to four days; 16 to 24 hours before the termination of the culture, ^{3}H-thymidine is added to it. After harvesting the culture, the cells are washed, collected on a strip of glass filter paper, and dried on a hot plate. Each disc from the strip is then placed in a scintillation vial, scintillation fluid is added, and the amount of radioactivity in the sample is determined by liquid scintillation spectrophotometry. The results are expressed either as an *index* (ratio between the mean counts per minute incorporated in experimental and control cultures—the latter being set up identically to the experimental cultures except for the omission of the antigen) or as *delta values* (the difference between the mean counts per minute of experimental and control cultures).

In vitro responsiveness of lymphocytes to antigens is controlled by class II genes of the major histocompatibility complex. In animals (e.g., the mouse), lymphocytes of certain strains carrying certain class II genes respond readily to a given antigen in culture, while lymphocytes of other strains carrying certain other class II genes are low responders or nonresponders. There is a good correlation between responsiveness to a given antigen as measured by the T-lymphocyte proliferation assay and by antibody detection assays (i.e., responses controlled by the classical *Ir* genes; see Chapter 8). Presumably, the two tests measure principally the same phenomenon—activation of T-helper cells by antigens. In the antibody assay, the helpers instruct B lymphocytes to produce antibodies to a given antigen; in the proliferation assay, it is the entrance of cells into the synthetic phase that signifies activation. The class II gene control of this response probably takes place at the recognition level. The macrophage presumably presents the antigen to the T lymphocyte in the context of class II molecules; if the T cells recognize the particular combination of antigen and class II molecule, they are activated and the strain from which the lymphocytes derive appears as a responder; if, on the other hand, the T cells fail to recognize the particular antigen-class II molecule combination, they fail to be activated and the strain of the T-cell origin appears to be a nonresponder.

12.5 MIXED LYMPHOCYTE REACTION

12.5.1 Discovery; Definition of Basic Terms

In 1961, while trying to find morphological differences between cultured leukocytes from normal and leukemic individuals, R. Schrek and W. J. Donelly observed in one of their five-day-old cultures "a small number of large cells with large clear nuclei and prominent nucleoli"; a few of these cells were in mitosis. The authors noted that the culture was a mixture of blood from two patients, but they failed to follow this hint and so missed discovering the mixed lymphocyte reaction. The discovery was made three years later by two groups of investigators—Barbara Bain and her co-workers, and Fritz H. Bach and Kurt Hirschhorn—who demonstrated in a series of carefully controlled experiments that co-cultivation of leukocytes from unrelated individuals leads to blast transformation and proliferation similar to that observed upon addition of mitogens. Later studies by several laboratories demonstrated that the basis of this reaction was the activation of T cells of one individual by cell-surface molecules of another. Co-culturing of blood leukocytes from two individuals is referred to as *mixed leukocyte culture* (*MLC*) and the reaction as *mixed leukocyte reaction* (*MLR*) or *interaction* (*MLI*); co-culturing of cells obtained from lymphoid organs is designated *mixed lymphocyte culture* or *mixed lymphocyte reaction*. But since even in the mixed leukocyte reaction, the participating cells are peripheral blood T lymphocytes, there is no difference between the two types of culture; in fact, immunologists often use the two terms synonymously and indiscriminately.

In the original experiments of the Bain group and of Bach and Hirschhorn, in which untreated leukocytes of two donors, X and Y, were co-cultured, the X cells responded to molecules on the Y cells and the Y cells responded to molecules on the X cells. In such a culture, referred to as *two-way MLC*, it is impossible to assess the contribution of each of the two cell populations to the reaction and so to study the genetics of the reaction. To avoid mutual responsiveness of the two cell populations, one of the populations must be made unresponsive and the culture turned into *one-way MLC*, in which cells from one donor are the *responders* and cells from the second donor are the *stimulators*. The most common way of making stimulating cells unresponsive to the responding cells is by blocking their ability to synthesize DNA (and thus the ability to transform and proliferate). The blockade can be achieved, for example, by exposing the cells to X-irradiation or by treating them with mitomycin C. The X-irradiation does not kill the cells immediately, but breaks polynucleotide chains in the DNA and thus prevents duplication of the genetic material that is a normal prerequisite for cell division. Mitomycin C, an antibiotic produced by *Streptomyces caespitosus*, crosslinks DNA chains by bonding to two sites, one on each of the complementary strands and so prevents their separation during replication. If stimulating cells are of an F_1 hybrid and the responding cells of P_1 origin (P_1 = one parent of the F_1 hybrid), no treatment is necessary, for the hybrid cells are unable to respond for genetic reasons (see section 12.9).

12.5.2 The Assay

The MLR is a relatively simple test, yet it exists in so many variants that one wonders whether any two laboratories do it the same way. Here are some of the variables: the cultured cells can be derived from peripheral blood, spleen, lymph nodes, or even the thymus; the cell number can vary by several orders of magnitude; the stimulating cells can be inactivated by one of several treatments (see above) and the culture medium can be one of many; the medium can, but need not be supplemented by serum proteins; if serum is added to the culture, it can be of autologous, syngeneic, allogeneic, or xenogeneic origin, and the cultivation can go from four to seven days; the degree of stimulation can be determined from the uptake rate of ^{3}H-thymidine or of radiolabeled amino acids, or by counting blasts and dividing cells; if radiolabel is used, it can be added from four to 24 hours before harvesting the culture; and the variations in terms of culture vessels seem to be unlimited.

In a typical test (if there is such a thing in the MLR)—say, in the mouse—cells are teased out from lymph nodes under aseptic conditions, washed, and divided into two aliquots—responders and stimulators (Fig. 12.7). After X-irradiation of the stimulators, both cell types are suspended in medium supplemented with fetal calf, normal mouse, or human serum (for reasons not completely understood, it is easier to culture lymphocytes in the presence, rather than the absence, of normal serum), and dispensed into wells of tissue culture plates in 0.2-ml aliquots (0.5 × 10^6 viable responding cells and 1 × 10^6 stimulating cells per well), each responder-stimulator combination in triplicate or quadruplicate. The plates are covered with loose-fitting plastic lids that allow gas exchange along the edges and incubated for four days at 37°C in a humidified atmosphere of 5 percent CO_2 and 95 percent air. Twenty-four hours before termination of the culture, ^{3}H-thymidine is added to the cells (2 μCi in about 50 μl solution per well). After the termination of the incubation period (accomplished by transferring the plates to a refrigerator), the cells are aspirated from the wells with a semiautomatic sample collector and dried on filters, and their radioactivity is determined by liquid scintillation spectrophotometry. The incorporation of the label in each culture is expressed as counts per minute, and for each responder-stimulator combination a mean or median value is calculated from replicate determinations. Since even cultures in which no specific MLR has occurred display some "background" radioactivity (resulting from mitogenic effect of the normal serum), the presence of the response must be determined by comparing the average in the experimental (allogeneic, xenogeneic) mixtures (E) with the average of the control (autologous, syngeneic) mixtures (C). The degree of stimulation is expressed either as a Δ value (Δ = E − C) or as stimulation index (SI = E/C).

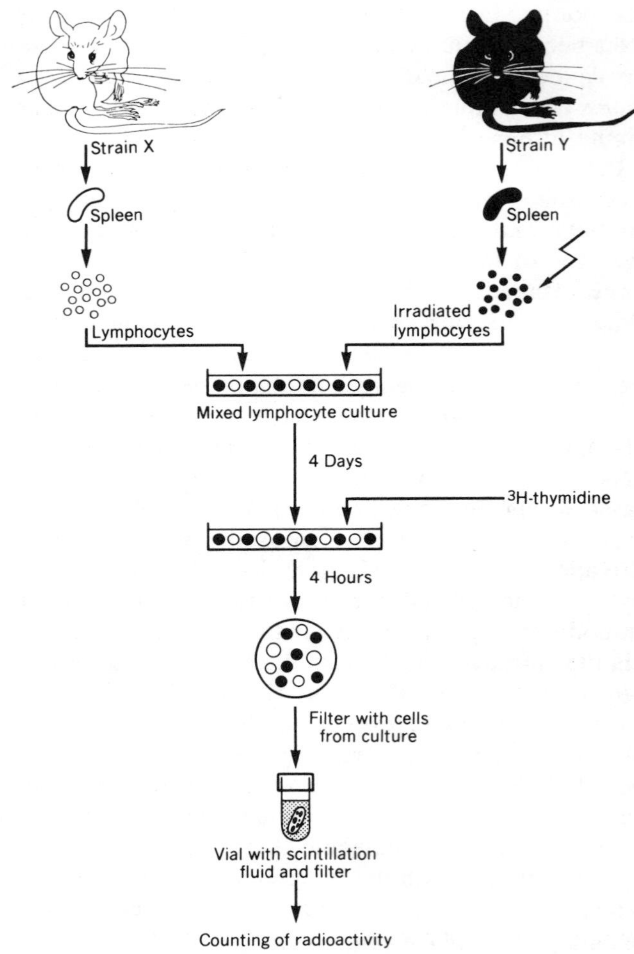

Figure 12.7. An assay for measuring mixed lymphocyte reaction.

12.5.3 Nature of Responding and Stimulating Cells

The majority of the responding cells in the MLR are T lymphocytes; the contribution of other cells to the reaction is not yet fully understood. Macrophages are clearly needed, for the reaction does not occur at all or its strength is sharply reduced when all the "adherent cells" are removed from the mixed culture. What their role in the reaction might be is not clear, but it probably does not require a high degree of specificity, since macrophages derived either from the responding or stimulating animal sustain the reaction. For the same reason, it is also unlikely that macrophages function as antigen-presenting cells in MLR—a function they may perform in other T-cell responses; they probably provide some soluble factors necessary for T-cell activation. B lymphocytes, when present in mixed culture, can also be stimulated to proliferate and may contribute to the mixed lymphocyte reaction. However, the nature of B-cell stimulation is probably different from that of T-cell stimulation. B cells are not stimulated unless T cells are stimulated first, probably because stimulated T lymphocytes must first produce a soluble factor (lymphokine). The factor then provides a second signal to those B cells that have bound, via their Ig receptors, the alloantigen of the stimulating cells. The stimulated B cells then differentiate into plasma cells and secrete antibodies directed against alloantigen. The factor can be produced even by the mitomycin C-treated stimulating cells, which react, despite the block of DNA synthesis, with the responding cells. This *back stimulation* could explain the observation that, in some instances, F_1 hybrid stimulators are—despite the genetic dogma that states they should not be—activated by parental responding cells. (The explanation would be that the responding F_1 cells are B lymphocytes.)

The stimulating cells are primarily B lymphocytes and macrophages or dendritic cells; the role of T lymphocytes in MLC stimulation remains controversial, despite—or perhaps because of—many studies in a number of laboratories. The reason for the controversial nature of these studies is that in those instances in which positive results were obtained, the possibility that the activation was caused by contaminating macrophages could not be completely excluded. However, when one makes a balance sheet of the various pros and cons, one is inclined to accept the stimulating role of certain T cells in certain genetic situations (see below). An MLR stimulatory role has also been claimed for epithelial and some other tissues, but it now appears that the observed stimulation might have been caused by the presence of the macrophagelike Langerhans cells in these tissues.

The stimulating cells must be alive to provide the activating signal; stimulation in *primary* mixed lymphocyte culture does not occur when cells killed by ultraviolet irradiation, cells treated with various inhibitors of RNA and protein synthesis, or cellular fragments are used. Apparently, stimulation depends on certain metabolic activities of the stimulating cells, and when these activities are disturbed, the cells fail to provide the stimulating signal. However, once stimulated, T lymphocytes can be restimulated by metabolically inert cells or cell fragments.

12.5.4 Nature of the Stimulating Molecules

The gist of what we have said about MLR stimulation is that the activation signal is provided by cell-surface molecules of B lymphocytes, macrophages, and probably some T lymphocytes. But what are these mysterious stimulating molecules? The answer to this question is still far from complete. Immunologists generally agree that the major MLR stimulus is provided by class II MHC molecules; the controversy revolves around the role of class I MHC and non-MHC loci in MLR stimulation.

Molecules Controlled by Class II MHC Loci

In 1971, Edmond J. Yunis and D. Bernard Amos, working with human cells, and Fritz H. Bach and his co-workers, working with mouse cells, demonstrated that, contrary to expectations, strong MLR occurred even in mixtures in which the responding and stimulating cells shared class I loci. This observation suggested that the MLR was governed by loci separate from class I loci, previously shown to play a major role in graft rejection. Several investigators then mapped the MLR-stimulating loci outside the *A* and *B* loci in the human and between the *K* and *D* loci in the mouse—in the region where the serologically detectable class II loci map.

The Human. Three main approaches are used in detecting MLR-stimulating determinants in humans. In the first approach, *direct MLR typing*, unrelated individuals phenotypically identical in their class I loci are selected and mixed cultures are set up between these individuals in all possible combinations. Absence of MLR between any two individuals is taken as evidence that they are identical at the MHC *D* locus, coding for the MLR-stimulating molecule; occurrence of MLR, on the other hand, suggests that the two individuals differ in determinants responsible for MLR induction. By comparing different responder-stimulator combinations, one can identify individual *D*-locus determinants and assign numbers to them.

In the second approach, based on the use of the so-called *homozygous typing cells*, one finds a family in which the parents share one *HLA* haplotype (the identity is determined by serological typing for class I antigens but the assumption is that it also extends to the *D*-locus determinants). One then types all members of the family for MLR in all possible combinations and searches for a child who neither stimulates nor is stimulated by cells of the parents. As Figure 12.8 shows, this child is a *D*-locus homozygote and hence can be used as a source of homozygous typing cells for testing unrelated individuals. The possible results of such a testing are these:

Responder	Stimulator	Result
D^3/D^4	D^1/D^1	+
D^1/D^3	D^1/D^1	–

where D^1, D^3, and D^4 are different *D*-locus alleles. Hence, whenever a given responder shares at least one

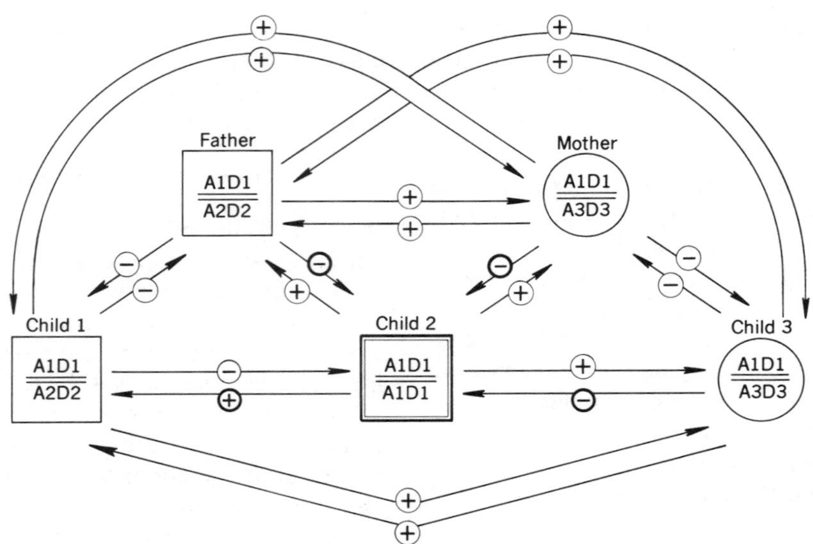

Figure 12.8. The principle of the homozygous typing cell test. The arrows indicate the direction of response (responder at the base, stimulator at the arrowhead). +, Positive mixed lymphocyte reaction; −, negative MLR; A1, A2, and A3, alleles at class I loci; D1, D2, and D3, alleles at class II loci of the human major histocompatibility complex (*HLA*).

D allele with the stimulator (i.e., with the homozygous typing cells), its cells fail to respond in MLR.

In reality, however, the human MLRs are rarely totally negative and so a distinction must be made arbitrarily between *weak* or *typing responses* and *strong responses*. It is the typing response that is considered to be an indication of *D*-allele sharing between responder and homozygous typing cells.

The third approach, the *primed lymphocyte typing test*, is based on somewhat different principles, which will be considered below. The combination of MLR typing methods has led to the identification of 11 *D*-locus determinants (see Table 8.8).

The Mouse. MLR studies with intra-*H*-2 recombinants demonstrated that, in the mouse, the most strongly stimulating molecules are controlled by the *A* loci (probably mostly A_β) and the less strongly stimulating by the *E* loci (again, mostly by E_β). While the *A*-locus determinants are expressed predominantly on B lymphocytes and macrophages, there is some evidence that at least some of the E determinants might be present on thymocytes. No designations have yet been given to the mouse MLR determinants.

In both human and mouse the loci coding for MLR-stimulating determinants map in the vicinity of class II loci coding for serologically detectable determinants. The question of the genetic relationship between the two types of locus is now finally, after a long debate, resolved: the serologically detectable molecules are the MLR stimulators.

Molecules Controlled by Class I Loci

Some immunologists deny an MLR stimulatory role for class I molecules in both the human and the mouse. However, studies with *H*-2 mutants clearly indicate that molecules controlled by the mouse class I molecules can, in some instances, induce MLR. This class I-induced reaction is often weaker than the class II-induced MLR, and in some combinations might be absent altogether. In humans, where *HLA* mutations have not yet been detected and where one usually works in situations that are genetically not very precisely defined, evidence for an MLR role of class I loci has not yet been reported.

Molecules Controlled by Non-MHC Loci

The mouse genome contains, in addition to the MHC, one other locus—the mixed lymphocyte-stimulating, or *Mls* locus—which is clearly involved in the control of MLR. The *Mls* locus, discovered in 1966 by Hilliard Festenstein, is on chromosome 1, closely linked to the *LyM*-1 locus coding for serologically detectable, B cell-restricted alloantigen. (There is some uncertainty as to the relationship of the two loci, but the latest evidence indicates that they are probably separate.)

Table 12.1 Alleles at the *Mls* Locus

Allele	Inbred Strain	Strength of MLR Stimulation
a	AKR, CBA/J, DBA/2	++
b	BALB/c, C57BL/6, C57BR, DBA/1, 129	+
c	A, CE, C3H/An, C3H/He, RF, SJL	−

Source. Based primarily on the work of H. Festenstein and his colleagues.

The *Mls* locus has four alleles (Mls^a through Mls^d) and when some of these are paired, strong MLR results (Table 12.1). The *Mls* determinants are expressed predominantly or exclusively on B lymphocytes.

Some investigators have reported that, in addition to the *Mls* locus, other non-MHC loci, particularly some minor *H* loci (see section 12.9), are also active in primary MLR. Other investigators have been unable to demonstrate any MLR outside the MHC and *Mls* loci.

12.5.5 Secondary MLR

Before 1974, lymphocytes could not be maintained in culture for more than about a week, after which rapid deterioration and cell death set in. In 1974, Leif C. Andersson and Pekka Häyry improved the culture conditions and extended the growth period of lymphocytes in vitro to about three weeks. They observed that after the first week, the blasts began to disappear from the culture and were replaced by small cells. But after three weeks even in these improved culture conditions, lymphocytes started to deteriorate unless restimulated. When fresh stimulating cells were added to the culture, the lymphocytes underwent a new burst of activity, more rapid than that following the first stimulation: the number of blasts in this *secondary MLC* peaked at about three days after restimulation, instead of the usual four days in the primary MLR. Furthermore, in the secondary MLR more than 90 percent of the cells remaining from the primary MLC transformed into blasts (in contrast to only about 5 percent of transformed cells in the primary culture). Apparently, during the prolonged cultivation, only the stimulated lymphocytes survived and the unstimulated ones died out. The restimulation can be repeated over and over and a series of consecutive peaks of blast transformation obtained. Andersson and Häyry started their experiment in January and carried the cultures through some 30 blast transformation cycles until June, when they went on summer vacation.

When the restimulation is discontinued, the cultured lymphocytes die after about three weeks; the culture conditions are simply not congenial for the quiescent (resting) lymphocytes. However, the lymphocytes can be injected into syngeneic T cell-deprived hosts and then recalled on demand at any time thereafter. Immunologists refer to this procedure as *parking*—since they use the lymphocytes as a car that can be parked and then started again. Parked lymphocytes have been maintained in vivo for 20 weeks (longer periods have not been attempted), but during this time, the lymphocytes gradually lost their memory characteristics (capability to respond promptly in secondary MLC).

The secondary MLR is the basis for one of the tests that define MLR-stimulating determinants in humans. In this *primed lymphocyte typing* or *PLT test*, family members are HLA-typed and pairs sharing one *HLA* haplotype are selected (usually a parent-child combination). In each pair one member is taken as a responder and the other as a stimulator, primary MLR is induced, and the activated responding cells are aliquoted and frozen; some stimulating cells are also frozen. At the time of typing, the frozen responding cells are thawed and restimulated in the secondary MLR by a panel of cells from unrelated individuals, as well as by the original stimulating cells. Individuals whose cells restimulate the PLT cells as strongly as the original stimulators are presumed to share MLR-stimulating determinants with the stimulating cells; individuals whose cells cause weaker reactions (most individuals cause some reactions) are thought to lack this determinant.

12.5.6 Interpretation

To sum up, the MLR is a response of T lymphocytes to alloantigens controlled largely by Class II MHC loci and, to a lesser degree, by Class I and some non-MHC loci. Although some Lyt-1^+Lyt-2^+ cells, if present, respond in the MLC, the majority of the responding cells are of the Lyt-1^+Lyt-2^- category—the helper cells. The stimulated cells transform into blasts, proliferate, presumably with the help of macrophages or macrophage-produced factors, secrete soluble mediators into the medium, and then transform back into small lymphocytes. The major unresolved question is the nature of the alloantigen-recognizing receptor. No one has isolated this receptor, so nothing is known about its chemical nature or physiological function. There are three main possible models of receptor function. First, the receptors are, even under physiological conditions, directed against alloantigens, and as such are distinct from receptors for other antigens. T cells thus possess two kinds of receptor, one for MHC alloantigens and the second for all other antigens. The second possibility is that the receptor used by the MLR responding cells for the recognition of alloantigens is, in fact, the receptor that the cells normally use for the recognition of other antigens. The repertoire of these receptors is so broad that it covers practically all antigens, including those controlled by the MHC. The third possibility is a kind of compromise between the first and second. The T-cell receptor may be constructed so that it normally recognizes two things—self and nonself. In a physiological situation it recognizes antigens as nonself and the individual's own MHC molecules as self. In the MLC it recognizes determinants differentiating the two individuals as nonself and the shared determinants as self. In other words, it treats the allogeneic determinants as other antigens and the shared determinants as self, so that the only difference from physiological recognition is that in MLR, self and nonself happen to be on the same molecule.

12.6 CELL-MEDIATED LYMPHOLYSIS

12.6.1 Discovery

In 1960, A. Govaerts described an experiment in which he transplanted a kidney from dog X to dog Y (Fig. 12.9). When the kidney was rejected, he obtained thoracic duct lymphocytes from the recipient and added them to a culture of kidney (epithelial) cells donated by dog X. He observed that within 48 hours after the addition of lymphocytes, lesions began to appear in the monolayer of kidney cells: the lymphocytes killed the epithelial cells of the kidney.

This experiment was one of the first direct demonstrations of lymphocytes' turning into killer cells and attacking targets against which they were sensitized. Govaert's procedure, in which lymphocytes are sensitized in vivo and their killing effect tested in vitro, was then adapted and worked out by several other investigators, in particular by K. Theodor Brunner, Jean-Charles Cerrotini, and Boris D. Brondz. The former two investigators made two important improvements in the assay: they used tumor cells as targets for cytotoxic lymphocytes (one of these tumors, a mastocytoma P815 derived from a DBA/2 mouse, proved a particularly superior target and is still used in many laboratories), and they adapted the ^{51}Cr-labeling technique to the study of target cell destruction. In this technique, radioactive chromium is bound to the cytoplasm of the target cells following the addition of sodium chromate to the cell suspension, and it is released only when the cells die and the cytoplasm leaks out.

In 1965, Haim Ginsburg and Leo Sachs took the first step toward transferring the killer cell assay completely into culture. They demonstrated that normal rat lymphocytes cultured on a monolayer of mouse embryo fibroblasts transformed into blasts, which then lysed target cells of the monolayer. However, a real breakthrough occurred in 1970, when two groups of investigators—Pekka Häyry and Vittorio Defendi, and Richard J. Hodes and Erik A. J. Svedmyr, working independently—demonstrated that cytotoxic lymphocytes capable of lysing tumor cell targets arise in mixed lymphocyte culture. This observation made it possible to carry out the test under controlled, in vitro conditions. One difficulty, however, remained: there were only a few suitable target cell types. Many different cells, including normal lymphocytes, could be labeled with ^{51}Cr, but the release of radioactive chromium in the experimental combinations was usually only slightly higher than that in the control combination. In 1971, James Lightbody and his collaborators resolved this difficulty when they discovered that

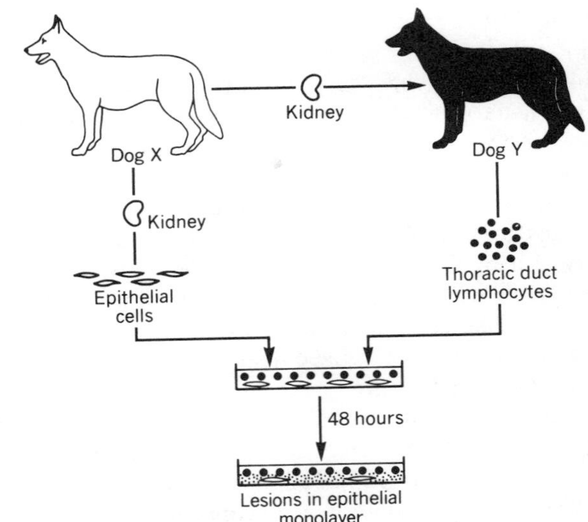

Figure 12.9. Govaert's experiment demonstrating the generation of cytotoxic lymphocytes in dogs transplanted with allogeneic kidneys.

mitogen-stimulated blasts, labeled well with ^{51}Cr, displayed a relatively low spontaneous release of radioactivity, and were highly susceptible to specific lysis by cytotoxic cells. (To this day it is not entirely clear why normal lymphocytes are such poor targets and blasts such superior ones for the cytotoxic lymphocytes.) Thus, in 1971 a rapid and reasonably simple technique became available for the production and testing of cytotoxic lymphocytes: the cells were produced in mixed lymphocyte culture, mitogen-stimulated blasts were used as targets, and killing was measured by the release of radioactive chromium from the labeled cells. This technique, usually referred to as the *cell-mediated lympholysis* or *cell-mediated lymphocytotoxicity* (*CML*) *assay*, is now used routinely by many laboratories.

In the original CML assay, the targets of the lymphocyte attack were MHC molecules of the target cell. Immunologists, however, gradually realized that CML can occur against many other molecules that are either naturally integrated into the cell membrane (e.g., minor histocompatibility antigens, tumor-specific antigens, or virus-specific antigens) or artificially attached to the membrane by chemical means (e.g., haptens). These studies culminated in 1974 and 1975, when Rolf M. Zinkernagel, Peter C. Doherty, Michael J. Bevan, Gene M. Shearer, Elizabeth Simpson, and their coworkers demonstrated that CML to non-MHC molecules was restricted by the MHC (in other words, that the minor H antigens, tumor-specific antigens, virus-specific antigens, and haptens were recognized in the CML in the context of the MHC molecules on the presenting cell). There are thus two principal kinds of CML—that directed against allogeneic MHC molecules and not restricted by any other molecules, and that directed against non-MHC molecules but restricted by the MHC. We shall refer to the two types as *nonrestricted* and *restricted*, respectively.

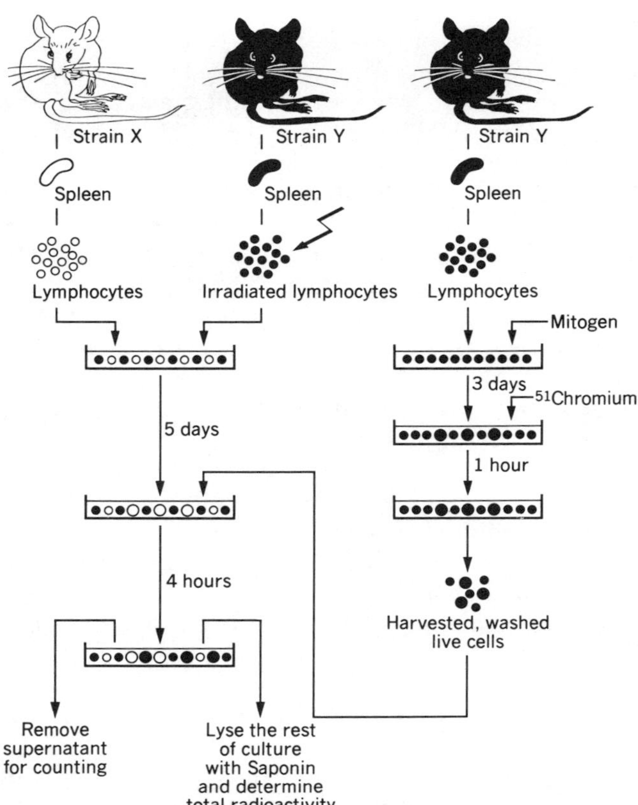

Figure 12.10. The principle of the cell-mediated lymphocytotoxicity (CML) assay.

12.6.2 The Assay

CML to MHC Molecules (Nonrestricted CML)

In the standard CML assay (Fig. 12.10), lymphocytes are incubated for 70 to 90 hours in a one-way mixed culture, and at the end of the incubation period the surviving activated cells are added to target cells, which are lymphocytes cultured for three days in the presence of PHA or Con A and labeled with ^{51}Cr. After four hours' incubation at 37°C, the cultures are centrifuged and the amount of radioactivity released in the supernatant is determined. The results are expressed in counts per minute (cpm) per culture, as a percentage of release, or as a percentage of specific ^{51}Cr release calculated from the formula

$$\frac{\text{release with sensitized lymphocytes} - \text{spontaneous release}}{\text{maximum release} - \text{spontaneous release}}$$

where maximum release is obtained after nonspecific lysis of control cells by detergent.

CML to Non-MHC Molecules (Restricted CML)

Of the large variety of CML assay systems for non-MHC cell-surface molecules, we shall give only one example—that used for the detection of antigens encoded by lymphocytic choriomeningitis (LCM) virus.

The Pathogenesis of LCM. The virus is transmitted through the fetus and persists in the tissues of adult mice, usually without causing disease. However, fatal disease (lymphocytic choriomeningitis) can be induced artificially by injecting the virus into the brains of adult mice. The injected mice show signs of severe neurological impairment from six to eight days after inoculation and die with characteristic convulsions. Death coincides with severe inflammation of the meninges (meningitis) and cellular infiltration of the choroid plexus and ependyma.

The exact pathophysiology of the disease is not known. According to one hypothesis, the virus infects the cells lining the brain and spinal cavities (the ependyma, meninges, and choroid plexus epithelium) and the cells then express viral antigens on their surfaces. The antigens sensitize cytotoxic T cells, which then attack the lining cells, reducing the integrity of the blood-brain barrier and increasing the flow of serum proteins into the tissues surrounding the brain. The overall effect of the increased extracellular protein in the brain is osmotic imbalance, resulting in decreased resorption of fluid by capillaries, swelling of nervous tissues, acute brain edema, characteristic convulsive seizures, and death. Thus, in this particular case, the defensive action of T cells is detrimental, rather than beneficial to the host.

Detection of LCM-Specific Antigens. The assay (see Fig. 7.5) consists of inoculating the LCM virus into the brains of the recipient mice, killing the mice seven days after the inoculation, removing the spleens, plating the spleen cells on a monolayer of ^{51}Cr-labeled, LCM virus-infected fibroblasts or macrophages, and measuring the release of cytoplasmic radioactivity. Thus, in this system sensitized lymphocytes are generated in vivo and tested in vitro—and this arrangement is also used in most of the other CML systems that detect non-MHC antigenic differences.

12.6.3 Kinetics

The kinetics of CML is determined primarily by the ratio of *effector cells* (i.e., cells that actually carry out the killing) to target cells. Measurable cytotoxicity is usually obtained only with an excess of effector cells over target cells, possibly because not all the cells in the effector-cell suspension are killers. Cytolysis requires direct cell-to-cell contact: target cells separated from effector cells by a Millipore membrane are not killed. The killing process, therefore, does not seem to be mediated by any diffuse, long-range, soluble substances such as lymphotoxins. Lysis starts immediately after contact between effector and target cells is established, and is based on single-hit kinetics (a single contact between an effector and a target cell is sufficient to kill the latter). Most investigators agree that effector cells are not damaged extensively during the interaction with target cells, although claims to the contrary have been made. One effector cell is able to kill more than one target cell. The lytic process proceeds in two steps: in the first, specific interaction between determinants on effector and target cells occurs; in the second, nonspecific lytic reaction is activated. The first, but not the second step is energy-dependent.

12.6.4 Generation of Cytotoxic Cells

In the mouse, the cell carrying out lympholysis is of the Lyt-1$^-$Lyt-2$^+$ type, but Lyt-1$^+$Lyt-2$^+$ and Lyt-1$^+$Lyt-2$^-$ cells may also participate in target cell killing in some situations. Binding of an antigen via a specific receptor activates the Lyt-1$^-$Lyt-2$^+$ cells but does not convert them into killers; for that to occur, a second, nonspecific signal is necessary. In the culture, the nonspecific signal can be provided by one of the following sources: by mitogens contained in the fetal calf serum supplementing the culture medium; by stimulated Lyt-1$^+$Lyt-2$^-$ cells, which proliferate in the culture together with Lyt-1$^-$Lyt-2$^+$ cells and secrete a soluble factor (interleukine-2) into the medium; and by interleukine-2, produced in another culture and added secondarily to the CML culture. In the last instance, the interleukine-2 can be produced by the proliferation of T helper cells as a consequence of either mitogen or alloantigen stimulation; factors produced in these two types of culture are interchangeable and probably identical. For proliferation, the helper cells themselves require a second signal in the form of a soluble factor, interleukine-1, produced by macrophages.

In a physiological in vivo situation, the sequence of events leading to generation of cytotoxic lymphocytes can be envisioned as follows (Fig. 12.11): an antigen is picked up by a macrophage and the macrophage is stimulated to produce interleukine-1; the factor acts on an antigen-stimulated Lyt-1$^+$Lyt-2$^-$ T helper cell, enticing it to proliferate and produce interleukine-2; this second factor acts on antigen-stimulated Lyt-1$^-$Lyt-2$^+$ cells and converts them into cytotoxic cells. In the in vitro situation, cytotoxic cell generation can be initiated at different points of the sequence, depending on the culture conditions.

The changes a precursor lymphocyte undergoes to become a killer cell are not known. It almost certainly passes through a stage of blast transformation and proliferation but the extent of proliferation has not been determined. How the cell kills its target is not known either. It seems to give the target a mere "kiss of death," triggering a sequence of events in which its own participation is no longer necessary. In contrast to the complement system, in which the membrane-attack complex is assembled on the membrane from components in the serum, the lytic mechanism in the CML is

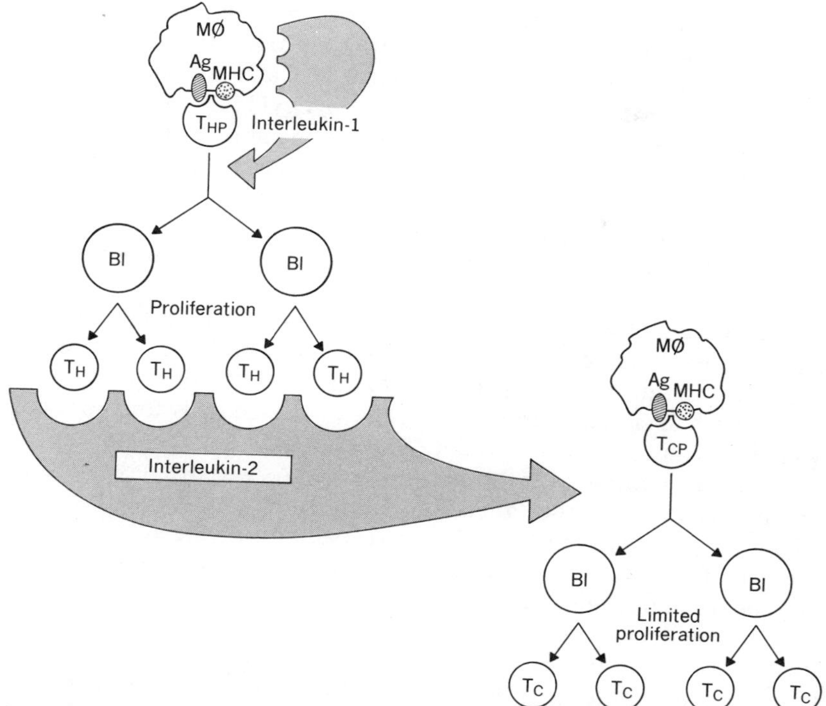

Figure 12.11. Cellular interactions leading to the generation of cytotoxic T lymphocytes. Ag, antigen; Bl, blast cells; MHC, major histocompatibility complex molecules; MØ, macrophagelike cell; T_C, cytotoxic T cells; T_{CP}, precursor of cytotoxic T cell; T_{HP}, precursor of T helper cell; T_H, T helper cell.

apparently built into the membrane; all the cytotoxic cell does is activate it. The participation of MHC molecules in the lytic process is possible, but apparently not necessary: cytotoxic cells can lyse any cell, regardless of which MHC molecules they carry, in a totally nonspecific way if they are "glued" to their targets by lectins, such as concanavalin A or PHA. But mere contact between cytotoxic and target cells does not suffice for the induction of the lytic process since some lectins agglutinate the two types of cell without causing lysis. Several lytic mechanisms have been postulated, of which three examples follow.

The adhesion of cytotoxic lymphocytes to target cells induces local changes in the target cell membrane, which result in leakage of intracellular K^+, influx of Na^+ and water, and thus cell lysis.

The adhesion of cytotoxic and target cells causes tangential shear forces on the target cell membrane similar to those implicated in laser beam-induced hemolysis.

The attachment of the cytotoxic cell activates a target cell membrane enzyme, phospholipase A (see Chapter 13), which converts membrane lecithin into lysolecithin and free fatty acids; lysolecithin is a strong detergent and potent cytolytic agent.

Other hypotheses exist and there are pros and cons to each of them. Their diversity is a witness to our ignorance and to the sparsity of experimental data that would set limits on speculation. An interesting but unresolved question is why the cytotoxic cells themselves are not killed during the triggering of the lytic process. Cytotoxic cells are not resistant to lysis, as is evidenced by the fact that another set of cytotoxic cells can be generated against them; but when attacking their targets, they are somehow protected from self-destruction.

12.6.5 Nature of the First Signal

In MHC-induced (unrestricted) CML, both class I and class II molecules can initiate lymphocyte differentiation into cytotoxic cells. Class I molecules induce CML more easily than class II molecules; in fact, immunologists erroneously believed for some time that only class I molecules could initiate cytotoxic cell differentiation. In the mouse, CML-inducing molecules are encoded by all three known class I loci (K, D, and L), at least two class II loci (A_α and E_β), and at least two *Qa* loci (*Qa*-1 and *Qa*-2). The involvement of *Qa* in CML induction underscores the relatedness of these loci to the MHC. Why class I loci are better inducers of CML than class II loci is not known.

In situations in which the stimulating and responding cells differ in both the class I and class II loci, cooperation in CML induction often occurs between the two. Class II molecules provide a strong proliferative stimulus; the proliferating T helper cells produce interleukine-2, which then acts on cytotoxic T cells stimulated by class I molecules. In this manner, class II molecules amplify the response to class I molecules nonspecifically. This cooperation is often seen in suboptimal cultures in which the medium itself (or rather, the fetal calf serum) fails to provide the nonspecific proliferative stimulus for the T helper cells. However, simultaneous disparity at class I and class II loci is not an absolute requirement for the generation of cytotoxic cells; in good culture conditions, the difference at class I loci suffices to generate a strong allogeneic CML.

There has been a protracted debate among immunologists concerning the relationship of the loci coding for the CML-activating molecules and loci coding for the serologically detectable class I and class II molecules. This controversy is now resolved: the experimental data support the conclusion that the two types of locus are identical. Hence, the same class I or class II molecules can activate both B and T lymphocytes; the activated B cells secrete antibodies that can be used in serological definition of the MHC molecules; the activated T lymphocytes differentiate into killer cells detectable by the CML (and MLR) assay. What still remains controversial is what parts of the class I and class II molecules the B and T cells recognize. We know from Chapter 8 that antibodies identify several determinants on each MHC molecule. Studies with *H*-2 mutants demonstrate that an analogous dissection of the class I molecule into a series of determinants can also be achieved by using cytotoxic cells instead of antibodies, and that one can construct a determinant chart resembling the serologically defined *H*-2 chart. The question is: are the determinants defined by serological methods and those by CML methods the same? Here the same arguments used in the discussion of the relationship between T cell-defined and B cell-defined determinants in general (see Chapter 7) apply. A sensible interpretation seems to be that some of the determinants may overlap, while others may prove to be distinct.

In the CML induced by non-MHC molecules (restricted CML) the inducing molecules can vary from simple haptens to complex membrane glycoproteins. What makes a molecule a suitable CML inducer (and target) is, again, not known. Perhaps the stimulating capacity depends on the molecule's ability to be "seen" by T lymphocytes in the company of the restricting MHC molecule. Molecules that restrict this form of CML are all encoded by class I loci; no convincing evidence has yet been obtained for CML-restricting ability of class II loci. But CML to these is not restricted by class I loci, and class II loci play a restricting role in helper cell function.

12.6.6 Nature of the Receptor

Cytotoxic T cells probably use the same receptor for MHC recognition as the responding cells use in the MLR. The relationship of this receptor to that used by the cytotoxic cells for the recognition of conventional (non-MHC) antigens in the restricted CML is not known. As was discussed in Chapter 7, two views have been put forward regarding the nature of target cell recognition in the restricted CML. According to the *altered-self hypothesis*, one receptor recognizes the conventional antigen and the MHC molecule simultaneously; according to the *dual-recognition hypothesis*, there are separate receptors for conventional antigens and for MHC molecules (see Fig. 7.7).

Whatever the nature of the cytotoxic T-cell receptor, there is clear evidence that it is distributed clonally. For example, when one plates cytotoxic lymphocytes on a monolayer of target cells, the activated cells attach transiently but specifically to these targets and remain in the culture dish after the decantation of the nonattached cells. One can then demonstrate that the suspension of nonattached cells no longer reacts with the particular targets but that it can still be activated against a third strain, unrelated to the original targets. On the other hand, cells mechanically detached from the monolayer kill target cells carrying the same MHC as the target but do not kill third-party cells. The conclusion from this experiment is that the suspension of cytotoxic lymphocytes contains clones of cells specific for the particular target but unable to recognize target cells carrying other MHC molecules.

12.6.7 Secondary CML and Cytotoxic Cell Lines

The cytotoxic activity of a primary mixed lymphocyte culture peaks five to seven days after the culture's initiation, declines thereafter, and disappears completely at about day 10. However, when such a culture is maintained for two to three weeks, its cytotoxic activity can be recalled by the addition of appropriate allogeneic cells. In this *secondary CML*, the cytotoxic activity peaks at about day three after the addition of allogeneic cells—a day or two earlier than in the primary CML. Third and fourth additions of allogeneic cells result in tertiary and quarternary CML, in which the activity appears even more promptly than in the secondary CML and which shows lower target-to-effector cell ratios than in the primary CML. But after the fifth and subsequent stimulations, cytotoxic activity gradually disappears; the lymphocytes respond by blast transformation but cytotoxic cells are no longer generated. Secondary cytotoxic activity can also be recalled nonspecifically with T-cell mitogens or with culture supernatants from secondary mixed lymphocyte cultures.

The secondary and tertiary cultures contain a mixture of T-cell clones directed against different determinants and different MHC molecules. To study the T cell's behavior, it is advantageous to work with pure *T-cell clones* consisting of cells that presumably express the same receptors. T-cell clones can be obtained in one of two principal ways. In the first method, one induces primary CML, leaves the cells in culture for two or three weeks, and then restimulates them once or twice with allogeneic cells. After the second restimulation, one grows the cells in a medium containing interleukine-2 (T-cell growth factor). The cells remain in the blast stage and proliferate, and so can be propagated over long periods. However, the culture is still a mixture of many clones. To separate them one uses the so-called *limiting dilution technique*, in which one serially dilutes a cell suspension in a row of test tubes or wells of a culture plate until one reaches an average concentration of one cell per well *or less* (the dilution becomes a limiting factor). At limiting dilution many of the tubes or wells will contain no cells at all, but those that do contain cells will have no more than one cell per tube (well). This procedure is the next best thing to actually dispensing single cells into tubes—a tedious and technically difficult undertaking. From the Poisson distribution one can determine that the suspension must be diluted so that it will give, on the average, 0.33 cells per well. At this low concentration, lymphocytes do not grow without other cells—the so-called *feeder cells*—present. For the lymphocyte cloning purpose, the feeders are usually peritoneal exudate cells, X-irradiated to prevent their own proliferation. When grown in the presence of interleukine-2, the clones retain the capability of growing over an extended period and of remaining cytotoxic.

In the second cloning method, one grows a monolayer of feeder cells on the bottom of a culture dish, X-irradiates the cells, overlays them with a highly concentrated (dense) agar solution containing tissue culture medium and interleukine-2, and pours another layer of less concentrated (soft) agar containing the cytotoxic cells on top. The density of cells in the top agar layer is such that the individual cells are clearly separated from one another. When these cells divide, they stay together and form a colony visible with the help of a microscope. One can then pick up individual colonies in a Pasteur pipette, transfer each separately into a liquid medium with interleukine-2, and culture them as individual clones.

12.7 DELAYED-TYPE HYPERSENSITIVITY

The T-cell responses discussed so far were based on in vitro assays. Although parts of the assays could be carried out in vivo, the actual response was measured in tissue culture. In the following sections we shall deal with T-cell responses that are measured in vivo. The first of these is delayed-type hypersensitivity (DTH).

12.7.1 Discovery and Definition

Although the discovery of DTH is usually attributed to Robert Koch (see Chapter 2), the first description of this phenomenon can be found in Edward Jenner's *Inquiry*, published in 1798. Jenner observed that persons inoculated with cowpox for the second time or persons who had had smallpox before, developed a red, indurated, painful swelling at the inoculation site in the skin, reaching a maximum at 24 to 72 hours and then disappearing without passing through the pustular stage. Robert Koch observed a similar phenomenon in 1890 after he injected tuberculin subcutaneously into persons with tuberculosis; normal persons gave no reaction, even after the injection of 10 times greater doses of tuberculin than that injected into tuberculous patients. This *tuberculin reaction* became a standard diagnostic test for tuberculosis. Later, other microbiologists demonstrated a similar reaction to culture fluids from bacteria other than *Mycobacterium tuberculosis*—*Salmonella typhi*, *Brucella abortus*, and *Pfefferella mallei*—and to proteins of nonbacterial origin (e.g., eggwhite or horse serum albumin). In all these instances, the course of the reaction was principally the same. The first exposure of a patient or animal to a given microorganism or to a nonbacterial protein produced no visible change, but the immune status of the recipient was clearly altered. The sign of this alteration was the fact that the recipient reacted differently to a second injection of the same antigen than it had to the first one. The first injection makes the animal hypersensitive to renewed antigen exposure; the major sign of this condition is the development of a characteristic skin lesion at the injection site—a lesion not seen after the first antigen exposure. Since the response to the second antigen inoculum is delayed by 24 to 48 hours, the reaction is referred to as *delayed-type hypersensitivity* (DTH). The adjective "delayed" was originally used to distinguish this type of reaction from immediate hypersensitivity, in which the response occurs within minutes (rather than hours) of the injection (see Chapter 13). Both types of reaction, however, were believed to have enough properties in common to group them in a single category of hypersensitivities. Only later did immunologists realize that the two reactions occurred by different mechanisms. But by then the two terms were so entrenched in immunological literature that it was too late to change them. When using this term, however, one must keep in mind its historical connotation: DTH is nothing more than a second-set (anamnestic) reaction, which, like other secondary reactions, has a time course and other characteristics different from the primary response. The characteristic manifestations of this particular form of second-set response (skin lesions) are the result of the particular way antigen is brought in contact with the sensitizing cell (in the skin) and the type of cells involved in the reaction. In the following paragraphs we shall learn that DTH is a T-cell response that differs from other such responses only in the specifics of its manifestation.

12.7.2 Methods of Detection

DTH reactions can occur only in an individual previously exposed (sensitized) to a given antigen. In humans, this sensitizing antigen derives from the microorganisms responsible for the disease (e.g., tuberculin from *Mycobacterium tuberculosis*, typhoidin from *Salmonella typhi*, and abortin from *Brucella abortus*), and sensitization occurs as a result of a chronic infection. In animals, sensitization is achieved by the injection of a given antigen emulsified in complete Freund's adjuvant into the skin. In both humans and animals, hypersensitivity is tested by the injection of the antigen dissolved in physiological salt solution into the skin (either intradermally or subcutaneously). In the guinea pig, a favorite experimental animal in DTH research, one tests the reaction as follows: one shaves or uses a depilatory on the area to be injected and injects the antigen in 0.1 ml volumes intradermally. One then periodically measures the thickness of the skin fold at the injection site with calipers and compares it with that of another site injected with physiological salt solution. Thickening of the antigen-injected site in comparison with the control site is taken as evidence of DTH reaction.

The mouse and rat have a peculiar skin structure (see below) that makes measurement of DTH reaction of the flank difficult. In these species, therefore, one injects the test antigen into one footpad and, using calipers, measures its thickening in comparison with another footpad injected with physiological salt solution. Or one injects the antigen into the skin of one ear (pinna) and physiological salt solution into the other ear, injects the animals intraperitoneally with radioactively labeled ^{125}I-deoxyuridine, kills the mice 24 hours later, cuts off the ears, determines their radioactivity, and expresses the results as the ratio of radioactivity in the antigen-injected ear to that in the control ear. This test is based on the observation that during the DTH reaction, replicating cells (labeled by the incorporation of deoxyuridine into DNA) from the blood stream infiltrate the site of antigen deposit (see below).

Important information about the mechanism of DTH can be gained by the transfer of the reaction from sensitized to normal individuals. To this end, one removes lymph node, spleen, or thoracic duct cells from the sensitized recipient about a week after sensitization and injects them intravenously into an unsensitized individual, preferably of the same strain as the first recipient. One then challenges the second recipient with an intradermal injection of the antigen about 24 hours after the transfer.

Although the sensitization for DTH is always done in vivo, the actual testing of the reaction can be carried out in vitro. One in vitro test is based on the observation that DTH effector cells produce factors, such as lymphotoxin, which kill innocent bystander cells (i.e., cells that happen to be within the factor's action range; see below). In this test, lymphocytes removed from mice one week after the sensitization are added, together with antigen, to a culture of target fibroblasts. After 72 hours of incubation—the time needed for the release of the factor by the lymphocytes and killing of the fibroblasts—target cell survival is compared with that of a control culture. Another test measures the production of macrophage-inhibiting factor, using an assay system described in Chapter 7. Still another in vitro test for DTH is the T-cell proliferation assay that is based on the finding that T cells derived from sensitized animals and cultured with the sensitizing antigen undergo a burst of proliferative activity at which time they incorporate labeled precursors into their replicating DNA. We described this assay in section 12.4. (You may recall that the assay was first used with cells obtained from tuberculous patients and with tuberculin as the stimulating antigen.)

12.7.3 Conditions for DTH Induction and Detection

DTH can be induced by a wide variety of natural and synthetic proteins; firm evidence for DTH induction by other substances is not available. Claims of DTH elicited by polysaccharide injection have been made, but in none of these experiments has the presence of contaminating proteins been rigorously excluded, and whenever a pure polysaccharide was used, no DTH could be obtained. Synthetic polypeptides containing L-amino acids (optical isomers present in natural proteins) do induce DTH, whereas those composed of D-amino acids (optical isomers absent in natural proteins) do not.

To induce DTH, a protein must be presented to the organism in a particular way. In a natural situation, there are infectious diseases that are accompanied by DTH and others that are not, but what exactly causes this difference in the host response is not known. The diseases that are accompanied by DTH are of a chronic type frequently associated with the formation of granulomatous tissues. Presumably, the microorganism or parasite must lodge in a particular way, in a particular tissue, and provide the host with a particular type of antigenic stimulus. In an experimental situation, DTH sensitization occurs only when the sensitizing injection is given in adjuvant, preferably the complete type, with bacilli of tuberculosis. Primary injection of the antigen in physiological salt solution usually fails to generate conditions for DTH induction: although such injection probably does stimulate an immune response, it apparently does not create the particular conditions necessary for the manifestation of this specific form of immune response.

12.7.4 Manifestation

DTH can manifest itself as either focal or systemic. The most characteristic *focal manifestation* of DTH is the *skin reaction*, exemplified by the tuberculin test. The course of the reaction differs somewhat, depending on the mode of tuberculin injection—subcutaneous, used originally by Robert Koch, or intradermal, introduced by Charles Mantoux in 1910. A few hours after the subcutaneous injection, the injected area becomes red, warm, and swollen. In contrast to the soft, fluid-filled swelling that accompanies some of the immediate-type hypersensitivities, the swelling in the DTH skin reaction is firm, because it is caused by dense accumulation of cells at the injection site. In humans, the redness and swelling peak at about 48 hours, and in guinea pigs at about 24 hours after the injection of the tuberculin. The diameter of the induration at the reaction peak is about 10 mm, but with antigens more diffusable than tuberculin the afflicted area can be larger. In succeeding days, the skin in the swollen area becomes necrotic and eventually sloughs, leaving a shallow ulcer that heals quickly. Following an intradermal injection of tuberculin, the area assumes a characteristic cocarde appearance, with a central nodule separated from a peripheral halo by an intermediate zone; otherwise, the course of the reaction is similar to that induced by the subcutaneous injection.

Histological examination of the swollen area reveals an accumulation of mononuclear cells, especially around small blood vessels. About 80 to 90 percent of the mononuclear cells are monocytes (the rest being lymphocytes) and this massive monocyte infiltration of the skin lesion is one of the most characteristic features of DTH. Although granulocytes can also be found in the swollen area, they are usually only minor components of the classic DTH reaction. The mononuclear cells are brought into the skin by the blood stream. Histological sections of the lesions at later stages of the reaction reveal extensive tissue damage.

Another focal manifestation of DTH is the appearance of milky white opacity in the cornea of the eye. In guinea pigs, this *corneal reaction* appears about 24 hours after the injection of antigen into the sensitized animal and it correlates well with the development of the skin reaction.

Whole body (systemic) reactions occur particularly in cases in which large quantities of the antigen enter the blood stream. The symptoms of the systemic reaction are fever, malaise, backache, pains in the joints, and reduction in the number of circulating lymphocytes (lymphopenia). Severe cases of the systemic reaction may result in shock, and even death, several hours after the antigen injection (as opposed to immediate hypersensitivity, in which shock occurs within minutes of antigen administration). The events leading to the shock may be initiated by a combined action of immune cells and antibodies. Unsensitized individuals tolerate antigen doses many thousands of times higher than do sensitized individuals.

12.7.5 Mechanism

The precise mechanism of DTH response is still not known, but a rough scenario of the main events in the response can be outlined as follows (Fig. 12.12). The first exposure of an organism to the antigen results in sensitization of lymphocytes carrying the corresponding receptors on their surfaces. In the mouse, these

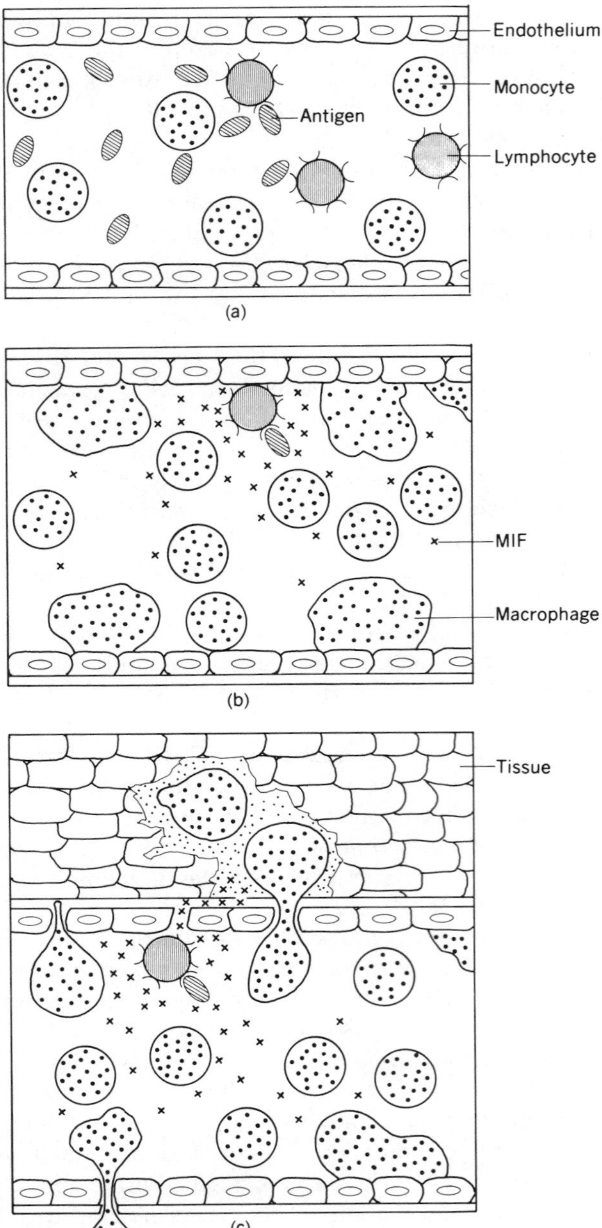

Figure 12.12. Initial events in the generation of delayed-type hypersensitivity lesions. (*a*) A sensitized lymphocyte binds antigen in a blood vessel (the antigen is probably presented to the lymphocyte by a macrophagelike cell but this step is omitted). (*b*) An activated lymphocyte produces a migration inhibitory factor (MIF), which stops the flow of monocytes by making them adhere to the endothelial lining. (*c*) Monocytes transform into macrophages, and macrophages force themselves through the endothelium and vessel wall and begin to release hydrolases, which attack the tissues surrounding the vessel.

lymphocytes can be of either the Lyt-1^+Lyt-2^- or Lyt-1^+Lyt-2^+ category. In what way the sensitized and nonsensitized lymphocytes differ is not clear. Some immunologists believe the difference to be merely of a quantitative character: the sensitization results in the expansion of clones specifically reactive with a given antigen, so that a second exposure of the host to the same antigen is met with a larger number of reactive cells than the first one and the secondary response is more vigorous than the primary response. Others consider sensitized lymphocytes qualitatively different from unsensitized ones. The manner of presentation of the antigen to the T cells is not known either but it is presumably mediated by macrophages. Sensitized lymphocytes circulate through the body via the pathways described in Chapter 5.

Following the second intradermal injection, the antigen diffuses through the skin and enters the small veins. There, a few sensitized lymphocytes that have reached the injection site by chance recognize and bind the antigen, and this binding restimulates these cells. The restimulated lymphocytes release soluble factors, the most prominent of which is the macrophage-inhibiting factor. The MIF acts on monocytes in the blood, making them sticky, and the sticky cells then adhere to the endothelial lining of the vein. MIF may also act on the endothelial lining, causing direct damage that may attract more monocytes.

The invading monocytes force themselves through the endothelium of the vessel wall and enter the surrounding tissue. There, some of the cells transform morphologically into macrophages, while others remain morphologically indistinguishable from blood monocytes. The result is an accumulation of monocytes and monocytelike cells at the site of injection—the mononuclear cell infiltration.

During their emigration from the blood vessel, the activated monocytes and macrophages release lysosomal hydrolases that attack and destroy the vessel wall and surrounding subcutaneous tissue. (The specifics of the attack on the tissue resemble those observed in immediate hypersensitivities, which will be described in Chapter 13.) Additional damage can be caused, as was already mentioned, directly by the MIF, lymphotoxin, and other factors released by restimulated lymphocytes.

This scenario provides the explanation for the three characteristic features of the skin reaction: the hard swelling of the injection site, caused by cellular infiltration; the reddening, caused by the damage to the underlying blood vessels and seepage of blood into the tissues; and the necrosis, caused by enzymes and factors released by activated monocytes and lymphocytes. The DTH reaction thus has two components—a minor specific component consisting of a few sensitized lymphocytes that, upon restimulation by the antigen, start the reaction, and a major nonspecific component, triggered by the products of the stimulated lymphocytes and responsible for most of the tissue damage. The delay in the manifestation of DTH is probably attributable to the extra time necessary for the amplification of the reaction from a few sensitized cells to a full-scale attack on the tissue.

Following the second exposure to the antigen, the host is sometimes unable to respond to a third antigen injection, especially if the third injection is given shortly after the second and if the antigen dose used for the second injection was high. Presumably, the antigen provided by the second injection engages most of the sensitized lymphocytes so that very few are left to respond to a new injection of fresh antigen. However, this state of *desensitization* is only transient, and sensitivity returns after a few days or weeks.

This account of the course of the skin reaction is undoubtedly an oversimplification. The actual process also involves other cells in addition to those mentioned—in particular, granulocytes. In some forms of DTH, some of these other cells (e.g., basophils) may take over the reaction and play a dominant role in it (see below). Furthermore, this mainly cellular response is often accompanied by the induction of humoral immunity and the end result is often a combined attack by both cells and antibodies. Antibodies may contribute particularly to the systemic manifestation of DTH.

12.7.6 Basophilic Cutaneous Hypersensitivity

The mechanism and manifestation of DTH may vary, depending on the specific circumstances of DTH induction. An extreme example of this variation is the *basophilic cutaneous hypersensitivity*, also known as the *Jones-Mote reaction*. Described in 1934 by T. D. Jones and J. R. Mote, it is characterized by massive infiltration of basophils at the injection site. Here basophils, presumably attracted by an as yet unidentified, lymphocyte-produced factor, can constitute up to 50 percent of the infiltrating cells. The reaction occurs following the injection of certain antigens in a certain manner (intradermal injection of the antigen in incomplete Freund's adjuvant or even in physiological salt solution). It is milder than the classic DTH and characterized by only slight skin thickening, which disappears after 48 hours.

12.7.7 Specificity

Most of the information about the specificity of DTH reactions derives from studies by Samuel B. Salvin, R. F. Smith, P. G. H. Gell, Baruj Benacerraf, and B. B. Levine. These immunologists used various conjugates of small molecules (haptens) with large proteins (carriers) to induce delayed- and immediate-type hypersensitivities in the guinea pig—the former as a measure of cell-mediated immunity, the latter as an indicator of humoral immunity. The main conclusions from these studies are the following.

First, DTH is directed against the carrier, the antibody response against the hapten. Although antibodies can be produced against the carrier when the carrier is injected without the hapten, the hapten-carrier conjugate usually induces antibodies against the hapten and not against the carrier.

Second, DTH can be induced to hapten-carrier conjugates in which the carrier is the animal's own protein. For example, immunization of guinea pigs with dinitrophenyl (DNP) attached to guinea pig albumin results in both DTH and antibody response. In this instance, however, the DTH is directed against the link between the hapten and the carrier (or to a determinant on the carrier generated by the attachment of the hapten), since neither the hapten (DNP) nor the carrier (guinea pig albumin) alone induces DTH in guinea pigs sensitized by hapten-carrier (DNP-GPA) conjugates.

Third, the region of the carrier recognized by sensitized lymphocytes often appears to be larger than that recognized by antibodies. This conclusion is suggested by experiments in which a guinea pig is sensitized by a hapten-carrier conjugate and then tested with the same hapten separated from the carrier by a spacer molecule. The separation has no effect on the antibody response, but significantly reduces the DTH response, suggesting that the lymphocytes recognize not only the hapten but also the link between the hapten and the carrier. (An implication of this observation is that the binding of the T-lymphocyte receptor with the antigen requires greater binding forces than the antigen-antibody reaction.) However, this conclusion is subject to criticism, as was discussed in Chapter 7.

Fourth, the degree of crossreactivity of lymphocytes and antibodies with substances related, but not identical to the immunizing conjugates depends on the particular conjugate used. Sometimes the lymphocytes appear more crossreactive than the antibodies; at other times, just the opposite is true.

Fifth, denaturation of proteins has a more profound

effect on antibody production than on DTH response. Immunization with various heat-denatured proteins provokes a state of delayed hypersensitivity but drastically reduces antibody production to the native protein, as if primary protein structure were more important in T-lymphocyte recognition than tertiary structure.

Sixth, DTH is a more sensitive immunological method than antibody production. Only minute amounts of protein (a few thousand micrograms) are necessary for DTH sensitization of a guinea pig, while a much larger dose is needed to elicit antibody production.

12.7.8 Genetic Control

Not all individuals of a given species respond to a given antigen in the delayed-type hypersensitivity assay. One of the most striking examples of individual differences in DTH responsiveness was provided by Baruj Benacerraf and his colleagues, who immunized guinea pigs of two inbred strains, 2 and 13, with DNP conjugated to the synthetic polypeptide, poly-L-lysine (PLL). Only the strain 2 guinea pigs produced DTH to this conjugate, and breeding experiments provided evidence that the responsiveness was controlled by a single immune response (*Ir*) gene, residing in the major histocompatibility complex (see Chapter 8). This demonstration was, in fact, the first clear evidence of the existence of *Ir* genes. Later studies revealed that the genetic control concerned the recognition of the carrier, rather than of the hapten. The nonresponder animals were unable to recognize the particular carrier, but when the carrier itself was placed on another carrier and thus forced to play the role of a hapten, the nonresponders became responders.

In later *Ir* gene studies, immunologists turned to the production of antibodies and away from DTH as an assay for the detection of differences in responsiveness, but the results of these two assays proved to be largely superimposable, suggesting that even the control of antibody production operates via carrier recognition mechanisms (see Chapter 8).

The mechanism of genetic control of DTH is suggested by transfer experiments. Studies in mice indicate that upon transfer, sensitized cells initiate DTH only in hosts compatible with them at class II or class I MHC loci, depending on the antigen. This requirement for MHC compatibility probably means that lymphocytes recognize the antigen in the context of a particular MHC molecule (presumably when the antigen is presented to them by a macrophage) and can be restimulated by this antigen only in the context of this molecule. The nonresponder situation arises when the particular T cell cannot, for whatever reason, recognize the particular antigen-MHC combination.

12.7.9 Role of DTH in Disease Pathogenesis

So characteristic is the association of DTH with certain infectious diseases, especially tuberculosis, that a test for DTH (tuberculin reaction) is used to diagnose some of them.[1] Yet the association might seem paradoxical: the sensitization of T cells is presumably a defense reaction, but the DTH reaction damages the host's own tissues rather than the invader. One should realize, however, that the testing of infected individuals, especially skin testing, is an experimental situation that does not occur spontaneously. To what extent the sensitized lymphocytes damage the infected individuals in nonexperimental situations is not clear. Some of the lesions occurring in tuberculous tissues might, in part, be caused by a misguided action of immune T cells, but until this point is definitely established and the balance between detrimental and beneficial effects of the immune status determined, it is premature to call DTH, as some immunologists have done, an "immunological mistake."

12.8 CONTACT SENSITIVITY

12.8.1 Discovery

In 1896, the dermatologist Josef Jadassohn described a patient, a young man in good health, who developed massive dermatitis (skin inflammation, from Gr. *derma*, skin; suffix *-itis*, inflammation) after he had used an ointment to get rid of pubic lice. Some time later, the patient returned to Jadassohn with a skin ulcer, which the dermatologist treated with another ointment. When the patient again developed severe dermatitis, Jadassohn suspected that the patient's skin was reacting to some substance contained in the ointments. Since both ointments contained mercury, Jadassohn decided to test mercury's involvement by applying a small patch of mercury-containing plaster to the patient's healthy skin. When, the next day, he found the skin under the plaster all inflamed, Jadassohn concluded that the patient's trouble was indeed caused by a reaction of the skin to contact with mercurous substances.

A number of other dermatologists had experiences similar to Jadassohn's: they too observed patients de-

[1] The association is not absolute, and occasionally patients with tuberculosis fail to give a positive tuberculin test.

veloping skin inflammation following contact with a variety of drugs and other substances. They referred to this type of inflammation as *contact sensitivity*, *contact dermatitis*, or *contact eczema*. To determine whether a person had contact sensitivity, they used the *patch test*, first described by Jadassohn (see also Chapter 13). As we shall see later, contact sensitivity is a form of delayed-type hypersensitivity in which the target organ is the skin and the inflammatory response is produced by application of the sensitizing substance to the skin surface. The differences between the two reactions are all attributable to the inducing antigen and to the way the antigens are presented to the organism. Hence, rather than discussing contact sensitivity in detail, we shall merely point out how this reaction differs from the classic form of DTH.

12.8.2 Inducing Agents

All contact sensitivity-inducing substances have at least two features in common: they have a low molecular weight, which allows them to diffuse through the skin, and they can combine with amino acid side chains and thus form protein conjugates. They themselves are usually not antigenic, but when combined with proteins they are capable of stimulating lymphocytes (or rather, the conjugate is). They are not limited to drugs but are also present in the excretions of certain plants and in industrial products, such as chromate, nickel, turpentine, varnish, various resins, cosmetics, and hair dyes. One of the best-known examples of contact sensitivity-inducing plant products is urushiol from poison ivy, *Rhus toxidendron* (Fig. 12.13). Poison ivy is a climbing or creeping plant from the family *Anacardiacae*, distributed all over North America. The plant has three-lobed leaves that turn brilliant red in the fall, inconspicuous greenish-white flowers in loose clusters, and small, hard berries that may be white, cream-colored, or pale green. The leaves secrete an oil, the urushiol (from Jap. *urushi*, lacquer and L. *oleum*, oil; a similar oil is also secreted by the Asiatic lacquer tree, *Rhus vernicifera*), which is a mixture of nonvolatile catechol derivatives. Other urushiol-secreting plants are the primrose, *Primula obconica*, and poison oak (Fig. 12.13). When one touches poison ivy or primrose leaves, some of the oil sticks to and then diffuses into the skin, initiating the reaction. The irritation can often be prevented by washing the skin with a strong soap that contains oil-absorbing detergents.

For experimental induction of contact sensitivity, immunologists usually use various nitro- or chloro-substituted benzenes that combine easily with proteins—for example, picryl chloride, 3,4-dinitrochlorobenzene (DNCB), or dinitrofluorobenzene (DNFB; see Chapter 10, Fig. 10.5).

12.8.3 Induction and Manifestation

In humans, contact sensitivity arises from prolonged or repeated contact with the inducing substance. In ex-

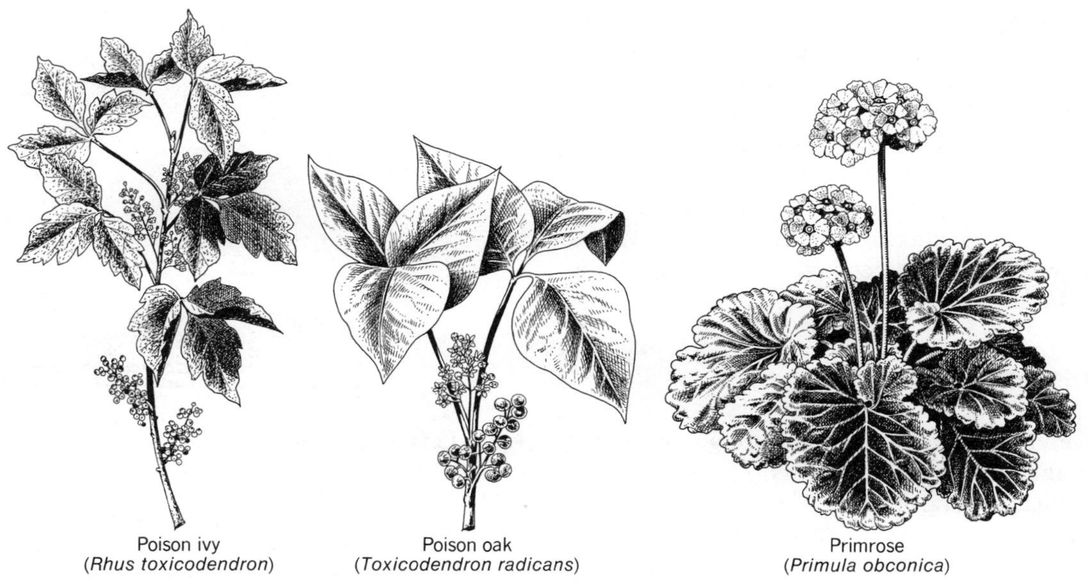

Figure 12.13. Plants responsible for contact sensitivity reactions in humans.

perimental situations, immunologists usually induce contact sensitivity by topical application (skin painting): they remove the animal's (usually guinea pig's) hair over an area of approximately 2 to 3 cm^2 and place a few drops of 2 percent alcohol solution of DNCB on the clear skin surface. They then stroke the fluid into the skin with a glass stirring rod and repeat this procedure for seven consecutive days. After letting the animals rest for two or three weeks, they shave them again, apply two drops of 0.1 percent alcohol solution of DNCB to the area of previous application, and rub the solution into the skin. Four, 24, and 48 hours after the application, they measure the size of the inflamed area with a millimeter ruler. The first few applications with a relatively high dose of the chemical, each of which is toxic and irritating to the skin, serve to sensitize the animal; the last, low (nonirritating)—dose application serves to test the reaction. However, sensitization can also be accomplished by intradermal, subcutaneous, intravenous, intraperitoneal, and oral administration of the sensitizing chemical. The noncutaneous routes usually produce good sensitization only when the chemical is applied in complete Freund's adjuvant.

A mild form of contact sensitivity is characterized by reddening of the skin (erythema), and swelling (edema). More severe cases of contact sensitivity result in the formation of blisters (vesiculation), which may break and leave raw, weeping areas. In humans the blisters may cover the whole body except for palms and soles, which are spared because the thickness of the cornified epithelium interferes with the penetration of the sensitizing chemicals. In contrast, the eyelids and genital regions, with relatively thin skin, are usually the most susceptible areas. The lesions reach their maximum at 24 to 48 hours and subside over a period of several days. The severe forms of contact sensitivity are sometimes referred to as *allergic contact dermatitis*, or *allergic eczematous contact dermatitis*. Prolonged exposure to the sensitizing substance may lead to a chronic condition characterized by thickening of the skin, scaling, and lichenification (leathery induration).

12.8.4 Mechanism

As the sensitizing chemical diffuses through the skin, it reacts with the body's own proteins, forming hapten-carrier conjugates (Fig. 12.14). The attachment of a small molecule to a protein changes the protein's antigenic properties: it is no longer a self component, but foreign matter. The conjugated proteins are probably picked up by macrophages, processed, and presented to lymphocytes, which then recognize them as antigens in the context of major histocompatibility complex molecules carried by the macrophage. Sensitization of the lymphocytes follows and the rest of the reaction sequence occurs according to the scenario described for the classic form of DTH. The identity of all the proteins to which the small chemical binds covalently has not been established. One of them is serum albumin (the chemicals apparently diffuse all the way into the blood capillaries), but several others are very likely involved. The nature of the determinants recognized by lymphocytes on conjugated proteins is also not completely clear. In some instances, the determinants seem to be present on the link between the protein and the small molecule, but in other instances, the binding possibly induces the appearance of a new determinant on the protein itself.

The principal difference between contact sensitivity and classic DTH is that in the former, the sensitizing hapten-carrier conjugates form locally in the skin, whereas in the latter they are injected into the or-

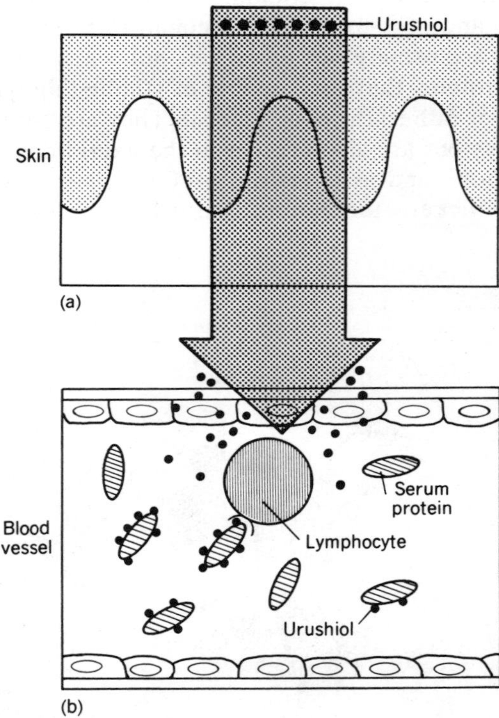

Figure 12.14. Initiation of a contact sensitivity reaction to urushiol from poison ivy. (*a*) Urushiol diffuses through the skin into a blood vessel. (*b*) In the vessel urushiol binds to serum proteins and the altered proteins activate lymphocytes (probably via a macrophagelike cell but this step is omitted for simplicity's sake). The steps that follow this initial phase are similar to those occurring in delayed-type hypersensitivity (see Fig. 12.12).

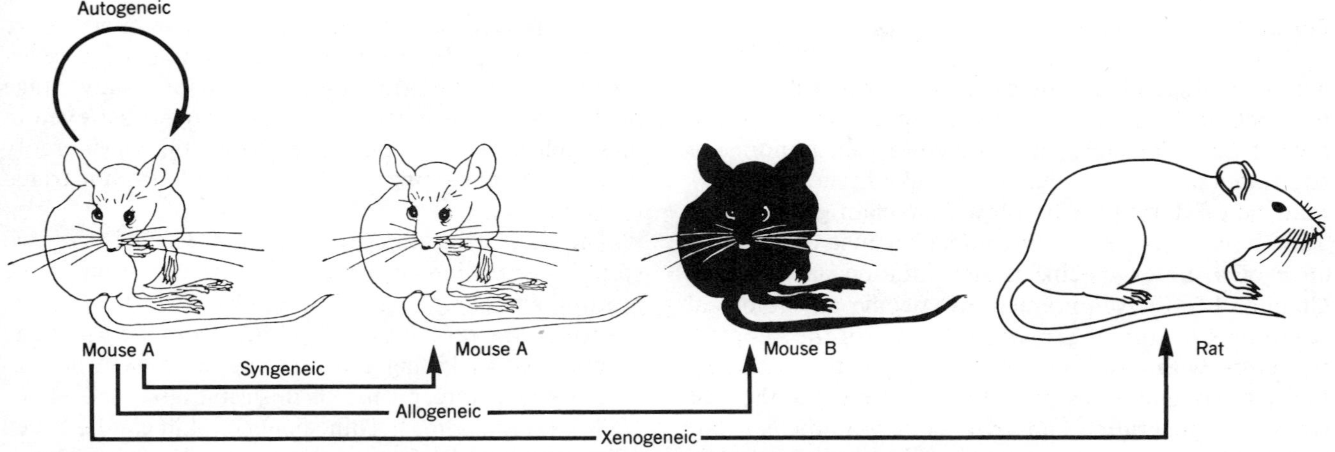

Figure 12.15. Types of graft. The direction of grafting is indicated by arrows.

ganism, ready-made. As in the case of DTH, partial or complete desensitization of sensitive individuals can be accomplished by a systemic or parenteral application of the sensitizing chemicals. However, as in DTH, the desensitization is only short-lived.

12.9 ALLOGRAFT REACTION[2]

12.9.1 Terms and Definitions

Transplantation, or *grafting*, is the transfer of living cells, tissues, or organs from one part of the body to another or from one individual to another. The transferred cell, tissue, or organ is the *graft* or *transplant*. Grafts placed in the same anatomical position normally occupied by the transplanted tissue are called *orthotopic*, and those placed in an unnatural position are called *heterotropic*. An example of a heterotropic graft is a piece of skin taken from the tail of a donor mouse and placed on the recipient's dorsum. Grafts taken from and placed on the same individual are called *autogeneic* (*autografts*); grafts transplanted between genetically identical individuals (for instance, between mice of the same inbred strain) are called *syngeneic* (*syngrafts* or *isografts*); grafts transplanted between genetically different individuals of the same species (for example, between two different inbred strains) are called *allogeneic* (*allografts* or *homografts*); and finally, grafts transplanted between individuals of two different species are referred to as *xenogeneic* (*xenografts* or *heterografts*; see Fig. 12.15).

[2] Based, in part, on J. Klein: *Biology of the Mouse Histocompatibility-2 Complex*. Springer-Verlag, New York, 1975.

The fate of a graft is determined by the genetic relationship between the donor and host. Each species has a set of *histocompatibility* (*H*) *genes* coding for *histocompatibility antigens* that determine compatibility or incompatibility of tissue transplants. In general, grafts exchanged between animals that do not differ in the histocompability genes are *accepted* (i.e., they heal in and survive indefinitely), whereas those transplanted between individuals differing in the *H* genes are *rejected* (destroyed). The rejection is brought about by the *allograft reaction*, the specific immune response against histocompatibility (transplantation) antigens. The complex of immunological phenomena leading to the rejection of grafts in unsensitized recipients is the *first-set reaction*; immunological response to a graft by a sensitized recipient is the *second-set reaction*.

In most situations, the allograft reaction is a one-way process: the host reacts against the graft, but the graft cannot react against the host (*host-versus-graft reaction* or HVGR). However, grafts containing significant numbers of immunocompetent lymphoid cells are capable of mounting a *graft-versus-host reaction*, GVHR, which may occur simultaneously with HVGR.

12.9.2 Transplantation Methods

Experimental Transplantation

Theoretically, a graft can be derived from almost any part of the body and can consist of either normal or neoplastic tissue. Because tumor grafting played an important role in the formulation of the genetic theory of transplantation (see Chapter 1), it will be considered first.

Tumor Transplantation

The advantage of the tumor method is that it is rapid and technically simple; the disadvantage is that it is not always specific. Only some newly arisen tumors are transplantable; others may never take in new hosts, or may die off during the first few transplant generations. Tumors may not be transplantable because of the presence of a tumor-specific transplantation antigen (see Chapter 14), the requirement of specific physiological conditions for tumor growth, infection of the neoplastic tissue with bacteria, or some other factor. Some tumors may undergo a period of adjustment in the first transplant generation and grow only sporadically, but later they become consistently lethal to their syngeneic hosts. Once established, transplantable tumors can be maintained indefinitely by serial transfers (*passages*) on individuals of the same strain. Some mouse tumors have been maintained by serial transplantation for over half a century.

However, with successive passages from host to host, the tumors may change progressively: they may undergo morphological alterations or shifts in chromosome number, and display variations in growth rate and invasiveness; they may also change their antigenic characteristics. Many tumors become less specific in later transplant generations and may override histocompatibility barriers that would cause rejection of normal tissues.

Tumor transplants can grow either as *solid* tissues or as *ascites* (i.e., a suspension of single cells growing in the fluid-filled peritoneal cavity). Many solid tumors can be converted into ascitic forms either directly or by repeated selection. Ascitic tumors can be transplanted by suction of the ascitic fluid from the peritoneum of tumor-bearing mice and intraperitoneal inoculation of the cells into the new host. Solid tumors can be transplanted either as small pieces with a special needle (trocar) or as a cell suspension, obtained by mincing the solid tissues. The latter technique is advantageous in that an accurately measured number of cells can be administered. The cell suspension can be inoculated in almost any part of the body, the more commonly used methods being subcutaneously on the flank, intramuscularly into the thigh, or intraperitoneally. The ultimate indication of graft acceptance is the tumor's causing the death of the host; the ultimate indication of rejection is the host's survival.

Transplantation of Normal Tissues

Skin Grafting. Skin grafting is by far the most popular experimental technique for normal tissue transplantation. Its advantages include great sensitivity, easy assessment of the graft survival, and relative resistance to transplantation trauma. A major disadvantage of this technique is its relative laboriousness; even in its simplest version, the technique is still considerably more time-consuming than, for example, tumor transplantation.

The standard skin-grafting technique consists of two steps: preparation of the graft and preparation of the grafting site (*graft bed*). The graft can be taken from the trunk, the tail, or the ear. Grafts from the trunk can be obtained by killing and skinning the donor and cutting the skin into pieces of desirable size and shape (*full-thickness grafts*). Thin sheets of skin can be sliced off with a scalpel from a living donor (*split-thickness grafts*), or the skin can be lifted up into a conical elevation with the forceps and cut free at the base with a scalpel (*pinch grafts*). Grafts from the tail can be obtained by slicing off thin sheets of skin with a scalpel, or by amputating the tail, skinning it, and trimming the skin to the required size. Grafts from the ear are easily produced by cutting off the pinna at its base and peeling away the thin skin from the underlying cartilage. Full-thickness grafts consist of epidermis and complete—or almost complete—dermis; split-thickness grafts consist of epidermis and only superficial dermal layers; and pinch grafts are comprised—at least in the center—of not only the epidermis and dermis, but also the underlying layers of fat (*panniculus adiposus*) and muscle (*panniculus carnosus*).

The usual grafting site in the mouse is the dorsal or lateral skin of the trunk, which has the advantage of being relatively inaccessible to the animal's teeth and having the firm support of the ribs. The graft bed can be prepared by cutting off the skin in small pieces with scissors until the desired shape and size of the area is cleaned off, or by pinching off the skin with a scalpel. During the cutting, care must be taken not to damage the *panniculus carnosus* and the blood vessels overlying it. The bed can be of the same size as the graft (*fitted grafts*), or it can be larger (*open-fit grafts*). The grafts are protected from misplacement and from physical damage by a gauze dressing and bandage, both of which are removed from seven to 10 days after grafting.

In the first few days after transplantation, incompatible skin grafts are grossly and microscopically indistinguishable from compatible grafts. In the first two days after the operation, the graft depends on diffusion of nutrients from the host through intercellular spaces. Blood supply is reestablished two to three days after grafting, primarily by the linking (anastomoses) of the host and graft capillaries, but also by an ingrowth of new capillaries into the graft. At about five or six days after transplantation, the compatible graft contains considerably more blood vessels than normal skin, and this hypervascularity causes the graft's characteristic pink color. The increase in vascularity is accompanied by intense mitotic activity in the epidermis, reaching its peak six to eight days after grafting and then slowly declining over a period of several weeks. At six days the graft epidermis is at least three times thicker than normal skin, and this *epidermal hyperplasia* causes the graft to appear swollen and soft to the touch. Later, the upper layer of the original epidermis hardens and eventually peels off as a "ghost graft." The hair follicles, damaged as a result of transplantation trauma, regenerate and begin to grow a new hair crop after the reestablishment of a blood supply. The space between the surfaces of the graft and the graft bed is filled with healing tissue, so that the six-day graft is already firmly attached to the host. When the compatible graft has merged imperceptibly with the host's skin and remains in that condition throughout the life of the recipient, it is said to be permanently *accepted*.

Incompatible grafts differ from compatible ones in that they induce an allograft reaction that damages or destroys the transplanted tissue. The destruction (*rejection*) can be either acute (its duration being relatively short, usually not more than a week) or chronic (prolonged over a period of several weeks or months), depending on the strength of the histocompatibility barrier. The onset of the allograft reaction is determined by the strength of H antigens, with strong antigens causing rejection as early as five or six days postoperatively.

The earliest sign of *acute rejection* is dilation of blood vessels and their engorgement with erythrocytes, followed by hemorrhages, and by invasion through the vesel walls of a mixed population of lymphoid cells, primarily small lymphocytes (*lymphocytic* or *round cell infiltration*). This inflammatory reaction spreads upward through the dermis, around the blood vessels, toward the epidermis. In addition to cells, large quantities of fluid also pass through the damaged vessels, causing the graft to swell and change color, from pink to red and then to yellow or brown. The cells of vessel walls become pycnotic and lose their cytoplasm, and their nuclei fragment into small pieces. Necrosis and breakdown of the remaining tissue quickly follow, and the graft transforms into a scablike mass that ultimately sloughs.

A *second-set reaction* across strong H differences usually follows the same pattern as the first-set reaction, only in an accelerated and more pronounced manner. Occasionally, however, when the reaction is very strong and begins very early, the graft fails to establish the initial blood anastomoses and degenerates without the transient period of healing in. Such *white grafts* do not show any lymphocytic infiltration in histological sections. Some believe that the white-graft phenomenon is associated with the presence of humoral antibodies directed against the donor-tissue antigens.

Chronic rejection is extremely variable in appearance and duration, its signs being gradual hair loss, scaliness of the graft surface, scar formation, thinning of the epidermis, and weakening of the attachment to the dermis. Histologically, chronic rejection is usually accompanied by mild inflammatory reactions in the graft dermis. The rejection may be complete, followed by the replacement of the graft with the host tissues, or partial, followed by recovery of the graft. Grafts of the latter type are said to have undergone a *cosmetic crisis*.

Skin grafts can be appraised visually (by naked-eye observation) or histologically. For first-set grafts, particularly those with relatively long survival times, the former usually suffices; for second-set grafts transplanted across a strong H barrier, the latter is often imperative, as naked-eye observation may not distinguish between the late effects of surgical trauma and the early effects of allograft reaction. The visual scoring is based on observation of macroscopic changes in the graft, such as variations in color, thinning or loss of the hair crop, swelling, wetness, ulceration, and scar formation. The grafts must be scored once a day in the early post-transplantation period (first four weeks) and once a week thereafter. The histological scoring is based on sections of grafts removed at varying intervals after transplantation. Although the histological scoring must take into account the whole status of the graft, two main criteria are used in appraising the sections: the survival of epidermis (expressed as percentage) and the degree of lymphocytic infiltration (expressed in arbitrary units, usually on a scale from one to four).

Even when transplanted under exactly the same conditions, across the same H difference, and to genetically homogeneous recipients, all grafts are not rejected at the same time. The rejection process is influenced by many environmental factors, which cause some grafts to be rejected sooner than others. The range of individual survival times can vary from a few days in the case of strong H antigens to several months in the case of weak H antigens. It has become customary to express the length of the graft duration in terms of the *median survival time* (MST), which is the time that passes between transplantation and rejection of 50 percent of the grafts.

Transplantation of Lymphoid Tissues. Lymphoid tissues can be transplanted in the form of single-cell suspensions prepared by homogenization of the donor organ (bone marrow, lymph nodes, spleen, thymus, or fetal liver) and inoculated intraperitoneally or intravenously. The recipient can be either untreated or irradiated with X-rays or gamma rays. The irradiation provides *Lebensraum* (space to live in) for the transplanted cells by destroying the recipient's lymphoid tissue, and decreases the host's capability for immunological response to the graft. The survival of the transplanted cells can be monitored radiologically (in cases where the donor and the host cells differ in their capability to incorporate radioactive isotopes), cytologically (provided that the donor and the host differ in the morphology of their chromosomes), serologically (for example, when the donor cells secrete immunoglobulins that are immunologically distinguishable from those of the host), or electrophoretically (when the donor and host differ in an allozyme, serum protein, or hemoglobin).

Transplantation of Other Normal Tissues. Any other normal tissue can be transplanted heterotopically, most commonly either subcutaneously or under the kidney capsule. Orthotopic transplantation of whole organs is feasible only in large animals.

Clinical Transplantation

While the experimentalist uses transplants only as a tool for answering certain basic questions regarding the allograft reaction, for a clinician, the transplant is a "spare part" with which he tries to replace the sick tissue or organ of a patient. The clinician therefore places technical requirements on tissue and organ transplantation that are different from those of the experimentalist. Where a researcher may be satisfied with a few beating heart cells, the clinician will regard transplantation as successful only when the whole new heart takes over all the functions of the old one. In other words, for a clinician, transplantation of a particular organ is a surgical problem first and an immunological one only secondarily: if transplantation of a particular organ is technically impossible, it is irrelevant, whether the organ would or would not be rejected by the host. Owing to the effort of Alexis Carrel, Norman E. Shumway, Roy Y. Calne, David M. Hume, Thomas E. Starzl, and other surgeons, transplantation is technically feasible with all major organs except the brain, testes, liver, and lung. The surgeons have done their job: the rest is up to the immunologists.

12.9.3 Mechanism of Graft Rejection

Variables Influencing Graft Survival

Graft rejection is a complex process that may assume various forms depending on specific circumstances. Some of the variables determining the specific form of allograft reaction are as follows.

The Establishment of Blood Supply. In an organ transplant where the surgeon connects the host's blood vessels directly to those of the transplant, blood supply to the graft is established almost immediately. In this case it is by means of the blood that the host immune system first learns of the presence of the transplant; and of all the lymphoid centers, it is the spleen that first gets the message. In tissue transplants such as skin grafts, the reestablishment of the blood supply may take two to three days, and during this time the host immune system may already have received the information about the presence of foreign matter by means of lymphatics that carry cells and debris from the graft. The lymphatics carry the information first to the nearest (regional) lymph node so that the defense reaction is initiated from these, rather than from the spleen. Since lymph nodes and spleen differ in their cell compositions, these two organs may initiate different forms of allograft reaction.

Content of Passenger Lymphocytes. At the time of transfer, the transplant contains lymphocytes in the lymphatics, blood vessels, and tissues. These cells probably emigrate from the graft and, via the host circulatory system, reach the spleen and lymph nodes, where they are recognized as foreign and attacked by the host's immune cells. This direct "walking in" of foreign cells to the defense centers may be the most efficient way of stimulating allograft reaction, and rapidity, vigor, and other parameters of the reaction may be determined by the passenger lymphocyte content of the graft.

Grafting Site. Some *privileged sites*, such as the anterior eye chamber, brain, and the cheek pouch of hamsters, permit prolonged or permanent survival of incompatible grafts. The privileged status of these sites is probably a result of paucity or complete absence of draining lymphatics in tissues surrounding them. The only way cells, including lymphocytes, can get to the grafts at privileged sites is via the blood stream, and hence via the spleen. Processing of the stimulus in the spleen may then lead to dominance of immune mechanisms that allow prolonged graft survival.

The Role of Cells and Antibodies

Congenitally athymic (*nu*/*nu*) mice, which lack functional thymocytes, fail to reject allogeneic and xenogeneic grafts. However, the ability to reject grafts returns when such mice are inoculated with T lymphocytes from a normal donor that is genetically compatible with the athymic recipient.

These experiments indicate that B lymphocytes alone are incapable of rejecting a graft; however, the experiments do not exclude B lymphocytes from participation in the graft rejection process. Alloantigens of the grafted cells clearly stimulate B lymphocyte differentiation into antibody-secreting cells, but the role of the antibodies in graft rejection remains controversial. Some immunologists have discovered that, in certain situations, antibodies alone could destroy a graft; other investigators could not find evidence for a significant contribution of antibodies to graft rejection. Probably whether antibodies participate in allograft rejection depends on the particular circumstances of grafting—the type of graft, the grafting site, and the properties of the host complement. The involvement of antibodies can help swing the host response to the graft either way—toward rejection but also toward survival of the graft. Antibodies can contribute to the rejection process by binding to the graft itself, initiating the complement cascade, and thus killing the grafted cells. Antibodies and complement are probably responsible for *hyperacute organ transplant rejection*, the signs of which a surgeon can often see while he is still suturing the transplant. Or, once bound to the allogeneic cells, the Fc regions of the antibodies may be recognized by receptors on K cells, which then kill the targets via the *antibody-dependent cell-mediated cytotoxicity* (ADCC) phenomenon (see Chapter 5).

Certain types of antibody, rather than contributing to graft rejection, protect the graft from being destroyed by cellular responses. Immunologists refer to this prolongation of graft survival by antibodies as *immunological enhancement*, or simply *enhancement*. The phenomenon was discovered in 1907 by Simon Flexner and J. W. Jobling, who noticed that pretreatment of rats or mice with disrupted (homogenized and freeze-dried) allogeneic cells promoted, rather than prevented, growth of a tumor derived from the same strain as the cells: while normal rats or mice rejected the graft and survived, the pretreated animals, paradoxically, were killed by the growing tumor. Later studies by Albert E. Casey, Nathan Kaliss, and George D. Snell demonstrated that the tumor-enhancing substance was an antibody. (The capability of enhancing a graft can be transferred with serum of pretreated individuals to normal individuals; enhancement by transferred antibodies is referred to as *passive*, in contrast to *active enhancement* induced by tissue pretreatment of the host.) What makes an antibody enhancing and how the enhancing antibodies act in preventing tumor (or normal tissue) rejection are not known. Some immunologists believe that the antibodies act on the graft, altering it in such a way that it evades the host's immune response (*efferent inhibition hypothesis*); others contend that the antibodies combine with antigenic material released from the tumor and thus prevent the material from sensitizing the host (*afferent inhibition hypothesis*); still others believe that the antibodies or antigen-antibody complexes act on the lymphoid centers, preventing them from mounting a cellular response against the tumor (*central inhibition hypothesis*). The actual mechanism may involve a combination of any two or even all three postulated events.

Three Phases of Allograft Reaction

The cellular reaction can be divided formally into recognition, amplification, and effector phases (Fig. 12.16).

Recognition Phase. No matter how carefully one manipulates the graft, some damage to the cells and tissues always occurs. The damaged cells and cell debris are processed by phagocytosing cells, particularly macrophages, and displayed in such a way that they can be recognized by lymphocytes. Where this recognition occurs is not clear; the site probably varies, depending on the particular grafting conditions. In some instances, the initial encounter of lymphocytes with the antigen may occur directly in the graft (*peripheral recognition*); in others, it may occur in the circulatory system on the way to the lymphoid centers or in lymphoid centers themselves (*central recognition*). The two modes of recognition may have different consequences for the type of ensuing immunity, since the graft and the lymphoid center present completely different conditions for cell interaction. Central recognition can occur either in the spleen or in regional lymph nodes, and these two manners of recognition again may stimulate somewhat different responses.

Amplification Phase. The initial recognition of alloantigen involves only a few cells, which alone cannot deal with such a massive foreign body as the graft. Hence, the reaction must be amplified. The activated lymphocytes proliferate and multiply; they also release substances that affect migration of other cells and activate them. The activated cells interact in a complex way and set different defense mechanisms in motion. Everything is mobilized—macrophages, T lymphocytes,

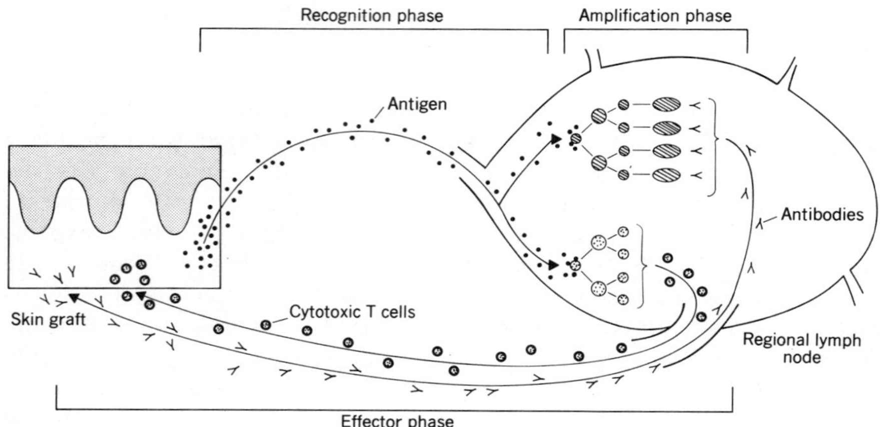

Figure 12.16. The three phases of allograft reaction.

granulocytes, B lymphocytes, natural killer cells, and perhaps other cells we do not yet know. As a result of this general mobilization, whole armies of cells become ready to attack the "enemy."

Effector Phase. What maneuvers the armies of cells use to destroy the foreign graft are not known. According to one hypothesis, the armies reach the graft via blood vessels, infiltrate the tissues of the graft, and destroy them in hand-to-hand combat, so to speak—that is, by direct cytotoxic killing. According to another hypothesis, the cell armies primarily attack the endothelial lining of the blood vessels in the graft, clog the disrupted vessels, cut off the blood supply, and lay siege to the graft. Deprived of nutrients, the grafted cells die of starvation and are removed by the body's scavenger cells. It is likely that both mechanisms play a role in graft rejection and that specific circumstances determine which of the two prevails. The actual killing of graft cells (either in blood vessels or in the graft parenchyma) can be mediated by effector cells (e.g., cytotoxic T lymphocytes, K cells, and activated macrophages), by soluble factors (e.g., lymphotoxin), or by antibodies and complement. Part of the killing is specific, directed against cells carrying foreign antigens; the other part is nonspecific and may include the host's own cells (innocent bystanders).

12.9.4 Genetics of Graft Rejection

Transplantation Laws

The primary genetic rule of transplantation is that *a graft is rejected whenever it possesses H antigens absent in the recipient.* This rule can be expanded into five *laws of transplantation* (Fig. 12.17):

Grafts within an inbred strain (syngeneic grafts) succeed.

Grafts between different inbred strains (allografts) fail.

Grafts from either inbred parent strain to the F_1 hybrid succeed, but grafts in the reverse direction fail.

Grafts from F_2 or subsequent F generations to F_1 hybrids succeed.

Grafts from either inbred parent strain succeed in some members of an F_2 generation, but fail in others. Also, grafts from one inbred parent strain succeed in some members and fail in others of a backcross generation produced by crossing the F_1 hybrid to the opposite parent strain.

The laws are based on the assumption that *H* genes are codominant, and that an F_1 hybrid expresses both alleles at each *H* locus. This assumption is supported by a large body of experimental data.

There are many exceptions to the laws, the most important being that they do not apply to transplantation between individuals of different sexes. Since both the Y and X chromosomes determine H antigens, the

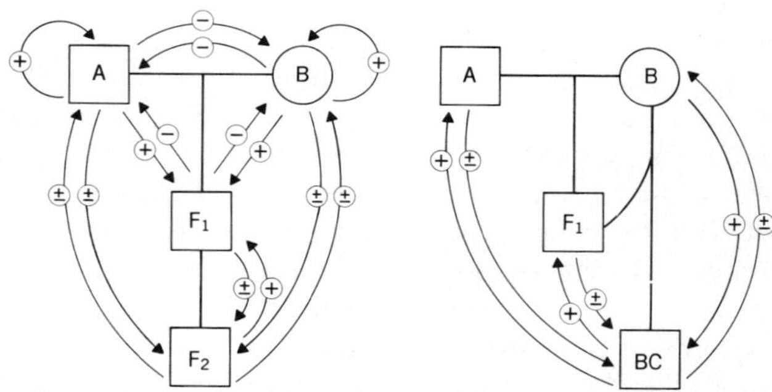

Figure 12.17. Laws of transplantation. A and B are individuals of two inbred strains. F_1, F_2, and BC are individuals of the first filial, second filial, and backcross generations, respectively. The arrows indicate the direction of grafting; + and − signify acceptance and rejection of a graft, respectively. ± indicates that some grafts are accepted while others are rejected.

presence or absence of sex-linked histocompatibility genes must be taken into account in a grafting experiment. The outcome of transplantation across the sex-linked histocompatibility barrier is shown diagrammatically in Figure 12.18. To provide for the sex difference, the transplantation laws must be modified as follows:

Within an inbred strain, grafts from females to males succeed, whereas grafts from males to females may be rejected.

Grafts from the female parent to a male or female F_1 recipient succeed, whereas grafts from the male parent to a male or female F_1 recipient may be rejected.

Histocompatibility Loci

Having discussed the response that the products of histocompatibility loci induce, we now turn our attention to the loci themselves.

Number of Histocompatibility Loci. There are several methods one can use to determine this number; here we shall describe only one, based on genetic segregation analysis. We shall explain this method by describing what results to expect when two strains differ in one, two, three, or more *H* loci.

Consider first two inbred strains differing in one *H* locus, *H-*1. If one strain is *aa* and the other *bb* (where *a* and *b* are alleles at the *H-*1 locus), the following segregation occurs in the F_2 generation:

		F_1 parent one	
		a	*b*
F_1 parent two	*a*	*aa*	*ab*
	b	*ab*	*bb*

If the F_2 mice are now grafted with skin from the *aa* strain, the *aa* and *ab* segregants will accept the grafts, and the *bb* segregants will reject them. Thus, three-quarters, or $(\frac{3}{4})^1$, of the F_2 mice accept the grafts from one of the two inbred grandparents.

If two inbred strains differ at two *H* loci (*H-*1 with alleles *a* and *b*, and *H-*2 allelex *x* and *y*), and if the strains' genotypes are *aaxx* and *bbyy*, then the F_2 animals segregate as follows:

		F_1 parent one			
		ax	*ay*	*bx*	*by*
F_1 parent two	*ax*	**aaxx**	**aaxy**	**abxx**	**abxy**
	ay	**aaxy**	*aayy*	**abxy**	*abyy*
	bx	**abxx**	**abxy**	*bbxx*	*bbxy*
	by	**abxy**	*abyy*	*bbxy*	*bbyy*

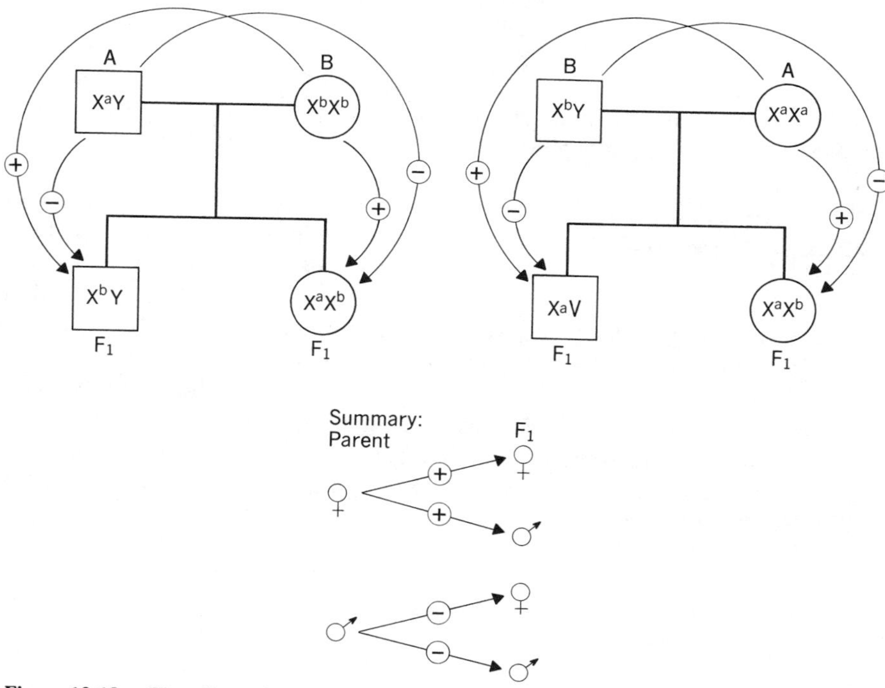

Figure 12.18. The effect of sex on the outcome of grafting. A and B, two inbred strains; F_1, first filial generation; X and Y, the two sex chromosomes (*a* and *b* indicate their origin from A or B parent, respectively). Direction of grafting is indicated by arrows. + and −, acceptance and rejection of a graft, respectively.

After grafting with skin from the *aaxx* strain, only those F_2 segregants carrying both the *a* and *x* alleles (boldface in the table above) accept grafts; all the others reject them. Thus, nine-sixteenths, or $(\frac{3}{4})^2$, of the F_2 mice accept the parental graft.

Following this approach, we can demonstrate that for three *H* genes the proportion of accepted grafts is $(\frac{3}{4})^3$, for four genes $(\frac{3}{4})^4$, and for *L* genes $(\frac{3}{4})^L$. The relationship between the number of successful grafts (*S*) and the number of *H* loci (*L*) in the P → F_2 grafting combination can therefore be expressed as

$$S = (\tfrac{3}{4})^L$$

and from this, *L* can be calculated:

$$L = \frac{ln\ (S)}{ln\ (\frac{3}{4})}$$

where *ln* is the natural logarithm.

Applying this method, investigators demonstrated that two inbred mouse or rat strains differ at a minimum of 15 *H* loci. Other approaches provided an estimate of some 30 loci, and still others of several hundred *H* loci. Since in the mouse, over 40 *H* loci (designated *H*-1 through *H*-40) have already been identified (with the help of congenic lines differing at these loci), the other approaches clearly provide a more realistic estimate. Evidently there is a large number of *H* loci, but whether this number reaches into the hundreds remains to be seen. (One difficulty in determining the number of loci is the fact that only polymorphic loci can be detected. If a given locus has only one allele and all individuals of a given species carry this allele, there is no simple way of identifying this locus.)

Major and Minor Histocompatibility Loci. In 1956 Sheila Counce and her co-workers described marked differences in the intensity of the allograft reaction directed against the antigens controlled by the first three *H* loci identified in the mouse—*H*-1, *H*-2, and *H*-3. For example, a tumor of C57BL/10 origin transplanted in a dose of 1000 cells per mouse to the B10.D2 congenic line that differs from C57BL/10 at the *H*-2 locus, was rejected by all the recipients; however, the same tumor in the same dose killed 90 percent of B10.LP mice that differed from the C57BL/10 mice at the *H*-3 locus. In the former case, the *H*-2 locus apparently was such a strong histocompatibility barrier that the tumor was unable to overcome it; in the latter case, the *H*-3 barrier was much weaker and so was overcome by the tumor in a large number of the inoculated mice. The distinction between a "strong" *H*-2 locus and a "weak" *H*-3 locus was confirmed by the results of a skin-grafting experiment. Skin grafts exchanged between mice differing in the *H*-2 complex survived an average of 8.5 days, whereas grafts exchanged between mice differing at the *H*-3 (or *H*-1) locus survived an average of 24 days or more. On the basis of these results, Counce and her co-workers defined a strong *H* locus as "a locus such that a difference between donor and host at this locus will prevent the progressive growth of nearly all tumor homotransplants and cause the rapid rejection of skin homotransplants," and a weak *H* locus as "a locus such that a difference between donor and host at this locus will permit the progressive growth of various tumor homotransplants and fail to cause the rapid rejection of skin homotransplants." At first, researchers thought the dividing line between major and minor loci to be rather arbitrary, but we now know that the two types of locus are fundamentally different in the way their products stimulate cytotoxic T cells: MHC-encoded molecules can be recognized by T cells alone, and they serve as restricting elements for the recognition of antigens; minor *H* locus-encoded molecules, on the other hand, are recognized by T lymphocytes only in the context of MHC molecules.

We need not say much here about the MHC (see Chapter 8), except that, at least in the mouse, both class I and class II molecules, alone or in combination, are capable of inducing strong allograft reaction. Instead, we shall devote the rest of this section to the minor histocompatibility loci.

Properties of Minor *H* Loci. The strength of minor *H* loci, as defined by the median skin-graft survival times (MST), is extremely variable. The grafts can be rejected as early as three weeks after transplantation or as late as 300 days; some may never be rejected. In general, the weaker the *H* barrier, the greater the interval between the onset and completion of graft rejection, and the broader the range of rejection times of individual grafts. The variability in rejection times of individual grafts is caused by environmental, rather than genetic factors.

Small skin grafts are often rejected more rapidly than large ones. It is conceivable that large grafts confront the host with a larger antigen dose and thus induce transient tolerance in the host, particularly in very weak combinations. Antigen dose is probably also responsible for the slower rejection of grafts from heterozygous, as opposed to homozygous, donors.

Antigenic strength is not so much a function of a particular *H* locus as of its particular allele. Alleles at the same locus are known to differ considerably in their effect on skin-graft survival, and may often be arranged in hierarchical order of decreasing immunological potency. For example, alleles at the *H*-1 locus can be arranged in the following order—$H\text{-}1^c \xrightarrow{15} H\text{-}1^b > H\text{-}1^b \xrightarrow{25} H\text{-}1^a > H\text{-}1^a \xrightarrow{100} H\text{-}1^b > H\text{-}1^b \xrightarrow{250}$ H-1^c—where numbers above the arrows indicate MSTs in days. The effect of individual *H* loci is additive, which means that a graft differing from the host at two loci is often rejected faster than a graft differing at either one of the two.

Nature of Minor Histocompatibility Loci. Little is known about the molecules encoded by minor histocompatibility loci. They are probably membrane-bound and present on several tissues (although minor H molecules specific, for example, for skin cells have also been described). Although claims have been made from time to time of successful serological detection of minor histocompatibility antigens, a routine, reproducible method of such detection is not available. Why it is so difficult to produce antibodies to minor H antigens is not known.

The function of minor H antigens is also unknown, but it is unlikely that they are primarily concerned with transplantation *per se*. They may be a diverse group of molecules participating in various cellular housekeeping functions and their antigenicity may come only incidentally, perhaps as a result of their expression in the plasma membrane.

12.9.5 Organ Transplantation in Humans

How do these findings, made with experimental animals, primarily mouse inbred strains, apply to an essentially outbred species such as the human? An immunologist would predict that, with the exception of a few privileged types of graft, all transplants made between unrelated human individuals would fail unless a way of suppressing the allograft reaction were found. There are so many different *HLA* haplotypes in the human population and individuals differ in so many minor *H* loci that the chances of finding genetically matched donor-recipient combinations are extremely small. Ignoring this pessimistic prediction, clinicians went ahead and attempted transplantation of all the organs they could lay their hands on. Their justifications for this decision were first, that they could, by HLA typing, attempt at least partial matching of MHC loci; second, they could try to control the remaining histoincompatibility by immunosuppressive drugs; and third, they could hope that some of the strict requirements for skin graft-recipient matching would not apply to organ transplantation. It is difficult to evaluate—even now, after the organ transplantation fever of the Seventies has subsided—whether this decision was right. On the one hand, transplantation of organs, such as the kidney, has clearly prolonged for several years the life of countless patients and proved that there were unexplained variables in organ transplantation, often defying genetic restrictions. On the other hand, transplantation of other organs, such as the heart, gave unspectacular results, so that these transplantations are now attempted only rarely. Furthermore, even successful organ transplantation procedures usually allow merely prolonged, rather than permanent, graft survival. When one adds to these difficulties the widespread shortage of organs available and suitable for transplantation, one must conclude that the problems of replacement surgery are far from being solved.

What role does *HLA* (*tissue*) *typing* play in clinical organ transplantation? We shall cite statistics below to demonstrate that, for some organs, at least, even partial HLA matching improves the chances of transplant survival. Despite these positive indications, surgeons often do not follow the recommendations of tissue-typing laboratories and choose genetically less favorable donor-recipient combinations for transplantation. Why? The selection of an organ donor is a complex decision, requiring the surgeon to take many parameters into account. The genetic disparity between donor and recipient is only one of these; others are the patient's disease, the patient's general health status, the prospects of survival, and age. When the surgeon weighs these parameters against each other, he is often forced to go against the advice of the tissue typist.

We shall now briefly evaluate the results obtained with individual organs. We begin with kidney transplantation, which, of the nonprovileged organs, has been the most successful and widely practiced form of organ grafting.

Kidney Transplantation

Kidneys for transplantation are donated either by the patient's relatives (parents, siblings) or by unrelated individuals. The former are provided by living donors, the latter by cadavers. The impact of HLA matching on graft survival in these two situations differs considerably. When the donor is a sibling who shares a complete set of HLA antigens with the recipient, more than 90 percent of the transplants survive for more than two

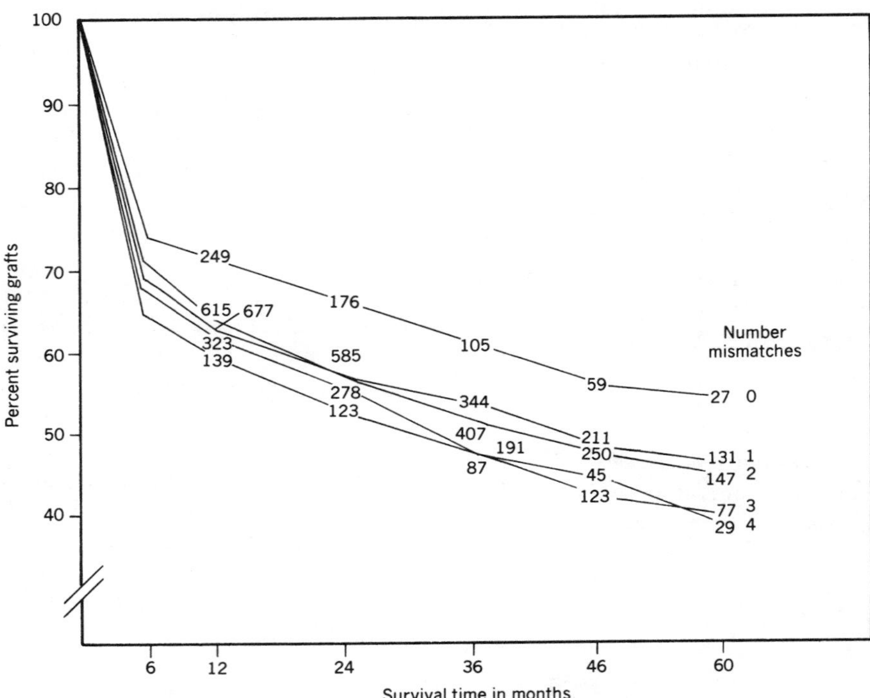

Figure 12.19. Kidney graft survival in human recipients matched with their donors for different numbers of HLA antigens. (From J. J. van Rood, G. G. Persijn, E. Goulmy, and B. A. Bradley: *Behring Inst. Mitt.* **63**:66–79, 1979.)

years, as compared to less than 50 percent survival in the mismatched group of patients (Fig. 12.19). The high survival rate of the matched transplants extends for more than six years. When the donor is an unrelated individual, the difference in survival between matched and mismatched groups is far less pronounced. One group of data (Fig. 12.19) shows that five years after transplantation, only about 15 percent of grafts with no HLA-A and HLA-B mismatches do better than grafts mismatched for three or four antigens. Figure 12.19 also shows that about one-third of the transplants fail within the first three to six months after transplantation, and that 40 percent of the completely mismatched grafts function well after five years. In other words, complete matching for HLA antigens does not guarantee long survival, and by contrast, complete mismatching does not always mean rapid graft rejection. These two points signify the importance of factors other than HLA antigens in the determination of graft survival. However, the primary reason for the striking difference in the behavior of grafts transplanted between a related and unrelated individual must be genetic. When two related individuals are serologically typed as HLA identical, they are truly identical. But two unrelated individuals typed as sharing all four HLA-A and -B antigens need not be identical: currently available serological methods simply may not be sensitive enough to detect minor genetic variations in the HLA-A and -B molecules—variations that could play an important role in the induction of cellular immunity. Furthermore, HLA-A- and -B-identical siblings are probably also identical at all other *HLA* loci; such is not the case, however, with unrelated individuals. Finally, siblings can also be expected to differ in fewer minor histocompatibility loci than unrelated individuals.

Originally, HLA typing of unrelated individuals involved only *HLA-A* and *-B* loci; later, the typing tests were extended to include HLA-D and HLA-DR antigens. Matching for one or two DR antigens improves the chance of graft survival to about 80 percent at one year (as compared to about 60 percent when matching involves only HLA-A and HLA-B antigens). Some improvement of graft survival was also obtained after matching for ABO blood groups. This result is surprising, since blood group antigens are polysaccharides, which would not be expected to induce cellular immunity.

One of many variables affecting kidney transplant survival is blood transfusion. Paradoxically, kidney grafts in patients who have received one transfusion before transplantation often survive longer than those grafted into patients who have received no transfusion. One would expect that the transfusion would induce immunity to allogeneic cells, but instead, it assumes a protective role. The mechanism of this protection remains to be defined.

Cornea Transplantation

The cornea, the transparent membrane of the eye, is normally not perfused with blood and does not contain lymphatics, so is not easily accessible to immune cells; when transplanted, it enjoys the status of a privileged graft. Furthermore, corneas can be preserved at low temperatures and stored in *eye banks* for future use. Corneal transplantation is a relatively simple procedure and since tests for early detection of graft rejection are available, prompt treatment is possible. All these factors make transplantation of the cornea a highly successful technique. However, even in this favorable situations, graft rejection sometimes occurs, presumably because of damage to the grafting site inflicted by surgery.

Skin Transplantation

Although one of the oldest forms of tissue transplantation, skin grafting has the least favorable prognosis for success. In humans it seems to be subject to the same genetic restriction as in animals so that allografts invariably fail, even between related individuals. Only autografts are successful.

Heart Transplantation

Of the several hundred heart-transplanted patients, only about two dozen have lived as long as four years following transplantation. At best the success rate of heart transplants approaches that of kidney transplants from unrelated cadaver donors (for obvious reasons, related donors are usually not available). However, in comparison to kidney transplantation, heart transplantation is handicapped by the absence of an artificial heart, which, like the artificial kidney, would keep the patient alive until a suitable donor were found or if the first transplant failed. Heart transplantation is usually the last resort, employed when other possibilities have been exhausted. At this terminal stage, the patient is often so sick that the operation itself carries with it a high mortality risk.

Bone Marrow Grafts

Bone marrow transplantation is a relatively simple procedure (bone marrow cells are obtained with a needle from large bones of the donor and injected intravenously into the recipient) and so has enormous potential. Unfortunately, this form of transplantation has a low success rate, not only because the graft itself is highly vulnerable to immune attack, but also because the bone marrow cells, being immunologically competent themselves, can attack the host. However, the success rate has been improving steadily over the last few years and even more pronounced improvement can be expected as new ways of reducing the HVGR and GVHR are found.

Transplantation of Other Organs

Many other organs, in addition to those mentioned, have been transplanted in humans: liver, lung, spleen, pancreas, intestine, tendon, bone, cartilage, blood vessels, and the larynx. The success rate has been variable but generally not very encouraging. The transplantation of some organs (e.g., liver or lung) still faces major surgical problems.

12.9.6 The Fetus as an Allograft

In a mating between an *aa* mother and *bb* father (where *a* and *b* are two alleles at a histocompatibility locus), the *ab* fetus represents an allograft because it bears alloantigens that the mother lacks (those controlled by the *b* allele). Why is the allograft not rejected? Several hypotheses have been proposed, and a discussion of some of the principal ones follows.

Barriers Separating Fetal and Maternal Tissues

From the earliest stage, the embryo is separated from the mother by special tissues that may shield it from an immune attack by the mother's defense mechanism (Fig. 12.20). In the primary follicles of the ovary, the maturing ovum is surrounded by follicular cells, which secrete a thick, translucent, extracellular mucopolysaccharide and mucoprotein coat—the *zona pellucida* (L. *pellucidus,* translucent). The ovum remains enveloped in the zona when it leaves the follicle and the ovary, and during fertilization the sperm must first penetrate this protective layer before it can reach the ovum. The zona is shed just prior to the embryo's implantation. It is possible that one of its functions is to shield the antigens of the embryo until other protective layers develop. Favoring this notion is the observation that an embryo transplanted to a heterotopic site becomes susceptible to an immune attack, presumably because it has lost its zona pellucida prematurely.

At implantation, the embryo acquires a new protec-

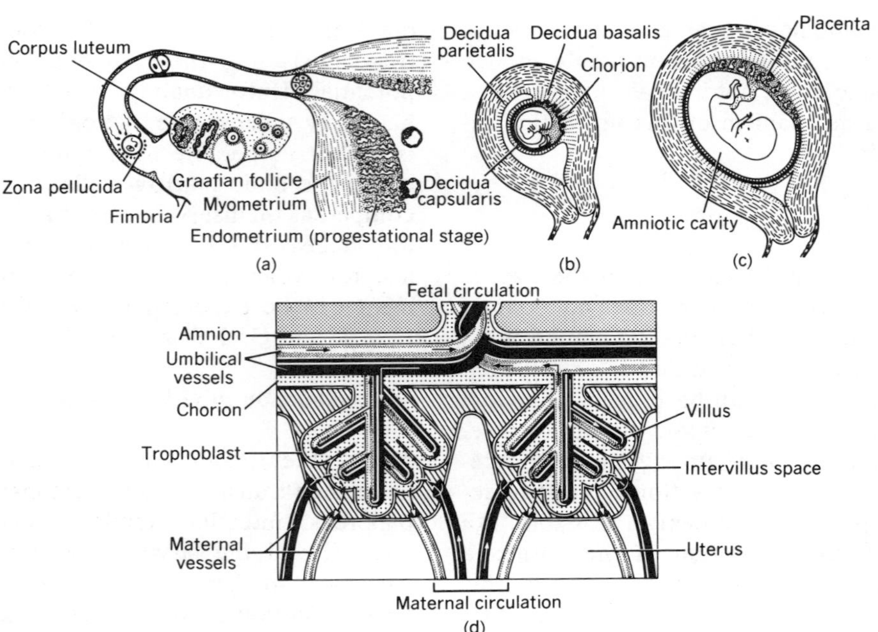

Figure 12.20. Membranes that may play a role in protecting the embryo from being rejected by the mother's immune system. (*a*) A fertilized oocyte protected by the zona pellucida moves through the oviduct toward the uterine lumen and implants itself. (*b*) Development of the chorion and decidua. (*c*) Development of the placenta. (*d*) Detailed view of placental circulation. (*a, b,* and *c* modified from J. Langman: *Medical Embryology*, 3rd ed. Williams and Wilkins, Baltimore, 1975; *d* from *Blood Group Antigens and Antibodies as Applied to Hemolytic Disease of the Newborn.* Ortho-Diagnostic, Raritan, New Jersey, 1968.)

tive layer. At this stage, the uterine wall consists of two main layers—the thick layer of muscles, or *myometrium* (Gr. *mys*, muscle, *metra*, uterus), and the inner mucous membrane, the *endometrium* (Gr. *endon*, within) (Fig. 12.20). Within a few hours after the embryo has contacted the uterine surface, the epithelial cells at the implantation site begin to loosen and degenerate. At the same time, active growth commences in the mucosa, and shortly an appreciable swelling develops. The swollen mucosa is referred to as *decidua* because it is eventually shed again (L. *decidus*, falling off). The thick decidual coating of the maternal uterus may act as a temporary immunological barrier during the time of implantation. But if it does, the protective action must be limited to the embryo, since other grafts transplanted onto the decidua apparently are rejected. (The uncertainty about this conclusion stems from the fact that these experiments are technically difficult because of the short duration of the decidual reaction—often shorter than the graft's normal median survival time.)

When it reaches the uterine cavity, the embryo has the appearance of a hollow sphere (blastocyst), differentiated into a knot of cells (inner cell mass) at one pole with a layer of *trophoblast cells* making up the rest of the sphere's wall (Fig. 12.20, see also Chapter 4). As the trophoblast contacts the uterine cell wall, the trophoblastic cells proliferate rapidly and form a multinucleate mass in which no cell boundaries are discernible. As the embryo sinks into the uterine wall, it becomes completely closed by the trophoblast, which forms an interface between the maternal and embryonic tissues. The trophoblast is uniquely qualified by its location to act as an anatomical barrier between the mother and the conceptus, provided it is nonantigenic to the mother itself. The antigenicity or nonantigenicity of the trophoblast has been the subject of prolonged and still unresolved controversy. Clearly, some cells of the multilayered trophoblast do carry histocompatibility antigens, while others either completely lack or have only very low levels of them. The contention that the poorly antigenic cells form an effective barrier between the mother and the fetus has not yet been proved.

At later stages of embryonic development, the outermost fetal membranes (trophoblasts, chorion, allantois) fuse with part of the uterine mucosa to form an organ of metabolic exchange between fetus and mother, the *placenta* (the Latin name for a cake, used in reference to the organ's characteristic shape). In the placenta, fetal and maternal blood vessels are apposed yet clearly separated: fetal and maternal blood do not mix (Fig. 12.20). Electron microscopic studies reveal that many cells on the fetal side of the placenta, particularly the giant trophoblastic cells, are surrounded by a layer of amorphous, electron-dense *fibrinoid material*, varying in thickness from 0.1 to 2 μ and composed of mucoproteins and mucopolysaccharides rich in hyaluronic and sialic acids. Some immunologists believe that the fibrinoid layer of the placenta masks histocompatibility antigens of the embryo, preventing their recognition by maternal immune cells. Supporting this interpretation is the observation that dissolution of the fibrinoid by neuraminidase increases the antigenicity of trophoblastic cells. However, the barrier between the fetus and the mother is not impenetrable. Using chromosomal markers or radioactively labeled cells, investigators have repeatedly demonstrated the presence of fetal cells in the mother's blood and maternal cells in the fetal circulation; so some limited exchange of cells, particularly blood elements (erythrocytes, leukocytes, and platelets), must occur across the placenta. Additional evidence for such exchange of cells is the fact that the serum of multiparous women often contains antibodies to red blood cell (Rh) and leukocyte (HLA) antigens (see Chapter 14). Production of such antibodies is presumably induced by cells or cell fragments that originate in the fetus and are brought by blood into the mother's lymphoid organs. However, despite this leakage, the placenta is an effective barrier between the mother and the fetus—a barrier that may also isolate the two organisms immunologically.

Antigenic Immaturity of the Fetus

The fact that alloantigens controlled by the major histocompatibility complex are either completely absent or present only in small amounts on cells of the early embryo has led some immunologists to suggest that this poor MHC antigenicity might be the main reason that the embryo is not rejected. It is now clear, however, that after implantation, the MHC antigenicity of the embryo steadily increases, as can be demonstrated by a variety of methods, including the induction of allograft reaction by embryonic tissues injected into adult recipients. Furthermore, many minor histocompatibility antigens are probably already present in midterm embryos. Antigenic immaturity alone, therefore, cannot explain the mother's immunological tolerance of the embryo.

Altered Immunological Responsiveness of the Mother

Another possibility is that the embryo transiently lowers the mother's immunological responsiveness. The lowering may be either specific, affecting only responsiveness to paternal antigens, or nonspecific, affecting general immune responsiveness. It is known, for example, that immune response can be influenced by hormones, and since the hormone levels change during pregnancy, the changes could conceivably reflect on the ability of the mother to react against the fetal allograft. However, experiments designed to demonstrate altered immune responsiveness in pregnant females have given equivocal results. Some investigators have reported prolonged survival of paternal allografts placed on pregnant females in comparison with grafts transplanted on nonparous females, while other investigators found no difference in the mean survival time of the graft in the two groups. Furthermore, even in experiments in which prolongation was observed, the effect was usually only marginal, clearly insufficient for the maintenance of the fetal allograft through the entire pregnancy. The marginal immunosuppression of pregnant females can be explained by a variety of mechanisms such as immunological enhancement, presence of blocking antibodies, or induction of a temporary state of immunological tolerance. The significance of this immunosuppression for the maintenance of the fetal allograft is doubtful. In no instance has convincing evidence been presented for a general immunological unresponsiveness of pregnant females.

Interpretation

Despite much speculation and experimentation, the question of why a pregnant female does not reject her fetus remains largely unanswered. Of the three main hypotheses discussed, clearly the one presupposing immunological isolation of the embryo is the most attractive. After all, we know that an organism can effectively isolate certain organs, such as the brain or testes, in such a way that antigens expressed by these tissues and organs remain inaccessible to the immune system. There is no reason that it cannot wall off the embryo in a similar way. The hypothetical barrier must lie in the protective membranes surrounding the embryo, but what its exact nature might be remains to be determined. The other factors mentioned (lowered antigenicity of the embryo and reduced immunological responsiveness of the mother) may contribute to the isolation, but it is unlikely that they play a major role in the maintenance of the graft.

12.9.7 Physiological Meaning of the Allograft Reaction

What does a mouse or human being need the allograft reaction for? Theoretically there are three possible answers to this question. First, the function of the allograft reaction might indeed be to protect an organism against allografts. Although the fetus is the only natural mammalian allograft known and an immune response against the fetus is not desired, one can argue that other allografts are not normally found *because* the allograft reaction is so effective in destroying allogeneic cells before they can establish themselves in the body. Possible candidates for such natural allografts are tumor cells. If the allograft reaction did not exist, would tumors be a contagious disease? Some immunologists have thought so and cited as evidence for their contention the so-called *venereal tumors* in dogs—tumors of the genital tract transmitted from one individual to another by sexual intercourse. However, inbred animals, which are not separated from one another by any histoincompatible barriers, have not shown any evidence of spontaneous tumor transmission between individuals. In fact, the experimental work on tumor transplantation has revealed that it is difficult to transfer a newly arisen tumor to another individual with an inoculum that consists of only a few cells, even when the individual is completely compatible with the donor. It is thus unlikely that the function of the allograft reaction is to protect mammals from allografted tissues. The venereal tumors in the dog are an exception that has no bearing on the function of the allograft reaction, for these tumors transgress histocompatibility barriers and the allograft reaction fails to protect new hosts against them.

Second, one can argue that the allograft reaction is a biological leftover (atavism) from the time when the vertebrate ancestors still led a sedentary life and needed a mechanism to prevent the fusion of individuals crowded into a small habitat (see Chapter 1). However, if such were the case, one would expect the allograft reaction to be the strongest among invertebrates and on the wane in vertebrates, where it is no longer needed. In fact, just the opposite is true. Although most invertebrates display some form of tissue incompatibility, one finds evidence for true allograft reaction only in the most advanced invertebrate phyla, the annelids and tunicates (see Chapter 1). And even in vertebrates, the vigor of the allograft reaction increases from cyclostomes to mammals—a trend opposite that expected if the allograft reaction were retreating in its functional significance. These observations make the atavism hypothesis a highly unlikely explanation for the biological function of the allograft reaction.

That leaves us with the third possibility—that the allograft reaction is an experimental artifact. According to this hypothesis, the T cells responding to an allograft are meant for something else and they react with alloantigens because they confuse them with that something. One can imagine, for example, that there are sufficient similarities between MHC antigens and certain other antigens for a T cell to confuse the two. In other words, T cells may react with alloantigenic determinants because to them they look like other determinants of the antigenic universe. However, other versions of the artifact hypothesis are also possible and it remains for the experimentalist to prove which of the versions is correct.

12.9.8 Prevention of the Allograft Reaction

The allograft reaction is the transplant surgeon's greatest source of frustration: no matter how skillful his work, the reaction manages eventually to spoil its fruits. To minimize the effects of this undesired form of the body's defense reaction, the surgeon enlists the help of *immunosuppressive agents*, capable of lowering the immune response. An ideal immunosuppressive agent would be one that would reduce the vigor of the allograft reaction but would not affect other forms of the immune response. However, such a specific immunosuppressive agent has not yet been discovered. And what is more, immunologists even have a hard time coming up with an agent that would *nonspecifically* affect cells of the *immune system* but not other cells. Most of the agents now in use not only lower general body resistance to infection but also have other undesirable side effects. When used at a high dose, these agents are toxic for immune cells and many others; when used at too low a dose, they do not have the desired biological effect on the immune cells. So the surgeon always walks a thin line between administering too much or too little of a given agent.

We shall first discuss some of the available chemical immunosuppressive agents, then the physical agents (ionizing radiation), and finally ways to suppress the immune response by immunological means.

Chemical Immunosuppressive Agents

The four main groups of chemical immunosuppressives are alkylating agents, antimetabolites, corticosteroids, and antibiotics. Since the four groups differ in their properties and modes of action, we shall discuss them separately.

Alkylating Agents. These compounds transfer alkyl groups (radicals with the general formula C_nH_{2n+1}, derived from saturated aliphatic hydrocarbons by the removal of one hydrogen atom; examples of alkyl groups are methyl, $-CH_3$ or ethyl CH_3CH_2-) to other substances. According to the number of groups a single molecule can donate, alkylating agents can be monofunctional [e.g., $H_2N(CH_2CH_2Cl)$], bifunctional [e.g., $HN(CH_2CH_2Cl)_2$], or trifunctional [e.g., $N(CH_2CH_2Cl)_3$]. They often require chemical activation or enzymatic conversion before they can donate alkyl groups. When taken up by a cell, alkylating agents can act on the DNA, RNA, or proteins. DNA contains several sites vulnerable to attack by the alkylating agent, of which the most open is the nitrogen at position 7 in guanine:

O
C 6
N 7
HN 1   5 C
8 CH
H_2N—C 2   4 C
3 N   9 N
H

The alkylation of DNA can have one of the following consequences. First, the addition of the methyl or ethyl groups to guanine can cause it to behave as a base analogue of adenine and thereby produce pairing errors. Second, alkylated guanine may loosen its bonds with the sugar-phosphate backbone and leach out, thereby producing depurinated gaps in the DNA chain. The gaps, in turn, may interfere with DNA replication or cause shortening of the nucleotide chain. Third, bifunctional agents may bind simultaneously to both strands, crosslink them (Fig. 12.21), and so again block DNA replication. The consequences of RNA and protein alkylation remain to be determined.

Alkylating agents were the first drugs shown to interfere with immune reactions. A hint that they exert this effect was provided by grisly circumstances during World War I, when Germany employed one of these agents, sulfur mustard, as a means of chemical warfare. Autopsies of the poisoned soldiers revealed a characteristic dissolution of the lymphoid tissues, including bone marrow. When later immunologists localized immune-response capability to lymphoid tissues, they remembered this observation and thought of some more humane use for these drugs.

Alkylating agents disturb cell growth, mitosis, and differentiation. They preferentially affect rapidly proliferating cells, so lymphocytes are particularly susceptible to their action. Some agents induce doubling of cell volume with immediate arrest of cell division, while others, like X-rays, permit cells to undergo one or more divisions before they stop proliferating. Because of the many similarities between the biological action of alkylating agents and those of ionizing radiation (induction of hematological changes and intestinal lesions, suppression of antibody formation, induction of fetal abnormalities in pregnant females, inhibition of cell proliferation), the former are sometimes referred to as *radiomimetic agents* (Gr. *mimētikos*, imitative).

Alkylating agents act on both T and B cells but more

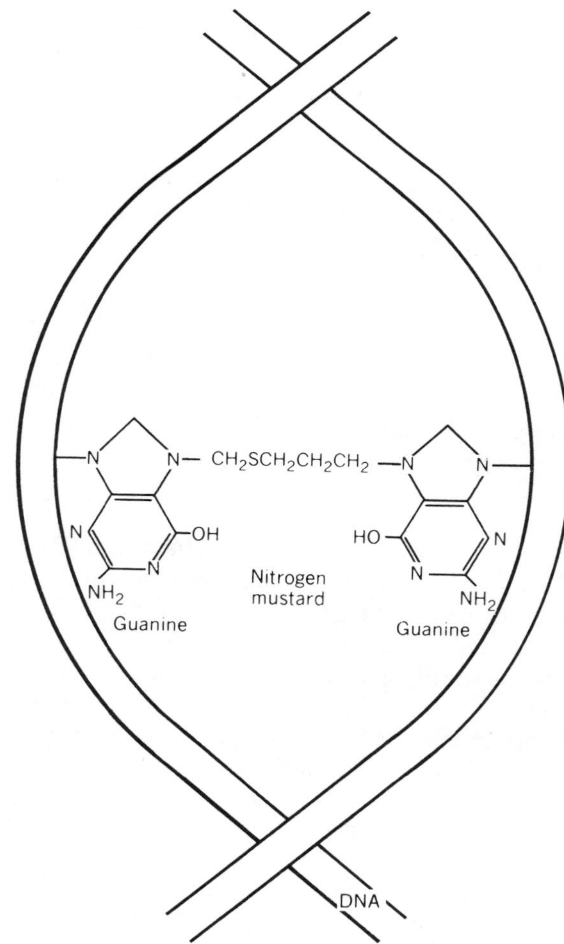

Figure 12.21. Crosslinking of two DNA chains by the reaction of nitrogen mustard with guanine in each chain.

strongly on B cells, especially in high doses, perhaps because the latter are metabolically more active than the former. To affect B cells without doing too much damage to T cells, one gives the host a high dose of the agent over a short period. Chronic treatment affects T cells as much as B cells, if not more so. As a consequence of a high-dose, short-term treatment, the host becomes depleted of lymphocytes in the regions of the lymph nodes normally occupied by B cells. Because of the preferential effect on B lymphocytes, alkylating agents are one of the most powerful inhibitors of antibody production; their effect on cellular immunity is not so pronounced.

The two alkylating agents most often used are cyclophosphamide and chlorambucil; a less frequently used drug is nitrogen mustard (Fig. 12.22). *Cyclophosphamide* (cytoxan, endoxan) must be metabolized in the liver and converted into an unidentified derivative before it is able to act on cells. For this reason it can safely be administered perorally and parenterally, but is ineffective when applied to cells in vitro. *Chlorambucil* has an advantage in that it causes fewer side effects than cyclophosphamide. *Nitrogen mustard* is too toxic for oral administration.

Antimetabolites. The idea behind the use of antimetabolites is to flood a cell or an organism with molecules, most of them synthetic, which resemble natural metabolites but are unable to perform the metabolites' function. Once these impostor molecules replace the natural metabolites, a blockage of a particular metabolic step follows; and if the fooled cell is a lymphocyte a way is found of suppressing the immune response. The three main groups of antimetabolites are molecules that function as antagonists of folic acid, pyrimidines, and purines.

Folic Acid Analogues. Folic acid is a broadly distributed vitamin first found in spinach leaves (L. *folium*, leaf); a deficiency results in a failure to grow. The folic acid molecule consists of three structural building blocks: a pteridine compound, *p*-aminobenzoic acid, and glutamic acid (Fig. 12.22). Its derivatives are involved in many one-carbon transfer reactions, notably in the synthesis of thymidilic acid required for DNA synthesis. Some of the enzymes involved in the production of folic-acid derivatives have a higher affinity for certain analogues of folic acid, notably aminopterin and amethopterin, than for their natural substrate. The analogues therefore compete successfully with the natural substrates for these enzymes, preventing normal synthesis of folic-acid derivatives and the growth of cells.

The two frequently used folic-acid analogues are amethopterin and aminopterin (Fig. 12.22). *Amethopterin* (methotrexate) inhibits a variety of chemical reactions and, through them, cell proliferation. It is better known as a cancer drug than as an immunosuppressive agent; it causes temporary remission of certain leukemias and choriocarcinomas. The latter are tumors derived from fetal membranes growing in the mother. They can thus be regarded as transplanted neoplasms; and it was this notion that inspired immunologists to test the effect of amethopterin on organ transplants. The tests revealed that the drug chiefly suppresses cellular immune responsiveness, although an effect on humoral response can also be demonstrated. The effects on antibody response vary with the species: the drug suppresses the response strongly in rats, mice, guinea pigs, and dogs, less strongly in humans, and weakly in rabbits. *Aminopterin* is structurally very similar to amethopterin (Fig. 12.22) and has similar effects, but its therapeutic index[3] is lower. Aminopterin also suppresses cellular immune response in rabbits.

Pyrimidine Analogues. Pyrimidines are nitrogenous bases found in nucleotides and nucleic acids. Three pyrimidines are commonly found—uracil (found in RNA), thymidine (found in DNA), and cytosine (found in both RNA and DNA; see Fig. 12.22). Synthetic analogues resembling naturally occurring pyrimidines act in one of two ways: they are incorporated into nucleic acid and cause structural disturbances, or they compete with the natural pyrmidines for enzymes involved in nucleotide synthesis and thus block metabolic reactions. An example of a pyrimidine analogue is the *cytosine arabinose* (ara-C; Fig. 12.22), an analogue of cytosine that blocks enzymatic formation of phosphorylated deoxycytidine derivatives from ribose-containing precursors. The drug must be phosphorylated intracellularly before becoming biologically active. It causes tumor regression, and depression of antibody formation and some forms of cellular immunity. Many other pyrimidine analogues are also available and sometimes used as immunosuppressive agents.

Purine Analogues. Purines, like pyrimidines, are nitrogenous bases of nucleotides and nucleic acids. The two main purines are adenine and guanine (Fig. 12.22). Purine analogues act in a way similar to that of

[3] *Therapeutic index* is the ratio of LD_{50} (*lethal dose*, one that is fatal to 50 percent of the test animals) to ED_{50} (*effective dose*, one that produces the desired effect in 50 percent of the test animals.

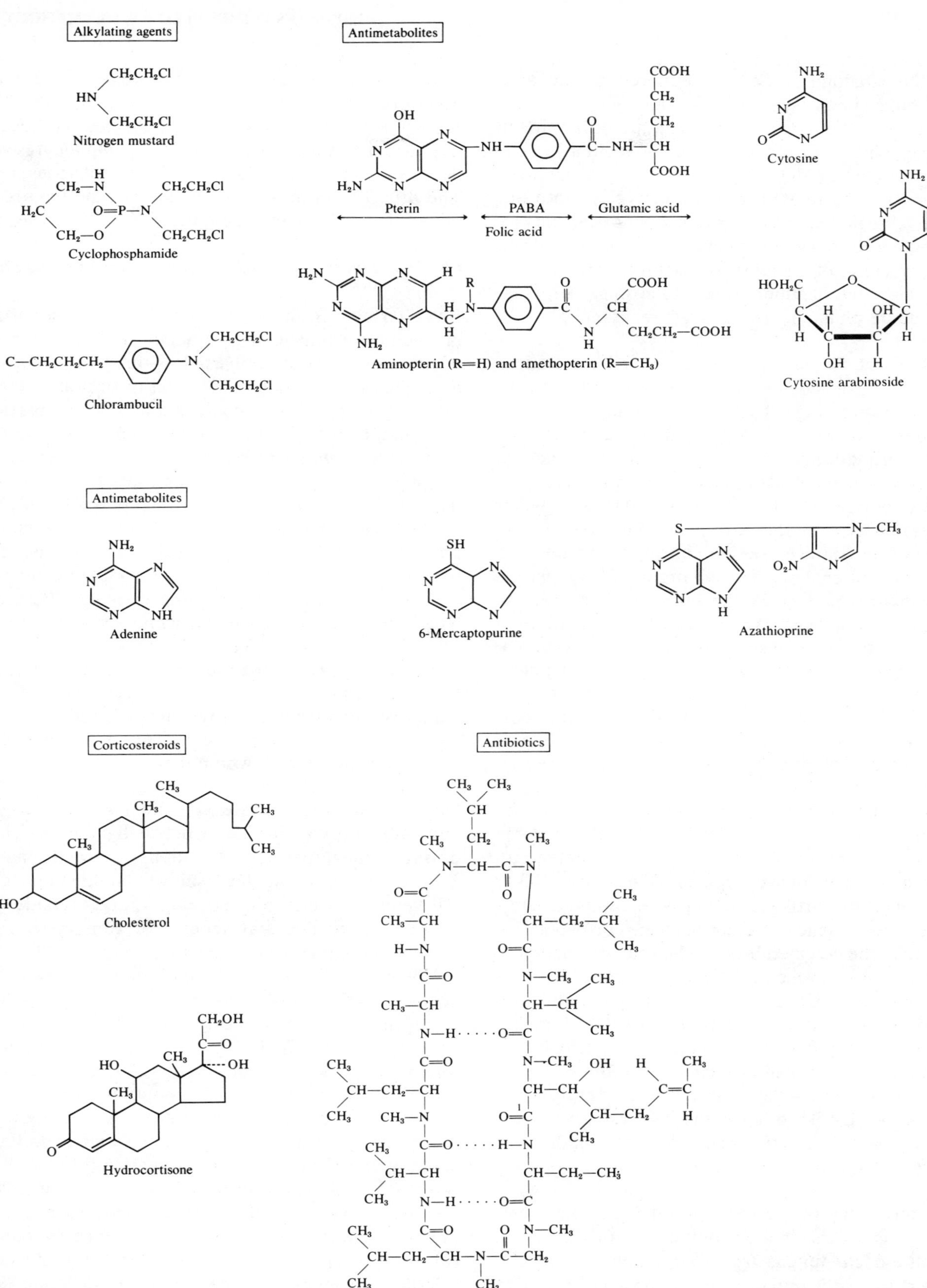

Figure 12.22. Structural formulas of some of the immunosuppressive agents.

pyrimidine analogues. Several hundred purine analogues have been synthesized, but only 3,6-mercaptopurine, 6-thioguanine, and azathiopurine are in wide use, chiefly in the treatment of leukemia. The precise manner of the drugs' action is still unclear. 6-*Mercaptopurine* (6-MP) must be converted into nucleotide to be biologically active. *Azathiopurine* acts by being catabolized slowly to 6-mercaptopurine. Both drugs preferentially suppress primary antibody response, although azathiopurine also strongly suppresses the acute phase of the allograft reaction.

Adrenocortical Steroids. Also called adrenocorticosteroids and corticosteroids, these are fatlike (cholesterol-derived; Fig. 12.22) compounds produced by the outer layer (cortex) of the adrenal gland (L. *ad*, toward, *ren*, kidney; i.e., glands located above the kidneys). Corticosteroids influence carbohydrate, protein, and purine metabolism; electrolyte and water balance; function of the cardiovascular system; and function of the kidneys, skeletal muscles, and nervous system. The adrenal cortex is an organ of homeostasis that maintains balance in the body, with respect to various functions and the chemical composition of fluids and tissues. It is responsible for the adaptation of the mammalian body to the constantly changing environment.

Of the more than 20 isolated steroids, the best known is *cortisone* (Fig. 12.22). Its two primary effects on the immune system are dissolution (lysis) of susceptible lymphocytes and anti-inflammatory action. The former effect is quite rapid: within an hour of administration, the nuclei of susceptible cells become pyknotic (they thicken and condense) and disintegrate, and the cells shed their cytoplasm. The susceptibility or resistance to cortisone action is apparently determined by the presence or absence of the corresponding receptors in the cell membrane. The selective action of cortisone is most pronounced in the thymus where, as was mentioned in Chapter 5, there are populations of cortisone-sensitive and cortisone-resistant lymphocytes. In its anti-inflammatory function, cortisone suppresses the development of local heat, redness, swelling, and tenderness—the characteristic symptoms of inflammation. Unlike other immunosuppressives, cortical steroids are effective regardless of whether the cells are in the replicative cycle.

Antibiotics. One of the most promising immunosuppressive agents is the antibiotic *cyclosporin A*, a metabolite of the fungus *Trichoderma polysporum*. Cyclosporin is a cyclic polypeptide composed of 11 amino acids. One amino acid has not been discovered in any other organisms and another occurs as a D, rather than the usual L optical isomer. The antibiotic is most active against antigen-stimulated T lymphocytes and does not seem to interfere with B-cell activities at all. The drug is still in a testing stage but the results obtained thus far are encouraging.

Physical Immunosuppressive Agents (*Ionizing Radiation*)

Basic Terms. Radiation can be of two types, particulate and electromagnetic. *Particulate radiation* consists of various subatomic particles—protons, neutrons, electrons, beta particles (identical to orbital electrons but originating in the nucleus), and alpha particles (helium nuclei consisting of two protons and two neutrons). *Electromagnetic radiation* is wavelike in nature, although it can also be viewed as consisting of discrete quanta of energy (photons). The name is derived from the fact that the waves have both electrical and magnetic components. Based on their wavelengths, electromagnetic radiation can be arranged into an *electromagnetic spectrum* of progressively increasing length and decreasing energy: gamma rays—X-rays—ultraviolet radiation—visible light—infrared light—short radio waves—long radio waves (Fig. 12.23). The two sorts of radiation in the shortest region of the spectrum (gamma rays and X-rays) are referred to as *ionizing radiation* because they can cause ejection of electrons from atoms with which they collide and the conversion of these atoms to ions. *Gamma rays*, which have the shortest wavelength and highest energy of any radiation classified as electromagnetic, originate during radioactive disintegration of atomic nuclei. *X-rays* are emitted as the result of a sudden change in the velocity of electrons striking a target (anode) in a vacuum tube. The wavelengths of gamma rays and X-rays overlap to a certain extent (Fig. 12.23).

The effect of ionizing radiation on living matter depends on the dose, which can be measured in roentgens or rads. One *roentgen* (R), the unit of administered radiation, is the amount of radiation required for the formation of 2.083×109 ion pairs per cubic centimeter of air at standard temperature and pressure (0°C and 760 mm Hg); expressed on an energy basis, this value is 83 erg/g. One *rad*, the unit of radiation actually *absorbed* by the living matter (the name derives from *r*adiation-*a*bsorbed *d*ose), is the energy imparted to matter by the particles per unit mass of irradiated material (1 rad = 100 erg/g). Since direct measurement of the absorbed dose is difficult, it is usually calculated from measurement of ionization in air using

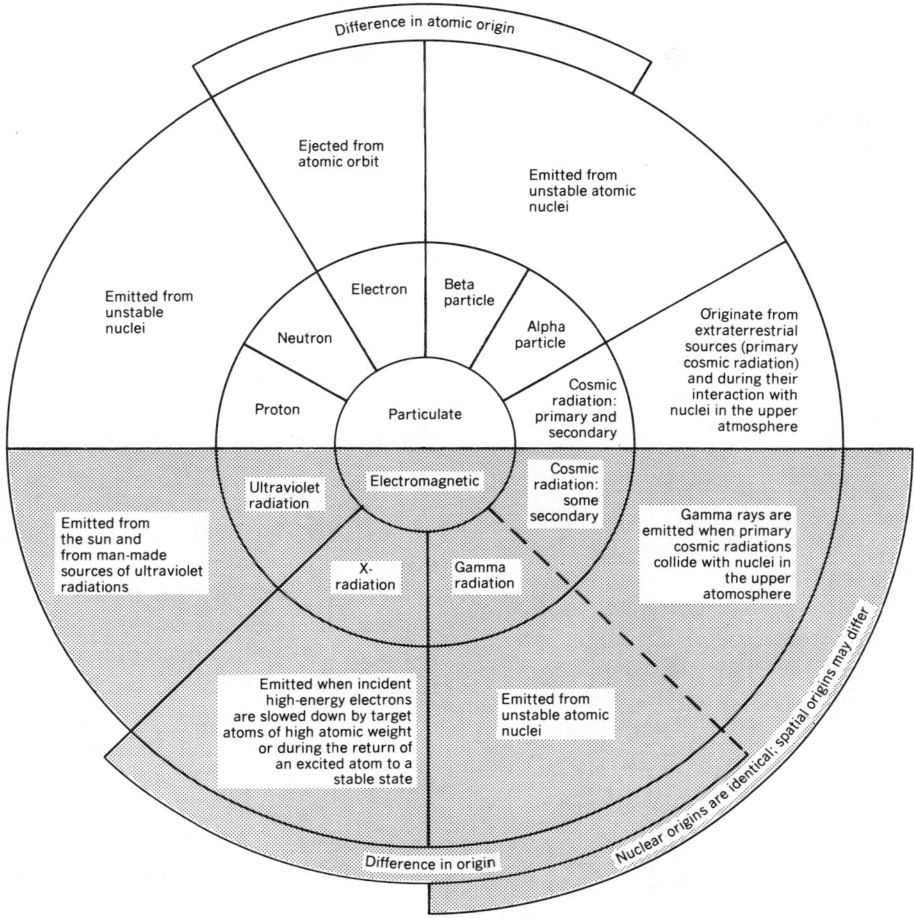

Figure 12.23. Types and origins of ionizing radiation. (From B. C. Block: *Man, Microbes and Matter*. McGraw-Hill, New York, 1975.)

the formula $Dm = fm \times R$, where D is the absorbed dose of medium (m), f the absorbed dose in rads per roentgen of administration dose, and R the administration dose in roentgens. The f value of various media can be found in standard tables.

Sensitivity of Different Cells to Ionizing Radiation. The use of ionizing radiation as an immunosuppressive agent stems from the original observation by E. Benjamin and E. Sluka in 1908 that exposure of rabbits to a certain dose of X-rays impairs these animals' ability to produce antibodies without seriously endangering the recipients' well-being. This observation, later confirmed by many other investigators, suggested that lymphoid and hematopoietic cells were more susceptible to the effect of ionizing radiation than were other cells in the body. However, the selective effect of ionizing radiation on cells is strictly dose-dependent. In the mouse, the lowest dose after which damage to the lymphoid system can be detected histologically is about 25 R. Animals recover from the effect of this *minimal dose* within one or two days after irradiation. Doses between 250 and 600 R cause extensive damage to the lymphoid system (decrease in the number of circulating lymphocytes and destruction of lymph node germinal centers), but usually do not cause death. Animals irradiated with this *sublethal dose* usually recover within one to three weeks after irradiation. Irradiation of mice with a dose of 750 to 1000 R results in massive destruction of lymphocytes in lymphoid organs and hematopoietic cells in the bone marrow, and death of the animals because of lack of hematopoiesis. This *lethal dose* of radiation, however, still does not seriously injure other cells, and the irradiated animal can be saved by the injection of normal bone marrow cells. Irradiation of mice with a dose greater than 1000

R causes irreparable damage to the gastrointestinal, nervous, and other organ systems. Animals exposed to this *supralethal radiation dose* can no longer be saved by bone marrow transplantation. Generally, rapidly proliferating cells are more radiosensitive than are nondividing cells. In the lymphohemopoietic system, the most radiosensitive are lymphocytes and hematopoietic cells; plasma cells are considerably less sensitive, and macrophages are relatively radioresistant.

Nature of Radiation Damage. The effects of ionizing radiation on cells are complex and variable. The main targets of radiation damage within a cell are the nucleus and the membrane system. In the nucleus, ionizing radiation causes alterations in DNA structure similar to those described for alkylating agents. The defects in DNA structure then result in faulty reading of the messenger RNA and thus in metabolic disturbances. Structurally altered DNA also fails to replicate normally, preventing the cells from dividing. In the membrane compartment, the high energy of ionizing radiation alters the atoms and results in membrane rupture, changes of membrane permeability, fluid mixing, and loss of osmotic balance. The rupture of lysosomal membranes leads to the release of hydrolases, which then attack the cell's own components. The destruction of mitochondrial membranes results in a dramatic depression of adenosine triphosphate (ATP) synthesis and, in turn, reduction of the overall rate of cell metabolism because of a lack of necessary energy. Defects in the rough endoplasmic reticulum cause slowing of protein synthesis and of intracisternal movement of molecules. The net result of all these lesions is swift cell death.

Radiation Chimeras. An animal that has recovered from the effects of a lethal radiation dose by virtue of cell transplantation is referred to as a *radiation chimera* because it carries hematopoietic and lymphoid cells of one individual and all other cells of anoher individual.[4] Radiation chimeras can be produced by inoculation into the lethally irradiated mice of bone marrow, fetal liver, or even spleen cells—that is, of cell populations containing hematopoietic stem cells. Depending on the genetic relationship between the donor and host, one can distinguish three types of radiation chimera: syngeneic, allogeneic, and xenogeneic. In *syngeneic chimeras*, the transplantation of bone marrow cells from a genetically identical individual prevents a failure of hematopoiesis in the irradiated host, but does not ameliorate the damage caused by irradiation to other tissues, particularly the gonads, lens epithelium, and melanocytes of the skin. Consequently, the chimeras usually become sterile, blind (the eye lens looses its transparency, a phenomenon referred to as *cataract*), and grey. Another delayed effect of radiation is nephrosclerosis, an induration of the kidney from an overgrowth and contraction of the interstitial connective tissue. These and other effects shorten the life span of radiation chimeras by about two-thirds in comparison to normal animals.

In *allogeneic chimeras*, produced by bone marrow transplantation from genetically dissimilar individuals of the same species, the initial repopulation of the host's hematopoietic tissues is as successful as in syngeneic chimeras. In mice, the irradiated animals survive the 14-day period during which virtually all the noninjected control mice die because of hematopoiesis failure. Survival beyond the two-week period depends largely on the degree of donor-recipient histoincompatibility. Most chimeras made between individuals incompatible at the major histocompatibility complex die between 30 and 60 days after irradiation; chimeras made between individuals compatible at single minor histocompatibility loci survive longer (Fig. 12.24). The death of the allogeneic chimeras is preceded by characteristic symptoms, called the *secondary* or *homologous disease*. The name "Secondary" derives from the fact that biologists once thought that the symptoms represented a secondary phase of radiation injury (the first phase being damage to the hematopoietic system); the name "homologous" goes back to the time when it was thought that the symptoms resembled those occurring in nonirradiated recipients injected with homologous (allogeneic) cells. The onset of the secondary disease is highly variable: sometimes it starts in the first week after irradiation but usually not for 30 days.

During the first week after irradiation, the mice lose weight sharply, then, during the next week, they begin to recover, and the syngeneic chimeras eventually reach normal weight after several weeks. In allogeneic chimeras, on the other hand, the weight begins to drop again about three weeks after irradiation and may become as low as 50 percent of the normal weight. Concurrently with weight loss the animals acquire chronic diarrhea, assume a characteristic hunch posture, and begin to lose hair. Postmortem examination of mice

[4] To the ancient Greeks, a chimera was a mythical, fire-breathing monster, whose anatomical features were a blend of lion, she-goat, and serpent.

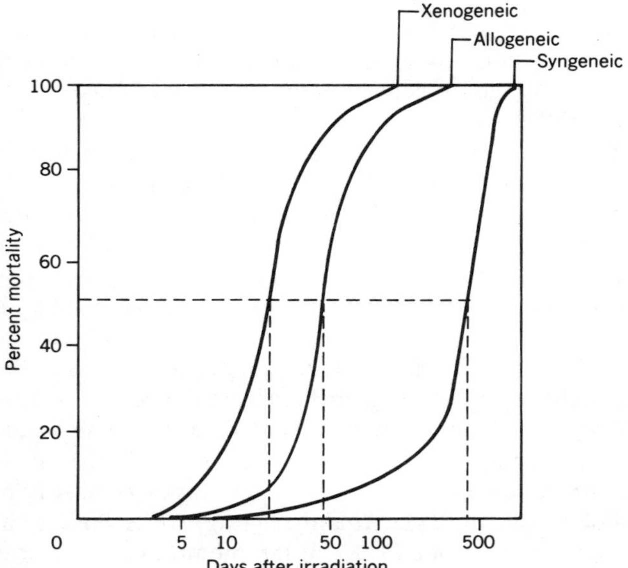

Figure 12.24. Survival rates of lethally irradiated mice injected with syngeneic, allogeneic, and xenogeneic bone marrow. (Based on the data of D. W. H. Barnes, J. F. Loutit, and H. S. Micklem: *in* M. Hašek, A. Lengerová, and M. Vojtíšková (Eds.): *Symposium on Mechanisms of Immunological Tolerance*, pp. 371–377. Czechoslovak Academy of Science, Prague, 1962.)

that have died of the secondary disease shows dramatic depletion of lymphocytes in lymphoid organs—lymph nodes, spleen, and thymus.

There has been a long debate about the disease's causes. It is now clear that it results primarily from the attack on the host tissues by the grafted allogeneic lymphocytes (graft-versus-host reaction; see Section 12.10). The attack disturbs the body's normal physiology and leaves the animal vulnerable to many infections. The ill effects of the secondary disaese can be reduced by eliminating T lymphocytes from the bone marrow prior to its inoculation into the irradiated host—a trick introduced into radiation chimera studies by Harald von Boehmer. In *xenogeneic chimeras*, produced by inoculation of cells from another species, the life spans of the irradiated animals are even shorter than in the allogeneic chimeras (Fig. 12.24). Here, in addition to immunological disparity, the two types of tissue may also be physiologically incompatible. Xenogeneic chimeras can be produced only between related species, such as the rat and mouse, and even in these combinations most of the animals die within three weeks of irradiation.

Clinical Use. In a clinical situation, lethal, whole-body irradiation is used only in extreme cases, where little hope exists that the patient's life can be prolonged in some other way. More common is the use of fractionated, small doses distributed over a long period. A rationale for this radiation regimen is the assumption that after each small radiation dose the non-hematopoietic, nonlymphoid cells will have enough time to repair the damage before the next dose is administered. There are reports that this treatment may also favor the induction of specific unresponsiveness to an allogeneic transplant. To minimize the damage to them, sensitive nonlymphoid organs must be shielded with protective lead casing.

Immune Reagents

Immune reagents can suppress defense reactions either specifically or nonspecifically. An example of a *nonspecific immunosuppressant* is the *antilymphocytic serum* (ALS), a xenogeneic serum specific for lymphocytes, particularly T cells (see Chapter 5). The serum or its gamma globulin fraction (antilymphocytic globulin, ALG), when injected into a host, affects lymphocytes regardless of their antigenic specificity, so it acts in a manner similar to that of the immunosuppressive drugs. The exact mechanism of ALS action is not known; one effect seems to be removal of mature T lymphocytes from circulation. ALS treatment of the recipient often significantly prolongs transplant survival, but the benefits of such treatment are frequently counteracted by severe side effects: since the antiserum acts on lymphocytes nonspecifically, the treated subjects become highly susceptible to infection.

Specific suppression can be achieved by the administration of antigens or antibodies. The rationale for the administration of antigens is the observation that a certain dose of the antigen, when given in the right form at the right time, can swing the immune interactions toward unresponsiveness. The antigen treatment thus prepares the ground, so to speak, for acceptance of the subsequent organ transplant. *Antigen-induced suppression* can occur via several mechanisms—for example, the antigen can elicit antibodies which then induce immunological enhancement, it can activate suppressor cells, or it can bind to the antigen-specific receptors and block the receptor-bearing cells. Which of these mechanisms dominates depends on the specific circumstances of antigen administration.

The *antibodies used for immunosuppression* can be directed against either the alloantigens or the immune receptors. The former class of antibodies (*alloantibodies*) can enhance graft survival via one of the as yet undefined afferent, central, or efferent mechanisms. The *receptor* (*idiotypic*) *antibodies* bind to lymphocyte clones specific for a particular alloantigen and somehow inactivate them.

All the different forms of specific immunological reagents have been tried, at least in experimental situations, with a variable degree of success. The major drawback of these techniques is their poor reproducibility: there are simply too many variables involved that immunologists have not yet learned to control. At present there is no immunological treatment that guarantees long-term survival of an allograft.

12.10 GRAFT-VERSUS-HOST REACTION

In Section 12.9, we based our considerations on the assumption that the graft is incapable of reacting immunologically against the host. This assumption is correct only in situations in which the graft does not contain any immunologically competent cells. Often, however, the grafts are full of lymphocytes, and in such instances one can expect an immunological response of the graft against the host. Normally this *graft-versus-host reaction* (GVHR) remains unnoticed because the host-versus-graft reaction (HVGR) prevails and all the transplanted cells are rejected before they can do any harm to the recipient. But when the host is *unable* to mount host-versus-graft reaction, the consequences of GVHR become clearly visible.

12.10.1 Discovery

The first unwitting description of GVHR dates back to 1916 and a paper by James B. Murphy on transplantation of neoplastic cells into chicken embryos. At that time many biologists believed neoplasia to be a return of cells to an undifferentiated, embryonic state, and they hoped to find a clue to neoplastic transformation by comparing the behavior of neoplastic and embryonic cells. To grow neoplastic cells in an embryo, Murphy carefully cut out a rectangular opening in the shell of fowl eggs, inoculated the exposed chorioallantoic membrane (see Fig. 5.17) with the neoplasm, placed the cutout pieces of shell back into position, sealed the openings with wax, and incubated the eggs for several days. At the end of the incubation period, he opened the eggs for observation and noted that, in addition to nodules of growing neoplastic cells, the chick embryo displayed two other characteristic changes. First, the membranes of the embryo were sprinkled with white-grey semitranslucent nodules (pocks, lesions), varying in size from that of a pinpoint to a pinhead. Histological examination of the nodules revealed them to consist predominantly of leukocytes. Second, the spleen of the embryo was greatly enlarged in comparison to that of a noninjected chicken, and again, the enlargement seemed to be caused primarily by leukocytes. To Murphy's great surprise, similar changes also occurred in embryos injected with normal spleen cells or spleen fragments, indicating that they had nothing to with the neoplastic nature of the inoculum. In 1916, scientists knew nothing about the mechanism of host-versus-graft reaction, so the thought of graft-versus-host reaction did not even cross Murphy's mind. Instead he put forward some vague explanation assuming stimulation of host spleen cells by the inoculum, subsequent proliferation of host lymphocytes in the spleen, and migration of splenic lymphocytes to various sites in the membranes. We now know that the pocks were initiated by the response of grafted lymphoid cells to histocompatibility antigens of the host. The stimulating antigens may be provided either by the cells composing the embryonic membrane, or more likely, by the host's lymphocytes brought into the membrane via the circulatory system. The pocks are accumulations of proliferating donor and host cells, but the initial stimulus to pock formation is provided by the inoculated donor lymphocytes; so pock formation is a consequence of graft-versus-host reaction.

Murphy discovered GVHR without kowing it. Paradoxically, two investigators who, 37 years later, thought they had discovered GVHR, were probably observing the HVGR instead. In 1953, Morten Simonsen and W. J. Dempster, working independently, described histological changes occurring in heterotopically transplanted dog kidney allografts. Two to four days after the transplantation, the cortex of the graft became infiltrated with a large number of pyroninophilic cells of the plasma cell series. Initially, the cells accumulated around small blood vessels, but later they flooded the entire cortex. Since at this stage there was no infiltration of the kidney medulla, both Simonsen and Dempster thought that the pyroninophilic cells were of renal (donor) origin and that the reaction represented an immune response of the graft to the host. However, from what we know about kidney graft rejection today, it seems more likely that the plasma cells seen by the two investigators were of host origin.

In 1956, Rupert E. Billingham and Leslie Brent discovered the graft-versus-host reaction for the third time, and again without specifically looking for it.

These two immunologists wanted to induce tolerance (see Section 12.12) in mice of one strain to tissues from another strain, so they injected donor spleen cells into the veins of newborn mice and later grafted the adult mice with the skin from the same donor. They observed that while tolerance could be induced in a high proportion of injected mice in some strain combinations, the injected animals in other combinations stopped growing and runted, as if suffering from a mysterious *runt diasease*. Billingham and Brent interpreted the runt disease as being a consequence of an immunological attack by grafted cells on the immunologically immature recipient. In the same year, Morten Simonsen came to a similar conclusion, working with domestic fowl embryos and mice. This time, both the observations and their interpretations were correct.

12.10.2 Detection

Conditions for GVHR Detection

GVHR can occur when the following three conditions are fulfilled: the host possesses histocompatibility antigens that the graft lacks; the graft contains immunologically competent cells (lymphocytes); and the host is immunologically incompetent (i.e., unable to react immunologically against the graft). Although, as has already been stated, GVHR proably also occurs in immunologically competent recipients, its effects in such a case are overshadowed by the more powerful host-versus-graft reaction.

Histocompatibility antigens capable of inducing GVHR appear to be identical to MLR-inducing antigens, so the strongest GVHR stimulus is provided by MHC-controlled class II antigens; MHC class I antigens produce a somewhat weaker stimulation, while the role of minor histocompatibility antigens is still largely unclear. Allogeneic cells are usually better GVHR inducers than are xenogeneic cells, and the degree of GVHR induction by xenogeneic cells correlates, to some extent, with the phylogenetic distance between the graft donor and the host: the further apart the donor and host are, the weaker the reaction.

GVHR can be induced by a transfer of thoracic duct lymphocytes, lymph node cells, peripheral blood leukocytes, and spleen cells into the recipient; bone marrow cells and thymocytes are usually poor GVHR inducers. The ability of a given inoculum to induce GVHR thus correlates with the content of mature T lymphocytes; numerous experiments have demonstrated convincingly that T lymphocytes are, in fact, the cells that initiate GVHR, though later in the reaction, many other cells may become involved. Immature T lymphocytes are unable to initiate the reaction.

Immunological incompetence of the host can be secured by using immunologically immature animals (fetuses, newborn animals within a few hours of birth), by using animals rendered tolerant to the antigens of the graft, by injecting F_1 hybrids with parental cells (the hybrid is unable to recognize parental cells, but the parental cells recognize F_1 hybrid antigens derived from the opposite parent), or by destroying the host's immunocompetence through X-irradiation.

Methods of Detection

Some of the assays for the detection of GVHR are listed below (see also Fig. 12.25); in each method, the effects on a group of animals injected with immunocompetent, incompatible cells are compared with effects on control animals injected with syngeneic cells.

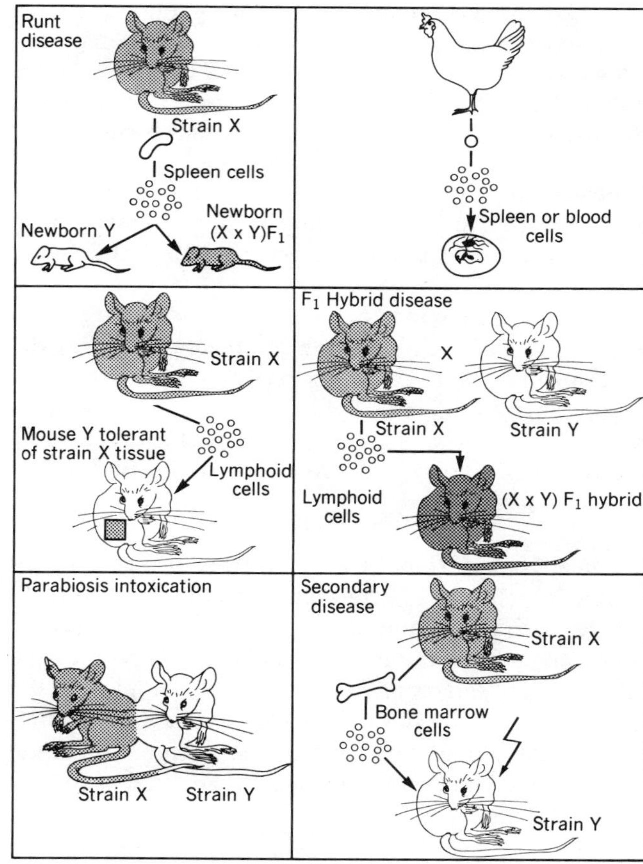

Figure 12.25. Experimental situations leading to the induction of graft-versus-host reaction.

Mortality Assay. The GVHR may be so severe as to cause death of the host, so the simplest way to measure the GVHR is to determine how many animals die after the injection of immunocompetent cells. The time of death depends on the strength of the histocompatibility barrier between the graft and host, with strong incompatibility causing death within the first three weeks after the injection. Death of the animals is usually preceded by characteristic GVHR symptoms, described below.

Weight Assay. A sign of GVHR in newborn and young animals is the runt disease: if mice are used, they stop growing (this effect can best be determined by weighing the animals daily), they suffer from diarrhea, grow only sparse fur, and assume a hunched posture and peculiar, mincing gait.

Organ Enlargement Assay. Another characteristic sign of GVHR in young animals is the pathological enlargement of certain organs, particularly spleen (*splenomegaly*), liver (*hepatomegaly*), or lymph nodes. The enlargement is determined by weighing the organs from six to 10 days after inoculation, and comparing the weight with that of control animal organs. The results are expressed in the form of indices. For example, the *spleen index* is calculated from a formula:

$$\text{spleen index} = \frac{\text{spleen weight/body weight of experimental animals}}{\text{spleen weight/body weight of control animals}}$$

An index of 1 indicates no change in spleen weight, an index of 2 indicates doubling of spleen weight in the experimental animal, and so on. The use of relative spleen weight (spleen weight divided by body weight) is necessary because, in young animals, absolute spleen weight increases proportionately with body weight.

Popliteal Lymph Node Assay. In this assay, parental lymphoid cells are injected into the hind footpad of F_1 hybrid recipients, and the draining popliteal lymph nodes are removed and weighed seven days after the inoculation. Enlargement of the lymph nodes is detected only in the draining nodes; contralateral popliteal nodes remain unaffected. The degree of enlargement shows a linear relationship to the number of parental cells injected.

Phagocytosis Assay. GVHR is accompanied by activation of macrophages and increased phagocytosis. The latter can be measured by intravenous injection of colloidal carbon into animals undergoing GVHR and determination of the rapidity of carbon clearance by the host's reticuloendothelial system. To this end, the animals are bled periodically, the blood cells lysed with 0.1 percent Na_2CO_3, and the carbon concentration in the lysate measured spectrophotometrically.

Chorioallantoic Membrane Assay. This was the original assay by which GVHR was discovered. Here, one injects 12-day old chicken embryos with immunocompetent cells and four or five days later counts the number of white pocks on the chorioallantoic membrane.

Liver Infiltration Assay. One to three days after intravenous injection of young mice with immunocompetent cells, histological liver sections reveal a characteristic mononuclear cell infiltrate around interlobular vessels. The degree of infiltration is a measure of GVHR.

12.10.3 Mechanism

GVHR is a complex process, involving many different cell types and soluble mediators. The details of this process are unknown but the general reaction sequence is probably this. Following their inoculation into the immunoincompetent host, donor lymphocytes home to and settle in the spleen and lymph nodes. A small proportion of lymphocytes then begins to undergo blast transformation, which resembles transformation of lymphocytes in MLC. The blasts divide repeatedly for several days, expanding the initial small clones of proliferating cells. Eventually, however, the blasts become smaller after each division and give rise to a population of small lymphocytes, which are then disseminated throughout the organs and tissues of the host. The new generation of small lymphocytes differs from those in the initial inoculum in that they have a killer capacity—they are committed to carrying out the destruction of the host tissue. However, this destruction begins even before the killer cells are generated, since the blast cells themselves have the capacity to injure the tissues in which they proliferate. The proliferation of the donor cells and the damage these cells inflict on the host tissue set in motion a complex response from the host. The most promiment features of this response are inflammation at the site of donor cell proliferation, increased phagocytic activity, and increased proliferation of the reticuloendothelial and lymphoid cells in the spleen and liver. The proliferation of host cells enlarges the spleen and often the lymph nodes. In the meantime, however, the donor-derived cytotoxic cells begin to attack the lymphoid tissue of the host, destroying large populations of cells and causing atrophy of spleen and lymph nodes, anemia, and lymphopenia. These effects weaken the host's resistance to pathogens and as a result, secondary complications begin to appear and the animal develops a typical runting (wasting) syndrome. In the most severe cases of GVHR the animal eventually dies; in less severe cases it may recover fully.

The specific manifestations of graft-versus-host reactions vary, depending on the conditions of its induction. Some of the forms the GVHR can assume are these.

Runt disease occurs when one injects strain-X lymph node or spleen cells into strain Y or $(X \times Y)F_1$ hybrid newborn animals. The disease is characterized by splenomegaly, failure to grow, diarrhea, and general wasting. Susceptibility to runt disease decreases with increasing age, presumably because of the maturation of the host's immune system.

Homologous disease occurs when a large number of strain-X lymphoid cells presensitized to strain-Y alloantigens is inoculated into adult strain-Y recipients. The inoculated cells overwhelm the host and the GVHR takes over the host-versus-graft reaction. Homologous disease also occurs when a large number of allogeneic cells is injected into tolerant hosts or when parental cells are injected into F_1 hybrid recipients (the latter form of GVHR is also called *F_1 hybrid disease*). The characteristics of homologous disease are spleen and lymph node enlargement, followed by rapid disappearance of lymphocytes from follicular areas and chronic involution (atrophy) of lymphoid organs; liver enlargement; appearance of lesions in the gastrointestinal tract; skin lesions (apparently caused by specific immunological attack by the infiltrating donor cells); and a host of hematological phenomena (anemia, positive antiglobulin test, leukopenia, drop in platelet count, drop in complement component concentration and Ig levels, and decreased bone marrow cellularity).

Secondary disease occurs in allogeneic radiation chimeras one to two months after the cell transfer, when the host has recovered from the primary effects of radiation. We described this form of GVHR in the section dealing with the effects of ionizing radiation.

Parabiosis intoxication occurs in individuals whose circulation systems have been fused naturally or joined surgically (the word *parabiosis* derives from Gr. *para*, alongside, and *biosis*, life). If one of the individuals is an F_1 hybrid and the other a parental strain, the former is "poisoned" (intoxicated) by the latter.

12.11 REGULATORY REACTIONS

The last category of T-cell responses we shall discuss are responses regulating (enhancing or suppressing) the reactions of other cells—macrophages, B lymphocytes, and other T cells. In this chapter we shall deal mainly with T-T interactions; in the next chapter we shall describe the T-B interactions. First we shall discuss the enhancing (helper) effect of T lymphocytes, and then their suppressor function.

12.11.1 Enhancing (Helper) Effects

Discovery

The first evidence of T-T interactions came, as is true in many other important discoveries, from a study of an unrelated phenomenon—the study of hemolytic anemia in New Zealand Black, or NZB, mice (see Chapter 14). In an effort to find the cause of the disease, researchers subjected the NZB mice to all kinds of tests and discovered, among other things, that the sick animals lose the ability to mount graft-versus-host reaction as the disease progresses. Since the disease is characterized by a higher than normal proliferation of hematopoietic cells in the spleen, the impairment of graft-versus-host reactivity could be explained as a kind of dilution effect, in which the hematopoietic cells take the place of the GVH reactive lymphocytes. This explanation was put to the test in 1970 by Harvey Cantor and Richard Asofsky. They reasoned that if GVHR impairment were indeed the consequence of dilution, it should be possible to replace the diluted old cells by an admixture of young cells (the disease increases progressively with age). They therefore performed a series of mixing experiments and discovered, to their surprise, that the GVHR induced by a mixture of old and young cells was stronger than some of the reactions caused by the two cell types injected separately. They observed, for example, that 10^6 young cells alone and 10^6 old cells alone did not produce any measurable GVHR. But the mixture resulted in a spleen index higher than the sum of the indices produced by 2×10^6 young or old cells. In other words, the two cell populations, when mixed, gave a *synergistic effect* rather than the expected additive effect. The synergistic effect suggested that the enhanced GVHR was the result of interaction between the two popula-

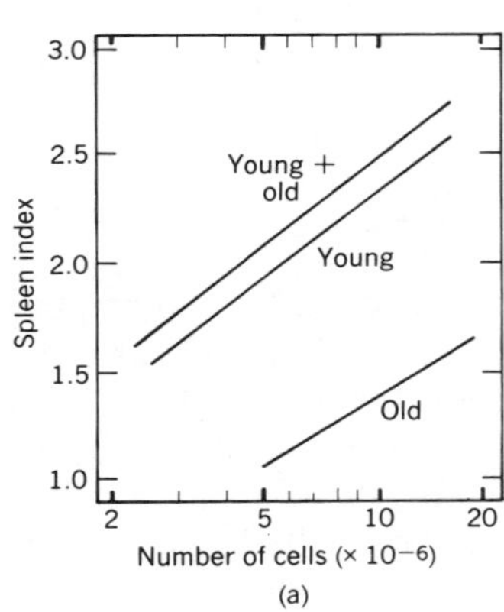

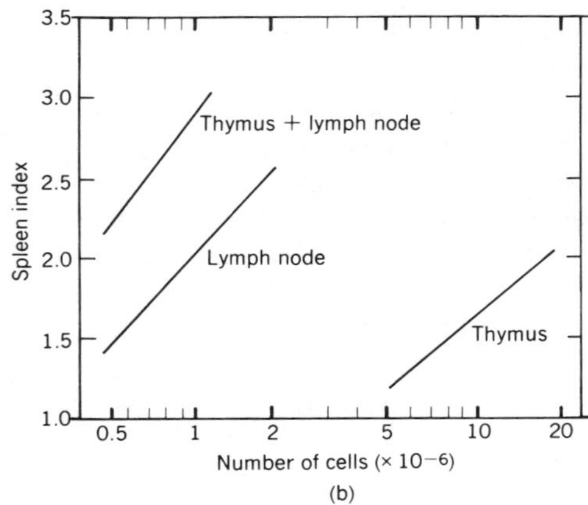

Figure 12.26. Synergistic effect of mixtures of T lymphocytes in the induction of graft-versus-host reaction. (*a*) Reactivity of old and young NZB lymphocytes injected separately or mixed into C57BL/6 mice. Mixtures were composed of equal numbers of old and young cells. (From H. Cantor, R. Asofsky, and N. Talal: *J. Exp. Med.* **131**:223–234, 1970.) (*b*) Reactivity of BALB/c thymus and lymph node cells and of mixtures of the two injected into (C57BL/6 × BALB/c)F_1 hybrid mice. (From H. Cantor and R. Asofsky: *J. Exp. Med.* **131**:235–246, 1970.)

tions. When Cantor and Asofsky did control experiments with normal mice of other strains, they realized that synergism was a general phenomenon, operating whenever populations of young and mature cells were mixed. In normal mice, young cells can be obtained from the thymus and mature cells from lymph nodes. Figure 12.26 depicts one such experiment with normal thymus and lymph node cells: the mixture is 10 to 100 times more effective in inducing splenomegaly in newborn F_1 hybrids than either of the two cell types alone. Since treatment with anti-Thy-1 serum and complement of either thymus or lymph node cells abolishes the synergistic effect, the interacting cells must be T lymphocytes. The effect is thus an example of T-T interaction.

Experimental Systems for the Study of T-T Interactions

The synergistic effect of different T-cell populations has been demonstrated in virtually all forms of T-cell response discussed on the preceding pages. A brief survey of some of the systems used in T-T interaction experiments follows.

Mixed Lymphocyte Reaction. The original demonstration of T-T interaction in MLC was similar in design to the Cantor-Asofsky experiment. Thymocytes alone were demonstrated to be poor responders in MLC, but when mixed with a low number of lymph node cells, they boosted the response of the latter.

Cell-Mediated Lymphocytotoxicity. As has already been discussed, T lymphocytes respond in CML to class I MHC alloantigens, but this response can often be augmented significantly through simultaneous stimulation by class II alloantigens. The T cells responding to class II antigens thus enhance the response of T cells that respond to class I antigens.

Delayed-Type Hypersensitivity. Guinea pigs injected with a hapten-amino acid conjugate (e.g., azobenzenearsonate conjugate of *N*-chloracetyl tyrosine) in complete Freund's adjuvant, and then with hapten-protein (i.e., azobenzenearsonate protein) in incomplete Freund's adjuvant give stronger delayed-type hypersensitivity reactions to the protein than animals immunized only with the hapten-protein conjugate. Apparently, the first injection mobilizes cells that then enhance the action of DTH inducers.

Graft-Versus-Host Reaction. The system used to demonstrate T-T cell cooperation in GVHR is that described originally by Cantor and Asofsky.

Helper Effect in Antibody Synthesis. The differentiation of B lymphocytes into antibody-secreting plasma cells is influenced by T helper cells (see Chapter 13). There is also evidence that the amplifying action of the T helpers can, in turn, be augmented by other T cells. For example, inoculation of an (X × Y)F_1 hybrid with parental X or Y lymphocytes prior to or simultaneously with a carrier protein improves the helper effect of the T cells isolated from these hybrids. Presumably, the parental cells mount a graft-versus-host reaction against the F_1 host and so somehow augment the helper ability of the host cells.

Other Regulatory Effects of T Cells. Regulatory action of T cells is not restricted to lymphocytes (T or B); T cells also stimulate macrophages, monocytes, and other inflammatory leukocytes to participate in delayed-type hypersensitivity responses (see section 12.7), induce osteoclasts to resorb bone, and induce colony-forming cells to differentiate into mature erythroid elements. And there may be other cells influenced by T cells that remain to be identified.

Nature of Regulation

There are at least two kinds of T cell exerting an augmenting effect on the immune response. In the mouse, the first kind is the cell usually referred to as a helper cell, characterized by the presence of Lyt-1 and the absence of Lyt-2 molecules. These cells act on B lymphocytes, precursors of cytotoxic T cells, and possibly on macrophages. Their function is to provide a second signal for lymphocyte activation and differentiation, the first being supplied by antigen, lectin, or some other lymphocyte-stimulating substance. The function is mediated by cell-to-cell contact or by soluble factors, which the lymphocytes begin to secrete when they are stimulated by antigen or some other means.

The second kind of enhancing T lymphocyte, sometimes referred to as *regulatory cell in the strictest sense*, is characterized by the expression of both *Lyt* loci (i.e., they are Lyt-1$^+$Lyt-2$^+$). These still poorly characterized cells may regulate immune response in two ways: they may serve as a precursor pool from which at least some of the Lyt-1$^+$ and Lyt-2$^-$ cells derive; and they may possibly exert immunoregulatory effects on other cells. The first function (regulation through supply of precursor cells) is reasonably well-documented, whereas the second function (direct regulation by Lyt-1$^+$Lyt-2$^+$ cells) is mostly hypothetical. We shall return to the complexities of regulatory cell interactions in Chapter 13.

12.11.2 Suppressor Effects

Discovery

The opposite of augmentation is suppression. It would seem logical, therefore, for helper cells to be counteracted by a system of suppressor T cells. Indeed, in the 1950s, after the discovery of helper effects, several immunologists described phenomena that, in retrospect, can be interpreted as manifestations of suppressor cell activity. But a conclusive demonstration that suppressor cells existed as a distinct subpopulation of T lymphocytes proved to be extremely difficult. For many of the observations, alternative explanations were possible, and for some time investigators could not make up their minds which explanation to accept. The credit for convincing immunologists that suppressor cells are real is due mainly to Richard K. Gershon. He and K. Kondo stumbled upon immune suppression accidentally, while attempting to induce unresponsiveness to sheep red blood cells (Fig. 12.27). The

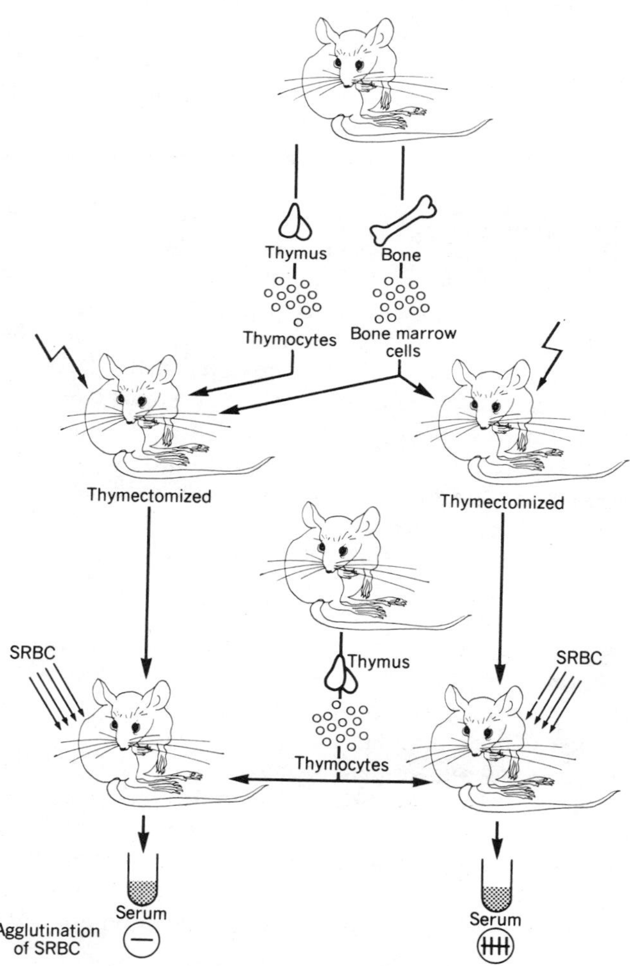

Figure 12.27. The experiment demonstrating T cell-mediated suppression of antibody response to sheep red blood cells (SRBC). (Based on R. K. Gershon and K. Kondo: *Immunology* **18**:723–737, 1970.)

specific question these investigators wanted to answer was whether tolerance to sheep red blood cells could be induced more easily in the absence of T lymphocytes than in their presence. So they lethally irradiated two groups of thymectomized mice, injected both groups with syngeneic bone marrow cells, and, in addition, injected one group (but not the other) with a small number of thymocytes. They then injected both groups repeatedly with large doses of sheep red blood cells, inoculated the two groups with syngeneic thymocytes (to provide cooperating T cells) four days after the last erythrocyte injection, and still later tested the mice for the presence of antibodies to sheep red blood cells. The result was just the opposite of what they expected: the mice that received no thymocytes at the time of bone marrow inoculation produced antibodies, whereas the sera from mice that received thymocytes failed to agglutinate sheep red blood cells altogether. Thus, in the absence of thymocytes the mice did not become tolerant to sheep red blood cells at all. It seemed as if interaction of sheep red blood cells with thymocytes during tolerance induction resulted in turning off the B cells so that they were no longer susceptible to the help of added T cells, or in turning off the added T cells, or both. However, when the unresponsive mice were injected with horse red blood cells, they began to produce antibodies to both horse and sheep red blood cells. Apparently the interaction of sheep red blood cells with thymocytes during the period of tolerance induction resulted in the production of a substance that specifically suppressed the helper function of thymocytes. When the thymocytes were stimulated by an unrelated antigen (horse red blood cells) the suppressive effect was abolished.

From these pioneering experiments it was still a long way to the attainment of respectability for the suppressor cell concept. The main reason that skepticism persisted for so long was the frustration accompanying any attempts to isolate pure populations of suppressor cells. The breakthrough occurred when Donal B. Murphy and his colleagues discovered a marker characterizing the suppressor cell populations—the alloantigens controlled by the *J* locus of the mouse major histocompatibility complex. Although this marker still did not completely solve the problem of suppressor cell isolation, it identified these lymphocytes as distinct from the cytotoxic T cells with which they share the Lyt-1^-Lyt-2^+ phenotype.

Model Systems

In their original study, Gershon and Kondo made use of the T-B collaboration assay system for antibody production. Later, Gershon and his colleagues, as well as other investigators, developed several other systems for the study of immune suppression. To illustrate the diversity of these systems we shall describe some of them.

Suppression of Lectin Stimulation of Antigen-Activated Spleen Cells. The in vitro stimulation of lymphocytes by PHA can be inhibited by the addition of syngeneic spleen cells from animals immunized against conventional antigens (e.g., sheep red blood cells, bovine gamma globulin, or bovine serum albumin). The inhibition can be augmented by the addition of the antigen to the culture. Presumably, the immunization activates suppressor cells, which then depress the response to the lectins. The suppressor activity disappears within one week after immunization.

Suppression of Antigen Stimulation by Lectin-Stimulated Cells. Incubation of lymphocytes in vitro with an antigen, such as sheep red cells, can result in the secretion of antibodies into the culture medium (see Chapter 13). The antibody response is severely depressed by the addition, at the start of the culture, of lymphocytes stimulated by optimal lectin doses. When lectin-stimulated lymphocytes are added to the culture later, or when the lymphocytes are stimulated by low lectin doses, the added cells enhance, rather than suppress the immune response.

Suppression of Mixed Lymphocyte Reaction by Lectin-Stimulated Lymphocytes. Spleen cells activated in vitro or in vivo by Con A and added to the mixture of alloantigen-disparate responding and stimulating cells (the Con A-stimulated cells being syngeneic with the responding cells) decrease the mixed lymphocyte reaction significantly.

Suppression of Mixed Lymphocyte Reaction by Alloantigen-Activated Lymphocytes. MLR of strain-X responding cells against strain-Y stimulators can also be inhibited by spleen cells from strain-X mice injected four days earlier into the hind footpad with strain-Y splenocytes. Interestingly, in this same system, draining lymph node cells of the preimmunized mice have the opposite effect: they enhance the MLR.

Suppression of Graft-Versus-Host Reaction by Spleen Cells from Mice with a Potential for Autoimmune Disease. Spleen cells from young (six weeks old) NZB mice, when injected into newborn allogeneic mice, induce a weak graft-versus-host reaction, as measured by the splenomegaly assay. Under the same circumstances cells from 25-week-old NZB mice induce a strong graft-versus-host reaction. But when the cells from young mice are mixed with cells from old mice, the GVHR-inducing ability of the latter is depressed. Apparently, spleens of young mice contain suppressor cells capable of inhibiting GVHR mediated by the old cells. The abundance of suppressor cells in young NZB mice may be related to the autoimmune disease these mice eventually develop (see Chapter 14).

Suppression of Contact Sensitivity by Cells from Tolerant Mice. Mice sensitized to picrylchloride fail to manifest sensitivity to this compound if the sensitization by skin painting is accompanied by injection of lymph node cells from syngeneic donors made tolerant to picrylchloride by repeated intravenous injections of this substance.

Suppression of Cell-Mediated Lymphocytotoxicity from Cells of Allografted Individuals. Lymphocytes isolated from individuals carrying kidney allografts, when harvested at a certain specific time and added to mixed culture of allogeneic lymphocytes, often suppress the cell-mediated lymphocytotoxicity that the culture would normally exert.

Mechanism

In all the situations described above, and in many similar situations not mentioned, inhibitory activity can be abolished by the treatment of the purported suppressor cell populations with mouse anti-Thy-1 serum (or a homologous antiserum in other species) and complement. This finding is one of several pieces of evidence identifying suppressor cells as T lymphocytes. As was mentioned earlier, the suppressor T cells of the mouse carry Lyt-2 antigens and antigens controlled by the *J* locus of the major histocompatibility complex. In many of their other characteristics, the suppressor cells resemble the cytotoxic Lyt-1^-Lyt-2^+ T cells.

It follows from the description in the preceding paragraphs that suppressor T cells can be derived from normal individuals, animals with an autoimmune disease, tolerant individuals, and animals in which allograft reaction is taking place. Suppressor activity of lymphocytes can be increased by their stimulation with lectins, conventional antigens, and alloantigens. A particularly rich source of suppressor T cells is the spleen, so that spleen cells sometimes suppress an immune response that is either enhanced or unaffected by cells from other lymphoid organs of the same individuals.

Suppressor T cells appear to be most effective early in the course of the immune response, although they do not seem to prevent antigen recognition by lymphocytes. In many instances they seem to act by restricting T-cell proliferation at the stage of clonal expansion. Their targets seem to be other T cells, particularly helper cells, although some may also act on B lymphocytes and on macrophages (see Chapter 13). The many instances in which specific suppression of a response to a given antigen occurs suggest that the suppressor cells carry antigen-specific receptors and are capable of antigen recognition. Although there are instances in which the suppressor cells appear to act nonspecifically (for example, after lectin activation), in these cases, the possibility that the nonspecific stimulus activates many clones, of which a few suppress the responses to a given antigen in a specific manner, has not been ruled out. The suppression would then only *appear* to be nonspecific because the different clones would inhibit responses to different antigens.

How the suppressor T cells act is not clear. In many experimental models evidence is available for the release, by the activated suppressor cells, of suppressor factors that mediate the inhibitory action. The properties of some of these factors will be described in Chapter 13.

Nothing is known about the identity of suppressor cells in the different experimental systems. Are different kinds of suppressor cells operating in different systems, or is there principally only one kind of suppressor cell, which, depending on the circumstances, mediates different effects? The answer to this and many related questions must be provided by future research.

12.12 UNRESPONSIVENESS

Up to now we have been discussing the manner in which T cells recognize nonself; now it is time to turn our attention to the recognition of self. There are obviously a great many substances in the body that a lymphocyte must learn not to attack (become unresponsive to). Of these, the T cells are primarily concerned with cell surface molecules, particularly those controlled by the major histocompatibility complex. In fact, it may be the MHC molecules around which the recognition of self revolves. For this reason, we shall concentrate in this chapter on self recognition of MHC-controlled molecules; we shall discuss recognition of other self molecules in Chapter 13.

To study self recognition is not easy, mainly because its result in unresponsiveness (*tolerance*)—that is, a negative characteristic. There are two principal ways one learns about a cell's tolerance of a molecule. One is to force a cell to tolerate a molecule (e.g., an

MHC-controlled alloantigen) that it would normally consider as nonself, and then to apply the knowledge of this artifactual situation to a physiological self recognition. It is this approach that has so far provided most of the available information about tolerance of MHC molecules, and it will be on this approach that we base our discussion in this chapter. The second way is to study situations in which the natural tolerance has broken down (for example, in various autoimmunity states), hoping that the pathology of the process will shed some light on the corresponding physiological mechanism. We shall discuss this approach in Chapter 14.

12.12.1 Discovery

Although immunologists were concerned with the problem of self recognition as early as the end of the nineteenth century (as in so many areas, most succinctly in the ideas of Paul Ehrlich), serious investigation of this question did not begin until the 1950s. The impetus came from a chance finding made during the study of an unrelated research problem. Though the description of this discovery will be a slight diversion from the main course of this narrative, and though it was mentioned in Chapter 2, we shall tell the story here in full. It will give us an opportunity to catch our breath before we resume the barrage of facts. This time the unexpected finding was made not in the mouse or human, but in cattle.

Like humans, cattle are occasionally born as twins, either monozygotic (derived from a single fertilized ovum and hence genetically identical) or dizygotic (derived from two separate zygotes and hence no more alike than siblings). Monozygotic twins are always of the same sex, whereas dizygotic twins can be either of the same or different sexes. Cattle breeders have known for a long time that in twins of different sexes, the males are usually completely normal, whereas the females are often masculinized. The affected animals develop female external genitalia, but have only a rudimentary uterus and oviduct and instead possess some male secondary sex organs, such as seminal vesicles and the epididymal duct. They are always sterile, and this fact might perhaps be the reason that they have been called *freemartins* (free, possibly from Scot. *fearr*, a sterile cow, and martin, from *Martinmas*, a November event when cattle, especially the sterile ones and those not producing milk, were slaughtered). The observation that the twin partners of freemartins were always males suggested that something, probably a hormone, from the male was being passed to the female and rerouting her development in a male direction. This passage hypothesis was supported by the observation, made in 1916 by F. R. Lillie, that at birth, all freemartins had their blood vessels connected with the vessels of their partners. In cattle, placentas of twin fetuses are located so closely together that they often fuse, and so apparently, do fetal blood vessels, allowing exchange of blood between the twins. All these observations made freemartins an interesting object of endocrinological research, but there was no reason for immunologists to get excited about cattle twins until a chance observation, made in 1945 by Ray D. Owen, revealed a new aspect of this area of inquiry.

At the time when no National Institutes of Health existed and there were no NIH grants, scientists often supported their research by tying it to a service function paid for by this or that branch of industry. Owen obtained money from dairy cattle breeders to type the blood groups of their animals and so provide the farmers with useful information in their attempts to improve the quality of their breeds. The typing provided Owen with the opportunity to study some basic genetic questions in which he was intersted. As he looked over hundreds of typing results, he observed that, surprisingly, many of the animals typed as monozygotic twins. This observation contradicted the actual experience of the farmers, who found the occurrence of monozygotic twins to be extremely rare. When considering the possible explanation for this discrepancy, Owen eventually remembered Lillie's observation on the exchange of blood between dizygotic twins and the idea occurred to him that some of the twins might be red blood cell chimeras that carried not only their own erythrocytes, but also erythrocytes of their partners. To test this idea, he exposed red blood cells typing positive for antigens X and Y to an anti-X serum and complement and then tested the lysate for the presence of intact red blood cells carrying antigen Y. He reasoned that if the twins had two erythrocyte populations, only one should be lysed by an antiserum monospecific for a given antigen. The results of these tests fully confirmed these expectations: some of the twins were indeed erythrocytic chimeras.

That the chimerism may also involve cells other than erythrocytes was demonstrated in 1952 by Peter B. Medawar and his colleagues. Like Owen, Medawar too got into cattle studies completely by chance, when he was asked by some agricultural workers to advise them on how to distinguish monozygotic from dizygotic cattle twins. Medawar thought this to be a simple problem: the monozygotic twins should permanently accept skin grafts exchanged between them, whereas dizygotic twins should reject the exchanged grafts. To Medawar's great surprise, however, there were many clearly dizygotic twins that accepted the skin grafts as if they were monozygotic twins. An obvious explanation for this disconcerting observation was that the anomalous twins were chimeric in many tissues, including those involved in the immune response, and that because of the coexistence in a single individual of genetically disparate tissues, the tissues somehow grew tolerant of each other.

However, the most ironic twist in the study of tolerance was saved for Milan Hašek. He set out to test whether acquired characteristics, as claimed originally by Lamarck and disputed by most biologists since, could be inherited, after all. He thought that if such a form of inheritance existed, it should be transmittable from one individual to another—for example, by blood. To achieve blood exchange, Hašek resorted to the technique of chicken embryo parabiosis we have already mentioned several times (see Chapter 2 and Fig. 5.17). He could not demonstrate the inheritance of acquired characteristics in this system, but the experiment paid unexpected dividends in a completely different way. By typing birds hatched from parabiotic eggs for their blood group antigen, Hašek discovered that the birds, like Owen's cattle, were erythrocytic chimeras. And they too were immunologically tolerant of each other in that they did not make antibodies against tissues injected from their partners nor did they reject their partner's skin grafts.

Inspired by Owen's observation, Macfarlane F. Burnet and Frank Fenner put forward in 1949 a hypothesis that stated that foreign substances presented to an embryo early enough in life come to be regarded as self, and a fully grown individual is then unable to react immunologically against them. Burnet and Fenner attempted to prove this hypothesis of immunological tolerance experimentally, but Destiny had one final ironic twist up her sleeve: they used the wrong antigen—only they did not know it then—and the experiment failed.

Destiny's duplicity held sway until 1953, when Rupert Billingham, Leslie Brent, and Peter B. Medawar intentionally induced tolerance in mice and in domestic fowl. These three immunologists inoculated a mixture of strain-X spleen, kidney, and testes cells into strain-Y fetuses (Fig. 12.28). When the inoculated mice matured, the experimenters challenged them with two skin grafts, one from strain X and the other from an unrelated strain-Z donor. The former grafts either survived permanently or their survival was significantly prolonged in comparison with uninjected controls; the strain-Z grafts were rejected with the same speed as in control mice. The inoculated mice thus became specifically tolerant of the alloantigens to which they were exposed during their embryonic life, while they still regarded all other alloantigens as foreign.

12.12.2 Methods of Induction

Originally, immunologists thought that tolerance could be induced only in immunologically immature animals, but later they realized that even adult recipients can become immunologically unresponsive when suitably treated. So there are two principal ways of inducing immunological tolerance—in immunologically mature and immature animals.

Manipulation of Immature Animals

Maturing animals go through a period of responsiveness to tolerance induction (*tolerance-responsiveness period,* for short) in which they readily become tolerant when exposed to an antigen. Tolerance induction beyond this point is still possible, but more difficult than in the earlier period. The responsiveness period terminates at different times in different species: in some (e.g., cattle, sheep, humans, and other mammals with relatively long gestation periods) it terminates well before birth; in others (e.g., rabbits, mice, domestic

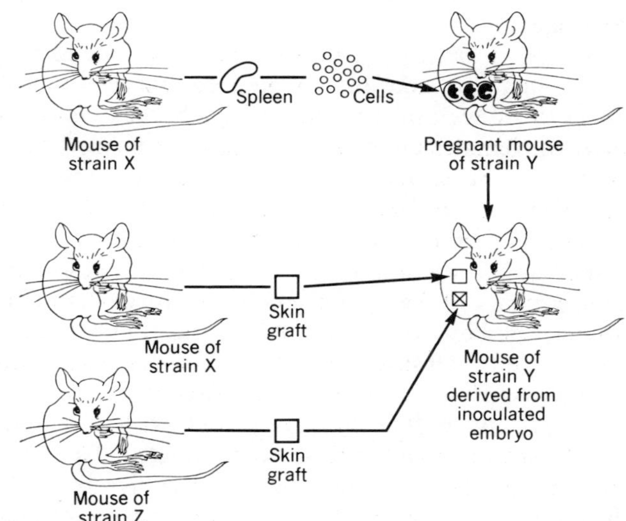

Figure 12.28. An experiment demonstrating the induction of immunological tolerance of skin grafts in mice. (Based on R. E. Billingham, L. Brent, and P. B. Medawar: *Phil. Trans. Soc. Lond.* **239**:357–414, 1956.)

fowl) it terminates within a few hours after birth, and in still others (e.g., rats and ducks) it terminates within the first two weeks of life. However, the time of termination is influenced to a large degree by the type of antigen inoculated. For example, for a weak antigen like H-Y, the tolerance responsiveness period in mice does not end until more than two weeks after birth, while for the strong H-2 antigens, the period ends right after birth. Furthermore, tolerance of weak antigens can be induced with relatively small doses of antigen presented by almost any route, whereas a high antigen dose inoculated intravenously is needed for the induction of tolerance to H-2.

The usual way of inducing tolerance to MHC antigens in mice is by the intravenous inoculation of a mixture of spleen, lymph node, and bone marrow cells into newborn mice within a few hours after birth. The cells are injected with a fine needle into the veins of the baby animal's head—a feat that requires some practice. The intrauterine injection method originally used by Billingham and his colleagues is usually associated with high mortality and a low yield of mature animals, so it is seldom employed. To avoid graft-versus-host reaction, the injected cells should be of F_1 hybrid origin whenever possible and the recipient should be one of the two parental strains of this hybrid.

A completely different way of obtaining tolerant animals is depicted in Figure 12.29. The method was originally developed by Andrzej K. Tarkowski and Beatrice Mintz for the study of embryonic differentiation, but it can also be used for the analysis of immunological tolerance. The starting point of each experiment is two females, X and Y, injected with hormones so that they produce a large number of ova (superovulation) and then mated to normal males. When the developing embryos reach the eight-cell stage, the females are killed, the embryos flushed from the uterus, the protective zona pellucida is enzymatically digested, and one embryo derived from mother X is placed in tissue culture next to an embryo from mother Y. During the subsequent short-term (18-hour) culture, many of the opposed embryos fuse, each pair forming one large embryo in which the X and Y cells intermingle. Each fused embryo is then deposited into the uterus of a pseudopregnant female of another strain (a female that has copulated with a vasectomized male) and allowed to come to term. The mice born to such females are referred to as *tetraparental* (they have four parents: the father and mother of embryo X and the father and mother of embryo Y), or as *allophenic* (Gr. *allos,* other, *phainō,* to display). Because of the intermingling of X and Y cells in the early embryos, the fetuses—and later the adult animals—have some parts of their bodies derived from strain X and others from strain Y. They are thus experimentally induced chimeras. The two types of tissue live in the chimera in perfect harmony, each tolerating the other, even if strains X and Y differ in MHC and other antigens.

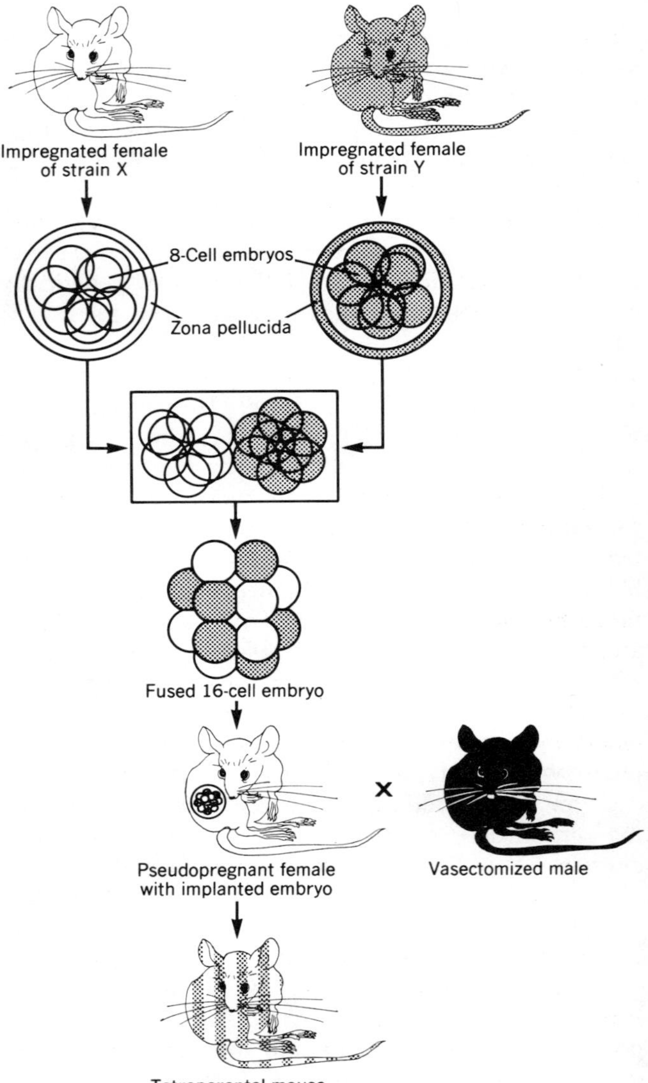

Figure 12.29. Method of producing a tetraparental mouse.

In birds, chimeras can be induced by the parabiosis method used by Hašek. Natural chimeras occur in several species of mammals other than cattle, including humans.

Manipulation of Mature Animals

As noted above, induction of tolerance in adult animals is possible but difficult. It usually requires massive antigen doses and treatment over a prolonged period. It is facilitated by artificially reducing the host's capability of immune response by sublethal X-irradiation, treatment with immunosuppressive drugs, thoracic duct lymphocyte drainage, and treatment with antilymphocytic serum or lectins. The usual way of inducing adult tolerance is by repeated injections of large numbers of spleen, lymph node, and bone marrow cells into the host. However, tolerance can also be induced by parabiotic fusion of two adult individuals and by injecting thymectomized, lethally irradiated individuals of strain X with T cell-depleted bone marrow cells derived from strain Y (radiation chimeras). The mechanism of tolerance in these different situations may not be the same.

The usual way of determining whether an animal is tolerant is by placing a skin graft on the host. Alternatively, one can measure tolerance by the host's inability to mount mixed lymphocyte reaction, cell-mediated lymphocytotoxicity, and antibody responses to tolerated antigens. The correlation between these different measurements is not always absolute. Some animals may be tolerant of skin grafts and show no MLR and CML, but others may give positive MLR and CML and yet, at the same time, retain skin grafts indefinitely.

12.12.3 Conditions for Tolerance Induction

Tolerance can be induced by the inoculation of live cells of the erythropoietic, myeloid, and lymphoid series (lymph node cells, splenocytes, peripheral leukocytes, bone marrow cells, and thymocytes). An important condition is the cell's ability to proliferate; X-irradiation abolishes their tolerance-conferring capacity. Apparently the cells must survive in the host for a long time and thus turn the host into a chimera. Induction of tolerance with other cells, such as kidney, liver, or epidermal cells, is extremely difficult; it requires massive treatment of the host and is usually possible only across weak antigenic differences, and the induced tolerance is of a short duration. Antigenic extracts usually fail to induce tolerance to histocompatibility antigens.

The cell dose required for the tolerance induction depends on the strength of the antigenic disparity between the donor and the host. Usually the greater the barrier, the more cells are needed to induce tolerance across it. The use of too low a cell dose may have an effect opposite from that expected: it may induce immunity instead of tolerance.

Often the induced tolerance is only *partial* (rather than *complete*), and after a period it turns into immunity, which then leads to elimination of the antigen (rejection of the graft). Sometimes one can also observe a *split tolerance,* in which some of the inoculated antigens are tolerated while others induce an immune reaction. An example of split tolerance is the situation in which an X host made tolerant of (Y $\times$ Z)F_1 tissue tolerates Y graft but rejects Z grafts.

12.12.4 Genetics

A condition of special importance in tolerance induction is the genetic relationship between the donor of the cell inoculum and the host. In the mouse, tolerance to antigens controlled by a single minor histocompatibility locus is relatively easy to induce and the induced tolerance is of long duration. However, such differences occur only in special combinations of congenic lines. Two ordinary inbred strains, whether carrying the same MHC alleles or not, differ at many minor histocompatibility loci. Tolerance induction across such barriers is difficult and when induced, the tolerance is often only partial.

Tolerance induction across an isolated H-2 barrier is relatively easy in some combinations and difficult in others, depending on the particular *H-2* haplotype involved and on the overall genetic background. The most striking example of background gene effect is the difference between strains A and C57BL: tolerance induction is far easier in congenic lines carrying different *H-2* haplotypes on the A-strain background than in lines carrying the same haplotypes on the C57BL background. The reason for this difference could be that C57BL mice mature more rapidly and thus have a shorter tolerance-responsiveness period than A mice, although experimental evidence supporting this explanation is lacking. Of the two main classes of MHC loci, class II seem to present a far less formidable barrier to tolerance induction than do class I loci. There is, however, some evidence to indicate that tolerance inducibility to class I-locus antigens could somehow be influenced by the *J* locus.

At this point we shall interrupt the narrative and postpone the rest of the discussion of tolerance until after we have learned about B cells since B cells participate in tolerance induction in an important way.

12.13 SYNTHESIS

Having acquainted ourselves with the various forms of T-cell response, we must now ask: how do these forms relate to one another? Do they have anything else in common besides the fact that they are all initiated by T lymphocytes? How does MLR, for example, relate to DTH? On the surface of it, there does not seem to be much that ties these two reactions together, but could this unrelatedness be only seeming while in actuality both reactions operate on the same principle? And how do these forms relate to the natural function of T lymphocytes? Proliferation of cells in culture, formation of skin induration, rejection of allografts, and destruction of host tissue by transplanted cells are obviously artifactual situations for which the body cannot possibly have any use. But is it possible that for each of these situations there is a natural correlate?

Although not all the answers to these questions are available yet, we now have a reasonably complete general view of what the function of T lymphocytes in the body's defense is. With regard to the first set of questions, it appears that there are indeed only a few basic T-cell response mechanisms and that the individual forms described on the preceding pages are merely different manifestations of these mechanisms. The diversity of forms is an illusion that arises because of the different methods immunologists use to investigate T-cell reactivity.

This point can best be explained by using an analogy. A photographer who is looking at a locomotive through a telephoto lens may get different impressions of the machine, depending on which part of the engine he views. Aiming his camera at one part, he sees only turning wheels, aiming at another, he sees smoke spewing from the stack, and still another shot reveals a stoker feeding the furnace. To an immunologist, the different methods that he uses for the detection of the T-cell response are like the telephoto lens that takes different shots of the same machine. The MLR is one such shot of the T-cell machine, the allograft reaction is another, DTH still another, and so on. Each of these responses probably involves mechanisms that are also involved in other responses, but of these, the immunologist sees only a few at a time because they are the ones toward which he aims his lens. For example, we know that the MLR involves not only proliferation of T helper cells, but also generation of cytotoxic cells, and the production of helper and suppressor factors. However, the test system is normally such that it measures only T-cell proliferation and nothing else, and similar observations apply to other types of T-cell response. Our assays give us close-up shots of the mechanisms; to get the whole scene into the frame, we w have to focus our lenses on infinity.

Differences between the responses also arise fro the particular circumstances of antigen presentatio which may favor dominance of one form over the ot ers. This point can be illustrated by the difference b tween some of the in vivo and in vitro responses. I dissecting out cells from the body and transferri them into tissue culture, one not only completely d stroys the homeostasis of the T-cell network (s Chapter 13), but also makes certain forms of respon impossible. So although a mixed lymphocyte and delayed-type hypersensitivity reaction probably ha many things in common, they appear to be differe because in the culture, in contrast to the living bod there are simply no monocytes and basophils that t proliferating cells can recruit. Similarly, there a many common characteristics between cell-mediat lymphocytotoxicity in vitro and graft rejection in viv but again, in the culture, elements such as ma rophages, which play an important role in vivo, cann enter the picture because they are simply not prese in sufficient numbers.

The main function of T lymphocytes in the natur in vivo situation is to act as guardians of self; T ce are indeed the Januses of the body. Of the trinity immune cells, only T lymphocytes are equipped f such a function, since macrophages lack specificity recognition, and B lymphocytes can use their specifi ity only when directed in their action by T cells (s Chapter 13). In this respect, T cells are the centr elements of the specific immune response, since th are probably the only cells that can discriminate b tween self and nonself.

This discrimination must have been a difficult pro lem to solve. There is no principal difference betwe self and nonself—the two are both parts of the san antigen universe. An individual happens to possess small selection of determinants from this universe a it is the presence of these particular determinants th identifies them as self. Other individuals may rega the same determinants as nonself simply because th happen to lack them. Vertebrates have apparent solved the problem by delegating the function of mar ing self to the molecules of the major histocompatib ity complex and by setting up training centers in whi T lymphocytes learn to regard these MHC molecul as self. When it comes to actual recognition, the T ce are somehow (and we are totally in the dark about *ho* weighing nonself, represented by a foreign antige against self, represented by the individual's MH molecules. It is this mysterious weighing up of self a nonself that tells the T cell whether the antigen is fo eign. This requirement for linked recognition places certain restrictions on the T cell's cognitive potential. Since foreign particles, such as viruses or bacteria, do not carry MHC molecules, they are ignored by T lymphocytes until a macrophage has digested some of them and displayed their fragments in its membrane next to MHC molecules. Only then do the T lymphocytes recognize the combination of foreign fragments and the macrophage's MHC molecules, and become activated. However, even the activated T lymphocytes cannot attack the viruses or the bacteria specifically, again because to launch an attack they must recognize the particle and the self MHC molecule simultaneously. So, instead, the lymphocytes instruct other cells (primarily B lymphocytes) to carry out the attack. We shall describe in the next chapter how this instruction is given and to what form of attack it may lead. Of the various T-cell responses described in Sections 12.3 through 12.9, antigen-induced proliferation of T cells in vitro and the MLR probably come closest to this natural T-cell function.

There are, however, at least two situations in which the T cells themselves attack the carriers of nonself determinants. One occurs when a virus or some other intracellular parasite infects a cell and displays some of its components in the plasma membrane next to MHC molecules. The activated T cells identify such a cell as nonself and kill it. The second situation occurs when, for whatever reasons, a cell within a body changes its surface characteristics. Some of the altered membrane components may then be identified as foreign by T lymphocytes and the cell is killed. In the experimental situation, this killer activity of T lymphocytes is manifested in the cell-mediated lymphocytotoxicity assay. We shall describe specific examples of T-cell killer responses in Chapter 14.

REFERENCES

General

Beer, A. E. and Billingham, R. E.: *The Immunobiology of Mammalian Reproduction*. Prentice-Hall, Englewood Cliffs, New Jersey, 1976.

Billingham, R. and Silvers, W.: *The Immunobiology of Transplantation*. Prentice-Hall, Englewood Cliffs, New Jersey, 1971.

Calne, R. Y.: *Organ Grafts*. Arnold, London, 1975.

Elkins, W. L.: Cellular immunology and the pathology of graft-versus-host reactions. *Progr. Allergy* **15**:78–187, 1971.

Häyry, P: Anamnestic responses in mixed lymphocyte culture-induced cytolysis (MLC-CML) reaction. *Immunogenetics* **3**:417–453, 1976.

Klein, J.: *The Biology of the Mouse Histocompatibility-2 Complex. Principles of Immunogenetics Applied to a Single System*. Springer-Verlag, New York, 1975.

Ling, N. R. and Kay, J. E.: *Lymphocyte Stimulation*, 2nd ed. North-Holland, Amsterdam, 1975.

Loor, F. and Roelants, G. E. (Eds.): *B and T Cells in Immune Recognition*. Wiley, Chichester, 1977.

Micklem, H. S. and Loutit, J. F.: *Tissue Grafting and Radiation*. Academic, New York, 1966.

Möller, G. (Ed.): *Transplantation Tolerance. Immunological Reviews*, Vol. 46. Munksgaard, Copenhagen, 1979.

Simonsen, M.: Graft-versus-host reactions. Their natural history and applicability as tools of research. *Progr. Allergy* **6**:349–467, 1962.

Snell, G. D.: Recent advances in histocompatibility immunogenetics. *Adv. Genet.* **20**:291–355, 1979.

Snell, G. D., Dausset, J., and Nathenson, S.: *Histocompatibility*. Academic, New York, 1976.

Turk, J. L.: *Delayed Hypersensitivity*, 3rd ed. Elsevier/North-Holland, Amsterdam, 1980.

Zinkernagel, R. M. and Dotherty, P. C.: MHC-restricted cytotoxic T cells: studies on the biological role of the polymorphic major transplantation antigens determining T-cell restriction—specificity, function, and responsiveness. *Adv. Immunol.* **27**:51–177, 1979.

Original Articles

Andersson, L. C. and Häyry, P.: Generation of T memory cells in one-way mixed lymphocyte culture. I. Selective recovery of activated cells and their reversion to "secondary" lymphocytes. *Scand. J. Immunol.* **3**:461–469, 1974.

Benjamin, E. and Sluka, E.: Antikörperbildung nach experimenteller Schädigung des hämatopoietischen Systems durch Röntgenstrahlen. *Wien. Klin. Wochenschr.* **21**:311–315, 1908.

Bevan, M. J.: Cross-priming for a secondary cytotoxic response to minor H antigens with *H-2* cytotoxic cells which do not cross-react in the cytotoxic assay. *J. Exp. Med.* **143**:1283–1288, 1976.

Billingham, R. E., Lampkin, G. H., Medawar, P. B., and Williams, H. L.: Tolerance to homografts, twin diagnosis, and the freemartin condition in cattle. *Heredity* **6**:201–212, 1952.

Billingham, R. E., Brent, L., and Medawar, P. B.: Quantitative studies on tissue transplantation immunity. III. Actively acquired tolerance. *Philos. Trans. R. Soc. Lond.* (*Biol.*) **239**: 357–414, 1956.

Cantor, H. and Asofsky, R.: Synergy among lymphoid cells mediating the graft-versus-host response. *J. Exp. Med.* **131**:235–246, 1970.

Counce, S., Smith, P., Barth, R., and Snell, G. D.: Strong and weak histocompatibility gene differences in mice and their role in the rejection of homografts of tumors and skin. *Ann. Surg.* **144**:198–204, 1956.

Dempster, W. J.: Kidney homotransplantation. *Br. J. Surg.* **40**:447–465, 1953.

Flexner, S. and Jobling, J. W.: On the promoting influence of heated tumor emulsions on tumor growth. *Proc. Soc. Exp. Biol. Med.* **4**:156–157, 1907.

Gershon, R. K. and Kondo, K.: Cell interactions in the induction of tolerance: the role of thymic lymphocytes. *Immunology* **18**:723–737, 1970.

Ginsburg, H. and Sachs, L.: Destruction of mouse and rat embryo cells in tissue culture by lymph node cells from unsensitized rats. *J. Cell. Comp. Physiol.* **66**:199–220, 1965.

Gordon, R. D., Simpson, E., and Samelson, L. E.: *In vitro* cell-mediated immune responses to the male specific (H-Y) antigen in mice. *J. Exp. Med.* **142**:1108–1120, 1975.

Govaerts, A.: Cellular antibodies in kidney transplantation. *J. Immunol.* **85**:516–522, 1960.

Häyry, P. and Defendi, V.: Mixed lymphocyte cultures produce effector cells: model in vitro for allograft rejection. *Science* **168**:133–135, 1970.

Hodes, R. J. and Svedmyr, E. A. J.: Specific cytotoxicity of *H*-2-incompatible mouse lymphocytes following mixed culture in vitro. *Transplantation* **9**:470–477, 1970.

Jadassohn, J.: Zur Kenntnis der medikamentösen Dermatosen. *Verh. Dtsch. Dermatol. Gesellsch.* **5**:103–129, 1896.

Jones, T. D. and Mote, J. R.: The phases of foreign protein sensitization in human beings. *New Engl. J. Med.* **210**:120–123, 1934.

Lightbody, J., Bernocco, D., Miggiano, V. C., and Ceppellini, R.: Cell mediated lympholysis in man after sensitization of effector lymphocytes through mixed leukocyte cultures. *J. Bacteriol. Virol. Immunol.* **64**:243–254, 1971.

Lillie, F. R.: Theory of the free-martin. *Science* **43**:611–613, 1916.

Mantoux, C.: L'intradermo-réaction à la tuberculine et son interprétation clinique. *Presse Med.* **18**:10–13, 1910.

Murphy, D. B., Herzenberg, L. A., Okumura, K., Herzenberg, L. A., and McDevitt, H. O.: A new subregion (*I-J*) marked by a locus (*Ia-4*) controlling surface determinants on suppressor T lymphocytes. *J. Exp. Med.* **144**:699–712, 1976.

Murphy, J. B.: The effect of adult chicken organ graft on the chick embryo. *J. Exp. Med.* **24**:1–6, 1916.

Pearmain, G., Lycette, R. R., and Fitzgerald, P. H.: Tuberculin-induced mitosis in peripheral blood leukocytes. *Lancet* **1**:637–638, 1963.

Schreck, R. and Donnelly, W. J.: Differences between lymphocytes of leukemic and non-leukemic patients with respect to morphologic features, motility, and sensitivity to guinea pig serum. *Blood* **18**:561–571, 1961.

Shearer, G. M., Rehn, T. G., and Garbarino, C. A.: Cell-mediated lympholysis of trinitrophenyl-modified autologous lymphocytes. Effector cell specificity to modified cell surface components controlled by the *H-2K* and *H-2D* serological regions of the murine major histocompatibility complex. *J. Exp. Med.* **151**:1348–1364, 1975.

Yunis, E. J. and Amos, D. B.: Three closely linked genetic systems relevant to transplantation. *Proc. Natl. Acad. Sci. U.S.A.* **68**:3031–3035, 1971.

Zinkernagel, R. M. and Doherty, P. C.: Restriction of *in vitro* T cell mediated cytotoxicity in lymphocytic choriomeningitis within a syngeneic or semiallogeneic system. *Nature* **248**:701–702, 1974.

(See also references 4, 6, 8, 12, 13, 40, 72, and 87 in Chapter 2.)

CHAPTER 13

RESPONSES DOMINATED BY B LYMPHOCYTES

Secretion of antibodies is the only known function of a B lymphocyte. To prepare for performing this function, the bone marrow-derived lymphocyte precursor undergoes a series of differentiation steps that culminate in the expression of immunoglobulin receptors on the cell surface (see Chapter 5). First, it expresses receptors of the IgM isotype, then of the IgM and IgD types, and finally, of the IgM, IgG, IgA, or IgE type, with or without IgD. The mature B lymphocyte settles down in a B-dependent area of a lymphoid organ and waits for an antigen to come by, like a Venus flytrap waiting for an insect. In this resting period the cell is in the G_0 phase, performing only housekeeping functions. When it encounters the right antigenic molecule, the V-region tentacles of the immunoglobulin receptor grasp the molecule at the complementary site—the "fly" has been caught. This interaction with the antigen sends the cell on a new differentiation course: the triggered lymphocyte leaves the G_0 phase and transforms, through a complex series of events, into a plasma cell that secretes antibodies having the same V-region specificity as the cell surface receptor of the original B cell. The secreted antibodies enter the blood or other bodily fluids and participate in the various forms of humoral immunity.

In this chapter we shall follow the general outline of B-cell function as described above. In the first part of the chapter we shall discuss the conditions leading to antigen binding by B cells, summarize the present knowledge of B-cell triggering, and introduce a few general principles of antibody production in vitro and in vivo; in the second part of the chapter we shall deal with specific forms of IgM, IgG, IgA, and IgE immunity; and in the last part we shall concern ourselves with the regulation of B-cell and antibody reactivity and with the conditions resulting in B-cell unresponsiveness.

13.1 CONDITIONS OF ANTIGEN RECOGNITION BY B LYMPHOCYTES

13.1.1 Carrier Effect

The reader will recall from Chapter 10 that the introduction of an unconjugated hapten into the body fails to stimulate antibody production. The introduction of a hapten attached to a carrier stimulates the production of both antihapten and anticarrier immunoglobulins, whereas the introduction of carrier alone leads to the production of carrier-specific antibodies. The contribution of the carrier to the stimulation of hapten-specific antibodies was investigated in 1963 by Zoltan Ovary and Baruj Benacerraf, who immunized three groups of rabbits with dinitrophenyl (DNP, used here as a hapten) attached to bovine gamma globulin (BGG, used here as a carrier; see Fig. 13.1). Following the first immunization, they reinjected the animals in the first group with DNP-BGG (the same hapten on a homologous carrier; Fig. 13.1*a*), those in the second group with DNP-ovalbumin (DNP-OA, the same hapten on a heterologous carrier; Fig. 13.1*b*), and those in the third group with BGG alone (the carrier without the hapten; Fig. 13.1*c*). Testing of the rechallenged recipients for DNP-specific antibodies revealed that only the first group (animals reinjected with the same hapten on the same carrier) responded strongly to the second injection; in the remaining two groups low antibody titer was probably a fading-away response to the first injection, and there was no evidence that the second injection had augmented this response. The experiments proved that an augmented antibody response to the second injection of a hapten occurs only when the hapten is presented on the same carrier in both the first and second injections—a phenomenon referred to as *carrier effect*.

At first, immunologists thought that the carrier effect was caused by the simultaneous recognition of the hapten and part of the carrier, so that when the hapten was presented to the stimulated cell on another carrier, the cell could not recognize it. But later studies proved this explanation to be wrong. In one study, for example, animals were immunized with a given hapten-carrier conjugate and rechallenged by the same conjugate but with the haptens separated spatially from the carrier by spacer molecules. The insertion of the spacer made it impossible for the antibody-secreting cells to recognize the hapten together with a portion of the carrier, yet the reinjected animals responded as if rechallenged with unseparated hapten-carrier conjugates. Experiments of this kind suggested that during an antibody response the haptenic and carrier portions of a hapten-carrier conjugate are recognized separately, but that both types of recognition must occur simultaneously for response to be initiated. This suggestion was borne out in 1969 by the experiments of N. Avrion Mitchison and his colleagues.

Mitchison immunized mice with hapten-carrier conjugate NIP-OA (where NIP is a hapten 4-hydroxy-3-iodo-5-nitrophenylacetic acid, and OA is a carrier, chicken ovalbumin) and then injected spleen cells of these mice into three groups of irradiated syngeneic recipients (Fig. 13.2). One group of recipients received NIP-OA (Fig. 13.2*a*) in addition to the cells, while the second and third groups received NIP-BSA (the same hapten conjugated to a heterolo-

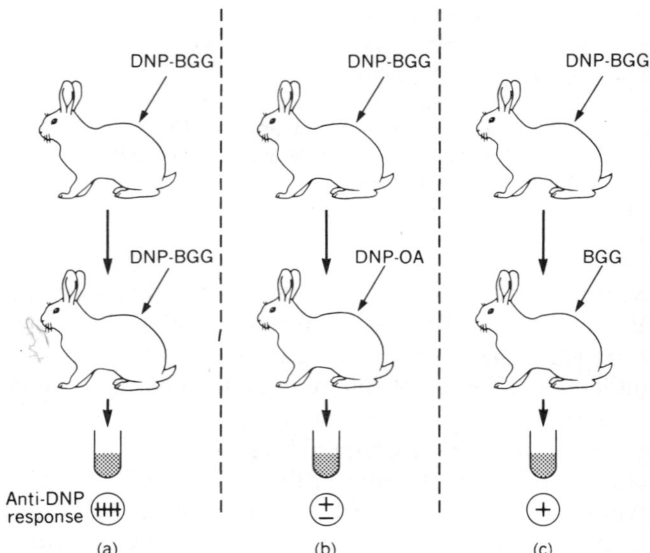

Figure 13.1. An experiment demonstrating the carrier effect. Explanation in the text. BGG, bovine gamma globulin; DNP, dinitrophenyl; OA, ovalbumin.

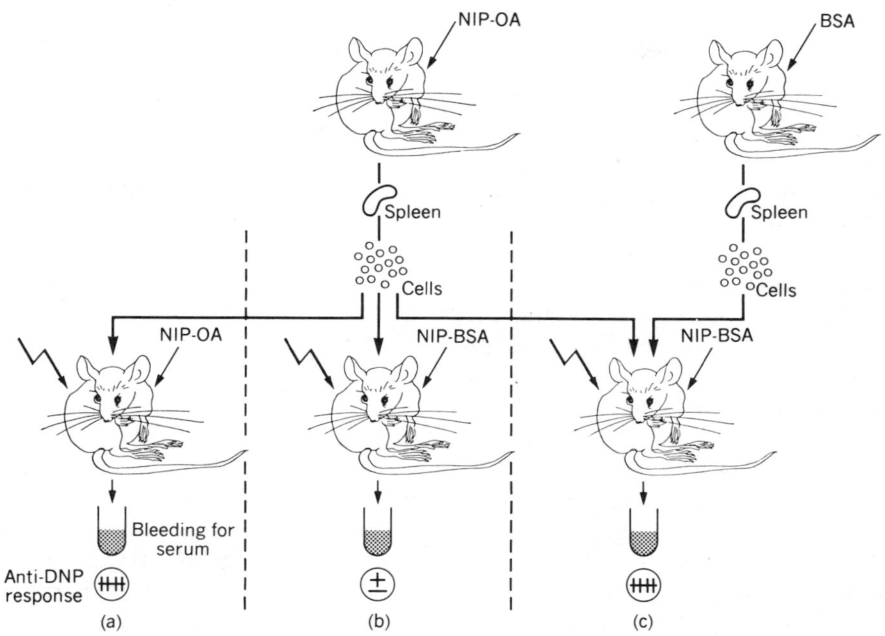

Figure 13.2. An experiment demonstrating that, in an antibody response, hapten and carrier are recognized by different cells. Explanation in the text. BSA, bovine serum albumin; NIP, 4-hydroxy-3-iodo-5-nitrophenylacetic acid; OA, ovalbumin.

gous carrier, bovine serum albumin; Fig. 13.2*b* and *c*). The third group also received spleen cells from syngeneic mice immunized against BSA (carrier alone without a hapten; Fig. 13.2*c*). Testing of the secondary recipients revealed augmented antibody response in the first and third, but not the second group. The result obtained in the first and second groups established that the carrier effect also operates following cell transfer (the immunizing hapten presented to the transferred cells on a heterologous carrier fails to induce augmented secondary response); the third group demonstrated that the carrier effect could be overcome by the addition of cells sensitized to the homologous carrier. The latter result suggested that the hapten and carrier might be recognized by different cells, and that the antibody response might be the result of a cooperative effort of at least two cell types. This conclusion was consistent with other investigators' findings indicating participation in the antibody response of both bone marrow- and thymus-derived cells.

13.1.2 T-B Collaboration

In 1966 Henry N. Claman and his co-workers described what is now regarded as one of the classical experiments in cellular immunology. These investigators lethally irradiated three groups of mice and inoculated them with an immunizing antigen (sheep red blood cells) and cells from a normal syngeneic donor (Fig. 13.3). One group received thymus cells (Fig. 13.3*a*), the second bone marrow cells (Fig. 13.3*b*), and the third group a mixture of thymus and bone marrow cells (Fig. 13.3*c*). When antibodies to sheep red blood cells could be found only in the group inoculated with

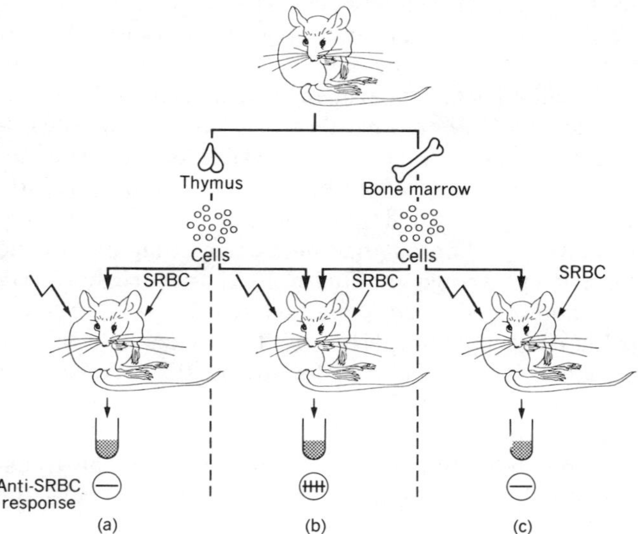

Figure 13.3. An experiment demonstrating collaboration between T and B cells in antibody response. Explanation in the text. SRBC, sheep red blood cells.

the thymus/bone marrow mixture, Claman and his co-workers concluded that at least two cell populations are required for antibody formation—one derived from bone marrow, the other from the thymus.

Experiments performed by Anthony J. S. Davies and his co-workers and by Graham F. Mitchell and Jacques F. A. P. Miller then (in 1967) demonstrated, through the use of chromosome or antigenic markers, that thymus cells proliferated in response to antigen but did not make antibodies, and that bone marrow cells in the absence of thymus cells neither proliferated nor produced antibodies. But when the two cell populations were injected together into a host and challenged with an antigen, antibodies were formed by the bone marrow-derived cells. The two cell types were later identified as thymus-derived (T) and bone marrow-derived (B) lymphocytes.

In 1970 Martin C. Raff brought the two lines of investigation together by demonstrating in the mouse that the carrier-specific cells were T lymphocytes because they were sensitive to the treatment of anti-Thy-1 serum and complement (the treatment abolished a cooperative effect in hapten-carrier recognition). The combined data from this series of experiments led to the conclusion that B lymphocytes recognize, via their Ig receptors, the haptenic portion of an antigen but alone cannot respond to the antigen. To be triggered, they need the help of T lymphocytes, which recognize—again via a specific receptor—a different region of the antigen, the carrier region. Antibody formation is, then, the result of cooperation between hapten-recognizing B lymphocytes and carrier-recognizing T helper cells. The carrier effect results from the fact that T helper cells sensitized to the carrier of one hapten-carrier conjugate cannot help B cells reacting with the same hapten on a different carrier. In their cell transfer experiments, Mitchison and his colleagues could overcome the effect because the sensitization of helper T cells by a carrier occurs independently of the hapten, and because these independently generated helper cells can interact with B cells sensitized by a different hapten-carrier complex. In the experiment shown in Figure 13.2, the original NIP-OA-immunized mice contained sensitized B cells capable of recognizing NIP and T cells capable of recognizing OA. Upon transfer in the third group, the expanded clones of OA-specific T cells were of no use because the NIP was now presented on the BSA carrier; but their function was taken over by the transferred helper T cells sensitized to the new carrier—the BSA.

Subsequent experiments performed by Richard W. Dutton, Anneliese Schimpl, Eberhard Wecker, David H. Katz, Michael J. Taussig, and others have revealed that T lymphocytes can be replaced in their helper function by soluble, T cell-secreted factors and that these factors are either specific or nonspecific for the antigen that induced T-cell proliferation leading to their production. We described these *T helper factors* and the experiments defining them in section 7.1, which the reader should reread before continuing further.

13.1.3 Allogeneic Effect

A different way of overcoming the carrier effect was discovered independently in 1970 by J. A. Hirst and Richard W. Dutton and by William E. Paul and his co-workers. The latter team immunized guinea pigs of strain X against DNP-OA conjugate, and three weeks later divided the animals into two groups, injecting one group with syngeneic (strain-X; Fig. 13.4*a*) and the other with allogeneic (strain-Y) lymphoid cells (Fig. 13.4*b*). Six days after the cell inoculation, they injected both groups with DNP-BGG (the same hapten on a heterologous carrier), and seven days later determined the level of DNP antibodies in both groups of guinea pigs. As expected (because of the carrier effect), the first group had a low level of antibodies; but surprisingly, the sera of the animals in the second group contained a high concentration of DNP antibodies. The latter result indicated that the injected allogeneic cells had overcome the carrier effect—a phenomenon named, by David H. Katz and his co-workers, the *allogeneic effect*.

Later studies revealed that the allogeneic effect is most pronounced under conditions favoring the development of graft-versus-host reaction, so the effect is explained as follows: the inoculated allogeneic T cells recognize histocompatibility antigens of the host and are activated by them; the proliferation results in the expansion of many T-cell clones, among them, clones reactive with a given carrier; the expanded T clones then help B lymphocytes to mount the response to the hapten.

In summary, there are two ways of overcoming the carrier effect—a specific way, in which only T-cell clones reactive with a given carrier are expanded, and a nonspecific way, leading to the expansion of many T-cell clones, among them clones specific for a given carrier.

13.1.4 MHC Involvement in T-B Collaboration

During the investigation of T-B collaboration in the late 1960s, investigators obtained several hints that molecules controlled by the major histocompatibility com-

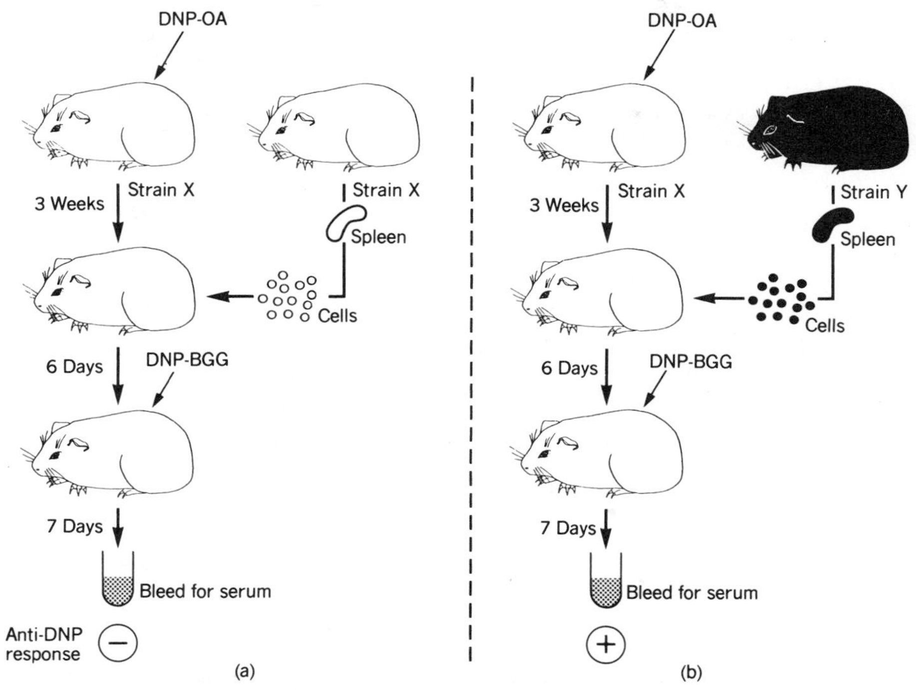

Figure 13.4. An experiment demonstrating the allogeneic effect. Explanation in the text. BGG, bovine gamma globulin; DNP, dinitrophenyl; OA, ovalbumin.

plex (MHC) might, in some important way, participate in this collaboration. But it was not until 1972 and 1973 that immunologists began to entertain seriously the notion of incorporating the MHC into their T-B collaboration models.

In 1972 Berenice Kindred and Donald C. Shreffler made the following observation. To make congenitally athymic mice produce antibodies to sheep red blood cells, they inoculated these mice with thymocytes of normal donors. They reasoned that, since the mice have B cells, the injection of T cells (and antigen) should result in normal T-B collaboration and antibody production. This expectation was indeed fulfilled by the experiment, but only when the thymocyte donor shared its MHC haplotypes with the athymic recipient; when the donor and recipient differed at the MHC, no collaboration occurred and no antibodies were produced.

In 1973 David H. Katz and his co-workers had a similar experience using a much more complicated experimental system (Fig. 13.5). They injected spleen cells from X-strain mice immunized against BGG into normal unimmunized (X × Y)F_1 hybrids (Fig. 13.5*b*); 24 hours later, when the injected cells reached their destination in the lymphoid organ, the recipients were lethally irradiated. The irradiation killed all the lymphocytes in the recipients except those T cells immune to BGG (the authors had shown previously that carrier-primed T cells are relatively radioresistant). Shortly after the irradiation, they injected the recipients with B cells from mice immunized against DNP-keyhole limpet hemocyanin (KLH; see Fig. 13.5*a*), and boosted the recipients with DNP-BGG. (The B cells were obtained by treatment of a spleen cell suspension with anti-Thy-1 in the presence of complement.) The recipients produced relatively high titers of DNP antibodies, indicating that the BGG-specific T cells cooperated with the DNP-specific B cells (KLH functioned as a carrier for the DNP hapten). The authors then repeated the experiment, using X-derived T cells and Y-derived B cells (or vice versa) instead (Fig. 13.5*c*). This time they failed to detect a significant level of DNP antibodies in the serum, indicating that the carrier-primed T cells did not cooperate with the histoincompatible hapten-primed B cells. One may ask why the B cells were not activated nonspecifically through the allogeneic effect. The authors explained the absence of the allogeneic effect as being the result of the restricted number of carrier-primed T cells (all the other T cells were presumably killed by the irradiation), and of the fact that the hapten-primed B cells in the F_1 recipient constituted but a small portion of cells against which the carrier-primed cells could react (the parental T cells

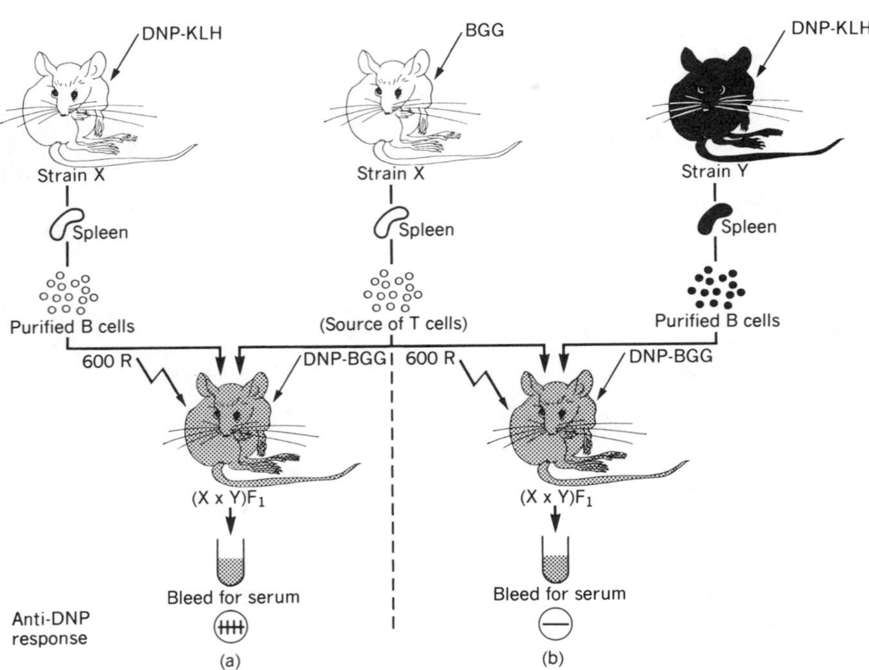

Figure 13.5. An experiment demonstrating the involvement of the MHC in T-B collaboration. Explanation in the text. BGG, bovine gamma globulin; DNP, dinitrophenyl; KLH, keyhole limpet hemocyanin.

could react against the cells of the F_1 host). Using a series of congenic mouse strains, Katz and his coworkers then demonstrated that the compatibility requirement is restricted to the MHC class II loci: T and B cells compatible at these loci cooperated, whereas class II-incompatible cells did not.

These experiments suggested that helper T cells, like the cytotoxic T cells described in Chapters 7 and 12, have dual specificity: they recognize the antigen (the carrier portion of the antigen, in the case of helper T cells) *and* the MHC molecules. The two types of T cells differ in which MHC molecules they recognize: cytotoxic T cells recognize antigens mostly in the context of class I MHC molecules, whereas helper T cells recognize antigens largely in conjunction with class II MHC molecules. It should be mentioned, however, that not every immunologist agrees with this interpretation. There are reports in the literature claiming that the requirement for MHC compatibility is an experimental artifact, and some of those who accept this requirement favor other, in my view, more complicated and less probable explanations.

13.1.5 Thymus-Independent Antibody Responses

The requirement for T-cell help in antibody synthesis by B cells is not absolute. There are substances—the so-called T-independent antigens and many lectins—that activate B lymphocytes in the relative absence of T lymphocytes as, for instance, in congenitally athymic or thymectomized mice. The emphasis in this last sentence is on the word *relative*, since in no instance has the participation of a low number of T cells or of T-cell precursors been rigorously excluded. There is, however, a clear difference between thymus-dependent antigens, the response to which is abolished by thymectomy, and thymus-independent antigens, which induce antibody response even in thymectomized animals. The division of antigens into T-dependent and T-independent is an operational one, for there is no single physicochemical property characterizing one or the other of the two groups (see also Chapter 10). Although the majority of T-independent antigens consist of identical units arranged into a more or less linear repetitive sequence, this feature is probably neither sufficient nor absolutely necessary for relative thymus independence. Some other characteristics common to many T-independent antigens are these: they persist for a long time in the injected animals; most are mitogenic for B lymphocytes and activate polyclonal antibody synthesis; they elicit mainly IgM production and far less IgG synthesis; memory in T-independent responses is either absent or poorly developed; and the responses are relatively independent of macrophage participation. It must be emphasized, however, that all these characteristics are relative; exceptions exist to all the above statements.

13.1.6 Mechanism of Antigen-Driven B-Cell Activation and Differentiation

Despite an intensive research effort in many immunological laboratories, there are still many loose ends and gaps in our understanding of the process that leads to antibody secretion. From the experiments we have discussed and from others not mentioned here, one can arrive at the following highly tentative scheme of events leading to antibody formation (Fig. 13.6).

An antigen entering the body is processed by macrophages and presented to helper T cells along with the macrophage's own class II MHC molecules (Fig. 13.6*a*). The helper T cell recognizes, via its antigen-specific receptors, the carrier portion of the antigen in the context of class II molecules and is thereby activated. The clone of activated T helper cells is expanded by multiple division (probably with the help of

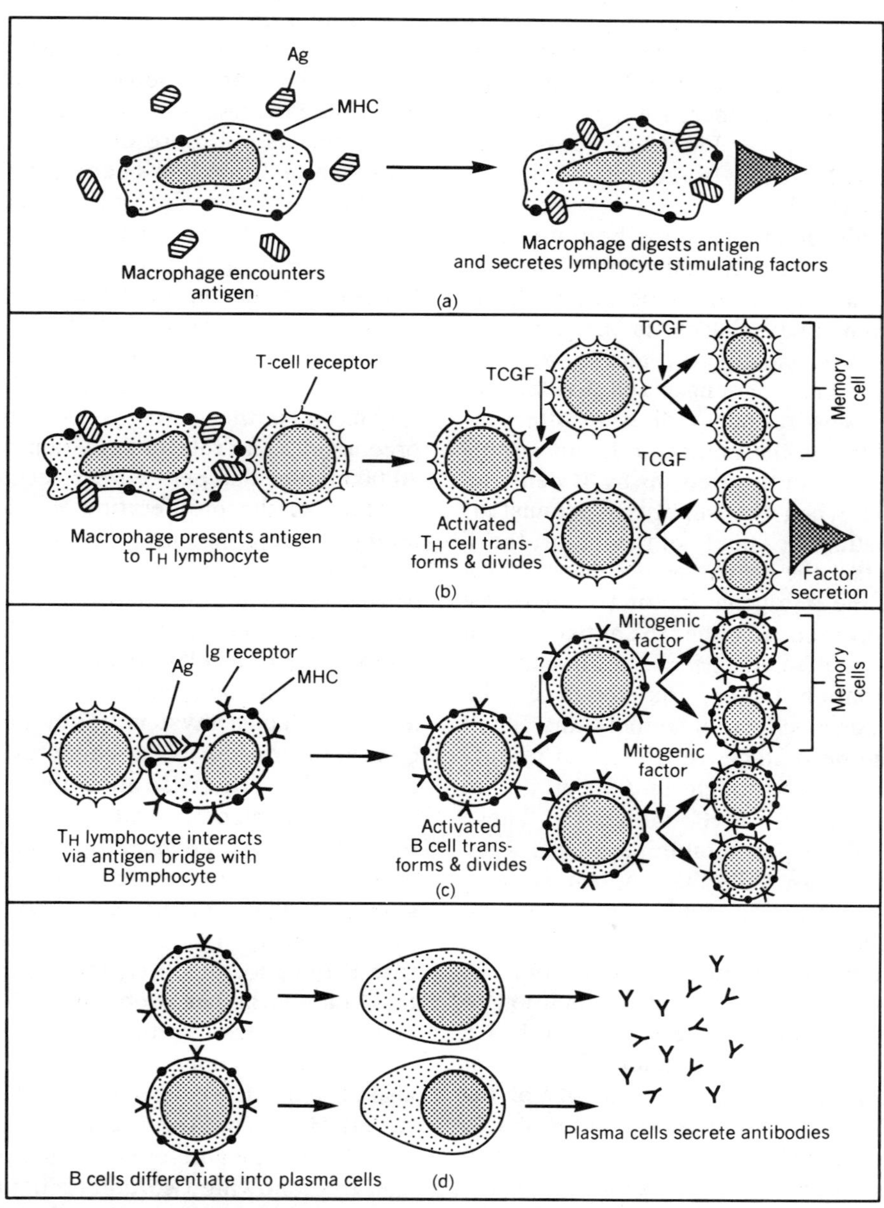

Figure 13.6. Postulated main steps leading to B-cell activation and differentiation into antibody-producing plasma cells. Explanation in the text. TCGF, T-cell growth factor.

macrophage-derived soluble factors), and during this expansion it, in turn, produces soluble T helper factors capable of interacting with B lymphocytes (Fig. 13.6*b*). The activated helper T cells then interact with B lymphocytes via an *antigen bridge*, in which the carrier portion is bound to the T-cell receptor and the haptenic portion to the B-cell Ig receptor; simultaneously, the T cell also recognizes major histocompatibility complex molecules, presumably also on the B-cell surface (Fig. 13.6*c*). Alternatively, the B cell may interact with the T helper factor. The simultaneous interaction with antigen and helper T cells starts a train of events that causes the B cell to leave the G_0 phase and enter the G_1 phase, in which it transforms morphologically into a blast: the cell enlarges; the nucleolus swells; polysomes and microtubules form; rates of macromolecular synthesis increase (the by now familiar *blast transformation*; see Fig. 13.6*c*). It is at the blast stage that the B lymphocyte requires additional help, probably from the T cell or possibly from the macrophage. The train of events stops here unless a helper factor (that may be identical to the one that helped set the train in motion, or some other factor, perhaps derived from macrophages) is present. The helper factor has a mitogenic effect: it allows the blast to enter the DNA synthetic (S) phase and divide. The cell then undergoes one round of division after another, but only as long as the mitogenic factor is present. The factor is apparently used up by B cells, so division cycles stop when the supply is exhausted. Therefore, by regulating the supply of the factor, the T helper cell can control the extent of B-cell proliferation. The action of the mitogenic factor is apparently independent of the presence of either the antigen or the class II molecule on the B-cell surface. So, in contrast to that of the initiation factor, the action of the mitogenic factor is nonspecific (polyclonal—any B cell that has reached the blast stage, regardless of its IgG receptor specificity, can be brought to division by the factor) and not restricted by MHC molecules. These two facts mean that, during an immune response, some bystander B cells—that is, cells that happen to be in the right stage of differentiation, not because of activation by a given antigen but for some other reason—are also brought to antibody secretion, so that some irrelevant antibodies may be produced, in addition to specific ones. However, the mitogenic factor has a short range of action and so the activation of bystander B lymphocytes is limited to the close vicinity of the producing helper T cells. The mitogenic, and probably the initiation factors as well, can be replaced to a certain degree by certain lectins and by the mitogenic portions of at least some T-independent antigens. The different B-cell lectins are largely interchangeable in the sense that a B cell brought to division cycle by one lectin can be brought into a second cycle by another lectin.

Following antigenic stimulation, the B lymphocytes differentiating toward plasma cells progressively lose their Ig receptors and thereby become less susceptible to antigen-mediated control (Fig. 13.6*d*). Cells approaching the plasma cell stage are essentially devoid of Ig receptors. The antibody-secreting cell is an end cell that cannot differentiate any further. It has been estimated that, from activation to the fully differentiated stage, a B cell undergoes from six to 10 rounds of cell division.

The question of whether IgM- and IgG-producing cells derive from separate, pre-existing antigen-inducible precursors or whether the latter derive from the former is still unresolved. (Although IgG-bearing cells derive from IgM-bearing cells, the question of whether the IgM-to-IgG switch occurs before or after the contact with an antigen remains; see Chapter 6.) When exactly a B cell begins to secrete antibodies (whether in the terminal plasma cell stage of differentiation or before) is not known either. Each plasma cell secretes antibodies of only one class (IgM or IgG) and one specificity—generally the same class and specificity as the Ig receptors displayed by its B-cell precursors. The rate of secretion ranges from 3000 to 30,000 molecules per cell per second.

Many of the proliferating B cells differentiate into antibody-secreting plasma cells, but some return to the morphology of a small lymphocyte and become *memory cells*, capable of rapid response to a repeated encounter with the same antigen. What decides whether the product of a cell division will be a plasma or memory cell is unknown, and the memory cells themselves are shrouded in mystery. They are thought to be, in contrast to resting B lymphocytes, long-lived and circulating, but otherwise almost nothing is known about them. Most memory cells express IgG receptors, so that when activated again by a second antigenic exposure, they give rise to IgG-secreting cells, though instances of IgM memory have also been recorded. This predilection for IgG secretors suggests that more mature B lymphocytes (i.e., those expressing IgG receptors) have a higher probability of becoming memory cells than do less mature cells.

The circumstances of memory cell generation are also obscure. If we designate, with Eli E. Sercarcz and Albert H. Coons, the precursor cells X, the memory cells Y, and the antibody-forming cells Z, we can envision the following two differentiation pathways in the generation of memory cells following primary immunization:

$$X \rightarrow Y \rightarrow Z \quad \text{or} \quad X \begin{smallmatrix} \nearrow Y \\ \searrow Z \end{smallmatrix}$$

(Linear pathway) (Branched pathway)

According to this scheme, the Y cells are either an arrested stage in the development of Z, or Y and Z derive by asymmetrical division from a common precursor.

When pre-existing Y cells are already present, new memory cells can be generated following secondary immunization in one of two ways:

$$Y \rightarrow Y \rightarrow Z \quad \text{or} \quad Y \begin{smallmatrix} \nearrow Z \\ \searrow Y \end{smallmatrix}$$

Most of the available data favor the branched pattern of differentiation, but the factors determining whether a cell becomes a Y or a Z are not known. One possibility is that Y cells are generated when the number of active T helper cells drops to a certain level, insufficient for the generation of T-dependent Z cells. Or possibly the dividing cells are channeled toward Y by a high ratio of antigen to T helper cells; low antigen/Th ratios would then favor production of Z cells (*signal balance model*; see below).

Let us return for a moment to the initial events in B-cell activation and consider what their nature might be. Most immunologists agree that at least two things must happen on the B-cell surface before the activation: the B cell must interact with a hapten via the Ig receptor and also with another factor (T cell, helper factor) via some other cell-surface structure. Immunologists differ, however, in the degree of significance they attribute to these interactions. According to one school of thought, the most vocal proponents of which are Göran Möller and Antonio Coutinho, the hapten binding by Ig receptors serves merely to focus the antigen into such a position that it can then interact with a second, unidentified receptor. It is the interaction with this second receptor that initiates B-cell triggering. Since it is the interaction with the hypothetical receptors—not the interaction with the Ig receptors—that results in an activation signal, this view is referred to as the *one-signal hypothesis* of B-cell activation. According to the second school of thought, represented, for example, by Melvin Cohn and Peter A. Bretscher, both interactions generate signals for the cell (hence the designation *two-signal hypothesis*). The lines between the contrasting views are sharply drawn on the basis of only a few facts—not a very helpful situation for the solution of the problem.

The manner of ligand-receptor interaction on the cell surface has been the subject of many speculations. Some immunologists believe that the interactions lead to a crosslinking and rearrangement of receptors similar to that observed during antibody-induced patching and capping of cell-surface components, but evidence supporting this hypothesis is lacking. The nature of the signal or signals transmitted from the cell surface to the nucleus is totally unknown. Many of the cell-surface and intracellular events in B-cell activation are probably similar to those occurring during T-cell activation, which we discussed in the preceding chapter.

The T-independent responses can be explained by postulating that a certain proportion of B cells expressing low-avidity IgM receptors can be induced to differentiate into IgM-secreting plasma cells, by multivalent, persisting (T-independent) antigens and by polyclonal B-cell activators, such as LPS. This "baseline" response is generated in the absence of T-cell help. Similar small fractions of low-affinity cells may also exist among the IgG-bearing lymphocytes, since certain T-independent antigens—for example, TNP-Ficoll—can also induce IgG antibody production. All other IgM- and IgG-bearing (higher affinity) B lymphocytes differentiate into antibody-secreting cells only in the presence of T cells.

13.2 IgM- AND IgG-DOMINATED RESPONSES

Of the five immunoglobulin classes, only four (IgM, IgG, IgA, and IgE) are known to be secreted by B lymphocytes in significant amounts and to participate as antibodies in defense reactions; the fifth class, IgD, is predominantly a cell-surface component presumably involved in B-cell differentiation. Since the M, G, A, and E immunoglobulins are all secreted under different circumstances, we shall deal with the four types of responses separately. We begin with the IgM-G responses, in vivo and in vitro.

13.2.1 Antibody Formation in the Whole Animal

Exposure to Antigen

Natural Immunization. From birth—and sometimes even earlier—to the death of an organism, the immune system is bombarded by quanta of the nonself world—the antigens. Studied at any point, the immune system of an organism bears witness to past encounters: the history of immunological warfare is imprinted on the organism's lymphocytes. One can best judge the effect of nonself stimuli on the immune system by comparing individuals living in conventional conditions with individuals raised in relative isolation from the outside world. The isolation can be accomplished by delivering fetuses through cesarean section, maintaining the maturing individuals in sterile boxes or rooms, and feeding them antigen-free food. These *germ-free* or *axenic* animals (Gr. *a*, negative, *xenos*, foreign) differ from conventional animals in several ways: they synthesize immunoglobulins at about $\frac{1}{500}$th the normal rate; they have exceedingly low levels of serum immunoglobulin (especially IgG); they have markedly underdeveloped secondary lymphoid tissues; and they lack the so-called natural antibodies.

Natural antibodies are serum immunoglobulins reacting with antigens that have not been deliberately introduced in the individual being tested; they are contrasted with *immune antibodies*, produced in response to deliberate introduction of an antigen, or *immunization*. The commonly occurring natural antibodies are those against erythrocytes of the same species (e.g., antibodies against blood group substances A and B in humans; see Chapter 10) or of a different species (e.g., mouse antibodies to sheep red blood cells), and against various bacteria and viruses. In many instances one can demonstrate antibody-secreting cells in the spleen, a condition that indicates that the antibodies are produced continually throughout the life of an individual. The original stimuli for the production of natural antibodies are thought to be provided by microorganisms indigenous to the organism (for example, bacteria living in the animal's intestine) or accidentally introduced during an infection. The antibodies apparently cross-react with certain antigenic determinants of other microorganisms and of mammalian erythrocytes. It is this cross-reactivity that constitutes the basis for the detection of natural antibodies.

There is no principal difference between natural and immune antibodies although the former are usually present in lower concentrations and have a lower affinity (probably because they are detected by cross-reacting antigens) than the latter.

Deliberate Immunization. Like other experimenters, immunologists do not want to leave anything to chance; they want to control the conditions of an experiment as much as possible. In the study of antibody formation, they exert this control by choosing an antigen and introducing it into experimental animals—in other words, they perform *deliberate immunization*. To this end, immunologists can use any of the antigen introduction routes that lead to natural immunization, but the preferred routes for the induction of IgM and IgG responses are into the blood stream (intravenously), the peritoneum (intraperitoneally), or the skin (subcutaneously or intradermally). Most of the discussion in the rest of this chapter will be based on observations obtained following deliberate immunization.

Handling of Antigen by the Body

Even when injected in a large dose, the antigen constitutes only a small fraction of the total body volume—a few sailboats in a vast sea. Therefore, the first task of bodily defense is to locate the antigen and trap it in a place where it can be destroyed. And the first question an immunologist studying antibody formation must ask is what happens to the antigen after it has entered the body. To answer this question, a researcher first labels the antigen by attaching colored substances, such as fluorescein, or radioactive material to it and introduces the labeled antigen into the body. Then, at different times after the injections, he determines the tissue distribution of the antigen, using immunofluorescence or autoradiography, respectively. Much of our present knowledge obtained in this manner has come from studies performed by the Australian immunological school, in particular by Gustav J. V. Nossal and Gordon L. Ada.

The fate of an antigen in the body is influenced by many factors, among them, the route of administration, physicochemical characteristics of the antigen (soluble versus particulate antigen), and the immune status of the recipient (presence or absence of specific antibodies). Of these, the administration route is often the most important factor, the two principal routes being through the skin and via the bloodstream. The fate of the antigen is somewhat different in each situation.

When injected into the *skin*, the antigen is picked up by the lymph and carried by afferent lymphatics into regional lymph nodes. As the lymph percolates through the lymph node, the antigen enters the macrophage-lined afferent sinusoids, then passes through the fine-laced reticular cell matrix of the cortex, and finally ends up in the medulla (Fig. 13.7). On its way "down" in the lymph node, the antigen is either picked up by macrophages or retained on the fine web of the dendritic reticular cell processes, particularly in the region of the primary follicles. The lymph node thus serves as an efficient filter that retains more than 90 percent of the entering antigen; the remaining 10 percent leaves the medulla via the efferent lymphatics, enters the bloodstream via the venous system, and is then filtered through the spleen, liver, kidney, and other organs of the reticuloendothelial system. Most of the antigen taken up by macrophages is degraded in phagosomes into nonantigenic components, while a small portion is processed for a surface display and for presentation to the T lymphocytes (see Chapter 11). The antigen retained by reticular cells in primary follicles is available for interaction with B lymphocytes.

When injected into the *bloodstream*, only a small portion (less than 1 percent) of the soluble antigen becomes involved in the induction of the immune response; the rest is removed from the body by *natural clearance*. The process of antigen degradation in the plasma can be differentiated into three phases (Fig. 13.8).

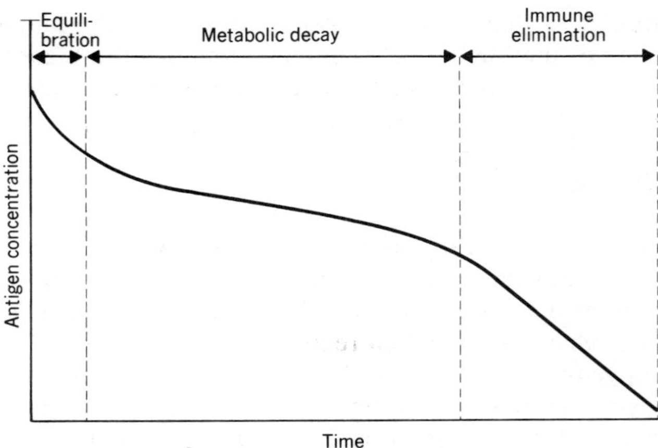

Figure 13.8. Three phases of antigen degradation in the plasma. Time and concentration units are left unspecified to indicate the variability encountered with different antigens under different conditions. Explanation in the text.

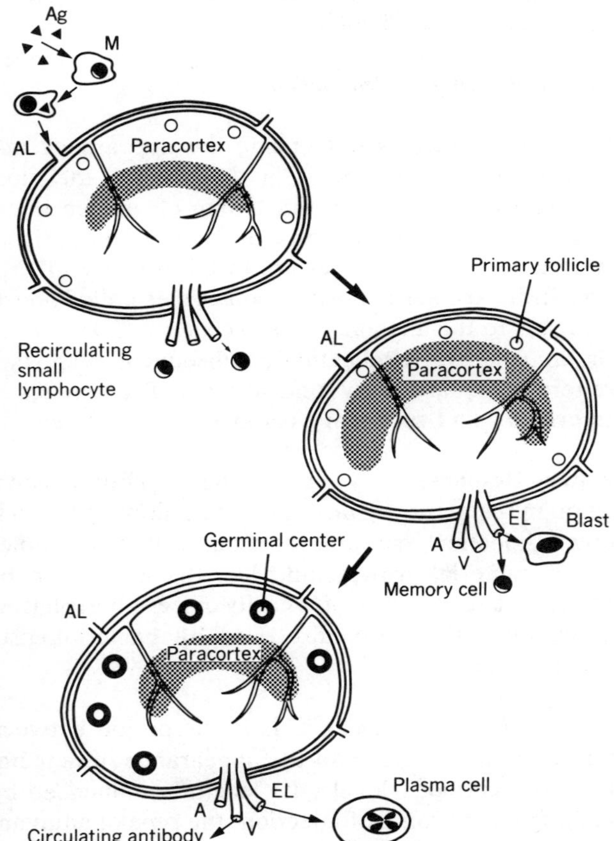

Figure 13.7. Sequence of events in a lymph node following the entrance of an antigen. From top to bottom: antigen (Ag) is taken up by macrophages (M) and brought into the lymph node by afferent lymphatics (AL). The antigen interacts with dendritic macrophages (DM) in the cortex and paracortex. The paracortical region and the primary follicles enlarge and germinal centers appear in the follicles. Antigen-activated cells leave the node via the efferent lymphatics (EL). A, arterial, and V, venous blood supply to the node. (From R. A. Thompson: *The Practice of Clinical Immunology*, 2nd ed. Arnold, London, 1978.)

Equilibrium Phase. The injection of a soluble antigen is followed by a rapid diffusion of the antigen into extravascular spaces and the initial high concentration of the antigen in the plasma drops rapidly. (Particulate antigens, such as bacteria or erythrocytes, do not diffuse into extravascular spaces and hence their clearance shows no equilibrium phase.)

Metabolic Decay Phase. The antigen circulating in the bodily fluids is gradually degraded and its concentration drops slowly.

Immune Elimination Phase. As soon as antibodies against the antigen begin to be produced, they bind the antigen and the ensuing soluble antigen-antibody complexes are taken up and digested by macrophages. Rapid decline in the concentration of free antigen follows. If antibodies are already present in the plasma at the time of injection, the concentration of the antigen drops rapidly from the beginning without a discernible metabolic decay phase.

As a part of this natural clearance, there are traps in the reticuloendothelial system set up for the antigen all over the body. The major entrapment sites of the blood-borne antigen are spleen, liver, bone marrow, lungs, lymph nodes, and kidney. In these organs, where veins connect to arteries, the antigen passes through narrow sinusoids lined with phagocytic cells, which act as a pack of wolves cornering their victim in a valley. In the spleen, antigen is processed in a way similar to that in lymph nodes. Spleen, as the major filter of the blood-borne antigen, contains the highest antigen concentration, although the greatest amount of antigen is found in the liver.

Histology of Antibody Response

The major sites of antibody formation are the lymph nodes and the spleen. In these organs, macrophages present the antigen to the helper T cells as these pass through as a part of their regular migratory circuit. The antigen-reactive T cells become activated, interrupt their migration, and settle down. They are thus rapidly removed from the circulation and the animal goes through a period when it has almost no T cells reactive with a given antigen in the circulating lymph: all the cells are either in the lymph nodes or in the spleen. The lymphocytes enter the lymph nodes through postcapillary venules, and upon encountering the antigen-charged macrophages somewhere in the diffuse cortex (the T-cell domain), they transform into blast cells, divide, and form clones of effector and memory cells. Some of the T cells migrate into the primary follicle, where they encounter the B lymphocytes. The latter, being more sedentary than T cells, show no pronounced retention from circulation after antigen stimulation; most of them are already in the lymph node, waiting for the antigen. Most of the T-B interaction probably occurs in the primary follicle. After stimulation by the antigen and by T helper factors, B cells, too, transform into blasts and begin to divide. The accumulation of dividing B cells, some T cells, and macrophages leads to the formation of germinal centers, which compress the follicle into a crescent (Fig. 13.7; see also Chapter 5). The appearance of germinal centers four to five days after antigen injection transforms the primary follicle into a secondary one. The germinal centers are pronounced for several days and then disappear. The progeny of activated B cells differentiate into plasma cells and memory cells, both of which leave the follicle and descend toward the medulla. Plasma cells are retained in the lymph node; they settle down between the sinuses, form medullary cords, and secrete antibodies. Memory B cells and T cells, on the other hand, enter the efferent lymph and are carried via the major lymphatic ducts into the bloodstream and other lymphoid tissues.

Activated T cells in the lymph node secrete soluble factors that have the following effects: some cause local vessel dilation and so allow leakage (transudation) of plasma from vessels into extravascular spaces; others attract macrophages and granulocytes into the node, which then plug some of the medullary sinuses, causing a slowing down of lymph drainage into efferent lymphatics. The accumulation of fluid and cells is responsible for the lymph node enlargement characteristic of an infection. Eventually, as most of the antigen is processed, the lymph nodes return to their normal size.

Secreted antibodies are transported via efferent lymphatics into the venous system and circulate with blood through the body. Antibodies of the IgG class can also traverse blood vessel walls and enter extravascular tissue spaces. Normally, IgG divides about half and half between blood and extravascular bodily fluids. IgM (and also IgA, IgE, and IgD), on the other hand, usually cannot pass through blood vessel walls and so is largely confined to the bloodstream and to a few special local sites. Circulating antibodies bind the offending antigens and participate in many other effector functions (see Chapter 6).

Kinetics of Antibody Production

Of the many factors influencing the appearance and concentration of antibodies in the plasma, the most important is the number and timing of antigen injections. The first exposure of a recipient to an antigen, referred to as *priming*, results in the *primary* (1°) *response*; the second exposure, sometimes called *boosting*, leads to the anamnestic or *secondary* (2°) *response* (Gr. *anamnesis*, recollection); subsequent responses are tertiary, quarternary, and so forth. The kinetics of the primary and secondary responses are different.

Primary Response. By plotting the antibody concentration in the serum against the time following the first antigen injection, one obtains a curve that resembles that of bacterial growth, and like the latter, can be divided into four (not always easily discernible) phases, known by names originally used by bacteriologists (Fig. 13.9*a*).

The Lag (Latent) Phase. This is the period between antigen administration and the appearance of detectable serum antibody levels. Its length is influenced by the antigen, the route of injection, the type of adjuvant used, and the recipient. It can be as short as three hours and as long as several weeks (Table 13.1).

The Log (Logarithmic, Exponential, Growth) Phase. This is the period during which the antibody concentration in the serum increases at an exponential rate (the curve forms a straight line in this region and can be expressed using natural logarithms). The *doubling time*, the time necessary for a twofold increase in anti-

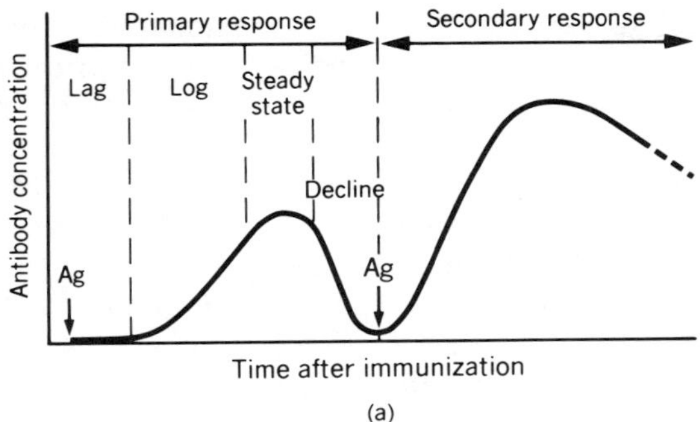

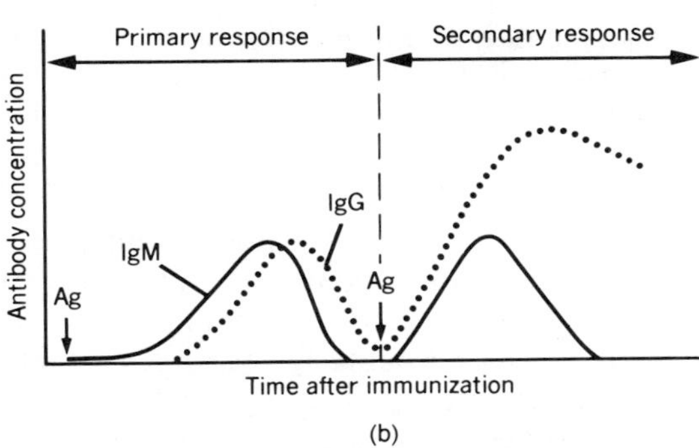

Figure 13.9. Changes in antibody concentration following the first and second injections of antigen (Ag). (*a*) Total antibody. (*b*) IgM and IgG antibody. Time and concentration units are left unspecified to indicate the variability encountered with different antigens under different conditions.

body concentration, determines the slope of the curve; it depends on the antigen dose, the type of antigen injected, and many other factors.

The Steady-State (Plateau) Phase. The period of no net increase or decrease in serum antibody level is called the steady-state phase. The time required to reach it, the height, and its length vary, depending again primarily on the antigen used (Table 13.1). The phase may be missing in some responses, while in others it may last for several weeks.

Table 13.1 Timetable of Primary Responses to Different Antigens

Antigen	Duration of Lag Phase	Attainment of Peak Response
Erythrocytes	3–4 days	4–5 days
Soluble proteins	5–7 days	9–10 days
Bacteria	10–14 days	2–3 weeks
Toxoid	>3 weeks	<3 months

The Decline (Decreasing) Phase. This phase covers the time in which the immunoglobulin degradation rate begins to prevail over the synthetic rate and the serum antibody concentration progressively drops. The length of this phase, once again depending on the circumstances, may range from a few days to several weeks.

Secondary Response. The second antigen injection elicits a response that differs from the primary response in several aspects (Fig. 13.9*b*): shorter lag phase (about half as long as in the primary response); more rapid increase in antibody concentration (the increase is still exponential but the curve is steeper); earlier attainment, greater height, and greater length of the steady-state phase; longer persistence of the decline phase (longer persistence of antibody synthesis; lower threshold antigen dose eliciting detectable response; prevalence of IgG over IgM response; and higher affinity and higher homogeneity of antibody affinity.

The magnitude of the secondary response depends on the interval between the two injections, the response being low when this interval is too short (the still-present antibody binds with the antigen and the resulting antigen-antibody complexes are rapidly cleared) or too long (although the memory cells are long-lived, they are not immortal and the memory eventually fades away).

The capacity for a secondary response may persist for many months (in mice) or years (in humans), long after the last of the antibodies in the blood has vanished. It is this capacity that provides animals with long-lasting protection against an infection once withstood. There is also a difference between primary and secondary response in the requirement for concomitant administration of an adjuvant: significant primary response to many protein antigens can be induced only when the antigen is injected emulsified in an adjuvant, while boosting can be achieved with aqueous antigen solution. Furthermore, primed cells respond to lower antigen concentrations than do unprimed cells, suggesting that memory B cells may have greater avidity.

Changes During Antibody Response

Antibodies at the outset of a response are not the same as those produced at the end of the response: immunologists like to say that the response *matures*. The changes characterizing the maturation of the immune response concern immunoglobulin class, antibody affinity, and antibody specificity.

Changes in Immunoglobulin Class. A simple test for studying the antibody class during antibody response involves treatment of the serum with reducing agents, such as β-mercaptoethanol. When measured by a test based on cell lysis or agglutination, the pentameric IgM antibodies are shown to be much more efficient than IgG. But when dissociated by β-mercaptoethanol into its 7S subunits, IgM has roughly the same activity as IgG. Therefore, when an antiserum containing predominantly IgM antibodies is treated with β-mercaptoethanol, the activity of the antiserum is greatly reduced; in contrast, treatment of IgG-dominated antiserum has little effect on this serum's reactivity.

Studies of the immunoglobulin class during antibody response have revealed that IgM and IgG are usually produced during both the primary and secondary response, but that IgG production in the primary response starts later than does IgM production, and that the secondary response is dominated by IgG production (Fig. 13.9*b*). In both responses, the concentration of IgM in the serum declines rapidly, so that the antibody ceases to be detectable after one or two weeks; in contrast, the IgG antibodies persist in the serum for a long time (but when the antigen is administered in an adjuvant, production of both IgM and IgG may continue for many months). However, as was mentioned earlier, the so-called T-independent antigens often stimulate IgM responses predominantly or exclusively (e.g., horse antibodies to pneumococcal capsular polysaccharide III, rabbit antibodies to the Forssman erythrocyte antigen, or rabbit antibodies to salmonella endotoxin are mostly of the IgM type).

Why IgM is detected earlier than IgG in the primary response is not known, but there are two possible explanations. First, secretion of IgM and IgG may start at the same time, but at the low concentration the more efficient (more avid) IgM is detected earlier than IgG (remember that one IgM molecule has 10 combining sites compared to two sites on the IgG molecule). Indeed, when methods favoring IgG detection were used, low avidity IgG was detected as early as IgM in some instances. The second possibility is that secretion of IgM starts earlier than secretion of IgG. The reason for the delay in IgG secretion could be either that IgM-bearing cells are activated first and IgM-IgG-bearing cells later, or that activated IgM cells later switch to IgG production.

Changes in Antibody Affinity. To study changes in antibody affinity (the strength of the union between antigen and antibody; see Chapter 10), one collects an antiserum at a specified time after immunization, adds a small amount of antigen to it, removes the precipitate, and determines the binding constant of the precipitated fraction. At low antigen concentration, only antibodies with the highest affinity will form antigen-antibody complexes, enabling them to be removed and leaving other antibodies in the solution. Next, the addition of a small amount of antigen to the once precipitated antiserum will precipitate an antibody with the next highest affinity, and so on, so that by repeating this procedure one can separate the antiserum into fractions of decreasing antibody affinity. Studies of this sort, carried out by Herman N. Eisen, Gregory W. Siskind, and others, demonstrated that, first, at any point an antiserum is a heterogeneous mixture of antibodies with different affinities; second, that after immunization, antisera become more homogeneous in terms of antibody affinity with time; third, that the average affinity (avidity) of an antiserum increases during the course of immunization (the increase can be 10,000-fold with some antisera); fourth, that the increase in affinity is particularly pronounced with IgG antibodies and less so or none at all with IgM. These changes are sometimes called *affinity maturation*. The degree of maturation depends on the priming antigen dose and many other parameters. The increase in affinity is most striking after primary immunization with a low dose of antigen; after a high antigen dose, the increase is slow or not detectable at all.

Affinity maturation has been explained by the so-called *antigen-selection hypothesis*, proposed by Gregory W. Siskind and Baruj Benacerraf in 1969. Its principal assumption is that the antigen-binding properties of a cell's membrane Ig receptors and those of the antibodies secreted by the cell's progeny are the same. In other words, a cell with high-affinity receptors synthesizes high-affinity antibodies, whereas cells with low-affinity receptors synthesize low-affinity antibodies. The hypothesis postulates further that, at low antigen concentration, there is competition among B lymphocytes for the available antigen, and that only those cells most fit in terms of receptor affinity are activated to antibody secretion, since they have the highest probability of reacting with the antigen. At the beginning of the response, there is enough antigen to bind not only with high-, but also with low-affinity receptors; but later, as the antigen concentration declines rapidly, the low-affinity receptors cannot compete with the high-affinity receptors, and so fewer and fewer cells with low-affinity receptors are activated. The restriction of activation to cells with high-affinity receptors restricts the heterogeneity of the antiserum in terms of antibody affinity, and the total avidity of the antiserum increases.

This hypothesis has been criticized for being too simplistic, and, indeed, there are several observations that do not fit into this picture of affinity maturation. First, in some instances, the initial rise in antibody affinity may be followed by a later fall; in other instances, alternating waves of high and low affinity have been observed; and in still other instances, antibodies remain functionally homogeneous from the inception of the response. Second, there is some evidence that at least some animals continually synthesize low-affinity antibodies in substantial amounts throughout the immune response, but the demonstration of these antibodies requires special techniques. And third, in accord with the last observation, there is evidence that animals producing relatively homogeneous high-affinity antibodies carry, in their lymphoid organs, heterogeneous populations of both high- and low-affinity memory cells. These observations contradict the antigen-selection hypothesis and suggest that, in fact, there are dynamic changes in antibody affinity throughout the immune response. These changes are probably controlled by many factors that are also involved in the regulation of antibody synthesis (see Section 13.5.4). During the response, cells with low-affinity receptors probably persist along with high-affinity cells and may actually increase their avidity, for example, by increasing their receptor density.

Changes in Antibody Specificity. Since an antigen often has several determinants, and since different determinants have different lag phases for antibody formation, more and more antibody species are produced as the response progresses. The antisera, relatively monospecific at the beginning of the response, become more complex and more cross-reactive with time. And since there is also often a simultaneous increase in antibody affinity, one comes to a seemingly paradoxical conclusion—namely, that high-affinity antibodies become more cross-reactive than low-affinity antibodies. Some immunologists refer to this observation as the *degeneracy of the immune response*.

B-Cell Memory

Although immunologists originally had some doubts about it, it is now clear that B cells do possess memory. For example, one experiment revealed that rabbits immunized with DNP-BGG and rechallenged one year later with DNP-hemocyanin responded in a characteristic secondary fashion, indicating that, in this instance, the memory was stored in the DNP (hapten)-recognizing B cells. However, since secondary response largely affects the IgG antibodies and since IgG production is T cell-dependent, the secondary antibody response usually involves both memory B and memory T cells.[1] It appears that memory B cells can be *generated* in the relative absence of T cells (e.g., in congenitally athymic mice), but that the *expression* of memory characteristics requires helper T cells. (In this respect T-independent antigens may induce memory B cells but the memory may not be expressed, because, for some reason, helper T cells cannot interact with these cells.) The requirement for T-cell participation is more pronounced in the secondary than in the primary response.

Memory probably involves both quantitative changes (e.g., increase in the precursor pool size) and qualitative alterations (e.g., there are reports that memory B cells have altered mobility in an electric field). Memory B cells are believed to carry IgG receptors on their surfaces and there is some evidence that they may also carry surface IgM; whether there is IgD on these cells is a question that is still unresolved. A discussion of B-cell memory would not be complete without mentioning two special instances of memory—the so-called original antigenic sin and nonspecific secondary responses.

Original Antigenic Sin. Thomas T. Francis and his co-workers observed in 1953 that adult humans vaccinated against influenza virus produced antibodies against antigens of the immunizing strain but, paradoxically, produced antibodies of higher titer against the antigen of a virus strain they had encountered during childhood. It was as if humans lived with an immunological memory of experiences acquired in the age of innocence—the way humankind is supposed to live, according to the Old Testament, with Adam's original sin. For this reason, immunologists refer to the phenomenon as the *original antigenic sin*. The phenomenon has been reproduced in laboratory animals and demonstrated to occur also with antigens other than those of the influenza virus. In influenza research, however, original antigenic sin has been used to define serotypes of extinct viruses from past epidemics in a kind of serological archeology (see Chapter 14). The phenomenon can be explained by postulating that memory cells elicited by the original antigen persist in the body and are restimulated by the new antigen, which cross-reacts with the original one. This *cross-stimulation* then results in augmented production of antibodies to the original antigen. Experimental evidence

[1] IgM memory is usually inconspicuous but may become apparent in the relative absence of IgG, as, for example, in some immunodeficiency states.

indicates that the original antigenic sin is a property of B cells.

Nonspecific Secondary Response. There are recorded cases of patients who, while suffering from an illness caused by one kind of bacteria, developed a high titer of antibodies directed against an unrelated bacterium. This observation can be explained by the bystander effect, described earlier in this chapter: T cells activated by one antigen release factors that act nonspecifically on memory B cells generated in response to an unrelated antigen.

13.2.2 Antibody Formation In Vitro

There is an obvious advantage to studying antibody formation in tissue culture, in that the experimental conditions are simpler and more amenable to the manipulation than in the whole animal. However, until 1966 all attempts to develop a culture system for in vitro antibody production were unsuccessful. In that year Robert I. Mishell and Richard W. Dutton described a relatively simple technique for culturing mouse spleen cells in vitro. As it turned out, there was no single magic trick in developing the culture system; instead, a combination of many apparently trivial factors—such as low oxygen tension, gentle agitation of the culture, the use of appropriate fetal bovine serum, adequate cell density, daily feeding of the cultures, and the use of an antigen that gives a high antibody response—proved to play an important role. Following the Mishell-Dutton discovery, several other in vitro techniques were reported; a description of some of the more widely used techniques follows.

Mishell-Dutton Assay

In this assay (Fig. 13.10*a*), one prepares a cell suspension from spleens of unimmunized mice, mixes the suspension with sheep red blood cells, places the mixture in a small Petri dish, and grows the cells for four to six days in culture medium containing fetal bovine serum, under low oxygen tension with gentle agitation. At the end of the culture period, one harvests the cells and tests them for antibody production to sheep red blood cells in the so-called hemolytic plaque assay (see below). The number of antibody-forming cells rises above the background level at two days and peaks at four to six days of culture, at which time the culture contains about 10^3 antibody-forming cells per 10^6 spleen cells.

The antibody formation in Mishell-Dutton cultures cannot be regarded as a full-fledged immune response, comparable to that occurring in vivo. For one thing, sheep red blood cells are virtually the only antigen against which these cultures produce antibodies, while most other antigens stimulate only very meager, poorly reproducible responses. Further, IgM is virtually the only antibody class produced in the Mishell-Dutton cultures; IgG antibodies are either not produced at all or are produced only in small quantities. Finally, the addition of fresh sheep red blood cells to the culture after six days of incubation fails to induce secondary response; instead, the ongoing response wanes and the cells in the culture die. However, secondary antibody response can be induced in vitro by antigen stimulation of cells from an animal immunized to sheep red blood cells in vivo. An assay system for a complete in vitro response—that is, a response inducible by a variety of antigens and leading to the production of both IgM and IgG antibodies and involving a memory element (in other words, a re-

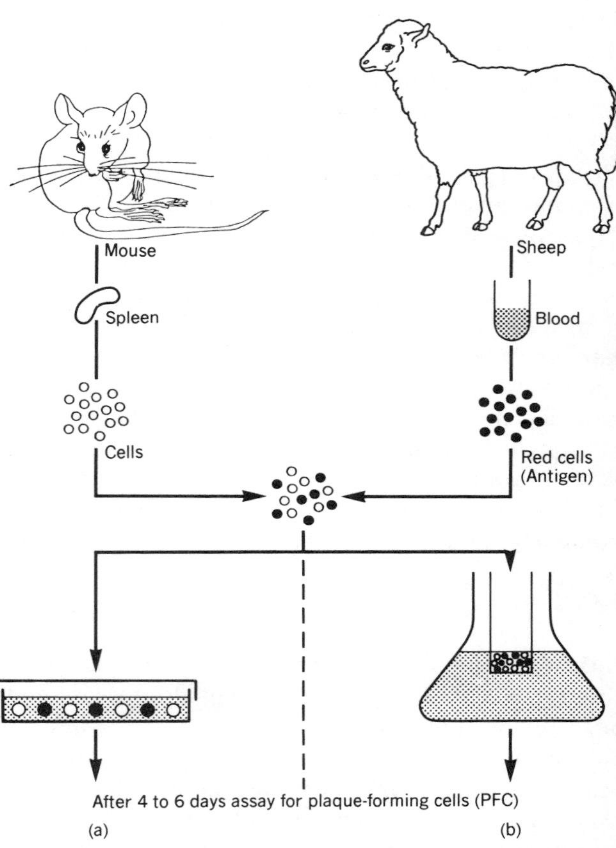

Figure 13.10. Two assays for in vitro antibody production. (*a*) Mishell-Dutton system. (*b*) Marbrook system. Explanation in the text.

sponse with all the principal characteristics of in vivo antibody formation)—has not yet been developed. However, despite these imperfections, the Mishell-Dutton culture system has been an extremely useful tool for studying a host of questions related to the interplay of cells and factors in the antibody response. Why sheep red blood cells are so unique in stimulating in vitro responses is not known. They may possess intrinsic mitogenic and other stimulatory properties that make up for the deficiencies of the in vitro system. Alternatively, there may be something special about the precursors of B lymphocytes that respond to sheep red blood cells, in that they might already be presensitized or preconditioned in some other way for the response.

At least three cell types interact in the Mishell-Dutton system to produce sheep red blood cell-reactive antibodies—B lymphocytes, as the precursors of antibody-forming cells; T lymphocytes, providing help in B-cell differentiation; and macrophages, providing conditions necessary for the growth of cells and for T-B interaction. The precise role of T cells in the response remains to be elucidated, but the observation that the addition of T cell-replacing factor (see Chapter 7) to the culture suffices for antibody production points to a relative T independence of the response's early phases, since the T cell-replacing factor is thought to act only in the final steps of the B-cell differentiation pathway. This relative T independence of antigen recognition is another property distinguishing the Mishell-Dutton system from many of the in vivo responses.

The requirement for macrophages in the Mishell-Dutton system was first demonstrated by Donald E. Mosier, who observed in 1967 that normal mouse spleen cells can be separated into two populations, one adhering to glass or plastic surfaces, the other nonadherent. Neither population, when stimulated in vitro with sheep red blood cells, was able to give rise to antibody-forming cells, but when the two were recombined, a good response comparable to that of an unseparated spleen-cell population ensued. Later studies demonstrated that the nonadherent population contained the actual antibody-forming cells, whereas the adherent population played an accessory role in the response. Still later, the *adherent* or *accessory cells* were identified as macrophages. The precise role of macrophages in the Mishell-Dutton system is, once again, unknown, but the fact that they can be replaced by β-mercaptoethanol or other thiols suggests a nonimmunological role pertaining to general cell survival in the culture. (The stimulatory effect of β-mercaptoethanol on the in vitro immune response was first demonstrated by Robert E. Click and his co-workers in 1972.)

Marbrook Assay

In 1967, J. Marbrook introduced a variant of the Mishell-Dutton system in which the mixture of spleen cells and sheep red blood cells is placed into a glass tube with a dialysis membrane at one end and the tube is immersed in the medium in a larger flask (Fig. 13.10*b*). After four to six days of incubation, the suspension in the tube is tested for the presence of cells producing antibodies to sheep red blood cells. In this arrangement, the nutrients of the medium can diffuse freely to the cells and the metabolites away from the cells into the medium.

Assays for Identification and Enumeration of Antibody-Producing Cells

The antibodies produced by the cultured cells are secreted into the medium and one can detect their presence by testing the culture supernatants by one of the serological methods described in Chapter 10. However, one can also test the in vitro antibody synthesis by assaying directly for antibody-producing cells. The two major tests used to identify such cells are the Jerne plaque assay and the rosetting technique.

Jerne Plaque Assay. This assay is named after Niels K. Jerne, who, with A. A. Nordin, introduced it in 1963. Cells obtained from a culture or from an immunized animal and producing antibodies to sheep red blood cells are mixed with an excess of sheep red blood cells in warm agar, and a thin layer of the agar is poured on a glass slide or into a Petri dish (the glass surface is usually precoated with a supporting agar layer; see Fig. 13.11). The agar is then allowed to solidify and the slide is incubated for one hour at 37°C. The immune cells in the suspension continue to produce antibodies, which diffuse through the agar and bind to the surrounding sheep red blood cells. After incubation, the top of the agar layer is covered with complement (normal guinea pig serum) and the slide is incubated for about 40 minutes. As the complement diffuses through the agar, it binds to antibodies coating the erythrocytes and lyses the latter. As a result, a clear area—a plaque—forms around each antibody-producing cell, now referred to as *plaque-forming cell*, or PFC. Since, at a certain low density of spleen cells, one plaque corresponds to one PFC, one can count the

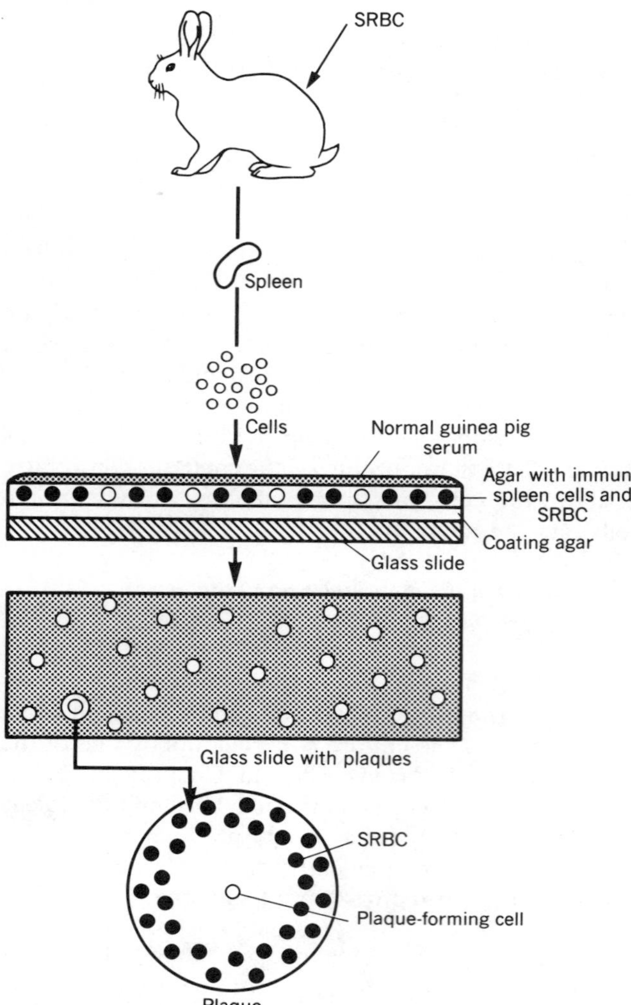

Figure 13.11. Jerne plaque assay. Explanation in the text. SRBC, sheep red blood cells.

plaques and estimate the number of antibody-producing cells in the suspension. In this *direct plaque assay*, the only antibodies detected are of the IgM type, since the IgG antibodies are not efficient enough in complement binding to mediate cell lysis under these experimental conditions. To detect IgG antibodies one must resort to the *indirect plaque assay*, in which one incubates the agar plate—prior to the addition of complement—with a xenogeneic antiserum specific for the coating antibodies (e.g., if the coating antibodies are of mouse origin, one uses a rabbit anti-mouse IgG serum). The xenogeneic immunoglobulin molecules crosslink the coating antibodies and generate conditions for efficient complement binding and hence for cell lysis.

Rosette Test. The rosette test was described in 1964 by O. B. Zaalberg. Here, cells producing antibodies to sheep red blood cells are detected by their ability to bind sheep erythrocytes via these antibodies. The cells become surrounded by the adhering erythrocytes, each forming a *rosette*—a cluster consisting of one central antibody-producing cell, here referred to as the *rosette-forming cell* (RFC), and at least four adhering erythrocytes (see Fig. 5.18).

Assays for Precursors of Antibody-Forming Cells

Both the plaque and rosette techniques detect cells that are already secreting antibodies; to detect the precursors of these antibody-producing cells, Joan L. Press and Norman R. Klinman used the so-called *focus-forming assay* (Fig. 13.12). In one version of this

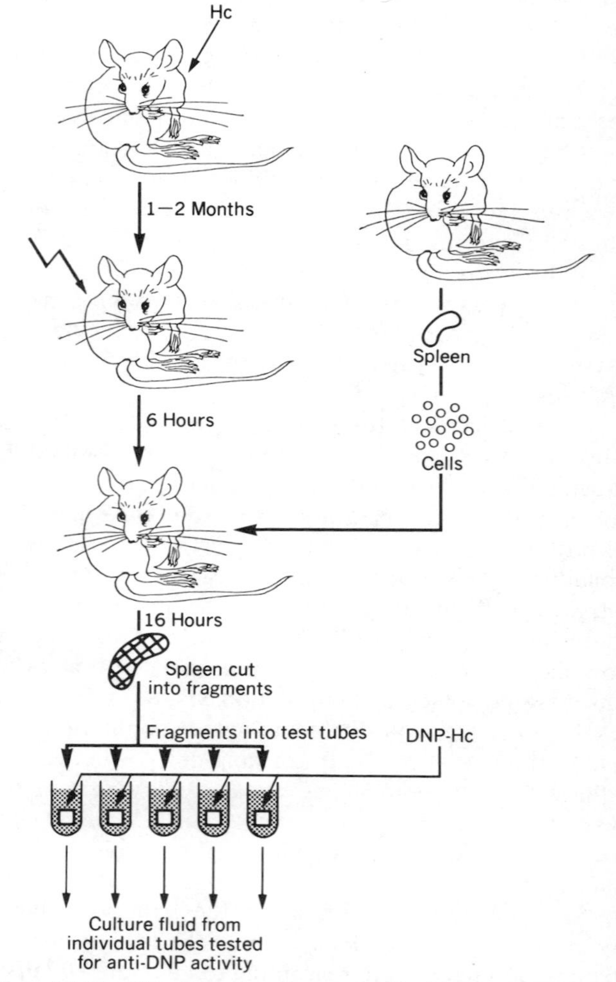

Figure 13.12. The focus-forming assay. Explanation in the text. DNP, dinitrophenyl; Hc, hemocyanin.

assay, mice are immunized against a carrier molecule (e.g., hemocyanin) and lethally X-irradiated one or two months later. The X-rays kill all the lymphoid cells in these mice except the primed helper T cells, which are, as we already know, relatively radioresistant. Six hours after the irradiation, the recipients are inoculated with a low number of spleen cells from an unimmunized syngeneic donor, and the injected cells are allowed to lodge in the spleen and other lymphoid organs. Then, 16 hours after the inoculation, the mice are killed, their spleens cut into small fragments, and each fragment is cultured separately in a test tube or the well of a plastic tray in the presence of hapten-carrier conjugates (e.g., DNP-Hc). Because the spleen is only sparsely populated by the inoculated cells and because of the low frequency of precursors capable of differentiating into cells producing antibodies to a given hapten, it is unlikely that any fragment that produces antibodies in a culture contains more than one precursor cell. So the count of foci (where a focus is a spleen fragment producing antibodies) gives the frequency of precursor cells for a given antigen per number of inoculated cells. The experiments based on the use of this assay have indicated that adult mouse spleen contains approximately two to five precursors of cells capable of making antibodies to a given hapten per 10^5 spleen cells. The advantage of the focus-forming assay is that each culture well contains homogeneous antibodies produced by a single cell clone derived from a single precursor B lymphocyte. One can therefore analyze these antibodies for their affinity, their isoelectric point, and other physicochemical characteristics, and so obtain information about affinity maturation and changes in the diversity of a response to a given antigen.

13.3 IgA-DOMINATED RESPONSES

Before we discuss IgA-mediated immune responses, we must digress a bit to describe the anatomical setting in which these responses take place. Readers familiar with basic anatomy may want to skip this section.

13.3.1 Bodily Surfaces and Secretions

Bodily surfaces (Fig. 13.13) are protected by a special tissue that has two main components, the externally located *epithelium* and the underlying *connective tissue* (see also Chapter 4). These bear different names, depending on the surface they cover. The epithelial tissue covering external surfaces is called *epidermis*, the underlying connective tissue is the *dermis*, and both components together form the *skin*. The surface layer of the respiratory, digestive, and genital systems is referred to as the *epithelium*, the underlying connective tissue as the *lamina propria*, and the combination of these two tissues as the *mucosa* or *mucosal membrane*. The epithelial tissue lining the abdominal cavity, internal organs, and the membranes of the heart and lungs is known as the *mesothelium*, the connective tissue as the *submesothelial layer*, and the combination of the two as the *serosa*. And finally, the lining of blood vessels and the heart is called the *endothelium*, the underlying tissue the *subendothelium*, and the entire complex either the *intima* (in vessels) or the *endocardium* (in the heart). Most of the coating tissues contain cells and groups of cells (glands) that specialize in the elaboration of secretory products. *Glands* releasing secretions into the bloodstream are termed *endocrine* (Gr. *endon*, within, *krino*, to separate); all the others are called *exocrine* (Gr. *exo*, outside). Only the latter will interest us here. The morphology of the exocrine glands varies considerably, depending on their location in the body and on the products they secrete. Some glands consist of isolated granular cells strewn over the epithelial surface (e.g., so-called mucous goblet cells in the epithelium of the intestine), others consist of cell clusters (e.g., intraepithelial glands of the urethra) or carpets of secretory epithelium (e.g., epithelium of the stomach), and still others are true glands with a secretory portion in the shape of a small tube, sac, or berry, and an excretory branched or unbranched duct. The products of the exocrine glands are called *secretions*. The composition, consistency, and the chemical na-

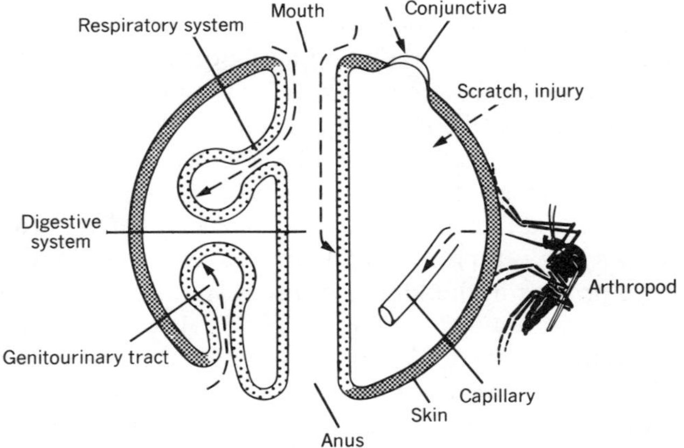

Figure 13.13. Bodily surfaces and sites of antigen entry (indicated by broken arrows). (From C. A. Mims: *The Pathogenesis of Infectious Disease*. Academic, London, 1977.)

ture of the individual secretory products vary, depending on the particular surface and type of glands present. Some secretions are watery and high in protein (enzyme) content, while others are viscous and rich in mucopolysaccharides or mucoproteins. The former are referred to as *serous* and the latter as *mucous*. Serous secretions bathe the particular surface and fill the particular gland cavity or organ, whereas mucous secretions often form sticky layers covering the mucosa. However, in addition to the products of exocrine glands, secretions often also contain some *exudate* (L. *ex*, out, *sudare*, to sweat)—that is, the fluid seeping from blood and lymph vessels into tissues and from there into the cavities. Immunologists refer to the secretions containing a high level of exudate (mainly serum) as internal because they fill internal body cavities, and to those composed mostly of exocrine gland products as external. Examples of *internal secretions* are the fluids filling the interior chamber of the eye (aqueous humor), bathing the brain and spinal chord (cerebrospinal fluid, or CSF), filling the joint cavity (synovial fluid), bathing the lungs (pleural fluid), bathing the jaws and gums (gingival fluid), filling the abdominal cavity (peritoneal fluid), and surrounding the fetus (amniotic fluid). Examples of *external secretions* are saliva, tears, and nasal, tracheobronchial, intestinal, and genitourinary secretions. The external secretions will interest us most.

13.3.2 The Concept of Local Immunity

Since about the second decade of this century, immunologists and epidemiologists have suspected that the system of bodily secretions may have its own defense mechanism relatively independent of antibodies circulating in the blood. They observed repeatedly that certain infections, such as cholera or influenza, produced few, if any circulating antibodies (*systemic immunity*), but were accompanied by the presence of antibodies in specific parts of the body (*local immunity*). For example, in the case of cholera, antibodies to cholera toxins were demonstrable in the feces of the infected individuals (so-called *coproantibodies*, from Gr. *kopros*, dung); in influenza, specific antibodies were present in the mucus of the respiratory tract (so-called *mucoantibodies*), and so forth. However, it was not until the late 1950s and early 1960s that the notion of a local or *secretory immune system* began to be taken seriously, mainly because of the work of W. Burrows, S. Fazekas de St. Groth, Thomas B. Tomasi, and others. The notion attained full respectability in 1963, when W. B. Chodirker and Tomasi demonstrated that

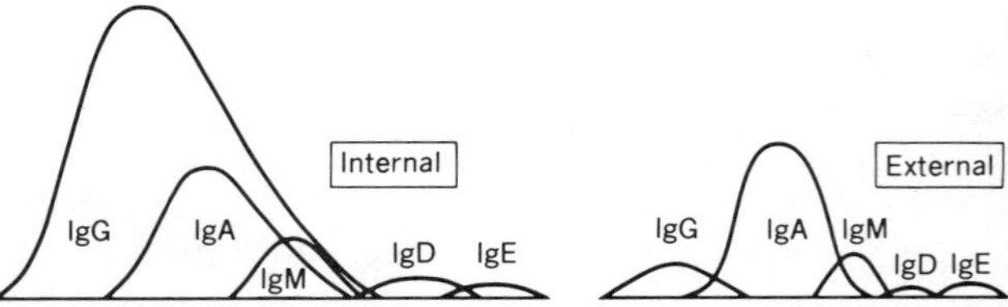

Figure 13.14. Comparison of immunoglobulin content in external and internal secretions. The relative concentrations of the various immunoglobulin classes are proportional to the areas under the corresponding curve. (From T. B. Tomasi: *The Immune System of Secretions*. Prentice-Hall, Englewood Cliffs, New Jersey, 1976.)

IgA was present at higher levels in secretions than in serum. Comparison of external with internal secretions revealed a higher IgA content in the former than in the latter (Fig. 13.14). Presumably, IgA of internal secretions is derived mostly from the serum, whereas IgA of external secretions is produced by the mucosa.

In the remainder of this section we shall consider briefly the main body surfaces and the mechanisms available for their protection. In doing so we shall once again digress slightly from the main theme of this chapter—the IgA response; the digression is necessary since this is the only place where we have the opportunity to discuss the defense reactions occurring at the body's surfaces.

The Skin

The outer layer of the epidermis, the *stratum corneum*, is composed of either dead or dying cells in various stages of hardening (cornification). The dead cells slough off as scales or squamae through normal wear and tear and are continually replaced by cells from deeper, germinal layers of the epidermis—the regions of active cellular proliferation. It has been estimated that an average person sheds about 5×10^8 squamous skin cells per day. The dry, horny stratum corneum is a relatively impermeable barrier between the body and the outside world. In many species this insulation is augmented by fur or other cornified derivatives of the skin. Although the skin surface is colonized by a number of viruses, bacteria, fungi, and even small arthropods, most of these organisms are normally harmless as long as their growth is confined to the stratum corneum. But when breaks occur in the skin's continuity, potentially pathogenic microorganisms may penetrate to the germinal layer and begin to cause damage. Such breaks may occur as a result of bites (by insects or biting mammals), abrasion, burns, or any other kind of wound.

The Conjunctiva

The continuity of the skin is naturally interrupted at several places by openings serving for the reception of light, sound, smell, air, and food, for disposal of wastes, and for sexual intercourse. These are Guillaume Apollinaire's celebrated nine gates to the body. The eye is exposed to the outer world by about one-sixth of its surface—the transparent cornea covered by a mucous membrane, the conjunctiva. The membrane is kept moist by the continuous flow of secretions from lachrymal (tear-producing) and other glands: every few seconds the lids pass over the conjunctiva and, like a car's windshield wiper, wash away particles that might have soiled the conjunctival surface. This mechanical cleansing is supplemented by the antimicrobial action of lysozyme and other agents in secretions. The combined mechanical and chemical actions of the secretions normally keep the conjunctival surface clean; complications arise only when the conjunctiva is damaged or when defects occur in the secretory mechanisms. Infection of the conjunctiva is referred to as *conjunctivitis*, and one of its most severe forms is *trachoma* (Gr. *trachoma*, rough, harsh) caused by *Chlamydia trachomatis*, a gram-negative microorganism resembling ricketsiae and marked by the formation of minute greyish or yellowish translucent granules beneath the eyelids (see Chapter 14). Trachoma, which can damage the cornea and cause partial or complete blindness, is as common as the common cold in some parts of the world.

The Respiratory System

The human respiratory system begins with the nose and its cavities, including paranasal sinuses—the hollow spaces in the bones of the skull that connect with the nose. The nasal cavities connect with the pharynx—a large, single cavity in the back of the mouth; the pharynx connects with the voice box (larynx), which connects with the windpipe (trachea). The single tube of this upper respiratory tract then divides into the treelike structure of the lower tract. The branches of the tree are called, in order of their increasing refinement, primary, secondary, and tertiary bronchi, and bronchioli. Bronchioli end with small sacs called alveoli. The bronchial tree, together with some other tissue, form the paired lungs.

Air entering the respiratory system contains suspended particles of all kinds—smoke, soot, dust, pollen, and microorganisms. There are more than 1000 million tons of particles in the earth's atmosphere and an average human being inhales some 10,000 microorganisms daily. But owing to several efficient cleansing mechanisms, the lungs normally remain sterile, despite this bombardment of particles. The mucosa of the lower tract contains ciliated and mucus-secreting (goblet) cells in the epithelium and mucus-secreting glands in the subepithelial layers. The secreted mucus entraps particles not retained by the hair in the nose and the cilia then move the particles upward from the lungs to the back of the throat. In the upper tract a similar mucociliary lining moves entrapped particles downward to the throat, where they are then swallowed. Particles not removed by this *mucociliary escalator* may reach the alveoli, which have no cilia or mucus but are lined by macrophages. Most of the *alveolar macrophages* ingest and degrade the particles by phagocytosis in situ, but others move with the particles upwards into the throat, using the mucociliary escalator. If macrophages alone cannot handle the invasion, the body quickly mobilizes the *granulocytic system* so that within hours of infection a large number of neutrophils and other granulocytes enter the lungs and begin to eliminate the offending microorganism. IgA becomes involved in the defense when some of the macrophages process the antigen and present it in an appropriate form to T and B cells of the bronchially associated lymphoid tissue.

When the cleansing mechanisms are functioning properly, most microorganisms have no chance to initiate an infection; but a few microorganisms possess special devices for avoiding these mechanisms. For example, the surfaces of influenza viruses possess hemagglutinin, which reacts with sialic acid groups on the glycoproteins of epithelial cells, and by firm attachment to these cells the viruses avoid being swept by the mucociliary escalators. When the cleansing mechanisms are damaged by destructive lesions of the respiratory system caused, for example, by viral infections, heavy smoking, or very dry air, the chance of infection increases.

The Digestive System

The digestive system is a tube passing through the body from the anterior opening, or mouth, to the posterior opening, or anus. The successive parts of the human digestive system are the mouth, pharynx, esophagus, stomach, small intestine (consisting of duodenum, jejunum, and ileum), large intestine (consisting of cecum with vermiform appendix, colon, and rectum), and anus.

Microorganisms entering the digestive system during eating and drinking are attacked by various enzymes (e.g., lysozyme in the saliva of the mouth, pepsin in the stomach juice, and trypsin in the small intestine), acids (e.g., hydrochloric acid in the stomach), and bile (in the duodenum). Even if they somehow escape the chemical attack, microorganisms do not have a great opportunity to settle down, for, in contrast to the respiratory system, everything is always in motion in the digestive system. In the small intestine, where the motion is most intense, at least three kinds of movement can be recognized: segmentation (rhythmic contractions involving localized regions of the intestine), peristaltic (contractions travelling short distances along the length of the intestine), and mucous membrane movement (increase or decrease in mucosa folding and motility of the villi). The combined action of these three movements results in constant mixing of particles in the intestinal lumen and a continual passage of the intestinal contents toward the anus. In the large intestine the movement slows down, and it is here that many microorganisms have a chance to settle and grow. Most of them are harmless, and in fact, many are beneficial in helping to digest the food. In humans, one finds some 10^{11} bacteria per gram of colon or rectum content, and in the rectum, bacteria constitute about one-fourth of the fecal mass. The intestinal flora may even contain some potential pathogens but these, as well as most other microorganisms, normally cannot penetrate the mucosa to enter the body. The mucus covering the mucosa provides a mechanical, as well as immunological barrier to the passage of bacteria through the intestinal wall. Furthermore, most epithelial cells of the digestive tract are capable of phagocytosis, although on a smaller scale than macrophages. Foreign particles that manage to enter the intestinal wall are picked up by macrophages in the lamina propria and processed, and their antigenic material is presented to the T and B cells of the gut-associated lymphoid tissue.

Because of their openness and despite the high efficiency of their protective mechanisms, the respiratory and digestive systems are the most vulnerable regions of the body in terms of invasion by pathogens. And so most acute infectious illnesses are either respiratory or dysenterylike in nature.

The Genitourinary System

The urinary system consists of two kidneys, each drained by one ureter, one urinary bladder into which the two ureters discharge their contents, and one urethra, which drains the bladder. The main components of the male genital system are two testes, a transport system delivering the sperm from the tes into the urethra (i.e., epididymides, vas deferens, a ejaculatory duct), and accessory glands producing cretions that maintain the viability of the spermato (i.e., two seminal vesicles, bulbourethral gland, a prostate gland). The female genital system is co posed of two ovaries, two Fallopian tubes, uterus, a vagina.

The urinary tract is flushed with urine every hour two so that most of the invading microorganisms washed out during urination. To avoid being wash out, a microorganism must be able to attach firmly the epithelium within a short time. Fortunately for few microorganisms have learned how to form a fi union with epithelial cells, so that most of the urina system, particularly its upper part and particularly males, remains sterile (in males, the urethra is lon and hence the bladder is less accessible than in males). Among those that have learned the attachm trick, the most stubborn is the gonococcus responsi for an inflammation of the genital mucous membrane a disease known as gonorrhea (Gr. *gone,* seed, *rho* flow).

The major protective mechanism of the vagina provided by the symbiotic bacterium *Lactobacill* which colonizes the vaginal epithelium and produ lactic acid; this substance then prevents the growth most other bacteria.

13.3.3 Mechanism Leading to IgA Secretion

Exposure to Antigen

Natural Immunization. To stimulate local immuni an antigen must reach a particular mucosal surfa traverse the epithelium, and be picked up by m rophages in the subepithelial layer. By what mech nism and in what form the antigen crosses the epit lial layer is not known, but it is unlikely—for reaso discussed in the preceding section—that the passa involves the whole microorganism. More probab the killed particle is partially degraded by agents pr ent in the secretions and some of the components th travel across the barrier. The conditions of crossing barrier are apparently important in determin whether an antigen will induce local immunity, s temic immunity, or both; but what these conditic are remains obscure.

Deliberate Immunization. The most reliable way inducing local immunity is by delivering the antig directly to the mucosal surface, but even then one us ally obtains both local and systemic responses. A ministration of an antigen by any other means gives unpredictable results. For example, when given parenterally, most antigens produce serum antibodies, predominantly of the IgG class; only a few antigens also stimulate local IgA synthesis. The different behavior of the two groups of antigen probably depends on their ability to reach the secretory tissues in a form capable of stimulating a response, but once more, the specific properties influencing this behavior remain undefined. The dose of the administered antigen is also important. For example, a low dose of influenza virus vaccine administered parenterally induces systemic immunity but little or no secretory IgA, whereas a higher dose also leads to the production of influenza antibodies in nasal fluids. In some instances, an antigen may first enter the blood and then be delivered to organs of local immunity.

Histology of the Response

The subepithelial layers of most bodily surfaces are interwoven with a network of lymphoid tissue, which the antigen must reach to stimulate local immunity. The tissue is most strongly developed in the lamina propria of the gut and lungs; in the former, it is referred to as the *gut-associated lymphoid tissue*, or GALT, and in the latter, as *bronchial-associated lymphoid tissue*, or BALT (see also Chapter 5). The gut, which is the major IgA secretor, contains as much lymphoid tissue as the spleen and probably synthesizes more IgA than any other lymphoid organ. The major components of the GALT are the Peyer's patches, appendix, mesenteric lymph nodes, and the tonsils. Most of the B lymphocytes present in the GALT bear IgA receptors, presumably because most IgA-bearing cells specifically home for the lamina propria, even in the absence of an antigen. If no antigen comes along, the cells die; if stimulated, they expand.

The mechanism of B-cell differentiation in the GALT and BALT is probably similar to that seen in regional lymph nodes or in the spleen (Fig. 13.15). Antigen probably gains access to GALT through the specialized microfold (M) epithelial cells overlying the Peyer's patches. The antigen is processed by macrophages, presented to the T cells, and the T cells then, together with the antigen, activate the B lymphocytes. In the GALT, most of the macrophage-T cell and T cell-B cell collaboration probably take place in Peyer's patches. The stimulated B cells then undergo blast transformation, leave the Peyer's patches with lymph without producing any antibodies, and migrate to mesenteric lymph nodes. Once in the lymph nodes, the cells complete their differentiation (combined with clonal expansion) into plasma cells and some of them begin to secrete antibodies. Thereafter they enter the efferent lymphatics and the thoracic duct and, via the blood circulation, either return to the gut or are disseminated to other secretory sites, primarily the lungs, but also, for example, the mammary, lachrymal, or salivary glands. In the gut, the cells settle down in the lamina propria and begin to synthesize antibodies.

Activation of B cells in the BALT occurs in a similar fashion and some B cells activated in the BALT end up in the gut, so that there is apparently a two-way traffic between these two major secretory sites. The migration of cells between different secretory sites suggests that all these sites may constitute a single system of *mucosal-associated lymphoid tissue*, or MALT. The system may include, in addition to the gut and lungs, the mammary, salivary, and lachrymal glands, and possibly the genitourinary system. How the B cells find the other secretory sites is not known; the recognition could involve specific receptors on epithelial cells, or alternatively, chemotaxis. The migration seems to be under hormonal control.

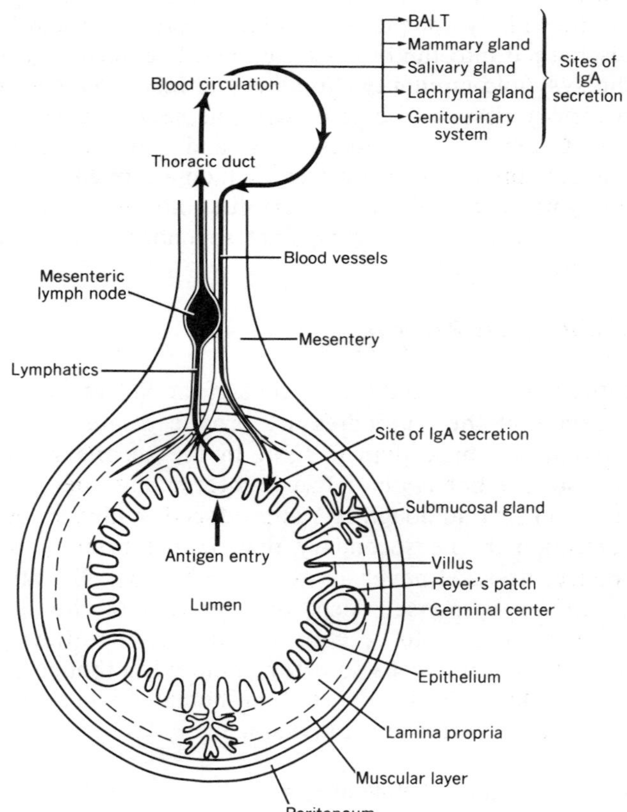

Figure 13.15. Histology of the IgA response in the gut and the migration pattern of activated IgA-bearing B lymphocytes. Explanation in the text. The figure shows a cross section through the small intestine. Direction of cell migration is indicated by arrows.

Once they reach the other secretory sites, the stimulated B lymphocytes differentiate into plasma cells and begin to produce IgA antibodies. An obvious advantage of this seeding process is that newborns of many species receive ready-made antibody-producing cells right after birth via the colostrum and milk. The cells seeding the gut of the newborn are those that the newborn needs most—cells sensitized to antigens of the gut flora, antigens it is likely to encounter first in the postpartum period. Seeding is also advantageous in situations where a single microorganism infects two sites simultaneously (for example, gonococcus affects the pharynx and the genital tract); here, seeding assures the simultaneous production of antibodies at both sites.

The migration patterns of the MALT T cells are presumably similar to those of B cells. Some immunologists also postulate the existence in the MALT of special T cells, adapted to serving the needs of local immunity. Indeed, cells that appear to be halfway between T lymphocytes and mast cells have been described in secretory tissues.

Plasma cells residing in the lamina propria produce the bulk of IgA that appears in secretions; the IgA produced in lymphoid tissues of nonsecretory organs is discharged into the bloodstream and becomes part of the systemic immunity. Some of the IgA produced in secretory tissues associates with the secretory pieces (see Chapter 6), becomes sIgA, and ends up in the mucosa; the rest forms dimers, which are released via the lymphatics and the thoracic duct into the systemic circulation and may be brought secondarily into the secretory organs.

Kinetics of the Response

Little is known about the kinetics of the IgA response, except that the antibodies are produced later in the immune response than is IgM. In the secondary response, the behavior of IgA is intermediate between IgM and IgG: although IgA is produced in higher concentration in the secondary than in the primary response, its level never approaches that of IgG in the secondary response. Also, the duration of the IgA memory appears to be generally shorter than that of the IgG (a few weeks to a few months), although instances have been reported in humans where the memory lasted for several years.

13.3.4 Biological Role of IgA

The secretory system (local immunity) is sometimes referred to as the *first line of defense*, in contradistinction to the *second line of defense* constituted by the systemic immunity. These designations derive from the postulate that the secretory system deals with the offending antigens first and that systemic immunity becomes involved later. In this division of defense into first- and second-line, local immunity is considered in broad terms as including not only humoral but also cellular immunity, and in the former, not only IgA- but also IgG-, IgM-, and IgE-mediated responses. (Some of the IgG, IgM, and IgE found in secretions derive from the serum but some are also secreted locally by mechanisms about which we know next to nothing.) The actual mechanisms by which IgA carries out its function as one of the most important elements of the first-line defense are surprisingly poorly understood. Although a considerable amount of specific data are available, they are often contradictory or incomplete, so generalizations are difficult to make. We shall consider separately the role of IgA in two phases of an animal's life—the postnatal and mature phase.

Role of IgA in Newborns

The presumed three main functions of local immunity in the newborn are the establishment of balanced normal bacterial flora, protection from pathogenic microorganisms, and protection from flooding with nonviable antigens.

Establishment of Normal Bacterial Flora. At the time of birth, mammals are virtually free of microorganisms; however, within a matter of hours the newborn begins to be colonized by many species and strains of bacteria, particularly in the gastrointestinal part of the digestive system. Only some bacteria entering the digestive tract—those that are either harmless or beneficial to the host—are allowed to colonize it. The selection of the colonizing bacteria is influenced by many factors—among others, probably the secretory IgA, which is known to be able to prevent the growth of certain microorganisms.

Protection from Infection. Some mammals—for example, cows or sheep—are born without any antibodies, apparently because in these species immunoglobulins cannot pass through the placenta. In other mammals—humans, for example—some antibodies are passed transplacentally to the fetus from the mother, but even in these species, the immunoglobulin concentration is not sufficient to protect the newborn from infection. In both groups, the necessary protection is provided by secretory immunoglobulins, particularly secretory IgA, present in the mother's colostrum (the first milk secreted at the termination of pregnancy). The crucial role of sIgA in this phase of life is evident from the observation that if one withholds colostrum from calves, many succumb to infection within a short time. Colostrum contains about the same level of sIgA as other external secretions and this predominance of IgA persists even after colostrum has been replaced by milk. However, the longer the mother nurses the young, the more other immunoglobulins appear in the milk.

Protection from Nonviable Antigens. In many species the gastrointestinal tract of the newborn is highly permeable to ingested macromolecules. Each species has a characteristic period of high permeability, which can vary from two to three days, as in cows, to 18 to 20 days, as in mice and rats. The permeability of the tract then gradually decreases with age, although some small but significant amount of antigenic macromolecules may pass the wall of the tract, even in adults. In some species—for example, in humans—the gastrointestinal tract is already largely impermeable at birth. Free passage of macromolecules through the gastrointestinal wall in this critical period is prevented by a number of mechanisms (for example, the mechanical barrier formed by the mucous coating or the degradation of ingested particles by proteolytic enzymes). One of these mechanisms might be binding of antigens by IgA. This protective role of IgA is indicated by the observation that IgA immunodeficient individuals have high titers of antibodies against various milk antigens. The protection may be restricted to small amounts of antigen that escaped elimination by other means.

Role of IgA in Adults

In general terms, IgA and other secretory immunoglobulins are thought to protect the adult organism from colonization of the mucosa by pathogenic viruses and bacteria. However, the precise mechanism by which this protection is accomplished is not known. Some of the mechanisms proposed to play a role in IgA defense are enumerated below.

Trapping of Microorganisms at Mucosal Surfaces. The reaction of specific antibodies with antigens on the surface of a microorganism presumably facilitates entrapment of the particle in the mucous coating. IgA antibodies to microorganisms have been found both in the mucus and in the fluid filling the lumen of a gland or organ.

Inhibition of Adherence to Mucosa. To colonize a mucosal membrane, a microorganism must attach to the membrane's epithelial cells. IgA may, theoretically at least, prevent colonization either by coating the interaction sites of the particle or inhibiting the growth of a particle already attached. The latter is probably accomplished through an interplay with ancillary factors, such a lysozyme or lactoferrin.

Inactivation of Microorganisms or Their Products. By binding to some vital region of a virus or a bacterium, IgA may block some essential step in the reproductive cycle of the microorganism. It may also combine with such bacterial products as toxins and inactivate them.

Lysis of Bacteria or Viruses. Direct killing of microorganisms requires the participation of complement, but the interaction of complement components with IgA remains controversial. IgA is definitely not able to fix components of the classical complement pathway, but the possibility that it activates the alternative pathway remains open.

Opsonization. To facilitate phagocytosis, immunoglobulins must bind to the corresponding receptor on the surface of a macrophage. Normally, IgA is incapable of a cytotropic attachment to macrophages, but it is possible that some attachment can be accomplished by some indirect means. Moreover, both bacteriolysis and opsonization can be mediated by other antibodies present in secretion—by IgG, for example.

13.4 IgE-DOMINATED RESPONSES

As far as can be determined, the main physiological function of IgE-mediated responses is to combat parasites. The response can be divided into five phases: an IgE-bearing B cell is exposed to an antigen (phase 1) and activated to secrete IgE antibodies (phase 2); the produced antibodies bind to mast cells and basophils in tissues (phase 3, antibody fixation), activate these cells, and cause the release of chemical mediators stored in their granules (phase 4, degranulation); and finally, the mediators induce a complex tissue response aimed at the expulsion of nonmicrobial parasites from the body (phase 5). Part of the expulsion mechanism is an attack on the tissue that harbors the parasite—that is, on self. To excise a tissue with a parasite without damaging the rest of the body is a delicate act comparable to that of a knife-thrower's outlining his partner's body against a board. The knives, when thrown with skill, end up in the board, but a single inaccurately aimed knife may turn a glorious act into a catastrophe. In a certain way, the mediators released by activated mast cells and basophils are like the knives launched to cut an outline. They, too, can cause considerable harm if released at an inappropriate time or launched at an inappropriate target. To achieve the required precision in the launching, the reaction must be closely controlled and stopped immediately after its goal has been achieved. As long as this control is functioning there is no danger that healthy parts of the body will be damaged, but should the controls fail, the beneficial reaction will turn into a harmful one. In humans, about 90 percent of all individuals have no difficulty in using their IgE only for defensive purposes; but the remaining unlucky 10 percent carry a genetic defect of the control mechanism that permits the stimulation of IgE responses by antigens that have nothing to do with parasites. At first it was thought that this defect was limited only to humans, but similar defects were discovered later in several other mammals. The inappropriately stimulated IgE responses cause a plethora of diverse diseases, grouped under the name *allergy* or *atopy*.

So the IgE system is a double-edged sword: it protects with one edge and harms with the other. In fact, it was the harmful side that was discovered first, and for a long time immunologists puzzled over the adaptive significance of this so obviously deleterious mechanism (see Chapter 2). It is only now, after the discovery of the role IgE plays in defense against parasites, that we are beginning to comprehend the apparent uselessness of the allergic reactions. But because immunologists previously knew only about the pathological side of the IgE-dominated responses, they have learned disproportionately more about allergies (though still not enough to cure them) than about the role of IgE in defense against parasites, and this fact naturally influences the selection of material to be covered in this section. Here we shall first discuss the five phases of IgE response and then some of the specific forms of this response, with emphasis on pathological forms.

13.4.1 Phases of IgE Response

Exposure to Antigen

Natural Immunization. Nonallergic individuals mount significant IgE responses only when exposed to parasites, particularly those infecting the digestive, respiratory, and genitourinary systems. While the serum IgE level in healthy individuals is extremely low (see Chapter 6), the level in individuals infested with parasites increases and stays high for as long as the infestation lasts, without any obvious harmful effects on the body. Certain nonparasitic antigens probably activate some B cells bearing the corresponding receptors, but this limited response is quickly extinguished, probably by regulatory T cells, before it can get out of hand: the flame is put out before it can develop into a conflagration. In individuals with regulatory defects, these limited responses enlarge uncontrollably to a full-scale attack on the individual's own tissues and the individual experiences an allergic reaction. The group of antigens capable of inducing an allergic reaction (the symptoms of which we shall describe later) are called *allergens*. Below we shall first give some examples of common allergens and then attempt to determine whether they have any common characteristics distinguishing them from other antigens.

As we shall see, most IgE responses occur in the subepithelial layers of the bodily surface. Hence, to act as an allergen, a particle or substance must be delivered on the mucosal membrane—in other words, it must be either inhaled or ingested. *Inhaled allergens* can be of plant, animal, or industrial origin. In persons breathing through the nose, these materials end up on the moist surfaces of the nasal membrane; in mouth-breathing persons, the allergenic particles land in the pharynx, larynx, or trachea (most are too large to enter the lungs).

Among the *plant-derived allergens,* the most common are carried by the pollen of herbs, grasses, or trees; a less common source of allergenic material is molds and fungi. Most plants depend on insect pollination and produce only enough pollen to assure its spread by the attachment to the insect's body. However, a small number of species depend on wind for crosspollination and produce large quantities of light, dry pollen, easily borne long distances by air currents. It has been estimated, for example, that 2.5 km^2 of ragweed, one of the principal sources of pollen allergens in the United States, may produce some 16 tons of pollen. The exposure to pollen is limited to a few weeks at a particular time of the year, depending on the flowering season of the particular plant.

Most pollen particles are surrounded by a tough wall that must be dissolved enzymatically (for example, by the lysozyme in nasal secretions) before the particle can become allergenic. Each particle contains a large number of constituents, only a few of which act as allergens. To identify the allergenic substance, biochemists prepare a pollen extract, which they then fractionate by chemical methods, testing each fraction for its ability to induce allergy. The individual fractions are usually designated by capital letters or by some other convenient symbols. Because of differences in plant distribution in each region, different plants are

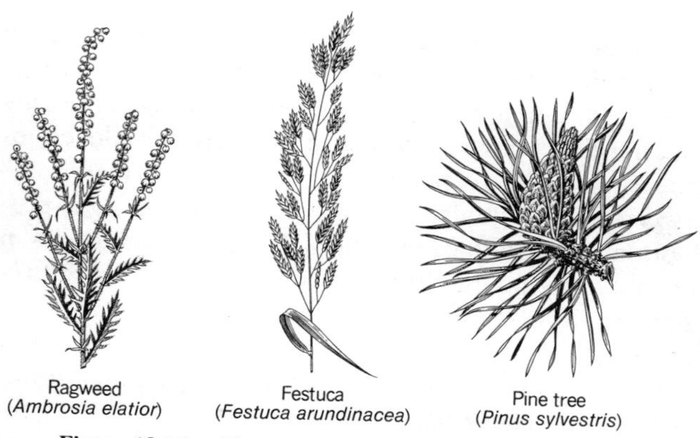

Figure 13.16. Plants most commonly causing allergies.

the common cause of allergy (Fig. 13.16). In the United States it is ragweed (*Ambrosia elatior*) and barley, in Central Europe barley and grasses (timothy, ryegrass, fescue), in Scandinavia the birch tree and so on. *Ragweed pollen* contains at least 13 substances capable of inducing IgG or IgM responses, but only four of these act as allergens. Two of them (E and K) evoke allergic reaction in all or most allergic patients and are therefore considered *major allergens*, whereas the other two (Ra_3 and Ra_5) are important only in a small number of patients (*minor allergens*). Allergen E is responsible for 90 percent of the allergenic activity of the total extract, although it constitutes only 6 percent of the total protein content. Both E and K have a molecular weight of about 40,000 daltons; Ra_3 and Ra_5 have molecular weights of 11,000 and 5000 daltons, respectively.

Among lower plants, the most common source of allergens is molds and fungi, which are widespread in nature and propagate by microscopic spores blown about by the wind. Spores of such omnipresent molds as *Cladosporium herbarum* and *Penicillium notatum* cause allergies in many parts of the world.

The main source of *animal allergens* are animal hair and dander, which is shed, desquamated skin epithelium. Allergy to dog epithelium is frequent among people keeping dogs as household pets; horse riders often develop an allergy to horse dander; and allergy to rat or mouse hair is found mostly among laboratory workers who handle these rodents. Parasites themselves can be the cause of allergy, particularly among persons and animals who are predisposed to an allergic condition. Another source of inhaled allergens is *house dust*, which is a heterogeneous mixture of fungi, molds, vegetable debris, bacteria, remains of food, epithelial fragments, small parasites or their eggs, and inorganic particles. The most frequent allergen of house dust is associated with an ascarian mite, *Dermatophagoides pteronyssinus*, a minute (0.3 mm in length) parasite living in epithelial scales.

Finally vapors of industrial products, such as phthalic anhydride, chloramine T, tannic acid, phenylmercuric acetate, or platinum acetate, can cause allergy when inhaled. In this instance, however, the compounds probably do not induce allergy directly but via tissue proteins to which they bind. Similar indirect mechanisms are also postulated in allergies caused by *drugs*, such as antibiotics (penicillin and streptomycin), sulfonamides, aspirin, local anesthetics, heparin, vitamin B_{12}, dextran, and others. Some of these compounds, however, might cause symptoms resembling allergy but with an underlying mechanism that does not involve IgE participation.

The most common sources of *ingested allergens* are milk, eggs, and fish. Allergenic activity of cow milk is contained in the lactoglobulin fraction, but sometimes also in α lactalbumin; the active compound in eggs is ovomucoid. Allergy to fish, especially to cod, is frequent in countries such as Norway, where fish is a major component of diet; it was one of the first allergies studied experimentally (see Chapter 2). The major cod allergen (M) is a member of Ca^{2+}-binding parvalbumins (molecular weight of 12,300), present in abundance in most vertebrate skeletal muscles.

After this overview of main allergens, let us now pose the question, *What makes an antigen an allergen?* In other words, why do some antigens stimulate IgE-bearing B cells, while others do not? Immunochemists have attempted to find the answer to this question by characterizing and comparing as many allergens as possible, hoping to find some common characteristics—perhaps a similar size, charge, or particular residue or sequence. However, they have come to the tentative conclusion that allergens are as diverse as antigens in general and that there is no single obligatory feature that imposes allergenic characteristics on a molecule. Allergenicity might be the result of a *combination* of characteristics of not only the introduced molecule, but also of the recipient and of the environment in which this recipient lives. Some of the characteristics *predisposing* a molecule toward allergenicity are these.

Chemical Nature. All allergens are proteins or protein-bound substances. Immunologists still argue whether in some special situations substances other than proteins, namely carbohydrates, may induce IgE production, but to this day no one has come forward with completely convincing evidence for the existence of a nonprotein allergen.

Origin. As was stated earlier, most allergens are derived from plants or animals. On the other hand, viruses and bacteria apparently cannot induce allergy. Why this is so, nobody knows.

Size. Many allergens have a molecular weight below 70,000 daltons and most have a molecular weight between 15,000 and 40,000. Simple haptens such as dinitrophenyl and benzylpenicilloyl are capable of inducing high IgE titers when administered on an appropriate carrier. Haptenic conjugates of T-independent antigens usually do not stimulate IgE responses—an observation probably related to the failure of bacteria and viruses to do so.

Charge. Many allergens are extremely polar compounds, but there are also many important exceptions to this rule.

Structural Characteristics. Many purified allergens are brownish in color and contain an enolized sugar-lysine residue (which forms the basis of the so-called *ripening* or *Mailliard reaction*). The lysine-sugar site and the *N*-glycosidic linkage were therefore thought to be involved in the induction of the allergic reaction. But later studies revealed many exceptions to this observation.

Multivalency. The presence of two or more determinants available for IgE binding is thought to be important for the crosslinking of receptors and initiation of the allergic reaction (see below). Spacing of the determinants on the allergenic molecule is probably also important.

In summary, many molecules that induce IgM, IgG, and IgA responses either do not induce significant IgE responses at all or induce only very poor IgE responses. Why this is so is not clear, except that a combination of several properties is probably required to make a molecule a good IgE inducer. In situations where the same molecule induces both IgG and IgE responses, chemical treatment of the molecule (e.g., with formalin or glutaraldehyde) can often separate the two, in the sense that it reduces IgE formation while having little effect on IgG formation. This observation indicates that, on a given molecule, some determinants induce IgG and others IgE responses preferentially.

Deliberate Immunization. Induction of IgE responses, more than the induction of any other antibody response, is dependent on the conditions of immunization—the antigen dose, the type of adjuvant employed, the immunization schedule, the genetic constitution of the recipient, the species, and other factors. High antigen doses and certain strong adjuvants usually give poor responses; extremely low doses induce reasonable responses but only in genetically predisposed individuals. The predisposition to IgE production is controlled, to a large degree, by the genes in the major histocompatibility complex. The induced responses are often transient, without a clear secondary response. Some species (e.g., the rat) are particularly poor producers of IgE antibodies in experimental immunization. These observations contrast with the generally good IgE responses of most individuals to natural parasitic infestations and underscore the importance of regulatory processes in IgE synthesis. Immunizations with isolated parasite antigens give better responses than with other antigens but not so good as those observed in natural parasitic infestations. The special conditions required for the induction of allergic IgE responses will be described in Section 13.4.2.

IgE Secretion

Precursors of IgE-secreting cells and the IgE-secreting plasma cells are found mostly on secretory surfaces such as the bronchi and the bronchioli of the respiratory system, mucosa of the gastrointestinal tract, the urinary bladder, nasal polyps, and the tonsils. Presumably, sensitization and most other phases of the IgE response occur in the organs of local immunity, although only a small amount of IgE antibody is released into the secretions; the antibodies do their job mostly in the tissues coating bodily surfaces.

Considering how much is known about the manifestation of IgE-mediated allergies, there is an embarrassing lack of knowledge about the cellular events following B-cell activation by allergens. Where, exactly, do the precursors of IgE-producing cells meet the antigen? In what form and by what mechanism is the antigen presented to them? Do the IgE precursors migrate as the precursors of the IgA-secreting cells do? What kind of cellular interaction regulates the IgE response? Where does the actual secretion take place? These are some of the questions that future immunologists will have to answer before they are able to claim any degree of understanding of what happens during IgE responses.

The activation of IgE precursor B cells is known to be T-dependent, presumably in a fashion similar to other precursor B cells. T cells are thought to control the differentiation of IgE precursor B cells into plasma cells, generation of IgE memory cells, and the degree of clonal expansion. Helper factors acting specifically on IgE responses have been identified. An important role in IgE responses is thought to be played by suppressor T cells, which normally keep the responses from turning against the individual's own tissues. Special classes of helper and suppressor T cells acting specifically on IgE-bearing B-cell precursors have been postulated, but direct evidence for their existence is lacking.

Tissue Fixation

Secreted IgE has affinity for tissue mast cells and basophils, found in close association with capillaries in connective tissue throughout the body. Most of the IgE antibodies bind to these cells immediately after secretion, so very few get into the circulation and serum. Furthermore, serum IgE has a relatively short half-life and so its level stays low, even when it is produced in considerable amounts, as is the case in allergic patients. When IgE is administered passively into the skin or some other tissue, there is a lag period of some 72 hours before cell-bound IgE can be detected, indicating that the binding is relatively slow; but then the bound IgE persists in the tissue for weeks or even months.

The binding of IgE to mast cells and basophils occurs via special receptors located in the cells' plasma membrane. Each cell has from several hundred thousand to more than a million receptors, which are glycoproteins containing about 10 to 15 percent carbohydrate and are embedded deeply in the membrane with only a small portion exposed to the exterior. The IgE molecules bind to the cell by inserting the two cylindrical domains of their Fc regions into the receptor (Fig. 13.17). The molecule can bind only to target cells of the same or a closely related species—in other words, it is *homocytotropic*.

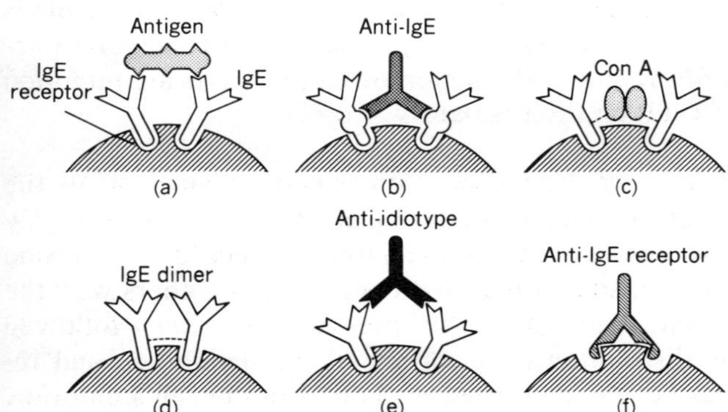

Figure 13.17. Various ways of activating a mast cell or basophil. Explanation in the text.

Degranulation of Mast Cells and Basophils

Activation and Granule Exteriorization. As far as is known, the combination of IgE with its receptor does not do anything to the receptor-bearing cell; it is only after the bound antibody combines with its corresponding antigen that things begin to happen in the mast cell or basophil. The antigen-antibody interaction initiates a sequence of events resulting in emptying of cellular granules to the exterior. This *degranulation*, however, can also be induced by means other than antigen-antibody interaction (Fig. 13.17*a*)—by the attachment of tissue-fixed immunoglobulins specifically recognizing the Fc region of the bound IgE (Fig. 13.17*b*); by the interaction of mitogens such as Concanavalin A or phytohemagglutinin with the bound IgE (Fig. 13.17*c*); by dimerization of the receptor-bound IgE molecules (because of membrane fluidity and mobility of membrane receptors, membrane-bound IgE molecules may accidentally "bump" into each other and stay together, held by weak binding forces; see Fig. 13.17*d*); by the binding of idiotypic antibodies recognizing the combining sites of cell-bound IgE molecules (Fig. 13.17*e*); and finally, by the attachment of non-IgE antibodies specific for the IgE receptors (Fig. 13.17*f*). In all of these six situations, a bridge connecting two IgE receptors is formed, and it is this bridging of receptors that is presumably essential for activation of the target cell.

IgE is not the only antibody homocytotropic for mast cells and basophils. Some IgG antibodies, particularly of the IgG4 subclass, are also known to cause degranulation of basophils. Furthermore, there is a whole array of other factors, nonimmunoglobulin in nature, that can activate mast cells (Table 13.2). The mechanisms of activation brought about by these various factors are probably not the same; also, the mechanism of mast cell activation may be different from that of basophil activation. Here, we shall limit our considerations to activation of mast cells by the formation of an antigen bridge connecting two or more cell-bound IgE molecules. This activation can be divided into several steps, the sequence of which is not yet certain; each step is delineated by the fact that it can be blocked by a distinct inhibitor.

Methylation of Membrane Phospholipids. This step is similar to that occurring during lymphocyte activation (see Chapter 12). Methylation of phospholipids

Table 13.2 Substances Capable of Mast Cell Activation and Degranulation

Antigen in combination with IgE or homocytotropic IgG antibodies
Complement factors (C3a, C5a, cobra venom factor)
Basic peptides:
Compound 48/80 (*p*-methoxy-*N*-methylphenylethylamine polymer)
Band-2 protein of polymorphonuclear leukocytes
Synacthen
Polymyxin B
Mast cell-degranulating (MCD) peptide from wasp venom
Dextran
Mitogens (concanavalin A, phytohemagglutinin)
Ionophore A 23187 (antibiotic isolated from *Streptomyces chartreusensis*
Exogenous adenosine triphosphate (ATP)
Enzymes:
Chymotrypsin
Phosphatidases
Phospholipases
Sodium fluoride

Source. Slightly modified from A. L. De Weck: *Schweiz. Med. Wochenschr.* **110**:175–179, 1980.

changes the viscosity of the plasma membrane, and the increased membrane fluidity facilitates lateral movement of receptors, a step necessary for further progression of the sequence. Methyltransferases can be inhibited by S-isobutyryl-3-diazoadenosine.

Calcium Ion Influx. One of the consequences of changed membrane fluidity is the opening up of Ca^{2+} channels. As a result, larger than normal quantities of Ca^{2+} ions begin to pour into the cell.

Activation of Serine Esterase. The influx of Ca^{2+} ions allows the uncovering of the active site of a proesterase, which is probably also associated with the membrane. Additional proesterase is then activated autocatalytically by the activated enzyme. The activated esterase has a chymoctrypsin-like activity and may be required for a microfilament-mediated granule alteration or membrane fusion. This step is inhibited by diisopropylfluorophosphate (DFP).

An Energy-Requiring Step. The source of energy is glucose and the energy is released by glycolysis. What the energy is needed for is not known; perhaps it is for microfilament-mediated movement of granules alongside the microtubules or plasma membrane. This step is inhibited by glucose deprivation, accomplished, for example, by the addition of metabolic inhibitor 2-deoxyglucose (2-DG).

Second Ca^{2+}-Dependent Step. Midway through the activation process, the need for additional Ca^{2+} ions arises independently of the initial Ca^{2+} influx into the cell. Intracellular Ca^{2+} ions are probably needed for the activation of the contractile proteins that form the cytoskeleton. This step is modulated through phosphorylation by a cyclic AMP-dependent kinase (see below); it is inhibited by the addition of ethylenediamine tetraacetate (EDTA).

Change in the Level of Intracellular Cyclic AMP. This is the most important regulatory step in the entire activation sequence. It determines whether the sequence proceeds further and if so, how extensively degranulation will occur. An increase in the level of intracellular cyclic AMP slows down or stops the sequence, whereas a drop in the cAMP level generally allows the completion of the sequence and degranulation. Similar modulation of the activation process may also occur via cGMP, and it might be the interplay of these two compounds that determines the degree of degranulation. The levels of intracellular cAMP and cGMP are, in turn, determined by signals from outside the cell, so that the two components serve as "second messengers," relaying the signals brought into the cell by such "first messengers" as hormones or neurotransmitters. We shall return to this point later in this section.

The production of cAMP from ATP is catalyzed by *adenylate cyclase*, a complex enzyme consisting of at least two components—the regulatory protein and the catalytic protein (Fig. 13.18). The complex is activated by the binding of GTP to the regulatory protein. But since the bound GTP is rapidly hydrolyzed to GDP by the enzyme GTPase, the complex normally displays only low cyclase activity. The increase in cyclase activity requires the action of factors favoring retention of GTP on the regulatory protein.

Release of Mediators. As a consequence of all the preceding steps, the granules—bags filled with highly active substances, or mediators—begin to move inside the cell, some fusing with one another, others with the plasma membrane. The latter type of fusion is followed by dissolution of a portion of the membrane and release of the contained mediators to the cell's exterior. Recent studies by Ann M. Dvorak and Harold F. Dvorak suggest that, at least in the basophils, the granules of even a nonactivated cell are communicating with the cell exterior. These experimenters observed small pinocytic vesicles pinching off the plasma membrane, migrating through the cytoplasm, and fusing with granules, and a similar transport of tiny vesicles has also been observed in the reverse direction: vesicles bud off granule membranes, travel to the cell surface, and discharge there. This continual communication between intracellular granules and the cell surface may play a role in the regulation of normal physiological processes by the mediators contained in the granules. Upon activation of a basophil or mast cell, the exteriorization of cytoplasmic granules speeds up greatly with the discharge of entire granules, the fusion of granules and discharge of the fusion complexes, and the formation of channels by the linear fusion of individual granules.

Regeneration of Granules. After complete extrusion of granules, the cell fills up again with vesicles and vacuoles. Some of the vesicles originate from the cell surface and are formed by endocytosis from the plasma membrane; they have been observed collecting and bringing back into the cell some of the released mediators. Other granules pinch off from the Golgi apparatus and become filled with de novo synthesized mediators. Eventually the morphologies of the mast cells or the basophils return to their preactivation state and the cells become ready for another round of degranulation.

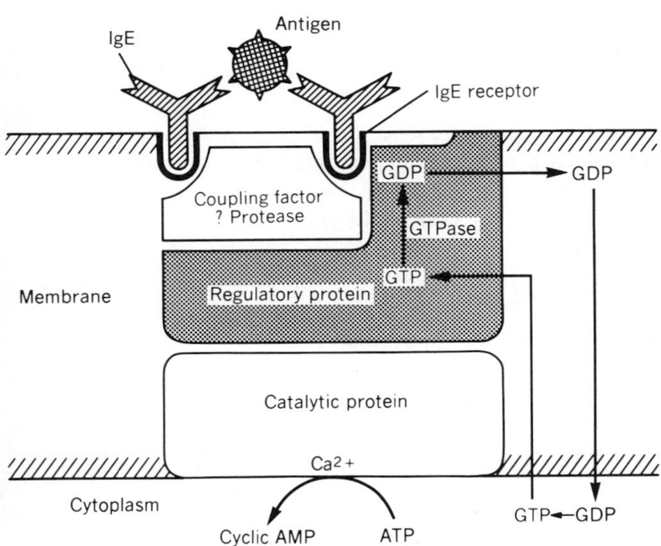

Figure 13.18. Possible interaction of the IgE receptor with the adenylate-cyclase complex in the plasma membrane of a mast cell. [Modified from S. T. Holgate, R. A. Lewis, and K. F. Austen *in* M. Fougereau and J. Dausset (Eds.): *Immunology 80*, pp. 846–859. Academic, London, 1980.]

A possible sequence of events in the entire mast cell activation process might be this. The binding of antigen to the IgE molecule and of IgE to the IgE receptor leads to methylation of phospholipids, opening of Ca^{2+} channels, influx of Ca^{2+} into the cell, and increased membrane fluidity. The IgE antigen-occupied receptors interact with the adenylate cyclase complex via a coupling factor (Fig. 13.18), which might be identical to the serine protease. The activated cyclase begins to convert ATP into cAMP and this second messenger then participates in a series of intracellular reactions leading to assembly of microtubules. The activated components of the cytoskeleton transport granules toward the plasma membrane, the granules fuse with the membrane and discharge their contents into the extracellular milieu.

Characteristics of Mediators. Degranulation floods the immediate surrounding of a cell with a number of pharmacologically active compounds capable of exerting a great variety of effects (Table 13.3). Some of these compounds, the primary mediators, were produced prior to degranulation and stored in granules until their exteriorization; others, the secondary mediators, are synthesized only after activation, or they result from processes occurring during degranulation.

Primary mediators are stored in the granule's matrix, bound electrostatically or otherwise to the matrix, or in soluble form. The electrostatically bound mediators are released in exchange for ions (primarily Na^+) present in high concentration in the extracellular milieu. The release of nonelectrostatically bound mediators must occur by some other mechanism; the soluble mediators simply diffuse from the matrix. We shall now discuss the main primary mediators one by one (Fig. 13.19).

Histamine, or β-imidazolylethylamine, is, as the name indicates, a derivative of the amino acid histidine (Fig. 13.19). The derivation consists of decarboxylation of the amino acid taken up by cells; histamine is degraded either by oxidative deamination or by methylation and oxidative deamination. Histamine is present in platelets, as well as in mast cells and basophils. It is stored in granules bound to heparin by electrostatic forces (see below); in this form it is protected from enzymatic degradation. When released from granules, histamine binds to target cells (smooth muscle cells, endothelial cells of blood vessels) via specific receptors. The binding can be inhibited by a variety of substances called *antihistamines*, which compete for histamine receptors. Antihistamines distinguish two

Table 13.3 Chemical Mediators of Immediate Hypersensitivity

Mediator	Structural Characteristics	Assays	Functions	Inactivation
		Primary		
Histamine	β-Imidazolyl-ethylamine M.W. = 111	Contraction of guinea pig ileum; specific radio-labeling by histamine *N*-methyltransferase	Increased vascular permeability; elevation of cyclic AMP; chemokinesis	Histaminase; histamine methyl-transferase
Serotonin	5-Hydroxytrypt-amine (5-HT)	Biological and enzymic assays	Increased vascular permeability	5-HT deaminase
Eosinophil chemotactic factor of anaphylaxis (ECF-A)	Hydrophobic acidic tetrapeptides M.W. = 360–390	Chemotactic attraction of eosinophils and neutrophils	Eosinophil and neutrophil deactivation	Aminopeptidase; carboxypeptidase
Intermediate-molecular-weight eosinophil chemotactic factor (IMW-ECF)	M.W. = 1500–3000	Chemotactic attraction of eosinophils and neutrophils	Eosinophil deactivation	
High-molecular-weight neutrophil chemotactic factor (HMW-NCF)	M.W. ≧ 750,000	Chemotactic attraction of neutrophils	Neutrophil deactivation	
Heparin	Macromolecular acidic proteoglycan M.W. ~ 750,000	Antithrombin III activation; metachromasia	Anticoagulant; anticomplementary activity	
Chymase	M.W. = 25,000	Hydrolysis of BTEE	Proteolysis	
N-Acetyl-β-glucosaminidase	Protein M.W. = 150,000	Hydrolysis of *N*-acetyl-β-glucosamine paranitro-phenyl substrate		
β-Glucuronidase	M.W. = 280,000	Hydrolysis of phenolphthalein-β-glucuronide		
Arylsulfatase A	M.W. = 115,000	Hydrolysis of *p*-nitrocatechol	Inactivation of SRS-A	
		Secondary		
Slow-reacting substance of anaphylaxis (SRS-A)	Leukotriens C-1 and D	Contraction of antihista-mine-treated guinea pig ileum	Contraction of human bronchiole; increased vascular permeability	Arylsulfatases A and B
Platelet-activating factors (PAFs)	Lipidlike MW ~ 300–500	Release of (^{14}C)5-hydroxytryptamine from platelets	Aggregation	
Lipid chemotactic factor	Lipidlike products of arachidonate metabolism	Chemotactic attraction of neutrophils	Neutrophil deactivation	
Lipid chemokinetic factor	(Lipidlike products of arachidonate metabolism)	Chemokinetic attraction of neutrophils		

Source. From K. F. Austen: *J. Immunol.* **121**:793–805, 1978.

kinds of receptor, H_1 and H_2. The H_1 receptors can be blocked by the so-called classical antihistamines (the first group discovered), whereas binding through H_2 receptors (not to be confused with *H-2*, the major histocompatibility complex of the mouse) is inhibitable by a newer group of antihistamines, such as the thiourea derivatives burimamide and metiamide. The two kinds of receptor have different tissue distributions, so that

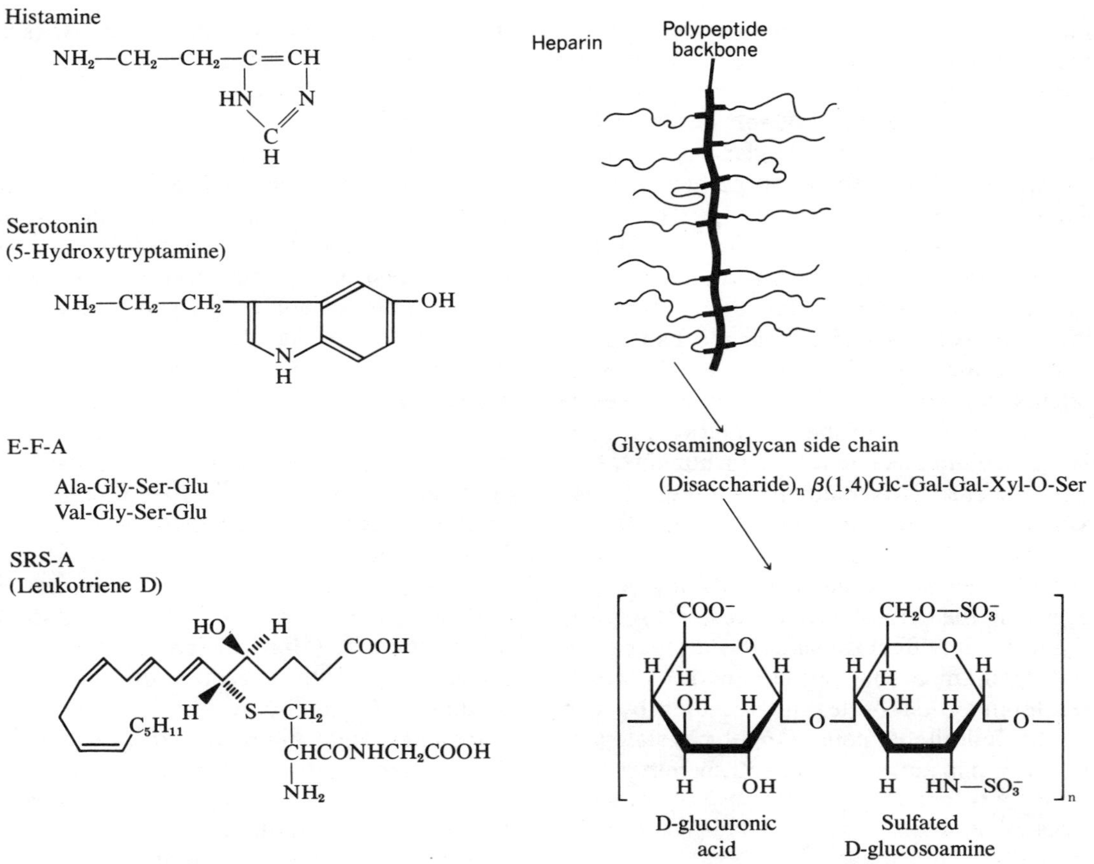

Histamine

$NH_2—CH_2—CH_2—C=CH$ (imidazole ring: HN, N, C–H)

Serotonin
(5-Hydroxytryptamine)

$NH_2—CH_2—CH_2$– (indole ring, N–H) –OH

E-F-A

Ala-Gly-Ser-Glu
Val-Gly-Ser-Glu

SRS-A
(Leukotriene D)

HO, H, COOH, H, C_5H_{11}, $S—CH_2$, $CHCONHCH_2COOH$, NH_2

Heparin

Polypeptide backbone

Glycosaminoglycan side chain

(Disaccharide)$_n$ β(1,4)Glc-Gal-Gal-Xyl-O-Ser

COO^-, $CH_2O—SO_3^-$, H, OH, H, O, $HN—SO_3^-$, n

D-glucuronic acid

Sulfated D-glucosoamine

Figure 13.19. Some of the mediators released during mast cell degranulation.

the effect of histamine on some tissues (endothelial cells, smooth muscle cells) is mediated by the H_1 receptors, while the effect on other tissues (stomach glands) is mediated by the H_2 receptors. The two receptors also mediate opposing effects of histamine on inflammation (described in Chapter 14): the binding of histamine through H_1 receptors enhances inflammation, whereas binding through H_2 receptors inhibits it. The three main targets of histamine are the blood vessels, smooth muscles, and exocrine glands. The effect on the vascular system varies, depending on the size of the vessels and on the animal species. In general, large blood vessels and arterioles are constricted by histamine, whereas minute vessels, capillaries, and venules are dilated. The histamine-induced arteriolar constriction is strong in rodents and slight in cats; in dogs, monkeys, and humans, histamine causes arteriolar dilation. These observations are important to bear in mind when considering the variability of IgE responses in different species. The dilation of fine blood vessels is brought about by some direct, as yet unidentified action of histamine on the musculature of the vessels, independent of innervation. Vasodilation is accompanied by an increase in permeability, leading to the seepage of plasma proteins and fluids into the extracellular spaces, and so to the formation of a swelling (edema). In larger vessels, histamine increases permeability by causing the cells of the endothelial lining to separate, thereby generating intercellular spaces through which plasma can escape. When injected intravenously, histamine affects almost all capillaries in the body, but the response in humans is most conspicuous in the skin over the face and upper part of the body, the so-called blushing areas, which become hot and red. The dilation of arterioles and capillaries results in a fall of systemic blood pressure. The mechanism of histamine action on smooth muscles is not understood either, but this action, too, is apparently independent of innervation. It is believed that histamine promotes movement of Ca^{2+} ions into muscle cells and that the ions then initiate the contraction. (Histamine has no effect on muscle cells in Ca^{2+}-free medium.) Muscles particularly sensitive to histamine are those of the uterus and bronchioli. In most species, these muscles contract upon exposure to histamine; but in some species (e.g., the rat), histamine produces the opposite effect, muscle relaxation. Of the exocrine glands, the most strongly affected are those of the stomach. Histamine probably acts directly on the gland cells, inducing them to intensify their secretion of highly acidic gastric juice.

Serotonin, or 5-hydroxytryptamine, is derived from the amino acid tryptophan by the introduction of one hydroxyl group into position 5 and decarboxylation (Fig. 13.19). It derives its name from the fact that it remains in the serum after blood has been allowed to clot. In rodents (e.g., rat, mouse) serotonin is present in mast cells, platelets, and in special enterochromaffin cells of the gastrointestinal mucosa; in humans, it is absent in mast cells. This mediator evokes a wide range of responses that vary not only between species, but also between individuals of the same species. It acts, in particular, on smooth muscle cells and nerves, affecting primarily the cardiovascular, respiratory, and digestive systems. Its effect on smooth muscle can be either direct or indirect via nerves. In the vascular system, serotonin produces leaking venules by partially disjoining endothelial cells. Under physiological conditions, serotonin acts as a neurotransmitter (see below); it plays a role in the IgE responses of rats and mice, but not of humans (because of its absence in human mast cells).

Among the released mediators are at least three *chemotactic factors*, which act on granulocytes and cause their migration to the site of response. They are the *eosinophil chemotactic factor of anaphylaxis* (ECF-A), the *intermediate-molecular-weight eosinophil chemotactic factor* (IMW-ECF), and the *high-molecular-weight neutrophil chemotactic factor* (HMW-NCF). Of these, the ECF-A has been studied most extensively, in particular by K. Frank Austen and his collaborators. Its active components are two tetrapeptides, Val-Gly-Ser-Glu and Ala-Gly-Ser-Glu, capable of interaction with eosinophil surfaces via their terminal amino acids. The amino-terminal valine or alanine interacts with a hydrophobic region of the plasma membrane and initiates concentration gradient-dependent chemotaxis. The highly charged carboxy-terminal glutamic acid interacts with an ionic domain of the membrane and causes the so-called *deactivation of eosinophils*—the cells' unresponsiveness to further stimuli. The deactivation results in the expression of a large number of C3b receptors on the cell surface, indicating that the function of ECF-A is to attract eosinophils chemotactically to the site of IgE response, trap them at this site by deactivation, and prepare them for involvement in immune reactions. (Expression C3b receptors makes the cell available for immune a herence—the first step in its engagement in immu reactions.)

Heparin is an intracellular proteoglycan compos of a peptide backbone and side chains of glucosamir glycan. (The side chains are attached to the serine the polypeptide via a characteristic trisaccharic with the rest of the chain consisting of repeated dis charide units of sulfated D-glucosamine and D-gluc ronic acid; see Fig. 13.19.) This structure accou for the characteristic metachromatic staining granules (see Chapter 5). It forms a skeleton on whi rest other constituents of the granule (e.g., histami or serotonin). The substance is so named because of abundant occurrence in the liver (Gr. *hēpar*, liver). T three main functions of heparin are, first, inhibition Hageman factor-dependent clotting fibrinolysis; se ond, augmentation of histamine inactivation diamine oxidase; and, third, suppression of compl ment function. (Heparin inhibits C1q binding to i mune complexes, interaction of C1s with C4 and C binding of C2 to C4b receptors, formation of C5b,6 complexes, and formation of the C3-cleaving enzym These three functions afford to the mast cell a capaci to regulate events leading to and following its own a tivation and degranulation.

Among the primary mediators are also several e zymes that probably play a role in degradation of pr teoglycans and their glucosaminoglycans. The mo prominent among these are chymase, *N*-acetyl- glucosaminidase, and arylsulfatases. *Chymase* is chymotrypsin-like neutral protease that sits on t heparin side chains in an inactive form; dissociati from heparin activates this enzyme. *N-acetyl-β-gluc saminidase* is an enzyme that cleaves, as the na indicates, *N*-acetyl-β-glucosamine, and in this capa ity is capable of degrading bacterial cell walls in soluble fragments. *Arylsulfatases* cleave phe sulfates, including cerebroside sulfates.

The *secondary mediators* are not stored in granule instead they are generated only after the immune eve either by the mast cell or by secondary cell types in t immediate environment. (Some may be released fro membrane phospholipids of these secondary cells up the action of primary mediators.) Here we shall me tion only two of the large array of these mediators, t slow-reacting substance of anaphylaxis and t platelet-activating factor.

The *slow-reacting substance of anaphylaxis* (SRS- was discovered as a compound causing a slow (slow than histamine), prolonged contraction of certain is lated smooth muscle preparations. For a long time the chemical nature of the substance remained unelucidated, but the substance has recently been identified as a mixture of the leukotriens C-1 and D. The leukocyte-produced luekotriens are unique among small, biologically active molecules in that they are a combination of peptides and fatty acids (Fig. 13.19). The peptide portion of the molecule is composed of three amino acids—glycine, glutamic acid, and cysteine, linked to a long-chain fatty acid derived from arachidonic acid and related to prostaglandins (see Chapter 11). SRS-A is inhibited by arylsulfatases, present among the primary mediators.

Platelet-activating factor (PAF) is also released by leukocytes during their activation. It activates platelets, as manifested by their aggregation and the release of amines from them. It probably represents a heterogeneous collection of chemically and biologically active materials, most of which are phospholipid derivatives.

Effector Phase

The discharge into the tissue of so many active compounds initiates a complex series of interactions, only a few of which have been elucidated. The specific interactions vary, depending on the circumstances of the response. Here we shall outline some of the known and postulated interactions accompanying parasite infestation; in the following section we shall mention interactions occurring during pathological IgE responses; and in the next chapter we shall discuss the involvement of mediators in self-repair processes, such as wound healing and inflammation.

A simplified view of what might be happening when a protozoan or metazoan parasite invades a vertebrate and lodges in the host tissue—say, in the intestine—is depicted schematically in Figure 13.20. The parasite inadvertently releases some of its antigens into the tissues (for example, by shedding). The antigens are picked up by macrophages; some of them are delivered to regional lymph nodes, where they stimulate IgM and IgG production, while some are presented to helper T cells and IgE-bearing B cells directly in these tissues. The tissue T and B cells become activated, and the B-cell progeny begin to secrete IgE antibodies specific for the stimulating antigen. The cytotropic antibodies bind to mast cells and basophils in the tissues surrounding the parasite, and when more of the same antigen comes along, the target cells are activated and they degranulate and release mediators into the tissue.

Some of the mediators cause leakage of serum proteins, including parasite-specific IgG and IgM antibodies, from the intestinal blood vessels and the antibodies then attack the parasite. Other mediators act as chemotactic factors. They attract granulocytes, particularly basophils and eosinophils, into the tissues surrounding the parasite and immobilize them there. Basophils bind IgE antibodies cytotropically, become activated, and release more mediators. Eosinophils become involved in the immune response in a variety

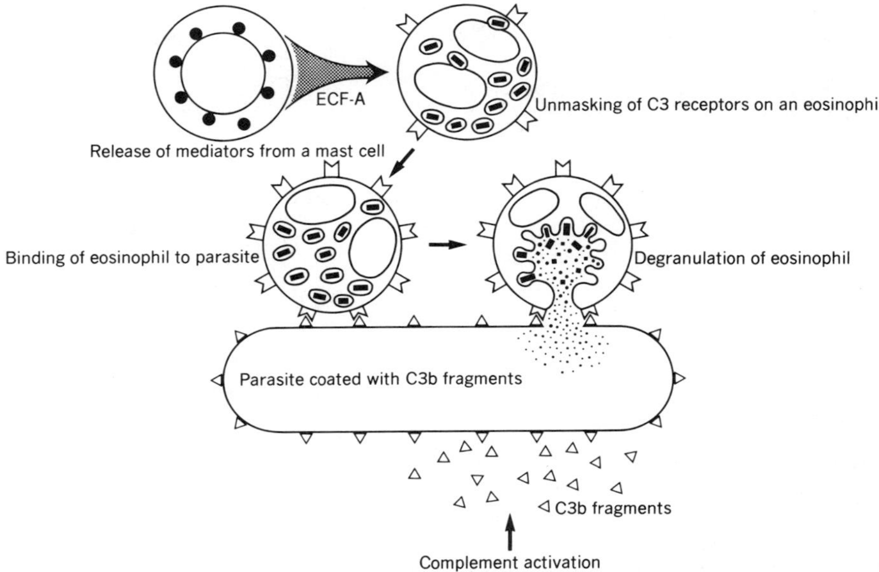

Figure 13.20. Mast cell-triggered attack of eosinophils on a parasite. Explanation in the text.

of ways. First of all, they attack the parasite directly, either via a C3b-dependent cytotoxicity mechanism or via IgG antibody-dependent cell killing. They exert some phagocytosis and they engulf soluble antigen-antibody complexes by pinocytosis. And finally, the eosinophils themselves release factors that regulate the function of the mast cells and basophils. The combined effect of all these events is the killing of the parasite and its expulsion from the tissue.

Some of the other interactions occurring during the response are described below (see also Fig. 13.21).

The Complement System. The antigen-IgG complexes activate the classical complement pathway, and the generated C3b and C5a fragments activate additional mast cells and basophils without the participation of additional antibodies. Parasites themselves may activate the alternative complement pathway, which then also leads to the release of anaphylatoxin and mast cell activation. Some of the complement fragments also act as chemotactic factors for granulocytes. On the other hand, heparin may exert negative feedback by inhibiting the generation of the amplification convertase.

Interaction Between Mediators Released by Mast Cells and Eosinophils. Eosinophils release several compounds that inhibit the action of mast cell-derived mediators: arylsulfatase B inactivates SRS-A; phospholipase D inhibits PAF; and diamine oxidase (histaminase) inhibits histamine. In fact, eosinophils have been seen taking up entire mast cell granules, thus becoming metachromatic. This detoxification of the released granules and biodegradation of mast cell mediators may be an important part of the regulatory role played by eosinophils.

Platelet Involvement. Activation of platelets via a variety of factors may lead to the release of arachidonic acid, prostaglandins, thromboxan, and serotonin, all of which may then interact with other mediators released during the response (see Chapter 14).

As has already been mentioned, the actual attack on the parasite is carried out primarily by eosinophils. An eosinophil can damage a parasite in at least two ways. The first, *IgG-antibody-dependent cytotoxicity*, was described in Chapter 5. In the second, *C3b-dependent cytotoxicity* (Fig. 13.20), the C3b produced by the activation of either the classical or alternative complement

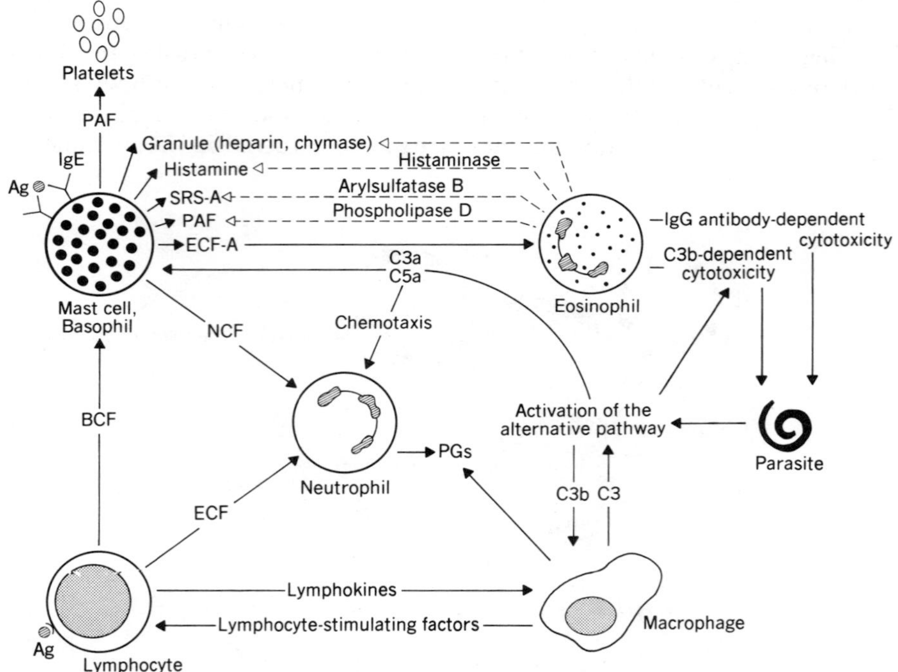

Figure 13.21. Role of mediators in cellular interactions during host defense against a helminthic parasite. Solid arrows indicate stimulatory effect, broken arrows inhibition. Ag, antigen; BCF, basophil chemotactic factor; ECF, eosinophil chemotactic factor; ECF-A, eosinophil chemotactic factor of anaphylaxis; NCF, neutrophil chemotactic factor; PAF, platelet-activating factor; PGs, prostaglandins; SRS-A, slow-reacting substance of anaphylaxis.

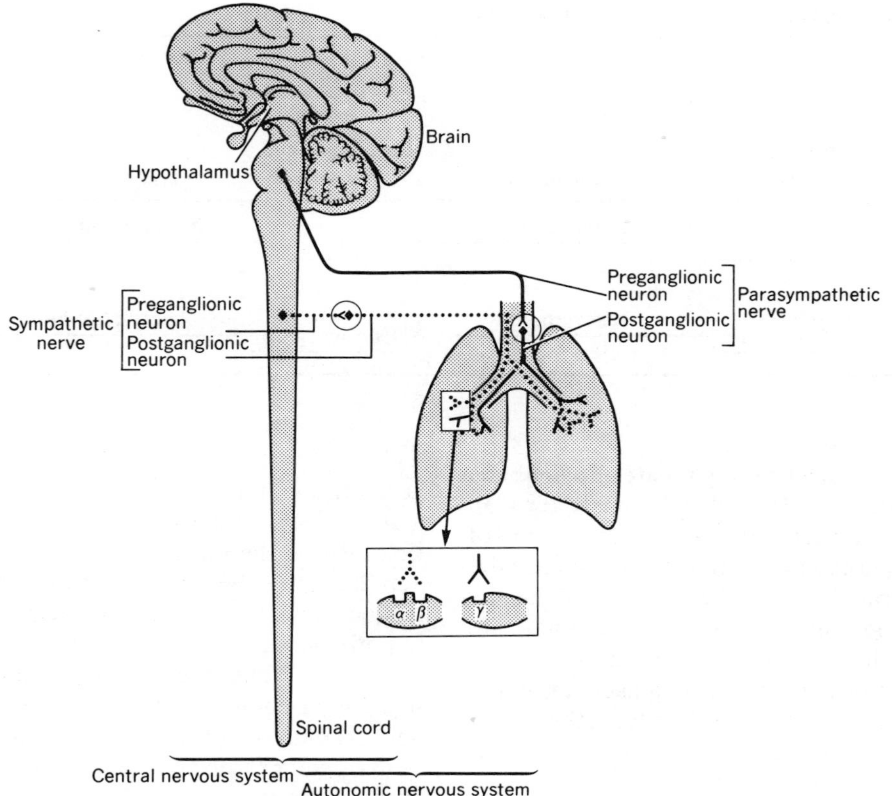

(a)

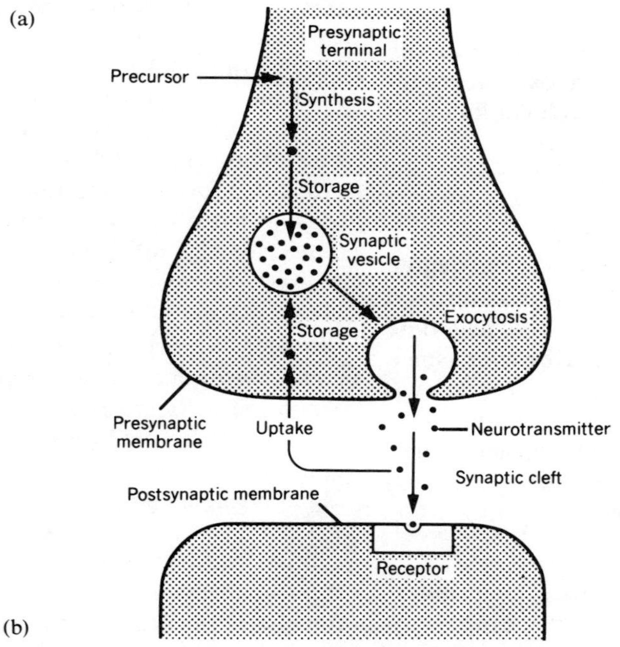

(b)

Figure 13.22. Neurohormonal regulation of IgE responses. (*a*) The autonomic nervous system. (*b*) A synapse of two neurons.

Table 13.4 Functional Organization of the Autonomic Nervous System

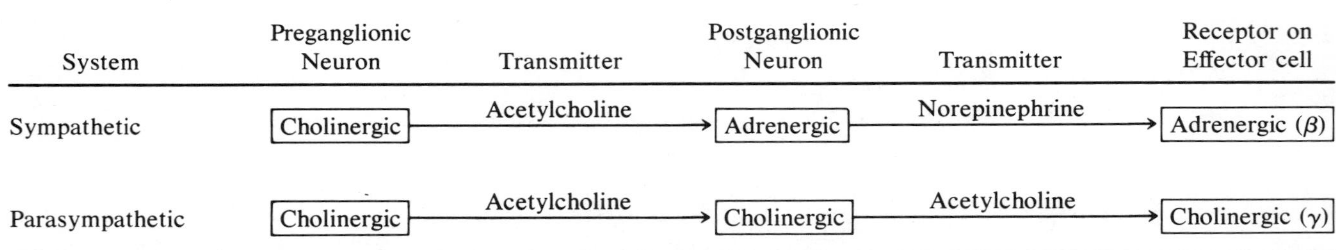

System	Preganglionic Neuron	Transmitter	Postganglionic Neuron	Transmitter	Receptor on Effector cell
Sympathetic	Cholinergic	Acetylcholine →	Adrenergic	Norepinephrine →	Adrenergic (β)
Parasympathetic	Cholinergic	Acetylcholine →	Cholinergic	Acetylcholine →	Cholinergic (γ)

pathway coats the surface of the parasite. Eosinophils then bind to the coating C3b molecules via their C3b receptors, which have been unmasked by the action of ECF-A. The attached cells are activated and release the contents of their granules onto the parasite. What the components of the granules actually do to the parasite is not known. The eosinophils granules contain peroxidases, arylsulfatases, phospholipases, arginine-rich cationic proteins, and other highly active compounds (see Chapter 5), which apparently somehow wreak havoc on the parasite surface.

There is an interesting difference between the action of neutrophils and eosinophils: while the former are specialized in phagocytosis, intracellular degranulation, and intracellular killing of invaders (bacteria), the eosinophils display very little phagocytosis, degranulate extracellularly, and exert an extracellular killing of parasites.

Modulation of IgE Responses

We mentioned in the preceding section that the degree of mast cell and basophil degranulation is controlled hormonally and via the nervous system. It is now time to have a closer look at this control. However, since we cannot discuss this subject without a basic knowledge of the autonomic nervous system, we must first make a brief excursion into the realm of neurology. Readers familiar with the workings of the nervous system are advised to skip this section.

The Autonomic Nervous System. This system innervates the heart, blood vessels, respiratory organs, digestive system, and other internal organs over which we have no willful control—we cannot, for example, voluntarily speed up or slow down the heartbeat or dilate or constrict blood vessels. The system is composed of two kinds of nerve, *sympathetic* and *parasympathetic* (Fig. 13.22), which always have an antagonistic effect on the innervated organ: if one speeds up its activity, the other slows it down. The system is controlled by a portion of the brain called the hypothalamus, but most of the nerves actually composing the system begin in the spinal cord. Each sympathetic or parasympathetic nerve (in contrast to other nerves) consists of only two neurons—a *preganglionic neuron*, the cell body of which is located in the spinal cord, and a *postganglionic neuron*, with the cell body located outside the spinal cord. In the sympathetic system, the cell body of the postganglionic neuron is close to the spinal cord, whereas in the parasympathetic nerves, the cell body of the postganglionic neuron lies with the organ it innervates.

The area of contact between two neurons is called the *synapse* (Fig. 13.22*b*). At the synapse, one cell process often forms a buttonlike enlargement (*presynaptic terminal*) resting on the body (the *postsynaptic membrane*) of the other neuron. The two plasma membranes, the presynaptic and postsynaptic, are often separated by a gap—the *synaptic cleft*. The synapse provides the organism with the opportunity to influence or stop an *impulse* traveling along a nerve fiber. Since the cells are not in direct contact, the impulse must be transmitted through the synaptic cleft by special *neurotransmitters*, which are like ferryboats carrying messengers across a river. The autonomic nervous system uses *chemical neurotransmitters*, compounds synthesized in the presynaptic terminal and stored in the so-called *synaptic vesicles*. The arrival of a nerve impulse at the presynpatic terminal entices some of the synaptic vesicles to move toward the presynaptic membrane, attach to the membrane, open up, and discharge their contents into the synaptic cleft. The neurotransmitters then diffuse through the cleft and

Increase in Intracellular	Effect on Mediator Release	Effect on Bronchial Smooth Muscle	Effect on Endothelium of Arteries	Receptor	Stimulation by		
					Epinephrine	Norepinephrine	Isoproterenol
cAMP	Decrease	Relaxation	Constriction	α	+	++++	+
cGMP	Increase	Constriction	Dilation	β	+	+	++++

interact with receptors on the postsynaptic membrane of the contact cell. The interaction of neurotransmitters with membrane receptors results in an influx of Na^+ ions into the cell, depolarization of the postsynaptic membrane, and regeneration of the impulse, which then travels further along the processes of this second neuron. At the end of transmission, neurotransmitters are often taken back into the presynaptic terminal and stored in vesicles for further use; the lost neurotransmitters are regenerated by de novo synthesis. The transmission of the nerve impulse from the nerve's ending to the muscle or gland cell is similar to that across a synapse.

The autonomic nervous system uses two compounds as neurotransmitters—acetylcholine and norepinephrine (noradrenaline). *Acetylcholine* is the acetic acid ester of choline originally isolated from ergot; *norepinephrine* is a catecholamine hormone. Transmission via acetylcholine is described as *cholinergic*, and transmission via norepinephrine as *adrenergic*. Corresponding to the two types of transmitter are two basic types of receptor, identically named. Each type can be distinguished further according to its response to various other substances. There are at least two *cholinergic receptors*, M and N: in the M type the effects of acetylcholine are mimicked by muscarine and the receptor is blocked by tropine, whereas in the *N type*, the effects of acetylcholine are mimicked by nicotine and the receptor is blocked by muscarine. Similarly, there are at least two *adrenergic* receptors, α and β (the cholinergic receptor is sometimes designated γ), where the *α receptor* responds primarily to norepinephrine, far less to epinephrine and isoproterenol, and is blocked by phenoxylbenzamine, and the *β receptor* responds primarily to isoprotenol, less to epinephrine or norepinephrine, and is blocked by propranolol. As Table 13.4 shows, the different synapses and nerve endings in the sympathetic and parasympathetic systems use different neurotransmitters and different receptors. As has been mentioned, the sympathetic and parasympathetic nerves work in opposition to each other, but the kind of action they stimulate depends on the particular tissue, the neurotransmitter, and the type of receptor involved (Table 13.4). In the bronchial muscle cells, for example, cholinergic stimulation via acetylcholine results in constriction, whereas adrenergic stimulation via epinephrine induces muscle cell relaxation. In a physiological situation, the muscle cell receives constantly alternating signals for constriction and relaxation, and this oscillation of responses maintains the muscle tone.

The conversion of a nerve signal into action in an effector cell (e.g., a muscle cell) is accomplished via cyclic AMP. When the membrane receptor receives the signal, it transmits it to another membrane protein called the *transducer* or *transmitter*. This protein, in turn, activates the membrane-associated enzyme *adenylate cyclase*, which then begins to convert cytoplasmic ATP into cyclic AMP, the *second messenger*. The cyclic AMP molecules act on a cytoplasmic enzyme called *protein kinase* and activate it by removal of an inhibitory subunit from the proenzyme. Activated protein kinase has been implicated in the initiation of many intracellular functions: glycogenesis and glycogenolysis; lipogenesis; DNA, RNA, and protein synthesis; and microtubule assembly.

Neurohormonal Regulation of Mast Cell Degranulation. Mast cells and basophils have both adrenergic (α, β) and cholinergic (γ) receptors on their surfaces, and can therefore respond to stimuli that activate or block these receptors. Stimulation through adrenergic β receptors (via the sympathetic system) results in an increase in the level of intracellular cyclic AMP, and

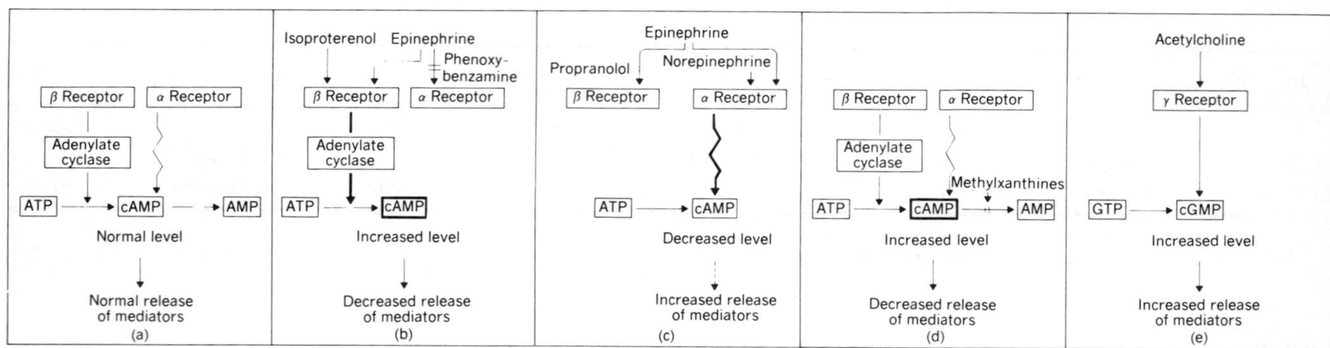

Figure 13.23. Control of mediator release from mast cells. (*a*) Normal status. (*b*) Blockade of α receptors by phenoxybenzamine. (*c*) Blockade of β receptors by propranolol. (*d*) Blockade of cAMP conversion into AMP by methylxanthines. (*e*) Stimulation of γ receptors by acetylcholine. [Based on R. P. Orange and K. F. Austin *in* R. A. Good and D. W. Fisher (Eds.): *Immunobiology*. Sinauer, Sunderland, Massachusetts, 1971.]

hence in the decrease of mediator release. Stimulation through cholinergic (γ) receptors (via the parasympathetic system) results in an increase of cyclic GMP level and so also in the increase of mediator release (Fig. 13.23*e*). Under normal circumstances, the balance between adrenergic and cholinergic stimulation of activated mast cells and basophils maintains the balance between cyclic AMP and cyclic GMP levels and keeps the mediator release under strict control (Fig. 13.23*a*). Deviation from this norm may lead to a failure to respond to one or the other stimulus, and the unregulated degranulation may turn the beneficial IgE response into an injurious one. That the nervous system influences IgE responses has been known for some time. Many pathological IgE responses (allergies) are known to be affected by the psychological condition of the patient, and in guinea pigs, the removal of the anterior hypothalamus (known to control the parasympathetic system) reduces the symptoms of experimentally induced IgE-mediated tissue injury, whereas the removal of the posterior hypothalamus (known to control the sympathetic system) enhances these symptoms.

In reality, the modulation of degranulation is probably much more complex than has just been described. One level of complexity is introduced by the fact that there are at least two cholinergic and two adrenergic receptors, and that each of these responds to and is blocked by different compounds. The actual response is, then, the result of an interplay between the various stimuli. It has been demonstrated in an experimental situation that both adrenergic receptors, α as well as β, play a role. When the α receptors are blocked by phenoxybenzamine, the stimulation of β receptors by isoproterenol and epinephrine is enhanced and the mediator release is decreased (Fig. 13.23*b*); when the β receptors are blocked by propranolol, the stimulation of α receptors by norepinephrine or epinephrine (the latter can interact with both α and β receptors) is enhanced and the release of mediators is increased (Fig. 13.23*c*).

Mediator release can also be controlled by cyclic AMP metabolism. This second messenger is normally broken down to 5-adenine monophosphate (5-AMP) by a cytoplasmic enzyme, phosphodiesterase. When this enzyme is inhibited by methylxanthine, the level of cyclic AMP increases and mediator release decreases (Fig. 13.23*d*).

Levels of intracellular cyclic AMP and cyclic GMP can also be influenced by many other substances, such as prostaglandins, kinins, and the mediators themselves (e.g., histamine). Most, if not all, of these substances act via specific receptors on the mast cell or basophil surface. Many of the substances are released by eosinophils trapped in the sites of IgE responses, and eosinophils, in addition, modulate IgE responses by releasing factors that inactivate or enzymatically degrade mediators (see preceding section).

13.4.2 Pathology of IgE Response

Despite the multitude of control mechanisms, the IgE response frequently derails and turns against the individual's own tissue. Two principal situations lead to pathological manifestation of the IgE response. In one, the circumstances of the response (antigen dose, the manner of antigen presentation, the length of exposure to antigen, and so forth) are such that they favor the formation of IgE antibodies over other antibodies in a given individual. If the right antigen then comes along in the right form and at the right time, mediator release that has no adaptive value and is, in fact, harmful to the body, may be induced. There is nothing wrong with the control mechanism in such individuals; they are victims of circumstance. The potential for the development of this form of the pathological response exists in any individual of a given species, and the pathological response can theoretically be induced by almost any antigen. In nature, this form of pathological response is rare, but it can be induced with relative ease by an experimenter.

In the second situation, the affected individual has a defect—usually of a hereditary nature—in the system regulating IgE responses. Because of this defect, the responses get out of hand and become injurious. These situations occur only in some individuals of a given species (those carrying the particular defect), and the pathological reactions are particularly striking in response to certain antigens that exploit the defect most efficiently.

We shall refer to the former condition as *anaphylaxis* and to the latter as *atopy*; we shall designate as *allergy* any condition leading to pathological responses characterized by degranulation of mast cells and basophils; in other words, the term "allergy" includes anaphylaxis, atopy, and certain degranulation phenomena not associated with IgE responses. But we must emphasize that the terms anphylaxis, atopy, and allergy have been and still are used by other immunologists with somewhat different meanings, which we must now discuss briefly.

Of the three terms, *anaphylaxis* is the oldest. It was introduced in 1902 by Paul J. Portier and Charles R. Richet to refer to the fact that dogs exposed to sea anemone toxin developed what then seemed to be *decreased* resistance to this substance (Gr. *ana*, away from, *phylaxis*, protection; see Chapter 2). This observation went against the prevailing concept that antibodies and immunity in general had a prophylactic function: they were supposed to heighten, rather than lower, the resistance of an organism to toxins and bacteria. The response described by Portier and Richet did not seem to make sense, but the puzzle became even greater when immunologists later realized that the reaction was not one of lowered resistance but of increased sensitivity, or *hypersensitivity*.

Shortly after the Portier-Richet observation on dogs, several other instances of unusual reactivity were described in other species, including humans. It then seemed as if immunity or increased resistance to infections was only one aspect of the host response to foreign matter; increased sensitivity seemed to be the other, nonprophylactic aspect. There seemed to be a need for a term that would encompass both immunity and hypersensitivity, and such a term—*allergy*—was introduced by Clemens P. von Pirquet in 1906 (Gr. *allos*, other, *ergon*, work). The original meaning of the word was "an altered reaction," a state—that is, any state—of an organism induced by the introduction of an antigen. But this meaning of the term lasted only a short time. Soon after its introduction, immunologists began to restrict its usage, first to phenomena resulting from circulating antibodies, and then to the states of increased sensitivity, including anaphylaxis.

The term *atopy* (Gr. *atopia*, strangeness) was introduced by Arthur F. Coca in 1923 to denote certain strange forms of human hypersensitivity characterized by leakage of proteins and fluids from blood vessels, and by strong hereditary predisposition. From the beginning, the term had a narrower meaning than "allergy" since it did not include anaphylaxis and certain other forms of allergy (i.e., those not mediated by IgE antibodies). It comes closest to what the layman usually understands by "allergy."

The confusion in terminology still persists. Virtually all possible variants of a relationship among the three terms can be found in immunological literature: anaphylaxis is equated with allergy, allergy is equated with atopy, atopy is restricted to IgE-mediated reaction or used in a broader sense, and so forth. The confusion is further aggravated by the fact that certain symptoms can apparently be induced by different pathological conditions; for example, hay fever (see below) can be of allergic origin (i.e., caused by pathological degranulation of mast cells), but it can also be caused by nonallergic conditions. This confusion will probably persist as long as the precise meaning of the individual forms of IgE response remain unclarified.

Allergy is often considered as one possible manifestation of *immediate hypersensitivity* (the other forms being, for example, the Arthus phenomenon or serum sickness), a condition characterized by promptness of response. Immediate hypersensitivity manifests itself within minutes of the application of antigen to a sensitized individual—as opposed to the hours or days necessary for the development of the delayed-type hypersensitivity (see Chapter 12). In the classification of immune responses used in this book, the term "immediate hypersensitivity" is largely superfluous.

Before we close this section on terminology, we should emphasize again that the puzzle of injurious immunological responses stems from a historical misconception caused by a lack of knowledge about the physiological function of IgE. Even today, the pathological forms of IgE responses are overemphasized in textbooks, while the physiological responses are hardly mentioned at all. To a clinician, anaphylaxis and atopy are, of course, very important; but to the biologist, they are insignificant curiosities. From a biologist's point of view there is no paradox of injurious antibodies (see Chapter 2), for in nature, the instances in which antibodies turn against an individual's own tissues are rare. As one immunologist remarked in 1947, "The guinea pig is extremely easy to kill by an immunological reaction we call anaphylaxis, but it may be doubted if many guinea pigs under natural conditions ever die of anaphylatic shock. When we perform such an experiment we are setting up conditions which are essentially artificial. . . . we are 'stacking the cards' against the guinea pig."[2]

Anaphylaxis

Definition. We shall use the term "anaphylaxis" to mean sensitivity inducible in any individual of a given species by appropriate antigenic challenge, and expressed by characteristic changes upon another challenge with the same antigen; the changes include the contraction of smooth muscles and dilation of capillaries and are caused by the release of pharmacologically active substances from mast cells and basophils after the combination of cell-fixed antibodies with the antigen. The antigenic challenge inciting increased sensitivity is called *sensitization* (equivalent to "immunization" in responses mediated by antibodies other than IgE), and the sensitizing substance is variously referred to as *sensitizing antigen*, *sensitizer*, *inducer*, *allergen*, or *anaphylactogen*; the substance actually evoking anaphylactic symptoms is called the *elicitor*; and the immunized animal is referred to as *sensitive*, *hypersensitive*, or *allergic*.

Conditions of Sensitization. Animals are constantly being exposed to antigens, yet only seldom do they become hypersensitive. Obviously, the hypersensitive state develops only when the antigen is presented to the recipient in a certain way. What is implied by this "certain way" is still poorly understood, and must be determined empirically most of the time, but some of the important factors of sensitization are the following.

Route of Antigen Administration. Sensitization can be accomplished by almost any route, but for actual induction of the response, the antigen must be administered in such a way that it comes into contact with the sensitized tissue suddenly. The best results are achieved when the inducing dose is given intravenously or directly into the heart.

Form of Antigen. To be effective, the antigen must be in a soluble form. Cellular antigens, such as sheep red blood cells or bacteria, cause only weak anaphylaxis.

Antigen Dose. The amount of antigen required for sensitization varies widely, but for a particular situation it must fall within certain limits: too small a dose produces no response and too large a dose may result in protection instead of sensitization (see below). For the induction of anaphylactic symptoms, the *shock-inducing dose* must be considerably larger than the minimal dose needed for sensitization.

Time Factor. It is important to allow enough time to elapse between the sensitizing and inducing dose. However, the actual length of this interval varies greatly, depending on all the other conditions.

Desensitization. An animal that has survived the administration of the shock-inducing dose is often temporarily refractory in that further administration of the antigen does not produce anaphylaxis. This *desensitized state* can also be induced by administering repeated injections of small doses, closely spaced in time, instead of a single, large, shock-inducing dose. Each individual dose is too small to produce anaphylactic symptoms, but the repeated exposure gradually exhausts the supply of reactive antibodies. In some situations, desensitization may be caused by the preferential induction of blocking IgG, instead of IgE, antibodies (see *Atopy*). The desensitizing state is only temporary and, in most instances, lasts only about two weeks, after which time the state of increased sensitivity returns.

Species Differences. The ability to become anaphylactic has been demonstrated in birds, amphibians, and fish, in addition to various mammals, and probably exists in all vertebrates, but the specific form of anaphylaxis varies from species to species. The main factors responsible for the interspecies variation are different tissue distribution of mast cells and different composition of granules. The species in which anaphylaxis can be induced most easily and which has, therefore, been used in most of the experimental work on this condition is the guinea pig.

Forms of Anaphylaxis. The particular manifestation of the hypersensitivity state varies greatly, depending

[2] W. C. Boyd: *Fundamentals of Immunology*, 2nd ed., p. 308. Interscience, New York, 1947.

Table 13.5 Classification of Anaphylactic Reactions

- Anaphylaxis
  - In vivo
    - Generalized
      - Active
      - Passive
        - Normal
        - Reversed
    - Local—Cutaneous
  - In vitro
    - Active
    - Passive

on the manner in which sensitization has been achieved and tested. The various forms can be classified according to whether sensitization occurs in vivo or in vitro, actively or passively (Table 13.5). The main forms are described below.

Active Systemic (Generalized) Anaphylaxis. This condition ensues when one injects an animal intravenously, intraperitoneally, or intradermally with an antigen, and after the latent period challenges the recipient with an intravenous shock-inducing dose of the same antigen. The first injection induces cytotropic IgE antibodies, which then bind to tissue mast cells and basophils; the second injection provides antigen for bridging of cell-bound IgE molecules, activation of mast cells, and mediator release, leading to smooth muscle contraction and vasodilation. The consequences of the mediator release are strongest in the tissues containing the largest quantities of mast cells. These differ in different species, so that each species has a particular *shock organ* or organs in which the pathological changes are most pronounced. But in addition to the shock organ, several additional organs are almost always involved (Table 13.6), which is why this form of anaphylaxis is called "systemic" or generalized." The manifestation of systemic anaphylaxis is also dependent on mast cell distribution and composition. In guinea pigs, the shocking injection induces restlessness, ruffling of the skin, sneezing, coughing, itching, uncontrolled discharge of urine and feces, breathing difficulty, and often violent convulsions—the *anaphylactic shock,* and finally death. The main pathological findings in such animals are constriction of bronchioles and hyperinflation of the lungs.

Passive Systemic Anaphylaxis. To induce this form of anaphylaxis, an animal is sensitized intraperitoneally against a given antigen, and its serum is injected intravenously into another animal, which is then challenged intravenously with the sensitizing antigen. The manifestations of passive systemic anaphylaxis are similar to those of active anaphylaxis. A variant of this form is *reversed passive anaphylaxis*, in which an animal is injected intraperitoneally with the antigen and is challenged 30 to 60 minutes later intravenously with serum containing IgE antibodies. The manifestations of this reaction are often shock and death.

Passive Cutaneous Anaphylaxis. PCA is a frequently used form of local anaphylaxis. Here, an animal is sensitized to an antigen and bled after the latent period. The antiserum is then injected intradermally into another animal, and four to six hours later this animal is injected intravenously with the antigen and a dye, such as Evans blue. Ten minutes later, blue spots appear in the skin at the injection site. In this instance, the passively administered IgE binds to mast cells in the skin and the antigen delivered by the bloodstream binds to the tissue-fixed immunoglobulins. The subse-

Table 13.6 Comparison of Anaphylaxis in Different Species

Species	Shock Organ	Principal Mediators	Principal Manifestations
Guinea pig	Lungs (bronchioles)	Histamine, SRS-A	Bronchiolar constriction, breathing difficulties, hyperinflation of lungs
Rabbit	Heart, pulmonary vessels	Histamine, serotonin, SRS-A, PAF	Heart failure, liver and intestine congestion
Dog	Hepatic veins	Histamine	Liver congestion, vomiting, diarrhea
Rat	Intestine	Serotonin, histamine	Circulatory collapse, augmentation of peristaltic activity, intestinal bleeding
Mouse	Intestine, lungs	Serotonin, histamine	Intestinal hyperemia, breathing difficulty, hyperinflation of lungs
Human	Lungs (bronchioles), larynx	Histamine, SRS-A	Breathing difficulty, abnormally low blood pressure, rash and itching, laryngeal swelling, circulatory collapse

quent mast cell degranulation and mediator release cause an increase in capillary permeability and leakage of serum albumin with the attached dye through the dilated blood vessels, and the area of reaction stains blue.

Active In Vitro Anaphylaxis. This form, also called, after its discoverers, *Schultz-Dale reaction* (see Chapter 2), can be accomplished as follows. An animal is injected with an antigen and killed after 14 days. An organ containing a great deal of smooth muscle (e.g., small intestine, lung, tracheal ring, or uterus) is dissected out and placed in a bath with buffered saline solution. One end of the organ is attached to the bottom of the bath and the other end is connected to a lever (Fig. 13.24). An antigen solution is then added to the bath and muscle contraction is recorded on a kymograph or polygraph.

Passive In Vitro Anaphylaxis. In vitro sensitization can be obtained by placing the intestine, lung, or uterus from a nonsensitized animal into a bath containing serum of a sensitized animal and incubating the bath for a period that allows fixation of antibodies to the tissue. Exposure of the washed muscle to antigen solution then induces contraction of the stretched organ.

In healthy humans, true anaphylaxis, as defined here, rarely occurs. However, a reaction resembling experimentally induced animal anaphylaxis is not infrequent in allergic individuals. The manifestation of this "anaphylaxis" probably requires hereditary predisposition, so the reaction is more of the atopic than of true anaphylactic type. Nevertheless, clinicians often use the term "anaphylaxis" as if it were equivalent to the experimentally induced reaction. The most common causes of human anaphylactic reactions are drugs and insect venoms. The reaction usually affects several organs simultaneously—skin (flushing, redness, rash, swelling), lungs (spasmodic narrowing of bronchi and laryngeal swelling), gastrointestinal tract (abdominal pains, nausea, vomiting, diarrhea), and the circulatory system (fall in blood pressure and shock as a result of increased vascular permeability); severe cases of anaphylaxis may result in death.

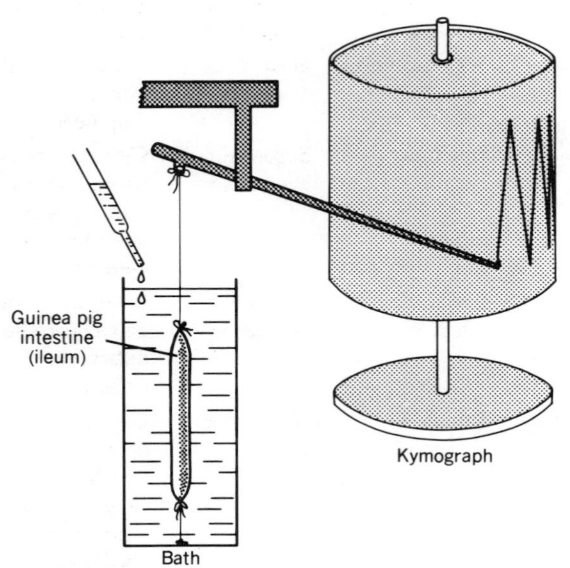

Figure 13.24. Method for measuring anaphylaxis in vitro. Addition of chemical mediators to the bath causes contraction of smooth muscles (guinea pig ileum), which is recorded on a kymograph drum.

Atopy

Definition. By *atopy* we mean a condition that affects only genetically predisposed individuals of a species, and is characterized by smooth muscle contraction and dilation of capillaries caused by the release of pharmacologically active substances from mast cells and basophils after the combination of cell-fixed IgE antibodies with the antigen. The distinguishing feature of atopy is its restriction to individuals with a particular genetic defect; it is this defect that is responsible for the loss of control over the physiological IgE response and the response's becoming pathological. To express the highly variable symptoms of atopy, the individual carrying the defective genes must first be *sensitized*. In contrast to that of anaphylaxis, atopic sensitization usually occurs by natural exposure to *allergens*. This exposure can occur by inhalation or ingestion of an allergen or by its contact with the exterior bodily surface. The condition cannot be induced in normal individuals.

Nature of the Genetic Defect. The hereditary predilection for atopy remains unspecified. One possibility is, as we have already discussed, that the T suppressor cells, which normally regulate the IgE response, do not function properly in atopic individuals, so that the response is uncontrolled. Another possibility is that the defect occurs in the receptors that normally receive regulatory signals in the form of neurotransmitters, hormones, and various other pharmacologically active substances. A defect may also occur in any of the many other regulatory pathways governing IgE responses, and it is possible that different forms of atopy and atopies in different individuals may be the consequence of different defects.

Diagnosis. The usual way of establishing that an individual suffers from an atopic condition is by patch, scratch, or intracutaneous skin testing. In the *scratch*

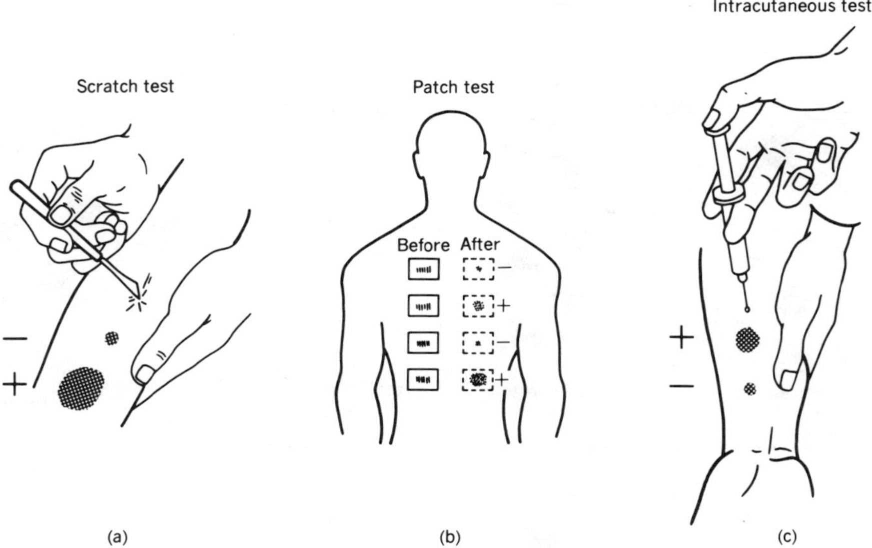

Figure 13.25. Tests for atopic sensitivity.

test (Fig. 13.25*a*), several shallow scratches are made on the skin and a small amount of the substance suspected of causing atopy is placed on each. The scratch that becomes itchy, red, and swollen (*wheal-and-flare reaction*) indicates atopic sensitivity of the individual to the applied allergen. In the *patch test* (Fig. 13.25*b*), the test substance is placed on a piece of paper or cloth, which is then fixed to the skin with tape. Skin irritation after removal of the patch 24 hours later suggests sensitivity to the applied substance. In the *intracutaneous test* (Fig. 13.25*c*), a diluted solution of the test substance is injected into the skin; irritation at the site of injection again indicates atopic sensitivity to the test substance.

Another way to detect an atopic condition is by demonstrating IgE antibodies in the patient's serum. The demonstration is based on the classic *Prausnitz-Küstner* (*PK*) *test* (see Chapter 2), in which serum from an atopic individual is injected intradermally into a nonatopic recipient and the injection site is challenged, 24 to 48 hours later, with the appropriate allergen. A wheal-and-flare reaction at the injection site indicates atopy to a given allergen. Since human IgE antibodies also bind to monkey cells, monkey skin, small intestine, or lungs can be used for testing of atopic sensitization by passive cutaneous anaphylaxis in vivo or by the Schultz-Dale reaction in vitro.

Atopy can also be detected by establishing increased levels of IgE in the patient's serum. To this purpose, however, highly sensitive techniques of Ig detection must be used, for even the increased IgE levels are still below the threshold of detection by most serological assays. Most of these testing procedures are based on the radioimmunoassay described in Chapter 10. In one such assay, one makes xenogeneic antibodies against human IgE (a myeloma protein), conjugates these antibodies to agarose beads, and then mixes the beads with a standard amount of radioactively labeled IgE and the human serum to be tested. The unlabeled IgE in the human serum competes with the labeled IgE for binding sites on the beads, and the radioactivity of the washed beads decreases proportionally to the IgE concentration in the serum (Fig. 13.26*a*). In another assay (Fig. 13.26*b*), the allergen is coupled to agarose beads, and the conjugated beads are incubated first with the patient's serum containing IgE antibodies to the allergen, and then with radiolabeled xenogeneic antibodies to human IgE. Radioactivity of the washed beads is then proportional to the amount of IgE in the patient's serum.

Blocking Antibodies and Desensitization. Repeated injections of an allergen into nonatopic volunteers results in the production of non-IgE antibodies (mostly IgG), which can bind to the allergen but are incapable of reacting with mast cells in the human skin. The binding of non-IgE antibodies with the allergen, however, blocks the allergen's ability to react with IgE antibodies, and so blocks the induction of an atopic reaction. The production of blocking antibodies is probably responsible for the *desensitization* of an atopic patient that results from injecting the patient with increasing doses of allergen. At the beginning of such treatment, the level of specific IgE antibodies first increases and then falls, and the treated person remains temporarily unresponsive to the allergen.

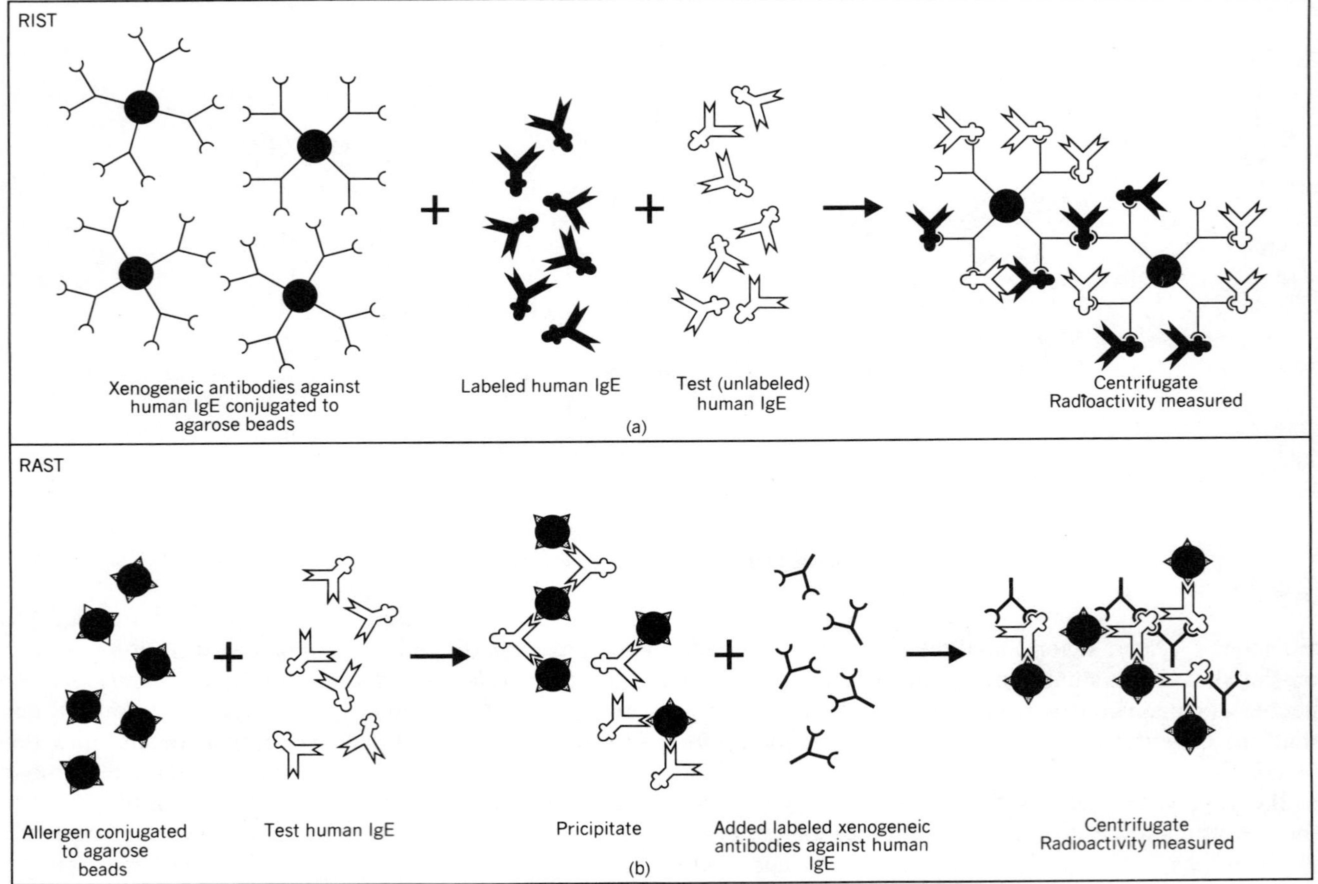

Figure 13.26. Two assays for the measurement of serum IgE levels. (*a*) Radioimmunoabsorption test (RIST), based on the competition between labeled and unlabeled (test) human IgE antibodies for the combining sites of xenogeneic antibodies directed against human IgE. (*b*) Radioallergosorbent test (RAST).

Specific Forms of Atopy. The manifestation of the atopic condition depends on the allergen, the route of sensitization, the nature of the defect, and probably on many other factors. According to the specific symptoms, several disease states can be distinguished; the four more common ones, two affecting the respiratory system and two the skin, are discussed below. It must be emphasized, however, that in almost every case, similar symptoms can be induced by mechanisms other than pathological IgE responses. Furthermore, the expression of each atopic condition can also be influenced by psychological stress, infections, and endocrine disturbances.

Allergic Rhinitis. This disease (Gr. *rhin*, nose, suffix *-itis*, inflammation), better known as *hay fever*, is one of the most common atopic conditions: more than 20 million people in the United States alone suffer from it. The designation "hay fever," first used in 1812 by the English physician John Bostock, is a misnomer since the condition is associated with neither hay nor fever. There are two varieties of hay fever, seasonal and nonseasonal. The more common *seasonal hay fever* occurs during the spring and summer, when the air is full of pollen from weeds, grasses, and trees. In the United States, weed pollen causes hay fever from the middle of August to October. Its most common source is ragweed, over 60 forms of which grow in the United States (see Fig. 13.16), and which, in one form or another, occurs all over the country. Grass pollen causes atopies from the last half of May to the first part of July and accounts for about 35 percent of all cases in the United States. The more common sources of grass allergens are timothy, Bermuda grass, and bluegrass. Tree pollen causes most seasonal atopies occurring in April and May; it is responsible for some 10 percent of all seasonal hay fever cases and causes relatively mild atopy. Seasonal hay fever manifests itself primarily in the eyes and nose, the two organs in which pollen grains are deposited in large quantities and in which local IgE sensitization occurs. The eyes itch, burn, appear congested, and are often abnormally sensitive to light. The nose also itches, burns, and becomes partially or completely obstructed; the nasal mucous membranes swell and produce a watery discharge, and the patient sneezes frequently. The *nonseasonal* or *perennial hay fever* is an atopic reaction to house pets, house dust, foods, and other agents to which the individual is exposed all year. Its symptoms tend to be less severe than those of the seasonal variety. In its mildest form nonseasonal hay fever manifests itself in slight nasal congestion (and, as a result, mouth breathing), sniffling, and a tendency to have an itchy nose and postnasal drip.

Bronchial Asthma. In this condition the patient experiences difficulty in breathing (the Greek word "*asthma*" actually means "difficult breathing") caused by obstructions to the air flow into and out of the lungs. Aside from bronchial asthma, there are other forms of asthma (cardiac and renal), each evoked by a different disease and affecting a different organ (heart or kidney). Bronchial asthma is a condition of the lungs characterized by a widespread narrowing of airways caused by constriction of smooth muscles, swelling of the mucosa, and the presence of mucus in the lumens of the bronchi and bronchioles. An attack of asthma is characterized by shortness of breath (*dyspnea*, from Gr. *dys-*, bad, *pnoe*, breathing), wheezing, coughing, and in severe attacks, by sharp spasms (paroxysms) and convulsions accompanied by the development of a bluish tint to the skin. Attacks of atopic bronchial asthma (there are also nonatopic forms) occur during the pollen season, in the presence of animals, and on exposure to house dust or other allergens. The deposit of allergens on the bronchial mucosa apparently triggers IgE-mediated mediator release in the mucosa and submucosa. The mediators then activate the autonomic reflex mechanism through the appropriate receptors and the resulting efferent cholinergic impulses cause bronchial muscle contraction. Some physiologists believe that the source of trouble in asthmatic patients is the abnormal sensitivity of the β-adrenergic receptors to stimulation, so in this instance, the basic defect might be physiological rather than immunological in nature and may represent a disturbance of a homeostatic bronchodilation mechanism.

Atopic Urticaria and Angiodema. *Urtica* is the Latin word for the nettle, a weed whose leaves produce a stinging sensation when the skin comes into contact with them. Urticaria, also called *nettle rash* or *hives*, is a skin condition characterized by the appearance of transient but intensely itching, circumscribed eruptions caused by swellings of the dermis; in contrast to eczema (see below) the epidermis is not involved in this condition. The elevations (wheals) vary in size from small, pimplelike papules to much larger, patchlike welts. The duration of the rash varies, depending on its cause, from hours to years, although individual eruptions do not persist longer than two days; atopic urticaria caused by a single exposure to a single allergen usually does not last longer than one or two weeks. The condition results from widening (vasodilation) and increased permeability of small blood vessels, notably the venules of the dermis. One reason for these effects is IgE-related release of mediators, but other agents—for example, antigen-antibody complexes (see below) and even nonimmunological factors—can be responsible. Mediator-triggered urticaria can be caused by drugs (penicillin, aspirin, and histamine-releasing drugs such as polymyxin, codeine, or morphine), foods (fish, eggs, milk) and substances added to food, pollen, parasites, insect stings, animal bites, and many other agents. One kind of urticaria can also be caused by physical factors such as cold, heat, and trauma. In *cold urticaria*, for example, hives appear either during the cold exposure or after rewarming. In this form of the disease, cold is thought to induce—directly or indirectly—changes in the skin that then induce the IgE response. *Contact urticaria* develops upon contact of the skin with cat hair, sheep wool, horse dander, pollen, and various other substances.

A condition closely related to urticaria but differing from it in that the affected blood vessels are deeper in the skin, so the resulting swelling is much more diffuse, is *angiodema* (Gr. *angeion*, vessel, *oidema*, swelling). It also goes under many other names, such as giant urticaria, Quincke's edema (described by H. Quincke in 1882), and Bannister's disease. It is characterized by a single or multiple circumscribed, evanescent swelling, which, in contrast to that of urticaria, usually does not itch. The swelling can occur in any part of the body—face, scalp, trunk, limbs, palms, soles, genitalia; sometimes it can also occur in the gastrointestinal tract (and is then accompanied by colicky abdominal pains, vomiting, and diarrhea) or in the respiratory system (involvement of the larynx results in hoarseness and dyspnea). Occasionally it is also accompanied by various neurological complications. Only some angiodemas are the result of faulty IgE responses; in these cases, the manifestations of the condition are largely affected by the entry site and the amount of the sensitizing allergen.

Atopic Dermatitis or Allergic (Endogenous) Eczema. This is another skin condition characterized by reddening of the skin followed by the appearance of minute blisters and vesicles which then grow in size, break, and discharge fluid (Gr. *ekzeo*, to boil over). The blistering, which can cover any area of the body, is accompanied by intense itching. The symptoms often begin in infancy and the condition is then called *infantile eczema*. Atopic dermatitis may be caused by food allergy but also by exposure to house dust, animals, and various environmental allergens. It is one of the most severe atopic conditions known.

Allergylike Reactions

For the sake of completeness, we shall mention three phenomena that involve IgE antibodies only indirectly but resemble IgE-mediated allergies superficially. The underlying mechanism of these phenomena, as we shall see shortly, is different from those of most of the IgE-mediated responses.

Arthus Reaction. In 1903 N. Maurice Arthus and Maurice Breton repeatedly injected normal horse serum subcutaneously into rabbits, with an interval of several days between the individual injections. After the fifth or sixth injection, they observed a skin reaction characterized by firm induration, persisting swelling, abscess formation, and eventual necrosis. It was not necessary that the site of the last injection coincided with those of previous injections; the reaction could be observed at any site where the last injection was made. The phenomenon, now referred to as the *Arthus reaction*, is peculiar to rabbits, but similar reactions were also observed in guinea pigs, rats, dogs, and humans. The reaction is explained as follows. The repeated injections induce the formation of antibodies specific for horse serum proteins. The antibodies combine with their corresponding antigen and insoluble antigen-antibody complexes form locally in and around the walls of venules at the injection site. The complexes activate complement, and the chemotactic and immune adherence factors liberated from the complement cascade begin to attract neutrophils and platelets to the reaction site. The cytotropic antibodies bind to the basophils, combine with the antigen, and cause the release of mediators. These initiate an inflammatory reaction: some activate the kinin, clotting, and fibrinolytic cascades; PAF aggregates and activates platelets, which then release various proteases, cationic proteins, collagenases, elastases, and blood vessel-dilating amines; still other mediators act as chemotactic factors, increasing the influx of granulocytes into the inflammatory site. Additional degradation enzymes are released from the lysosomes of activated neutrophils. Tha amines cause parting of the endothelial cells lining the blood vessels and the exposure of the underlying basement membrane (Fig. 13.27). The gaps then act as pores of a filter, trapping the antigen-antibody complexes and transferring the inflammatory reaction directly to the basement membrane, which is attacked and damaged by the liberated elastases, collagenases, and other factors. The influx of cells causes induration, the seepage of fluids caused by increased vessel permeability leads to swelling, and the tissue damage manifests itself in necrosis.

Serum Sickness. The realization, at the end of the nineteenth century, that such infectious diseases as diphtheria can be cured by the injection of an antiserum produced in another species (for example, a horse) and specific for the corresponding bacterial toxin made injections of xenogeneic sera into human beings a relatively common practice. However, it was soon noticed that some of the serum recipients developed undesirable reactions, particularly when large

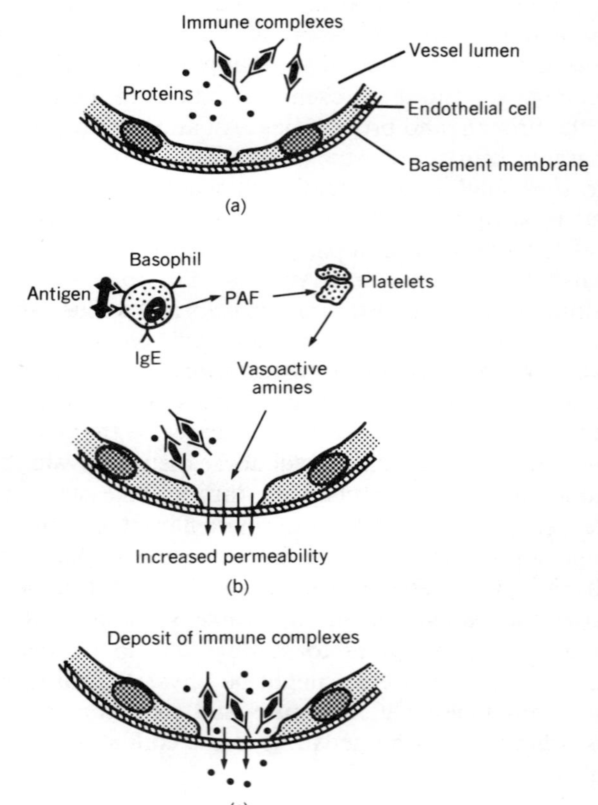

Figure 13.27. Damage caused by immune complexes to the endothelial cell lining and the basement membrane of a blood vessel.

quantities of sera were introduced (in excess of 10 ml). This *serum sickness* was characterized by the occurrence of rashes of the urticarial type, often commencing at the injection site; fever; glandular swelling, particularly in the lymph nodes near the injection site (one of the first symptoms); and pain in the joints. In the most severe cases, particularly when serum injections were repeated following the appearance of serum sickness, the recipients went into a state of shock, and some died. The mechanism of serum sickness is probably similar to that of the Arthus reaction, only more generalized. The immune complexes formed by the interaction of antibodies with the serum protein antigens are deposited in the blood vessels not only near the injection site, but also in the kidneys, heart, and joints; as a result, these organs too become involved in the reaction.

Studies on experimental animals, particularly the rabbit, led to the recognition of two forms of serum sickness, acute and chronic. *Acute serum sickness*, also referred to as *acute immune complex disease* (AICD), results from a single, intravenous injection of a large dose of xenogeneic protein antigen, such as bovine serum albumin (BSA; 250 mg/kg). As antibodies begin to form some seven days after the injection, they combine with the antigen still circulating in the blood, generating immune complexes with molecular weights of between 300,000 and 500,000 daltons (mostly of the Ag_2Ab type, though Ag_2Ab_2 or Ag_3Ab_2 complexes also occur). The circulating complexes can be detected by using radiolabeled antigen for the injection and precipitating it with immunoglobulins by ammonium sulfate at concentrations that do not precipitate free, uncomplexed antigen. Concurrently with the appearance of immune complexes in the circulation, characteristic lesions begin to develop in the kidney, blood vessels, joints, and skin (reaching a maximum at 12 to 13 days postinjection, when the antigen becomes practically undetectable in the serum). The lesions in the kidney consist of diffuse cellular proliferation of endothelial and mesangial cells in the glomeruli (see Chapter 14 for a review of kidney anatomy) and slight thickening of the basement membrane (*immune complex-induced experimental glomerulonephritis*). The lesions are accompanied by the appearance of proteins in the urine (proteinuria) between the eighth and eleventh day after the injection. The blood vessel lesions consist of endothelial cell proliferation, progressing to cell death, and the appearance of fibrinoid necrosis (the appearance of necrotic tissue that displays some staining reactions resembling fibrin), and followed by neutrophilic infiltration. This *arteritis* (inflammation of the arteries) affects primarily the heart arteries and branches of the aorta or pulmonary artery. All the lesions are initiated by the deposit of immune complexes at the particular site and by the humoral and cellular reactions that occur as a consequence of this deposit and that were described on the preceding pages. The immune complex deposits in the kidney or in the blood vessels can be demonstrated by immunofluorescent staining (see also Chapter 14 for further details). The disease wanes from two to three weeks after the injection of the antigen.

Chronic serum sickness (*chronic immune complex disease*) occurs when small doses of xenogeneic protein are injected into rabbits daily over a period of several weeks. The dose has to be manipulated so that immune complexes are maintained in circulation for some time, which is achieved when the rabbits produce antibodies in amounts too small to cause immediate clearance of the antigen but large enough to produce circulating complexes. (The injection of too small a dose of antigen into a rabbit producing a large quantity of antibodies would result in the formation of large complexes that would be cleared too rapidly to induce damage.) The main site of immune complex deposit and hence the principal target of injury is the kidney; arterial lesions, characteristic of the acute form, occur rarely in chronic serum sickness. The glomerulonephritis induced by low antigen doses is characterized mainly by the thickening of the glomerular basement membrane (*membranous glomerulonephritis*) often accompanied by intense proteinuria, whereas that induced by high antigen doses or prolonged immunization is characterized by diffuse cellular proliferation (*proliferative glomerulonephritis*), occasionally accompanied by local necrosis and kidney failure. As in the acute form, in chronic serum sickness immune complex deposits can be demonstrated in the kidney by immunofluorescent staining. As the disease subsides, antigen disappears first from the deposits (probably masked by antibodies), followed by immunoglobulin and complement.

Shwartzman Phenomenon. This reaction, described in 1928 by Gregory Shwartzman, is the least related to true allergy. It occurs, for example, in rabbits injected intradermally with a suspension of Gram-negative bacteria (e.g., *Salmonella typhi*) or a cell-free filtrate of bacterial culture. When, 24 hours after the first injection, another injection of the same or unrelated bacteria (filtrate) is administered intravenously, the animals develop bleeding and necrotic lesions at the site of the original intradermal injection within a few hours. This reaction is probably not even immunological in the true sense: it is nonspecific and develops faster than any known immunological reaction. The mechanism of the Shwartzman phenomenon is poorly understood, but it is thought to involve endotoxins of the bacterial membranes. The released endotoxins are believed to attract granulocytes to the injection site and to provoke the release of lysosomal hydrolases from the accumulated neutrophils, which then cause lesions in the walls of small blood vessels, aggregation of platelets, and other symptoms of an inflammatory reaction (see Chapter 14). When both injections are administered intravenously, a generalized reaction, characterized particularly by kidney lesions, develops. The Shwartzman phenomenon is an example of a reaction that simulates atopy but has little relation to it.

13.5 REGULATION OF B-CELL RESPONSES

When we introduced the topic of B-cell activation at the beginning of this chapter, we limited our considerations to basic mechanisms leading to antibody production. Now that we have acquired some knowledge of the various forms of B-cell response, we shall return to the principles of B-cell activation and view them in their entire complexity, as it is understood in 1981. In the simple scheme presented in Section 13.1.1, we envisioned three interacting cells as participating in B-cell stimulation: macrophage, helper T lymphocyte, and B lymphocyte. Here, we shall learn that each B-cell response, even to the simplest antigen, involves more than three cells, perhaps even a large number of cells. First, we shall realize that not one, but at least two helper T lymphocytes interact with the B cell; then we shall learn that there are probably whole legions of suppressor T cells regulating the T helper-macrophage, T helper-B cell, and T helper-T helper interactions; and finally, we will be astounded by the true complexities of the immunological networks formed by all these cells. We shall begin with a description of the intricacies of the T helper system.

13.5.1 Helper T Lymphocytes with Specificity for B-Cell Receptors

The T helper (Th) lymphocyte introduced in the preceding sections was a cell carrying a receptor with which it could recognize an antigen in the context of an MHC molecule—either on a macrophage (whereby it is stimulated) or on a B lymphocyte (whereby it stimulates). Since 1976 evidence has been accumulating for the existence of another helper T cell, capable of recognizing the immunoglobulin receptor on B lymphocytes.

Discovery

Clues pointing toward the existence of a second class of helper T cells have been obtained by Charles A. Janeway, Leonore A. Herzenberg, and their co-workers, but an experimental proof turning a postulate into a reality was provided in 1978 by R. Woodland and Harvey Cantor, whose work will be described here, and independently by Klaus Eichmann, Klaus Rajewsky, and their co-workers.

You may recall from Chapter 6 that when A/J mice are immunized with the hapten *p*-azophenylarsonate (Ars) coupled to a protein carrier, such as keyhole limpet hemocyanin (KLH), about 20 to 70 percent of the recipients' Ars-specific IgG antibodies carry the same idiotype, which can be detected with an antiserum produced in rabbits after their immunization with the IgG fraction of the A/J anti-Ars serum. It was this cross-reacting idiotype (CRI) that Woodland and Cantor studied in their experiments (Fig. 13.28). They immunized one group of mice with keyhole limpet hemocyanin and another group with *p*-azophenylarsonate bovine gamma globulin (Ars-BGG), and isolated Lyt-1$^+$ T cells from the former group and B

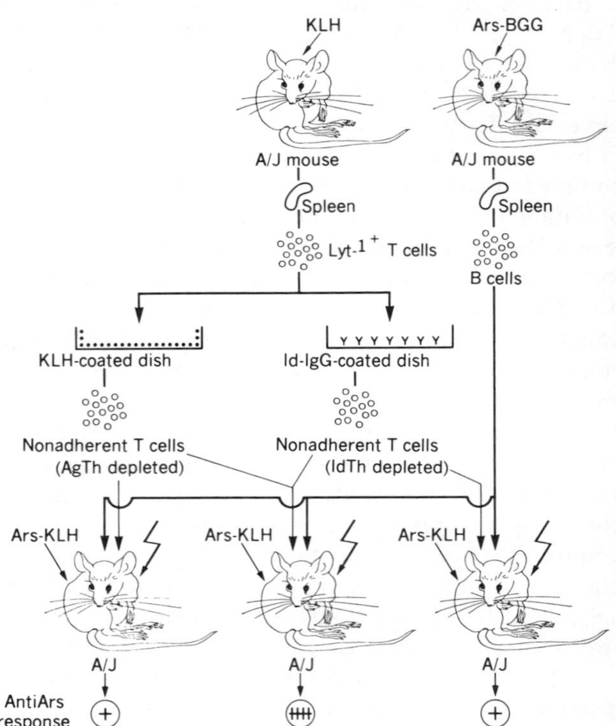

Figure 13.28. Woodland-Cantor experiment demonstrating the existence of idiotype-specific helper T lymphocytes. Explanation in the text.

cells from the latter. They then divided the purified T cells into two aliquots and incubated one aliquot in a dish coated with IgG molecules, almost all bearing the CRI idiotype, and the other aliquot in another dish coated with KLH.[3] Following the incubation, they isolated nonadherent cells from the two dishes, and injected into one group of lethally irradiated A/J mice the nonadherent cells from the Id-IgG dish, into another group the nonadherent cells from the KLH dish, and into a third group a mixture of cells from the two dishes. All three groups simultaneously received B cells isolated from the Ars-BGG-immunized mice and an injection of Ars-KLH. After seven days the three groups were tested for the production of antibodies to Ars and it was found that high antibody response occurred only in mice inoculated with the mixture of nonadherent cells; the unmixed populations conferred only low responsiveness on the recipients.

The authors interpreted this experiment as follows. There were two subpopulations of helper T cells—antigen-specific T helper cells, AgTh (Th1), and idiotype-specific T helper cells, IdTh (Th2)—in the original T-cell population. The AgTh cells bore receptors for the carrier (KLH) and were therefore retained on the KLH-coated dish; the IdTh cells bore receptors specific for the CRI idiotype of the B-cell receptors (i.e., the receptors that specifically recognize the hapten Ars) and hence were retained on the dish coated with antibodies carrying this idiotype. Among the nonadherent cells in the KLH-coated dish were the IdTh lymphocytes capable of recognizing the CRI idiotype, whereas among the nonadherent cells from the IgG-Id-coated dish were AgTh cells capable of recognizing the KLH. The AgTh or IdTh cells were unable to provide optimal help to B cells; only when combined did they confer high responsiveness on the irradiated animals. Obviously, for an optimal response, the B cell must receive two signals, one from the carrier-reactive T cell (AgTh) and another from the idiotype-reactive T cell (Fig. 13.29).

Properties

Little is known about the new class of helper T cells. In some systems, IdTh are capable of collaborating with B cells in the absence of antigen, but how general this capability is remains unclear. Some data suggest that IdTh bears two receptors, one for the idiotype and another for the antigen, and that the cell must be stimulated with antigen (not necessarily related to that used for B-cell priming) before it can perform its function. However, regardless of whether it recognizes the antigen or the idiotype, the helper T cell apparently always recognizes class II molecules simultaneously; in other words, the IdTh cells, like all other Th cells, are MHC-restricted.

The IdTh cells are apparently capable of reacting with the idiotype only after the B-cell receptors have combined with antigen, an arrangement that probably prevents these cells from being continually activated, even in the absence of antigenic stimulation. The circumstances of IdTh activation are obscure. The fact that the cell recognizes idiotypes on B-cell receptors does not mean that it is *activated* by these receptors. It might be that, like AgTh, the IdTh must first be activated by a macrophage presenting either the passively acquired idiotype or an antigen to it.

[3] The description given here does not correspond exactly to the original Woodland-Cantor experiment, but contains elements of later experiments.

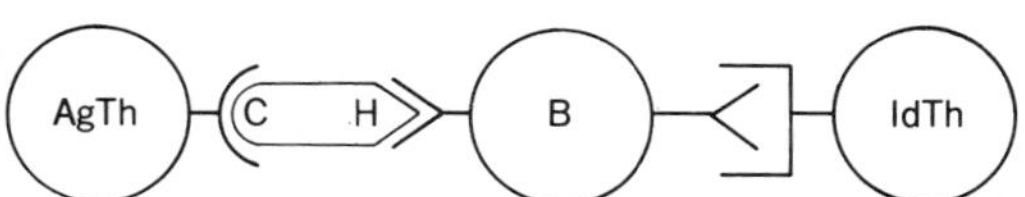

Figure 13.29. Presumed mode of interaction between a B lymphocyte (B), an antigen-specific helper T lymphocyte (AgTh), and an idiotype-specific helper T lymphocyte (IdTh). C and H represent carrier and haptenic portions of an antigen, respectively. For simplicity, recognition of major histocompatibility complex molecules is not shown in this diagram.

Function

The role of the IdTh in vivo might be to guide, together with other helper T cells, the B cells through the various stages of antigen-induced differentiation. There is some evidence that, in addition to idiotype-specific helper T cells, there are also Th cells specific for the allotype or isotype of the B-cell receptor. It is possible that all these cells act on B cells at the moment when the idiotypic, allotypic, or isotypic markers appear, and so advance the B cell one step further along the differentiation pathway. One such hypothetical scheme is depicted in Figure 13.30. Here the AgTh cell acts first, probably on the *virgin B cell*, and so advances the cell into the stage of the *mature B cell,* in which the receptor expresses its idiotype. The activated B cell is then acted upon by the IdTh cell and so advances into the *memory B cell* stage, in which it expresses its allotype and isotype. The memory cell can be acted upon by Ig-specific helper T cells, which advance the cell, perhaps through more than one step, into the stage where it can begin to secrete antibodies. However, it must be mentioned that some researchers consider the

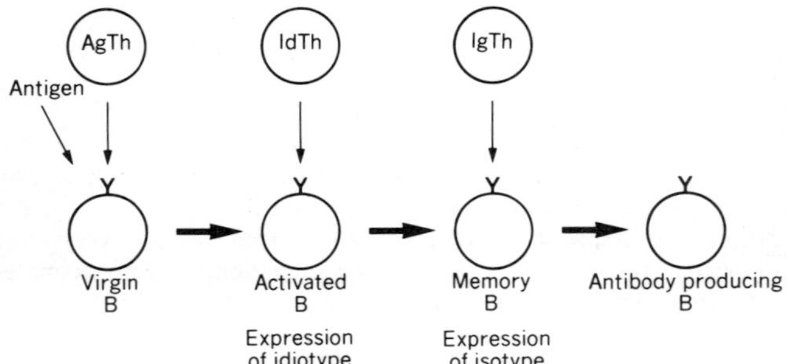

Figure 13.30. Regulation of B-lymphocyte differentiation by a series of helper T lymphocytes capable of recognizing the antigen (AgTh), the idiotype (IdTh), and the isotype (IgTh) on the B lymphocyte. The existence of the IgTh cell is hypothetical.

IdTh cells to be experimental artifacts that have little or no bearing on what is happening in an animal body.

13.5.2 Suppressor T Cells

Much of what we have said about suppressor T cells in relation to T cell-mediated immunity also applies to T suppressors involved in B-cell responses. The reader is therefore advised to reread the pertinent section in Chapter 12 before continuing further with this chapter.

Discovery

We narrated the story of the discovery of suppressor T cells in Chapter 12. Here it suffices to remind ourselves that it was the inability to induce tolerance to sheep red blood cells in mice deprived of their T cells that set Richard K. Gershon on the track of T-cell suppression. Since tolerance inducibility could be restored by T-cell restitution to such animals, the possibility arose that, in tolerant mice, B cells with the capacity to produce antibodies to sheep red blood cells were still present but could not make these antibodies so long as T cells were also present. This possibility was further supported by the observation that the transfer of T cells from tolerant mice to normal mice conferred on the latter a state of tolerance; when T cells were removed before transfer, tolerance was not transferred. The conclusion from these experiments was that T cells were needed to suppress immune response of tolerant mice to sheep red blood cells, and once tolerance was established, T suppressors were able to prevent antibody synthesis by nontolerant cells.

Experimental Systems

Although suppressor T cells can be studied in almost any B-cell response system, there are a few systems that have been used extensively and have provided most of the current knowledge about these cells. We shall now acquaint ourselves with some of these systems.

Allotype Suppression. In 1960, shortly after the discovery of rabbit allotypes (see Chapter 6), Jacques Oudin noted that most immunoglobulins in newborn rabbits often had the allotype of the mother and almost none of the father. Two years later, Sheldon Dray discovered that this *allotype suppression* was particularly pronounced in the offspring of mothers carrying antibodies against the allotype of the father. Still later, Leonore A. Herzenberg and Leonard A. Herzenberg

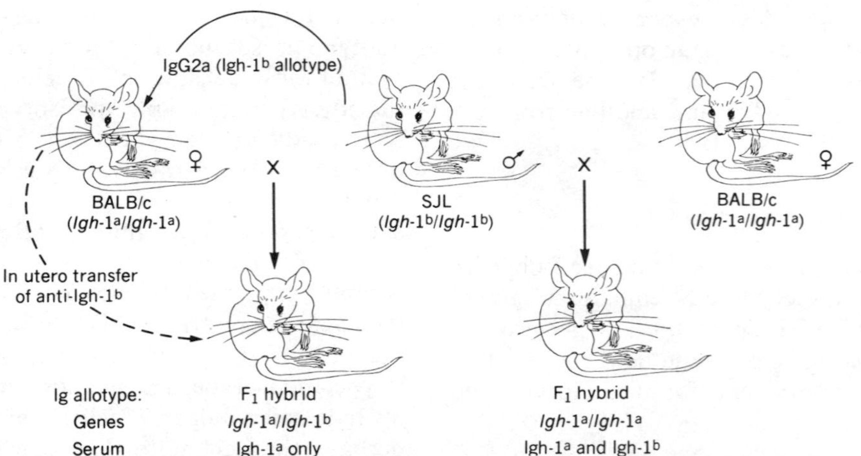

Figure 13.31. An experiment demonstrating allotype suppression in mice. Explanation in the text.

made a similar observation in mice; it is the Herzenbergs' mouse model on which most of the work regarding the mechanism of allotype suppression has been based.

In this model (Fig. 13.31), BALB/c female mice homozygous for the *Igh-*1^a gene are mated with the SJL males carrying the *Igh-*1^b gene. (Somehow these two strains are more suitable for this kind of experiment than others, perhaps because SJL mice have a number of immunological defects that, when passed on to the F_1 hybrids, make the hybrid more susceptible to allotype suppression.) Normally, the offspring produce IgG2a molecules carrying both the Igh-1^a and Igh-1^b allotypes, but if the mothers are immunized against the paternal allotype, the expression of this allotype is completely or chronically suppressed in more than half the F_1 hybrids by the time they are six months old. The suppression is incited by maternal antibodies to the Igh-1^b allotype that cross the placenta and enter the fetal circulation, and the suppression persists long after maternal antibodies have disappeared from the offspring's blood. Transfer of spleen cells from normal into suppressed F_1 hybrids has no effect on the appearance of the Igh-1^b allotype, indicating that the suppression is an active process. Transfer of T cells, together with a small number of normal F_1 spleen cells, from suppressed mice to irradiated F_1 mice results in the suppression of Igh-1^b secretion by the normal cells. Taken together with other observations that we shall discuss later in this chapter, these data suggest that the production of IgG2a (and other classes and subclasses of immunoglobulins) by B cells requires the action of special, allotype-recognizing helper T cells; interfering with this action is a group of suppressor T cells, which are activated by the passage of maternal antiallotype immunoglobulins into the fetal circulation.

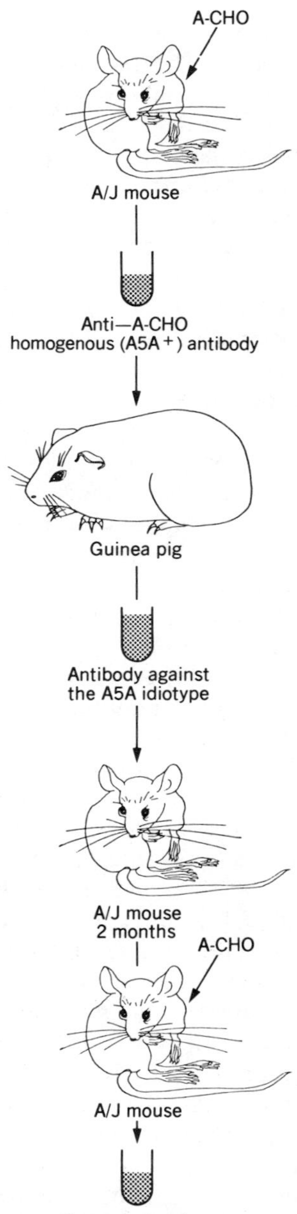

Figure 13.32. An experiment demonstrating idiotype suppression in mice. Explanation in the text.

Idiotype Suppression. Instead of antibodies to an allotype, one can also use anti-idiotypic reagents to activate suppressor T mechanisms. An example of an anti-idiotypic system is that introduced by Klaus Eichmann in 1975. In this system (Fig. 13.32), A/J mice are immunized with group A streptococcal carbohydrate (A-CHO) to produce antibodies that carry predominantly a single idiotype referred to as A5A (see also Chapters 6 and 7). The A5A-bearing immunoglobulins are isolated from the mouse antiserum and injected into guinea pigs to produce guinea pig antibodies to the A5A idiotype. The IgG1 fraction of the anti-A5A serum is then separated from the IgG2 fraction and the latter is injected into A/J mice. Two months later, the treated mice are injected with the A-CHO and their serum is tested for the presence of antibodies to A-CHO and for the presence of the A5A idiotype on such antibodies. The mice usually form plenty of antibodies to A-CHO but almost none of these carry the A5A idiotype, in contrast to untreated control mice, in which up to 90 percent of the anti-A5A immunoglobulin is A5A-positive. The interpretation of these experiments is similar to that of the allotype suppression experiments. The xenogeneic anti-A5A serum reacts with the corresponding idiotype on the receptors of suppressor T cells; this reaction triggers the T suppressors, which then act on helper T cells and prevent them from activating B cells that are capable of secreting A5A-positive antibodies specific for A-CHO. Hence, in contrast to the IgG1 fraction of the xenogeneic anti-A5A serum, which *enhances* antibody formation (see Chapter 7), the IgG2 fraction *suppresses* antibody formation.

Antigen-Triggered Suppression. In the two previous models the triggering was brought about by an antibody (antiallotypic or anti-idiotypic). However, there are also several experimental models in which the triggering element is the antigen. We described one such model, designed by Tommio Tada and his collaborators, in Chapter 7; here, we shall mention briefly one other model, designed by Judith A. Kapp and her co-workers in 1974. The antigen used in this model is a synthetic terpolymer of L-glutamic acid, L-alanine, and L-tyrosine, GAT. The antibody response to this polymer in mice is genetically controlled, with some strains (e.g., C57BL/6) acting as high responders and others (e.g., DBA/1) as nonresponders. The DBA/1 mice, although nonresponders, can be made to produce antibodies to GAT when immunized with GAT coupled to methylated bovine serum albumin (MBSA). However, when DBA/1 mice are first immunized with GAT and then injected with GAT-MBSA, no measurable anti-GAT response can be detected. The exposure to GAT alone apparently stimulates suppressor T cells, which then prevent helper T cells from augmenting the response of B cells to GAT-MBSA. When GAT-MBSA is injected without earlier pretreatment with GAT, the helper T cells recognize the MBSA as a carrier and the B cells recognize the GAT as a hapten, so that if any suppressor T cells are activated by the coupled GAT, they cannot prevent the helper T cells from providing help to B cells. The DBA/1 mice are nonresponders when injected with GAT alone, because the GAT, for some reason, activates suppressor T cells preferentially, rather than helper T cells in this strain.

Suppression Triggered by Other Factors. In addition to antibodies and antigens, suppressor T cells can also be triggered by all the other factors capable of activating T lymphocytes. We discussed these in Chapter 12, where we also described some experimental systems based on the use of such factors. The most commonly used of these nonantigen, nonantibody factors are the various T cell-specific lectins.

Properties

Although evidence for the suppressor function of T lymphocytes has been available since 1970, the existence of suppressor T cells as a separate T-cell subset has been doubted for some time. Some immunologists have argued that help and suppression might be two different functions of the same cell, and that which of the two prevails depends on the circumstances of the response. But by now, most immunologists are convinced that suppressor T cells do exist, mainly because of the markers these cells carry: in the mouse, mature suppressor T cells are Lyt-1^-Lyt-2^+, whereas the helper T cells are Lyt-1^+Lyt-2^-. This classification puts the suppressor T cells into the same lymphocyte category as the killer T cells, which often are also Lyt-1^-Lyt-2^+. The precursors of suppressor T cells carry special class II MHC molecules controlled, in the mouse, by the *J* locus. Little else is known about the suppressor T cells. They are difficult to separate from other T cells, and hence difficult to study morphologically and functionally.

Mechanism of Action

The primary target of suppressor T cells is the helper T cell. Although suppressor T cells that act directly on B lymphocytes or on macrophages may exist, the bulk of the suppressor action is directed against helper T cells. One piece of evidence supporting this conclusion is provided by experiments in which helper T, suppressor T, and B cells have been titrated out to determine which population is directly influenced by suppressor T cell depletion. The experiments demonstrated that T helper activity was lost proportionally to the suppressor T-cell dose, regardless of T helper and B-cell dose, suggesting a stoichiometric depletion of helper by suppressor cells. The result of suppressor T-cell action is functional depletion of helper T cells. It appears unlikely, however, that the helper T cell is actually eliminated physically by the suppressor T cell; rather, the suppressor T cell might emit signals that inactivate the helper T cell functionally—that is, make it unresponsive to further stimulation.

Since suppressor T cells can be activated by antigens, they must possess antigen-specific T-cell receptors; for the same reason, they must also possess lectin receptors. The activation by antibodies is believed to occur via an idiotype of the suppressor T cell receptor. But how do the suppressor T cells recognize their target helper T cells? Or is it that the helper T cell recognizes a suppressor T cell and is inactivated by such a recognition? One can imagine, for example, that the suppressor T cell—like the macrophage in other situations—binds antigen and presents it to helper T cells in the context of J molecules; the helper T cells then recognize both the antigen and the J molecules and are thus inactivated. This interaction may occur either directly, via an antigen bridge, or indirectly, via suppressor factors. Recent evidence indicates that the suppressor factors consist of two elements, a V_H chain and a J chain. The two elements are sometimes bound covalently, at other times, noncovalently. The V_H chain provides for the antigen specificity of the suppressor factor. Another possibility is that the suppressor T-cell receptor actively recognizes idiotypes of the T helper receptor, but in this case it is not clear where the J molecules come into the picture. But idiotype-specific suppressor T cells have been described by several laboratories; the cells are retained on dishes coated with antibodies carrying the particular idiotype.

13.5.3 The Feedback Loop

The evidence described so far indicates that helper T cells control the differentiation of B cells and are themselves controlled by suppressor T cells. However, there is also evidence that the differentiation of suppressor T cells is controlled by helper T cells, so that the three cell types form a regulatory system controlled by a feedback mechanism.

Discovery

We already know that coculturing of B and T lymphocytes in vitro in the presence of sheep red blood cells (Mishell-Dutton system) leads to the production of antibodies to sheep erythrocytes. The working of the system very much depends on how many sheep red blood cells are added: if too many erythrocytes are added, the system shuts off, and one can actually demonstrate that suppressor cells, rather than helpers, are generated. In other words, a high concentration of antigen in the Mishell-Dutton system favors development of suppressor T cells. Diane D. Eardley and her co-workers used this observation in 1978 in experiments that led them to the demonstration of the feedback loop (Fig. 13.33). These investigators cocultured purified Lyt-1^+-Lyt-2^- helper T and B cells with a high concentration of sheep red blood cells, then isolated Lyt-1^+Lyt-2^- cells from these cultures and added them to another culture of fresh Lyt-1^+Lyt-2^- cells, B cells, and a low concentration of sheep red blood cells. This second culture generated a normal anti-sheep red blood cell response without any evidence of suppression, a fact that indicated to the investigators that Lyt-1^+Lyt-2^- helper T cells cannot be converted into suppressor T cells and gave them the answer they were looking for. But not completely satisfied, the investigators carried out another experiment in which they again cultured purified Lyt-1^+Lyt-2^- cells and B cells with a high concentration of sheep red blood cells, and afterwards isolated the cultured Lyt-1^+Lyt-2^- cells and added them to another fresh culture of purified Lyt-1^+Lyt-2^- cells, B cells, and a low concentration of sheep red blood cells. But this time they added a few unselected, nonimmune T cells to the latter culture. Since in this case the response in the fresh culture was suppressed, the authors concluded that the Lyt-1^+Lyt-2^- helper cells from the original culture acted on nonimmune T cells added to the fresh culture and turned them into suppressor T cells, which then inhibited the anti-sheep red blood cell response. On the basis of these results, the investigators reasoned that helper T cells control the generation of suppressor T cells, which then turn on the helper T cells themselves and shut them off. The authors referred to the helper T cell as the *feedback inducer* (Tfi), in recognition of the fact that it stimulates a cell that will eventually turn off the activity of the feedback inducer itself. The existence of the feedback inducer has since been confirmed by several laboratories. Some investigators refer to this cell as the *T-suppressor inducer* (Tsi).

Function

It seems that suppressor T cells differentiate from precursor cells in a manner that in many ways resembles that of B lymphocyte differentiation; in both instances, the individual differentiation steps are apparently controlled by a set of helper T cells. The suppressor T cell differentiation, like that of B cells, might be antigen-

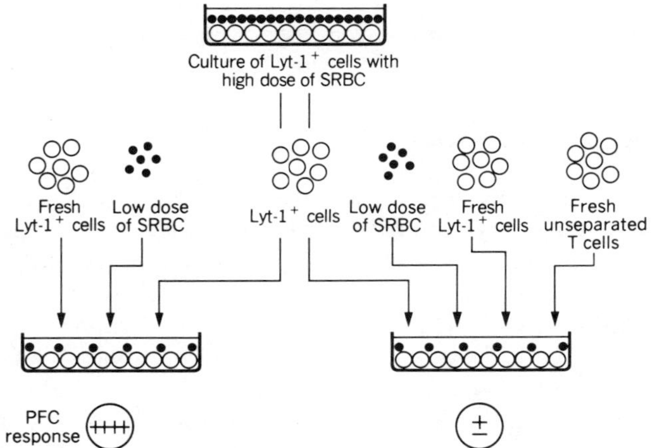

Figure 13.33. An experiment demonstrating the existence of feedback-inducer T lymphocytes. Explanation in the text.

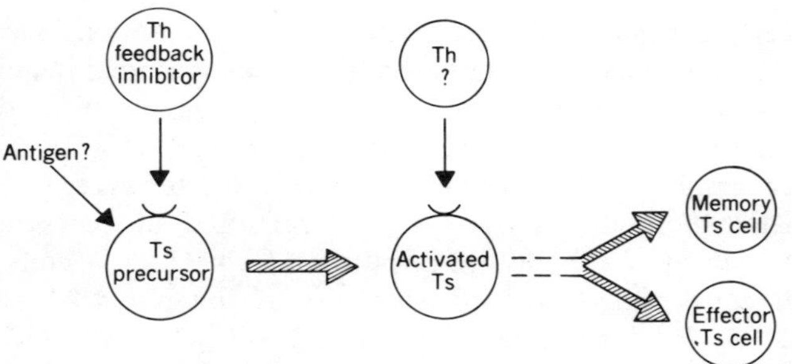

Figure 13.34. The presumed regulation of suppressor T-lymphocyte differentiation by helper T cells.

driven. It starts from a suppressor T precursor (virgin) cell and passes through an activated suppressor T cell to either a Ts memory cell or a Ts effector cell (Fig. 13.34). The number of stages and their exact sequence are not known. The T helper feedback inducer is thought to act in an early stage of the differentiation pathway, perhaps directly on the precursor cell; it has the Lyt-1^+Lyt-2^- phenotype in some systems and the Lyt-1^+Lyt-2^+ in others. Evidence exists to suggest that, in addition to the feedback inducer, at least one other helper T cell affects differentiation, perhaps in turning the memory cell into an effector cell; still other cells are presumed to exist. The Ts memory cells can persist for a long time in the absence of Th cells.

13.5.4 Coordination of Regulatory Elements

The picture emerging from the studies described above is that of a large number of elements interacting with one another in a complex fashion. But the interaction must follow some established rules—otherwise, the system would collapse in chaos. What are these rules? Even before the interacting cell types were discovered, Niels K. Jerne predicted, in 1974 that coordinated regulatory lymphocyte networks must exist in the body, and he suggested how such networks might operate.

The Network Hypothesis

The basic assumption of the network hypothesis is that each lymphocyte is a part of a complex system, in which each cell acts upon at least one other cell and is itself acted upon by at least one other cell. The interactions between cells occur via *paratopes* (the combining sites of cells' receptors) and idiotypes. A small section of such a network is depicted in Figure 13.35. If we start with the cell on the extreme left, we see that it carries a paratope αi2, capable of recognizing idiotype 2, associated with an anti-id4 paratope on another cell. The recognition may potentially activate the αi_2-bearing cell. But the αi2 is associated with an id1, which is recognized by an anti-id1 receptor carried by yet another cell, and this recognition inhibits the anti-id2-bearing cell from responding. And the same thing happens to every other cell in the network. Each cell has the potential of being activated by recognition of an idiotype on another cell, but this potential is counteracted by an inhibitory action of another cell recognizing the first cell's idiotype. The result is a *functional network*—a steady state in that all the cells have a potential for responding but are prevented from doing so by counterbalancing signals from other cells.

What happens when an antigen enters the network? The antigen carries an epitope (antigenic determinant) that resembles one of the idiotypes composing the network. The idea is that the immune system is able to recognize every conceivable antigenic determinant—in other words, for every epitope there must be a corresponding paratope (combining site) in the immune system. But because the system normally occupies itself with idiotypes instead of epitopes before the antigen enters, there must be as many idiotypes as there are paratopes, and for every epitope there must be a corresponding idiotype. Every

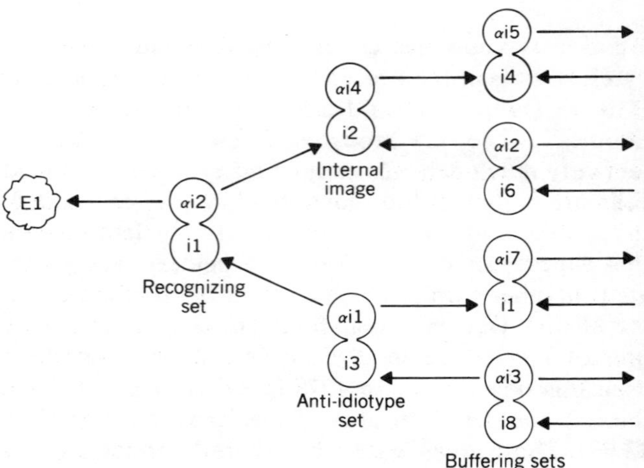

Figure 13.35. The network hypothesis of how the immune system is regulated. In this scheme, each lymphocyte is represented by a pair of joined circles, one circle indicating the paratope (the combining site) and the other the idiotype of the lymphocyte receptor. The paratope has specificity for an idiotype of another lymphocyte (indicated by "αi"). The arrow originating from a given lymphocyte always points to another lymphocyte whose idiotype the first lymphocyte is capable of recognizing. E1 represents an antigen (epitope) resembling idiotype i2. [Modified from N. K. Jerne: *Sci. Am.* **229** (July):52–60, 1973.]

epitope, therefore, has its own *internal image* in the body. In Figure 13.35, epitope E1 is recognized by paratope anti-i2, which normally recognizes the idiotype 2; idiotype-2 is thus the internal image of epitope E1. The recognition of E1 by anti-i2 provides an activating signal to the cell carrying this receptor. Since there is no counteracting inhibitory action on E1 (not being part of the system, the E1-bearing element cannot be suppressed), the balance between activating and inhibiting signals in the αi2 cell is temporarily disturbed in favor of activation, and the cell begins to differentiate in the direction of an antibody-secreting plasma cell. The disturbance is transmitted to the nearest neighbors of αi2 in the network, and these, too, are temporarily thrown off balance. But as the disturbance spreads from αi2, it becomes weaker and weaker, being buffered by the elements surrounding αi2. Eventually it trails off, so that it has no effect on distant regions of the network. As the stimulation by E1 ceases, the disturbed patch of the network regains its balance and returns to the steady state.

There are several variants of this basic model. The interested reader will find mathematical treatment of these models in Bruni, Doria, Koch, and Strom (1979) (see *References*).

Immunological Circuits

It is possible, however, that the network is not as homogeneous as suggested by the original Jerne model, but rather that it is divided into smaller groups of cells, each group connected in a circular series of interactions such that each cell regulates the cell preceding it and is regulated by the cell following it. An example of such a group, referred to as *immunological circuits*, is depicted in Figure 13.36. Here, two Th and two Ts cells are shown. Th1 recognizes the idiotype of Ts2 and also of a B cell; Ts2 recognizes the idiotype of Th2; Th2 recognizes the idiotype of Ts1; and Ts1 recognizes the idiotype of Th1. This mutual recognition connects the cells into a circuit, which can be locked temporarily into help or suppression, depending on the first cell to be activated or established. If Th1 is activated first, it allows the maturation of Ts2, which depletes Th2 in the circuit. The absence of functional Th2 means that Ts1 cannot differentiate, and in the absence of Ts1 there will be an increase of Th1, so that the circuit locks into a help position. If, on the other hand, Th2 is activated first, it allows differentiation of Ts1, which depletes Th1. In the absence of functional Th1, Ts2 cannot differentiate, and in the absence of Th2 there is no restriction on Ts2 differentiation, so the circuit locks into a suppression position. The individual circuits can be connected to macrophages or B cells and can be influenced in various ways by the antigen.

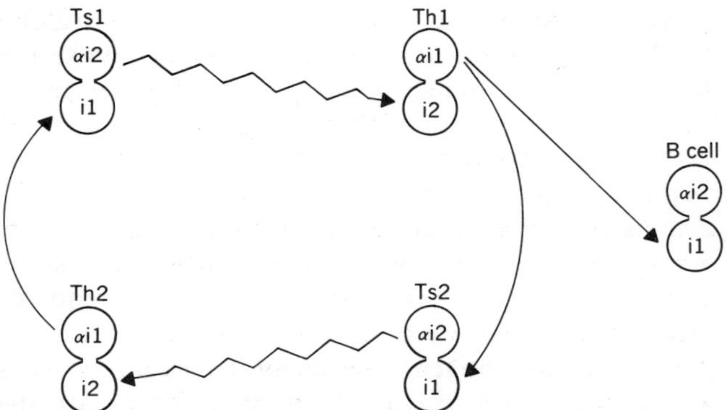

Figure 13.36. An immunological circuit. Each helper (Th) or suppressor (Ts) T lymphocyte is represented by a pair of joined circles with one circle indicating the idiotype and the other the combining-site specificity of the lymphocyte's receptor (the combining site recognizes the idiotype of the receptor of the next lymphocyte in the circuit). Straight arrows indicate help, wavy arrows suppression. (Based on L. A. Herzenberg, S. J. Black, and L. A. Herzenberg: *Eur. J. Immunol.* **10**:1–11, 1980.)

All of these speculations are unproved; at present, nobody really knows how immunoregulation occurs in the body. The theoreticians have provided us with some leads; it is now up to the experimentalists to prove or disprove these leads and come up with new ones. An important implication of the theory is that, in principle, there is no difference between self and nonself: self is merely an internal image of the external nonself. This realization provides a completely new angle from which to view immunological responses. It might be from this vantage point that a revolution in immunology will begin, a revolution that will force us to reinterpret old data and old theories. The concept of immunoregulation might prove to be the quantum theory of immunology.

13.5.5 Other Forms of Immunoregulation

In addition to the regulatory interactions just described, there are several other phenomena the mechanism of which is not known, but that also provide means of controlling the immune response. Here we shall mention two of these mechanisms—antigenic competition and immunoregulation by antibodies.

Antigenic Competition

This phenomenon was discovered in 1902 by Leonor Michaelis, who injected rabbits with foreign serum and found that the recipients produced antibodies to globulins but not to albumins. To obtain antialbumin serum, Michaelis had to inject albumin alone. He designated this phenomenon, in which the response to one *dominant antigen* (globulin) inhibited the response to a *suppressed antigen* (albumin), *antigenic competition*. Examples of antigenic competition were later found by many other investigators working with other antigen pairs. The phenomenon is of practical importance for vaccination, since vaccines often contain, in addition to the relevant antigen, a series of irrelevant antigens, which may compete with the former. There are two principal kinds of antigenic competition, intermolecular and intramolecular.

Intermolecular Competition. This is the type described originally by Michaelis—a type in which two competing antigens are present on two different molecules. In addition to the globulin-albumin pair, intermolecular competition has also been reported for ferritin versus albumin, diphtheria toxoid versus tetanus toxoid, and many other antigens. The two antigens can be administered simultaneously, as in Michaelis's experiment, or sequentially. When given in a mixture, the dominance or suppression of an antigen depends on the relative amounts of the two antigens. With a change in the ratio, the same antigen may become dominant or suppressed, or the competition can be eliminated altogether. The inhibition usually occurs only in the primary response; in the secondary response, antibodies to both antigens are usually formed (although in some instances, the inhibition also extends to the secondary response). Injection of large amounts of antibody specific for the dominant antigen or induction of tolerance to this antigen abolishes the inhibition of response to the suppressed antigen. The competition is thought to occur at the T-cell level in the early phase of the response, perhaps in the antigen-recognition stage.

In *sequential competition*, the animal responds to the antigen administered first but not to that given second. This form of competition is common in immunizations using two kinds of foreign red blood cells. For example, rabbits injected first with sheep erythrocytes and then with horse erythrocytes respond to the former but not to the latter. Not surprisingly, the occurrence of sequential competition depends on the interval between the two injections. An optimal interval for induction of competition is that in which the second antigen is administered at the peak of response to the first antigen. The underlying mechanism of sequential competition is believed to be stimulation of T suppressor-factor production by the first antigen and nonspecific inhibition of the response to the second antigen by this factor.

Intramolecular Competition. This type occurs when two competing antigenic determinants are carried by the same molecule. An example of this form of antigenic competition is the response of mice to rabbit IgG. When intact IgG molecules are injected, the mice mount a good primary response to the Fc portion of the immunoglobulin molecules, but a poor response to the Fab portion. A good anti-Fab response is obtained when the molecule is cleaved enzymatically and the Fab portion is injected alone. However, when the Fc and Fab portions are injected as a mixture, Fc again becomes dominant over Fab. Intramolecular competition also occurs with many synthetic antigens and with various haptens. This form of competition too can be abolished by the administration of antiserum specific for the dominant antigen or by making the recipient tolerant of the dominant determinants. The competition is thought to occur at the B-cell level. If B cells recognizing the first determinant are more numerous than those recognizing the second determinant, or if they bear receptors of higher affinity, they will successfully claim the antigenic molecule for themselves and exhaust its supply before B cells recognizing the second determinant can be stimulated in significant numbers.

Immunoregulation by Antibodies

The observation that an administration of antibodies can influence an ongoing response has been made repeatedly since the beginning of this century. The clearest demonstration of *suppression of antibody formation* by passive administration of antibodies was provided by Jonathan W. Uhr and J. B. Baumann in 1961. These two immunologists observed that the injection of horse diphtheria-specific antibodies into guinea pigs completely abolished the antitoxin response in these animals, while the administration of nonantitoxin horse γ-globulin had no effect on the response. Two years later, Göran Möller had a similar experience while producing antibodies to mouse antigens controlled by the major histocompatibility complex. For example, an A.CA anti-A serum (where A.CA and A are two congenic mouse lines differing at the *H*-2 complex), when injected into A.CA mice, suppressed synthesis of antibodies specific for A cells, injected simultaneously with the antiserum. The phenomenon of suppression by antibodies has, however, been most extensively studied using sheep red blood cells as the immunizing antigen and anti-SRBC serum as the suppressing agent.

Antibodies can be administered before, at the time of, or after immunization with the antigen. Administration later than 24 hours after immunization has little effect on primary IgM response, although the IgG and secondary responses may be affected. The duration of the suppression depends on the biological half-life, amount, and class of the injected antibodies. Both IgM and IgG can suppress antibody response, although IgM can sometimes have an opposite effect: it may increase the response of mice to suboptimal doses of sheep erythrocytes. Enhancement, rather than suppression, has also been noted in several other systems, and the decision as to what effect the antibodies will have depends on the circumstances of the particular response (the particular antigen, antibody, presence of antigen-antibody complexes, and so on).

The simplest explanation for the suppression phenomenon is that the injected antibodies combine with the antigen and make it unavailable for lymphocyte stimulation. However, the kinetics of the suppression suggests that the mechanism is not so simple. It is more likely that one of the following mechanisms operates. First, the antibodies combine with antigen on macrophages and prevent antigen presentation to T cells. Second, the antibodies interfere with the binding of antigen by B cells and thus with T-B collaboration. And third, the antibodies act in a feedback manner on the antibody-secreting cells. It is possible that inhibition occurs by different mechanisms in different systems.

Other examples of immunoregulation by antibodies are allotype suppression (discussed earlier in this chapter), T-cell activation and suppression by idiotypic antibodies (discussed in Chapter 12 and in this chapter), and immunological enhancement (discussed in Chapter 12).

Before we leave this topic, we shall mention one specific example of immunoregulation by antibodies, an example that is of great practical importance. It concerns the Rh blood group antigens (see Chapter 10). About 85 percent of all humans possess the RhD antigen, the original Rh antigen discovered by Karl Landsteiner and Alexander S. Wiener in 1940 with the use of rabbit anti-rhesus monkey sera. Individuals carrying this antigen are usually referred to as "Rh-positive," and this designation is justified because the D is the most prevalent of all the 30 or so Rh antigens. About 15 percent of all humans are "Rh-negative"—that is, they lack the D antigen. In situations where an Rh^- mother carries an Rh^+ child in her uterus, small number of fetal red blood cells may pass into the mother's circulation, particularly during delivery, when the placenta separates from the uterine wall. The fetal red blood cells may induce the formation of antibodies to RhD antigen in the mother. If a significant level of these Rh antibodies builds up, those of the IgG class may pass through the placenta during subsequent pregnancies, enter fetal circulation, and attack fetal Rh^+ erythrocytes. As a result of this *hemolytic disease of the newborn*, severe anemia develops. In an attempt to compensate for the loss of mature erythrocytes, the fetal hematopoietic system begins to pour immature erythroblasts into the blood—a condition known as *erythroblastosis fetalis*. Another consequence of the attack is the accumulation of excessive amounts of fluid in tissues, organs, and cavities, a condition referred to as *hydrops fetalis*. Still other symptoms are enlarged liver and spleen and generalized swelling. Some of the affected fetuses may be aborted, others may be delivered stillborn, and still others may be born alive but with severe defects, particularly in the central nervous system, where considerable damage is caused by the deposit of bilirubin in ganglia. Hemolytic disease of the newborn does not always develop in every Rh^- mother carrying an Rh^+ fetus. Usually the first pregnancy is not affected, but in later pregnancies, as the titer of Rh antibodies increases, the chances of hemolytic disease of the newborn also increase.

The disease can be prevented by giving the mother anti-RhD IgG fraction intramuscularly at the time of delivery (within 60 hours). These passively administered antibodies have the same effect as those in the experiments of Uhr, Baumann, and Möller: they prevent sensitization of the mother's lymphoid system and thus production of Rh antibodies. The passively administered antibodies are then eliminated by natural decay. This treatment reduces the risk of an anamnestic response during subsequent pregnancies by 95 percent—a truly remarkable achievement.

13.6 IMMUNOLOGICAL UNRESPONSIVENESS

Like T cells, B cells can exist in one of two opposite states—responsiveness and unresponsiveness. B cells are normally unresponsive (tolerant[4]) to self components and, by appropriate manipulation, can also be made unresponsive to many nonself components. B-cell responsiveness or unresponsiveness is normally influenced by the state of T cells, but B cells, as we shall see shortly, can also be made unresponsive in the absence of T cells (and vice versa), and T- and B-cell unresponsiveness can occur independently of each other. In this section, we shall deal with conditions that lead to the absence of B-cell response, regardless

[4] We shall treat the terms *immunological unresponsiveness* and *immunological tolerance* as synonymous. However, some investigators consider "unresponsiveness" a broader term than "tolerance"; in this sense, the so-called *classical tolerance* is only one specific form of immunological unresponsiveness.

of whether these conditions do or do not involve T cells. Conditions leading to the absence of T-cell response were discussed in Chapter 12, and since many features of T-cell unresponsiveness are shared with B-cell unresponsiveness, the reader is advised to reread Section 12.11.

13.6.1 Conditions Favoring Tolerance Induction

The establishment, extent, and duration of immunological tolerance depend on many factors, some of which are discussed briefly below.

State of the Lymphoid System

It is easier to induce tolerance in animals with immature lymphoid systems or with the lymphoid system damaged by irradiation, drugs, thoracic duct drainage, or antilymphocytic serum treatment, than in normal, mature animals. As was discussed in Chapter 12, the lymphoid system matures over a period of time, the length of which varies from species to species. The more mature the system is, the more difficult it is to make it unresponsive; this conclusion applies to both T and B cells. However, completely mature animals *can* be made tolerant, provided that one of two conditions is fulfilled. First, the animal's immunocompetence is inhibited temporarily by one of the treatments damaging the lymphoid system and antigen is given during that time; after the treatment has been discontinued, the system has recovered, and full immunocompetence has been regained, the animal remains unresponsive to the administered antigen. And second, the antigen is given in either a nonimmunogenic form or by a nonimmunizing route (see below).

Physicochemical Properties of the Antigen

An important feature contributing to the decision of whether a given antigen will induce responsiveness or unresponsiveness is the size of the molecule. The size effect is particularly conspicuous with antigens that occur in both polymeric and monomeric forms and with antigens that form aggregates. An example of the former is flagellin from *Salmonella adelaide* (see Chapter 10). Polymerized flagellin (POL), which has a molecular weight of 10^7 daltons, is a potent immunogen, inducing T-independent responses almost exclusively. Monomeric flagellin (MON), which has a molecular weight of 40,000, induces responsiveness when administered at low doses and unresponsiveness when administered at a high dose. The so-called fragment A, which is obtained by cyanogen bromide cleavage of MON and has a molecular weight of 18,000 daltons, is tolerogenic at all doses. The difference among the three forms is not in that they present the host with different determinants, since all three forms consist of the same repeating subunits, but exclusively in the size of the molecule.

Many serum proteins (e.g., albumin or γ-globulin) form aggregates spontaneously when left in an aqueous solution, and the speed of aggregation is increased by heating the solution. The aggregates can be removed by ultracentrifugation, so that one can obtain two forms of the protein preparation—aggregated and deaggregated. The two forms have different effects on the immune system of the recipient: aggregated proteins are strongly immunogenic, whereas deaggregated proteins promote the induction of tolerance. The difference probably stems from the way the two forms are handled by the host's reticuloendothelial system: aggregated proteins are removed rapidly from circulation and taken up by macrophages, and after processing, they are presented to lymphocytes in an immunogenic form. Deaggregated proteins stay in circulation for a long time and are only slowly processed by macrophages. However, previously immunized animals respond equally well to aggregated and deaggregated proteins, and an immunogenic dose of aggregated protein can be prevented from immunizing an animal when administered simultaneously with a large dose of deaggregated protein. On the other hand, deaggregated proteins can be made immunogenic by incorporation into suitable adjuvants.

Chemical Nature of the Antigen

Certain compounds are strong tolerogens by nature. A striking example is the D-amino acid polymers, which induce tolerance over a wide range of doses, in contrast to L-amino acid polymers, which are immunogenic at these same doses. Furthermore, pretreatment of animals with the tolerogenic form often prevents the formation of antibodies to haptens presented on an immunogenic carrier. For instance, mice injected with DNP conjugated to a polymer of D-glutamic acid and D-lysine (DNP-D-GL) fail to make antibodies to DNP when subsequently injected with DNP conjugated to the immunogenic carrier keyhole limpet hemocyanin. Often a slight modification of a molecule may convert it from an immunogen to a tolerogen. For example, following acetoacetylation, MON becomes tolerogenic, even at doses that normally induce immunity.

Particularly suitable for the study of immunological tolerance are serum proteins. The list of other frequently used antigens includes xenogeneic red blood cells, haptens, synthetic polymers, and bacterial and viral antigens.

Epitope Density

Variation in the number of antigenic determinants on a given molecule may sway lymphocytes from one state to another. For example, when DNP-POL is added to normal spleen cells in culture, the response of the lymphocytes will depend on the number of DNP groups per flagellin molecule. At a density of about 0.7 DNP groups per molecule, a good anti-DNP response is observed over a wide range of antigen concentrations; at a density of about 2.7 DNP groups per molecule, one observes good antibody response at intermediate concentrations and no response at high concentrations; and finally, at a density of 3.8 DNP groups per molecule, all antigen concentrations induce tolerance.

Antigen Dose

Testing of a given antigen over a wide range of concentrations reveals that low antigen doses often induce tolerance, intermediate doses induce immunity, and high doses induce tolerance (Fig. 13.37). There are thus two kinds of tolerance, low-zone and high-zone, which will be described later in this chapter. Some investigators also distinguish an ultra-low-zone tolerance, induced by minute quantities of antigen.

Mode of Antigen Presentation

The route of antigen administration probably plays a more important role when dealing with adult animals than with newborns. The route of injection determines accessibility of the antigen to macrophages, which, as has already been mentioned, is one of the most important factors deciding between tolerance and immunity. Macrophage-bound antigen is highly immunogenic: for example, only about 0.001 as much macrophage-bound bovine serum albumin as unbound antigen is required to immunize a mouse. Removal or paralysis of macrophages often facilitates tolerance induction.

A change in the route of administration may sometimes convert an immunogen into a tolerogen. For example, when aggregated serum proteins, which are normally immunogenic, are injected into the hepatic portal vein, they are quickly brought into the liver; there the aggregates are removed by Kupffer cells and the rest of the antigen passes, in an aggregate-free form, into the circulation, where it induces tolerance.

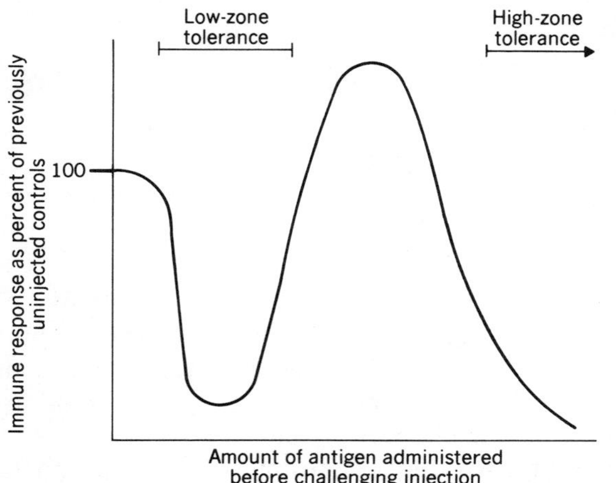

Figure 13.37. High-zone and low-zone tolerance. (Redrawn from H. N. Eisen: *Immunology*. Harper and Row, Hagerstown, Maryland, 1974.)

Genetic Make-Up of the Recipient

The genetic influence on the ease of tolerance induction is exemplified by the inbred mouse strains BALB/c and C57BL/10. The former strain is relatively resistant to tolerance induction by xenogeneic γ-globulin; the latter (and most other mouse strains) is relatively easy to make tolerant. In crosses between BALB/c and C57BL/10, tolerogenicity segregates among the offspring, indicating that it is genetically controlled.

13.6.2 Characteristics of B-Cell Tolerance

To determine the properties of tolerant T and B cells, Jacques M. Chiller, Gail S. Habicht, and William O. Weigle carried out the following experiment (Fig. 13.38). They inoculated newborn mice with deaggregated human γ-globulin (HGG) and so made them tolerant to this antigen. After a certain period, they killed the tolerant mice and transferred their bone marrow (as a source of B cells) or thymus (as a source of T cells), together with bone marrow or thymus cells of normal, untreated mice, into lethally irradiated syngeneic recipients. They then injected the chimeras with aggregated HGG and determined their response. By combining normal bone marrow cells with tolerant thymus cells, or vice versa, the investigators were able to determine which of the cell populations was necessary for the transfer of tolerance onto the irradiated host. And by varying the interval between the injection of deaggregated HGG and the killing of the injected bone marrow and thymus cell donors, they established the speed of induction and the duration of tolerance in

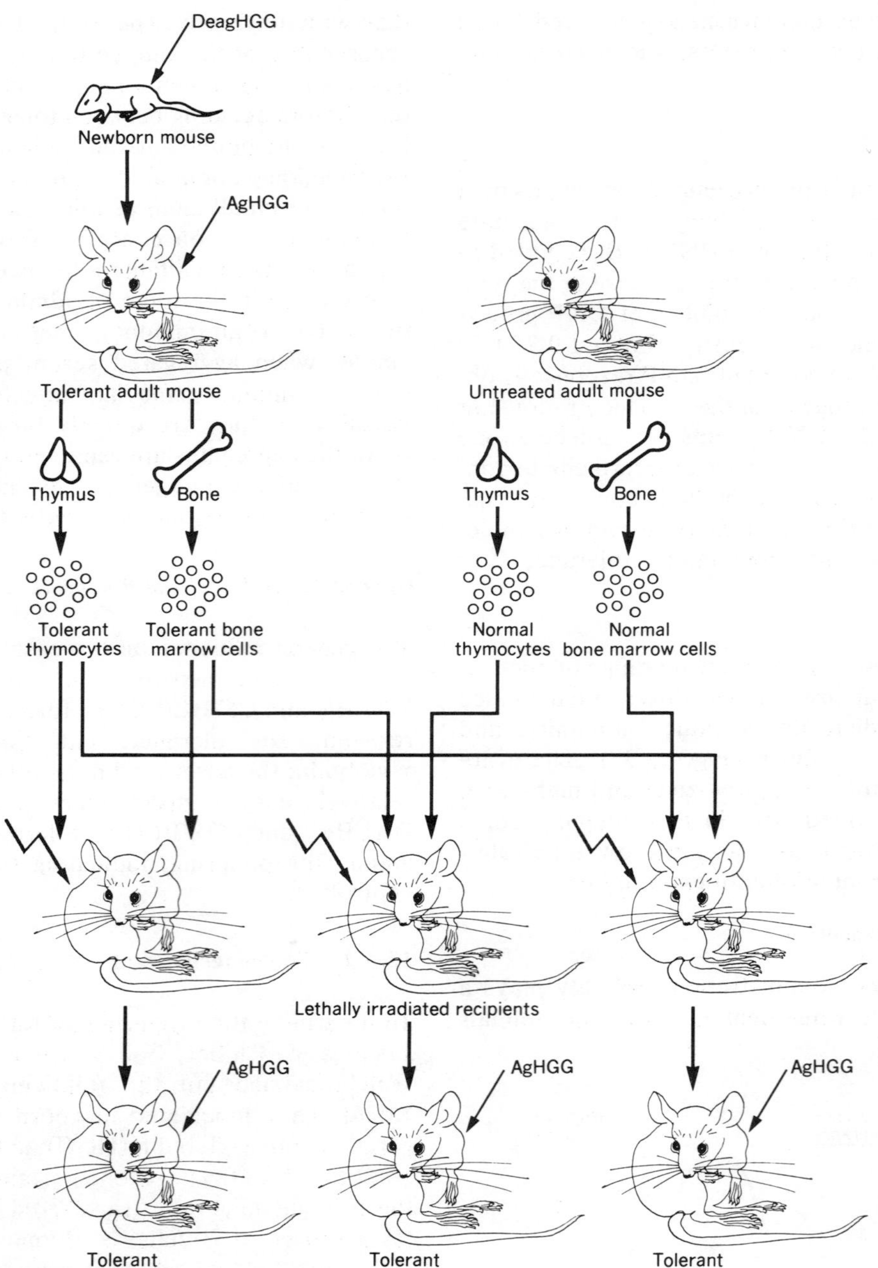

Figure 13.38. An experiment designed by Weigle and his co-workers to test T- and B-cell tolerance. Explanation in the text.

the T- and B-cell populations. In later experiments, Weigle and his co-workers used this same experimental design to test the inducibility of tolerance in mature T and B cells: they simply repeated the original experiment, but instead of using bone marrow and thymus cells, they used spleen lymphocytes, which they separated into T and B cells.

The conclusions derived from these experiments are summarized in Table 13.7. Thymus cells and splenic T cells can be made tolerant very quickly (within 24 hours of antigen injection), and they maintain their tolerant status for a long time (more than four months). Splenic B cells also acquire tolerance relatively quickly (within two to four days), but the duration of this unresponsiveness is only about 1.5 months, at least three times shorter than that of T cells. Immature bone marrow B cells, on the other hand, acquire tolerance only slowly (not earlier than one week after antigen administration) and, as in the case of mature B cells, the tolerance is of short duration.

The experiments demonstrate, first, that T and B cells may become tolerant independently of each other. (Two months after the injection of deaggregated HGG, most of the mice carry tolerant T cells and responsive B cells, but the animal as a whole appears tolerant because B cells need T lymphocytes to mount a response to an antigen.) Second, the experiments show that T and B cells possess different temporal patterns of tolerance induction. Further experiments have demonstrated that T and B cells also have different requirements in terms of antigen dose for the induction: in general, T-cell tolerance can be induced by lower antigen doses than B-cell tolerance. This observation, too, provides an opportunity to produce animals carrying tolerant T cells and responsive B cells. The opposite situation—coexistence of tolerant B cells and responsive T cells—is more difficult to demonstrate. Formally, such a situation occurs when T cells do not recognize an antigen and B cells do, but do not respond. For example, guinea pigs injected with DNP-poly-D-glutamic acid-poly-D-lysine fail to give an anti-DNP (B-cell) response, even if they have been sensitized previously to DNP-ovalbumin. One could argue that in this case T cells fail to recognize the poly-D-GL carrier and B cells do not respond because they are tolerant; but in actuality, the B cells do not respond because they do not receive the necessary T-cell help. Supporting this interpretation is the finding that, in general, tolerance to a carrier results in unresponsiveness to a hapten coupled to the same carrier, and that when the poly-DNP-D-GL is injected into DNP-sensitized guinea pigs undergoing a graft-versus-host reaction to injected foreign cells, antibodies to DNP are formed. Apparently, the helper T cells stimulated by the graft-versus-host reaction provide help nonspecifically to the B cells. However, B cells can be tolerized in the absence of T-cell involvement when the animal is treated with tolerogenic doses of T-independent antigens.

Table 13.7 Induction and Duration of Immunological Tolerance to Human γ-Globulin in A/J Mice

Site	Days of Induction	Days of Maintenance
Thymus	<1	120–135
Bone marrow	8–15	40–50
Spleen: T cells	<1	100–150
B cells	2–4	50–60
Whole animal	<1	130–150

Source. From W. O. Weigle: *Hospital Practice*, June 1977, pp. 71–80.

13.6.3 High-Zone and Low-Zone Tolerance

The observation that a high dose of an antigen makes an animal unresponsive to subsequent challenges by the same antigen was first made by L. D. Felton in 1949. He injected one group of mice with 100 μg and another with 10 μg of pneumococcal polysaccharide type III (SIII), and then challenged both groups with virulent pneumococcus bacteria. When only the latter group was protected from the disease, Felton speculated that, in the former group, the high dose of antigen somehow paralyzed the immune system. Since that time the phenomenon has been known as *immunological paralysis*. Felton was right in his interpretation of the phenomenon he discovered, for modern studies have revealed that the animals treated with the high dose of SIII are, in fact, only outwardly unresponsive. In reality, they produce antibodies, but these combine immediately with the persistent nondegradable polysaccharide and are neutralized; the paralyzed animals have about the same frequency of antibody-forming cells as the group of animals injected with the low dose of SIII. Immunological paralysis is therefore usually not considered to be a genuine tolerance, but a *pseudotolerance*. However, if Felton were to have increased the injected dose of SIII to some 250 μg, he would have discovered a true high-zone tolerance, for at this dose, SIII-reactive antibody-forming cells are no longer detected in the spleens of the injected animals.

The notion that true tolerance can be induced only with very high doses of antigen prevailed among immunologists for a long time. So it came as a surprise when N. Avrion Mitchison discovered in 1964 that tolerance can also be induced by subimmunogenic doses of antigen. In the particular protocol he used, Mitchison injected mice with soluble bovine serum albumin three times per week for up to 16 weeks. He then challenged the animals with an immunogenic dose of BSA and discovered that the animals made much less anti-BSA immunoglobulin than did control animals. This repeated treatment with low doses of antigen over a prolonged period has remained the standard method of inducing low-zone tolerance. In newborns, low-zone tolerance can be induced by a wide variety of antigens, whereas in the adult, only a few antigens are known to work. However, low-zone tolerance to many antigens can be induced in adults that have been irradiated, thymectomized, or otherwise compromised immunologically. In other words, damage to the lymphoid system facilitates low-zone tolerance induction. Low-zone tolerance is probably a T-cell phenomenon since T cells are apparently more susceptible to tolerization by low antigen doses than are B cells.

13.6.4 Completeness and Termination of Tolerance

Tolerance is seldom complete. Tolerant animals often produce small amounts of antibody, particularly if the tolerogen is a complex molecule. If one tolerizes with a mixture of proteins (e.g., normal serum) in which some proteins are present in a higher concentration than others, tolerance to some components of the mixture and immunity to others may be induced. However, even a single determinant is not recognized by one lymphocyte clone, but by several clones bearing receptors with different affinities. Since affinity of receptor-antigen binding probably influences tolerance induction, some of the clones might become tolerant and others not. The completeness of tolerance will then depend on the proportion of tolerant and nontolerant clones.

When tolerance is measured simultaneously by several parameters, it sometimes happens that it can be detected by one assay but not by another. Such a *split tolerance* has been observed, for example, in guinea pigs injected with tuberculoprotein and then with bacillus Calmette-Guérin (see Chapter 10). The animals were tolerant when tested by the delayed-type hypersensitivity assay but they produced antibodies to the tuberculoprotein. Split tolerance sometimes also occurs in regard to different immunoglobulin classes.

Induced tolerance is not a forever affair. After induction it gradually wanes and, if the animal lives long enough, is eventually lost. The duration of tolerance depends on many factors, among which one of the most important is the continual presence of the tolerogen. Although a single dose of serum protein may make newborn mice tolerant for several months, the tolerance eventually terminates spontaneously. To prolong the duration of the tolerant state, one must keep rechallenging the animal with the tolerogenic form of the antigen. However, replicating antigens—for example, cell-surface alloantigens in lymphoid chimeras—may induce tolerance for life.

Tolerance can also be terminated experimentally, most commonly by injection of an antigen that cross-reacts with that to which the host is tolerant. We shall give one example of such an induced termination—an experiment reported by the Weigle group. In this experiment, rabbits were injected at birth with 500 mg of bovine serum albumin, and demonstrated three months later to be tolerant by another injection of BSA. The tolerant animals were then injected with human serum albumin, which is known to cross-react with BSA to a small extent, and later also with BSA. After the HSA injection the animal produced antibodies to HSA-specific determinants; after the BSA injection it produced antibodies to determinants shared by HSA and BSA. Since the animal produced no BSA antibodies before the HSA injection (was tolerant to all determinants, including the shared ones), the administration of HSA must have *partially* terminated tolerance to BSA. However, the animal remained tolerant to BSA-specific determinants, even when repeatedly challenged with BSA. In fact, the production of antibodies to the shared determinants gradually decreased, and eventually the animal returned to a state of full unresponsiveness to all BSA determinants.

The mechanism of the partial tolerance termination is not known. It seems that the administration of HSA somehow leads to a bypassing of the T-cell block, which is responsible, in the tolerant animals, for the absence of help necessary for B-cell stimulation.

Cross-reactive antigens may also induce termination of natural tolerance of the body's own molecules. An example of this situation is the induction of antibodies to thyroglobulin, a hormone produced by the thyroid. Thyroglobulin, being a normal constituent of the body, is tolerated, and this tolerance resides solely in the T cells; B cells responsive to thyroglobulin are normally present in the body but fail to respond because there are no T cells capable of giving them the necessary help. However, when the animal is injected with a thyroglobulin from another species, it begins to produce antibodies to determinants shared by the two thyroglobulins—and hence, in fact, against self, against a molecule that is a part of its own body.

Tolerance can also be terminated by the administration of chemically altered antigens or by nonspecific stimulation accomplished by the administration of lectins, antigen-antibody complexes (e.g., tolerated antigen and xenogenic antibodies to cross-reactive antigen), and allogeneic cells capable of inducing graft-versus-host reaction. The nonspecific stimulants probably activate helper T cells, which then provide nonspecific help to immunocompetent B cells. For example, when one makes mice tolerant of HGG and 90 days later, at the time when T cells are still tolerant of HGG but the B cells are not, injects the recipients with HGG and

LPS (a B-cell mitogen that replaces T-cell help) simultaneously, the animals begin to produce HGG antibodies. Injection of either HGG or LPS alone has no effect on the tolerance status of the animals.

13.6.5 Mechanism

Tolerance has been known for more than a quarter of a century (see Chapter 12) and intensively studied for almost as long. Yet, despite its obvious importance to the understanding of how the immunological machinery works, tolerance research is still in a mostly descriptive stage. A number of phenomena pertaining to the induction, maintenance, and termination of tolerance have been described, but little insight has been gained into the mechanisms by which it is achieved. One reason we know so little about the mechanism of tolerance is the fact that unresponsiveness can probably be achieved by various means, and that at least some of the unresponsiveness phenomena have different underlying mechanisms. The second reason is that natural tolerance is probably tightly linked to immunoregulation, of which we are only now getting our first glimpse. A brief discussion of some of the hypotheses proposed to explain immunological tolerance follows.

Clonal Deletion

This process is part of Burnet's clonal selection hypothesis (see Chapter 7). According to this hypothesis, the differentiating immune system generates a large number of clones, with different clones specific for different antigens and all clones together covering the entire antigen universe, including self components. However, the differentiation of the clones is sensitive to the presence of antigen: whenever a differentiating clone encounters the corresponding antigen, its differentiation stops and the clone is eliminated. Since the only antigens the differentiating immune system of the fetus normally encounters are those constituting self, antiself clones are eliminated, whereas all other clones are permitted to complete their differentiation. In his original hypothesis, Burnet proposed that the antiself clones are truly deleted (physically eliminated); however, there is now considerable evidence that antigen-binding cells specific for self are still present in tolerant animals.

To save the clonal deletion hypothesis, some immunologists have argued that the clones, though physically present, are *functionally deleted.* According to one such hypothesis, in the process of maturation, T and B lymphocytes pass through a transient phase, during which any contact with antigen, endogenous or exogenous, results in specific inactivation of these cells. The inactivated cells are not removed but they fail to mature—they are aborted in their development. This *clonal abortion hypothesis*, like the clonal deletion hypothesis, is also contradicted by experimental data. There is no evidence for aborted development in tolerant animals; on the contrary, the tolerized cells appear to mature normally, but instead of reacting to positive signals, they receive and store negative tolerizing signals. The specific state of the tolerant cells has been called *clonal anergy* by Gustav J. V. Nossal and his colleagues (Gr. *an*, negative, *energeia*, energy, from *ergon*, work; here, absence of reaction). There has been much speculation about the nature of the negative signals; but since we know almost nothing about the positive signals sent between T and B cells, there is little on which to base such hypotheses.

Immunological Enhancement

As was explained in Chapter 12, immunological enhancement is an antibody-mediated prolongation of allograft (especially tumor allograft) survival. Several immunologists, notably Guy A. Voisin and his colleagues, have attempted to apply the enhancement concept (Voisin uses the term *facilitation*) as an explanation of immunological tolerance. According to this explanation, the self constituents induce the formation of enhancing antibodies, which then maintain a check on the corresponding lymphocyte clones. Indeed, sera of animals carrying tolerated skin allografts often do contain antibodies that enhance allogeneic tumors or skeletal muscle allografts when transferred into normal individuals. But the presence of enhancing antibodies is not sufficient for the maintenance of tolerance: sera of animals that no longer tolerate allografts often continue, upon transfer to normal individuals, to enhance allograft survival. This dissociation of tolerance and enhancement indicates that enhancement cannot be the sole explanation of tolerance.

Blocking Factors

In 1969, the Hellströms, Karl Erik and Ingegerd, reported that lymphocytes from mice bearing certain virally induced sarcomas killed these tumor cells in vitro; but when serum from tumor-bearing mice was added to the test system, the killing was specifically blocked. Evidence of specificity was the observation that sera from mice not bearing tumors did not block the reaction. The Hellströms ascribed the blocking to hypothetical *blocking factors*, produced by tumor-bearing animals. Later studies demonstrated that blocking factors can be dissociated at low pH into two components, one of a much larger size than the other. When tested separately, neither the small nor the large component blocks tumor-cell killing by lymphocytes, but when recombined, the blocking activity reappears. Blocking factors are now thought to be complexes of antibodies and antigens, or portions thereof. The Hellströms believed that blocking factors were of great biological importance, not only in tumor immunity but also in the maintenance of tolerance. Indeed, blocking factors can be demonstrated, at least by some investigators, in the sera of tolerant animals. Nevertheless, the blocking factor hypothesis is an extremely unlikely explanation of tolerance. At least three observations argue against it. First, there is no correlation between blocking activity in vitro and tumor growth in vivo; nonblocking sera are as effective in enhancing tumor growth as are blocking sera. Second, sera from tolerant mice without demonstrable blocking activity in vitro enhance tumor growth in vivo. And third, induction of tolerance is not facilitated by passive administration of blocking sera. In sum, like enhancing antibodies, blocking factors (immune complexes) probably play only an auxiliary role in the induction and maintenance of tolerance.

Suppressor Cells

The presence of suppressor cells in tolerant animals can be demonstrated by an *adaptive transfer of tolerance*: normal animals inoculated with lymphocytes from tolerant donors become specifically tolerant themselves. The problem with this kind of transfer is that the "normal" recipients are not really normal, but usually X-irradiated and otherwise treated to facilitate acceptance of the inoculum. One can therefore argue that this treatment itself favors the induction of suppressor cells. However, when the necessary controls are included, there remains little doubt that the transfer of suppression from tolerant animals is a real phenomenon. The presence of suppressor cells in tolerant animals is also supported by the observation that injection of a certain dose of normal cells into tolerant animals does not lead to rejection of tolerated grafts, presumably because the recipient's suppressor cells inactivate the transferred normal cells before they can mount an immune response against the graft.

In conclusion, the two mechanisms likely to be involved in tolerance induction are clonal inactivation and inhibition of lymphocyte activity by suppressor cells. These two mechanisms may, in fact, be different manifestations of one basic process, in the sense that the clonal inactivation may occur via suppressor cells. Other phenomena, such as immunological enhancement by antibodies and inhibition by blocking factors may contribute to the maintenance of a tolerance state, but probably do not play a decisive role in it. Tolerance, however, may not be a single phenomenon, and enhancing antibodies and blocking factors may play an important role in certain forms of tolerance.

Immunological tolerance probably cannot be understood without understanding how lymphocytes interact in their networks or circuits. The postulated homeostasis of the immunoregulatory system is, in fact, natural tolerance—a state that prevents the organism from attacking its own components while preserving the potential to respond to foreign substances. Therefore, the clue to tolerance lies in immunoregulation.

The above comments apply to the so-called classic tolerance—the kind of tolerance involved in the normal recognition of self. There are, however, experimental forms of immunological unresponsiveness that may be governed by principles other than those governing the classic tolerance. To these forms one of the following explanations may apply (and different explanations may apply to different phenomena).

Exhaustive Immunization. Facing a large excess of antigen, all cells capable of recognizing this antigen may be stimulated to differentiate into end-stage antibody-producing cells without the generation of memory cells. Such differentiation effectively exhausts the supply of B cells for a given antigen, so that there is no memory and no response to subsequent challenges with the same antigen.

Receptor Blockade. Binding of antigen or antibody to the B-cell receptor may prevent this receptor from functioning properly if the bound ligand is, for whatever reason, incapable of providing an activation signal. The receptor is blocked from further interaction with the antigen and the cell is unresponsive. Some sort of receptor blockade probably occurs in immunological paralysis, effected by high doses of polysaccharide antigens, and in tolerance induced by unnatural D-isomers of synthetic polypeptides. (The proteins probably bind to the receptors but fail to induce any action in the cell.) Blocking of receptors by antibodies may be responsible for the cases of *antibody-mediated tolerance* (e.g., the addition of POL, together with POL-specific antibodies to a culture of spleen cells, inhibits the in vitro response to this antigen).

13.6.6 Immunosuppression

Most immunosuppressive agents act nonspecifically on lymphocytes, and therefore affect both cellular and humoral immunity. Consequently, most of the agents used for suppression of antibody formation are the same as those described in Chapter 12 and used for suppression of T-cell responses. To this description we shall add only a few specific comments.

Antilymphocyte serum (ALS) is used primarily to suppress cellular responses, but it also acts on humoral immunity, reducing primary responses when administered shortly before the antigen. It has no effect when given after an antigen administration or when used for the treatment of secondary response.

X-irradiation affects primary antibody response far more than secondary responses, probably because memory cells are relatively radioresistant. Secondary responses can be abolished only by high doses of irradiation that have deleterious effects on cells other than lymphocytes. Sublethal doses of whole-body irradiation suppress antibody responses to most antigens for several weeks, but usually not permanently. The greatest suppression is achieved when the recipient is irradiated 24 to 48 hours before antigen administration, probably because, in this case, the antigen is eliminated from the body before the antibody-forming capacity is restored.

Alkylating agents have an effect similar to that of X-irradiation, but the recovery of the lymphoid tissues from the treatment is more rapid, so the drugs must be administered at more frequent intervals.

Corticosteroids are effective only in large doses that can be administered to animals but not to humans. However, they are used to inhibit the inflammation accompanying allergies, delayed-type hypersensitivity, and certain autoimmune diseases (see Chapter 14).

Antimetabolites are most effective when given about two days after antigen administration. This observation makes sense since antimetabolites act by inhibiting DNA replication and so exert their effect when cells begin to proliferate.

In vitro antibody responses can be suppressed by *chloramphenicol* and *actinomycin D.* The latter is most effective when added to the culture simultaneously with the antigen.

REFERENCES

General

Austen, K. I.: Biological implications of the structural and functional characteristics of the chemical mediators of immediate-type hypersensitivity. *Harvey Lect.* **73:**93–161, 1977.

Bach, M. K. (Ed.): *Immediate Hypersensitivity. Modern Concepts and Developments.* Marcel Dekker, New York, 1978.

Bruni, C., Doria, G., Koch, G., and Strom, R.: *Systems Theory of Immunology.* Springer-Verlag, Berlin, 1979.

Eichmann, K.: Expression and function of idiotypes on lymphocytes. *Adv. Immunol.* **26:**195–257, 1978.

Fougereau, M. and Dausset, J. (Eds.): *Immunology 80.* Academic, London, 1980.

Golub, E. S.: *The Cellular Basis of Immune Response. An Approach to Immunobiology.* Sinauer, Sunderland, Massachusetts, 1977.

Good, R. A. and Fisher, D. W. (Eds.): *Immunobiology.* Sinauer, Stamford, Connecticut, 1971.

Gupta, S. and Good, R. A. (Eds.): *Cellular, Molecular, and Clinical Aspects of Allergic Disorders.* Plenum, New York, 1979.

Jerne, N. K.: The immune system: a web of V-domains. *Harvey Lect.* **70:**93–110, 1975.

Katz, D. H.: *Lymphocyte Differentiation, Recognition, and Regulation.* Academic, New York, 1977.

Kazimierczak, W. and Diamant, B.: Mechanisms of histamine release in anaphylactic and anaphylactoid reactions. *Progr. Allergy* **24:**295–365, 1978.

Loor, F. and Roelants, G. E. (Eds.): *B and T Cells in Immune Recognition.* Wiley, Chichester, 1977.

Miescher, P. A. and Müller-Eberhard, H. J. (Eds.): *Textbook of Immunopathology,* Vols. 1 and 2, 2nd ed. Grune and Stratton, New York, 1976.

Nossal, G. J. V. and Ada, G. L.: *Antigens, Lymphoid Cells, and the Immune Response.* Academic, New York, 1971.

Phillips, S. M. and Colley, D. G.: Immunologic aspects of host responses to Schistosomiasis: resistance, immunopathology, and eosinophil involvement. *Progr. Allergy* **24:**49–187, 1978.

Samter, M. (Ed.): *Immunological Diseases.* Vols. 1 and 2, 3rd ed. Little, Brown, Boston, 1978.

Tomasi, T. B.: *The Immune System of Secretions.* Prentice-Hall, Englewood Cliffs, New Jersey, 1976.

Weller, P. F. and Goetzl, E. J.: The regulatory and effector roles of eosinophils. *Adv. Immunol.* **27:**339–371, 1979.

Original Articles

Arthus, M. and Breton, M.: Lésions cutanées produites par les injections de sérum de cheval chez le lapin anaphylactisé par et pour ce sérum. *Compt. Rend. Soc. Biol.* **55:**817–820, 1903.

Chiller, J. M., Habicht, G. S., and Weigle, W. O.: Kinetic differences in unresponsiveness of thymus and bone marrow cells. *Science* **171:**813–814, 1971.

Chodirker, W. B. and Tomasi, T. B.: Gamma-globulins: quantitative relationships in human serum and nonvascular fluids. *Science* **142:**1080–1081, 1963.

Claman, H. N., Chaperon, E. A., and Triplett, R. F.: Thymus-marrow cell combinations. Synergism in antibody production. *Proc. Soc. Exp. Biol. Med.* **122**:1167–1174, 1966.

Click, R. E., Benck, L., and Alter, B. J.: Immune responses *in vitro*. I. Culture conditions for antibody synthesis. *Cell. Immunol.* **3**:264–276, 1972.

Davies, A. J. S., Leuchars, E., Wallis, V., Marchant, R., and Elliott, E. B.: The failure of thymus-derived cells to produce antibody. *Transplantation* **5**:222–231, 1967.

Dray, S.: Effect of maternal isoantibodies on the quantitative expression of two allelic genes controlling γ-globulin allotypic specificities. *Nature* **195**:677–680, 1962.

Eardley, D. D., Hugenberger, J., McVay-Boudreau, L., Shen, F. W., Gershon, R. K., and Cantor, H.: Immunoregulatory circuits among T-cell sets. I. T-helper cells induce other T-cell sets to exert feedback inhibition. *J. Exp. Med.* **147**:1106–1115, 1978.

Eichmann, K.: Idiotype suppression. II. Amplification of a suppressor T cell with anti-idiotypic activity. *Eur. J. Immunol.* **5**:511–517, 1975.

Felton, L. D.: The significance of antigen in animal tissues. *J. Immunol.* **61**:107–117, 1949.

Francis, T. T., Jr., Davenport, F. M., and Hennessy, A. V.: Epidemiological recapitulation of human infection with different strains of influenza virus. *Trans. Assoc. Am. Physicians* **66**:231–239, 1953.

Hellström, I. and Hellström, K. E.: Studies on cellular immunity and its serum-mediated inhibition in Moloney virus-induced mouse sarcomas. *Int. J. Cancer* **4**:587–600, 1969.

Herzenberg, L. A., Herzenberg, L. A., Goodlin, R. C., and Rivera, E. C.: Immunoglobulin synthesis in mice. Suppression by anti-allotype antibody. *J. Exp. Med.* **126**:701–713, 1967.

Hirst, J. A. and Dutton, R. W.: Cell components in the immune response. III. Neonatal thymectomy: restoration in culture. *Cell. Immunol.* **1**:190–195, 1970.

Ingraham, J. S. and Bussard, A.: Application of localized hemolysis reaction for specific detection of individual antibody-forming cells. *J. Exp. Med.* **119**:667–684, 1964.

Jerne, N. K.: Towards a network theory of the immune system. *Ann. Inst. Pasteur (Paris)* **125c**:373–389, 1974.

Jerne, N. K. and Nordin, A. A.: Plaque formation in agar by single antibody producing cells. *Science* **140**:405, 1963.

Kapp, J. A., Pierce, C. W., and Benacerraf, B.: Genetic control of immune responses in vitro. III. Tolerogenic properties of the terpolymer L-glutamic acid^{60}-L-alanine^{30}-L-tyrosine^{10} (GAT) for spleen cells from nonresponder (H-2^s and H-2^q) mice. *J. Exp. Med.* **140**:172–184, 1974.

Katz, D. H., Hamaoka, T., and Benacerraf, B.: Cell interaction between histoincompatible T and B lymphocytes. II. Failure of physiologic cooperative interaction between T and B lymphocytes from allogeneic donor strains in humoral response to hapten-protein conjugates. *J. Exp. Med.* **137**:1405–1418, 1973.

Kindred, B. and Shreffler, D. C.: H-2 dependence of cooperation between T and B cells in vivo. *J. Immunol.* **109**:940–943, 1972.

Landsteiner, K. and Wiener, A. S.: An agglutinable factor in human blood recognized by immune sera for rhesus blood. *Proc. Soc. Exp. Biol. Med.* **43**:223, 1940.

Marbrook, J.: Primary immune response in cultures of spleen cells. *Lancet* **2**:1279–1281, 1967.

Michaelis, L.: Untersuchungen über Eiweisspräzipitine. *Dtsch. Med. Wochenschr.* **28**:733–736, 1902.

Miller, J. F. A. P. and Mitchell, G. F.: The thymus and the precursors of antigen reactive cells. *Nature* **216**:659–663, 1967.

Mishell, R. I. and Dutton, R. W.: Immunization of normal mouse spleen cell suspensions in vitro. *Science* **153**:1004–1006, 1966.

Mitchison, N. A.: Induction of immunological paralysis in two zones of dosage. *Proc. R. Soc. Lond. (Biol.)* **161**:275–292, 1964.

Mitchison, N. A.: *In* M. Landy and W. Braun (Eds.): *Immunological Tolerance*, p. 149–151. Academic, New York, 1969.

Möller, G.: Studies on the mechanism of immunological enhancement of tumor homografts. I. Specificity of immunological enhancement. *J. Natl. Cancer Inst.* **30**:1153–1175, 1963.

Mosier, D. E.: A requirement for two cell types for antibody formation *in vitro*. *Science* **158**:1575–1576, 1967.

Oudin, J.: Allotypy of rabbit serum proteins. II. Relationships between various allotypes: their common antigenic specificity, their distribution in a sample population; genetic implications. *J. Exp. Med.* **112**:125–142, 1960.

Ovary, Z. and Benacerraf, B.: Immunological specificity of the secondary response with dinitrophenyl proteins. *Proc. Soc. Exp. Biol. Med.* **114**:72–76, 1963.

Paul, W. E., Katz, D. H., Goidl, E. A., and Benacerraf, B.: Carrier function in anti-hapten immune responses. II. Specific properties of carrier cells capable of enhancing anti-hapten antibody responses. *J. Exp. Med.* **132**:283–299, 1970.

Press, J. L. and Klinman, N. R.: Enumeration and analysis of antibody-forming precursors in the neonatal mouse. *J. Immunol.* **111**:829–835, 1973.

Raff, M. C.: Two distinct populations of peripheral lymphocytes in mice distinguishable by immunofluorescence. *Immunology* **19**:637–650, 1970.

Schimpl, A. and Wecker, E.: Replacement of T-cell function by a T-cell product. *Nature New Biol.* **237**:15–17, 1972.

Shwartzman, G.: Studies on *Bacillus typhosus* toxic substances. Phenomenon of local skin reactivity to *B. typhosus* culture filtrate. *J. Exp. Med.* **48**:247–268, 1928.

Sercarcz, E. and Coons, A. H.: The exhaustion of specific antibody producing capacity during a secondary response. *In* M. Hašek, A. Lengerová, and M. Vojtíšková (Eds.): *Mechanisms of Immunological Tolerance*, pp. 73–83. Publication House of the Czechoslovak Academy of Science, Prague, 1962.

Siskind, G. W. and Benacerraf, B.: Cell selection by antigen in the immune response. *Adv. Immunol.* **10**:1–50, 1969.

Taussig, M. J.: T-cell factor which can replace the activity of T cells in vivo. *Nature* **248**:234–236, 1974.

Taylor, R. B. and Wortis, H. H.: Thymus dependence of antibody response: variation with dose of antigen and class of antibody. *Nature* **220**:927–928, 1968.

Uhr, J. W. and Baumann, J. B.: Antibody formation. I. The suppression of antibody formation by passively administered antibody. *J. Exp. Med.* **113**:935–957, 1961.

Woodland, R. and Cantor, H.: Idiotype-specific T helper cells are required to induce idiotype-positive B memory cells to secrete antibodies. *Eur. J. Immunol.* **8**:600–606, 1978.

Zaalberg, O. B.: A simple method for detecting single antibody-forming cells. *Nature* **202**:1231, 1964.

THE FOURTH MOVEMENT
Synthesis

CHAPTER 14

DEFENSE REACTIONS IN ACTION

The composers of great symphonies sometimes use the finale to achieve a grand synthesis of the concepts and images expressed in the preceding movements. The finale is often a return to the themes of the first, second, and third movements—a search for the meaning of the individual parts from the point of view of the whole. Beethoven did this in his *Ninth*, Bruckner in his *Fifth*, Mahler in his *Second*, and Franck in his *D Minor Symphony*.

We shall follow this example by attempting in this, the book's "finale," to integrate the principles we have learned in the previous movements, to develop a scheme that will explain how defense reactions might operate in the living body. We shall divide this synthesizing chapter into four parts—the first dealing with the ways the body reacts to an injury, the second summarizing the mechanisms activated by the attachment of another organism to the body, the third describing the options the body has in dealing with its own aberrant cells and tissues, and the fourth discussing what happens when the defense mechanisms turn perversely against the body's own components. This quartile division is reminiscent of the four threats to bodily integrity with which we opened this book. We shall close with a kind of a coda, a musical tailpiece that will present the author's highly personal, biased view of the present situation in and the future of immunology.

14.1 INFLAMMATION

14.1.1 Definition and History

The series of changes that occurs in a living body following an injury is referred to as *inflammation* (L. *in-*

flammare, to set on fire). The injuries can be caused by physical agents, such as excessive heat or cold, ultraviolet or ionizing irradiation, cuts or abrasions; by a wide variety of inorganic or organic chemical substances; or by biological agents such as viruses, bacteria, and other parasites. The classic macroscopical features of inflammation have been known to humankind for more than 2000 years: a description of the inflammatory process can be found on old Egyptian papyri and the physicians of ancient Greece and Rome wrote extensively on its various aspects. The most concise description of inflammation is attributed to Cornelius Celsus, who lived in the first century A.D. According to Celsus, *Notae vero inflammationis sunt quator: rubor et tumor cum calore et dolore* (There are four cardinal signs of inflammation: redness and swelling with heat and pain). To these, the second-century physician Galen added a fifth cardinal sign, *functio laesa*, loss of function of the affected part.

After the invention of the microscope, scientists began to ask questions about the mechanism leading to the five cardinal signs and about the adaptive value of inflammation. At first, pathologists, represented particularly by Rudolf Virchow, contended that inflammation was a local cellular reaction, and that the vascular system and blood vessels played only a secondary role in it. But following the classic experiments of Julius F. Cohnheim on inflammation in the thin tissues of the foot-web, mesentery, and tongue of the frog, it became apparent in 1882 that small blood vessels participated in an important way in the induction of inflammation. Pathologists first thought that inflammation was a deleterious phenomenon, a disease; but starting with John Hunter's classic treatise on "Gunshot Wounds, Blood and Inflammation," published in 1794, they began to realize that inflammation was, in fact, a defense mechanism. The adaptive value of inflammation was thoroughly documented by Elie Metchnikoff, who established that phagocytosing cells and phagocytosis constituted one of the principal factors of the inflammatory process.

14.1.2 Gross Morphology of the Inflammatory Process

To describe what happens in an injured tissue, we shall use as an example a small wound caused by the penetration of a sharp object (e.g., a thorn or splinter) into the skin. The injury triggers a complex series of events, many of which occur simultaneously and are interrelated in a variety of ways. To simplify the description of these events, we shall divide the inflammatory process into phases and stages, while keeping in mind that in the wound, many of the stages may occur concurrently with one another.

Degenerative Phase

The object penetrating the skin damages some cells, destroys their interconnection, severs blood vessels, and disturbs the tissue's normal metabolism. When the wound breaks open, the inner tissue of the body becomes accessible to microorganisms. The affected cells, primarily epidermal cells and fibroblasts, swell, their cytoplasms become vacuolized, and their nuclei enlarge and fragment. Some platelets in the damaged blood vessels disintegrate and release serotonin and other mediators, which then act on sympathetic nerve endings of the autonomic system. The stimulation induces a sudden contraction of the smooth muscle surrounding the blood vessels, so that within a few seconds after penetration, the broken vessels close, and so keep blood loss at a minimum. A visible consequence of this event is a marked paling of the afflicted tissue immediately after the injury. However, the blood vessel constriction is transient, lasting only a moment. Soon the smooth muscles relax again, the vessels open up, and blood floods the wound. The blood exerts a pressure on the wound and contributes to the degeneration of cells. Most of the events in this phase are passive, occurring as a direct consequence of the trauma. The sudden constriction of blood vessels oc-

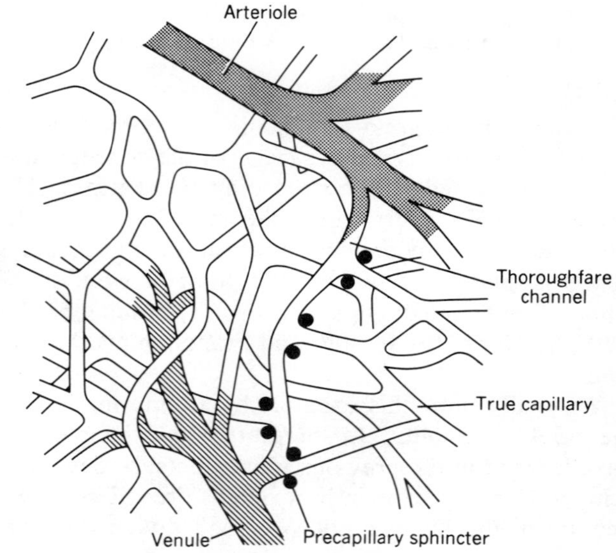

Figure 14.1. The microcirculation. The thoroughfare channel is the major connection between an artery and a vein. The true capillaries branch off from it but, at any one time, most of them are closed by the constriction of the precapillary sphincter muscle.

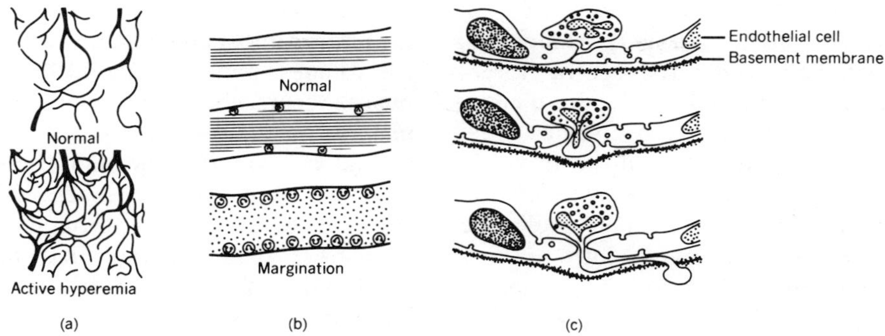

Figure 14.2. Vascular changes occurring during inflammation. (*a*) Opening and flooding of capillaries in the inflamed tissue. (*b*) Vasodilation, changes in the character of blood flow, and margination. (*c*) Emigration of neutrophils from blood vessels into the surrounding connective tissue. (Compiled from various sources.)

curs only in some injuries; it is absent in those caused by irradiation or other gradually acting stimuli.

Vascular Phase

Following the passive phase, an active, aggressive defense reaction sets in, characterized mainly by changes in the blood vessels, extensive migration and activity of the so-called *inflammatory cells* (granulocytes—particularly neutrophils, lymphocytes, monocytes, and macrophages), and the clearing of the degenerated cells and cellular debris.

Changes in Microcirculation. You may recall that *arteries*, the blood vessels carrying blood away from the heart, divide repeatedly, with the successive branches gradually diminishing in size. The smallest arterial branches, the *arterioles*, have diameters of about 150 μm or less and are normally invisible to the naked eye. In the tissues, the arterioles divide to form a network of *capillaries*, the smallest of all blood vessels (Fig. 14.1). Capillaries join to form *postcapillary venules*, which in turn, combine to give rise to larger *veins*, the vessels that bring blood back to the heart. Under normal conditions, only about 5 or 10 percent of all the capillaries in a resting tissue are open; the rest are closed by one of two mechanisms. First, each capillary has at its origin a thin layer of muscle, the *precapillary sphincter*, which, when constricted, prevents blood flow into the capillary. Second, fine arteries and arteriovenous capillaries are surrounded by a muscular cuff, the constriction of which closes them. (True capillaries have no smooth muscle and probably no nerve endings.) The surface of the capillary bed in humans is 6300 m^2, but a large portion of the bed is closed; if all the capillaries were opened, the normal blood volume would have to be increased by some 300 ml. At different times, different capillaries are open, and their opening and closing is probably controlled by the local concentration of oxygen, tissue metabolites such as lactate, and hydrogen ions.

This *microcirculation* (circulation of blood in the fine blood vessels) changes drastically following injury. Substances liberated in the injured tissue paralyze the precapillary sphincter, so that most of the capillaries in the inflamed area open and allow blood to flow into them. This flooding (congestion, engorgement) of the capillary network and the postcapillary venules with blood is called *active hyperemia* (Gr. *hyper*, above, over, *haima*, blood; thus, presence of an increased amount of blood in a particular tissue).[1] On microscopic inspection, one finds that many more capillaries are visible in a hyperemic tissue than in a normal tissue (Fig. 14.2a); on macroscopic examination, one observes that the inflamed tissue looks red, a condition referred to as *erythema* (Gr. *erythema*, flush).

The changes in microcirculation lead to changes in tissue temperature. The normal temperature of the hand skin is between 30 and 32°C, that of a resting limb muscle 34 or 35°C. The increased blood flow causes the temperature of the inflamed area to approach that of aortic blood: compared to the surrounding normal tissues, the wound seems hot.

Since the capillary bed, when fully opened, has a much larger cross-sectional area than either the arterioles or the venules, the blood flow in the inflamed area slows down: the effect is similar to that seen when a narrow river suddenly opens up into a wide delta.

[1] *Active* hyperemia is caused by the inflow of arterial blood, in contrast to *passive* hyperemia, caused by an obstruction in the blood flow.

The deceleration of blood flow affects the distribution of the blood vessels' content: normally, almost all blood cells are contained within the central three-quarters of the vessel (*axial flow*), while the quarter nearest the wall is occupied mostly by plasma (Fig. 14.2*b*). In the axial flow leukocytes tend to travel in the slower periphery and red cells in the faster central portion. Some of the leukocytes may enter the periphery of the bloodstream, bump into the endothelium from time to time, adhere to it momentarily, then detach again, and rejoin the axial flow. In the inflamed tissue, as the blood flow slows, leukocytes roll over the endothelium more slowly and take longer to detach from it, until finally some of them fail to detach at all, and instead, begin to wander about on the vessel wall. The endothelium gradually becomes paved with leukocytes—a phenomenon referred to as *leukocytic margination* (Fig. 14.2*b*). The reason for the increased adhesion of leukocytes is probably changes occurring in the endothelial wall as a consequence of the injury; the leukocytes themselves are no different from those in normal tissues. The pavement obstructs the blood flow and increases the pressure in capillaries, forcing some of the fluid out into the surrounding tissue. The loss of fluid results in an increased viscosity of the blood remaining in the vessels, and the blood flow slows even more. Since the hemoglobin in the red blood cells is partly deoxygenated, the inflamed area acquires a dusky red color. In contrast, the tissue surrounding the wound is, for reasons explained below, bright red, constituting the so-called *flare*.

Concurrently with these events, changes occur in the diameter of the blood vessels in the inflamed and neighboring tissue. The capillary wall is normally composed of flattened endothelial cells, with adjacent cells separated by a gap that is about 250 Å wide and is filled with glycoproteins secreted by the cells. Some of the cells are perforated by small tunnels, and these too are normally closed by the glycoprotein coating, through which only small molecules can pass, whereas proteins and other macromolecules are prevented from leaving the blood. Upon injury, the damaged tissue releases substances long known to be related to histamine and hence called *H substances*; they are, in fact, a mixture of histamine and serotonin released by disrupted tissue mast cells. The H substances stimulate sympathetic nerve endings in the smooth muscle surrounding the arterioles, causing an active dilation of blood vessels (*vasodilation*; Fig. 14.2*b*); passive dilation occurs because of the increased blood flow in the arterioles. The endothelial cells of the dilated vessel separate from one another and the gaps between them enlarge.

The dilation occurs in two phases. The first follows the injury almost immediately, affects mainly the smallest venules, and lasts about 30 minutes. The second phase occurs about an hour after the injury, affects mainly true capillaries, and lasts for hours or days. In the dilated vessels, the gaps between cells become large enough not only for macromolecules, but also for cells (see below) to pass through. As a consequence, a protein-rich fluid, the so-called *inflammatory exudate*, leaks out of the vessel into the surrounding tissues, causing tissue swelling—the *inflammatory edema*. The swelling immobilizes the tissue and is often responsible for the fifth cardinal sign of inflammation—the loss of function. The leakage of fluid serves to dilute bacterial toxins and toxic metabolites produced by the injured cells; it also contains substances that neutralize the toxins and aid in the destruction of the agent causing the inflammation.

Blood vessel dilation occurs not only directly in the inflamed area, but also in the surrounding tissue. It is mediated by nervous stimuli, referred to collectively as the *axon reflex*: an irritant stimulates the endings of the sensory branch of the nervous system, and afferent nerve fibers conduct this impulse centrally; the impulse is then transferred to another branch, without traversing a nerve cell body, and this branch then acts on smooth muscle and causes vasodilation. The rapid blood flow in the dilated vessels is responsible for the flare.

Cellular Changes. The margination process causes leukocytes to accumulate on the vessel walls in the inflamed area. The leukocytes, particularly neutrophils and monocytes, move about on the wall until they find a suitable gap through which they can leave the vessel. Although at least 10 times thicker than the openings, the cells manage to squeeze through them, first sending pseudopods into them and then pulling the rest of the body along (Fig. 14.2*c*). During this process, the cells enlarge the openings somewhat. This *leukocyte emigration* is an active process on which the migrating cell spends a considerable amount of its energy. Once through the endothelial layer, the cell walks on the underlying basement membrane until it again finds a suitable pore through which to cross. Once free, the emigrants move on into the perivascular structures and tissue spaces and attack the dead and dying cells, digesting them intracellularly by phagocytosis, or extracellularly by proteolytic enzymes released from their lysosomes when they themselves die. The stimuli for the leukocyte emigration apparently come from the injured tissue in the form of chemotactic factors.

The platelet is another cell type profoundly affected

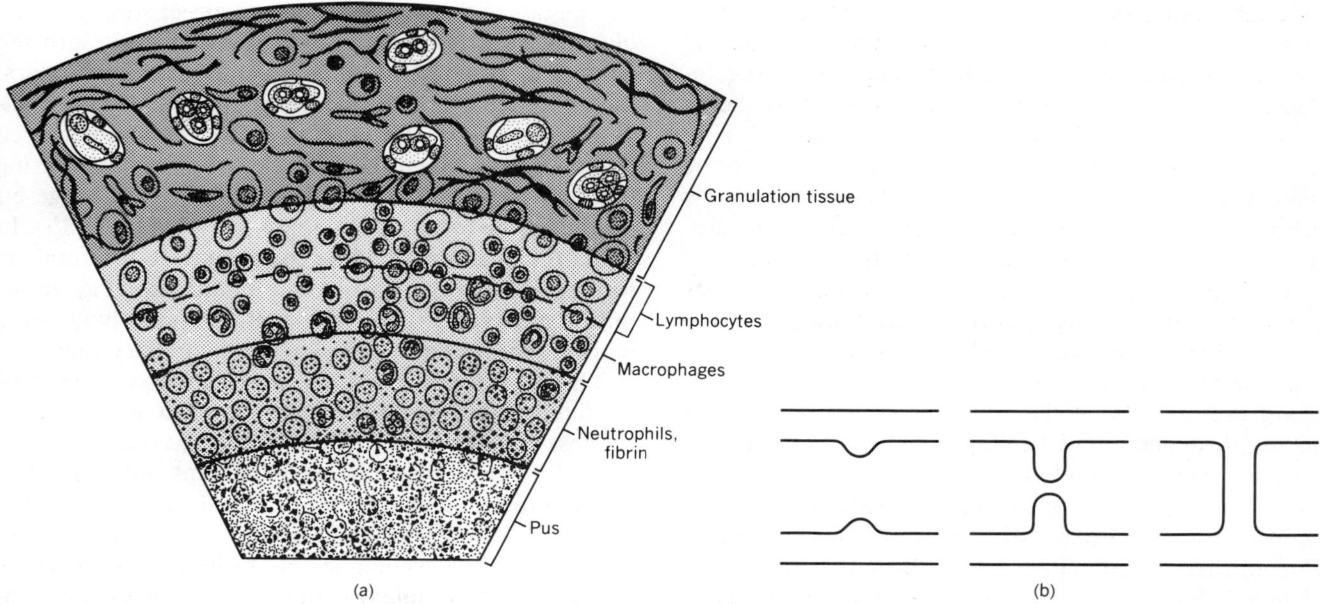

Figure 14.3. Repair phase of inflammation. (*a*) The formation of the pyogenic membrane (the shape of which is determined by the shape of the wound). (*b*) Three stages in the formation of a new capillary.

by tissue injury. Shortly after the injury, platelets, singly or in clumps, may be seen adhering to the vessel walls. At first the clumps are small; they often detach from the wall, after which the individual platelets separate from one another again. But later the clumps grow larger and adhere to the wall firmly. As more and more platelets accumulate, they form a solid plug that stops the flow of blood from the damaged vessel. In the early aggregates, each platelet retains its individual plasma membrane and its fine structure, but later, as the aggregates grow, the outlines of the individual cells become indistinct and the cells lose their granules. Simultaneously with the formation of aggregates, fibrin fibers begin to appear, forming a fine mesh that helps to trap cells.

Quite extensive formation of fibrin fibers also occurs outside the blood vessels and leads to clotting of the plasma in the inflammatory exudate: the fibrin reticulum traps the cells, debris, and fluid, and the retraction of the resulting clot pulls the edges of the disrupted tissue together.

Liquification of Injured Tissues. The intra- and extracellular digestion of necrotic tissue by neutrophils and monocytes produces a fluid, which then combines with the serous material extruded from the vessels. The resulting mixture is the so-called *pus*, and a circumscribed collection of pus is referred to as an *abscess* (L. *abscessus,* going away). The abscess cavity is lined by a *pyogenic membrane* (Gr. *pyon,* pus, suffix *-gen,* producing), which can be divided into four definite but ill-defined layers (Fig. 14.3*a*). The innermost part of the membrane contains predominantly neutrophils dispersed through a network of fibrin and protein-rich inflammatory edema. The middle portion of the membrane is composed of two layers, one consisting primarily of lymphocytes, and another dominated by macrophages. These cells fade into the outermost layer of *granulation tissue,* so designated because it forms minute, discrete grains on the surface of a healing wound. The granules represent fleshy connective tissue projections to the wound surface. The pyogenic membrane isolates the wound from the surrounding tissue and prevents spreading of the inflammation into other parts of the body. In wounds infected with bacteria, the pyogenic membrane prevents *septicemia*, the dissemination and multiplication of pathogenic microorganisms into the blood.

Healing Phase

The changes occurring in the first two phases of the inflammatory process either cause destruction of the foreign body (if it is an organism) or loosening of the tissue around the object (for example, a splinter), so that it then falls out by itself or can be pulled out more easily. Once the cause of inflammation has been removed, inflammation begins to subside; hyperemia gradually diminishes; leukocyte adhesion becomes less and less pronounced; individual blood vessels and the vascular pattern become normal once again; the inflammatory exudate diminishes, most of it being drained away by lymphatics into regional lymph nodes; and repair of the wound commences. The three main events in the repair process are formation of new connective tissue by proliferating fibroblasts, regeneration of epithelium, and outgrowth of new capillaries.

Even before the inflammation subsides, fibroblasts are seen to be moving into the injured area from the surrounding normal tissue where they exist in a dormant state. They migrate, by an ameboid movement, along the strands of the fibrin and distribute themselves throughout the healing area. At first they resemble tissue macrophages, but then they lose their oval shape, and passing through a stellate stage, finally acquire their characteristic elongated configuration. During their morphological transformation, they also change internally, in that they develop an extensive rough endothelial reticulum and several Golgi complexes. Once fixed into position in the injured tissue, they begin to synthesize collagen on ribosomes of the rough endoplasmic reticulum and secrete this protein through the channels of the Golgi apparatus. The synthesis requires ascorbic acid (vitamin C) for the conversion of proline and lysine into hydroxyproline and hydroxylysine, the two major constituents of collagen. This dependence on vitamin C explains why wounds do not heal in persons suffering from scurvy. The secreted collagen organizes itself into fibers, which are laid down somewhat haphazardly at first, but later form bundles oriented with their longitudinal axes in the direction of the greatest stress. As the collagen bundles grow in firmness, the fibroblasts gradually degenerate and attach closely to the bundles, and the injured area transforms into *scar tissue.* At first the tissue is rather dense but later it loosens and acquires the normal appearance of connective tissue (see Appendix 4.1).

Simultaneously with scar tissue formation, the intact epidermal cells on the edge of the wound begin to proliferate and move, as one sheet (the individual cells being held together by local plasma membrane thickening, the *desmosomes*), toward the center of the injured area. As the sheets meet in the center, they fuse and so completely cover the wound. Since the sheets grow into the clot filling the wound, part of the clot remains above the new epidermis, forming a protective *scab*, which sloughs off only when the wound has completely healed.

Nutrients for the growing scar tissue are supplied at first by the inflammatory exudate, but as the inflammation begins to subside, a need for a direct supply by the blood arises, and new vessels begin to grow into the wound. Stimulated by some as yet unidentified factors, the endothelial cells of the injured vessels begin to divide mitotically. The newly arising cells either force themselves between the existing ones, thus increasing the diameter or length of the vessel, or they bulge off and begin the formation of a new vessel (Fig. 14.3*b*). In the latter case, the dividing cells slip past one another, forming a bud that grows out of the existing vessel until it meets and fuses with another similarly growing bud of another vessel, producing a capillary loop.

This description provides an explanation for each of the five cardinal signs of inflammation except pain: the redness and heat result from hyperemia; the swelling is caused by the accumulation of inflammatory exudate in the interstitial tissue and of blood in the congested arterioles, capillaries, and venules; and the loss of function is the consequence of swelling. The causes of pain are more complex, with the following factors contributing to them: direct stimulation of nerve endings by H substances and by other pharmacologically active compounds released in the damaged tissue; increased tissue tension as a result of edema formation; increased osmotic pressure (macromolecules of dead cells break down into smaller fragments, making the fluid inside the wound more concentrated than in the surrounding tissue; as a result water is drawn into the wound and the pressure of the fluid increases, as is evidenced by the fact that the pus spurts out when an abscess is incised); and pH changes (the inflamed tissue has a high rate of glycolysis, leading to the accumulation of lactic acid and fall of pH; low concentration of H^+ then stimulates nerve endings).

14.1.3 Molecular Mechanisms

The cellular and tissue responses in inflammation are accompanied by the liberation into the injured region of a number of active compounds, which interact with one another in a complex manner. So far, only some of these complexities have been elucidated, and the sequence of events is only partially established.

Among the elements damaged by the injury are likely to be some mast cells, and some mediators are likely to be released in the very early stage of the inflammatory process. It might be these mediators that trigger the first phase of vasodilation, accompanied by the separation of endothelial cells and exposure of collagen fibers in the subendothelial layer. The fibers in the intercellular gaps trap platelets and trigger the release of mediators from these cells (Fig. 14.4). One of the earliest events in this triggering is activation of ade-

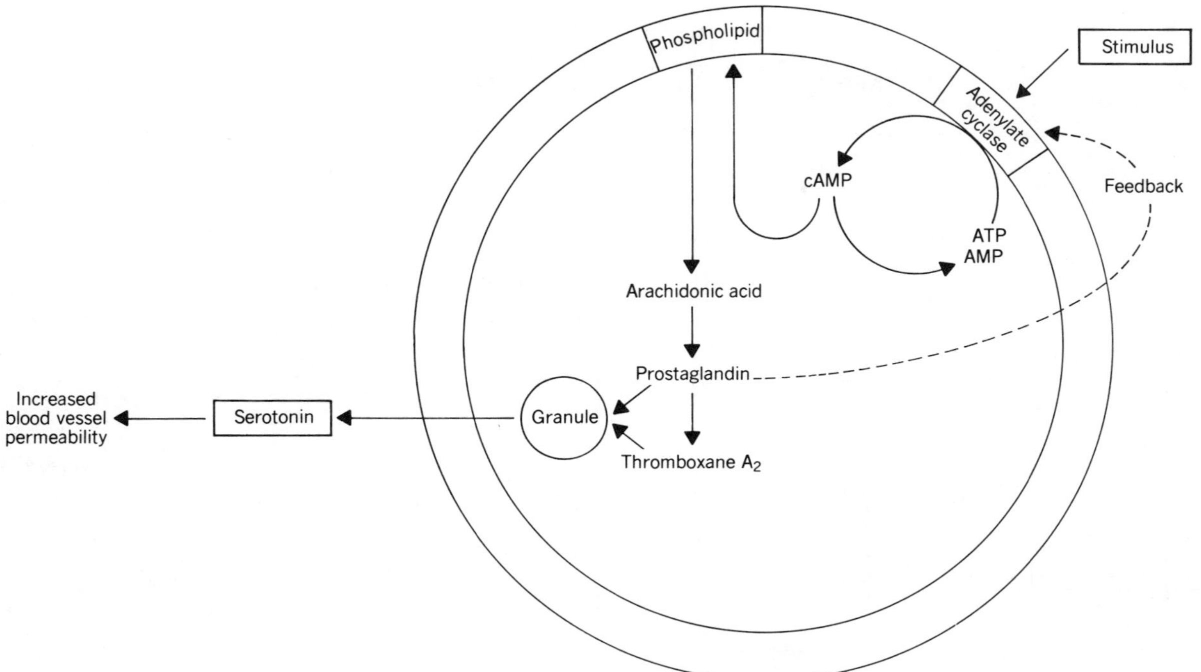

Figure 14.4. Reactions leading to serotonin release from platelets. The train of events begins with the action of a stimulus (e.g., a hormone) on membrane-bound adenylate cyclase and ends by serotonin-mediated dilation of blood vessels. The double circle represents the membrane of a platelet.

nylate cyclase in the platelet membrane and the generation of cyclic AMP from ATP. Increased levels of cyclic AMP allow the formation of arachidonic acid from membrane phospholipids and the conversion of the acid into prostaglandins and thromboxane A_2. These two compounds then act on platelet granules and trigger the release of serotonin, which then proceeds to increase blood vessel permeability and to participate in a series of other molecular interactions. The prostaglandin also acts in an inhibitory fashion on adenylate cyclase, competing with the triggering stimulus and thus regulating the platelet response.

In addition to platelets, the exposed collagen fibers also interact with proteins of the plasma that filters through the pores of the dilated vessel wall. One of these proteins is the precursor of the Hageman factor, the triggering factor of the blood-clotting cascade (Fig. 14.5). The interaction with collagen activates the Hagemann factor, initiates the cascade, and so leads to the generation of thrombin from prothrombin. The activated thrombin then plays a double role: it converts fibrinogen into fibrin, but it also activates plasminogen and converts it into plasmin. Fibrin fibers form dense networks, inside and outside the vessel, in which cells are trapped and a clot is formed. Plasmin, a component of the fibrinolytic cascade, degrades fibrin into smaller components and so contributes to the dissolution of the clot. But plasmin also has another function: it acts on the activated Hagemann factor, converting it into the prekallikrein activator and thus initiating the kinin-bradykinin cascade (Fig. 14.5; see also Chapter 9). The prekallikrein activator catalyzes the conversion of prekallikrein into activated kallikrein, which then assists in the generation of its own activators, and also catalyzes the conversion of kininogen into bradykinin. The latter substance then becomes involved in vasodilation, increase of blood vessel permeability, and chemotaxis. Bradykinin is inactivated by various hydrolytic kinases, which degrade it into smaller fragments.

This simplified description explains how three of the four main plasma activation systems become involved in inflammation. The fourth system, the complement cascade, can be activated by several stimuli: the injured blood vessels, the proteolytic enzymes released by the damaged cells, the membrane components of the participating bacteria, and the antigen-antibody complexes. Some of the activated complement components act as chemotactic factors, responsible for the influx of leukocytes into the inflamed area; others facilitate phagocytosis and participate in cell lysis.

The complexity of molecular interactions in the in-

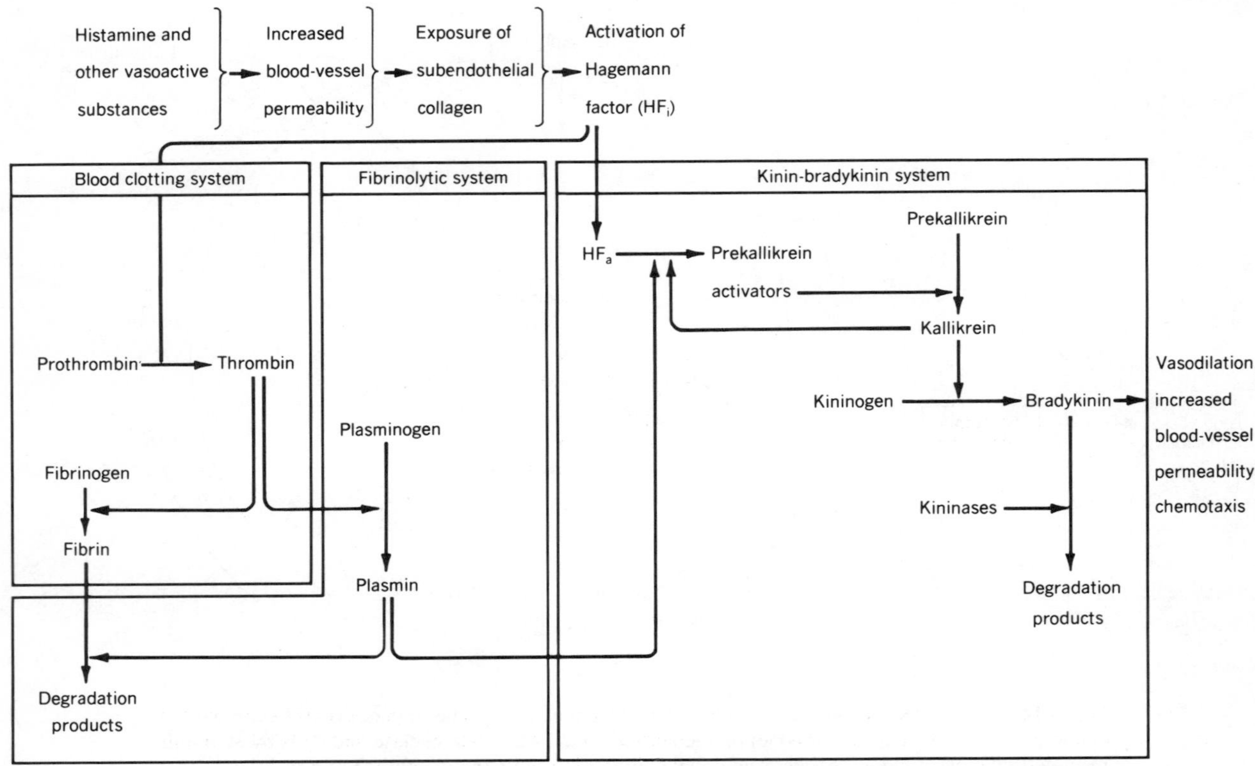

Figure 14.5. Reactions leading to the activation of the blood-clotting, fibrinolytic, and kinin-bradykinin cascades during inflammation. HF_a, activated Hagemann factor; HF_i, inactive factor.

flamed area is further increased by the participation of various mediators released by mast cells, basophils, and eosinophils. While mast cells are already present in the tissue at the time of injury, basophils and eosinophils are drawn into the injured tissue by the various chemotactic factors. The cells can be induced to release mediators by mechanical injury, proteases, complement components, or bacterial toxins. The released mediators then interact in the manner described in the preceding chapter.

Knowledge of the molecular interactions during inflammation is useful for the selection of *anti-inflammatory agents*—that is, agents that help to contain undesirable inflammation. The most commonly used anti-inflammatory agent is aspirin, which acts by blocking prostaglandin synthesis, as do indometacin and phenylbutazon. Steroids, another group of frequently used anti-inflammatory agents, probably act by influencing the stability of the lysosomal membrane.

14.1.4 Clinical Signs of Internal Inflammation

So far we have limited our description to an inflammatory reaction following an injury on the external body surface, where the consequences of the reaction are easily recognizable. However, inflammation can also result from internal injury, and then the signs of the reaction are indirect and less apparent. The three main changes accompanying internal inflammation are an increase in the erythrocyte sedimentation rate, appearance in the blood of C-reactive protein, and fever.

Increased Sedimentation Rate. When heparinized blood is placed in a capillary tube, the blood cells settle down with a certain speed, referred to as the *sedimentation rate*. In patients with an inflammatory disease, this rate is often higher than in healthy individuals. Presumably the inflammation leads to changes in plasma proteins, such as an increased concentration of gamma-globulins in relation to albumin, and so to more rapid erythrocyte sedimentation.

Appearance of C-Reactive Protein. The serum of patients with an inflammatory disease contains a new type of β-globulin, referred to as the *C-reactive protein* because it can be precipitated out of the serum by the C carbohydrate of pneumococcal bacteria (see Chapter 9).

Fever. In humans, the mean body temperature is 36.8°C (98.2°F), with a daily variation of about 1.3°C (2.3°F) and with a maximum at about 6.00 p.m. and minimum at about 3.00 a.m. When bodily temperature drops below from 28 to 30°C, people become unconscious; when it rises to 40.5°C, they become disoriented, and when it reaches 43.3°C or more, they become comatose. The *fever* accompanying inflammation is caused by the *endogenous pyrogen* released by macrophages or monocytes (see Chapter 10). The release is triggered by phagocytosis, bacterial toxins (endotoxins), and the various mediators liberated during inflammation. Endogenous pyrogen is present in the inflammatory exudate and plasma. It acts on the temperature-regulating center in the anterior hypothalamus, which then sends nerve signals that lead to an increased production of heat through increased metabolic rates. Whether fever serves any useful role in the inflammatory process is not known. Some physiologists have argued that it does, citing as supporting evidence the observation that persons suffering from syphilis or gonorrhea are often cured of these diseases when they contract malaria. Apparently, the high fever accompanying the malaria attacks (see Section 14.2.7) kills the bacteria responsible for syphilis and gonorrhea. However, this method of curing disease amounts, as the Czechs say, to exorcizing Satan with the devil, and is unlikely to play any significant role in natural situations.

14.1.5 Chronic Inflammation

The type of inflammation discussed on the preceding pages is referred to as *acute*, because it is of short duration, lasting only a week or two. But there is another type of inflammation that can last for months or even years. This *chronic inflammation* is caused by a low-grade but prolonged injury, the source of which can be any of the following:

persistent bacterial, fungal, or parasitic infections, exemplified by tuberculosis and leprosy (caused by mycobacteria), syphilis (caused by spirochetes), histoplasmosis (caused by fungi), and schistosomiasis (caused by parasites);

exogenous physical and chemical irritants, such as inhaled particles of silica, asbestos, dust, or fumes of, for example, berrylium compounds, as well as *endogenous irritants*, such as cholesterol crystals, unabsorbable sutures, or splinters;

hypersensitivity reactions accompanying, for example, tuberculosis or autoimmune disease, such as thyroiditis and gastritis;

unknown agents as, for example, in the case of *sarcoidosis* (Gr. *sarx*, flesh), a disease characterized by the appearance of granulomatous lesions in lymph nodes and various other organs, especially lungs, skin, spleen, or eyes. The disease somewhat resembles tuberculosis but is not caused by the tubercle bacilli; its causative agent has not yet been identified.

In situations where the body is unable to remove the inflammatory agent, it settles for the next best thing—a controlled surveillance of the effects of the agent: no large amounts of chemical mediators are released, no massive influx of neutrophils into the area occurs, and necrosis is maintained at a low level, being continually counterbalanced by an ongoing regeneration process. The most characteristic feature of chronic inflammation is the formation of *granulation tissue*, or *granuloma*. In the early stages, the tissue is highly cellular, consisting of fibroblasts, monocytes, macrophages, lymphocytes, epitheloid cells (plump, polygonal cells with a central nucleus and eosinophilic cytoplasm, probably derived from macrophages), and giant cells (large, multinucleated cells originating from the fusion of several epitheloid cells). It is well vascularized and contains only a few fine collagen fibers. But as the tissue ages, it matures into a tougher *fibrous tissue*, in which the cellularity and vascularity diminish greatly and the fibers thicken because of further collagen deposits. The term "granuloma" derives from the observation that the tissue often forms a lump grossly resembling a tumor (the suffix *-oma* usually being reserved for tumors).

When chronic inflammation occurs in hollow organs (e.g., the heart or small intestine), it may lead to the narrowing of orifices and tubes and to an obstruction, with all its consequences. In other situations it may result in shrinkage, scarring, and distortion of an internal organ, caused by the loss of parenchymal cells and their replacement with fibrous tissue. For example, when acute viral hepatitis is followed by chronic hepatitis, it leads to cirrhosis (Gr. *kirrhos,* tawny) or a fibroid induration of the liver, culminating in liver failure.

14.1.6 Amyloidosis

Inflammation is sometimes accompanied by the deposit in the tissues of a special substance, which Rudolf Virchow thought to be of polysaccharide composition and which he therefore called amyloid (Gr. *amylon*, starch, *eidos*, resemblance).

Discovery and Types

As a separate pathological condition resulting from the extracellular deposit of a waxy, translucent, homogeneous grey matter in the ground substance of the connective tissue, amyloidosis was first described by the Austrian pathologist Carl F. von Rokitansky in 1842. The form described by Rokitansky would be classified today as *secondary*, since it occurs secondarily to certain diseases, such as tuberculosis, leprosy, or rheumatoid arthritis. Later, three other types of amyloidosis were identified—primary, myeloma-associated, and tumor-forming. *Primary* or *atypical amyloidosis* occurs in the absence of discernible preceding or concurrent disease and is characterized by a predilection for involvement of mesenchymal organs, such as the cardiovascular system, muscles, and especially the gastrointestinal tract, in contrast to secondary amyloidosis, which involves mostly the liver, spleen, kidneys, and suprarenal glands. The cause of primary amyloidosis is not known.

Myeloma-associated amyloidosis develops in approximately 20 to 30 percent of patients with multiple myeloma and affects a wide variety of organs, including lymph nodes.

In *tumor-forming amyloidosis*, the accumulation of amyloid assumes such massive proportions that the affected organs (e.g., the tongue, portions of the intestinal tract, or the heart) look as if a tumor were growing in them.

This classification is highly artificial; there may be no principal difference between the four types of amyloidosis, and the apparent distinctions may arise merely as a consequence of specific circumstances of amyloid formation and deposit. A more natural classification may be possible only when the mechanisms of amyloid formation are elucidated.

Distribution and Methods of Demonstration

Most amyloid is deposited beneath the endothelium of capillaries, arterioles, and venules, forming a coating around them. The affected organs may become enlarged, firm, and tense and assume a pale, waxy, or glossy appearance. The progressively thicker coating of amyloid around blood vessels retards diffusion of nutrients and causes starvation of parenchymal elements. The parenchyme gradually atrophies and the organs malfunction, with fatal consequences. There is no inflammatory reaction to the amyloid, nor does the substance produce necrosis in the affected organs.

Amyloid stains dark brown with iodine, just as does starch, to which, however, it is totally unrelated. It can be demonstrated in vivo by the injection of a measured amount of a vital dye called Congo red (sodium diphenyl-diazo-*bis*-α-naphthylaminesulfonate) into the patient's blood. The dye is absorbed selectively by the amyloid, so that when, half an hour or an hour after the injection, one takes a sample of the patient's blood and determines colorometrically the amount of dye in it, one finds that at least 80 to 90 percent of the dye is unaccounted for, in comparison to normal individuals, in whom only about 50 percent has disappeared. When the tissue of a patient injected with Congo red is examined with a polarizing microscope, light polarized in one plane is retarded differently from light polarized in another plane. In other words, the amyloid presents different indexes of refraction—it is birefringent.

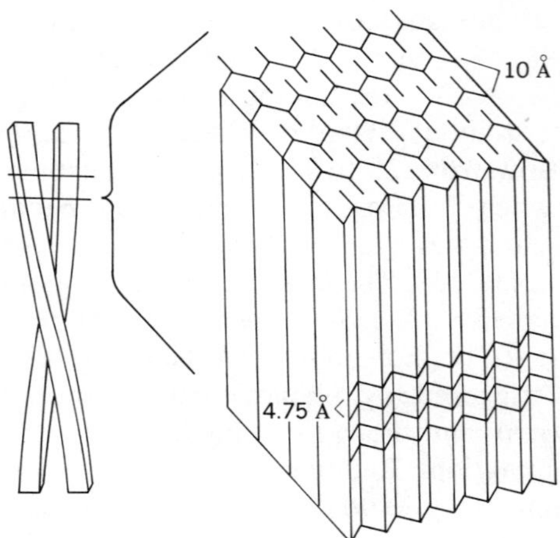

Figure 14.6. Structure of amyloid. (Modified from G. G. Glenner: *New Engl. J. Med.* **302:**1283–1292, 1333–1343, 1980.)

Physical Properties and Chemical Nature

When examined under the electron microscope, amyloid is seen to be composed of an array of rigid, linear, nonbranching, aggregated, hollow fibrils of indefinite length (Fig. 14.6). The orderly arrangement of the fibrils is responsible for the birefringence that becomes evident upon the examination with a polarized microscope. The fibrils are composed of polypeptide chains arranged into β-pleated sheets that run perpendicular to the fibrils' axes.

Chemically, two major types of fibril can be distinguished—AL and AA. The *AL-type fibrils*, frequent in primary or myeloma-associated amyloidosis, are derived from immunoglobulin light chains. They consist of the N-terminal fragment of the L chain, a complete L chain (rare), or a mixture of complete L chains and N-terminal fragments (also rare). All AL proteins contain the entire V_L region; the C_L is, however, usually absent. (The molecular weight of an AL protein ranges from 5000 to 30,000 daltons.) The L chain of the AL protein is not always the same as the normal chain: unusual amino acid sequences, substitutions, and deletions are often found in the abnormal chain. The chain can be of either the κ or the λ type and of a different subgroup, the frequently occurring subgroup being λ_{VI}. The AL protein is different in every patient, and so far no uniform peculiarity that could be used to identify a chain as amyloidogenic (fibril-forming) has been found. Also, antisera made against the AL protein have failed to reveal a common amyloid-specific antigenic determinant. When a patient has Bence-Jones proteins in the urine and amyloid in the tissue, the two proteins may be the same, but in most cases of primary amyloidosis, one finds only low serum or urinary levels of Bence-Jones proteins. The AL protein can be generated artificially by limited enzymatic degradation of Bence-Jones proteins. The artificially generated protein is indistinguishable from the natural AL substance, but only a small number of Bence-Jones proteins are capable of giving rise to amyloid. One may therefore assume that the naturally occurring AL protein is also derived by enzymatic splitting from immunoglobulin L chains.

The *AA protein* is frequent in secondary amyloidosis. It derives from serum protein, designated SAA, to which it is antigenically related. The SAA protein has a molecular weight of about 180,000 daltons and is composed of subunits with molecular weights of about 12,000 daltons. These subunits and the tissue AA proteins share at least the first 20 amino acids of their respective polypeptide chains. The tissue AA protein has a molecular weight of about 8500 daltons, contains 76 amino acids, and has no obvious relationship to immunoglobulin. Its N-terminal amino acid sequence is Arg-Ser-Phe-Phe-Ser-Phe-Leu-Gly-Glu. The protein is probably derived from the SAA protein by proteolytic digestion. In contrast to AL, AA proteins are similar in different patients. However, some microheterogeneity also exists among these proteins, especially near the C terminal. The AA protein occurs either alone or in combination with the AL protein.

In addition to these two major types of amyloid protein, several minor components have also been described. One of them is antigenically identical to normal serum prealbumin; normal homologues of the other proteins have not yet been identified. Furthermore, almost all amyloid deposits also contain a small amount (about 10 percent) of a nonfibrilar, pentagonal material called *P component*.

Mechanism

The amyloids are a variable group of proteins or protein fragments derived from normal proteins in the serum—immunoglobulins or others. The only thing these proteins have in common is a predilection for aggregation into fibrils with a β-pleated sheet structure. There are two conditions for amyloid formation and deposit. The first is abnormal prolonged stimulation of a protein-secreting cell, such as the plasma cell, so that the cell and its descendants produce large amounts of single protein; this condition is fulfilled, for example, by the continual presence of an irritating agent in chronic inflammation. The second is processing of the produced proteins, so that fragments capable of aggregating into fibrils with a β-pleated sheet structure are generated. Such processing may occur, for example, by proteolytic lysosomal enzymes of a macrophage. For some reason, immunoglobulin light chains are particularly prone to become the source of the amyloid protein, but at least one other serum protein, not yet identified functionally, is also involved in a major way. Since amyloid formation depends on the structure of the protein, there is a genetic component to amyloidosis in addition to the physiological one. The particular form of amyloidosis is thus dictated by a combination of genetic and nongenetic factors, which together determine whether the deposits will be local or systemic, which organs will become involved, which protein will be processed into amyloid, and so on. Consequently, amyloidosis is not a single condition, but a disease complex characterized by certain common features and diversified according to the specific conditions of its etiology.

14.2 DEFENSE AGAINST PARASITES

Parasitism (Gr. *parasitos*, a guest; from *para*, beside, *sitos*, food) is an association of two organisms in which one (the *parasite*) exploits the other (the *host*); the exploitation leads to the host's injury, or even death. The process of colonization of the host by the parasite is referred to as *infection*, and the illness caused by this colonization is an *infectious disease*. The parasite's ability to harm the host and to cause disease is its *pathogenicity* (Gr. *pathos*, suffering, *-gen*, to produce), which may vary greatly, depending on the circumstances of the association between the two organisms. The relative pathogenicity of a parasite is known as *virulence* (L. *virulentus*, poisonous)—its disease-evoking power; a parasite can be highly virulent, weakly virulent, or even avirulent (nonpathogenic). Sometimes two organisms may live in harmony under normal circumstances, but when one of them is injured or weakened the other may turn into an *opportunistic parasite*. A host that has recovered from an infectious disease may serve as a *carrier* or *vector* of the parasite for some time afterwards, spreading the parasite to other individuals.

The relationship between a host and its parasites is the result of a long evolution in which natural selection plays a decisive role. A parasite obviously tries to get the maximum from the host, but it cannot be oblivious to the consequences of the exploitation. If nothing else, the host must live at least as long as the parasite needs it, which usually means until the completion of the parasite's reproductive cycle. A parasite that kills the host too soon is not evolutionarily successful because it reduces the chances of its own multiplication. As a matter of fact, it is a disadvantage altogether when the host dies as a consequence of the parasite's actions. A parasite that killed every host it infected would eventually eliminate the entire host species and would itself die out as a species because of a lack of organisms in which to multiply. A profound injury to the host means one other disadvantage for the parasite: the injury is likely to provoke a strong defense reaction aimed at the elimination of the parasite.

The most evolutionarily successful parasite is therefore one that gets all it needs with a minimum of injury to the host. Obviously, a parasite does not plan its action intentionally in these terms; rather, the adaptation occurs because natural selection prefers mutations conforming to certain basic rules of the game the parasite plays with the host. If a new mutation increases the virulence of a given parasite, the mutated forms will gain temporary advantage over the less virulent forms and spread through a population. But soon the new form kills most of the available hosts and so, effectively, commits suicide. Alternatively, a genetic variant capable of coping with the virulent parasite arises in the host population, and so, after the parasite has killed all the susceptible hosts, it again ends up in a blind alley with no suitable organisms to live on. The less virulent forms, on the other hand, kill only some of the hosts, and so, because they do not threaten the existence of the host species, do not evoke any *extreme* counterreaction in the host population. One is almost tempted to say that parasites and their hosts live according to a sort of "gentlemen's agreement," which both sides constantly try to violate by inventing new ways of sneaking around it—a situation not unlike that in international politics. (We shall have more to say about the evasiveness in the host-parasite relationship later in this chapter.) According to this concept, mortal infectious disease is an evolutionary accident that is good for neither the host nor the parasite.

The word "parasite" is used in two ways: in the broader sense it includes both prokaryotic and eukaryotic parasites; in a more restricted sense, it includes only eukaryotic animals and so excludes most microorganisms. Here, we shall use the word in its broad sense and consider consecutively the following groups of parasites: viruses, rickettsiae, chlamydiae, toxoplasma, true bacteria, fungi, and animal parasites.

14.2.1 Viruses

The ancient Romans knew that the bite of a rabid dog transmitted to the afflicted human a potentially lethal substance, and since they thought that the substance was similar to that transmitted by a snake bite, they called it *virus*, which is the Latin word for poison. Although scientists realized more than 2000 years later that the "poison" in the saliva of a rabid dog was nothing like snake poison, they nevertheless retained the term *virus* for the causative agent of rabies and other similar diseases. For a while the agents were referred to as "filtrable viruses," since they, unlike most bacteria, are able to pass through fine filters. However, since some bacteria also pass through such filters and some viruses do not, the adjective "filtrable" was eventually dropped.

Structure and Composition

Viruses are intracellular parasites that cannot grow or multiply outside a cell. They differ from all other parasites and, for that matter, from all other forms of life, in that they are not organized into cells. Although far from the "naked genes" they were once considered to be, they are more primitive than the most primitive cell and are able to replicate only by diverting the biosynthetic pathways of a cell to virus production. In contrast to all other life forms—among which, in each group, there are always some forms that can lead nonparasitic lives—all viruses are parasites.

They range in size from 15 to 300 mμ or more, and in shape from spherical through polyhedral to rod-shaped. A *virus particle*, or *virion*, consists of one or more molecules of nucleic acid (single-stranded RNA, double-stranded DNA, or rarely, single-stranded DNA) contained within a protein coat, or *capsid* (the individual protein subunits of the capsid being called *capsomers*). The complex of nucleic acid and proteins, or *nucleocapsid*, can be either *naked* or enclosed by a lipoprotein *envelope*.

Viruses are classified according to the type of nucleic acid they contain, the capsid symmetry, the presence or absence of envelope, and other features. The main taxonomic groups of viruses are listed in Table 14.1 and the features on which this classification is based are depicted in Figure 14.7.

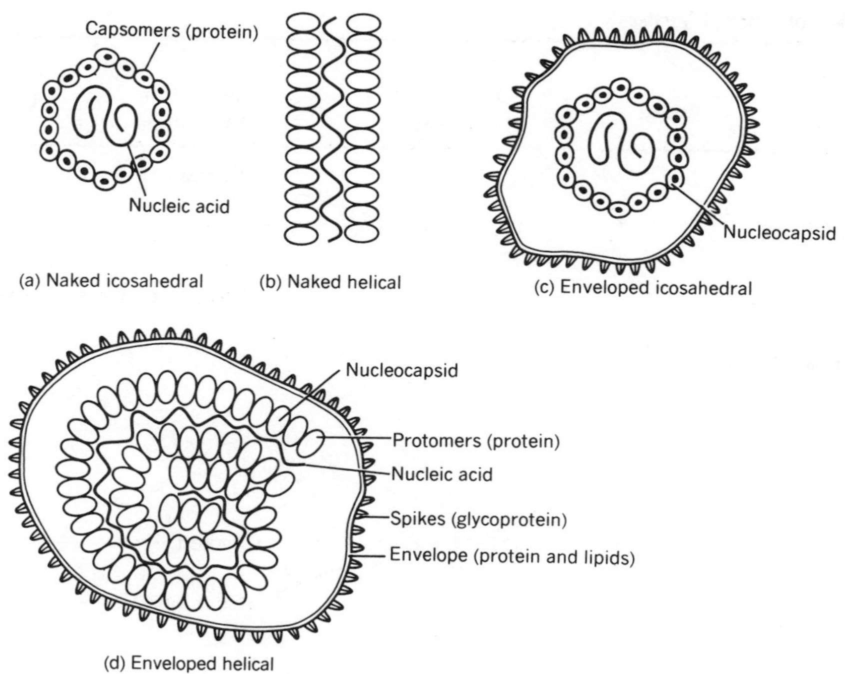

Figure 14.7. The main morphological types of virion. The naked polyhedral virions resemble small crystals; the naked helical virions resemble rods with protein protomers arranged in a helical pattern. In the enveloped polyhedral virions, the crystal-like nucleocapsid is surrounded by a membrane; in the enveloped helical virions, the nucleocapsid forms a coarse, often irregular core, surrounded by a membrane. (Slightly modified from B. D. Davis, R. Dulbecco, H. N. Eisen, H. S. Ginsberg, and W. B. Ward: *Microbiology*, 2nd ed. Harper and Row, Hagerstown, Maryland, 1973.)

Iultiplication Cycle

The multiplication cycle of a virus can be divided into wo phases, extracellular and intracellular. In the *ex-racellular phase*, the virus exists in the form of an nert, infectious virus particle. To be activated and so o initiate the *intracellular phase*, the virus must attach o a suitable cell via a specific membrane receptor and nter the cell's cytoplasm. Some enveloped viruses nay possibly gain entrance to the cell by direct fusion etween the viral membrane and the host's plasma nembrane; other viruses are probably first phago-ytosed or endocytosed and enter the cytoplasm from he phagocytic vacuole, perhaps, again, through mem-rane fusion. During its residence in the phagocytic acuole or following the entrance into the cytoplasm, artial or complete *uncoating* of the virus particle takes lace: the proteins of the capsid are either digested by ysosomal enzymes or shed, and the nucleic acid core s exposed. What happens next depends on the particu-ar type of virus. In DNA viruses (Fig. 14.8*a*) the ex-osed viral DNA enters the nucleus, and a part of it (the so-called *early genes*) is transcribed—either by the host DNA-dependent RNA polymerase, or, in the case of poxviruses, by viral transcriptase, contained in the virion. The transcript, an early messenger RNA, attaches to host-cell ribosomes and is translated into the enzymes needed for viral replication, which occurs with the viral DNA serving as a template. These events are followed by the transcription of *late viral genes* and translation of the messenger RNA into capsid proteins and other components of the viral particle.

In RNA viruses, three modes of replication occur. In the *double-stranded RNA-containing viruses*, one of the two strands is transcribed into an mRNA, which is then translated into proteins. The same mRNA is then used as a template for the synthesis of complementary RNA and the double-stranded RNA species are then incorporated into the forming virions (Fig. 14.8*b*). In the *single-stranded RNA-containing viruses*, the RNA replicates either via a double-stranded RNA (Fig. 14.8*c*) or a double-stranded DNA intermediate (Fig. 14.8*d*). The former mode of replication occurs in two variants. In the picorna viruses, the viral RNA func-

Table 14.1 Classification of Animal Viruses

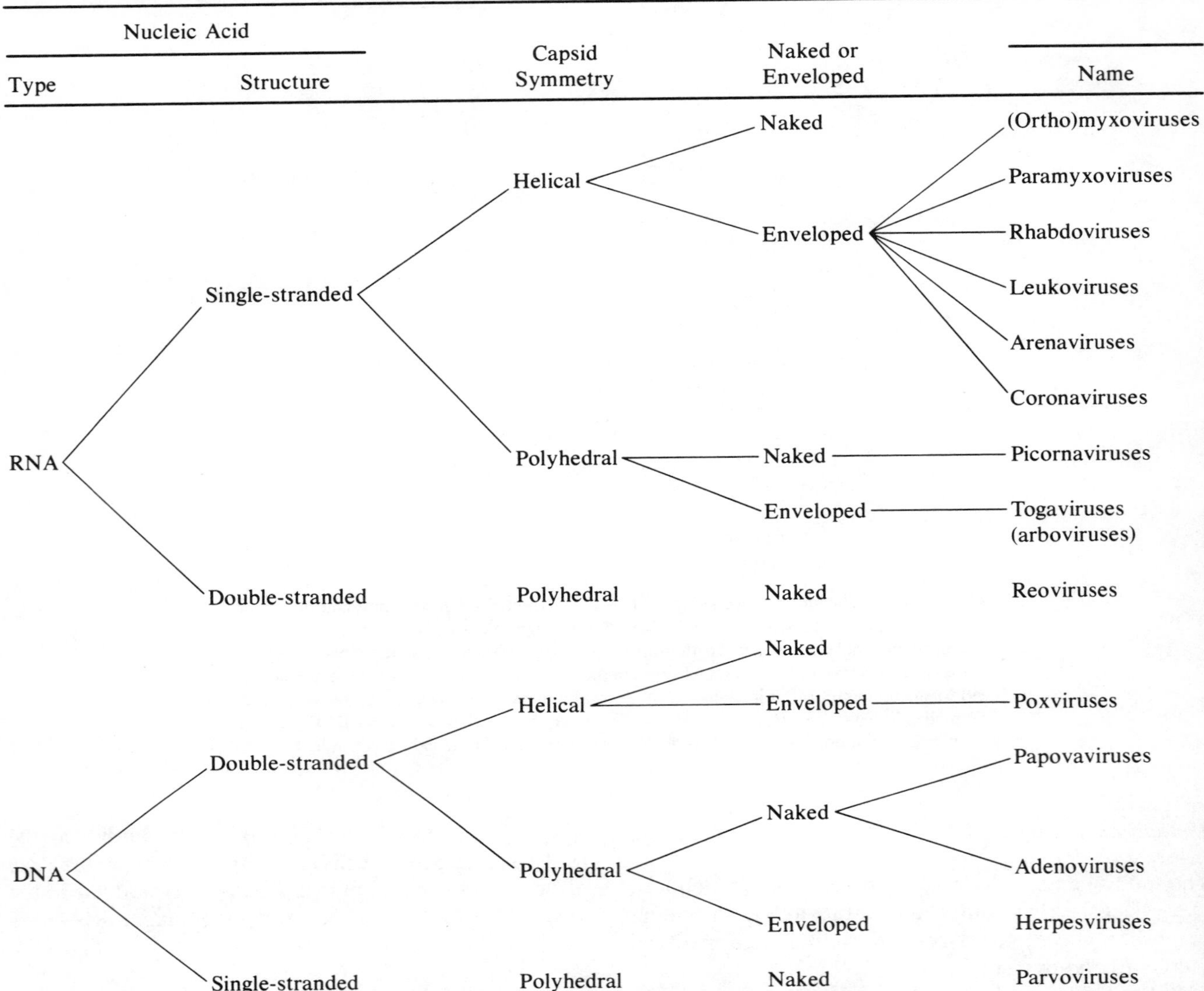

Nucleic Acid: Type	Nucleic Acid: Structure	Capsid Symmetry	Naked or Enveloped	Name
RNA	Single-stranded	Helical	Naked	
			Enveloped	(Ortho)myxoviruses
				Paramyxoviruses
				Rhabdoviruses
				Leukoviruses
				Arenaviruses
				Coronaviruses
		Polyhedral	Naked	Picornaviruses
			Enveloped	Togaviruses (arboviruses)
	Double-stranded	Polyhedral	Naked	Reoviruses
DNA	Double-stranded	Helical	Naked	
			Enveloped	Poxviruses
		Polyhedral	Naked	Papovaviruses
				Adenoviruses
			Enveloped	Herpesviruses
	Single-stranded	Polyhedral	Naked	Parvoviruses

Unclassified: human hepatitis virus

tions directly as messenger RNA, which is translated immediately after uncoating into a single giant polypeptide; this is then cleaved into the individual viral proteins. One of these proteins is a viral replicase (an RNA-dependent RNA polymerase), which then replicates the viral RNA after its release from the host ribosomes. The replication occurs in two steps: first, the original RNA strand (+) makes a copy (−) of itself, forming a double-stranded RNA molecule (+/−), and then the "−" strand of the double-stranded molecule serves as a template for the repeated synthesis of new virion (+) strands. In all other RNA viruses—excep the so-called leukoviruses—the virion RNA is acte upon by a virion-associated, RNA-dependent RNA polymerase, and RNA that is complementary to the virion RNA is produced. Individual genes are the translated separately from this complementary RNA and the RNA replicates in the same manner as that i picorna viruses. In leukoviruses, the virion contain its own polymerase, which acts on virion RNA, syn

Virus Family	
Derivation of Name	Examples
Gr. *orthos*, correct, *myxa*, mucus; true viruses with affinity for mucus	Influenza virus
Gr. *para*, alongside of; in some respect resembling myxoviruses	Mumps virus, measles virus
Gr. *rhabdos*, rod; rod-shaped	Rabies virus
Produce leukemias or leukoses	Leukemia-leukosis-sarcoma viruses, mammary tumor virus
L. *arena*, sand; electron-microscopic appearance of virions	Lymphocytic choriomeningitis virus
In electron micrographs appears as segmented rings suggestive of coronas	Mouse hepatitis virus
L. *picollo*, small, + RNA	Poliomyelitis virus, common cold virus
L. *toga*, cloak (*ar*thropod-*bo*rne)	Semliki Forest virus, yellow fever virus, rubella virus
Respiratory *e*nteric *o*rphan virus	Reovirus type 1
Pox, an eruptive disease	Vaccinia virus, ectromelia virus, variola virus
*Pa*pilloma-*po*lyoma-*va*cuole inducing agent	Rabbit papilloma virus, mouse polyoma virus, simian virus 40
Gr. *adēn*, gland	Human adenovirus
Gr. *hērpes*, spreading skin eruption	Herpes simplex virus, Epstein-Barr virus, Marek's disease virus, varicella virus
L. *parvus*, small	Latent rat virus

hesizing a complementary DNA strand. This RNA-ependent DNA polymerase is, therefore, also called he *reverse transcriptase*. The single DNA strand then eplicates to produce double-stranded DNA, from which both the messenger RNA and new virion RNA molecules are synthesized by DNA-dependent RNA olymerases.

With the single exception of the so-called oncogenic iruses (described in Section 14.3.3), the individual iral components synthesized in the cell assemble spontaneously into a nucleocapsid, which is then liberated from the cell by one of two mechanisms. Some nucleocapsids bud off through the plasma membrane, thereby acquiring an outer membrane envelope that is composed primarily of the host-cell membrane components but also contains some viral components inserted into the plasma membrane before the liberation began. This *steady-state form of liberation* may continue for many hours, and the host cell need not necessarily die in the process. Some of the infected cells

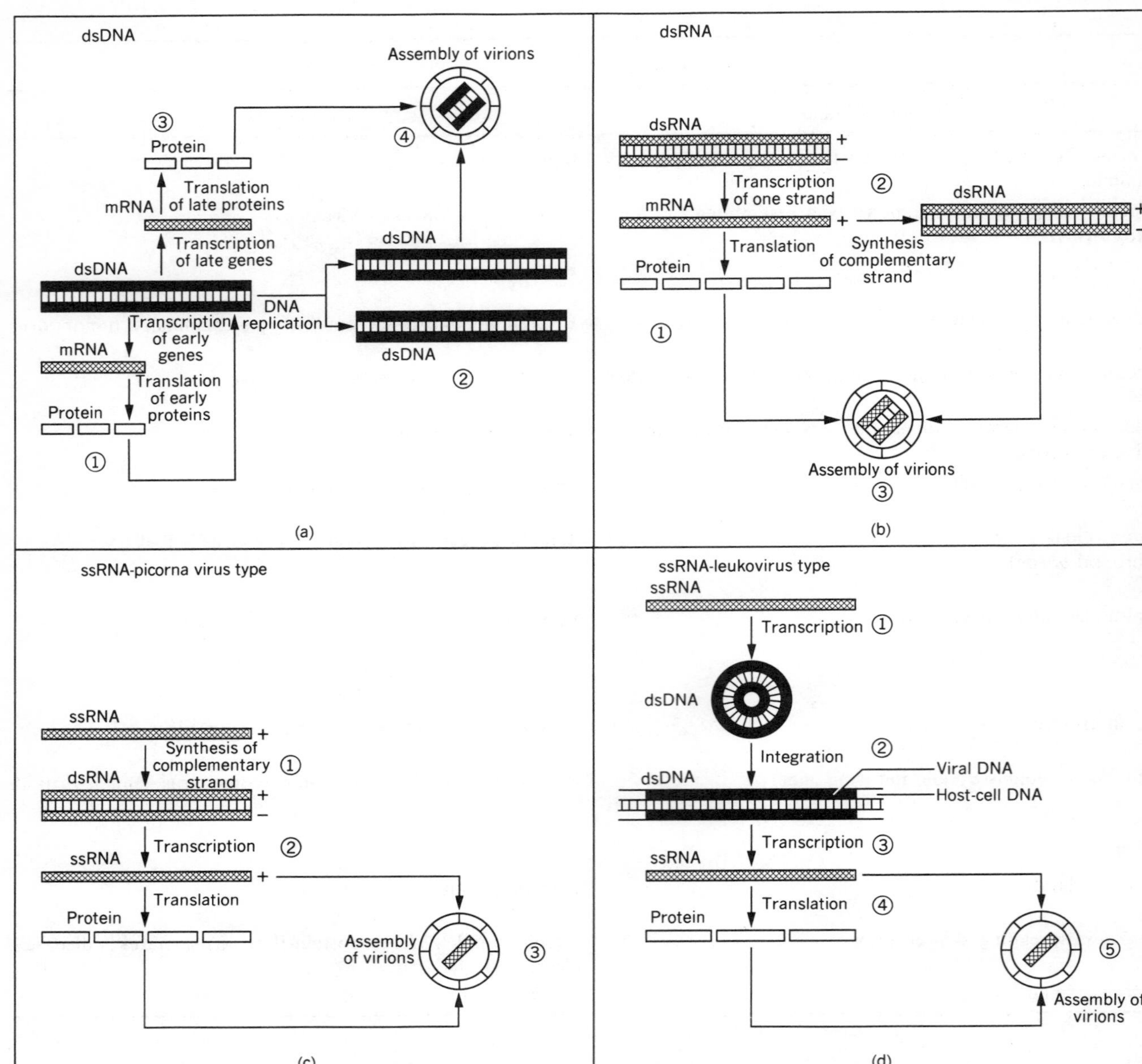

Figure 14.8. Four principal modes of viral multiplication. (*a*) Multiplication of viruses containing double-stranded DNA. (*b*) Multiplicatio viruses containing double-stranded RNA. (*c*) and (*d*) Multiplication of viruses containing single-stranded RNA. Encircled numbers indi approximate sequence of events. A variant of mode *a* occurs in DNA oncogenic viruses in which the viral DNA integrates into the host chromosome before entering the productive phase. A variant of mode *c* occurs in picornaviruses in which the uncoated viral RNA serve mRNA and is translated into proteins; some of the synthesized proteins then act as enzymes in the replication of the single-stranded RNA the double-stranded species.

may even divide and give rise to a clone consisting of cells that are all continually liberating virus particles, because each daughter cell acquires an intracytoplasmic virus during the division. In the second, the *cytolytic form* of liberation, the cell always dies and ruptures, and free virions burst out. This form is char terized by the sudden appearance of a large numbe virions.

Viruses can damage and kill cells in a variety ways, some of which are enumerated below.

Shutdown of Cellular Macromolecule Synthesis. The first thing most viruses do upon entering the cell is block synthesis of cellular RNA and proteins; DNA synthesis is then affected secondarily.

Cytopathic Effect of Viral Proteins. Viral capsids in a high concentration are often toxic for the animal cell, and since a great number of these toxins accumulate in the cell late in the multiplication cycle, the cell is killed by them.

Release of Lysosomal Enzymes. One of the consequences of a viral infection may be an increase in the permeability of lysosomal membranes, leading to the diffusion of lysosomal enzymes into the cytoplasm and degradation of cell components by these enzymes.

Changes in the Permeability of the Plasma Membrane. A virus-induced increase in the permeability of the plasma membrane leads to an influx of water into the cytoplasm and swelling and bursting of the cell.

Formation of Inclusion Bodies. Infected cells can often be identified histologically by their altered staining properties. The alteration is caused by the accumulation of the so-called *inclusion bodies*, which are "virus factories"—foci in which viral nucleic acids and proteins are being synthesized and virions assembled.

Cell Fusion. Certain viruses induce changes in the plasma membrane that favor fusion of neighboring cells. Although the mechanism of this virus-induced fusion is still unknown, the fusion has found an important application in biology as a tool for the production of somatic cell hybrids (see Appendix 6.2).

Viral Hemolysis. Paramyxoviruses contain hemolysins in their envelopes capable of lysing red blood cells.

Induction of Chromosomal Aberrations. Even if a cell survives a virus infection, its genetic apparatus may be so altered that the cell may not be able to reproduce properly. Chromatid breaks, fragmentation, and even "pulverization" of chromosomes are well-documented consequences of viral infections.

Types of Infection

Three major types of virus infection can be distinguished, depending on what the virus does to the host cell (Fig. 14.9): *cytolytic infections*, in which most of the infected cells are destroyed by viral multiplication; *steady-state infections*, in which only some cells are lysed by the virus, while others stay alive and keep producing viral particles; and the *integrated type of infection*, in which the genetic material of the virus incorporates into the genome of the host cell. (The last type will be discussed in the section on tumor immunology later in this chapter.) Each of the first two types can be divided further into localized and generalized.

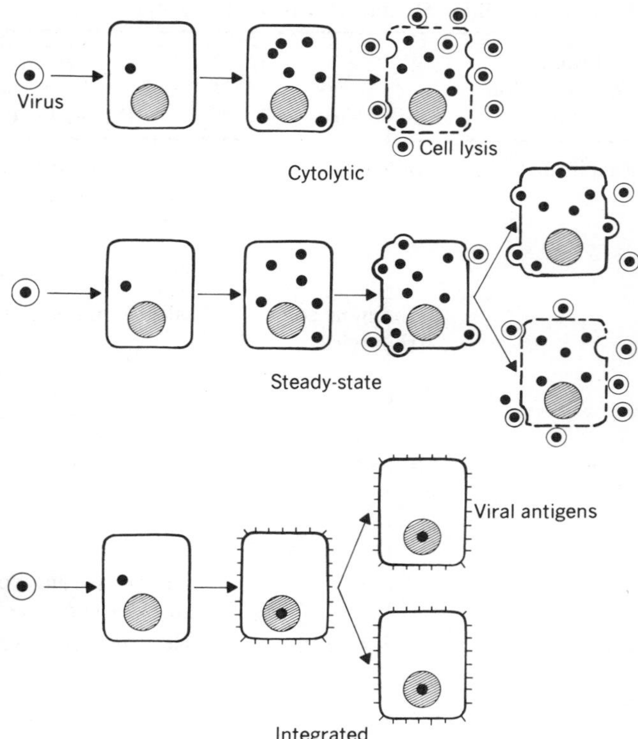

Figure 14.9. The three principal types of virus–host cell interaction.

In a *localized infection*, viral multiplication and cell damage remain localized near the site of entry, and the virus spreads from one cell to another in the same region by diffusion in intercellular spaces, cell contact, or secretions and excretions. The result is the formation of a single lesion or group of lesions in a particular organ. According to their target organs, localized infections are divided into *dermatropic* (affecting the skin), *neurotropic* (affecting the nervous system), *pneumotropic* (affecting the respiratory system), and so on.

In *generalized* (*systemic*, *disseminated*) *infections*, on the other hand, the virus spreads from the original site

Table 14.2 Major Human Diseases Caused by Viruses

Principal Transmission Route	Virus	Properties of Virus	Symptoms of Disease
Respiratory	Influenza	ssRNA, myxovirus group, host-derived envelope	Inflammation of epithelial cells lining respirato passages. Chills, fever, severe prostration, headache, muscle aches, dry cough. Sudden onset. Complications: secondary bacterial infections.
	Common cold (rhinovirus)	ssRNA, picornavirus group	Mild upper respiratory inflammation. Nasal obstruction and discharge, sneezing, scratch throat, mild cough, malaise. Complications: bronchitis.
	Measles (rubella)	ssRNA, paramyxovirus group, host-derived envelope	First signs: acute respiratory inflammation, cough, fever, and conjunctivitis. Later: oval eruption called Koplik's spot; measle rash, begins on the head and moves downward, eventually covering the entire body.
	Mumps	ssRNA, paramyxovirus group, host-derived envelope	Acute inflammation of the salivary (parotid) gland and the reproductive organs.
Enteric	Poliomyelitis	ssRNA, picornavirus group	First signs: fever, headache, gastroenteric disturbances. Later: inflammation of the gre matter of the spinal cord, stiff neck and bac flaccid paralysis of one or more muscle grou
	Infectious hepatitis	Largely unknown	Inflammation and necrosis of the liver, usua accompanied by jaundice. Short incubation period (from 15 to 40 days).
	Serum hepatitis	Largely unknown	Transmitted by injection of infected blood. Long incubation period (from 60 to 160 days otherwise symptoms similar to those of infectious hepatitis.
Direct contact, fomites	Herpes simplex	dsDNA, herpesvirus group, host-derived envelope	Eruption of one or more groups of vesicles c the lips or on reproductive organs.
	German measles (rubella)	ssRNA, togavirus group	Enlarged lymph nodes, fever, rash, usually mild.
	Chicken pox (varicella)	dsDNA, herpesvirus group, host-derived envelope	Sparse eruptions of papules, becoming vesic and then pustules. Occurs usually in childre only.
	Smallpox (variola major)	dsDNA, poxvirus group	Ulceration of mucous membranes, skin lesio and eruptions, fever. The virus is now virtua eradicated.
Animal bites	Rabies	ssRNA, rhabdovirus group, host-derived envelope	Inflammation of the brain accompanied by paralysis, delirium, and convulsions.
	Yellow fever	ssRNA, togavirus group	Headache, backache, fever, nausea, and vomiting; liver damage accompanied by jaundice.

of entry by blood and lymphatics to other organs, multiplies in these organs, spreads from them to still other organs, and so forth. The presence of viruses in the blood is referred to as *viremia*.

We shall now describe the major types of viral infe tion, using a few selected specific examples. Br characteristics of viruses causing major diseases a given in Table 14.2.

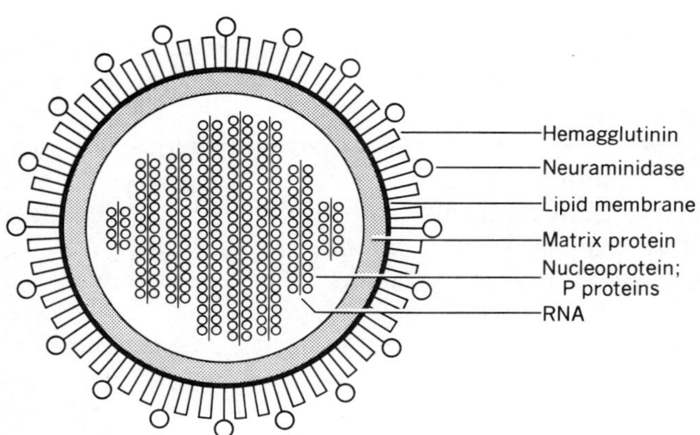

Figure 14.10. Schematic diagram of an influenza A virus. (Modified from P. Palese: *Cell* **10:**1–10, 1977.)

Influenza is an example of a cytolytic virus causing a localized infection. The virus is spherical in shape (Fig. 14.10) and about 900 to 1100 Å in diameter. Its surface is covered with evenly spaced spikes, which are of two kinds—one consisting of hemagglutinin molecules responsible for agglutination of erythrocytes, and the other consisting of the enzyme neuraminidase. The spikes project from an envelope that encloses a core of proteins and eight single-stranded RNA molecules. Immunologically, the influenza virus can be identified by means of four kinds of antigen carried by the spike hemagglutinin (H), the spike neuraminidase (N), the major structural proteins of the envelope (M), and an internal nucleocapsid molecule (S). On the basis of their S and M molecules, influenza viruses can be divided into three immunologically distinct types—A, B, and C—carrying distinct, noncross-reactive antigens. According to its H and N antigens each type can be divided further into subtypes, designated by subscript numbers [e.g., $A_1(N_1H_1)$, $A_2(N_2H_2)$, etc.]. We shall have more to say about the variation generating these subtypes later in this chapter.

The virus attaches to the surface of the cells lining the respiratory tract (nose, throat, trachea, lungs) by means of H spikes and plasma membrane receptors; the same receptors are apparently present on erythrocytes too, which explains why the virus can agglutinate these cells. After the attachment, the virus particle fuses with the host cell's plasma membrane, is engulfed by the cell, uncoats, and begins to multiply. During this period the virus temporarily loses its infectivity, a phase referred to as *viral eclipse*. The multiplication is so rapid that, in a matter of hours after entering the cell, one virus particle can give rise to as many as 1000 offspring. The new generation of virus particles escapes from the cell, thereby killing it, and the massive necrosis accompanying the particle release causes desquamation of the respiratory epithelium. The dried mucus and the virions are then released into the air, during sneezing and coughing, in the form of small droplets, which, when they dry, turn into so-called droplet-nuclei. Shedding of the virus starts about 24 hours after exposure to the infection and continues for about a week. In the droplet-nuclei the virus is capable of staying alive for many hours, provided it is not exposed to sunlight. The nuclei are carried about by air currents, and when inhaled by a susceptible person, they get into the nose or all the way into the lungs and start a new infection. The incubation time of the influenza virus is only two days, but it can range from one to seven days. The first symptoms of the disease are headache, a general feeling of illness, and either chills or feverishness. Within a few hours, the bodily temperature rises to about 39°C, or even higher, and the fever lasts for about three days. Other symptoms are short, dry cough, aching of the back and leg muscles, and sometimes pains in the joints. The fever, aches, and pain distinguish influenza from the common cold with which it is sometimes confused. The acute phase of the infection is over in three to five days, but malaise persists for another week. The viral disease may be accompanied by bacterial infection, leading to pneumonia. The disease is often fatal to a great number of people within a relatively short time, so that influenza virus has earned the dubious distinction of being the last great plague of humanity. The virus can also multiply in rodent and even bird cells.

The *ectromelia*, or *mouse pox*, is an example of a virus that causes a cytopathic disseminated infection. The virus closely resembles human vaccinia, or smallpox virus, described in Chapter 2, but as the name indicates, it is indigenous to the house mouse. The virus enters the skin through an abrasion and multiplies in the epidermal cells at the site of entry, causing local swelling, ulceration, and ultimately scarring of the tissue (the *primary lesion*; see Fig. 14.11). Some of the shed particles are then carried, via the lymphatics, into regional lymph nodes, where a second round of virus multiplication occurs. From the lymph nodes the particles spread into the blood (*primary viremia*) and are disseminated into various other organs—in particular, the spleen and liver. In these organs, the virus enters and multiplies in the parenchymal cells, causing focal necrosis. The new generation of virions then enters the bloodstream again (*secondary viremia*) and is delivered to the ultimate target tissue, the skin.

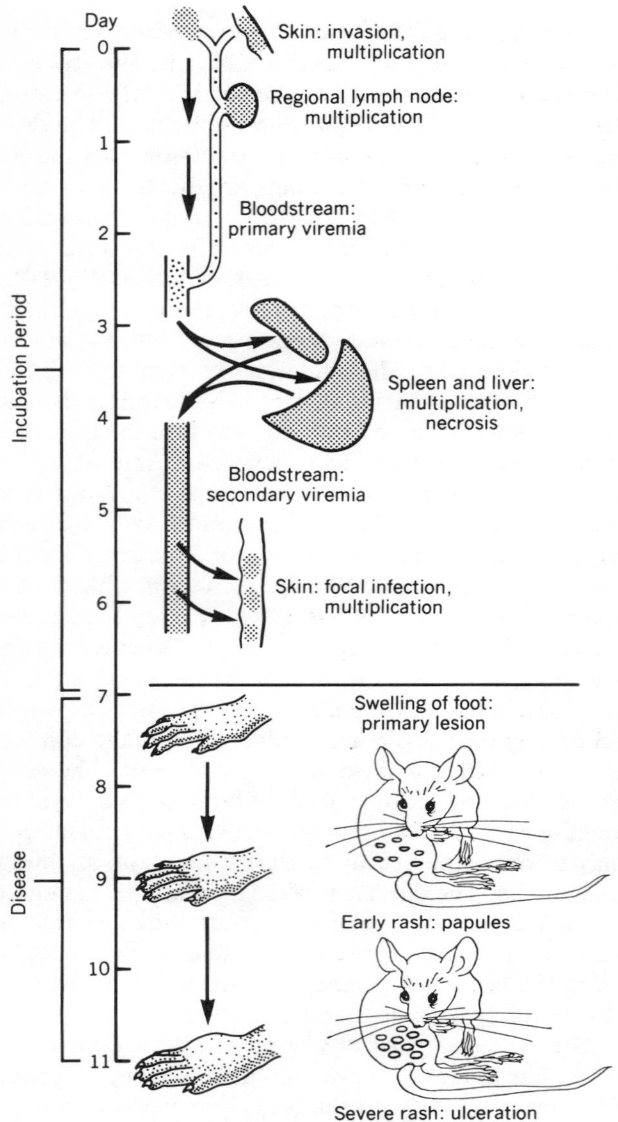

Figure 14.11. Sequence of events in an infection of mice with the mouse pox virus. (Modified from F. Fenner: *Lancet* **2**:915, 1948.)

This return of the virus to the skin marks the end of its *incubation period*, during which no conspicuous signs of the disease are visible. The virus again enters the epidermal cells, multiplies in them, and kills them, causing a rash of lesions all over the mouse body. The lesions are particularly pronounced on the feet and tail, where they are often accompanied by characteristic swelling and necrosis, caused by the obstruction of blood flow. The necrosis is sometimes so strong that the feet or tail fall off—a symptom from which the scientific name of the disease is derived (Gr. *ectrosis*, miscarriage, absence of a part, *melos*, limb). The mortality rate from the infection is as high as 50 to 100 percent, and so, for mouse breeders, it is ectromelia that is the great plague.

As an example of a steady-state infection, we shall describe that caused by the *herpes simplex virus*. The name derives from the fact that the virus causes spreading skin eruptions or shingles (Gr. *herpo*, to creep). The virion is about 1800 Å in diameter and consists of a DNA-containing core; an icosahedral capsid, composed of 162 elongated, hexagonal capsomers; a granular zone; and an envelope with short projections. (The basic structure of the virion is similar to that shown in Fig. 14.7c.) The virus enters the body through breaks in the skin or the mucous membranes of the mouth, throat, genitals, or eye. After fusion with the epidermal or epithelial cells, the virus enters an eclipse period of about five or six hours, during which it multiplies within the cell. The initial shedding of the virus leads to the formation of a lesion—a small blister or a cold sore. Fluid exudes from the sore and forms a crust, which eventually flakes off. The shed virus can be transferred to another inidividual by person-to-person contact or by contaminated eating and drinking utensils. Sometimes the infection also spreads to regional lymph nodes and causes their enlargement. The initial infection ordinarily occurs in children from six to 18 months of age, and causes a primary disease characterized by multiple vesicles. When the initial infection recedes, the virus persists in the body, producing a *latent infection*. It stays in the cell in the presence of immunity but does not cause disease. This steady state is readily upset by a number of factors, such as upper respiratory tract infection, fever, menstrual period, physical and emotional stress, or overexposure to sunlight. Any of these factors can trigger a recurrent disease and cause a reappearance of the sores.

Finally, we shall mention briefly one more virus, which is so unorthodox and so esoteric in its properties that it has not yet been seen, even in the best electron microscope. The virus causes a disease called *kuru*, which is confined to tribes living in the valleys of the mountainous interior of New Guinea. In the language of these tribes, *kuru* means shivering or trembling, which are the characteristics of the disease. The symptoms worsen progressively over a period of about a year, eventually leading to complete immobility and virtually always to death of the victim. The symptoms are caused by degenerative changes in the patient's central nervous system—a progressive vacuolization of nerve cells and overgrowth of glial cells, giving the grey matter of the brain a spongelike appearance. The changes are caused by slow multiplication of a virus that is unconventional in many respects: it is resistant to ultraviolet and ionizing irradiation, has an extremely long incubation period (months, years, or even decades), causes no inflammatory response, immunity, or interferon response (see below), is invisible by electron microscopy, produces no demonstrable viral antigens and no inclusion bodies, and contains no demonstrable nucleic acid—in short, it has all the characteristics of a phantom. But we know it does exist, since the infection is transmitted from one person to another by cannibalism. As part of a rite of mourning and respect for the dead kinsman, the tribesmen eat the deceased person's brain and so perpetuate the infection. There are several other examples of this kind of *slow-virus infection*, the best known of which is *scrapie*, a disease of sheep characterized by a progressive loss of the power of muscular coordination, wasting, and death.

Defense Against Viruses

The host has at its disposal a whole range of mechanisms aimed at preventing viral infection or, when infection has already occurred, at containing it. Which of these it employs depends on the circumstances of the infection; usually, however, several mechanisms are activated simultaneously. We shall discuss the main mechanisms in the order of their increasing specificity.

Mechanical Protection. To initiate an infection, a virus must reach the right bodily surface and be able to stay on it long enough to adsorb to the right cell. A respiratory virus must be inhaled with a droplet and land on the surface of the respiratory system; an enteric virus must be ingested with contaminated food or drink; an arbovirus must be injected into the blood by an insect sting; a dermatropic virus must be deposited on the skin by direct contact with an infected person or a contaminated object (fomite); and a neurotropic virus must enter the body—for example, through an animal bite. Viruses that have landed on the right bodily surface may be prevented from infecting the host by one of several mechanisms: they can be removed by the mucociliary escalator; they can be prevented from attaching by the movement of the intestines; they can be wiped off the corneal surface; or they can be flushed from the urethra with urine. Those viruses that manage to hold onto the surface must be able to penetrate the mucosal layer, which contains a number of antiviral substances, including antibodies (see below), and must find the receptors to which it will bind. If a virus that normally multiplies in epithelial cells gets this far, it has almost—but not quite—made it; all it has to do now is penetrate the epithelial cells. Viruses multiplying in other tissues must overcome several other obstacles before they get to their target organs. Because of the short duration of their journey to the target organ, viruses infecting the epithelial cells are highly successful parasites. Their success is further augmented by their effective use of a hit-and-run tactic: they enter epithelial cells, multiply rapidly in them, and exit by killing the cells. The whole attack is over within a few days, well before the body has had time to develop immunity against them. Furthermore, since the infection is limited to the epithelial layer and affects the underlying tissue very little, the defense is limited to primarily nonimmunological resistance mechanisms. Upon exiting from one focus of infection, the virus may be disseminated by the movement of the liquid or semi-liquid film on the mucosal surface, and fresh infectious foci may be established. Infections on wet surfaces, such as the mucosa of the respiratory system, are therefore usually more disseminated than infections on relatively dry surfaces, such as the skin.

Interferon. Even when inside the cell, the virus has not yet fully won the battle, for its multiplication then stimulates the production, by the infected cells, of a specialized protein called *interferon*, which will attempt to confine the infection to the few already invaded cells. Because of its importance in checking viral infections and the interest it has aroused in recent years, we shall have a close look at interferon before we proceed further in the discussion of other antiviral defense reactions.

Discovery. Virologists have known for some time that individuals suffering from one virus-caused illness virtually never contract another viral disease at the same time. But it was not until 1957 that Alick Isaacs and Jean Lindenmann discovered the basis for this *viral interference*. They cultured chicken cells in vitro, infected them with influenza virus, and demonstrated that, as expected, these cells were resistant to infection by other viruses. They then harvested the medium from the infected cultures, freed it from cells and viruses, added it to a culture of healthy cells, and challenged these with a virus. When the treated cultures remained uninfected, Isaacs and Lindenmann concluded that the virus infection in the primary culture had stimulated the cells to produce a soluble substance that interfered with further viral assault. They called the substance *interferon*.

Methods of Study. Interferon can be produced either in vitro or in vivo. The in vitro method is the one used by Isaacs and Lindenmann, in which the interferon source is the culture fluid of virus-infected cells. The fluid can be tested in vitro by observing, as Isaacs and Lindenmann did, whether it reduces the number of virus-produced plaques when added to fresh cells, or in vivo, by determining whether injection of the fluid into an animal prevents a virus-caused disease. In the in vivo interferon production method, one infects the animal and determines whether the treatment prevents infection of the same animal by another virus. Since cells produce only minute amounts of interferon, it is virtually impossible to isolate the substance from an infected animal, so most interferon studies have been done on a substance produced by cultured cells. The activity of an interferon preparation is expressed in relative units—for example, as *interferon* titer, which is the concentration of cultured fluid resulting in a 50 percent reduction in the number of viral plaques in comparison to a control. International standards to which one might compare one's preparation are not yet established.

Production. Interferon can be induced not only by viruses, but by other stimuli, some of which induce production both in vivo and in vitro (e.g., certain synthetic or natural polyribonucleotides), while others act only in vivo, presumably because they stimulate cells that are either absent or poorly represented in culture. To the latter category of stimuli belong certain bacteria and bacterial products (e.g., endotoxin), rickettsiae, protozoa, organic compounds (such as pyran copolymers, polyacrylic acid copolymers, vinyl copolymers, and polyvinylsulfate), antibiotics, polysaccharides, mitogens, and antigens. There may be two mechanisms of interferon induction—one specific, mediated primarily by viruses, and another more general, mediated by stimuli altering cell metabolism.

Interferon is produced by host cells, not by viruses, and the three main cell types capable of producing it are fibroblasts, T lymphocytes, and macrophages (monocytes). The capacity to produce the substance is probably present in all vertebrates; production by invertebrate cells has not been demonstrated, but whether this is because invertebrates do not produce interferon or because only a few suitable culture systems of invertebrate cells are available is not known. Prokaryotes definitely do not produce interferon, and plants produce a substance that resembles it functionally, but this resemblance may be superficial.

Specificity. With few exceptions, interferon is species-specific; so, for example, human interferon works in humans but not in most other vertebrate species, mouse interferon works in the mouse, and so on. An exception is the activity of human interferon on rabbit and mouse cells. Low cross-reactivity can sometimes also be demonstrated between cells of closely related species. But interferon is not virus-specific, so that the interferon induced by one type of virus makes cells resistant to others. Probably all viruses are sensitive to the substance, but not all to the same degree. The variation in sensitivity is independent of the inducing virus: a virus may be relatively resistant to the interferon that it itself has induced, but this very same interferon may act as a strong inhibitor of another virus.

Properties. There are at least three interferon (IFN) types, designated by the Greek letters α, β, and γ, and distinguished by their antigenic properties.

INF-α was originally discovered as a product of leukocytes and is therefore also referred to as *leukocyte interferon* (LeIF; other synonyms are classical or type I interferon). Human INF-α is a family of proteins with at least five different, though homologous, primary structures. The individual proteins are probably the products of different genes. Two of the proteins have been sequenced and shown to differ in about 17 percent of their amino acids.

INF-β was originally discovered as a product of virus-infected fibroblasts and so it is also referred to as *fibroblast interferon* (FIF). Although INF-α and INF-β may be structurally sufficiently similar for them to be recognized by the same receptor, they are encoded by different genes, have a different host-cell range, different dose-response curves when assayed for antiviral activity in cell cultures, and a varying degree of cytostatic action on cells. Furthermore, antibodies raised against one type do not neutralize the other. Both INF-α and INF-β are proteins containing about 166 amino acids and having molecular weights of approximately 20,000 daltons. Recent studies indicate about 45 percent sequence homology between them.

INF-γ, the so-called *immune interferon* (type II), is produced by mitogen- or antigen-stimulated T lymphocytes. It differs from INF-α and INF-β in that it is labile at pH 2 and in that it has more pronounced anticellular than antiviral activity (see below).

Mechanism of Action. The two main effects of interferon are inhibitory: it prevents virus replication and inhibits cell growth. The antiviral effect can be explained

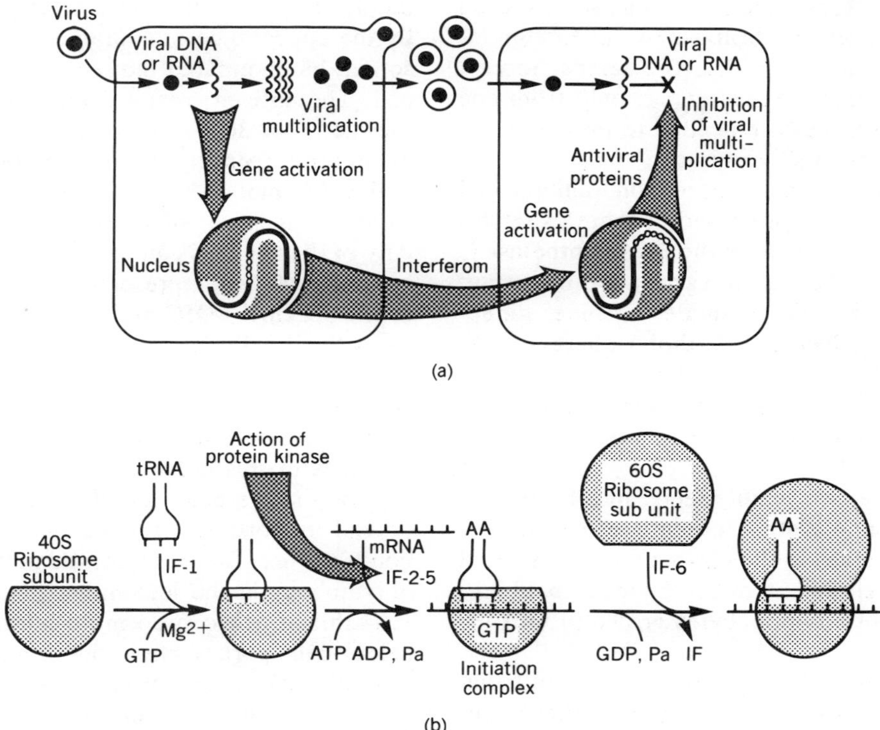

Figure 14.12. Interferon synthesis (*a*) and the postulated mechanism of action of interferon-induced protein kinase in the initiation phase of protein synthesis (*b*). AA_1, first amino acid of the polypeptide chain; ADP, adenosine diphosphate; ATP, adenosine triphosphate; GDP, guanosine diphosphate; GTP, guanosine triphosphate; IF, initiation factor.

as follows (Fig. 14.12*a*). The infecting virus adsorbs to the host cell, penetrates the cell membrane, releases its genetic material, and replicates in the cell. The new viruses leave the cell, enter the surrounding fluid, and penetrate another cell. During the early stages of infection, the virus causes a series of changes in the metabolism of the first cell, some of which lead to the activation of the interferon genes in the host's genome. The activated genes produce messenger RNA, which then leaves the nucleus and is translated in the cytoplasm by host-cell ribosomes into protein—interferon. Some of the interferon leaves the first cell and enters the surrounding fluid and then the second cell. Once synthesized, interferon itself stimulates the synthesis of two enzymes—protein kinase and 2-5A synthetase. The first of these, *protein kinase*, transfers a phosphate group to an initiation factor, IF-2, involved with other such factors in protein synthesis. IF-2 normally holds the initiation complex of protein synthesis (the strand of mRNA to be translated, the smaller of the two ribosome subunits, and the initiator tRNA) together (Fig. 14.12*b*). The phosphorylated form of IF-2 is no longer able to assist in the formation of the initiation complex, and the viral mRNA remains untranslated; it is then attacked by ribonucleases and degraded. The induction of protein kinase synthesis requires double-stranded RNA, probably supplied by viral mRNA, which, although single-stranded, loops back on itself to form double-stranded regions. The prsence of these regions in viral mRNA might be the basis for the specificity of protein kinase. If the host's mRNA molecules were to lack such regions, they would be protected from the action of this enzyme and host-cell protein synthesis would continue, while viral protein synthesis would be blocked.

The second enzyme, 2-5*A synthetase*, catalyzes the polymerization of adenine nucleotides into a long chain of adenine units called 2,5-oligoadenylic acid. This oligonucleotide activates ribonucleases, normally present in the cell in an inactive form, which then degrade viral mRNA.

Shortly after the first interferon is produced, yet another gene is activated and a regulatory protein is produced that eventually inactivates the interferon gene so that the production stops. Interferon thus serves as an intercellular messenger that brings news of foreign invasion to other cells and mobilizes the defense forces. It is an extremely effective messenger: only from one to 10 interferon molecules are needed to protect a cell against an interferon-sensitive virus.

The mechanism by which interferon inhibits cell growth is not known. One possibility is that this inhibition occurs via the 2-5A system: the 2-5A synthetase is capable of adding AMP to a variety of important metabolites, such as nicotinamide adenine dinucleotide (NAD) or adenosine 5′-diphosphate (ADP) ribose, and the dephosphorylated core of 2-5A is known to inhibit DNA synthesis. So, through the 2-5A system, interferon has access to mechanisms regulating normal cell growth.

In addition to the two main effects, interferon also modulates the immune system, potentiates natural killer cells, effects changes in the plasma membrane, and enhances the expression of major histocompatibility complex molecules on lymphocytes grown in vitro.

Phagocytosis. A virus that has crossed the epithelial layer of the body's surface on its way to distant target organs is like a soldier who has managed to get past the barbed wire line: it now faces the real defenders in their trenches—the macrophages of the subepithelial tissues. The macrophages will try to ingest the virus particles by phagocytosis and destroy them inside their phagocytic vacuoles. But macrophages do not always succeed in killing the invaders. There are viruses that not only avoid being killed inside the phagocytic vacuoles, but also manage to multiply within them. Viruses that have escaped the assault by the front-line macrophages are carried, with the lymph, into regional lymph nodes and filtered through a second macrophage entrenchment in the nodes' sinuses. The viruses that escape even this second macrophage defense line are carried by the blood to various organs (such as the liver) that are rich in reticuloendothelial system cells. Here macrophages and histiocytes get one more chance to catch the invader. The reticuloendothelial system is also the main site of capture for viruses entering the blood directly through insect stings or animal bites. In addition to their function in phagocytosis, macrophages also contribute to the neutralization of the viral infection by cleaning up the debris of the destroyed cells and presenting viral antigens to T lymphocytes.

T-Lymphocyte Responses. Once a virus infects a cell and disappears from intercellular spaces, it can no longer be recognized directly by immune cells. Fortunately, however, the virus often betrays its presence by the appearance of characteristic *viral antigens*, and so can be eliminated indirectly by killing the infected cell. The antigens result from insertion of newly synthesized, virally encoded proteins into the plasma membrane, from the production of new host-encoded molecules induced by the presence of the virus, or from modification of normal membrane antigenicity. Any of these forms can be recognized specifically by T lymphocytes when presented to T cells in the context of the species' MHC molecules. The recognition activates the T cells, turning some of them into killers and others into regulatory cells. The killer T lymphocytes attack the host cell that displays viral antigens and destroy it before the virus can mature in it. The disadvantages of this defense mechanism is that it attacks the body's own cells, and if these cells happen to be of crucial importance for normal functioning of the body—as are, for example, the neural cells in the case of lymphocytic choriomeningitis infection (see Chapter 12)—this attack can do more harm than good. The T helper cells participate in the production of antibodies to viral particles and produce factors that recruit, activate, and arm macrophages for combating the infection.

Antibody-Mediated Responses. Antibodies combat virus infection either immediately, at the site of virus entry, or later, when the infection spreads into the blood. At the portal of entry, the defending antibodies are mostly of the IgA class, whereas in the blood, other antibody classes take part in the defense. However, once a virus has gained access to the circulation, antibodies cannot prevent an infection; they merely help to contain it.

Antibodies act on viruses in two principal ways, directly or indirectly. In the direct way, antibodies cause *virus neutralization*—that is, an abolition of viral infectivity. Antibodies can bind directly to virus particles and prevent their adsorption to cellular receptors; they may interfere with the penetration of a virus into a cell; or they may hinder proper uncoating of the virion. The mechanism of virus neutralization is not understood, but the simplest explanation is that the antibodies interfere sterically with the normal viral function. Antibodies can be assisted in their neutralizing role by complement components, and furthermore, the interaction of virus-bound antibodies with the full array of complement components, including the late-acting ones, may lead to lysis of virus particles. But not all viruses are susceptible to antibody-mediated complement lysis.

In the indirect way, antibodies interact with viral

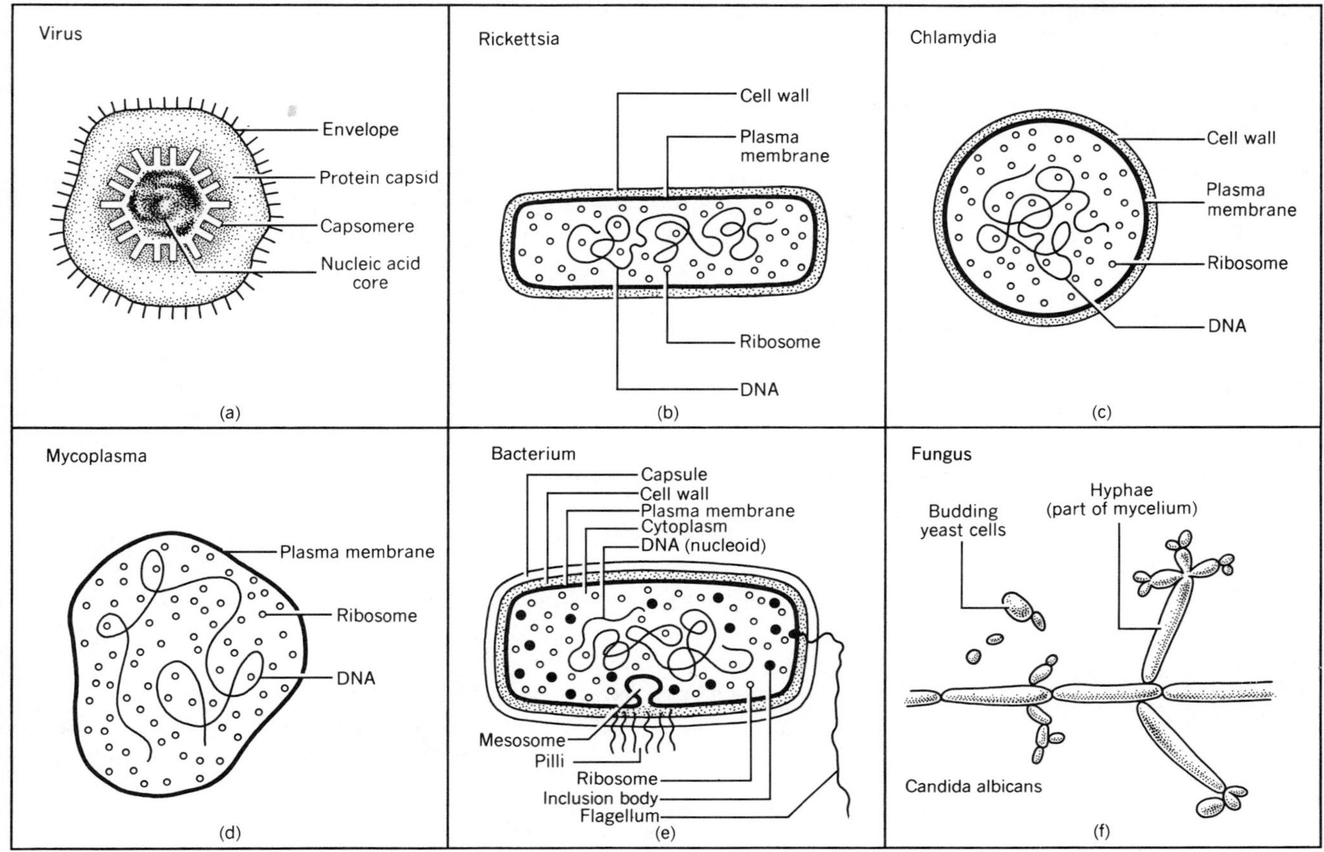

Figure 14.13. General structural features of microbial parasites.

antigens on the surface of the infected cell and mediate elimination of these cells, either through complement or through antibody-dependent cell-mediated lysis. Antibodies can also bind to macrophages and facilitate phagocytosis—that is, they have an opsonizing effect.

Exposure to some viruses (e.g., those causing smallpox, specific types of poliomyelitis, measles, mumps, and yellow fever) induces lasting immunity. Individuals who have once contracted diseases caused by these viruses suffer an attack of the same disease again only rarely (see description of smallpox infection in Chapter 2). On the other hand, exposure to certain other viruses (e.g., influenza, common cold, and certain other forms of poliomyelitis) does not protect individuals from subsequent bouts with the same illness. The reason for the absence of durable immunity to these viruses is that the viruses exist in several different genetic variants; the immunity to one variant does not prevent other variants from attacking the host (see the description of antigenic variation later in this chapter).

14.2.2 Atypical Bacteria

Rickettsiae

Rickettsiae, named after their discoverer, the American pathologist Howard T. Ricketts, were once thought to be midway between large viruses and small bacteria. They are now known to be atypical bacteria, possessing cell walls and membranes, both types of nucleic acid (DNA and RNA), and a complete machinery for protein synthesis (Fig. 14.13). Like viruses, however, all rickettsiae are intracellular parasites. They live in certain groups of arthropods (notably fleas, lice, and ticks) without causing any apparent disease. However, when transmitted by a bite to a vertebrate host, they cause severe, often fatal infection (Table 14.3). Rickettsiae are the cause of epidemic typhus, murine or endemic typhus, and Rocky Mountain spotted fever. *Epidemic typhus* is carried by the human louse, in which the rickettsiae multiply in the

Table 14.3 Major Human Diseases Caused by Atypical Bacteria

Microorganisms	Disease	Manifestations	Transmission
Rickettsiae			
Rickettsia rickettsii	Rocky Mountain spotted fever	Endothelial cell damage, lesions in small blood vessels, bleeding and necrosis. Fever, headaches. Rash on hands and feet.	Tick *Dermacentor andersoni*
Rickettsia prowazekii	Epidemic typhus fever	Obligate intracellular pathogen of epithelial cells. Fever, headache, muscular pains, rash.	Human louse *Pediculus humanus*
Rickettsia typhi	Endemic (murine) typhus	Similar to above but less severe.	Rat flea *Nosopsyllus fasciatus*
Rickettsia tsutsugamushi	Scrub typhus (tsutsugamushi fever)	A lesion called eschar at site of infection. Rash, headache, fever.	Chigger mite *Trombicula akamushi*
Rickettsia akari	Rickettsial pox	Lesion at site of infection. Rash, fever.	Tropical rat mite *Bdellonyssus bacoti*
Rickettsia quintana	Trench fever	Rash, headache, fever.	Human louse *Pediculus humanus*
Coxiella burnetii	Q fever	Mild pneumonia, hepatitis, headache, fever.	Tick *Dermacentor andersoni*
Chlamydia			
Chlamydia psittaci	Psittacosis	Obligate intracellular pathogen. Focal areas of necrosis in the liver and spleen, with a predominance of mononuclear cells. In the lungs, thickening of alveolar walls. Pneumonia, hepatitis, inflammation of brain and heart, skin rash.	Birds
Chlamydia trachomatis	Trachoma	Obligatory pathogen of epithelial cells of the eye. Chronic inflammation of conjunctiva, scarring of conjunctiva.	Infection limited to humans
Mycoplasmas			
Mycoplasma pneumoniae	Primary atypical pneumonia	Extracellular parasite. Damages epithelial cells of the respiratory system. Pneumonia. Fever, headache, fatigue, sore throat, cough.	Limited to humans

intestinal lining and escape with excrements. They enter the body through abrasions produced by scratching a louse bite. *Murine typhus* is a disease of rats and humans (the rat belongs to the family *Muridae*), transmitted to humans by rat fleas. *Rocky Mountain spotted fever* is transmitted by the bite of the wood or dog tick.

Chlamydia

Chlamydia (Gr. *chlamys*, cloak) is another group of small, atypical bacteria previously considered to be large viruses (Fig. 14.13). They resemble rickettsiae, from which they differ in that they are not transmitted through invertebrate hosts; they pass directly from one vertebrate to another. Like rickettsiae, chlamydia are obligatory intracellular parasites. They are responsible for psittacosis, lymphogranuloma, and trachoma (Table 14.3). *Psittacosis*, or parrot disease (Gr. *psittakos*, parrot, suffix *-osis*, condition), is an infectious disease of birds, especially parrots, characterized by diarrhea, loss of appetite, wasting, and feather ruffling. When transmitted to humans (through handling or by inhalation of dried bird feces), chlamydia cause a disease resembling pneumonia or influenza. *Lymphogranuloma* starts as a small ulcer at the site of infection, usually on the genital organ. The infection then spreads into the regional lymph nodes and causes their enlargement and chronic inflammation, leading to granulomalike lesions. *Trachoma*, as was already discussed in the preceding chapter, is an inflammation of the conjunctiva, originally caused by a virus followed by an infection of chlamydia. The chlamydia are responsible for the minute greyish or yellowish granules on the lid.

Mycoplasmas

Mycoplasmas (Gr. *mykes*, fungus, *plasma*, something formed) are distinguished from true bacteria in that they lack a rigid cell wall and consequently are rather formless—like some fungi (Fig. 14.13). Their cells are, however, bounded by a three-layered membrane. In humans, mycoplasmas are responsible for pneumonialike respiratory diseases (the causative agents were termed pleuropneumonia-like organisms, or PPLO; see Table 14.3). We shall discuss defense reactions to rickettsiae, chlamydia, and mycoplasmas together with those against bacteria.

14.2.3 True Bacteria

Characteristics

Bacteria (Gr. *bakterion*, diminutive of *baktron*, a staff; bacteria = small staff) are one-celled microscopic organisms that lack a well-defined nucleus and divide by fission (see below). The bacterial cell (Fig. 14.13) may be surrounded by as many as three layers—the cell (plasma) membrane, cell wall, and capsule. The innermost *cell* (*plasma*, *cytoplasmic*) *membrane* is similar to the plasma membrane of eukaryotic cells except that it contains little or no phosphatidyl choline and no sterole. The *cell wall* is a complex, semirigid structure that helps to maintain the shape and overall integrity of the cell. It surrounds the cell membrane, protecting it and the whole cell from adverse environmental changes, particularly changes in osmotic pressure. Based on the structure of the cell wall, bacteria can be divided into two main groups, Gram-positive and Gram-negative, described in Chapter 10. The *capsule* is the outermost, nonobligatory, low-density, viscous layer, composed of a gelatinous polymer of polysaccharide, a polypeptide, or both. When it is not well defined, it is referred to as a *slime layer*. Some bacteria possess, in addition, *flagella*—thin, filamentous appendages composed almost entirely of elastic protein (flagellin) and attached to both the cell wall and cell membrane by a granule, the basal body. A single bacterium may possess a single polar flagellum, two or more flagella at one pole of the cell, tufts of flagella at both ends of the cell, or many flagella distributed over the entire cell. Minute filamentous appendages, visible only by electron microscopy, are called *pili* or *fimbriae*. They are not only smaller, but also less rigid than flagella, and in contrast to flagella, which are organelles of motility, pili function mainly in attachment of the bacterial cell to surfaces or to other bacteria.

The *cytoplasm* of the bacterial cell contains granules of glycogen, proteins, and fat; ribosomes, but no mitochondria; and endoplasmic reticulum. There is a defined *nuclear region* (nucleoid), occupied by the cell's genetic material (DNA), but this region, in contrast to a typical nucleus, is not bounded by a nuclear membrane and it lacks discrete chromosomes, mitotic apparatuses, and a nucleolus. It contains one circular, double-stranded DNA molecule attached at one point to the cell membrane or its extension, the *mesosome*.

Bacteria reproduce by division (*fission*) of the parental cell. In rod-shaped bacteria, the cell elongates until it attains twice its original length, then constricts in the middle and splits into two identical daughter cells. The division is preceded by the replication of the DNA molecule, and each daughter cell inherits one replica of the original molecule. However, sometimes the DNA replication and cell division may get out of phase, so that one cell may contain more than one DNA molecule and so more than one nuclear region. The DNA molecule, in contrast to a typical chromosome, is "naked"—that is, devoid of protein.

On the basis of shape, one can distinguish three types of bacterium: bacillus, coccus, and vibrio. *Bacilli* (L. *bacillus*, diminutive of *baculus*, a rod) are rod-shaped, often motile bacteria. They possess the abilty to form *endospores* under certain environmental conditions. Endospores are intracellularly produced spherical or egg-shaped structures composed of a spore coat, a cortex, and a nuclear core. Generally, a single cell produces a single spore, and after it has done so, the cell sloughs off. When the conditions return to normal, the spore germinates to form one vegetative cell. *Cocci* (Gr. *kokkos*, berry) are spherical or ovoid in shape, and occur singularly (*Micrococcus*), in chains (*Streptococcus*, from Gr. *streptos*, twisted), in pairs (*Diplococcus*), in irregular bunches (*Staphylococcus*, Gr. *staphyle*, a bunch of grapes), or in cubical packets (*Sarcina*, from L. *sarcina*, a pack, bundle). In contrast to bacilli, cocci do not form spores and are nonmotile. *Vibria* (L. *vibro*, vibrate) have the shape of curved or bent rods; they are motile, but form no spores. Their representatives are comma-shaped *Vibrio*, helical *Spirillum* (L. diminutive of *spira*, a coil), and spiral-shaped *Spirochetes* (Gr. *speira*, a coil, *chaite*, hair).

Table 14.4 Major Human Diseases Caused by True Bacteria

Bacterium	Disease	Symptoms
Gram-positive cocci		
Staphylococcus aureus	Boils	Focal, pus-containing lesions.
	Osteomyelitis	Infection of the growing bone. Fever, chills, pain over the bone, muscle spasms around the area of involvement.
	Food poisoning	Severe cramping, abdominal pain, nausea, vomiting and diarrhea.
Streptococcus pyogenes	Pharyngitis and scarlet fever	Inflammation of the mucous membrane of the pharynx. Sore throat, fever, chills, vomiting, headache, malaise. Red flush over various parts of the body.
Streptococcus pneumoniae	Pneumococcal pneumonia	Inflammation of the respiratory tract, including lungs. Chills, pain in the chest, rusty sputum, rapid breathing, abdominal pain, jaundice.
Gram-negative cocci		
Neisseria gonorrhoeae	Gonorrhea	Infection of reproductive organs. Redness, swelling, penile or urethral discharge, frequent and burning urination.
Neisseria meningitidis	Meningitis	Infection of the respiratory tract, nervous system, and sometimes blood. Severe headaches, violent vomiting, high fever, delirium, and rigid neck and back.
Gram-positive bacilli		
Corynebacterium diphtheriae	Diphtheria	Infection of the respiratory tract. Sore throat, fever, vomiting, formation of ulcers and fibrous exudates (pseudomembranes) in the throat. Difficult breathing. Nerve and heart muscle degeneration.
Bacillus anthracis	Anthrax	Pustules in skin. Infection of blood and lymph. Bleeding and serous effusions in the organs and cavities of the body.
Clostridium tetani	Tetanus (lockjaw)	Toxins affecting the nervous system. Spasm of muscles and convulsions.
Clostridium perfringens	Gas gangrene	Infection of wounds. Gassy swelling of the wounds, foul odor.
Clostridium botulinum	Botulism	Toxins acting on the nervous system. Severe gastro-intestinal upset, vomiting, and diarrhea, fatigue, disturbance of vision, paralysis.
Gram-negative bacilli		
Escherichia coli	Urinary tract infections, infantile gastroenteritis	Urinary pains. Diarrhea and dehydration.
Salmonella typhosa, *Salmonella paratyphi*	Typhoid and paratyphoid (enteric) fever	Infection of lymphoid tissues, ulceration, bleeding, and perforations of intestinal walls. Fever, nausea, vomiting, severe abdominal pains, chills, and diarrhea.
Shigella dysenteriae	Shigellosis (bacillary dysentery)	Infection of intestinal tract. Fever, nausea, vomiting, severe abdominal pain, blood in the stool, diarrhea.
Bordetella pertussis	Whooping cough (pertussis)	Infection of mucous membranes of respiratory tract and eyes. Coldlike symptoms, with characteristic cough followed by a whoop.
Pasteurella pestis	Bubonic plague (pestis)	Infection of blood, spleen, liver, and lymph nodes. Enlarged inguinal lymph nodes (buboes). High fever, vomiting, hot, dry skin, thirst, black spots on skin.
Brucella abortus	Brucellosis (undulant fever)	General infection throughout the body. Periods of fever alternating with periods of normal temperature. Recurrent attacks, loss of weight, backache, weakness and insomnia.

Table 14.4 (*Continued*)

Bacterium	Disease	Symptoms
Acid-fast bacilli		
Mycobacterium tuberculosis	Tuberculosis (consumption, phthisis)	Chronic infection of lungs, bones, and other organs. Formation of tubercles. Cough, fever in the evening, fatigue, loss of weight.
Mycobacterium leprae	Leprosy	Chronic infection of skin, mucous membranes of mouth, and peripheral nerves. Lesions on the skin that cause mutilations.
Miscellaneous		
Vibrio cholerae	Cholera	Intestinal infection. Vomiting, diarrhea, fluid loss, shock.
Treponema pallidum	Syphilis (lues)	Infection of blood and nervous system. A hard, painless sore or chancre on the genitalia, variable types of skin eruption. Destruction of brain, heart, skin, bones, and viscera.

Individual bacteria cells can be seen only with the aid of a microscope, but often the rapidly multiplying cells stay together and form macroscopically visible *colonies*. When bacteria are seeded on a solid medium at a low density, each colony can be seen to originate from a single cell. Colonies of individual bacterial species have characteristic diameters, shapes (circular or ovoid), margins (regular or irregular), elevations (flat, raised, thin, or thick), colors (pigmented or nonpigmented), textures (rough or smooth), and light absorbencies (opaque, translucent, or opalescent).

Damage Caused by Bacterial Infections

Most bacteria remain outside the host cell throughout their lives, but a few have adapted to intracellular parasitism. Some of the intracellular bacteria (e.g., *Mycobacterium leprae*) can no longer multiply outside the cell—that is, they are *obligative* intracellular parasites; others (e.g., *Mycobacterium tuberculosis*) are *facultative* intracellular parasites that will live inside a cell whenever they have the opportunity, but when forced to, they can also survive outside the cell. Extracellular and intracellular bacteria cause different types of illness (Table 14.4): the infection by extracellular bacteria is of the *acute* type—that is, of short duration but very intense, whereas that caused by intracellular bacteria is of the *chronic* type—that is, of long duration but less pronounced.

The manner in which parasitic bacteria damage the host is complex and not yet completely understood. The mere presence of a large number of foreign bodies in an organ often interferes with its normal function. But bacteria may also produce substances that have an adverse effect on the host's body. Since these substances "poison" the body in a broad manner of speaking, they are referred to as *toxins*. They are all proteins but, apart from this fact and their toxicity, they differ from one another in most of their properties—size, structure, manner of production, and mode of action. They can be divided into two groups: endotoxins, which are associated with the cell wall and released only after the death of bacteria, and exotoxins, which are liberated by multiplying bacteria.

Endotoxins are an integral part of the cell wall of such Gram-negative bacteria as *Salmonella*, *Shigella*, and *Escherichia coli*. They are relatively heat-stable, complex macromolecules, containing phospholipid and polysaccharide, with toxicity residing in the phospholipid fraction and antigenicity in the polysaccharide moiety (see Chapter 10). Endotoxins exert many biological effects: they release pyrogens from neutrophils and so induce fever; they destroy neutrophils and so impair the organism's phagocytic ability; they initiate the clotting sequence and cause intravascular coagulation; and they cause dilation of the blood vessels and bleeding. Since the human intestine normally contains a large number of Gram-negative bacteria, a portion of which continually die off, small amounts of endotoxin are incessantly released, absorbed by the intestine, carried by the portal circulation into the liver, and degraded there by reticuloendothelial cells—mainly Kupffer cells. This low-grade exposure of the animal to endotoxin has no obvious pathological consequences, although it probably influences the development of the immune system, particularly in an immature individual. During an infection by Gram-negative bacteria, the amount of endotoxin entering the blood increases considerably and may lead to so-called *endotoxin shock*: the blood vessels dilate, blood collects in the peripheral regions of the body, circulation slows down, blood pressure falls drastically, and the patient collapses. Endotoxin shock is second only to myocardial infarction as a cause of death in many large hospitals.

Exotoxins are heat-labile proteins, produced primarily by Gram-positive bacteria. A great many exotoxins have been identified and characterized, at least to some degree, but we shall mention here only a few. *Cholera enterotoxin* is produced by *Vibrio cholerae*, which attaches to intestinal epithelium and multiplies in the lumen of the small intestine without invading the tissue (Gr. *enteron*, intestine). The toxin has a molecular weight of 82,000 daltons and is composed of seven polypeptide chains: A_1 (23,000 daltons), A_2 (5500 daltons), and five B chains (11,500 daltons), with A_1 and A_2 covalently linked by S–S bridges and the A_1A_2 dimers noncovalently associated with the five identical B subunits, which are also noncovalently associated with one another (Fig. 14.14). The B subunits form a ring around the A subunit, and this ring has the ability to recognize and attach to ganglioside G_{M1} on the surface of intestinal epithelial cells. The attachment apparently breaks the disulfide bond between the A_1 and A_2 subunits, and the A_1 subunit enters the membrane of the epithelial cell and enzymatically activates adenylate cyclase on the cytoplasmic side of the membrane. The activation is believed to occur as follows. In a normal cell, adenylate cyclase is activated when GTP binds to the regulatory protein of the cyclase system, and this binding then induces a change in this protein (see Chapter 13 and Fig. 13.18). But since, normally, GTP is rapidly hydrolyzed to GDP, the activation is only ephemeral; hence GTP alone results in little cyclase activity. However, the hydrolysis of the bound GTP is inhibited by ADP-ribosylation of the regulatory protein—a reaction catalyzed by the cholera toxin:

$$\text{GTP} - \text{regulatory protein} + \text{NAD}^+ \xrightleftharpoons{\text{cholera toxin}} \text{ADP-ribosyl-GTP-regulatory protein} + \text{nicotinamide} + \text{H}^+$$

As a result of the ribosylation, the cyclase activity persists so long as the toxin is present.

The activated adenylate cyclase converts ATP into cyclic AMP, and the level of intracellular cAMP rises and disturbs the passage of ions and water across the plasma membrane. Water and electrolytes leave epithelial cells and enter the lumen of the small intestine, leading to a watery diarrhea. The amount of water a patient loses is enormous—some 15 to 20 liters per day! The loss of fluid results in the reduction in volume of blood (so-called *hypovolemic shock*), a decrease of alkali in bodily fluids in proportion to the content of acid (so-called *metabolic acidosis*), the suppression of urine formation, and a total collapse of the patient.

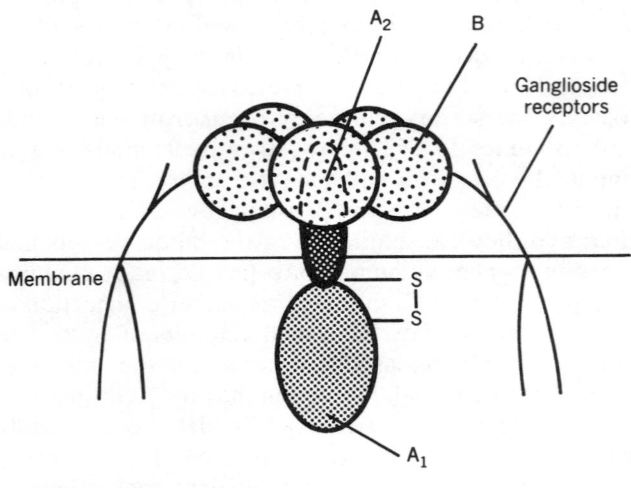

Figure 14.14. Postulated composition of the cholera toxin molecule. (Based on B. J. Wisnieski and J. S. Bramhall: *Nature* **289**:319–321, 1981.)

Shigella enterotoxin is produced by *Shigella dysenteriae*, another intestinal parasite, which, in contrast to *Vibrio cholerae*, not only attaches to, but also penetrates intestinal epithelial cells (in this case, of the *large* intestine). The infected cells die, and an eroded area or ulcer forms on the intestinal mucosa. The enterotoxin, which has a molecular weight of about 75,000 daltons, also induces fluid loss from the intestine, but the induction occurs by an unknown mechanism that does not operate via adenylate cyclase. The infection is accompanied by bleeding from small blood vessels in the intestine; the blood mixes with water, mucus, and pus from the ulcers, resulting in bloody diarrhea. The Shiga bacteria also produce a neurotoxin that diffuses into the blood and acts on the brain and spinal cord; this neurotoxin, however, might be the same as the enterotoxin.

Diphtheria toxin is the product of *Corynebacterium diphtheriae*, the bacillus that multiplies on the epithelial surface of the nose, throat, or skin (see Chapter 2). Although it does not penetrate deeply into the tissues, the bacillus causes necrosis of mucosal cells, production of an inflammatory exudate, and the formation of a

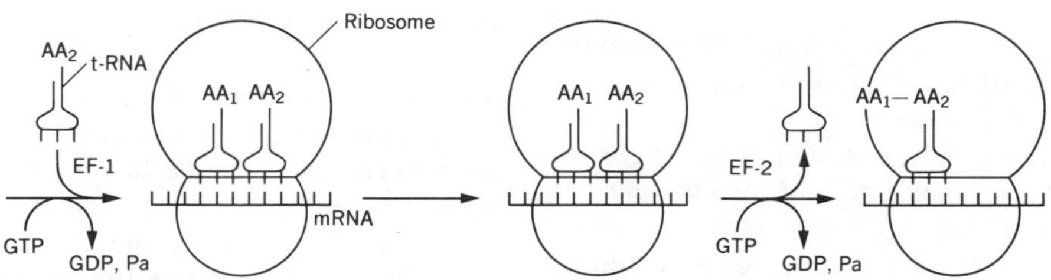

Figure 14.15. The chain-elongation step in protein synthesis—the step affected by diphtheria toxin.

thick false membrane that may spread into the larynx and create respiratory obstruction. The toxin probably assists bacterial colonization of the throat or skin by killing epithelial cells and neutrophils. Intact, it consists of a single polypeptide chain with a molecular weight of about 62,000 daltons and with two disulfide bridges. Trypsin treatment nicks the toxin in the region spanned by one of the two disulfide bridges. If the treatment is followed by reduction of the disulfides, this bridge breaks and the polypeptide splits into two fragments—A (24,000 daltons) and B (39,000 daltons)—held together by noncovalent bonds. The intact and nicked chains are toxic but enzymatically inactive (see below); the B fragment is nontoxic and lacks enzymatic activity, whereas the A fragment has enzymatic activity but is toxic only when delivered into the cell. The intact toxin binds, via its B fragment, to glycoprotein receptors on cell surfaces and is then interiorized into the cell, perhaps via receptor clustering and endocytosis. Inside the cell, the chain is cleaved proteolytically, and the released A fragment interacts with the protein-synthesizing ribosomes in the cytoplasm. The interaction occurs in the following manner. Normal protein synthesis on a ribosome requires the participation of elongation factor 2 (EF-2), a protein with a molecular weight of about 100,000 daltons. The protein is required for the translocation step, in which the peptidyl-tRNA is shifted from the acceptor to the donor site on the ribosome, mRNA is translocated by one trinucleotide codon on the ribosome, and GTP is hydrolyzed to GDP and inorganic phosphate (Fig. 14.15). The toxin acts in a way similar to the cholera toxin in that it catalyzes ADP-ribosylation of the elongation factor:

$$\text{NAD}^+ + \text{EF-2} \xrightarrow{\text{diphtheria toxin}} \text{ADP-ribosyl-EF-2} + \text{nicotinamide} + \text{H}^+$$

The ribosylated factor is then unable to carry out its function and protein synthesis is blocked. It is this inhibition of protein synthesis in a variety of cells that is behind the poisoning action of the diphtheria toxin. Particularly susceptible to this action are cells of the heart and of peripheral nerves, in which the toxin probably inhibits the synthesis of some specific proteins. The inhibition eventually leads to an inflammation of muscular walls of the heart (myocarditis) and of the nerves (neuritis) and to paralysis. Interestingly, the toxin is not a product of the diphtheria bacillus itself, but of a bacteriophage that lives in an integrated state in this bacillus; the evolutionary and functional implications of the fact that a diphtheria toxin is a product of a phage gene are not yet clear. Another interesting observation is that there is also another bacterium, *Pseudomonas aeruginosa*, completely unrelated to *C. diphtheria*, that produces a toxin with an identical mode of action. Although the two bacteria and the two toxins do not seem to have much in common, the toxins seem to act in the same way.

Botulinum toxin is the product of *Clostridium botulinum*, a long, rod-shaped bacterium that lives in the soil and in decaying organic matter or animal excreta. The bacterium's spores are highly resistant to temperature, withstanding boiling for several hours. The toxin occurs in at least six different types—A, B, C, D, E, and F—differing somewhat in their potency and antigenicity. The most potent type-A toxin is a globular protein, with a molecular weight of about 900,000 daltons, that consists of two major subunits—the smaller α, which possesses the toxic activity and has a molecular weight of about 150,000 daltons, and β, which contains hemolytic activity and has a molecular weight of about 500,000 daltons. Botulinum toxin has an affinity for nerve endings in muscle cells. It binds to the surface of the cholinergic nerve ending via specific receptors, and then somehow prevents the release of acetylcholine, and so also prevents the transmission of the nerve impulse to the muscle cell. The mechanism of this inhibition is not known; one possibility is that the toxin lodges in a critical site in the membrane or in the cell and prevents exocytosis of acetylcholine-containing vesicles; another possibility is that it binds to the vesicles themselves and impairs their function. In any case, the binding stops neurotransmission and paralyzes all neuromuscular and autonomic activity. The affected person suffers from double vision because of derangement of the eye muscles, from difficulty in speaking and swallowing because of gradual paralysis of the tongue and other muscles in the mouth, and from life-threatening paralysis of the diaphragm. The condition (*botulism*) is usually associated with the eating of improperly prepared home-canned food, infected with *C. botulinum*. The term derives from L. *botulus*, meaning "sausage," and refers to the observation that outbreaks of botulism were caused by improperly cooked sausage.

Tetanus toxin is produced by *Clostridium tetani*, an anaerobic bacterium found in the soil and in the animal intestinal tract. Spore germination and growth require anaerobic conditions, generated, for example, by the necrotization of a wound. The toxin produced in such a wound is transported, via the bloodstream and along the peripheral nerves, to the spinal cord, where it acts principally on the anterior horn cells. Investigators have not yet agreed on the structure of the toxin. According to some, the intracellular toxin consists of a single polypeptide chain with a molecular weight of about 150,000 daltons, and this chain, when secreted, splits into two disulfide-bonded subunits—one 55,000 daltons and the other 95,000 daltons. The toxin binds, via a ganglioside receptor, to the cells of the so-called inhibitory synapses, and probably interferes with the release of the inhibitor of neurotransmitter substance, presumably glycine. The inhibition leads to a spastic muscular contraction and paralysis with convulsions (Gr. *tetanos*, convulsive tension).

Streptolysin is a representative of cytolytic bacterial toxins, which act on the plasma membrane and disrupt it. There is a large number of such substances, produced by a variety of bacteria. Streptolysins O and S are the products of *Streptococcus pyogenes*, a species found in the human mouth, throat, and respiratory tract and in inflammatory lesions in which it causes the formation of pus (hence the designation *pyogenes*). Streptolysin O presumably consists of a single polypeptide chain with one disulfide bond and a molecular weight of about 68,000 daltons. Its membrane receptor is probably cholesterol, a critical constituent of plasma membranes of eukaryotic cells. Upon binding to cholesterol, the disulfide bond of the streptolysin breaks, and a lytic site on the toxin molecule is exposed. The binding inhibits the stabilizing interaction of cholesterol with neighboring phospholipids and leads to the formation of holes or channels around the toxin-cholesterol complex.

Defense Against Bacteria

The general strategy of the host defense against bacteria is the same as that against viruses—namely, first to prevent entrance of the microorganisms into the inner tissues of the body, and if the microorganisms are internalized, to confine the infection, prevent its spreading, and eliminate the microorganisms locally. For the parasite, the body is a fortress with several fortification rings that it must storm if it wants to reach the inner core. As we did with the virus, we shall describe what kind of resistance the bacterial parasite encounters as it storms one fortification ring after another, getting progressively closer to the core.

Anatomic Barriers and Secretions. A bacterium that has reached the bodily surface by being inhaled, ingested, or transmitted by contact must attach to this surface to gain a foothold in the host. The body uses the same mechanical devices against bacterial invasion as it does against viral attacks. A considerable degree of protection is also afforded by the various bodily secretions, such as the gastric juice that destroys many bacteria because of its acidity, or the lysozyme in tears, saliva, and nasal secretions, which degrades the mucopeptide layers of many bacterial cell walls. However, many species that do manage to colonize a bodily surface do not necessarily do any harm. They live extracellularly, using the body's wastes without provoking any defense reactions. Consequently, every vertebrate is a host to many species of *normal bacterial flora*—a complex ecosystem that, like any other ecosystem, exists in a dynamic but stable equilibrium maintained by a unique system of checks and balances. Present in the flora, however, are also some *potentially* harmful species, which, under circumstances adverse to the host, may become invaders. Such circumstances arise when the integrity of the skin or mucous membrane is disturbed. An example of an *opportune parasite* of this kind is *Staphylococcus aureus*, which normally colonizes human skin without causing disease. However, when the skin is damaged—by burning, for instance—the bacterium enters the tissue and causes a dangerous infection. Similarly, when the integrity of the respiratory epithelium is damaged by an influenza infection, *Staphylococcus aureus* uses the opportunity to invade the respiratory tissue and causes staphylococcal pneumonia, which seriously hinders recovery from the original infection. The adverse circumstances are, of course, also exploited by all obligatory parasites that happen to land on the body in this vulnerable time for the host.

Phagocytosis and the Inflammatory Response. A bacterium that has overcome the mechanical and anatomical barriers and has managed to invade deeper tissues of the body is immediately attacked by tissue macrophages, and the attack induces an inflammatory response, attracting additional phagocytic cells to the battlefield. Nonencapsulated bacteria are readily phagocytosed by macrophages, while those of the encapsulated sort often resist engulfment. Encapsulated bacteria are usually far more dangerous than the former because, to conquer them, the host must first make antibodies against them and opsonize them before they can be phagocytosed. But since some time is required to produce antibodies in sufficient quantities, the parasite may spread, relatively unchecked, through the body in the interim.

If the bacteria are not killed locally at the entry site, they are delivered, with lymph, into regional lymph nodes, which then become the second battlefield. A visible sign of this battle is enlargement of the nodes during bacterial infection. Bacteria that manage to progress further into the blood and cause *bacteremia* (Gr. *haima,* blood) face blood monocytes and neutrophils, and when carried further into the liver and the spleen, the reticuloendothelial system of these organs. When not overcome, the bacteria may invade the bone

Table 14.5 Mechanisms by which Microorganisms Interfere with Phagocytosis

Microorganism[a]	Type of Interference[b]	Mechanism (or Responsible Factor)
Streptococci	Kill phagocyte	Streptolysin induces lysosomal discharge into cell cytoplasm.
	Inhibit neutrophil chemotaxis	Streptolysin
	Resist phagocytosis	M substance
	Resist digestion	
Staphylococci	Kill phagocyte	Leukocidin induces lysosomal discharge into cell cytoplasm.
	Inhibit opsonized phagocytosis	Protein A blocks Fc portion of antibody.
	Resist killing	Cell wall mucopeptide
Bacillus anthracis	Kill phagocyte	Toxic complex
	Resist killing	Capsular polyglutamic acid
Haemophilus influenzae *Streptococcus pneumoniae* *Klebsiella pneumoniae*	Resist phagocytosis (unless antibody present) Resist digestion	Polysaccharide capsule
Pseudomonas aeruginosa	Resist phagocytosis (unless antibody present) Resist digestion	"Surface slime" (polysaccharide)
Escherichia coli	Resist phagocytosis (unless antibody present)	O antigen (smooth strains) K antigen (acid polysaccharide)
	Resist killing	K antigen
Salmonella typhi	Resist phagocytosis (unless antibody present)	Vi antigen
	Resist killing	
Cryptococcus neoformans	Resist phagocytosis	Polysaccharide capsule
Treponema pallidum	Resist phagocytosis	Cell wall
Pasteurella pestis	Resist killing	Protein-carbohydrate cell wall
Mycobacteria	Resist killing and digestion	Cell wall structure
	Inhibit lysosomal fusion	?
Brucella abortus	Resist killing	Cell wall substance
Toxoplasma gondii	Inhibit attachment to polymorph	?
	Inhibit lysosomal fusion	?

Source. From C. A. Mims: *The Pathogenesis of Infectious Disease.* Academic, London, 1977.

[a] Often it is only the virulent strains that show the type of interference listed.

[b] Sometimes the type of interference listed has been described only in a particular type of phagocyte (neutrophil or macrophage) from a particular host, but it generally bears a relationship to pathogenecity in that host.

and cause *osteomyelitis*, or the brain or kidney and cause abscesses in these organs. Some of the mechanisms by which bacteria resist phagocytosis are listed in Table 14.5.

Specific Immunity. While the invaders are combated by the nonspecific systems of immunity, the elements of the specific system are summoned to the battlefield. Although probably all elements of specific immunity are activated in all infections, the relative role of the individual elements varies with the type of invading microorganism. Extracellular parasites responsible for common, acute bacterial infections—such as those caused by staphylococci, streptococci, or pneumococci—stimulate primarily humoral response. This conclusion is supported by, for example, the observations that agammaglobulinemic patients are highly susceptible to these infections and that they acquire resistance by transfer of specific antibodies. The protective role of antibodies in extracellular bacteria infection manifests itself in three major ways—opsonization, complement activation, and toxin neutralization.

Opsonization is the body's way of making bacteria more palatable to the phagocytic cells. Antibodies produced against the parasite bind to the bacteria via their Fab regions and to the Fc receptors of macrophages via the Fc region, and this process facilitates phagocytosis. Antibodies bound to the bacterial surface also activate the *complement cascade*, and the assembly of the membrane-attack complex on the bacterial membrane culminates in bacteriolysis. Some of the complement fragments liberated during the activation act chemotactically, and so indicate the location of the bacteria to the phagocytic cells. The complement cascade, particularly its alternative pathway, is also activated independently of antibodies, by bacterial products, such as endotoxin. The union of antibodies with toxins *neutralizes* the latter, and the toxin-antitoxin complexes are then removed by phagocytosis. However, if too many complexes form in a short time, they may cause an immune complex disease and injure the host by one of the mechanisms described later in this chapter. In clinical situations, active immunization for protection against toxins is usually not carried out with the native molecules, but with toxins that have been treated—for example, with formaldehyde—so as to destroy their toxic properties but retain antigenicity. Such modified toxins are called *toxoids* (Gr. *eidos*, resemblance).

Gram-negative intestinal bacteria stimulate IgM production primarily, and these antibodies remain largely confined to the vascular system. They are particularly suited to agglutinating, lysing, and opsonizing bacteria. However, most bacteria that produce acute infections primarily stimulate production of IgG antibodies, which are good precipitins and, in addition, diffuse readily to extravascular spaces. They are, therefore, best suited for toxin neutralization. Certain localized infections, particularly those in the respiratory and gastrointestinal tracts, initiate predominantly the production of IgA antibodies, which then act against the bacteria on the bodily surface. An example is the coproantibodies produced in the gastrointestinal tract during cholera infection.

Intracellular bacteria—such as the various species of *Mycobacterium*, *Pasteurella*, *Brucella*, and *Listeria*—induce cellular immunity primarily. In chronic infections, such as tuberculosis (see Chapter 12) and leprosy, phagocytes engulf the bacteria, but they cannot degrade them. The infected macrophages induce T-cell immunity, which then purges the body of the bacteria. But in some individuals, particularly in those in which the cellular immunity systems are not functioning properly, the T cells fail to get rid of the invader. The host then begins the process of walling off the infected area, and a granulomatous tissue that is characteristic of these diseases develops. The persistent presence of cellular immunity in the infected individual is an aid in the diagnosis of the infection—as, for example, in tuberculosis.

14.2.4 Fungi

Fungi are plantlike organisms that lack the green pigment chlorophyll and grow on previously produced organic matter as *saprophytes*—that is, they use dead organic matter as a source of food (Gr. *sapros*, rotten, *phyton*, plant)—or as *parasites* that obtain food from living bodies. A few are one-celled but most are many-celled, forming masses (*mycelia*) of tubular branching filaments called *hyphae* (Gr. *hyphe*, a web). They reproduce asexually by generating one-celled spores, or sexually by fusion of male and female gametes. There are some 40,000 fungal species, including yeasts, molds, mildews, rusts, smuts, and mushrooms; some 35 to 40 of these are capable of producing disease in humans (Table 14.6). The infection is spread by spores in the atmosphere or soil. When a spore is inhaled or picked up from the soil by bare feet, it begins to germinate on moist bodily surfaces and gives rise to a mycelium, which may either colonize the surface or spread through the body, causing a systemic infection. Examples of fungi that cause localized infections are *Microsporum*, *Trichophyton*, *Epidermophyton*, *Candida*, and *Aspergillus*; representatives of systemically acting fungi are *Cryptococcus*, *Histoplasma*, *Coccidiodes*, and *Blastomyces*.

Table 14.6 Major Human Diseases Caused by Fungi

Fungus	Disease	Manifestation of Disease	Epidemiology
Candida albicans	Candidiasis	Member of normal flora of the mucous membranes in the respiratory, gastrointestinal, and female genital tracts. Turns into a parasite in immunologically compromised individuals. Produces either systemic disease or localized lesions in the skin, mouth, lungs, or vagina. Thrush, dermatitis.	Present in most individuals
Cryptococcus neoformans	Meningitis	Infection via respiratory tract. Inflammation of brain and spinal cord membranes, sometimes accompanied by lesions of the skin and lungs.	Bird feces are the main source of infection.
Blastomyces dermatitides	Blastomycosis	Infects lungs and disseminates into skin, bones, internal organs, brain and spinal cord membranes. Responsible for abscess formation and tuberclelike granulomas.	Soil fungus in the Americas. Acquired by inhalation of dust.
Histoplasma capsulatum	Histoplasmosis	Usually limited to lungs but may disseminate throughout the body. Lesions resemble tubercles.	Soil fungus in the Americas. Abundant in bird and bat feces.
Coccidioides immitis	Coccidioidomycosis	Infection of the respiratory tract. Symptoms resemble pneumonia or tuberculosis. Sometimes also red nodules in the skin and other organs.	Soil fungus; southwestern U.S.
Geotrichum candidum	Geotrichosis	Infection of the respiratory tract. Symptoms resembling chronic bronchitis; lesions in the mouth.	Probably member of normal mouth flora.
Epidermophyton sp.	Ringworm	Skin infection of varying severity.	Some species acquired from animals.
	Tinea cornis	Jock itch.	
	Tinea pedis	Ringworm of foot (athlete's foot).	
	Tinea corporis	Ringworm of smooth skin.	
Trichophyton sp.	Tinea capitis	Ringworm of scalp.	
Microsporum sp.	Tinea unguium	Ringworm of nails.	
Aspergillus fumigatus	Aspergillosis	Skin, respiratory, and general body infection.	Birds

The first three examples are representatives of *cutaneous fungi*, which have a predilection for such keratin-rich tissues as skin, hair, and nails. They appear to have the ability to degrade keratin and use its breakdown products as a nutritional source. They are found frequently in children and rarely in adults, perhaps because the attainment of puberty is marked by an increase in the secretion of saturated fatty acids with antifungal activity. They cause *dermatomycoses* affecting various parts of the body. *Microsporum audouini* is the causative agent of ringworm on the human scalp (*tinea capitis*), characterized by the appearance of one or more raised, round sores on the skin that seem to heal in the center while the edges continue to grow outwards—a characteristic growth pattern of many mycelia (L. *tinea*, worm, moth). *Trichophyton interdigitalis* is the cause of athlete's foot (*tinea pedis*), a condition characterized by painful itching or burning cracks in the skin, particularly between and underneath the toes. *Epidermophyton inguinale* is responsible for jock (or dhobie) itch (*tinea cruris*), characterized by eruptions on the inner and upper surfaces of the leg (the Latin word for leg is *crus*), groin, and genital region.

Candida and *Aspergillus* can cause either local or disseminated infections. Both are opportunistic organisms that normally exist in a stable relation with the host as a part of the normal flora, but which become parasitic following local abrasions or changes in the nutritive and chemical milieu. *Candida albicans* (Fig. 14.13) is a yeastlike organism causing thrush (*candidiasis*), a disease characterized by the appearance of discrete whitish patches (L. *albus,* white) on the tongue, mouth, or throat, or in the vagina (especially during pregnancy or in diabetes). In immunologically compromised individuals, the local infection becomes systemic and chronic (the so-called *chronic mucocutaneous candidiasis*, or *CMC*). *Aspergillus fumigatus* is a mold that may cause inflammatory and destructive disease of the bronchi and lungs. It also grows in several species of bird, causing a disease that often destroys whole flocks of domestic fowl or turkeys.

Histoplasma capsulatum is another yeastlike organism that occurs in the soil and grows abundantly in bird feces (in chicken houses) and bat guano (in caves). When acquired by the inhalation of contaminated dust, it grows in the lungs as an intracellular parasite, causing lesions that resemble tubercles (*histoplasmosis*). Most individuals contain the infection within two weeks, but in some the fungus spreads through the body and begins to grow in the spleen, liver, heart, and brain, causing dangerous chronic infection.

Coccidioides immitis is a soil fungus responsible for *coccidioidomycosis,* a disease common in the San Joaquin Valley of California and a few other places in the southwestern United States. When localized, it causes only influenzalike symptoms; when disseminated, it can attack almost any tissue of the body and the disease may become chronic.

Blastomyces dermatitidis is another soil inhabitant that can be acquired by inhalation of dust. It too may be limited to the lungs, or it may be widely disseminated to the skin, bones, viscera, and brain. The organism is responsible for small abscesses and tuberclelike lesions.

Resistance to fungal infections is mediated primarily by T lymphocytes and the entire cellular arm of specific immunity. Most individuals with well-developed T-cell immunity systems readily contain the infection: the fungus grows rapidly at the port of entry for a week or two, causing an acute infection; but after this period T cells become sensitized to fungal antigens and attack the cells in which the parasite grows. Individuals with T-cell defects, on the other hand, are unable to cope with the infection, which then becomes chronic. The same thing happens in individuals genetically susceptible to fungal infections, newborns with incompletely developed systems, or patients receiving immunosuppressive therapy. Antibodies often play only a secondary role in fungal infections.

14.2.5 Protozoal and Metazoal Parasites

Representative Parasites

So diverse are the animal parasites that we shall not even attempt to characterize them as a group; instead, we shall describe three representative examples to illustrate this diversity. Of the three selected parasites, two (*Trypanosoma* and *Plasmodium*) represent the protozoa and one (*Schistosoma*) represents the metazoa.

Trypanosoma. Trypanosomes are a group of one-celled, spindle-shaped organisms that swim by means of a wavy membrane and a flagellum. (The undulation of the membrane gives the cell the appearance of a drill—hence, the name, from Gr. *trypanon*, an auger or nave drill). They infect mammals but have an intermediate invertebrate host (Fig. 14.16). In mammals, they live in the blood plasma (that is, extracellularly), from which they obtain all the nutrients they need by osmosis. There are two major groups of trypanosoma—African and South American—which differ somewhat in their life cycles and which we shall therefore consider separately.

The *African trypanosomes* are represented by a number of species, subspecies, and variants, and the relationships among these various forms is not always clear. The two main species infecting human beings are *T. gambiense*, distributed from the west coast of Africa eastward to the lake district and southward to Angola and the southern border of Zaire, and *T. rhodesiense*, endemic in the highlands of central Africa. The third most important species, *T. brucei*, is pathogenic to many wild and domestic mammals in Africa, but not to humans. The three species are morphologically indistinguishable from one another, and since the two human species also infect other African mammals, it is possible that they derived from *T. brucei*. The intermediate hosts of the African trypanosomes are the tsetse flies of the genus *Glossina* (*G. palpalis* for *T. gambiense* and *G. morsitans* for *T. rhodiense* and *T. brucei*). The incubation time of the parasite within the fly is from 12 to 15 days; during this time the trypanosomes multiply by binary fission in the midgut of the fly, then migrate to the salivary glands, transform into infective forms, and are transmitted to humans in droplets of saliva as the fly sucks blood through human skin. After an incubation period av-

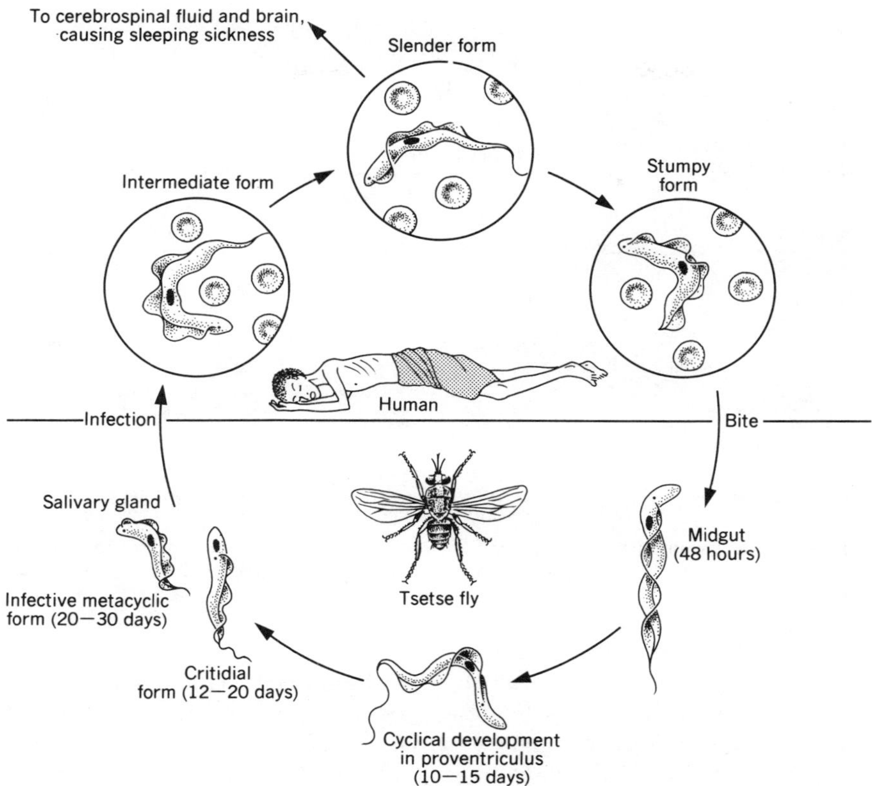

Figure 14.16. The multiplication cycle of *Trypanosoma gambiense* or *T. rhodesiense*, the parasites responsible for African sleeping sickness. (Compiled from various sources.)

eraging six to seven days, trypanosomes begin to appear in large numbers in human blood. Later, they invade lymph nodes, spleen, and eventually the lymph fluid surrounding the nerves and brain. The symptoms of *trypanosomiasis* are irregular fever, delayed sensation to pain, severe headaches, apathy, tremors, paralysis, and above all, profound sleepiness. It is for this last symptom that the disease is called *African sleeping sickness*. Rhodesian trypanosomiasis usually assumes an acute or subacute form, whereas Gambian sleeping sickness is usually chronic and long-lasting. Both forms are often fatal if untreated. As the number of parasites in the human blood begins to reach a plateau, short, stumpy trypanosomes with a larger and more elaborate mitochondrion and more developed Golgi apparatus and smooth endoplasmic reticulum than the slender forms begin to appear. It is at this stage that the parasites become infectious for the fly, and when ingested with blood, the trypanosomes lose their flagella, curl up, and begin the multiplication cycle in the intermediate host. *T. brucei* is nonpathogenic in wild antelopes and other wild herbivores, but highly fatal in domestic cattle, causing the *nagana disease*, which makes vast ranges of the African continent unsuitable for the production of livestock.

The South American trypanosomiasis is caused by *T. cruzi*, named after the Brazilian epidemiologist Oswaldo Cruz. Trypanosomiasis, also known as Chagas disease, after the Brazilian microbiologist Carlos Chagas, is endemic in most rural areas of Central and South America. The disease is transmitted to many mammals, including humans, by *Triatoma infestans* and other bugs of the order *Hemiptera*. The insect becomes infected by sucking the blood of a mammal, and the trypanosomes multiply in its intestine and pass out with its feces. Because the insects regularly defecate while sucking blood, the trypanosomes enter another mammal through the bite wound. Once in the mammal, the trypanosomes go through a complicated life cycle, which includes nonreproducing forms in the blood plasma and small, rounded, reproducing parasites without flagella and resembling the protozoa of the genus *Leishmania*, living intracellularly in the macrophages of the spleen, fibroblasts of the connective tissue, and muscle fibers of the heart. The disease

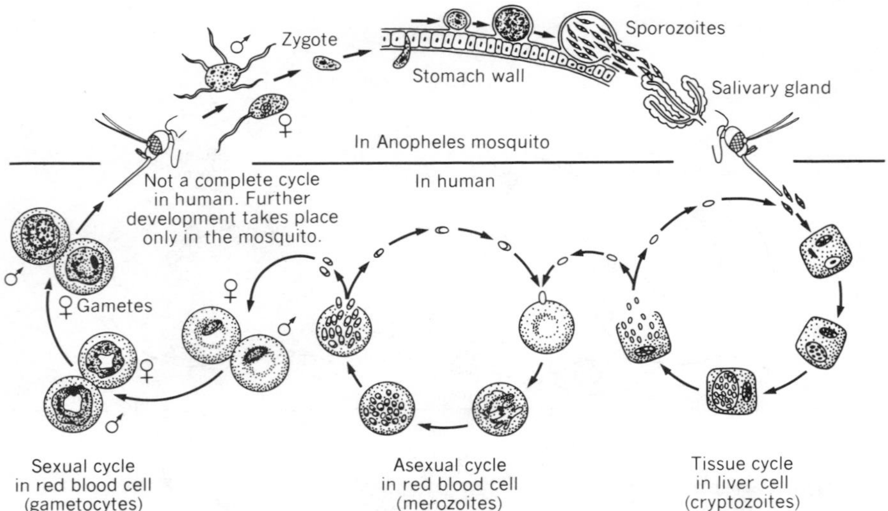

Figure 14.17. The multiplication cycle of *Plasmodium*, the parasite responsible for malaria. (Redrawn from R. D. Barnes: *Invertebrate Zoology*, 3rd ed. Saunders, Philadelphia, 1974.)

starts with the swelling of the eyelids, enlargement of lymph nodes near the ear and in the neck, and fever. The acute stage is then followed by a chronic phase, characterized chiefly by heart trouble. It has been estimated that some 35 million people worldwide suffer from trypanosomiasis.

Plasmodium. This protozoan belongs to the genus *Sporozoa*, characterized by the ability of its members to reproduce by nonsexual formation of spores. The *Plasmodium* parasites alternate between two hosts—a mammal (humans, monkeys) and an insect (mosquitoes of the genus *Anopheles*). It is only the blood-sucking female mosquito that transmits the protozoan; the male feeds only on plant juices. When the mosquito bites a human, it injects an infectious form of the parasite called *sporozoite* with its saliva (Fig. 14.17). The parasite enters the bloodstream, circulates in the blood for about 30 minutes, and then enters the liver and invades the parenchymal cells there. Within the cell, the parasite enlarges and its nuclei divide without a cell division. Then each nucleus surrounds itself with a portion of the cytoplasm, and the cell fragments into a number of *cryptozoites* (Gr. *kryptos*, hidden, concealed, *zoön*, animal). This form of nonsexual reproduction, in which the nucleus first divides into several parts and then the cell divides into as many parts as there are nuclei, is called *schizogony* (Gr. *schizo*, to split or cleave, *gone*, generation). The infected liver cell then bursts, and the cryptozoites leave and either infect another liver cell or enter the blood and infect red blood cells. Once in a red cell, the parasite undergoes a process similar to that in the liver cell: it enlarges so that it almost completely takes up the volume of the erythrocyte, and divides by schizogony, producing so-called *merozoites*, which are similar, if not identical, to cryptozoites (sometimes cryptozoites are also referred to as first-generation merozoites). The parasites then burst the erythrocyte and leave it to infect new erythrocytes and to produce new merozoites. By the repetition of the cycle, more and more parasites are produced, destroying more and more red blood cells. After several such cycles, the invading merozoites do not undergo fission in some erythrocytes, but instead, transform into either female or male *gametocytes*, which remain in the red cells until they are taken up by a mosquito. Once in the mosquito's stomach, the gametocytes leave the erythrocyte; male microgametocytes fuse with female macrogametocytes to form a zygote, which then enters the stomach wall and undergoes a meiotic division, accompanied by the reduction of chromosome number from diploid to haploid. The products of the division form rounded cysts in the stomach wall, and the parasites multiply rapidly within the cyst, giving rise to as many as 10,000 sporozoites in about three weeks. Mature sporozoites break out of the cyst and wander about the body of the mosquito host, many of them coming to rest in the salivary glands, ready to be injected with the next mosquito bite and start a new infection cycle.

Plasmodium causes *malaria* (It. *mala aria*, bad air), a disease so named because of an old superstition that it was produced by poisonous air from swamps. The parasites have a tendency to multiply synchronously in many of the infected red blood cells, so that large numbers of blood cells are simultaneously destroyed periodically, and metabolic products of the parasites, together with the remains of the parasitic cells, suddenly flood the blood, causing an attack of malaria. The attack begins with a shaking chill, which is then followed by a rapid rise of temperature, often to 40.5°C, general body aches, severe headaches, and a rapid pulse. After four or six hours, the temperature begins to drop and the patient begins to sweat profusely. Eventually the symptoms disappear but the patient remains weak and tired.

The frequency of the attack depends on the infecting *Plasmodium* species. In *P. vivax* and *P. ovale*, the fever occurs every two days and the attack lasts about one day, so that the disease has a three-day cycle (so-called *tertian malaria*). In *P. malariae*, fever occurs every three days and the attack lasts about one day, making a four-day cycle (so-called *quartan malaria*). And finally, in *P. falciparum*, there is less tendency for the rupture of infected red blood cells to occur simultaneously, and chills and fever may occur every day or be quite irregular (so-called *quotidian malaria*, from L. *quotidianus*, daily). However, even in tertian or quartan malaria, fever can occur daily when the parasites' multiplication cycle originates from several primary infections that overlap each other. In patients infected with *P. falciparum*, the erythrocytic multiplication phase of the parasite occurs in the blood vessels of internal organs, where the decaying blood corpuscles attach to each other and to the blood vessel walls, obstructing the blood flow and causing brain or heart damage. Malaria caused by this species is therefore the most dangerous of the different forms of this disease and may be fatal. In patients infected with *P. vivax* or *P. ovale*, the acute stage of the disease lasts, if the disease is not treated, for about two weeks, after which time the patient slowly recovers. There may, however, be relapses over many months or years, leading to *chronic malaria*, probably caused by parasites living in the cells of the reticuloendothelial system. Malaria is a worldwide disease, with most of the cases concentrated in Central and South America, north and central Africa, all countries bordering on the Mediterranean, and middle and far eastern Asia.

Schistosoma. Formerly called *Bilharzia*, after the German physician Theodor Bilharz, *Schistosoma* is a genus of helminthic worms infesting the small intestinal and portal veins of their host. The worms belong to the *Trematode* class of flatworms (*Platyhelminthes*) and are also called blood flukes. The adult worms of the human parasite *Schistosoma mansoni* are of separate sexes, living in a most unusual arrangement: the male's body is split longitudinally (hence the name, from Gr. *schistos*, split, *soma*, body) and in the groove thus formed resides the threadlike female (Fig. 14.18). Eggs deposited by the female in the blood contain small, rapidly developing larvae, which, by secreting digestive substances, aid the eggs in escaping from the blood vessels through the tissues into the lumen of the intestine and out of the body with the feces. Some eggs, however, enter the circulation and eventually become trapped in the lungs and liver, eliciting a granulomatous reaction from the host. If feces are deposited in water, the fully embryonated eggs hatch and develop into ciliated, free-swimming larvae called *miracidia* (Gr. *meirakidion*, a boy). To develop further, the larvae must find an intermediate host—a freshwater snail. The larvae do not display great host specificity—at least 17 different species of pulmonate snail belonging to three genera may serve as intermediate hosts for this parasite. The miracidium bores into the snail and, upon reaching the snail's digestive tract, develops into a *mother sporocyst* (Gr. *sporos*, seed, *kystis*, bladder)—a simple, saclike structure in which germinal cells bud off internally and develop into a number of *daughter sporocysts*. Eventually the sporocysts transform into fork-tailed *cercariae* (Gr. *kerkos*, tail), which leave the snail and live in the water until they chance upon a human who happens to be bathing or working in the infested pond. On contact, the cercariae penetrate the human skin by a boring action that also involves enzymatic digestion, enter the bloodstream, and let themselves be carried first to the lungs, then to the liver, and finally to the intestinal veins. During this journey, the cercariae are gradually transformed into adult *schistosomulae*.

The infection caused by *S. mansoni*, the so-called *Manson's schistosomiasis*, can be divided into three clinical stages—the incubation period, the acute stage, and the chronic stage. The *incubation period* spans the time between the penetration of the cercariae and the beginning of egg deposit. In this period, the worm causes local and systemic irritation and inflammation, coughing, late afternoon fever, watery skin eruptions (giant urticaria), and swelling, pain, and tenderness of the liver. Most of these symptoms are the result of an allergic reaction of the host to the parasite (see below and also preceding chapter). The *acute stage* is initiated with the beginning of egg deposit. The invasion of eggs into the intestinal wall and liver causes a

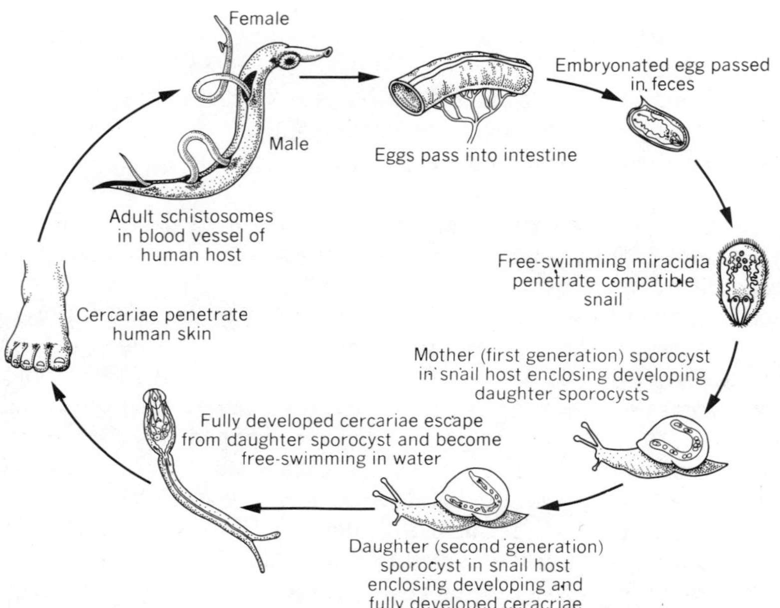

Figure 14.18. The multiplication cycle of *Schistosoma mansoni*. (Compiled from several sources.)

trauma, irritation, and bleeding, to which the host responds with an inflammatory reaction. In the *chronic stage*, which may last 20 years or more if the patient survives, the eggs and parasites are gradually walled off by fibrous tissue, the intestine gradually develops the elasticity of an old garden hose, the liver becomes fibroid and granular, and both organs eventually fail to function.

Schistosomiasis is a widespread helminthic infection in tropical and subtropical regions of Africa, the Middle East, South America, and the Caribbean. Other species of schistosoma parasitic to humans are *S. japonicum* and *S. heamatobium*. The former is the most pathogenic of the three human schistosomes because of the extremely large number of eggs each female produces, and it is also the most difficult to control; the disease it causes is characterized by dysentery and painful spleen and liver enlargement. *S. heamatobium* is common in the Nile delta; it invades the urinary tract, causing inflammation of the bladder and the appearance of blood in the urine.

Defense Reactions

Animal parasites continue to be the great scourges of humanity: some 35 million people in the world suffer from trypanosomiasis, 150 million from malaria, and more than 200 million are infested with schistosomes. In addition, there are several other widely distributed parasitic infections we have not discussed—*amebiasis*, one of the most frequent protozoan infections in humans, caused by *Entamoeba histolytica* and manifested by amoebic dysentery; *leishmaniasis*, caused by a protozoan flagellate related to trypanosomes; *toxoplasmosis*, caused by *Toxoplasma gondii*, another protozoan parasite in the bloodstream or within various cells, especially cells of the reticuloendothelial system; *ancylostomiasis,* caused by the hookworm, *Ancylostoma,* a nematode parasite of the duodenum; and *ascariasis*, caused by *Ascaris* roundworms of the small intestine (see also Table 14.7). An even greater number of parasites infest domestic animals and cause great economic losses.

Why are the protozoal and metazoal parasites so widespread? Are the parasites so successful because the host has failed to develop the proper defense mechanisms against them? For a while it almost seemed so, but now immunologists are beginning to realize that, were it not for powerful defense mechanisms, the parasites would have been even more successful than they are now. The main reason that it is so difficult for the host to handle the protozoal and metazoal parasites is that the parasites have perfected the art of evasiveness. The complex life cycle is itself a major problem for the host, for hardly has it had time to develop immunity to one form than the invader has already reached the next stage, so it takes a while for the host to catch up with the parasite. However, on top of all this, the parasite deliberately changes its "coat," so to speak, to escape the immune mechanisms (see Section 14.2.6).

Table 14.7 Major Human Diseases Caused by Protozoan and Metazoan Parasites

Organism	Disease	Symptoms	Transmission
Protozoa			
Entamoeba histolytica	Amoebic dysentery	Invasion of intestinal mucosa; ulceration of large intestine. May spread to liver, lungs, and brain; causes abscesses.	
Giardia lamblia	Giardiasis	Low-grade intestinal disease. Indigestion and dietary deficiencies.	
Balantidium coli	Balantidiasis	Mild diarrhea; severe ulcerations in mucosa of large intestine.	Pigs
Trichomonas vaginalis	Vaginitis (trichomoniasis)	Genitourinary infection in both sexes. Persistent vaginal or urethral discharge and inflammation.	
Trypanosoma gambiense	African trypanosomiasis	Blood (plasma) parasite.	Tsetse fly
Trypanosoma rhodesiense		Intense headache, fever, insomnia; drowsiness, tremors, delusions, lethargy.	*Glossina* sp.
Trypanosoma cruzi	South American trypanosomiasis	Blood (plasma) parasite. Swollen lymph nodes, fever, anemia.	Hemipteran bug *Triatoma* sp.
Leishmania donovani	Leishmaniasis (kala azar)	Blood parasite. Lesions on internal organs and skin.	Sandfly *Phlebotomus* sp.
Plasmodium sp.	Malaria	Red blood cell parasite. Chills and fevers at regular intervals, followed by profuse sweating.	Mosquito *Anopheles* sp.
Toxoplasma gondii	Toxoplasmosis	Blood parasite. Invasion of reticulo-endothelial cells, leukocytes, and epithelial cells. Fever and swelling of lymph nodes but may affect other organs as well. Transplacental infection.	Widely distributed in animals and birds
Metazoa—flatworms			
Schistosoma sp. (fluke)	Schistosomiasis (bilharziasis)	Enters through skin; develops in portal veins; multiplies in bladder or rectum. Inflammation of skin and bladder. Blood in urine.	Several species of snail
Opisthorchis sinensis (fluke)	Opisthorchiasis	Entry with contaminated food. Infection in bile passages. Irritation; secondary effects from toxic secretions.	Snail, fish
Paragonimus sp. (fluke)	Paragonimiasis	Entry with contaminated food. Lodging in duodenum and lungs. Tuberculosis-like symptoms. Coughing and blood-stained sputum.	Crabs, crayfish, snail
Taenia sp. (tapeworm)	Teniasis	Entry with contaminated food. Lodging in brain and liver. Gastrointestinal and nervous upsets. Anemia and malaise.	Cattle, pigs
Dibothriocephalus latus (tapeworm)	Dibothriocephaliasis	Entry with contaminated food. Lodging in intestine. Gastrointestinal and nervous upsets. Anemia, induced vitamin deficiencies. Diminished appetite, lowered vitality.	Fish
Metazoa—roundworms			
Ascaris lumbricoides	Ascariasis	Entry with food. Migration: intestine → blood → lungs → intestine. Inflammation of the lungs. Anemia, fever, restlessness.	

Table 14.7 (*Continued*)

Organism	Disease	Symptoms	Transmission
Ancylostoma duodenale	Hookworm disease (ancylostomiasis)	Enters through skin. Migrates from blood to lungs and then to intestine. Itching and localized eruption at site of entry. Anemia. Abscesses at site of intestinal attachment.	
Trichinella spiralis	Trichinosis	Enters with food. Migration: intestine → blood → muscles. Abdominal pains, nausea, vomiting and diarrhea, fever, edema, muscular pains, pneumonia.	Pig
Strongyloides stercoralis	Strongyloidiasis	Entry through skin. Migration: blood → lungs → intestine. Redness and intense itching, inflammation of lungs, abdominal pains, nausea, vomiting, diarrhea, and loss of weight.	
Enterobius vermicularis (pinworm)	Enterobiasis	Entry with food, lodging in intestine and perianal region. Rectal irritation and anal itching.	
Trichuris trichiura	Trichuriasis	Entry with food. Development in intestine. Nutritional and digestive disturbances. Anemia and eosinophilia. Muscular aches and dizziness. Abdominal pains.	
Wuchereria sp.	Filariasis	Entry through skin. Microfilariae in peripheral blood; adult forms in lymphatics and connective tissue.	Mosquito *Culex* sp.
Onchocerca volvulus	Onchocerciasis (filariasis)	Entry through skin, lodging in skin. Nodules on face and neck and itching skin.	Black fly *Simulium* sp.
Loa loa	Loiasis (filariasis)	Entry through skin; lodging in subcutaneous connective tissue. Itching and swelling at infection site. Skin and eye irritations.	Mango fly *Chrysops dimidiata*

How, then, does a mammalian species avoid being completely overtaken by parasites? The answer to this question is not yet available; parasitic immunology is a young science, currently generating a large body of individual facts and bits of information that cannot as yet be organized into an all-encompassing view. It is clear that the defense mechanisms are complex and that—as in responsiveness to other parasitic forms—all the defense elements available are mobilized in response to an invasion by an animal parasite. In the following sections we shall consider some of the options available to the host in its effort to confine the parasitic infestation.

Natural Resistance

Incompatibility of Conditions. If the chemical, physiological, and nutritional conditions provided by the host are not those required by the parasite, the parasite fails to survive or reproduce. An example of *chemical incompatibility* is the failure of *Plasmodium vivax* to infect erythrocytes lacking the Duffy blood group antigens. Apparently, the molecular configuration presented by the Duffy antigen is required for a successful interaction of the parasite with the erythrocyte membrane. *Physiological conditions,* such as pH, oxygen tension, or concentration of various metabolites, must be the reason that plasmodia can invade only cells that have reached a very specific stage of their development and that cells in other stages are resistant to the infection. The effect of *nutritional conditions* is apparent from an observation that mice kept on a milk diet are relatively resistant to murine malaria, apparently because they are low in *p*-aminobenzoic acid, which the parasite requires as a growth factor.

Natural Humoral Immunity. Various protozoan parasites, including trypanosomes and leishmanias, are killed when incubated in vitro with fresh serum of many mammalian species. Presumably, normal serum of certain mammal contains factors that can lyse certain protozoal parasites in vivo. However, this observation does not mean that whenever a parasite is killed in vitro by a serum of a given species, it cannot infect this species in vivo, for the parasite can escape the lytic action of the serum—for example, by hiding inside the cell. The *humoral resistance factors* are probably natural antibodies, complement components, or both. For example, *Leishmania enrietti* is killed by normal guinea pig serum because the serum contains natural antibodies directed against the β-D-galactosyl determinant of the parasite membrane, an antigenic configuration commonly found in nature.

Role of Macrophages. Protozoal parasites and certain intermediate developmental stages of metazoal parasites fall into the size range of particles ingestible by phagocytic cells, and phagocytosis undoubtedly plays at least an ancillary role in resistance to certain parasitic infections. However, some parasites resist degradation by phagocytes, even if they have been digested, and in fact, some parasites actually live in macrophages. The antiparasitic potential of macrophages can be enhanced nonspecifically, for example, by endotoxin or by concomitant infection with phylogenetically unrelated organisms. When they become activated as a result of infection, the efficacy of macrophages in killing parasites increases. Activated macrophages have been demonstrated in laboratory animals infested with a variety of protozoal parasites, and pretreatment of animals with agents, such as bacillus Calmette-Guérin (BCG), known to activate macrophages, has been shown to increase the resistance of some of these animals to some parasites.

Role of T Cells. An ability to kill parasites directly has not been demonstrated for T lymphocytes, and they may not have such an ability, since they need to recognize the target in the context of the species' own major histocompatibility complex molecules. However, several intracellular parasites are known to cause the expression of a parasite-specific antigen in the host-cell membrane, and such infected cells can serve as targets for T cell-mediated killing. In addition, T lymphocytes are definitely involved in resistance to animal parasites through their action as helper cells in the stimulation of antibody production.

Role of Antibodies. Antibodies contribute to antiparasite resistance in a variety of ways—the same ways described for antimicrobial immunity. Antibodies can bind to determinants on protozoal parasites, the antigen-antibody complexes can bind complement, and the lytic sequence of the complement cascade can kill the parasite. Antibodies can also bind to a protozoal parasite in the absence of complement and prevent it from infecting a host cell—a phenomenon akin to virus neutralization. Furthermore, antibodies can opsonize the parasite and facilitate its engulfment by macrophages. And finally, antibodies can mediate parasite killing by lymphocytes, in the absence of complement (through antibody-dependent cell-mediated cytotoxicity, ADCC). All four of these functions have been demonstrated to operate against at least some parasites and in at least some experimental conditions. However, with the exception of a few protozoal parasites, such as *Plasmodium*, IgM, IgG, and IgA antibodies do not play a *major* role in antiparasitic immunity.

Role of the IgE-Eosinophil System. The IgE-mediated reactions are probably the main defense mechanism in immunity to metazoal parasites. The reactions lead to the release of pharmacologically active mediators from eosinophils, basophils, and mast cells, and the mediators participate in the defense in at least three major ways. They are responsible for the local accumulation of neutrophils and other leukocytes; they activate these leukocytes and augment their ability to damage the parasite; they act on local tissue elements such as smooth muscle cells, induce local inflammation, produce an environment inhospitable for attachment and feeding of parasites, and aid in the expulsion of parasites already lodged in the tissue. However, eosinophils can also damage the parasite directly. They have been seen attacking a worm's surface, flattening out, and presumably releasing their contents—in particular, the major basic protein from the eosinophil crystaloid core. They cause small lesions in the tegument, and then migrate through these lesions into the interstitial tissue of the worm. After this attack, the tegument is pried off and the worm dies. Eosinophils themselves are drawn to the parasite by the signal from mast cells activated by IgG bound to the parasite (see Chapter 13).

14.2.6 Ways in Which Parasites Evade Immunity

To conclude this section on antiparasitic immunity, we shall describe some of the tricks parasites use to escape the immune response. During this discussion we should keep in mind that the parasite cannot afford to elude host immunity completely, for if it did, it would perish with the host on which it depends for survival.

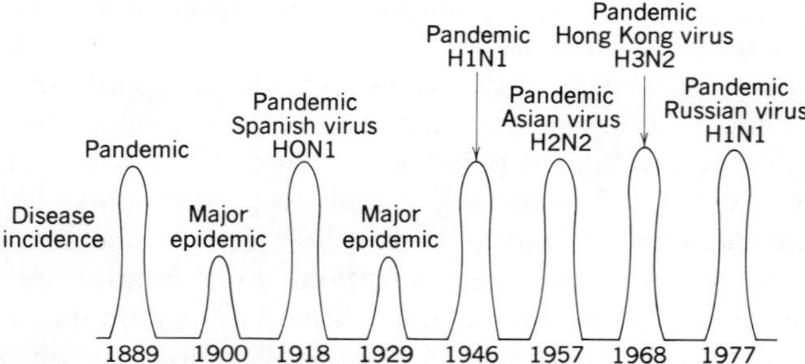

Figure 14.19. Major pandemics and epidemics of influenza in the human population since 1889. (Modified from the NIAID Director's Report for 1978.)

Herpes Virus in Hiding

If a herpes simplex virus manages to reach deep epidermal layers of the skin, it infects the cells but goes immediately into hiding. Nothing on the cell surface reveals its presence, and for good reason—the deep epidermal layers border tissues that are full of macrophages scanning the area for alien elements. The virus keeps this "low profile" for as long as it is in this danger zone. But as the infected cells divide and the daughter cells move toward the surface, and hence away from the combat zone, the virus—which multiplies along with the cells it inhabits—becomes bolder, its activity increases, and it even expresses viral antigens on the cell surface. So, in effect, the virus tricks the immune system, by hiding inside the cell when in the combat zone and surfacing when it is out of the dangerous area.

Antigenic Shifts and Drifts of the Influenza Virus

The influenza virus eludes the host's immune response by constantly changing its antigenic properties. These changes are of two kinds—antigenic drift and antigenic shift—and occur in the hemagglutinin (H) and neuraminidase (N) molecules on the surface of the virus particle. The changes can best be explained by following the evolution of the virus since 1918, the year of the Spanish flu that killed an estimated 20 million people worldwide (Fig. 14.19). The virus that caused this global outbreak (pandemic infection) was of type A and had certain antigenic characteristics (i.e., it reacted with certain specific antibodies directed against the H and N molecules), which were given the designation "subtype H0N1," where the numbers are arbitrary designations of the serotype. (Since the virus is related to a virus isolated in pigs in 1931, it is also referred to as subtype HswN1—"sw" for swine.) The H0N1 subtype persisted in the human population until 1946, when a second influenza pandemic occurred. When the virus causing this outbreak was isolated, investigators realized that it was still of the A type (it shared core proteins with the H0N1 virus), and furthermore, that it shared the N1 serotype with the H0N1 subtype but carried a completely different H molecule that did not react with any of the antibodies produced against the H0 molecule. This new molecule was designated H1, and the subtype of the new A-type virus was designated H1N1. This sudden, drastic change in antigenic properties of the viral molecule was called the *antigenic shift*. This new virus rapidly displaced the previous virus and circulated all over the world for more than a decade. Then, in 1956, another major antigenic shift occurred in both the H and N molecules, and a new "Asian" virus appeared, presumably spreading from Asia. The new H2N2 virus circulated in the population until 1968, when it was replaced by a new subtype, H3N2, the Hong Kong virus. Finally, the most recent antigenic shift of the virus occurred in 1977, with the re-emergence of H1N1 (Russian) virus.

Each antigenic shift finds the human population unprepared for the infection, since the antibodies directed against the preceding subtype provide little protection against the new subtype, so the virus spreads easily across the globe. How the new subtypes arise is not known, but some clues are beginning to be provided by the recent advances in molecular biology that have allowed the cloning of the H-encoding gene and elucidation of the primary structure of some of the H molecules. A comparison of two H molecules belonging to two different subtypes (Fig. 14.20) reveals so many differences between them that one subtype's evolving into the other by accumulation of point mutation within the period between the two pandemics can virtually be excluded as an explanation. The possibility that the new subtype derives by recombination between two different viruses is a more likely theory. You may recall that the influenza virion contains eight molecules of RNA carrying different genes. If a single cell is infected simultaneously by two viruses, the RNA molecules may reassort in such a way that a new virus, carrying some RNA molecules of one virus and other molecules of the other virus, arises. According to this hypothesis, the origin of the Hong Kong virus can be explained as follows:

$$\begin{array}{c} \text{H2N2} \times \text{H3NX} \\ \downarrow \\ \text{H3N2} \end{array}$$

JAP HA (H2, 1957)	M A I I Y L I L L F T A V R G D Q I C I G Y
X31 HA (H3, 1968)	M K T I I A L S Y I F C L A L G Q D F P G N D N S T A T L C L G H
29C HA (H3, 1968)	M K T I I A L S Y I F C L A L G Q D L P G N D N N T A T L C L G H
VIC HA (H3, 1975)	M K T I I A L S Y I F C L V F A Q D L P G N D N N S T A T L C L G H
	H A N N S T E J V D T B K E R B V T V T G A J D U K E J T G B G J K C K L N G
	H A V P N G T L V K T I T D D Q I E V T N A T E L V Q S S S T G K I C N — N P
	H A V P N G T L V K T I T D D Q I E V T N A T E L V Q S S S T G K I C N — N P
	H A V P N G T L V K T I T N D Q I E V T N A T E L V Q S S S T G K I C N — N P
	I P P L E L G D C S I A G W L L G N P E C D R L L S V P E W S Y I M E K E N P
	H R I L D G I D C T L I D A L L G D P H C D V F Q N E T W D L F V E R S K A
	H R I L D G I D C T L I D A L L G D P H C D V F Q N E T W D L F V E R S K A
	H R I L D G I D C T L I D A L L G D P H C D G F Q N E K W D L F V E R S K A

Figure 14.20. Partial amino-acid sequences of influenza H2 and H3 hemagglutinins. The sequences have been aligned to maximize homology (indicated by boxes). Amino acid symbols are explained in Table 6.15. (From M.-J. Gething, J. Bye, J. Skehel, and M. Waterfield, *Nature* **287**:301–306, 1980.)

Here, the Asian virus might have recombined with another, unknown virus in such a way that the new virus inherited the N-encoding RNA molecules from the Asian virus and the H-encoding molecules from the unknown virus. The big question now is where these unknown viruses come from. Since influenza viruses are present in many other mammals, including pigs and horses, and in many species of bird, it is possible that the new viruses are drawn from these animal reservoirs.

In addition to antigenic shifts, the influenza virus undergoes yet another type of change in the period between two pandemics. These changes, the *antigenic drift*, are far less drastic and are fully explainable by the accumulation of point mutations in the viral RNA genes. The drift generates new virus strains, designated by the virus type, the place of infection, the sequential number of the isolate, and the year of isolation. For example, A/Peking/4/77 is an influenza type-A virus responsible for an outbreak in Peking; it is the fourth isolate, and the isolation occurred in 1977. Different strains of a given subtype differ in their number of amino acid substitutions (Fig. 14.20), and one can use this observation to construct an evolutionary tree that shows the presumed relationship between the individual strains (Fig. 14.21). When any of the accumulating mutations affect the antigenic site of the molecule encoded by the particular gene, the site changes and may no longer react with some of the antibodies directed against it. The virus with the altered antigenic site may, therefore, possess a growth advantage, and may cause a local outbreak (endemic) of the disease until antibodies against the altered determinants are formed. Antigenic drift thus appears to be the result of selection of virus particles with altered antigenic determinants. Antigenic drift also occurs in

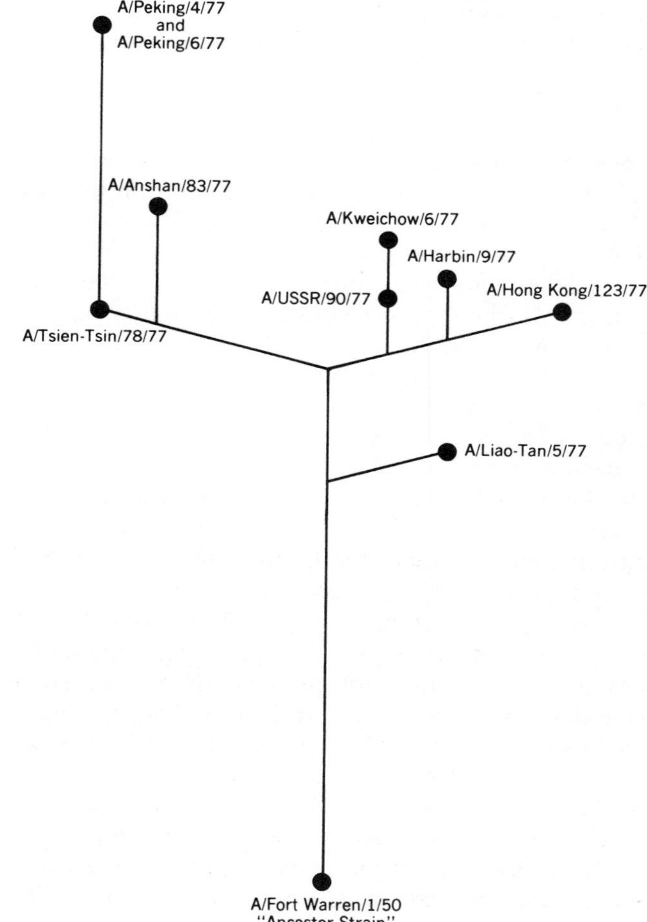

Figure 14.21. Evolutionary tree of different H1N1 influenza virus strains. The basis for the construction of the tree was data on the primary structure of the RNA molecules from the indicated virus strains. The length of the lines between isolates indicates relative genetic distance according to detectable point mutations. (According to J. F. Young, U. Desselberger, and P. Palese: *Cell* **18**:73–83, 1979.)

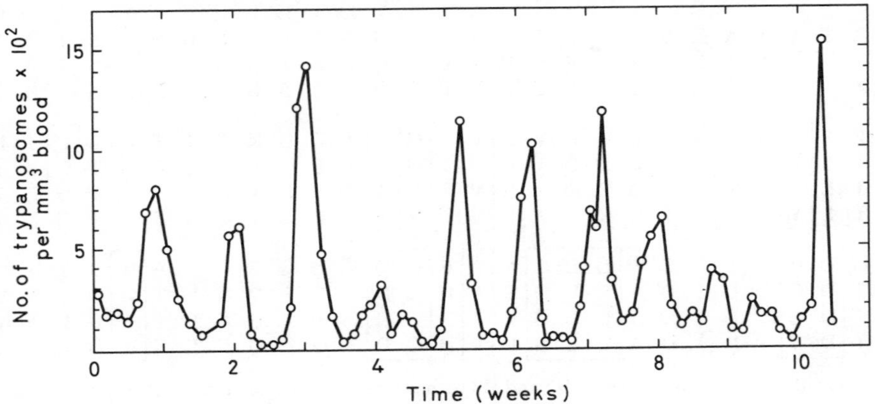

Figure 14.22. Number of circulating parasites in a patient with African trypanosomiasis. (From K. Vickerman: *Ciba Found. Symp.* **25**:53–80, 1974.)

the milder type-B virus; antigenic shifts, on the other hand, occur only in the type-A virus.

Antigenic Variation in Trypanosomes

Since the beginning of this century, parasitologists have known that, following an infection from the bite of the tsetse fly, the number of trypanosomes in the blood fluctuates periodically: the parasite population peaks about one week after the infection, then declines, peaks again two weeks after the infection, and so on for many months (Fig. 14.22). Later studies have revealed that this fluctuation is the result of a remarkable deadly game between the parasite and its host. The infecting parasite catches the host unprepared, so the trypanosomes multiply unchecked for about a week. But during this time, the host mobilizes its immune system and begins to produce antibodies against the antigen molecules that coat the parasite: the antibodies lyse or agglutinate the trypanosomes, and the size of the parasite population rapidly declines. But then, a few parasites emerge from the declining population; they are coated with molecules completely different from those of the preceding variant, and are therefore unaffected by the antibodies that the host has so laboriously produced. Unchecked by any defense mechanisms, the few multiply and flood the host, which must now start all over again with the production of a new kind of antibody. When it manages to redirect the antibody production and the antibodies begin to eliminate the second variant of the parasite, the trypanosomes change their coats again, and so the process goes on. Since the new coat is always completely different from all the preceding ones, the previously produced antibodies are of no use against the new parasite variants.

The coat that the trypanosome changes so ea consists of glycoprotein molecules, each with a mol ular weight of about 60,000 daltons, attached fr outside to the cell membrane of the parasite. The mc cules constitute from 5 to 10 percent of the tc protein and 30 percent of the soluble protein of a t panosome cell. Each cell is coated by about 7 × molecules, a number probably sufficient to cover entire surface of the parasite with a uniform homo neous glycocalyx. The variant glycoprotein molecu are composed of between 7 and 17 percent carbo drate; it resides in the C-terminal of the polypept chain, which is also the region of the molecule's atta ment to the membrane. Amino acid sequencing of N-terminal ends of glycoproteins isolated from f successive variants of *T. brucei* revealed essentially structural homologies; each polypeptide had a cc pletely unique sequence (Fig. 14.23). Since *antigenic variation* can also occur in clones of trypa somes grown from a single organism, each trypa some must contain the genetic information necess for the expression of all the variant antigens. The t

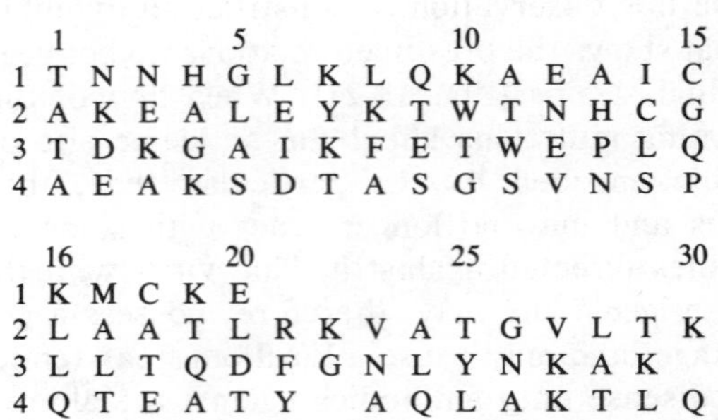

	1				5					10					15
1	T	N	N	H	G	L	K	L	Q	K	A	E	A	I	C
2	A	K	E	A	L	E	Y	K	T	W	T	N	H	C	G
3	T	D	K	G	A	I	K	F	E	T	W	E	P	L	Q
4	A	E	A	K	S	D	T	A	S	G	S	V	N	S	P

	16				20					25					30
1	K	M	C	K	E										
2	L	A	A	T	L	R	K	V	A	T	G	V	L	T	K
3	L	L	T	Q	D	F	G	N	L	Y	N	K	A	K	
4	Q	T	E	A	T	Y		A	Q	L	A	K	T	L	Q

Figure 14.23. N-terminal amino-acid sequences of four va antigens of *Trypanosoma*. (From P. J. Bridgen, G. A. Cross, a Bridgen, *Nature* **263**:613–614, 1976.)

number of variants that can be expressed by a single trypanosome clone probably runs into the hundreds. Although there seem to be no strict sequences in which the different variants appear, there may be a definite pattern that is predictable, at least to some extent. DNA cloning experiments indicate that the gene encoding a given variant antigen is, indeed, present in different trypanosomes, but that it is flanked by different DNA sequences in each case. This finding suggests that antigenic variation is preceded by some kind of gene rearrangement.

The role of antibodies in antigenic variation is not completely clear, although it is extremely unlikely that the antibodies induce the variation directly. The possibility that the different variants already exist in the parasite population and that, as the predominant variant is killed by the antibodies, another variant simply outgrows it has also been excluded. It is more probable that new variants arise continually with a low frequency of perhaps one per 10,000 individuals, and the host antibodies, by killing the predominant variant, enable the new variant to expand. The generation of new variants probably involves expression of new genes.

Plasmodium Jamming Immune Response

Patients with malaria have extraordinarily elevated levels of IgM, rising on occasion to 5 g per 100 ml. Yet paradoxically, fewer than 5 percent of the immunoglobulins react with antigens of plasmodium. Furthermore, such patients, when immunized against irrelevant antigens—such as those of *Salmonella* or tetanus toxoid—respond much less than do healthy persons. And spleen cells from plasmodium-infected animals usually give high backgrounds when tested in the Jerne-plaque assay for their response to sheep red blood cells—an observation strongly reminiscent of that made on mice treated with a polyclonal activator, such as endotoxin. It seems, therefore, that the parasite exerts polyclonal mitogenic activity on the host's lymphoid system, causing many clones of B lymphocytes to undergo division and differentiation. In this manner, the parasite jams the immune system and so depresses its protective potential. Similar depression of humoral immunity also occurs in patients infected with trypanosomes.

Disguising in Schistosomes

Schistosomes have learned yet another trick to avoid being killed by the host's immune response. Following the attachment to human skin, the cercariae discard the glycocalyx needed during their existence in fresh water and reveal the double-bilayer outer membrane, which carries parasite-specific antigens. The exposed antigens stimulate the host's immune response, but while the response is developing, the immature worm, the *schistosomulum*, makes its way to the blood vessels and there begins to cover itself with the host's molecules—red blood cell antigens and molecules controlled by the major histocompatibility complex. The blood plasma probably contains a low concentration of these molecules, which are continually shed from cells regenerating their surfaces. The schistosomulum somehow picks up the MHC molecules and completely coats its body with them, masking its own membrane antigens. By doing so, the parasite becomes effectively invisible to the host immune system, which, from then on, regards the schistosomulum as a part of self. If such a host is re-exposed to new cercariae, the developing new schistosomules will encounter the immune response stimulated by the first infection and be killed, while the adult schistosomes already living in the body will be untouched by the immunity. This mechanism prevents superinfection by new parasites, while allowing the old parasites to persist in the body for many years.

14.3 NEOPLASIA AND THE IMMUNE SYSTEM

All living cells have the potential to bear offspring (to *proliferate*) and to acquire characteristics and functions different from those of the original type (to *differentiate*). Normally, the expression of this potential is very carefully regulated and coordinated with the behavior of other cells and tissues in the body. Occasionally, however, a cell may escape these strict controls and begin to proliferate at a rate that greatly exceeds the normal requirements of the tissue of which this cell is a part. By an unregulated proliferation and differentiation of the aberrant cell, a body arises within the body that obeys its own laws without respect for the organism as a whole and without serving any useful function. In some instances, this new "formation," or *neoplasm*, although autonomous to some extent, is not autonomous enough to invade surrounding and distant tissues; in other cases, the neoplasm aggressively attacks and replaces normal tissues, and by doing so, sooner or later kills the organism. The former type of neoplasm is called a *tumor*, the latter a *cancer*. In this sense, a tumor is a less vicious form of neoplasm than cancer; but in practice, it is often difficult to decide what is the less and what is the more vicious growth, and so the three terms—neoplasm, tumor, and cancer—are often used interchangeably.

Neoplasia is undoubtedly the most universal of all diseases. Tumors have been found in plants, oysters, fruitflies, fish, amphibians, birds, and mammals. The potential for the emergence of neoplasms probably exists in all many-celled organisms, but most organisms do not live long enough to express it. Neoplasia is probably also the oldest disease—it may have existed from the time the first many-celled organisms appeared on earth, although this statement is impossible to document. Certainly neoplasia must have existed at least since the time of the dinosaurs, because dinosaur bones that bear marks interpreted as being caused by cancer have been found. Human cancer is mentioned in some of the oldest written records of humankind, as for example, the so-called Ebers Papyrus or the Edwin Smith Papyrus, produced in Egypt in about 5500 B.C. And indeed, X-ray analysis of mummies from the Egyptian Third, Fourth, and Fifth Dynasties reveals that some of the pharaohs suffered from and even died of cancer.

The word "cancer" was coined by Hippocrates in the fourth century B.C. According to some scholars, he used the name because cancer of the breast, with the congested veins radiating from the center to the periphery, reminded him of a crab with its many legs and claws (Gr. *karkinos*, crab); according to others, the name refers to the observation that cancer causes pain similar to that experienced from the bite of a crab. The word "tumor" first appears in the writings of Claudius Galen, known to his contemporaries as Clarissimus the Brilliant. Galen, the medical authority of the western world from the second century A.D. to the beginning of the Renaissance, distinguished three kinds of tumor—tumors according to nature, tumors exceeding nature, and tumors contrary to nature (this last category included true tumors as we define them today). Originally, therefore, the word "tumor" was used for any kind of swelling, including that resulting from neoplasia.

Cancer is second only to diseases of the heart and blood vessels as a killer of people in the western world. In the United States alone, more than half a million people develop cancer and 330,000 people die of it annually. Cancer causes 10 percent of all deaths in people between 40 and 80 years of age.

14.3.1 Terms and Definitions

We shall use the term *neoplasm* (Gr. *neos*, new, *plasma*, thing formed) to designate any abnormal tissue growth, autonomous in nature and occurring at the expense, rather than for the benefit, of the body. A neoplasm that attacks the surrounding tissue aggressively and replaces it with a disorganized mass shall be referred to as *malignant* (L. *maligno*, to do something maliciously); that which is not autonomous enough to invade surrounding tissues will be referred to as *benign* (L. *benignus*, kind). Malignant neoplasms (cancers) are characterized by the following features (Fig. 14.24): *aplasia*, a loss of normal appearance and the transformation of a tissue into a disorganized mass; *invasiveness*, the pushing forward of cancer cells into normal tissues and destruction of normal cells; and *metastasis* (Gr. *meta*, in the midst of, *stasis*, a placing, a stand, literally a removing), the release of cell clusters capable of colonizing distant organs.

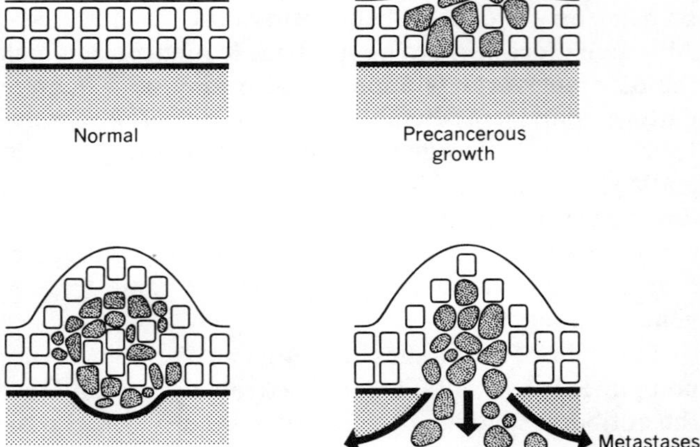

Figure 14.24. Schematic representation of normal tissue and various forms of abnormal cell masses. (From R. Weil: *Biochim. Biophys. Acta* **506**:301–388, 1978.)

Malignant neoplasms are usually resistant to treatment, recur after removal, and are often fatal. Nonmalignant, or benign, neoplasms (tumors) grow more slowly than the malignant ones, are usually surrounded by a capsule of compressed normal tissue, do not come back after removal by surgery or irradiation, do not infiltrate surrounding tissues, and do not metastasize. They can nevertheless be dangerous if they occur in vital locations such as the brain. However, it should be emphasized again that the distinction between cancers and tumors is made mostly by clinicians dealing with human tumors; experimental neoplasms are difficult to divide into these two categories, so many researchers use the terms "neoplasm," "cancer," and "tumor" as synonyms.

Neoplasms usually retain some resemblance to the normal tissue from which they arise, so that an experienced pathologist can determine the origin of a given neoplasm merely by examining histological sections made from it (Fig. 14.25). Neoplasms arising from dif-

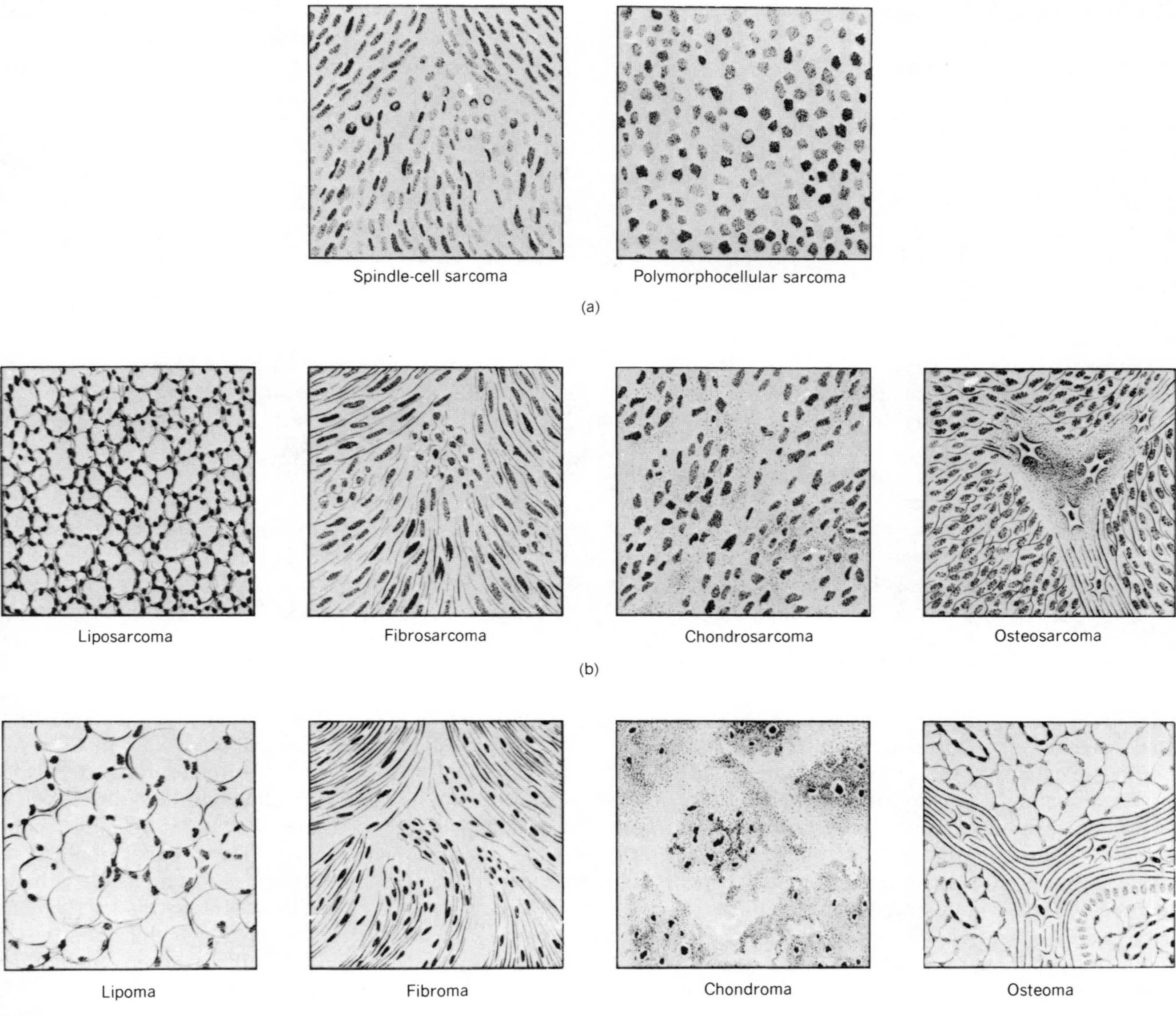

Figure 14.25. Histological appearance of some mesenchymal neoplasms. (*a*) Dedifferentiated sarcomas. (*b*) Sarcomas partially retaining the character of the tissue of their origin. (*c*) Benign tumors. (From M. Eder and P. Gedigk: *Lehrbuch der Allgemeinen Pathologie und der Pathologischen Anatomie*. Springer-Verlag, Berlin, 1975.)

ferent tissues bear different names, hundreds of them, since naming things is part of human nature. Most of these end in *-oma*, the suffix generally used to indicate a tumor. Neoplasms derived from epithelial tissues, such as the skin and the lining of the digestive or respiratory tract, are called *carcinomas*. The term is often attached to another word, and names such as *adenocarcinoma*, a cancer of glandular tissue (Gr. *aden*, gland), *hepatocarcinoma*, cancer of the liver (Gr. hēpar, liver), *bronchocarcinoma*, cancer of the lungs, arising from the bronchus, and *cervical carcinoma*, a cancer of the uterine cervix, are formed. Tumors derived from tissues of mesodermal origin, such as connective tissues, bones, or muscle, are referred to as *sarcomas* (Gr. *sarx*, flesh). These too may assume a variety of forms, referred to by different names—*osteogenic sarcoma*, or *osteosarcoma*, cancer of the bone, *fibrosarcoma*, cancer originating from connective tissue, or *lymphosarcoma*, cancer involving lymph nodes.

14.3.2 Experimental Induction of Cancer

Neoplasms arising in an animal that has not been treated in any way to cause the development of cancer are termed *spontaneous*, in contrast to *induced* neoplasms that have been produced purposely by a cancer-producing agent or *carcinogen* (Gr. *genesis*, generation). Carcinogens can be of physical, chemical, or biological nature.

Physical Carcinogens

It was noted early in the sixteenth century that most of the miners excavating silver, nickel, cobalt, uranium, and arsenic in Krušné hory, the mountain ridge in west Bohemia, developed, over a period of years, a progressive, fatal disease of the lungs. It was not until 1879, however, that the disease was identified as cancer, and it was only several decades later that the high incidence of lung carcinoma could be ascribed to the inhalation of radon, the gaseous emanation from radium.

Within a few years after the discovery of X-rays in 1895 and of radioactivity in 1896, a high frequency of skin burns and malignant skin cancers were noted on the hands of radiologists and other users of X-ray devices and radium. By 1914 a total of 104 cases had been recorded and analyzed, and the conclusion was reached that ionizing radiation can cause cancer.

Evidence implicating ultraviolet light as a cancer-inducing agent has also been gathered over many years. It was noted, for example, that sailors who were exposed to intense sunlight over long periods had a high incidence of skin cancer. Acting on this clue, researchers later demonstrated that irradiation of mice with UV light causes skin cancer. (Exposure of the whole body to ionizing irradiation, in contrast, induces mostly cancer of the hematopoietic and lymphoid systems.)

Despite years of intensive research, the mechanism of cancer induction by ionizing and UV radiation remains to be elucidated. The following hypotheses have been proposed to explain the carcinogenic effects of ionizing radiation.

The absorbed energy of the radiation activates a latent virus present in the irradiated cell, and this virus then transforms the normal cell into a cancerous one.

Radiation-induced depression in the body's immune reactivity increases the chances of infection by a carcinogenic virus.

Radiation induces mutations in somatic cells, and some of these mutations may result in the loss of control over the cell's proliferative abilities.

Radiation induces chromosomal rearrangement, some of which may predispose the cell to cancer.

The mechanisms of cancer induction by UV radiation are also unknown. In addition to the mechanisms listed above, this form of radiation may also act via metabolic products, the formation of which it stimulates. Researchers have demonstrated, for example, that the exposure of human skin to UV light leads to the synthesis of cholesterol-α-oxide, a compound known to have cancer-inducing properties.

Chemical Carcinogens

When my mother died I was very young,
And my father sold me while yet my tongue
Could scarcely cry "weep, weep, weep, weep,"
So your chimney I sweep & in soot I sleep.

So begins William Blake's moving description of the hardships of a chimney sweep in eighteenth-century England. In the history of child labor, there are few chapters more horrible than that dealing with the institution of chimney sweeps. They were very young boys who were forced by their masters to sweep chimneys by climbing through them, and often, when they seemed to be too slow, the master would make them move faster by lighting a fire under them. Blake's contemporary, the eminent English physician Sir Percival Pott, treated many of the unfortunate youngsters and noted that an unusual percentage of them developed a carcinoma of the scrotum. Pott's observation, published in 1775, was the first recorded example of a cancer induced by a chemical substance, for it later turned out that the most likely explanation for the high incidence of scrotum carcinomas was the retention of soot and tar in the wrinkles of the scrotum when other parts of the body were cleansed.

The first experimental evidence that compounds contained in tar can indeed induce cancer was provided in 1915 by Katsusaburo Yamagiva and Koichi Ichikawa. These two investigators painted the inner surfaces of rabbit ears with a crude tar dissolved in benzene every second or third day for almost a year. Their persistence paid off, for eventually, papillary growth that later became cancerous developed at the site of painting. The observation suggested that the prolonged action of some chemical substances in the tar induced cancer in the epithelial cells of the ear; the substances were later identified as polycyclic hydrocarbons. To this day, tar-painting has remained a favored experimental method of cancer induction in experimental animals.

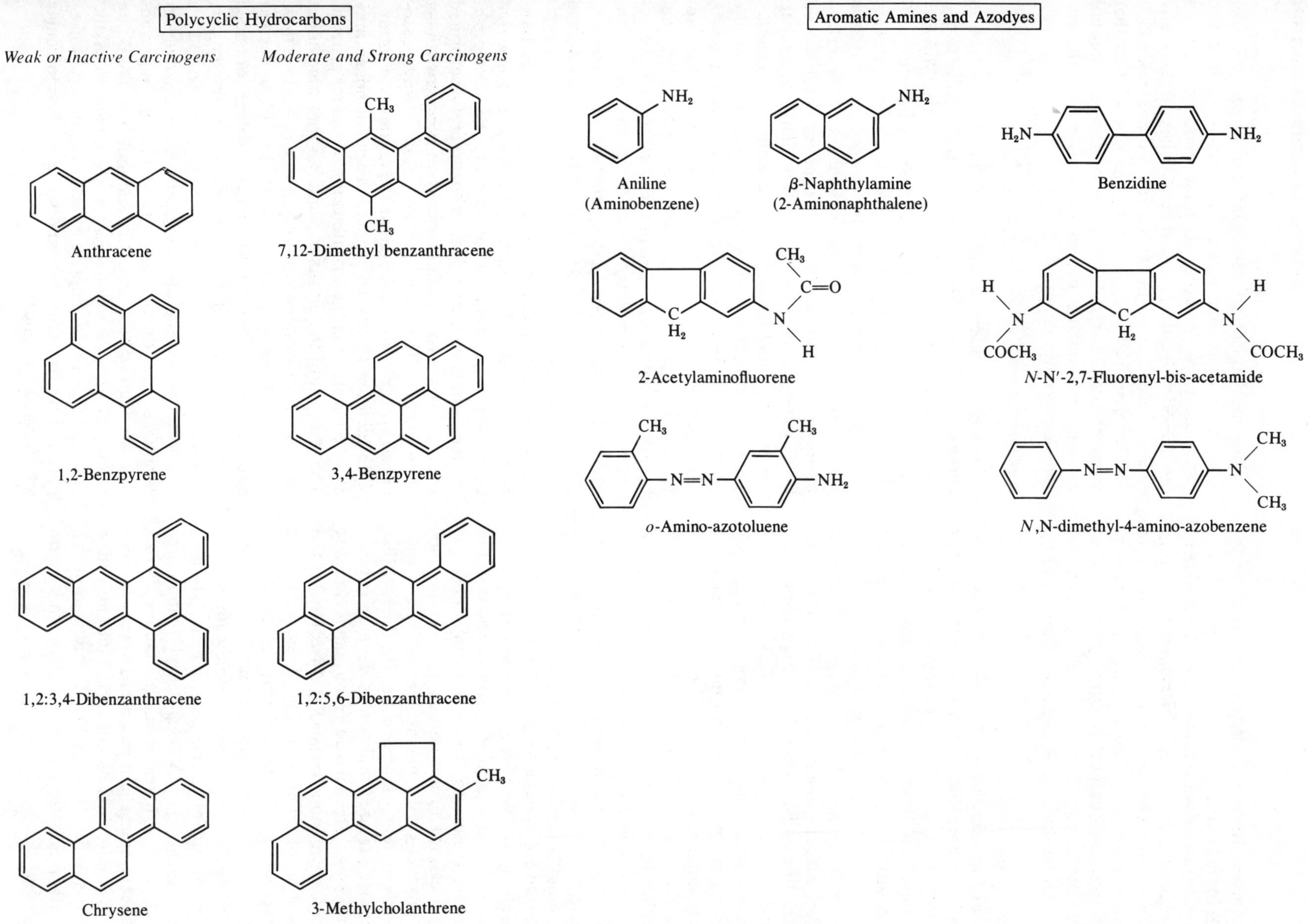

Polycyclic Hydrocarbons

Weak or Inactive Carcinogens *Moderate and Strong Carcinogens*

CH_3 CH_3

Anthracene

7,12-Dimethyl benzanthracene

1,2-Benzpyrene

3,4-Benzpyrene

1,2:3,4-Dibenzanthracene

1,2:5,6-Dibenzanthracene

CH_3

Chrysene

3-Methylcholanthrene

Aromatic Amines and Azodyes

NH_2

Aniline (Aminobenzene)

NH_2

β-Naphthylamine (2-Aminonaphthalene)

H_2N NH_2

Benzidine

CH_3 C=O N H C H_2

2-Acetylaminofluorene

H N $COCH_3$ C H_2 H N $COCH_3$

N-N′-2,7-Fluorenyl-bis-acetamide

CH_3 N=N CH_3 NH_2

o-Amino-azotoluene

N=N N CH_3 CH_3

N,N-dimethyl-4-amino-azobenzene

Figure 14.26. Examples of chemical carcinogens.

Yamagiva's and Ichikawa's discovery set off an intense search for substances with carcinogenic activity. Many such substances were found, some by accident, others by painstaking testing of thousands of compounds. The known chemical carcinogens are quite heterogeneous in terms of their structure and properties, and no unifying characteristic common to all of them has been found. The two main groups are polycyclic hydrocarbons and aromatic amines (Fig. 14.26).

Polycyclic hydrocarbons are benzene derivatives containing, as the name suggests, only hydrogen and carbon. Their carcinogenicity depends on the number of benzene rings present in their molecules: substances with fewer than four rings are not carcinogenic; substances with four rings are mildly carcinogenic; and substances with five or more rings (e.g., 3,4-benzpyrene and 3-methylcholanthrene) are often highly efficient cancer-inducing agents. They are structurally related to sterols, bile acids, and sex hormones, found normally in higher organisms. This fact has led to speculations that cancer-producing hydrocarbons may arise in organisms by the abnormal metabolism of these natural compounds, and may be responsible for some spontaneously developing neoplasms. Most of the polycyclic hydrocarbons are not carcinogenic themselves; to become cancer-producing, they must first be converted to their active forms by specific enzymes present in the cell. For example, 3,4-benzpyrene must be converted by a liver enzyme, aryl hydroxlase, into 5,6-epoxide (Fig. 14.27) before it can act as a carcinogen. The normal function of aryl hydroxylase is to detoxify aromatic hydrocarbons in the liver by turning them into harmless metabolites; but when given a chance to act on benzpyrene-like substances, it produces carcinogenic derivatives. Variation in the enzyme levels may account for the fact that not all carcinogen-treated individuals develop cancer.

Aromatic amines are derived from *aniline* (Arabic *an-nil*, indigo), an aminobenzene (Fig. 14.26) that is the parent substance of many synthetic dyes. In fact, it was the observation of a high frequency of bladder cancer among dye factory workers that first drew attention to aniline derivatives as possible carcinogens. And again, aniline itself is not carcinogenic, but its derivatives, such as *N,N*-dimethyl-4-aminoazobenzene, and other azodyes, β-naphthylamine, benzidine, and 2-acetylaminofluorene, are. However, these carcinogens too must first be converted into an active form by hydroxylation (Fig. 14.27). The oxidation can take place either directly on the aromatic ring or on the amino group.

The mechanism of chemical carcinogenesis, like that of physical carcinogenesis, is not known. Since carcinogens are known to act directly or indirectly on the DNA molecules, researchers believe that many cancers arise as a result of changes in these molecules. This contention is supported by the observation that many chemical carcinogens are also mutagens that are capable of inducing hereditary changes in the organism's genetic material.

Biological Agents

Of the great variety of biological factors involved in carcinogenesis, we shall mention here only two—hormones and viruses. The profound effect of *hormones* on some cancerous growths has been demonstrated in several experimental systems. Researchers have observed, for example, that in mice, spontaneous mammary carcinomas—that is, cancers of the breast tissue—grew rapidly during pregnancy and slowed down or even disappeared after the delivery, only to renew their rapid growth in a subsequent pregnancy. These observations led to the conclusion that the growth of mammary carcinomas is dependent on female sex hormones. This conclusion is further supported by another experiment, demonstrating that breast cancer in rats disapppears after surgical removal of ovaries, and by the observation that implantation of diethylstilbestrol, a synthetic crystalline compound possessing estrogenic activity, into an animal induces cancer.

In some instances, however, sex hormones hav just the opposite effect in that it is their absence that potentiates development of cancer. For example, hunters sometimes find deer with severely deformed antlers that are the result of incessant bone growth—a bone cancer. The condition is almost always associated with previous damage to the animal's scrotum.

In addition to sex hormones, other hormones may also be involved in the maintenance of cancer growth. The removal of the pituitary gland has the same effect on mammary carcinomas as ovariectomy—it stops their growth. Conversely, the implantation of a second pituitary gland under the skin, into the spleen, or under the kidney capsule of a mouse induces mammary carcinomas.

The second group of biological factors involved in carcinogenesis, the *oncogenic viruses*, is so important that we shall devote an entire section to it. By doing so, we shall once again digress somewhat from the main theme of this chapter, but this digression is necessary if we are to understand some of the molecular mechanisms of cancer induction.

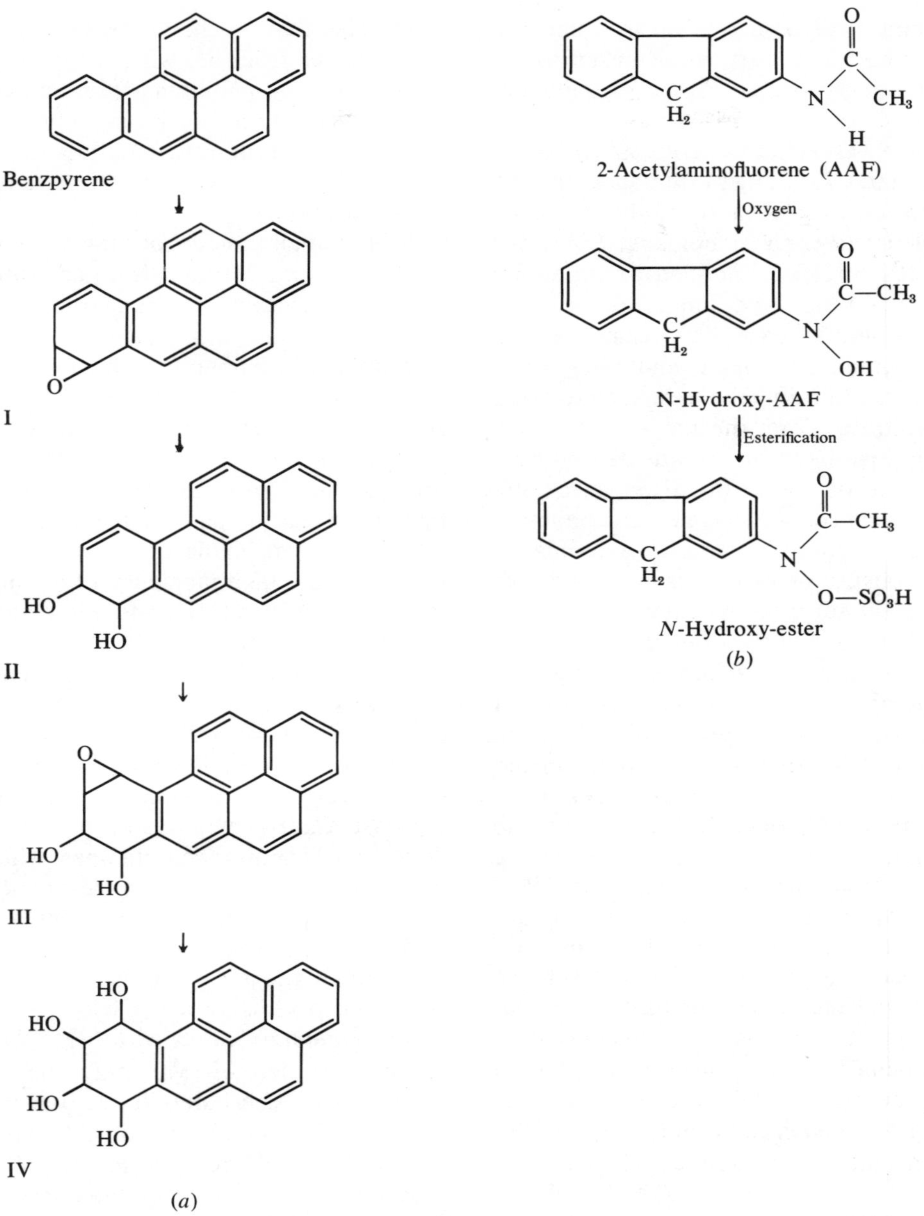

Benzpyrene

I

II

III

IV

(*a*)

2-Acetylaminofluorene (AAF)

Oxygen

N-Hydroxy-AAF

Esterification

N-Hydroxy-ester

(*b*)

Figure 14.27. Metabolic reactions converting precarcinogenic compounds benzpyrene (A) and 2-acetylaminofluorene (B) into potent carcinogens. The conversion is part of a metabolic detoxification process that normally occurs in the liver. Of the four intermediates of benzpyrene metabolism, the most strongly carcinogenic is compound III which can react with guanine residues in DNA molecules, intercalate between the two DNA strands and cause error-prone DNA repair leading to gene mutations. In the case of AAF, the most carcinogenic is the N-hydroxy-ester form of this azodye.

14.3.3 Oncogenic Viruses

Discovery

There are discoveries in science that catch on immediately and are, from the start, almost generally accepted; others must be repeated several times before the point they are making is understood and accepted. The discovery of virus involvement in cancer induction is an example of the latter. Over a period of some 50 years, various researchers repeatedly observed that certain neoplasms contained infectious agents capable of inducing the same type of neoplasm in other animals, and for over half a century these observations were either ignored or demeaned. Some of these observations are described briefly below.

The very first observation in this series was made by Vilhelm Ellermann and Oluf Bang in Denmark. In 1908 these authors reported on a disease of the domestic fowl that resembled leukemia in humans. Since the blood of the affected birds was flooded by immature erythrocytes (erythroblasts) and immature granulocytes (myeloblasts), the disease was termed erythromyeloblastic leukemia. Ellermann and Bang demonstrated that the leukemia could be passed on to other birds by cell-free filtrates from the blood of the sick chickens, and they postulated that it was caused by a virus. The publication of the work raised no excitement at all, mainly because, at that time, leukemia was considered to be an infectious rather than a neoplastic disease, so the demonstration of a virus as a causative agent came as no great surprise. Needless to say, the prevailing view of leukemia at the time of these experiments was wrong—leukemia *is* a form of cancer.

The second time around, in 1911, viral etiology of cancer was demonstrated by Peyton Rous, also on domestic fowl. Rous later told a story about an old farmer who came to him with a chicken bearing a strange lump, and how he then tried to transplant the lump to other chickens and was surprised when he succeeded. He then tried the same thing that Ellermann and Bang had tried before him: he passed material from the tumor through a bacterial filter impermeable to cells and bacteria, and injected the cell-free filtrate into young chickens. When the birds again developed what he had, in the meantime, diagnosed as sarcoma, Rous concluded that viruses were able to produce cancer in chickens. This time there was no excuse for ignoring the observation, but, in fact, very few people paid any attention. Recognition came to Rous 55 years later in the form of a Nobel Prize, awarded at a time when the *Rous sarcoma virus* was already a highly popular model in the study of virus-cell interaction.

A third cancer-inducing virus was discovered in 1933 by Richard E. Shope in wartlike growths or papillomas (L. *papilla*, a nipple) occurring in wild cottontail rabbits of Kansas and Iowa. Some of the warts were so large that hunters referred to them as "horns." Shope made an extract from the neoplasms, filtered off the cellular material, and rubbed the cell-free filtrate on the scarrified skin of wild and domestic rabbits. Papillomas appeared in both types of rabbit, but in the wild rabbit they appeared more slowly and attained larger size than in the domestic rabbit. Furthermore, only filtrates from the warts of wild rabbits were able to transmit the papilloma-forming agent to other animals; in the domestic rabbits, the agents seemed to have disappeared, although, in fact, later studies demonstrated that the virus in these animals had merely gone into hiding.

Still another cancer-forming virus was described in 1935 by John J. Bittner in mice. Bittner had noticed before that certain families of mice were more prone to developing mammary carcinomas than others, and he was able, by deliberate selection, to develop an inbred strain, C3H, in which such neoplasms occur spontaneously at a high frequency—almost 100 percent in female mice over one year old. In contrast, other strains, such as C57BL, developed almost no mammary carcinomas at all. When Bittner crossed the two strains, he made a curious observation: the F_1 hybrids had a high incidence of mammary carcinomas if the mother was C3H, and a low incidence when the mother was C57BL. In 1936, Bittner proposed a simple explanation for this observation—namely, that mother's milk contains a factor that promotes breast cancer. He showed that, by delivering C3H mice by caesarian section and foster nursing them on C57BL mothers, he could keep the mice free of neoplasms. In contrast, C57BL mice foster nursed on C3H mothers, developed mammary carcinomas. This time, however, it was Bittner himself who hesitated to ascribe viral etiology to the mammary carcinoma, and insisted on calling the transmitting factor the "milk-borne mammary tumor agent," even after it became clear that this agent was a virus.

The *mammary tumor virus* (MTV), also called the *Bittner virus*, is, however, only one of several factors necessary for the induction of breast cancer in mice. The other factors are hormonal stimulation and genetic susceptibility. Mice carrying MTV do not develop breast cancer unless a suitable hormonal environment, normally associated with pregnancy and lactation, is provided. For example, in A-strain mice, known to harbor MTV, only breeding females have a high incidence of spontaneous mammary carcinoma. However, in strains such as C3H, the incidence of breast cancer is high in both breeding and virgin females, indicating that here the hormonal influence is overridden by genetic factors. There are apparently several genes in the mouse genome that influence MTV carcinogenesis: there is one near the *A* locus in chromosome 2, another near the *b* locus in chromosome 4 (where *A* and *b* are coat-color loci), still another in the *H*-2 complex on chromosome 17, and there may be more.

The discovery of mouse leukemia virus is associated with the name of Ludwik Gross. As in the case of mammary carcinomas, researchers noticed that some mouse families were more susceptible to spontaneous leukemia than others, and were able to produce inbred, high-leukemic strains from these families. Two such strains are AKR and C58, in which up to 90 percent of the animals develop leukemia spontaneously. Attempts to transfer leukemia to adult animals of other inbred strains, such as C3Hf/Bi or C57BR, invariably failed. However, Gross demonstrated in 1951 that AKR leukemia could be transferred to C3Hf/Bi or C57BR mice by inoculation of *newborn* or suckling animals of these strains with extracts prepared from the leukemic organs of AKR animals. By comparison, mice of strains C57BL/6 or I/St were highly resistant to leukemia, even when inoculated early in infancy (three to five days after birth). The inbred strains thus fell into three categories with regard to susceptibility or resistance to leukemia: strains with a high incidence of both spontaneous and induced leukemia (AKR, C58), strains with a low incidence of spontaneous and a high incidence of induced leukemia (C3Hf/Bi, C57BR), and strains with a low incidence of spontaneous and induced leukemia (C57BL/6, I/St).

The virus isolated by Gross is now referred to as *Gross leukemia virus*. Later, Charlotte Friend, Frank J. Rauscher, John B. Moloney, and Judith R. Tennant isolated other leukemia viruses, and these too bear the names of their discoverers.

In the course of his studies on the leukemia virus, Gross discovered another virus, which also became widely used by investigators in a variety of specialties. Gross noticed that some of the C3H mice injected with the AKR leukemic extract failed to come down with leukemia, but instead developed small neoplasms in the neck, in the area of the parotid (salivary) glands. Gross followed this lead and, in early 1953, obtained unequivocal evidence that the AKR leukemic extracts contained two neoplasm-inducing viruses: one that induced leukemia and another that caused parotid neoplasms. The second virus was then isolated by Sarah E. Steward, who, in collaboration with Bernice E. Eddy, demonstrated that, once passed through a culture of mouse embryo fibroblasts, the virus was able to induce neoplasms in a surprisingly large variety of tissues—parotid glands, thymus, mammary gland, lungs, skin, bone, connective tissue, kidney, and nerve tissue. Furthermore, Stewart, and Eddy and their collaborators could demonstrate that the virus induced neoplasms not only in mice, but also in hamsters, rats, and rabbits. Because of this unusual behavior, the two investigators designated the new virus *polyoma*, which, translated literally, means "many neoplasm inducer." (The virus should not be confused with the poliomyelitis, or polio, virus; the two viruses have nothing to do with each other.) The polyoma virus is normally present in mice but causes only inapparent infections, probably because its spreading is checked by a potent antibody response; but once passed through a tissue culture and allowed to multiply in the absence of antibodies, it becomes a potent cancer producer.

A virus closely related to polyoma was discovered in 1960 by B. H. Sweet and Maurice R. Hilleman in cultures of rhesus monkey cells. Such cultures were used for the production of human polio virus vaccine, and it was therefore important to know whether they were free of cancer-producing viruses. A considerable number of viruses had already been discovered in these cells and had been assigned serial numbers SV1, SV2, SV3, and so on (SV being an abbreviation of "Simian virus"; L. *simia*, monkey). Sweet and Hilleman discovered one other virus—serial number 40—that differed from the other viruses in that it did not cause any significant change in the cells of its natural host (most other simian viruses lysed the rhesus monkey cells), but caused characteristic vacuolation of kidney cells derived from African green monkeys. Sweet and Hilleman described SV40 as "just one more of the troublesome simian agents to be screened and then eliminated from stocks and then from live virus vaccines." But when, a few years later, SV40 was demonstrated to induce neoplasms when injected into hamsters and to cause malignant transformation of cultured human cells, it quickly became the target of intense research in many laboratories around the world.

Classification

All the viruses described above have one thing in common—the ability to cause cancer. They are therefore lumped into a single group of *oncogenic viruses* (Gr. *onkos*, bulk, mass, here a tumor; *genesis*, production). The group is further divided according to the nucleic acid content and the morphology of the viral particle (Table 14.8). According to the former criterion, one distinguishes *RNA viruses*, also referred to as *oncorna viruses* (an acronym standing for *onco*genic *RNA* viruses), or *retraviruses* (*re*verse *tra*nscriptase-containing viruses), and *DNA viruses*. Representatives of RNA viruses are the Rous sarcoma virus, Gross virus, and all other mouse leukemia viruses; representatives of DNA viruses are the group of *papovaviruses*

Table 14.8 Classification of Oncogenic Viruses

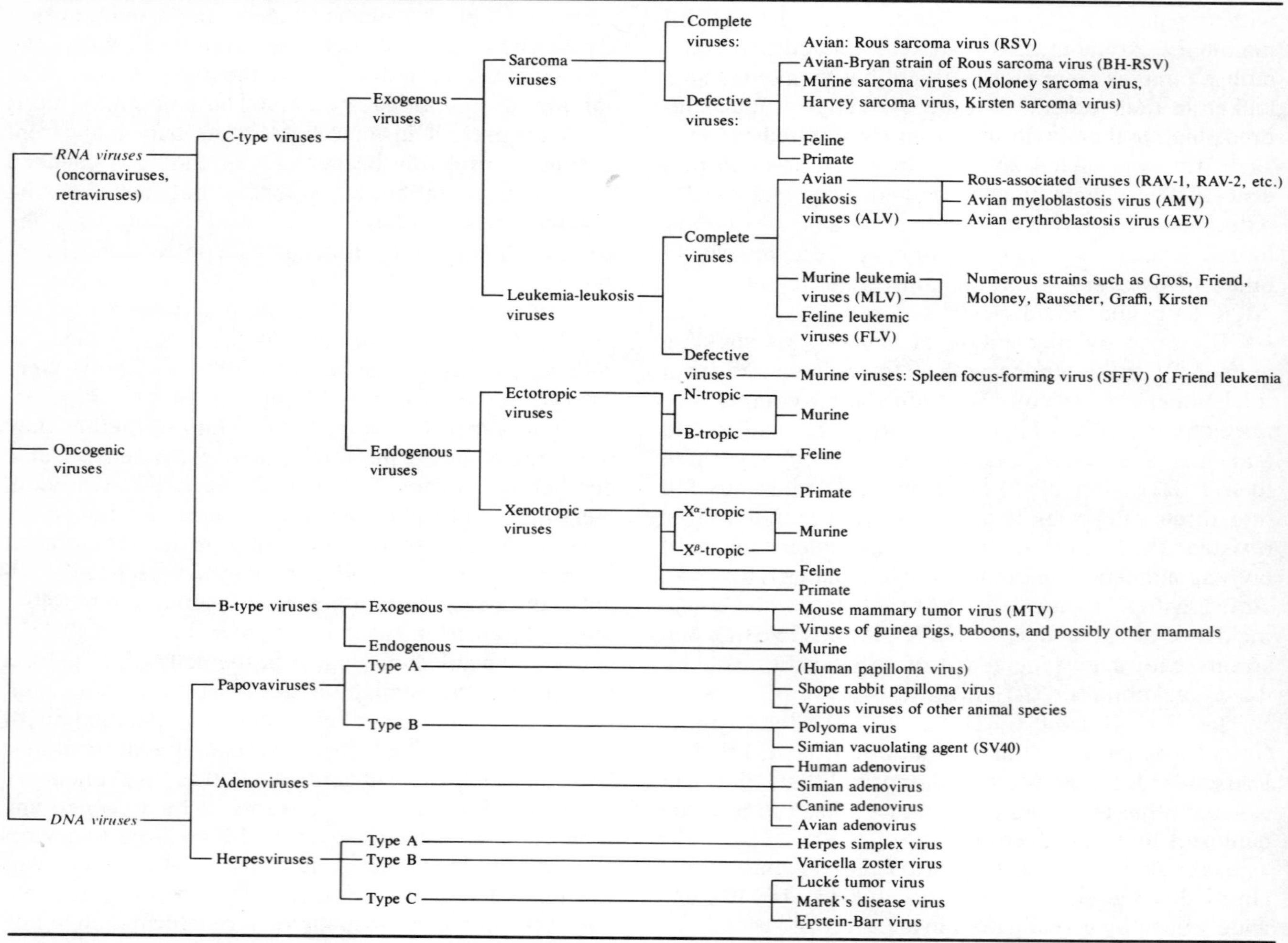

(another acronym, standing for *pa*pilloma, *po*lyoma, and *va*cuolating viruses), adenoviruses, and the herpesviruses (herpes simplex virus, Epstein-Barr virus, and Marek's disease virus).

The morphological classification is based on the appearance of virus particles examined by electron microscopy. Four types of particle were originally distinguished and designated A, B, C, and D, but only two of these designations, B and C, are still being used. The *B type*, found in mammary carcinomas, is an extracellular particle, with an excentrically located electron-dense nucleoid (Fig. 14.28). The C type, found in leukemias, is also an extracellular particle with loosely fitting envelope rings like the B type but with a centrally located nucleoid (Fig. 14.28).

RNA Viruses

These viruses store their genetic information in RNA molecules and transcribe it with the help of the enzyme reverse transcriptase. The group includes the B-type and C-type viruses, which are related to each other in the way their genetic information is organized and expressed but different in their mode of maturation, morphology, and pathogenesis. For lack of space, we shall say no more about the B-type viruses, and concentrate instead on the C-type; however, much of what will be noted about the C-type viruses also applies to the B-type.

Families of C-Type Viruses. Before we describe the properties of C-type viruses, we shall mention how

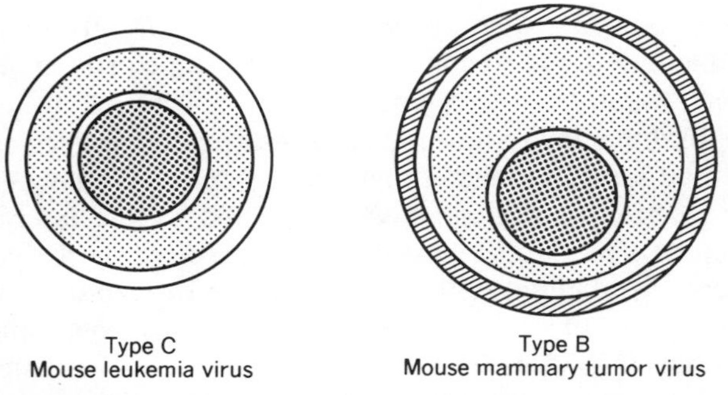

Figure 14.28. Appearance of mouse leukemia and mammary tumor virus on electron micrographs (scheme).

these viruses are divided into various groups and families. The division is rather complicated and the reader is therefore advised to consult Table 14.8 whenever he or she gets lost in the description below.

The two main divisions of C-type viruses are the *exogenous* and *endogenous viruses*. Although the genetic material of both groups can be integrated into the host genome (see section on the multiplication cycle below), the two groups differ in regard to the cell in which this integration occurs. Exogenous viruses integrate only in somatic cells, whereas the endogenous viruses are integrated in both somatic and germ cells. An exogenous virus infects a cell, multiplies in it, and as a part of the multiplication process, incorporates into the host's chromosomal DNA; but then it leaves the cell again to infect new cells. The length of the integrated period of the life cycle may vary, and the virus may, in fact, replicate harmoniously with the host cell for a while, but at the end it always leaves the cell or its progeny and converts into an infectious particle. In other words, it emphasizes the extracellular, infectious part of its multiplication cycle.

An endogenous virus, on the other hand, remains in the integrated state most of the time and produces infectious particles only occasionally, when it is induced to do so, for example, by ionizing radiation, inhibitors of protein synthesis, 5-bromo- or 5-iododeoxyuridine (which must be incorporated into DNA before they can act as inducers), chemical mutagens, carcinogens, allograft reaction, mixed lymphocyte reaction, and by prolonged culture of the virus-bearing cells in vitro. Often the efficiency of virus induction is enhanced by adrenal corticosteroid hormones. When activated, the virus can carry out the extracellular, infectious portion of its multiplication cycle, but it is rarely transmitted in the infectious state from one animal to another. At all other times, the virus behaves as part of the host genome, multiplying whenever the genome multiplies. An endogenous virus thus emphasizes the chromosomally integrated part of its multiplication cycle. Hence, in principle, the multiplication cycles of exogenous and endogenous viruses are the same (see below), but the length of time the two types spend in the different phases of the multiplication cycle differs: exogenous viruses exist most of the time as infectious particles, whereas endogenous viruses are virtually always integrated into the host genome. In all other respects, the two types of viruses are very similar: their overall genetic and morphological features are indistinguishable; the antigens of their virion structural components are usually strongly cross reactive when tested with antisera made in species not closely related to the normal host species, and their nucleic acids show extensive biochemical homology.

Exogenous viruses can be divided further into two groups, sarcoma viruses and leukemia viruses. *Sarcoma viruses* induce neoplasms of connective tissue in vivo, and in tissue culture they transform normal fibroblasts into malignant cells (see section on malignant transformation). *Leukemia viruses* do not induce sarcomas in vivo or transform cells in vitro, but do induce neoplasms of the hematopoietic and reticuloendothelial systems; as a consequence, the blood of the infected animals contains large numbers of circulating hematopoietic neoplastic cells (*leukemia*) or the neoplastic cells form solid masses in some organs (*lymphomas*). In the domestic fowl and in cattle, the leukemias and aleukemic neoplasms are often referred to as *leukoses*.

Sarcoma viruses are of two types, complete and defective. *Complete sarcoma viruses* contain all the genetic information necessary for their replication in the host cell. This group of viruses is thus far known only in birds, and its prototype in the Rous sarcoma virus (RSV). *Defective sarcoma viruses* are unable to replicate when present alone in the cell because they have lost the capacity to synthesize major structural proteins of the virion, particularly the envelope proteins (see the section on structure of viral particles). They can, however, replicate in the presence of a *helper virus*, which provides the missing structural components. Particles released from a cell superinfected by the two viruses, the defective and the helper virus, are of two kinds—typical helper virus particles, and the so-called *pseudotype particles*, consisting of sarcoma virus genomic RNA enclosed in components provided by the helper virus. The helper function is provided by some of the leukemia viruses, which thus have the ability to *rescue* the sarcoma virus genome from the superinfected cell. Cells infected by the defective sarcoma virus alone are *nonproducers*—they do not release infectious virus particles (but the cells continue to harbor the virus in the form of integrated viral DNA). In the notation for pseudotype viruses, the helper virus is indicated in parentheses. For example, MSV(RLV) indicates a pseudotype virus composed of Moloney murine sarcoma virus RNA and particle proteins derived from the Rauscher leukemia (helper) virus. Defective sarcoma viruses have been detected in birds and in various mammals (mice, rats, and primates). Type-C viruses from a given animal species can rescue defective genomes from a variety of other species. Defective type-C viruses, however, usually cannot be rescued by type-B viruses.

Most of the *leukemia viruses* are of the *complete type*, capable of replicating without the help of other viruses; a few, however, are of the *defective type*. An example of the latter category is one of the two Friend leukemia viruses, the so-called spleen focus-forming virus (SFFV; see Chapter 5). Complete leukemia viruses have been isolated from birds, mice, and cats. The murine leukemia virus (MLV) occurs in many strains and is designated by the name of its discoverer (Gross, Friend, Moloney, Rauscher, Graffi, Kirsten). Although leukemia viruses do not transform cells in vitro, their presence can be recognized because they induce the appearance of virus-specific, serologically detectable proteins in the cultured cells.

Turning now to the *endogenous viruses*, we must first emphasize that, although they are related to the exogeneous viruses, the two types are also clearly distinct antigenically and biochemically. There are two major classes of endogenous RNA tumor viruses, ecotropic and xenotropic. *Ecotropic*, or *E-tropic viruses* (Gr. *oikos*, home, *tropos*, turning), readily infect cells from which they were induced but do not infect cells of other species—that is, they can be grown only in cells of their "home" species. For example, mouse ecotropic viruses infect mouse cells, but not hamster or feline cells. *Xenotropic*, or *X-tropic* (Gr. *xenos*, foreign), cannot infect cells of the species from which they were induced, but can infect cells of other foreign species. For example, mouse xenotropic viruses do not infect mouse cells, but can infect hamster or other mammalian cells. The two classes have been studied best in the mouse, but they also apparently occur in the domestic fowl, rat, hamster, pig, guinea pig, and primates. In the mouse, sometimes a third class of *dualtropic* (*polytropic* or *amphitropic*) *viruses* is distinguished: these can infect both mouse cells and cells of other species. The virus tropism is apparently determined by the gene controlling an envelope protein (see section on genome organization).

In the mouse, the ecotropic endogenous viruses can infect some, but not other mouse cells. Which cells they infect is presumably determined by the interaction of a particular viral protein controlled by the *gag* gene (see below) with a particular cell receptor (controlled by the *Fv*-1 locus; see section on host genes influencing virus expression). Based on their host range, mouse ecotropic viruses can be divided into *N-tropic*, growing preferentially in NIH Swiss mice (and in mice of a few other strains), *B-tropic*, growing preferentially in BALB/c mice (and in mice of other strains), and *NB-tropic*, growing in cells derived from both groups of mice. (The NIH Swiss group of mice carries the *Fv*-1^n allele, the BALB/c group the *Fv*-1^b allele.) Mouse xenotropic viruses can also be classified into two groups, X^α and X^β, on the basis of relatedness between themselves and the ecotropic viruses. The X^α *viruses* derive from the BALB/c group of mouse strains, whereas the X^β *viruses* derive from the NIH Swiss group. The X^α xenotropic viruses are more closely related to ecotropic viruses than to the X^β

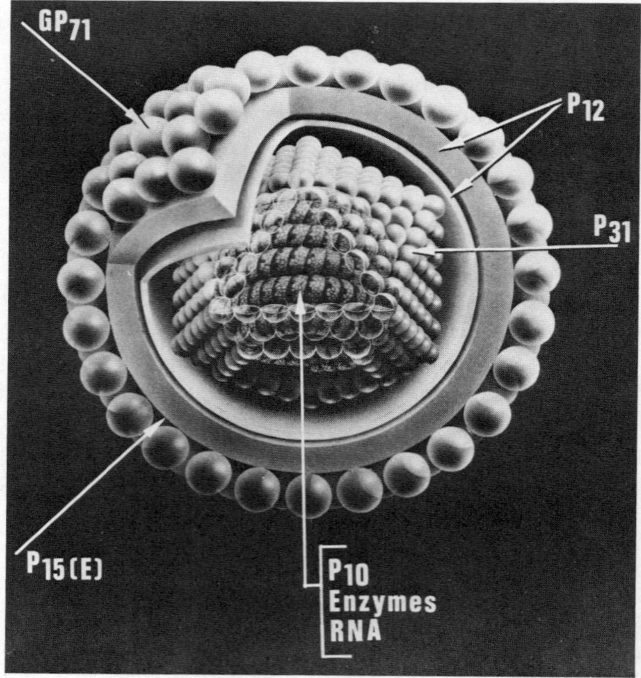

Figure 14.29. Structure of Friend leukemia virus (FVL). The cutaway view of the icosahedron permits visualization of the ribonucleoprotein. See text for further details. (From D. P. Bolognesi, R. C. Montelaro, H. Frank, and W. Schäffer: *Science* **199:** 183–186, 1978.)

xenotropic viruses. (Incidentally, the two groups of mouse inbred strains also differ in terms of the incidence of spontaneous leukemias and the number of endogenous virus genomes they contain: in strains of the NIH Swiss group, spontaneous leukemia does not occur and the mice appear to contain no ecotropic viruses, although they do contain xenotropic viruses; in strains of the BALB/c group, spontaneous leukemia does occur, although with low frequency, and the mice contain a number of both ecotropic and xenotropic viral genomes. High leukemia strains, such as AKR, also have several ecotropic and xenotropic viral genomes.)

Endogenous RNA tumor viruses are of the leukemia/leukosis type. They have been demonstrated in various species of mammal, bird, and reptile, and may be present in all vertebrates. However, their presence—and for that matter, the presence of any C-type viruses—in humans has not been demonstrated conclusively. Although several reports describing C-type particles by electron microscopy in human tissues have appeared, their validity has been questioned by other investigators.

Structure. The spherical mature C-type particle (Fig. 14.29) is enclosed by an *envelope*, which consists of a lipid bilayer with proteins, and is derived at least in part from the host cell. From the envelope project loosely attached *knobs*, which, in avian viruses, are connected to the envelope by thin spikes. Beneath the envelope is a thin layer of the *inner coat*. The center of the particle is taken up by the virus *core*, composed of an outer *shell* of hexagonally arranged subunits and an inner electron-opaque ribonucleoprotein filament arrangement into a spiral. The components of the virion are designated *p* (for protein) or *gp* (for glycoprotein), coupled with a number indicating their molecular weight. The major components of the virion are listed in Figure 14.30; their distribution is shown in Figure 14.29.

Organization of the Genome. The genetic information of a C-type virus is stored in a single-stranded RNA with an apparent molecular weight of about 10^7 daltons and a sedimentation constant of about 60S. Exposure to heat or mild denaturing conditions leads to dissociation of the RNA complex into 30S subunits, indicating that the genome consists of two identical subunits held together by hydrogen bonds.

Each RNA molecule of a complete sarcoma virus carries four genes (Fig. 14.30): *gag*, which codes for an internal structural protein of the virion; *pol*, which codes for RNA-dependent DNA polymerase (reverse transcriptase); *env*, which codes for a glycoprotein constituting the knobs and spikes on the outer surface of the envelope; and *src*, which codes for a nonstruc-

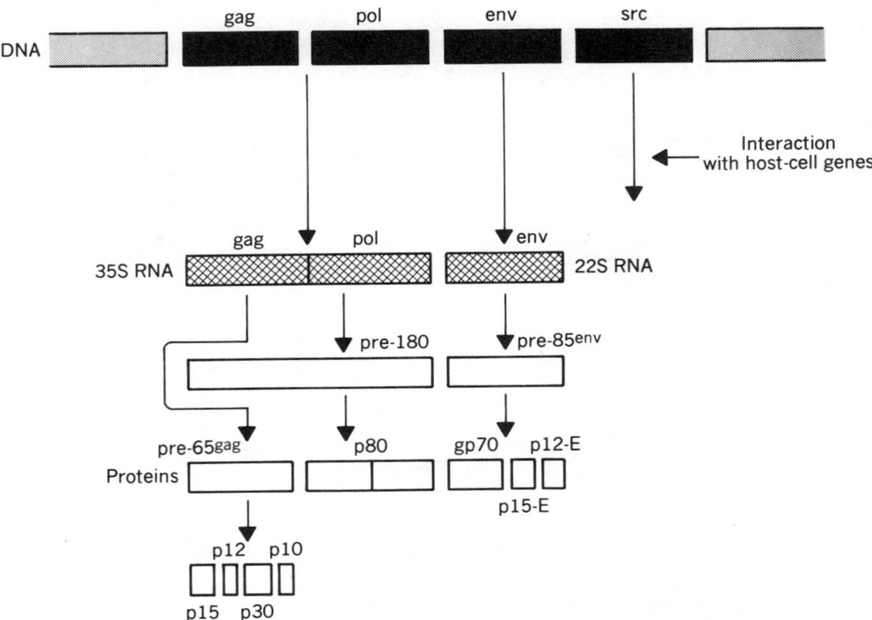

Figure 14.30. The mode of transcription and translation of an oncogenic RNA virus.

tural protein involved in neoplastic transformation of cells in both the tissue culture and in vivo. This gene is present in the sarcoma viruses and absent in leukemia viruses. The gene order is 5′-*gag-pol-env-src*-poly(A)-3′, and it appears to be the same in all C-type viruses studied thus far. The defective viruses have various segments of the RNA molecule deleted and sequences from the host inserted instead. The length of the deletions varies, depending on the virus. The terminal regions of the viral genome appear to be the most essential, since they are always retained, no matter what middle portion is cut out. The deletion and insertion of genetic material probably occurs by recombination at the time that the viral genome integrates into the host chromosomes and at the time of excision from these chromosomes, respectively. The recombination at the 3′ end of the viral genome seems to take place always in the same, highly conserved region [about 1000 base nucleotides from the 3′poly(A) end].

The viral genome seems to consist of two principal parts, replicative and infectious. The *replicative part*, located at both ends of the genome, is involved in the physical association and dissociation of the viral and host genome; if a virus loses this part, it also loses the ability to replicate and hence the ability to exist as a biological entity. The *infectious part*, occupying the middle regions of the genome, contains structural genes coding for virion components and those enzymes not supplied by the host cell. This part is essential for the extrachromosomal portion of the viral multiplication cycle; loss of this region may mean that the virus remains integrated in the chromosome, unable to leave it and form infectious particles.

Multiplication Cycle. There are two distinct phases—infectious and integrated—in the multiplication cycle of a C-type virus (Fig. 14.31). The *infectious phase* begins with the adsorption of the virus particle to the cell membrane of the host cell, accomplished by the interaction of the gp70 knob component of the virus and an unidentified glycoprotein membrane receptor of the host cell. The specificity of the interaction is prob-

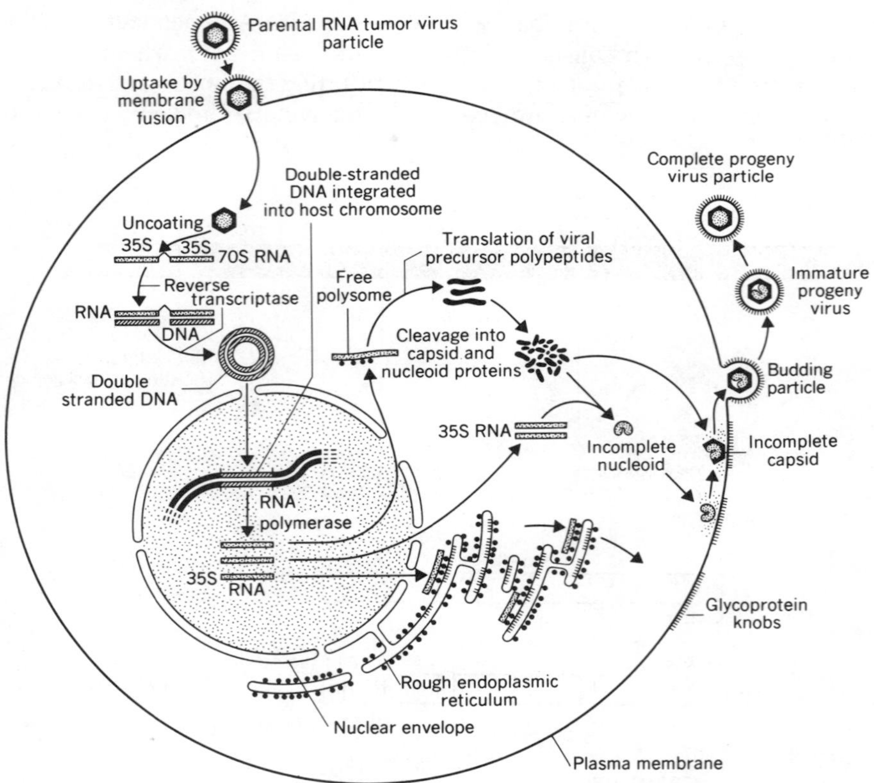

Figure 14.31. Multiplication cycle of an oncogenic RNA virus. (Redrawn and slightly modified from J. D. Watson: *Molecular Biology of the Gene*. 3rd ed. Benjamin, Menlo Park, California, 1976.)

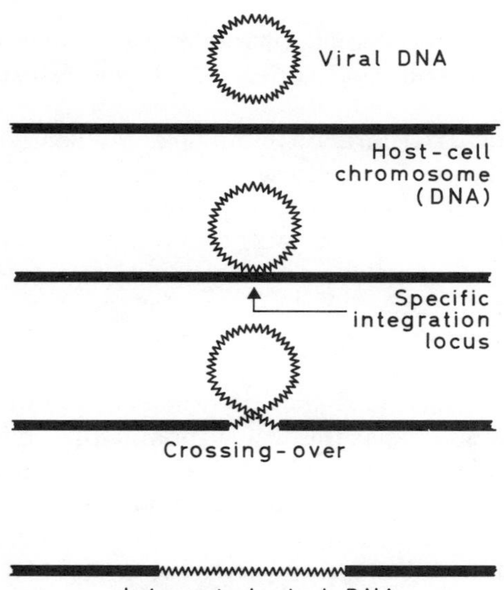

Figure 14.32. Integration of viral genome into the host-cell chromosome.

ably a major factor in determining the host range of a virus. The adsorption is followed by penetration, perhaps via membrane fusion, uncoating of the particle, and replication of the two RNA subunits, each containing a complete set of viral genetic information required for the reproduction of the virus. The single-stranded RNA molecules are first transcribed into a single-stranded DNA copy by the reverse transcriptase present in the viral particle. This single-stranded DNA is then converted by host enzymes into double-stranded circular DNA, which migrates from its site of synthesis in the cytoplasm to the nucleus, where it integrates into host chromosomal DNA, and the virus enters the *integrated phase* of its multiplication cycle. The number of integrated proviral genes per cell probably ranges from one to seven. During the integration, the DNA circle opens up in the region of the *gag* and *src* genes and inserts itself into the host chromosome at a particular locus (Fig. 14.32). The flanking host sequences in the integrated proviral DNA may have a role in regulating the expression of the proviral genes. The integrated DNA can replicate simultaneously with and by the same mechanism as the host DNA, and can thus be transmitted to all daughter cells. It resembles a host gene, but in contrast to such a gene it can give rise to complementary RNA that can be packaged into an infectious virus particle.

The early 35S transcripts of the integrated DNA serve as templates for the synthesis of viral proteins. The individual genes are translated in the following fashion (Fig. 14.30). The *gag* gene is translated into a precursor protein of 65,000 daltons (pre-65^{gag}), which is then cleaved, via intermediates, to give four proteins—p15, p12, p30, and p10. The *pol* gene is apparently never translated alone, but always with the *gag* gene, giving a precursor protein of 180,000 daltons (pre-180). Normally, about one molecule of pre-180 is synthesized per 10 molecules of pre-65. The pre-180 molecule is then cleaved, via intermediates, to produce the mature enzyme (p80), which consists of two subunits—α (60,000 daltons) and β (95,000 daltons), where the α subunit probably arises by the degradation of the β subunit. The *env* gene is translated from a separate 22 S mRNA, derived from the 35S mRNA by splicing. The 22S mRNA is translated into a precursor protein of 85,000 daltons (pre-85^{env}), which is then cleaved into polypeptide chains of gp70, p15-E, and p12-E (pre-85 is first cleaved to gp70, and some of the 15-E is then degraded into p12-E). The *src* gene is transcribed into a poorly characterized protein that has a phosphotransferase (kinase) activity.

As more RNA molecules are made, some RNA chains combine to form the core of a maturing particle, and the particles move toward the cell surface, pick up some of the synthesized viral proteins, and envelop themselves in the host membrane, into which gp70 molecules have been inserted by the virus. They then bud off from the membrane as complete virions. As has already been discussed, the duration of the infectious and integrated phases varies, depending on whether the virus particle is exogenous or endogenous.

Host Genes Influencing Virus Expression. The host plays a role in both phases of the viral multiplication cycle: at the integration phase, it provides the chromosomal locus for the incorporation of the viral DNA, and in the infectious phase, it provides the functions that the virus lacks and needs in order to replicate successfully. There are therefore two types of host gene that influence virus expression—structural loci, representing the integration sites of the virus, and regulatory loci, controlling virus behavior outside the chromosome. Both types of locus have been studied most extensively in endogenous viruses of the mouse.

Two groups of *structural loci* have been identified so far in the mouse—one using AKR mice, and the other using NZB mice. The AKR mice express high levels of infectious N-tropic virus spontaneously throughout their lives. In crosses between AKR mice and mice of an ectropic virus-negative strain, the ability to express infectious virus has been found to be controlled by two unlinked, autosomal, dominant genes—*Akv*-1 and *Akv*-2. Further studies have demonstrated that the two genes probably represent the sites of viral genome integration in the mouse chromosome. The *Akv*-1 locus is located on chromosome 7 between *Gpi*-1 (the locus coding for an enzyme) and *c* (one of the loci responsible for coat color). The *Akv*-2 locus has not been mapped yet. Crosses between an NZB strain containing relatively high levels of xenotropic viruses in its tissues and a xenotropic virus-negative strain indicate the existence of another two loci—*Nzv*-1 and *Nzv*-2, the presence of the former leading to high levels of the virus, that of the latter to only low levels. Both are presumably the sites of integration of ecotropic viruses in the NZB strain.

Of the large number of *regulatory loci* that undoubtedly exist, only a few have been identified. Some of these will be discussed in the section on tumor-specific antigens later in this chapter; here we shall mention only the *Fv*-1 locus, first defined as a locus governing susceptibility or resistance to Friend virus-induced erythroleukemia and to the formation of superficial spleen foci after the infection with this virus (see Chapter 5). The locus maps to chromosome 4, close to the *Gpd*-1 locus controlling an enzyme. It appears to interfere with infection of mouse cells by type-C viruses at a postpenetration step. As was mentioned earlier, the *Fv*-1 locus separates ecotropic viruses into two classes—N-tropic, which replicate 100 to 1000 times more efficiently in cells derived from NIH Swiss mice than in BALB/c mice, and B-tropic, which replicate 30 to 100 times more efficiently in BALB/c cells than in NIH Swiss cells.

Immunological Analysis of C-Type Viruses. Immunological techniques have played an important role in identification of C-type viruses and their components, and also in establishing the relationships between the individual viral groups. Two kinds of antibody have been employed in these studies—*virus-neutralizing antibodies*, recognizing the *env* gene products either on virus particles or on the surface of the virus-infected cells, and *cytolytic antibodies*, recognizing the products of the *env* and *gag* genes expressed on the infected cell surface. The serologically defined antigenic determinants carried by viral structural proteins are of three categories—*type-specific*, unique to a particular virus isolate; *group-specific*, shared by corresponding proteins of different virus isolates of a given species; and *interspecies-specific*, shared by corresponding proteins of virus isolates from different species. In the mouse, the type-specific envelope antigens divide the known viruses into two subgroups—*AKR*-Gross and *FMR* (Friend, Moloney, Rauscher).

Neoplastic Transformation In Vitro. When added to tissue culture, RNA viruses carrying the *src* gene, as well as some DNA viruses, cause a characteristic change in the properties of the cultured cells, a change referred to as *neoplastic* (*malignant*) *transformation*. The transformed cells have the following characteristics.

Loss of Contact Inhibition. Normal cells grow in culture only so long as they have room; close cell-to-cell contact hinders new mitoses—a phenomenon termed *contact inhibition*. As a result, normal cells in culture form only a single layer (a *monolayer*). Transformed cells, on the other hand, do not display contact inhibition, but grow on top of one another and form irregular, multilayered piles resembling small tumors.

Increased Growth Rate. Transformed cells often divide more rapidly than their normal counterparts and show signs of invasive growth, characteristic of neoplasms.

Tumor Formation. When implanted into an animal of the same strain as the cell donor, transformed cells continue to grow and develop into tumors.

Immortalization. Normal cells in culture usually go through a certain number of cell divisions and then stop growing. Transformation converts the cells into a *permanent line*, capable of unlimited passage in tissue culture.

Appearance of Virus-Specific Antigens. Cells transformed by an oncogenic virus display on their surfaces characteristic antigens absent in their normal counterparts.

Since transformation and production of virus particles are controlled by different portions of the viral genome, the two phenomena can occur independently of each other. Cells in culture can therefore exist in one of the following four states: they are transformed and produce virus particles; they are transformed but do not produce virus particles; they are not transformed but they do produce virus particles; they are not transformed and they do not produce virus particles, although they harbor the virus.

Origin of C-Type Viruses. Two hypotheses concerning the origin and possible function of C-type viruses have been proposed. According to the *oncogene hypothesis* of Robert J. Huebner and George J. Todaro, all cells contain *virogenes* in their chromosomes that carry the information necessary for the synthesis of RNA viruses. The virogene normally functions in a certain stage of cell differentiation, just as all other genes do. However, the virogene is special in that one part of it, the so-called *oncogene*, possesses the ability to transform cells. The oncogene is normally repressed, but when this repression is lifted by one or another of the carcinogenic factors, the cell is transformed into a neoplastic one.

According to the *protovirus hypothesis* of Howard M. Temin, genetic information normally flows not only from DNA to RNA, but also in the opposite direction. The RNA → DNA flow, mediated by the reverse transcriptase, allows the cell to incorporate new DNA into its chromosomes, and so provides the opportunity for the modification of the existing genome. Occasionally, however, the new DNA either incorporates at a wrong site or acquires, by mutation, a relative independence, which allows it to exist in an infectious form outside the chromosome. Each of the two hypotheses is supported by some data and contradicted by others.

DNA Viruses

Rather than describe the characteristics of the various oncogenic DNA viruses (which would take up too much space, since these viruses are more heterogeneous than the oncogenic RNA viruses), we shall select one of them, SV40, and use it as an illustrative example of this group. Other examples of oncogenic DNA viruses include Shope's papilloma virus and the polyoma virus we discussed briefly at the beginning of this section.

Structure of SV40. Simian vacuolating virus 40, or SV40, is one of the smallest DNA viruses, measuring only about 450 Å in diameter. The spherical virion consists of a protein shell (capsid) and a nucleoprotein core (Fig. 14.32). The shell is composed of three proteins, designated VP1, VP2, and VP3. The VP1 is the major protein component (molecular weight of 45,000 daltons), accounting for about 70 percent of the total mass of the virus particle. It forms 72 capsomeres on the outside of the shell; 60 of these—those composing the 20 faces of the icosahedron—contain six copies of VP1 each, whereas the remaining 12, located at the vertices of the icosahedron, contain five copies of VP1 each, so that the protein is represented a total of 420 times in each viral particle. The VP3 has a molecular weight of 23,000 daltons, represents about 10 percent of the total mass of the viral particle, and probably lines the inside of the capsid shell. The location in the virion of VP2, which has a molecular weight of about 32,000 daltons and is present in about 40 copies in each particle, is not known.

The core consists of four species of protein (VP4 through VP7) and one molecule of DNA. The proteins are host-derived and are identical to four of the five major chromosomal histones—VP4 = H3 (molecular weight, 14,000 daltons), VP5 = H2B (molecular weight, 13,000 daltons), VP6 = H2A2 (molecular weight, 12,000 daltons), and VP7 = H2A1 (molecular weight, 11,000 daltons). The fifth histone, H1, is also involved in the formation of virus particles but is not incorporated into the virion. The single, circular, double-stranded DNA molecule has a molecular weight of 3.6×10^6 daltons and contains a total of 5227 nucleotides. The complete sequence of these nucleotides is known. The molecule resembles a rosary, with "beads" (nucleosomes) connected by straight stretches of DNA. Each nucleosome is composed of a DNA segment, about 200 nucleotides long, wound around a core that consists of two molecules of each of the four histones. The segment interconnecting two nucleosomes is about 55 nucleotides long, so that the whole molecule has from 21 to 24 nucleosomes. Despite this regular spacing, nucleosomes are randomly distributed in terms of DNA sequence in a population of DNA molecules.

Lytic SV40 Infection. After adsorption and penetration, the virus particle is transported into the nucleus, where uncoating occurs. Part of the DNA molecule is transcribed into an early mRNA, which is then spliced in two different ways (Fig. 14.33). One splicing deletes an intervening sequence of 65 nucleotides from the primary transcript, the other 346 nucleotides. The larger spliced mRNA is translated into a polypeptide chain with a molecular weight of 90,000 daltons (translation terminates just before the 3′-end of the mRNA molecule). The protein carries the so-called *large T antigen*, so designated because antibodies against this antigen are present in sera of animals bearing SV40-induced tumors (the "T" stands for "tumor"). Of the smaller spliced transcript, only a short segment is translated into a polypeptide with a molecular weight of 17,000 daltons—the so-called *small t antigen*. Since large T and small t antigens derive from the same primary transcript, they share part of their amino acid sequences and are immunologically related. The large T-bearing molecules also carry an-

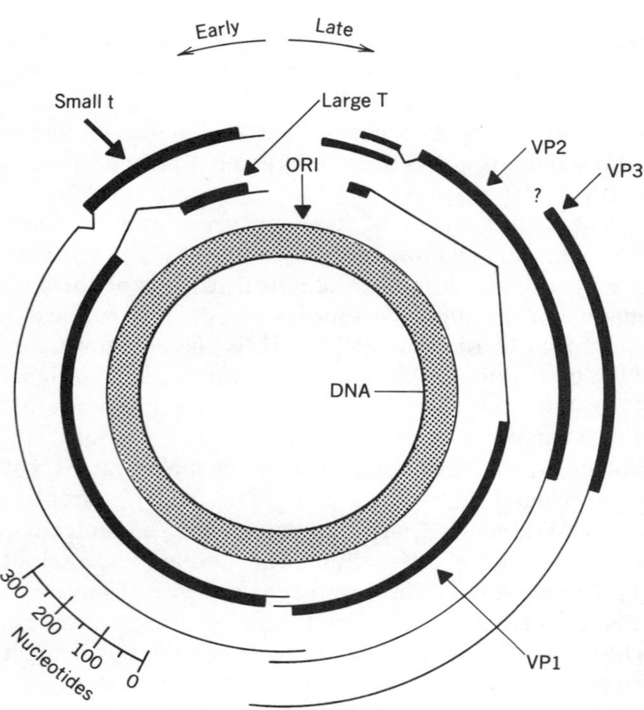

Figure 14.33. Map of the SV40 genome indicating regions coding for mRNA transcripts (thin line) and proteins (heavy lines). ORI, origin of DNA replication. Early mRNA species are transcribed counterclockwise on this map, and late species clockwise. Splicing is indicated by a ∧ sign. (Based on E. B. Ziff: *Nature* **287**:491–499, 1980.)

other antigen, the *U antigen*, detected by another antibody. The function of the small t protein is not known; the large T protein, which has ATPase activity, locally unwinds portions of the viral DNA duplex, allowing polymerases to bind and initiate replication. The T protein may also act on host DNA and stimulate host DNA synthesis.

The onset of viral DNA replication marks the end of the *early phase* of the SV40 multiplication cycle, which lasts about 12 hours. DNA replication is always initiated at the same specific site, close to the point where the transcription of the early mRNA starts, proceeds bidirectionally, and is completed when the two forks meet about 180° from the origin. The two interlocked replicating circles then separate into two newly synthesized viral DNA molecules, each consisting of one parental and one daughter strand. The transcription of early genes continues even after the onset of viral DNA replication, but now, in addition, the rest of the viral genome—the *late genes*—begins to be transcribed (the transcription of the late region cannot start without the DNA replication), and the infection enters the *late phase*. The late region is transcribed in at least two different ways—by reading the same sequence twice with a different frame each time. As a result, two different transcripts—16S and 19S—are produced. The 16S mRNA is translated into the VP1 component, the 19S mRNA into VP2 and VP3. (The primary transcript is spliced in two different ways; one derived transcript then serves as a template for VP2 and the other for VP3.) The replicated DNA molecules associate with cellular histones and then begin to gather the structural components around themselves and to assemble into complete virions inside the cell. The cell filled with mature virions bursts and the released virions are ready to infect new cells. In the cell culture, the foci in which cells are lysed appear as clear *plaques*.

Neoplastic Transformation. The *lytic form* of the multiplication cycle, which results in the *productive infection*, occurs only when the SV40 infects so-called *permissive cells*, such as African green monkey kidney cells. The same virus, when introduced into *nonpermissive cells*, such as secondary cultures of hamster, rat, or mouse embryo cells, causes *nonproductive infection*, which is not accompanied by cell disintegration and production of free virions. Although most of the virus particles go through the early phase of the multiplication cycle just as in productive infection, there is no viral DNA replication or expression of the late-phase genes: the infection is *abortive*. But some of the viral DNA manages to recombine with the cellular DNA and incorporate into the cellular chromosomes. This *integration* of the virus causes *transformation* of the nonpermissive cells, whereby the cells are not lysed, but change their properties in a way similar to that described for neoplastic transformation caused by oncogenic RNA viruses. Hence, in contrast to the lytic cycle, in which the viral DNA remains free throughout the cycle, in transformed cells, the viral DNA integrates into the cellular DNA and replicates synchronously with the cell chromosomes.

The pattern of SV40 DNA integration is complex. Sometimes the whole viral genome, at other times only a portion, integrates into the chromosome. (However, the transformed cell must always contain at least one intact copy of the entire early region of the SV40 genome.) Individual transformed cell lines may contain either a single copy or multiple copies of viral DNA. Integration may occur at many different sites of the viral genome, and within the host genome are many sites into which the viral DNA may be incorporated. The transformation can be stable, or it can be transient (abortive), in which case the cell returns to normal after a few generations. When the transformed cell is fused with an uninfected permissive cell, the somatic hybrid begins to produce viral particles. The fusion thus *rescues* the viral genome. What exactly causes the neoplastic changes in the transformed cell is not known.

14.3.4 Antigenicity of Tumor Cells

Once a tumor appears, the body seems to be helpless against it: cases of spontaneous disappearance of tumors are rare. Is it possible, however, that whenever we diagnose a tumor, we are witness to a battle already lost, and that only very infrequently do we become aware of the body's victories precisely because they cannot be diagnosed? In other words, could it be that cancer is much more frequent than our statistics indicate, but that cancerous cells are often eliminated before they have a chance to multiply and get completely out of hand? In fact, some cell biologists find it surprising that, given so many opportunities, in so many cell divisions, more aberrant cells than those detected do not arise. Can the body defend itself against those of its own cells over which it has lost control? And if so, what kinds of mechanism does the body use in this defense?

At the beginning of this century, when immunology began to flourish, the idea that the defense against cancer might be of an immunological nature was first expressed. A number of investigators tried to prove it by excising tumors from one animal and transplanting them to other individuals. And when, in most instances, the new host rejected the transplants, they had a ready explanation for the observation: the transformation of a normal into a cancerous cell is accompanied by the appearance of new molecules, which the body recognizes as foreign antigens (*tumor-specific antigens*, *tumor-associated antigens*); it mounts immunity against them, and destroys the tumor. This immunity, these scientists argued, is strongly expressed against a transplanted tumor, in contrast to the original tumor, because the former has not had the opportunity to become adapted and so resistant to the defense responses. Although the idea was correct, the interpretation of the observed facts was completely wrong. For as soon as inbred lines of mice and other animals became available, it became apparent that tumors were rejected only when they were transplanted to individuals genetically different from the original tumor; tumors transplanted between individuals of an inbred strain grew and killed the host. What the researchers considered to be a response against tumor-associated antigens turned out to be a response against the donor histocompatibility antigens. Once this fact was established, the opinion of many investigators shifted to the opposite extreme: since tumors grew so well when transplanted within an inbred strain, they could not carry any tumor-associated antigens, and so such antigens apparently did not exist. But a few immunologists thought that the original idea was right, despite the accumulating evidence to the contrary, and continue searching for the tumor-associated antigen. One of the first for whom this persistence paid off was E. J. Foley, who used a special trick to demonstrate tumor-specific antigens.

Discovery of Tumor-Associated Antigens

Foley strangled developing methylcholanthrene-induced tumors by a gradual tightening of threads wound around them, thereby inducing tumor necrosis and preventing the tumors from spreading further into the host. When he then rechallenged the hosts with live cells of the same tumor, he observed that the grafts were frequently rejected, while similar grafts to previously untreated mice killed the hosts. But immunologists, having burned their fingers once, remained skeptical about these results, and several independent demonstrations were necessary before the concept of tumor-associated antigens was generally accepted.

One of the most convincing demonstrations was provided by Richmond T. Prehn and J. M. Main in 1957. These authors first repeated and confirmed Foley's experiments and then went on to show that, while transplants of methylcholanthrene-induced tumors could immunize syngeneic mice against subsequent transplants of the same tumor, normal tissues from the very same mouse could not. Conversely, tumor transplants did not immunize syngeneic mice against skin grafts obtained from the very animal that had donated the tumor. By these experiments, Prehn and Main ruled out the possibility, then frequently cited as an argument against the existence of tumor-associated antigens, that the mouse strains employed were not completely inbred, and the tumor rejections were caused by residual heterozygosity at histocompatibility loci. Prehn and Main also obtained evidence that different methylcholanthrene-induced tumors carried different tumor-associated antigens, an observation suggesting great individuality of carcinogen-induced tumors.

In 1960, George Klein and his colleagues provided the final proof of tumor-associated antigens by demonstrating the rejection of a tumor by the host in which

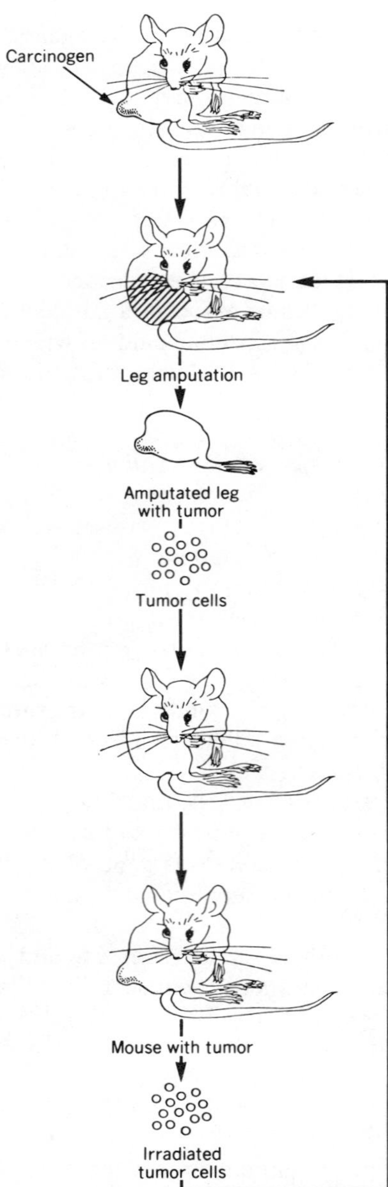

Figure 14.34. The experiment by which George Klein and his colleagues demonstrated the existence of tumor-associated antigens. Explanation in the text.

the tumor arose (Fig. 14.34). They induced a tumor in a leg of a mouse, then amputated the leg and transplanted the tumor to another mouse of the same strain. They then obtained cells from the transplanted tumor, irradiated them to prevent their proliferation, and injected them into the original tumor donor. After this immunization, they transplanted live tumor cells back to the original donor and demonstrated that the immunized mouse now rejected the tumor.

Source of New Antigens in Tumor Cells

Today, there is no doubt that tumor cells do indeed carry antigens that their normal counterparts lack. These *tumor-associated antigens* can be generated by several mechanisms.

Synthesis of New Molecules. Virtually all virus-induced tumors contain new antigens—in fact, the appearance of tumor-associated antigens is considered one of the signs indicating that neoplastic transformation by the virus has occurred. Some of these antigens are encoded by viral genes, others by host genes activated during transformation. It is conceivable that a similar activation of normally repressed genes also occurs in other tumors induced by agents other than viruses.

Unmasking of Normally Covered Antigens. Neoplastic transformation by certain viruses leads to the appearance of antigens that cannot be detected on the surfaces of normal cells unless these cells are first treated with proteolytic enzymes. Presumably, these antigens are normal components of the cell membranes, but are masked by other molecules. Both the viral infection and enzymatic treatment remove the masking molecules and uncover the antigens.

Loss of Molecules. Deletion of some molecules from the plasma membrane may alter the profile of adjacent molecules in a given membrane patch, and thus, in effect, generate a new profile that might become immunogenic to the host.

Modification of Existing Molecules. A membrane alteration accompanying neoplastic transformation may expose new, previously hidden regions of a molecule, or may result in addition of new structural features to an existing molecule. The modified regions of the molecule may then be recognized as new antigenic determinants by the host.

Release of Intracellular Molecules. Shedding and disintegration of tumor cells may expose the immune system to nuclear, nucleolar, or cytoplasmic components that are normally hidden in the cell, and of which the host is therefore tolerant.

Types of Tumor-Associated Antigens

Tumor-associated antigens fall into two broad categories—true tumor-associated antigens, which are antigens that cannot be detected on normal cells, and abnormally expressed normal antigens. We shall deal with the former category in the following section; here we shall concentrate on tumor antigens that are also expressed by some normal cells at some stage of differentiation, but are not expressed by normal cells from which the tumor derives. The two main groups of such antigens are the oncofetal and differentiation antigens.

Oncofetal Antigens. Normally, these are synthesized during certain stages of embryogenesis but are absent from normal adult cells or are present in these cells at a very low concentration. They reappear in tumor cells or in connection with tumor growth, perhaps as a result of derepression of certain host genes. There is a long list of such antigens, but here we shall mention only two—α-fetoprotein and carcinoembryonic antigen.

α-Fetoprotein (*α-FP*) was discovered by G. I. Abelev in 1963. It is an α-globulin secreted into the serum by normal embryonic liver cells. In the first trimester of human embryos, it comprises 90 percent of the total serum globulin, but its level declines rapidly after birth. The antigen reappears in patients with embryonal, pancreatic, and hepatic carcinomas; in most other tumors, the levels of α-fetoprotein remain low. However, increased production of α-fetoprotein has also been recorded in certain non-neoplastic diseases, such as acute viral hepatitis. α-Fetoprotein is a glycoprotein with a molecular weight of 70,000 daltons; its normal function is not known.

Carcinoembryonic antigen (CEA) was described by P. Gold and S. O. Freedman in 1965. These researchers obtained rabbit antiserum against a perchloric acid extract from a pool of human carcinomas. Following absorption with normal colon tissue, the antiserum formed a single precipitin line with extracts from other colon carcinomas. Later studies revealed that the antigen detected by the antiserum was shared by human colon cancer cells and by cells of fetal gut, pancreas, and liver up to the sixth month of gestation (hence the name). The antigen is carried by a glycoprotein molecule with a molecular weight of 200,000 to 300,000 daltons; the molecule contains from 50 to 70 percent carbohydrates, and is apparently a part of the mucous coating of the cell. Originally, clinicians hoped to use carcinoembryonic antigen for diagnosis of colon cancer, for the antigen was also detected in the serum of several cancer patients. Unfortunately, it later turned out that a large percentage of normal individuals and patients with non-neoplastic diseases often had higher levels of serum carcinoembryonic antigen than did colon cancer patients.

Differentiation Antigens. These are expressed in some adult tissues and absent in others; they reappear inappropriately in certain tumors. Several antigens of this category have been described in the mouse by Edward A. Boyse, Lloyd J. Old, and Elisabeth Stockert; here we shall mention only two, the Tla and G_{IX} antigens.

Table 14.9 Antigens Controlled by the Thymus-Leukemia Antigen (*Tla*) Locus

	Antigens in Normal Thymocytes					Antigens in Leukemic Cells				
Tla Allele	1	2	3	4	5	1	2	3	4	5
a	1	2	3	—	5	1	2	3	—	5
b	—	—	—	—	—	1	2	—	4	—
c	—	2	—	—	—	1	2	—	—	—
c	—	2	—	—	—	1	2	—	4	5
d	1	2	3	—	—	.	.	.	.	.

1, 2, etc., presence of antigen; —, absence of antigen; ., not known.

The *thymus leukemia antigen*, or Tla, is, as the name suggests, shared by normal thymocytes and certain leukemias. It is not a single antigen, but a complex of at least five antigenic determinants, designated Tla.1 through Tla.5. In inbred mice, four different alleles at the *Tla* locus have been identified, each coding for a particular combination of determinants present on normal thymocytes (Table 14.9). Leukemias derived from some strains express the same determinants as those found in normal thymuses of these mice; but leukemias of other strains expresss some of the determinants inappropriately. For example, leukemias of Tla^b strains express determinants 1, 2, and 4, while the corresponding normal thymocytes do not express any known Tla determinants at all. The *Tla* locus is closely linked to the *H*-2 complex, the major histocompatibility complex of the mouse, and may, in fact, be part of it. The Tla molecule is a cell-surface glycoprotein with a molecular weight of 44,000 daltons; it associates in the membrane with a smaller component, which, like the β_2-microglobulin of some of the H-2 molecules, has a molecular weight of 12,000 daltons.

The *G_{IX} antigen* was first identified using an antiserum from rats immunized with Gross virus-induced leukemia cells; hence the name. (The numerical designation refers to the fact that the antigen was originally thought to be controlled by a gene located in linkage group IX; it was later discovered that the gene was not in this linkage group, and the linkage group was shown to be carried by chromosome 17, so that the ''group IX'' designation was dropped anyway. The designation of the antigen, however, remained.) The G_{IX} antigen is present on normal thymocytes of some, but not all, inbred strains. Furthermore, strains that do express the antigen fall into three groups, according to the *quantity* of the expressed antigen. The antigen also appears on certain virally induced leukemias, including those originating in G_{IX}-negative strains. The genetic control of G_{IX} expression in normal tissues is a mystery. There seem to be at least two *host* genes involved in this control—*Gv*-1 and *Gv*-2, which are incapable of giving rise to infectious virus—yet biochemical studies have demonstrated that the G_{IX}-bearing molecule is a gp70, which is normally of viral origin.

True Tumor-Associated Antigens

True tumor antigens are those expressed only on tumor cells and not normal cells. They are often referred to as *tumor-specific antigens*, but since complete restriction of antigens to tumor cells is quite difficult to prove, we shall refrain from using this designation.

Methods of Detection. Tumor-associated antigens can be detected by a variety of methods based on both cellular and humoral immunity. The two commonly used cellular immunity methods are tumor transplantation in vivo, whereby the presence of the tumor-associated antigen is revealed when the tumor is rejected by syngeneic hosts, and cell-mediated lymphocytotoxicity in vitro, whereby the presence of the antigen is revealed by lysis of tumor cells mixed with immune lymphocytes. Antigens detected by the in vivo method are sometimes referred to as *tumor-associated transplantation antigens*, or TATA. To achieve rejection, the syngeneic host must first be immunized against the tumor-associated antigens, since the immunogenic stimulus provided by the tumor is weak and the tumor easily overrides the immunity it induces (which is the reason it is not rejected by the original host in the first place). The immunization can be achieved by tying or ligating the tumor, removing an actively growing tumor after it has reached an appreciable size, eradicating the tumor with chemotherapeutic agents, inoculating subthreshold doses of tumor cells, inoculating X-irradiated tumor cells, injecting tumor extracts, and—in the case of virally induced tumors—inoculating UV-irradiated viruses. In the in vitro CML assay, care must be taken that the target cells carry the same MHC genes as the tumor that stimulated the immunity, since tumor-associated antigens are recognized by T lymphocytes in the context of class I MHC molecules.

In situations where a tumor also induces humoral immunity, the tumor-associated antigens can be detected by one of the many available serological methods. Commonly used are methods based on membrane immunofluorescence and on complement-mediated cytotoxicity. Often, however, it is difficult to produce antibodies against tumor-associated antigens in titers sufficient for serological demonstration of the antigen.

Properties. The characteristics of tumor-associated antigens are very much dependent on the origin of the tumor carrying them. Antigens of *tumors induced by chemical carcinogens* are individually distinct, so that each tumor has a unique antigen or set of antigens. The distinctiveness of tumor-associated antigens from different tumors has been demonstrated, using methods based on transplantation immunity: immunity induced by one tumor protects the animal against the tumor, but not against other tumors of independent origin. Groups of some 30 different tumors induced by the same chemical have been tested in this fashion, and no two tumors have been found to carry the same tumor-associated antigens. How large the diversity of the tumor-associated antigens is is not known. The immunogenicity of the tumor-associated antigens carried by chemically induced tumors varies widely, and this variation is somewhat influenced by the type and dose of carcinogen used for induction.

In sharp contrast to the chemically induced tumors are *tumors induced by oncogenic viruses*. Here, tumors induced by the same virus have common tumor-associated antigens, although they may possess specific antigens in addition. The common antigens are almost always associated with the virus, whereas the individually specific antigens are not virus-related, at least not directly. The individually specific antigens are most easily demonstrated in virus-infected mice, presumably because the response to the stronger virus-associated antigen is suppressed in such mice.

Tumor-associated antigens on *spontaneous tumors*, particularly human tumors, are often difficult to demonstrate, probably because of the reaction of the cancer cell surface to the host immune response (see below). Whether the antigens are actually lacking in some of these tumors or are masked, modulated, or blocked is not yet certain. However, many spontaneous tumors clearly do express tumor-associated antigens.

The nature and origin of tumor-associated antigens are not known. Attempts to isolate and chemically characterize these antigens have encountered serious difficulties, many having to do with a lack of reagents suitable for precipitation of the antigen-bearing molecules from a solution. Some investigators believe that at least some of the tumor-associated antigens, even in the chemically induced and spontaneous tumors, are directly or indirectly related to viruses activated by the neoplastic transformation of the cell. A particularly attractive candidate for the role of tumor-associated antigens is the C-type virus-encoded gp70 molecule, which has been demonstrated to vary considerably from virus to virus.

14.3.5 Defense Against Cancer

Like many other stimuli, the tumor-associated antigens activate not one but a whole set of defense mechanisms—both specific and nonspecific, humoral and cellular—of which some play a more important role than others. The dominant role in in vivo resistance to tumor growth is played by *T lymphocytes*. These cells can recognize tumor-associated antigens presented to them by macrophages, be activated by this recognition, and upon activation and differentiation, attack and kill the tumor cells. An in vitro expression of this specific cellular resistance to tumors is the cell-mediated cytotoxicity reaction, frequently used for the demonstration of tumor-associated antigens. The activated T lymphocytes also secrete lymphokines and various other soluble factors, some of which may kill the tumor cells or inhibit their growth; other factors may stimulate noncommitted cells to join the attack on the neoplasm.

The main manifestation of *B lymphocyte* involvement in the resistance to cancer is production of antibodies specific for tumor-associated antigens. In addition to the induced antibodies, the host may also possess natural or spontaneously appearing antibodies that possess reactivity against a variety of tumor- and virus-associated antigens. The antibodies may mediate complement killing of tumor cells or they may produce antibody-dependent cell-mediated cytotoxicity (ADCC). There are also reports that activated B cells can, under certain circumstances, kill tumor cells directly, just as T lymphocytes do.

The role of *natural killer cells* is suggested by the observation that inoculation of mice with various tumor cells leads to a rapid, transient increase in these cells' activity, with a peak at three days. Furthermore, the levels of natural killer cell activity in different mouse strains correlate with the relative resistance of these strains to growth of transplantable tumor cells. Natural killer cells may also play a role in preventing the emergence of cancer in the first place (see below).

Macrophages may be drawn into the anticancer response in at least two ways. Antibodies to tumor-associated antigens may form a bridge between the tumor cells (to which they bind via the combining sites) and the macrophage (to which they attach via the Fc region and the Fc receptor on the macrophage). The bridging activates the cytolytic potential of the macrophages and leads to killing of the bound tumor cell. Macrophages can also be stimulated by the specific macrophage-activating factor (SMAF) released from immune T lymphocytes.

14.3.6 How Do Tumors Evade Immunity?

The fact that many individuals die of cancer indicates that the defense mechanisms are often ineffective, despite the involvement of so many components of the body's immune system. Apparently, the tumor uses some of the tactics parasites do to evade immunity and to grow unchecked. A brief description of some of these escape mechanisms follows.

Immunoselection

Although each tumor probably begins from a single cell and so represents a clone, the cells in this clone do not remain the same. As the tumor grows, additional changes occur, so that at any time, the tumor cell population is a heterogeneous mixture of different subclones. If some of the changes result in decreased antigenicity, the low antigenic variants may gain advantage under the selective pressure exerted on the tumor cells by the host's immunity. These variants may, therefore, take over and so increase the general immunoresistance of the tumor. The lower antigenicity of these tumor cells could result not only from deletion of the antigens, but also from a decrease in their density on the plasma membrane. If the density drops under a certain threshold level, the tumor may become "invisible" to the immune system.

Antigenic Modulation

Mice immunized against Tla antigens and containing high titers of cytotoxic Tla antibodies might be expected to resist syngeneic Tla-positive leukemias. Paradoxically, not only do such mice succumb to the tumors, but the tumors recovered before the host's death lose their sensitivity to Tla antibodies and their ability to absorb cytotoxic Tla antibodies in vitro. The loss is only temporary, because a single passage of the tumor in untreated syngeneic hosts leads to a complete reappearance of the Tla antigens. The phenomenon of temporary loss of antigens after exposure to specific antibodies has been termed *antigenic modulation*. The disappearance of antigens from the cell surface is thought to occur via patching, capping, and endocytosis, or shedding of the caps (see Chapter 6).

Stimulation of Suppressor Cells

In tumor-bearing individuals, such reactions as lectin-induced T-lymphocyte blastogenesis, in vitro generation of specific cytotoxic T cells, and in vivo antibody synthesis are often switched off, and this nonspecific suppression can be attributed to the presence of activated macrophages. How these "suppressor" macrophages function is not known. One proposed explanation is that the activated macrophages release prostaglandins, which then activate adenylate cyclase in the lymphocyte membrane, and the activated enzyme then increases the level of intracellular cyclic AMP, inhibiting proliferation. In addition to these nonspecific "suppressor" cells, tumor-bearing individuals probably contain typical suppressor T cells directed specifically against tumor-associated antigens.

Sneaking Through

Researchers have noted that animals challenged with a very low dose of tumor cells often develop tumors more frequently than those inoculated with larger doses. This observation led to the formulation of the "sneaking through" hypothesis, according to which a few isolated tumor cells contain too little antigen to sensitize the host, but by the time significant immunity does develop, the tumor is already so large that it is beyond the capabilities of the immune system. This simple hypothesis is very difficult to prove or disprove experimentally.

Enhancement

In experimental situations, treatment intended to increase the immune response of a host to a tumor sometimes leads to just the opposite effect—namely, to promoted tumor growth. This *immunological enhancement* usually occurs when animals are challenged with inactivated tumor cells before they are inoculated with live cells. The increased tumor growth is mediated by a special class of serum antibodies that act either on the tumor itself or on the immune system stimulated by the tumor (see Chapter 12 for further details). Enhancement is frequently encountered with allogeneically transplanted tumors; whether it also affects the growth of syngeneic tumors is less certain.

Blocking Factors

Cancer patients' sera sometimes have the capacity to abrogate lymphocyte-mediated killing in vitro. The inhibition is attributed to blocking factors, which, by combining with antigens on tumor cells, prevent sensitized lymphocytes or cytotoxic antibodies from attaching to them and inducing cytolysis (see also Chapter 13). The factors are presumably different from enhancing antibodies and may, in fact, represent antigen-antibody complexes. What role, if any, blocking factors have in vivo is not known.

Immunosuppression

Some tumors may invade lymphoid tissues and so interfere with normal immune response. Others may secrete as yet unidentified soluble substances, which may act as immunosuppressive factors by inhibiting lymphocyte proliferation. The result of both these actions is a depression of the individual's ability to mount immune response. Such a depression in tumor-bearing individuals has been demonstrated for a wide variety of antigens.

14.3.7 Immune Surveillance

From the preceding discussion it should be clear that the immune system does indeed try, though often unsuccessfully, to stop cancer growth once cancer is established. However, the question remains: does the immune system also resist the *emergence* of cancer cells? The idea that one of the main functions of the immune system might be to preserve uniformity of cell types and to prevent mutant cells from colonizing the body—in short, to prevent neoplasia—was first expressed by Lewis Thomas in 1959. The idea was then expounded and popularized by F. Macfarlane Burnet, who also introduced the term *immune surveillance* as an expression for the immune system's role in detection and destruction of aberrant cells. The concept of immune surveillance can best be explained by the following analogy.

Imagine a totalitarian city that George Orwell might have created for *1984*. The city has a strict code governing the appearance of its buildings and a squad of building inspectors who enforce this code. Suppose that one home owner has become dissatisfied with the appearance of his house and begins to remodel it to his liking. As long as he makes alterations inside the house, the building inspectors do not notice anything because they inspect only from the outside. But as soon as he touches the facade and alters it so that his house is different from all the other houses on the street, the inspectors become alarmed. They run to their headquarters with the news, mobilize a demolition squad, and return to the offending house, which they proceed to tear down. Some of the inspectors will take part in the demolition, while others will coordinate the squad's work to make it the most efficient with the least damage to the adjacent "conforming" houses.

According to the immune surveillance hypothesis, the cells of the immune system are like the building inspectors: they patrol the tissues of the body, searching for nonconforming alterations to the cell surfaces. They have learned in special schools how the surfaces should look and how to recognize any surface that deviates from the body's building code. When they spot a cell with an unfamiliar plasma membrane, they become activated and organize an all-out attack on the strange cell, destroying it before it can spread through the body.

So attractive is the idea of immune surveillance that one is almost tempted to accept it as self-evident. The difficulties arise when one attempts to prove it experimentally. The main prediction of the immune surveillance hypothesis is that abrogation of immunocompetence by neonatal thymectomy, irradiation, antilymphocyte serum treatment, or treatment with immunosuppressive drugs should increase the incidence of cancer in individuals so treated. Also, an increased incidence of tumors should be observed in individuals with inherited immunodeficiency. To a limited extent, this prediction has been borne out by experimental and clinical observations: in general, immunologically deficient individuals do develop cancer more frequently than do intact individuals. The difficulty, however, is that most of the tumors arising in such individuals are tumors of the lymphoid system. If the immune surveillance hypothesis were correct, one should observe a general increase of all kinds of tumor, not just lymphoid tumors. The preponderance of lymphoid tumors suggests that the increased incidence does not result from a failure of immune surveillance, but from the treatment the immunodeficient individuals receive. Supporting this argument is the observation that congenitally athymic mice, believed to have one arm of the immune system incapacitated, have the same tumor incidence as normal mice. Also arguing against the immune surveillance hypothesis is the "sneaking through" phenomenon, since here the surveillance apparently fails in a situation where it should be acting most strongly. However, to each of these arguments there is a counterargument: immunodeficient individuals do not survive long enough to show a greater than normal incidence of cancer; athymic mice are not completely devoid of T lymphocytes, and besides, have a fully developed complement of natural killer cells, which may either take over or even play a dominant role in immune surveillance; for every tumor that has sneaked through, there may be dozens of which we are not aware that have been stopped. Undoubtedly, the arguments will continue for awhile, before a consensus is reached about the role played by the immune system in controlling the emergence of cancer.

14.3.8 Prospects for Immunotherapy

There is no doubt that the immune system can eliminate at least some cancers but is often prevented from doing so by the evasive maneuvers of the tumor cells. Naturally, then, the question of whether ways could be found either to strengthen the immune response or to control tumor evasiveness arises. In other words, can effective anticancer immunotherapy be designed? In the following we shall list some of the approaches that have been attempted.

Lymphocyte Transfer

Experiments on animals have demonstrated that transfer of immune lymphocytes from one individual to another can protect the recipient against tumor challenge. In clinical trials, attempts have been made to immunize each of two cancer patients against a tumor of his partner and then to exchange leukocytes between the two patients. Unfortunately, no significant antitumor effects have been observed, and this failure has been explained by the fact that the transferred leukocytes, being allogeneic, were probably rejected by the host. However, similar exchanges between identical, and hence histocompatible, twins have also failed, probably because the tumors were already too advanced to be brought under control. Reinjections of the patient's own leukocytes after in vitro stimulation with mitogens such as phytohemagglutinin have resulted in a slight decrease in tumor size, but no long-term cure.

Antibody Transfer

In mice, the injection of a specific hyperimmune antiserum protects the host against a leukemia, but attempts to reproduce these results in humans have failed, probably because of a difference in the quality of antisera. For logistic and ethical reasons, highly specific cytotoxic antitumor sera are difficult to produce in clinical situations. Attempts to use specific antibodies as transport vehicles for attached nonspecific tumoricidal agents, such as diphtheria toxin, ricin, or high-energy isotopes, have also been unsuccessful. The idea behind these experiments was that the antibodies would bind specifically to the tumor, and the attached toxic agent would kill the cell. Although some localization of the agent to the tumor cells was observed, regression of the tumors was not seen.

Use of Adjuvants

Nonspecific stimulation of the immune system of tumor-bearing individuals has been attempted by the administration of adjuvants such as BCG and *C. parvum*. *Bacillus Calmette-Guérin*, or BCG, is a live, attenuated strain of *Mycobacterium bovis*. The injection of BCG into animals leads to enhanced antigen clearance and phagocytosis, increased humoral immunity, accelerated rejection of transplants, increased resistance to infection—and also retardation of tumor growth. In humans, the greatest success with BCG injections has been in the treatment of skin tumors—in particular, melanomas. In 25 percent of patients with postoperative recurrence of melanoma, and so very poor chances of recovery, BCG treatment has resulted in total tumor regression and complete cure. The mechanism by which BCG acts is not known. It was first thought that it stimulates lymphocytes, which then recruit and nonspecifically activate macrophages, which then attack the tumor. Later experiments, however, have suggested that there is antigenic crossreactivity between the BCG organisms and human melanomas, so that the action of the adjuvant might involve some degree of specificity.

Corynebacterium parvum is another bacterium capable of stimulating vigorous immune response and acting primarily on macrophages. In contrast to BCG, *C. parvum* is administered in a nonviable form (which is an advantage), preferably directly into the tumor site. It is most effective when used in combination with chemotherapy. In humans, some success of combined *C. parvum* immunotherapy and chemotherapy has been reported in patients with lung cancer.

Dinitrochlorobenzene (DNCB) Painting

Regression of skin and other superficial tumors can sometimes be achieved by sensitizing the patient against dinitrochlorobenzene and then painting the tumor with DNCB. The sensitization presumably induces delayed-type hypersensitivity, the target of which becomes the DNCB on tumor cells.

Immunization with Tumor Cells

Immunization with unmodified autologous or allogeneic tumor cells alone, without any further protective measure, is usually ineffective in enhancing antitumor immunity, and may actually have just the opposite effect in some instances. More promising is immunization with modified cells—for example, tumor cells treated with neuraminidase. The treatment presumably unmasks some normally hidden cell-surface antigens, which then become the target of the immune response. However, researchers have also noted that neuraminidase-treated tumor cells bind different immunoglobulin classes than untreated cells and have speculated that the treatment may provoke a shift in the host response toward protective immunity. Other treatments of tumor cells include attachment of small haptens or infection of the cells with a virus. Attempts are also being made to isolate tumor-associated antigens and use the purified antigens to produce antitumor immunity by their inoculation into the host.

Transfer Factor and Xenogeneic Immune RNA

Transfer factor is a dialyzable substance extracted from the lymphocytes of donors sensitive to tuberculin and purportedly capable of conferring tuberculin sensitivity to normal individuals (see Chapter 12). Attempts have been made to isolate tumor-directed transfer factor that would elicit only cell-mediated, not humoral immunity in the host, and thus avoid the danger of producing blocking or enhancing antibodies. The results of these attempts, however, have been unimpressive. It has also been claimed that RNA extracts from immune macrophages or lymphocytes, when added to nonimmune cells, have conferred immunity on these cells. This *immune RNA* seems related in some way to the transfer factor, and the two may actually be the same. Attempts to use the immune RNA in tumor immunotherapy were largely unsuccessful.

The balance sheet of the attempts to develop effective antitumor immunotherapy is a depressing sight. Almost everything one can think of has been tried, often quite extensively; yet in only a few instances have encouraging results been obtained. The difficulties lie in the complexity of the disease (it has often been stated that cancer is not a single entity but an extremely diverse collection of diseases), complexity of the immune response, which we still do not understand enough, the fine line between immunostimulation and immunosuppression, and above all, our complete ignorance of the molecular mechanisms of cancer induction. Tumor immunotherapy as practiced today is more witchcraft than science, and will remain so for as long as we remain in the dark about the basic processes underlying the emergence and spread of cancer.

14.4 AUTOIMMUNITY

To Paul Ehrlich and his contemporaries, the immune system seemed as foolproof in its ability to distinguish self from nonself as if it were guarded by some mysterious *horror autotoxicus*, the fear of self-poisoning. This view prevailed for almost half a century, despite the fact that here and there researchers observed what seemed to be instances of the immune system's attacking self components. It was only in the 1950s, and primarily because of the work of Ernest Witebsky and Noel R. Rose, that immunologists became aware of the immune system's imperfections. The system clearly was not foolproof, and its ability to distinguish nonself from self was not absolute. Occasionally the system broke down and turned against the body, generating an *autoimmune disease*. It has been only recently that researchers have begun to realize that apparently the *potential* for self injury is built into the immune system, that recognition of nonself is tightly linked to recognition of self, and that autoimmune diseases might be only the exaggerated expression of events that normally occur all the time in the body. However, before we discuss how it might happen that the immune system turns against itself, let us first consider a few selected examples of accidental all-out attacks on the body.

14.4.1 Examples of Autoimmune Disease

Autoimmune Hemolytic Anemia

Among patients who come to the doctor's office complaining of general weakness, some are found to have a lower than normal amount of erythrocytes in their blood and are thus diagnosed as anemic. Erythrocytes of some of these patients are found to be agglutinated by xenogeneic antisera to human immunoglobulin, or to human complement components C3 and C4. This positive direct *Coombs test* indicates that erythrocytes in the blood of the anemic individuals are coated with either immunoglobulins (presumably the patient's own antibodies reacting with some antigens on the erythrocyte surface) or with complement components. The coating antibodies sometimes activate the complement cascade, leading to rupture of the erythrocyte membrane, hemoglobin release, and the appearance of hemoglobin in the urine (*hemoglobinuria*). In less severe cases, the attached antibodies bind only some complement components, which then mediate immune adherence to macrophages, or the antibodies opsonize the erythrocytes. Both the immune and opsonic adherence result in either total phagocytosis of the sensitized erythrocytes or morphological changes, particularly in turning the doughnut-shaped erythrocyte into a ball-shaped, short-lived *spherocyte*. The end effect of the hemolysis, phagocytosis, or life span shortening of erythrocytes by autoantibodies is the same—the reduction in erythrocyte numbers, or *autoimmune hemolytic anemia*.

The coating antibodies can be eluted from the red blood cells and their properties studied in vitro. Such studies have revealed the existence of two kinds of autoantibody—warm, reacting with red blood cells at 37°C, and cold, with a reaction optimum close to 0°C.

The target of the *warm autoantibodies* appears to be the Rh antigens. Some of the antibodies detect alloantigenic Rh determinants (that is, determinants present in some humans and absent in others), others detect determinants common to all Rh molecules. (These *panagglutinins* react with all human red blood cells except those carrying the Rh null blood group.) Most of the warm autoantibodies are of the IgG class, and so possess good opsonizing and immune adherence ability. They therefore mediate preferentially either complete or partial phagocytosis, the latter resulting in the appearance of spherocytes.

The *cold autoantibodies*, or *cold agglutinins*, attach to red blood cells at cold temperatures and dissociate as the cells are rewarmed. They appear to be directed against either the I or the i blood-group antigens. The anti-I factors occur in the transient anemia accompanying virus or *Mycoplasma pneumoniae* infections; the i-specific antibodies are characteristic of the so-called *chronic cold agglutinin disease*, accompanying chronic lymphoproliferative diseases of the non-Hodgkin type. It is not the antibody that is cold-dependent, but the antigen it reacts with. The I and i determinants are carried by *glycophorin*, the major glycoprotein of human erythrocyte surfaces. The conformation of glycophorin is apparently temperature-dependent, and at cold temperatures it is such that the I and i determinants are exposed and available for interaction with antibodies; at 37°C, the determinants are hidden. Isolated glycophorin binds cold-reacting antibodies even at 37°C. Most cold autoantibodies are of the IgM type, and hence are capable of binding complement and mediating hemolysis. Nonetheless, hemolysis is minimal or mild in patients with cold autoagglutinins, probably because the temperature in most parts of the body is higher than 31°C, the maximal temperature at which these antibodies lyse cells. However, on exposure to cold, the temperature of blood circulating in the peripheral regions of the skin may drop below 31°C, and the patient may experience a more severe attack of the disease.

On rare occasions, the cold-reacting antibodies are of the IgG class. One example is the so-called *Donath-Landsteiner antibodies*, which bind to red blood cells in the cold and fix the early components of the complement cascade. Upon rewarming, the complement sequence is completed and massive hemolysis ensues, leading to the sudden appearance of hemoglobin in urine, fever, chills, pains in the joints and muscles, and jaundice—the characteristic symptoms of *paroxysmal cold hemoglobinuria* (Gr. *paroxyne*, to sharpen, here meaning a sudden onset of symptoms).

Some autoimmmune hemolytic anemias appear without any apparent cause; others accompany certain diseases (in addition to the diseases already mentioned, they may accompany other autoimmune diseases, such as systemic lupus erythematosus); still others are induced by the use of drugs. There are at least four possible ways in which the drugs can induce autoimmune hemolytic anemia: the drug incites antibody formation, and the formed drug-antibody complexes bind to red blood cells and fix complement; the drug conjugates spontaneously to proteins in the red blood cell membrane, forming hapten-carrier complexes, which then induce antibody formation (derivatives of penicillin, as you may recall from Chapter 10, are sometimes used as hapten because they bind easily to protein); the drug may make the red cell surface sticky to serum proteins, including immunoglobulins, and the nonspecifically bound antibodies may then enhance phagocytosis of the coated cells; the drug interacts directly with cell-surface antigens and alters them in such a way that they then become immunogenic. Evidence exists for the occurrence of the first two of these four mechanisms; almost none is available for the other two.

Autoimmune Endocrine Diseases

The organs of inner secretion are the target of several autoimmune diseases, but we shall describe only three, all affecting the thyroid. This butterfly-shaped endocrine gland is located in the neck, with the "wings" (lobes) on either side of the windpipe. The gland consists of a large number of small, spherical vesicles or follicles, lined with epithelium and containing colloid. The two hormones secreted by the thyroid, thyroxine and tri-iodothyroxine, are necessary for growth, development, and metabolism. The hormones are stored in the colloid of the follicles and released from there into the blood. The three diseases of the thyroid that we shall discuss are Hashimoto's thyroiditis, its counterpart in the domestic fowl—obese chicken thyroiditis, and Graves' disease.

Hashimoto's Thyroiditis. Named after the Japanese surgeon H. Hashimoto, but also going under the names of autoimmune thyroiditis, chronic lymphoid thyroiditis, or lymphoid goiter, this disease is one of the most common autoimmune conditions, occurring most frequently in women between 30 and 50 years of age. In the affected individuals, for reasons we do not understand, an as yet unidentified agent makes the thyroid the target of an inflammatory response. Inflammatory cells—mainly lymphocytes, mononuclear cells, and plasma cells—begin to infiltrate the gland and to destroy its normal architecture. The thyroid attempts to regenerate, and this regeneration process combined with the inflammatory infiltration leads to an enlargement of the gland—the *struma* (L. *struo*, to pile up, build) or *goiter* (L. *guttur*, throat). The gland at first continues to function normally, but, as more and more of the follicles are destroyed, the output of thyroid hormones diminishes, resulting in *hypothyroidism*. The extreme form of hypothyroidism is *myxedema* (Gr. *myxa*, mucus, *oidema*, swelling), characterized by infiltration of many bodily tissues with a mucuslike fluid, which causes puffiness of the skin and interferes with the normal function of certain internal organs. The skin becomes exceedingly dry; the hair and fingernails are brittle; the loose tissue of the face becomes puffy, giving the person the appearance of wearing a mask; the skin may become yellowish as a result of the body's inability to convert the vegetable pigment carotene into vitamin A; the tongue enlarges, sometimes so much that it prevents closure of the mouth; the changes in the vocal cords result in hoarseness of the voice; the heart may become enlarged; effects on the nervous system may lead to mental impairments; and heat production is slowed, so that the patient feels cold most of the time.

Concurrently with the destruction of the thyroid, the body begins to produce antibodies to certain components of the gland. So far, four such components have been identified.

Thyroglobulin. This is the thyroid hormone that constitutes about 75 percent of the gland's protein and contains most of the body's iodine. The thyroglobulin-specific antibodies are probably produced by plasma cells infiltrating the thyroid. They are mostly of the IgG class and can be detected in the serum by precipitation, radioimmunoassay, agglutination of thyroglobulin-sensitized latex particles, and passive agglutination with tanned red blood cells.

Microsomal Cytoplasmic Antigens. Microsomes are spherical vesicles derived from the endoplasmic reticulum after disruption of cells by centrifugation. The antigen is a lipoprotein carried by the microsomes of the thyroid epithelial cells. It can be detected by immunofluorescence on thyroid slices. Some of the antibodies are specific for the microsomes of the thyroid; others also react with microsomes of other organs.

Second Colloid Antigen. CA2 is a substance in the fluid filling the thyroid follicles. Like the microsomal antigens, CA2 can be detected by immunofluorescence.

Thyroid Cell-Surface Antigen. This antigen can be detected by immunofluorescence or mixed hemadsorption. A component of the plasma membrane, it may serve as a target for the destruction of the thyroid cells.

The question of whether antibodies against these antigens are the cause or the consequence of the disease remains unanswered. We have already mentioned that B lymphocytes of a normal individual are capable of reacting with thyroglobulin, and perhaps also with the other three antigens, but are prevented from doing so by the tolerance status of the T cells (see Chapter 13). In the disease, this block to B-cell responsiveness is presumably removed, although we do not know how the removal takes place.

Obese Chicken Thyroiditis. One strain of the domestic fowl, derived from the White Leghorns, develops spontaneous autoimmune thyroiditis characterized by subcutaneous fat deposits, particularly in the abdomen, and by abnormal sensitivity to cold. These obese chicken thyroiditis resembles Hashimoto's disease in that the bird's thyroid becomes infiltrated by lymphocytes and the bird's blood contains antibodies to thyroglobulin. The fact that almost all the obese strain (OS) chickens develop thyroiditis by the time they are seven weeks of age indicates that the disease is genetically controlled. Apparently, during the development of the strain, several genes that strongly predipose the birds to the disease were accidentally brought together. Noel R. Rose and his co-workers, who have studied chicken thyroiditis extensively, have been able to identify at least three groups of these predisposing genes—one effecting heightened immune responses, another causing disordered thymic maturation, and a third responsible for the abnormality of the thyroid itself. The heightened response is imposed onto the OS chicken by the presence of a particular allele at its major histocompatibility complex loci. The OS chickens segregate for two MHC alleles, B^{13} and B^{5}; chickens carrying the B^{13} allele develop much higher levels of autoantibodies to thyroglobulin and display more pronounced infiltration of their thyroids than chickens homozygous for the B^{5} allele. The OS chickens thus possess an *Ir* gene that predisposes them to high immune responsiveness to thyroglobulin.

The disordered thymus maturation presumably manifests itself in a premature release of effector T cells, or in the delayed departure from the thymus of suppressor T cells. Rose and his colleagues have hypothesized that this abnormal sequence of maturation may be one of the important factors promoting autoimmunity in the OS chickens.

The third genetic factor predisposing OS chickens to autimmune thyroiditis lies in the thyroid itself. It is manifested, for example, by a greater than normal uptake of radioactive iodine by thyroids of OS chicken embryos.

Graves' Disease. In normal individuals, the production of thyroglobulin is controlled by the thyroid-stimulating hormone (TSH) secreted by the pituitary gland. The TSH binds to specific receptors on the surface of thyroid cells and, via the by now familiar adenylate cyclase (cAMP) channels, activates the cell to synthesize and secrete thyroglobulin (Fig. 14.35*a*). Since the body normally maintains only a low level of TSH, the amounts of thyroglobulin produced are also low.

In patients with Graves' disease, this normal run of things is disturbed. The patients are apparently genetically predisposed to produce antibodies capable of binding, via their Fab regions, with the TSH receptors on thyroid cells. This binding has the same effect as the binding of TSH itself—stimulation of thyroglobulin production by the thyroid cells (Fig. 14.35*b*). Unlike the TSH, however, the action of the antibodies is not subject to normal hormonal feedback control, so the patient's cells continually produce thyroglobulin over long periods. This characteristic earned the autoantibodies the designation *long-acting thyroid-stimulating antibodies*, or LATS. The presence of the antibodies can be demonstrated by injecting the patient's serum into mice and measuring the release of labeled iodine from the animal's thyroid gland. Because of this fact, the antibody is sometimes also referred to as *mouse thyroid-stimulating autoantibody*, or MTS. A 4S protein, presumably the TSH receptor, has been isolated from the thyroid cell membranes; when this protein is injected into mice simultaneously with LATS, it blocks the antibodies and prevents their stimulation of the thyroid (Fig. 14.35*c*). However, Graves' disease pa-

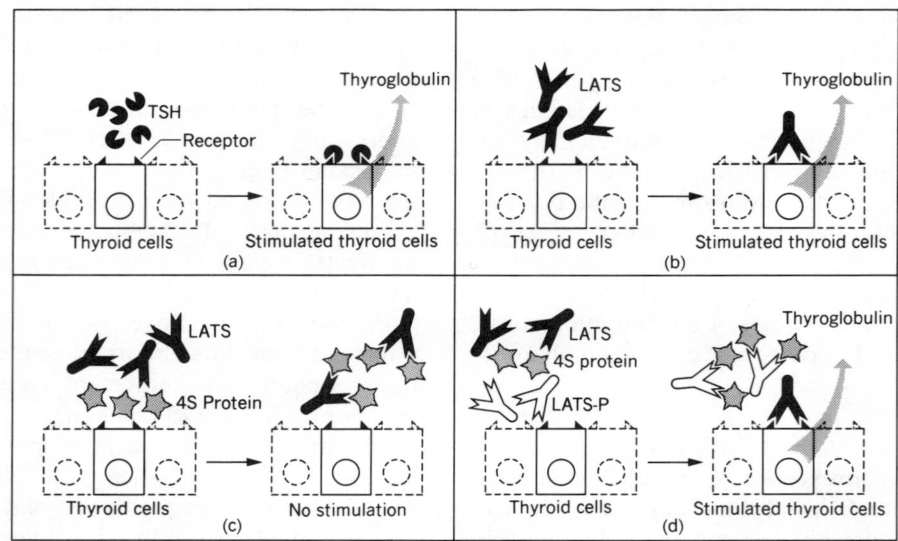

Figure 14.35. Action of hormones and antibodies on the thyroid. (*a*) Stimulation of thyroid cells by the thyroid-stimulating hormone (THS). (*b*) Stimulation of thyroid cells by long-acting thyroid-stimulating (LATS) antibodies. (*c*) Blocking of the LATS antibody action by the 4S protein. (*d*) Competitive inhibition of LATS antibody-4S protein binding by the LATS-protector (LATS-P).

tients also produce another autoantibody, presumably also binding to the TSH receptors and stimulating the thyroid cells via these receptors. Unlike the LATS, this second antibody binds only to human, not to mouse, thyroid cells. But it also binds to the isolated human 4S protein, so when injected into the mouse simultaneously with this protein and the LATS, it prevents LATS inhibition by competing with LATS for the 4S protein (Fig. 14.35*d*). Because of this behavior, this second antibody is referred to as *LATS-protector* (*LATS-P*) or the *human-specific thyroid-stimulating autoantibody* (HTS).

Binding of both the LATS and LATS-P to the thyroid cells has the same effect—continual stimulation of these cells and thus overproduction of thyroid hormones (*hyperthyroidism*). The elevated levels of thyroid hormones are then responsible for many of the symptoms associated with Graves' disease—increased basal metabolic rate, increased heartbeat rate, nervousness, heat intolerance, and sweating. The high thyroid hormone levels also stimulate the sympathetic nervous system and indirectly cause retraction of the eyelids—another sign of Graves' disease. The binding of autoantibodies to antigens in the thyroid initiates an inflammatory reaction, leading to the enlargement of this bland (goiter). The causes of the inflammatory reaction in the eye region are not yet completely clear. Since Graves' disease patients also produce autoantibodies to thyroglobulin, and since the thyroglobulin-antibody complexes seem to have affinity for extraocular muscle membrane, the extraocular myositis (muscle inflammation) accompanying the disease may be triggered by the deposit of immune complexes within the muscle. Since, furthermore, the adipose tissue of the retro-orbital region appears to be responsive to stimulation by TSH, it may also be responsive to LATS and LATS-P, and the constant stimulation by these two autoantibodies may cause proliferation of this tissue and the *exophthalmos*—the deposit of fatty tissues in the rigid orbital cavity of the eye.

Like many other autoimmune diseases, Graves' disease is more frequent in females than in males. The incidence of Graves' disease in western countries ranges from two to three per 30,000 individuals. One of the genes predisposing for the disease is associated with the genes coding for the antigens HLA-A8 and HLA-DW3, controlled by the human major histocompatibility complex.

Rheumatic Diseases

Complex diseases are like mountain ranges—each peak is easily identifiable, but its base fuses imperceptibly with that of a neighboring mountain. To a clinician, the complex of rheumatic diseases is such a mountain range: when all the symptoms point to one disease of the complex, the diagnosis is clear; but often they do not, and then the physician is at a loss as to where in the range to place the disease. So broad is the group of rheumatic diseases that, as someone once remarked, to know them is to know almost all of internal medicine.

Rheumatism (Gr. *rheuma*, flux, flow) is an indefinite term applied to various conditions characterized by pain radiating from the joints or other parts of the skeletal system, and often also by musclar soreness or stiffness. Since the joints play such an important role in this group of autoimmune diseases, let us briefly review their normal structure before we discuss how they are affected by the rheumatic condition. In a *joint* (Fig. 14.36*a*), the two bones are held together by a cuff of fibrous tissue, the so-called *capsule* (*capsular ligament*), lined by a *synovial membrane* (*synovium*, a word invented by the sixteenth-century Swiss physician Paracelsus, from Greek *syn*, together, and *oon*, egg). The opposing surfaces of the bones are covered by *articular cartilage*, and the space between the bones, the *joint cavity*, is filled with a small amount of *synovial fluid*, which normally consists mainly of mucin with some albumin, fat, epithelial cells, and leukocytes. The function of the synovial fluid is to lubricate the joint.

In a rheumatic condition, the joint becomes the target of an inflammatory reaction that may destroy the articular cartilage, the bones, and even the attached muscles. Sometimes the attack on the joint is only a secondary consequence of a primary attack on some other organ; at other times it is the joint that is the primary target of the disease. Examples of the former category of rheumatic disease are so-called rheumatic fever, affecting primarily the heart, and systemic lupus erythematosus, affecting a variety of organs; a representative of the latter category is rheumatoid arthritis. In the joint and other target organs of rheumatic diseases, the attack is directed against the connective tissue—more specifically, its collagen fibers. For this reason many rheumatic conditions are included in the category of *connective tissue* or *collagen diseases*. In the following, we shall consider the mechanisms leading to some of these diseases.

Rheumatic Fever. As the name implies, the two cardinal signs of this disease are pain in the joints and fever. The disease follows a throat and nose infection by one particular type of streptococcal bacteria, the group-A hemolytic *Streptococcus*; other infectious streptococci are not involved in this disease. Laboratory investigations have demonstrated that group-A streptococci possess, in their cell walls and cell membranes, antigens that are also present in human endocardium (the innermost tunic of the heart) and the myocardium (the middle muscle layer of the heart), cartilage, smooth muscle, skeletal muscle, and the glomerular basement membrane of the kidney. If the conditions are right (or wrong, from the patient's point of view), the patient's body begins to produce antibodies that are directed against streptococcal antigens, but crossreact with the host antigens; the antibodies bind to the host tissues, particularly in the heart and joints, and initiate an inflammatory response injurious to these tissues. The attack on the heart produces characteristic lesions of granulomatous tissue, so-called *Aschoff bodies*, named after the German

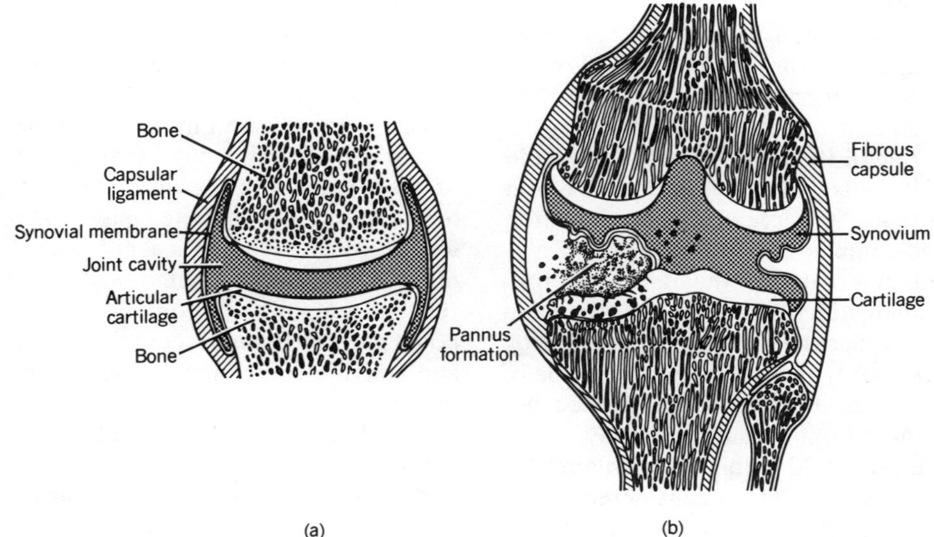

Figure 14.36. Structure of a healthy (*a*) and a rheumatoid (*b*) joint.

pathologist Ludwig K. A. Aschoff, and if the lesions are extensive, they may damage the organ permanently, particularly the valves. The inflammation in the joints manifests itself by swelling, redness, tenderness, and pain. The large joints are usually affected first, and when these heal, the infection may move to other joints.

The autoantibodies may also bind to nerves and skin, inducing inflammation of these tissues as well. Damage of the nervous tissue may lead to irregular, spasmodic, involuntary movements of the limbs or facial muscles—the so-called *chorea* or Saint John's (Saint Vitus') dance (L. *choreia*, a choral dance). Damage to the skin and to tissues lying beneath the skin manifests itself in the appearance of reddish areas (*erythema marginatum*, i.e., redness associated with leukocyte margination) and small lumps (*subcutaneous nodules*). Rheumatic fever usually develops in susceptible individuals between six and 19 years of age. The susceptibility appears to be genetically determined.

Rheumatoid Arthritis (Gr. *eidos*, resemblance, *arthron*, joint, *-itis*, inflammation). Also known as chronic polyarthritis (i.e., affecting many joints), chronic rheumatoid arthritis, chronic rheumatism, or arthropic arthritis, this disease is a chronic inflammation of joints; it is this disease that comes closest to what the layman usually understands by "rheumatism."

An important unanswered question about rheumatoid arthritis is how it begins. Family and population studies have revealed that the disease occurs either only or frequently in genetically predisposed individuals, but what exactly this predisposition means is not known. The disease is associated with some HLA antigens, notably DRW4 and DRW3, more frequently than with others, indicating that *HLA* genes themselves or genes closely linked to the *HLA* complex play a role in the emergence of the condition, but there must also be other genes involved. Physiological factors also play a role in the induction of rheumatoid arthritis, for the disease is almost symptomatic of old age. By retirement age, 80 percent of the population has some rheumatic complaint.

However, the direct stimulus of the disease is probably some as yet unidentified antigen. The two main possibilities are, first, that the antigen is provided by the body itself, presumably by the connective tissue of the joint that is the target of the reaction; or, second, that the antigen comes from outside the body in the form of an infectious agent. Mycoplasmas, chlamydia, clostridia, and viruses have all been considered at one time or another, but all were dismissed for lack of implicating evidence. The latest fad among immunologists is the Epstein-Barr virus, but no conclusive evidence has yet been provided for this agent either.

A common assumption is that presence of the hypothetical antigen provides continual stimulation to the body's immune system, particularly to B lymphocytes, and leads to persistent antibody production, either specific or of the polyclonal type. The secreted immunoglobulins then themselves become the target of an immune response, leading to the production of the so-called *rheumatoid factor* (RF), which is an antibody to the patient's own IgG molecules. How could the production of the RF be stimulated? Here too one has a choice of several possibilities. First, the antibodies produced against the hypothetical rheumatoid arthritis antigen bind to this antigen and this binding exposes new determinants on the participating IgG molecules; arguing against this possibility is the observation that the rheumatoid factor combines with IgG, even if it is not complexed with an antigen. Second, the high level of the original autoantibodies results in degradation of large quantities of IgG, and the degraded fragments express determinants that crossreact with the native IgG molecules. Third, the rheumatoid factor is normally present in all sera, but its production becomes exaggerated by the persistent antigenic stimulation. In view of the present knowledge about immune regulation, this third possibility seems to be the most likely. The determinant recognized by the rheumatoid factor (the Ga determinant) is located in the Fc region of the target IgG molecule. The factor itself is an IgM molecule, although other Ig classes may also occasionally display anti-Ig activity. The factor is present in high titers in the serum, as well as in the synovial fluid of the joint. Its occurrence, however, is not restricted to rheumatoid arthritis; the factor is also present in patients with many nonrheumatic diseases—in tuberculosis and leprosy, in diseases caused by viruses and animal parasites, and in renal transplant patients, particularly those receiving blood transfusions. The role of the rheumatoid factor in rheumatoid arthritis remains obscure. The factor may bind to the complexes formed by the hypothetical antigen and its corresponding antibodies, and thus facilitate phagocytosis of the antigen-antibody complexes. Alternatively, once bound to the immune complexes, the factor may fix and activate complement, and so contribute to the inflammation.

However, the main stimulus initiating the inflammatory response is probably the immune complexes; and since most of the complexes are apparently deposited on or in the synovium, this membrane becomes the primary target of the inflammatory reaction. The deposited complexes fix and activate complement, the activated complement components produce chemotactic factors, and the chemotactic factors attract inflammatory cells. The deeper layers of the synovium are infiltrated by lymphocytes (both T and B), plasma cells, macrophages, and occasionally neutrophils; the synovial fluid, on the other hand, contains mostly neutrophils, with some lymphocytes. The infiltrating cells elaborate antibodies, mediators of cellular immunity, complement components, enzymes, prostaglandins, and other effector molecules of the inflammatory reaction. Some of the factors dilate blood vessels, and by increasing vascular permeability, allow fluids to escape and accumulate in the joint cavity. This process turns the joint fluid into an inflammatory exudate.

The accumulation of fluid separates the synovial membrane from the underlying tissue and the membrane responds to this displacement by *cell proliferation*, increasing its original thickness from 10 to 20 times. The inflammatory reaction leads to the necrosis of thickened synovium and the replacement of the lost tissue by a granulation tissue, composed of young fibroblasts and exudative cells. Granular tissue is also deposited on the surface of the articular cartilage, forming a membrane called *pannus* (Fig. 14.36*b*).

The immune complexes, as well as factors produced by the immune lymphocytes, activate the clotting pathway, which leads to the production of fibrin. When the fibrin production exceeds the fibrinolytic capacity of the joint, large amounts of fibrin begin to be deposited in the joint space, synovium, pannus, and cartilage. In the synovial fluid, where it eventually accounts for up to 34 percent of the fluid's volume, fibrin is present either freely as rice-like bodies and flakes, or within phagosomes of neutrophils. In the synovium, pannus, and cartilage, it is present extravascularly, chiefly in the surface layers. The deposit of fibrin contributes to the swelling and proliferation of the synovial lining, pannus formation, fibrous thickening of the synovium, sustained emigration, degranulation, lytic degradation of neutrophils into the joint space, and induration of the synovium. The nutritional needs of the new tissues stimulate proliferation of small blood vessels, the blood flow into the joint increases, raising the intrajoint temperature to levels close to core body temperature, and the joint becomes warm and swollen.

Concurrently with these changes, large quantities of hydrolytic enzymes are produced throughout the joint. In the joint space, neutrophils break down and release elastase and cathepsin G from their azurophilic granules and collagenase from their specific granules. Additional enzymes are released from neutrophils during phagocytosis, when the granules fuse with phagosomes and discharge their contents into them. All these enzymes accumulate in the synovial fluid, and when their natural inhibitors become saturated, the enzymes begin to act unopposed on the superficial layers of the cartilage. In the inflamed synovium, the synovial cells produce the inactive form of collagenase and the plasminogen activator; the latter acts on plasminogen, seeping from the blood into the inflammatory effusions through capillary walls. This action produces plasmin, which then activates the collagenase.

With the aid of these enzymes, the synovium begins to eat into the cartilage from the side. The destructive process is highly polarized, being limited only to the region of the synovium bordering the cartilage. The reason that the synovium burrows into the cartilage but does not invade outwardly in a centrifugal direction might be the localized deposit of immune complexes in the cartilage, or it could be that the connective tissue of the joint capsule contains inhibitors of proteolytic enzymes. In the cartilage itself, the proximity of the inflamed synovium induces recruitment of cartilage cells (chondrocytes), which multiply and produce proteinases. These enzymes then begin to chew on the cartilage from the inside.

The cartilage is thus attacked from all sides. The attack is aimed primarily at the cartilage matrix, which consists of two major structural elements, collagen and proteoglycans. The enzymes first destroy the protein portion of the proteoglycans, leaving the carbohydrate that constitutes 90 percent of this molecule intact. With the proteoglycan lost, the collagen becomes accessible to proteolytic degradation by elastase and collagenase. Elastase cleaves nonhelical regions of collagen—that is, regions containing the interchain crosslinks. Collagenase cleaves helical regions at specific sites. Once the collagen framework is destroyed, the damage becomes irreversible because chondrocytes cannot regenerate normal cartilage.

The released enzymes and the breakdown products are recognized by the patient's immune system, and antibodies are produced against them. Antibodies to pepsin, neutral proteases, cathepsins, collagen, and nucleoproteins have been demonstrated in rheumatoid arthritis patients. These additional autoantibodies bind with their corresponding antigens, forming more immune complexes, and the deposit of these complexes in the tissues further perpetuates the disease.

At the same time, changes are also taking place in the bone below the cartilage. The bone loses its mineral components and becomes fibrous, and the degeneration then spreads to the cartilage. The concentrated attack on the cartilage converts it into a bloodless, fibrous tissue, leading to stiffness (*ankylosis*) of the joint. The fibrous ankylosis may then become bony, and this last alteration brings the whole process to an end: the inflammation stops, the pain disappears, the joint becomes immobile, and the patient is permanently crippled.

Simultaneously with the inflammatory process in the joint itself, changes also occur in the supporting structures. Because motion in the joint causes pain, the muscles operating the joint go into spasms, and since the muscle that bends the joint is stronger than the muscle that stretches it, the spasms bend the joint. It is in this bent position that the joint is then fixed, while the muscles eventually degenerate from disuse.

Although the joint is the main target in rheumatoid arthritis, other parts of the body may also be affected, chiefly because of inflammation-provoking immune complex deposits in these parts. One sometimes observes a scattered inflammation of arteries and veins (*vasculitis*), skin lesions, ulcers, nodules, skin reddening (*erythema*), lung lesions, and degeneration of peripheral nerves.

Systemic Lupus Erythematosus (SLE). The opinions on the origin of the designation "lupus erythematosus" (literally translated, it means "red wolf") differ. According to some, the designation was introduced because the pattern produced by the facial reddening that accompanies the disease reminds one of a wolf's head; according to others, the designation stems from the resemblance of the facial ulceration to a wolf bite. The adjective "systemic" is used to point out that the disease can involve almost any part in the body.

As in the case of rheumatoid arthritis, we are completely in the dark about the origin of systemic lupus erythematosus. According to some investigators, the disease begins in the skin of genetically predisposed and immunologically derailed individuals, with ultraviolet light being one of the major factors in its induction. According to this hypothesis, the UV radiation induces changes in the skin-cell DNA, which make the molecule antigenic when the cells, unable to function normally, break down. Speaking in favor of this hypothesis are two observations: first, SLE patients are abnormally sensitive to UV light, and second, antibodies to DNA are found in the patient's blood. But there may also be other ways in which the disease begins, such as activation of latent viruses (C-type RNA viruses, in particular, are suspect in this regard), and the action of hormones and drugs.

Nevertheless, circulating DNA antibodies are a typical feature of SLE. The antibodies are directed against the native, double-stranded form of DNA, against denatured single-stranded DNA, or against DNA complexed with histons (i.e., against the nucleoprotein). The DNA antibodies, and perhaps other autoantibodies as well, form complexes with their corresponding antigens, and these are then deposited in various tissues of the body. What follows is presumably the consequence of the deposit of immune complexes, and the protean nature of the disease stems primarily from the variety of places at which the complexes can be deposited. The role of immune complexes in the development of autoimmune diseases such as SLE has been demonstrated by two laboratories in particular, those of Henry G. Kunkel and Frank J. Dixon.

One of the organs in which the deposit of immune complexes causes extensive damage is the kidney. In a normal kidney (Fig. 14.37), blood is brought, via afferent arterioles, into a *glomerulus* (diminutive of L. *glomus*, a ball of yarn), a knot of capillary loops surrounded by epithelial tubuli, where it is filtered and then returned into circulation via efferent arterioles. During the filtering, toxic substances are removed from the blood; passed through the capillary wall of endothelial cells and basement membrane, and through the adjacent epithelial walls of the tubuli into the lumen of the tubuli; collected from the individual tubuli into the ducts; and excreted as urine from the body. The space between the individual capillary loops in the glomerulus is filled with *mesangial matrix*, containing scattered phagocytic *mesangial cells* (Gr. *mesos*, middle, *angeion*, vessel).

Among the substances removed from blood in the kidney are immune complexes that are constantly formed in small quantities in every healthy individual. The fate of the immune complexes depends on their size (which, in turn, depends on the antigen : antibody ratio) : large complexes formed in antibody excess are ingested by phagocytic cells, either directly in the capillary or in the mesangium; complexes with a molecular weight of about 500,000 daltons (formed in antigen excess) are deposited along the glomerular membrane; and finally, small, soluble complexes (formed at a 1 : 1 antigen : antibody ratio) either recirculate or are filtered into the urine. The kidney usually has no difficulty in handling the very large and the very small immune complexes if their concentration does not exceed certain tolerable levels; it is the medium-sized complexes that are the most troublesome.

In a normal glomerulus, some immune complex deposits are almost always found, but they are usually limited to the mesangial matrix, where they do not cause any harm. In contrast, in the glomerulus of an SLE patient, immune complex deposits form along the

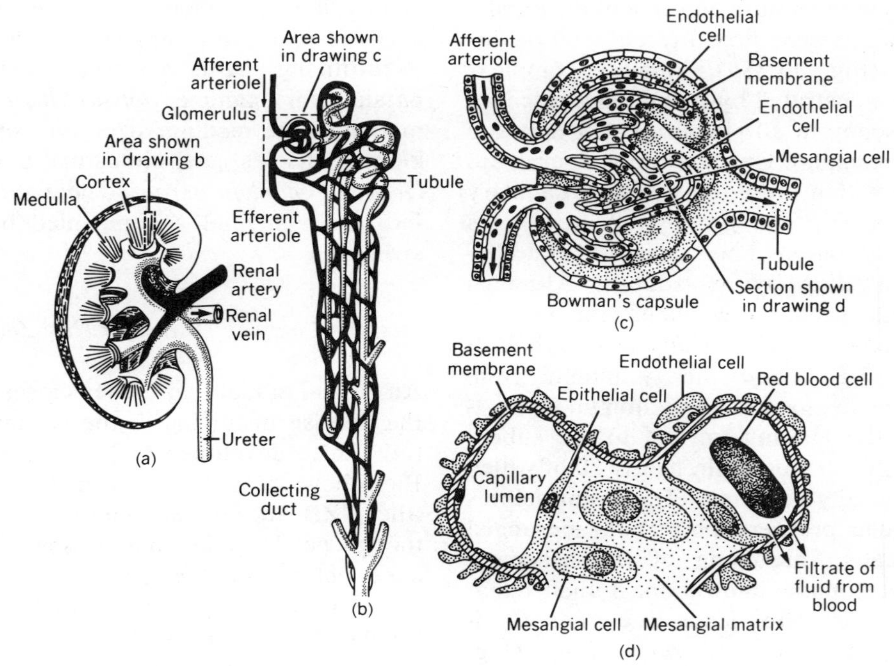

Figure 14.37. Anatomical organization of a kidney. [From D. Koffler: *Sci. Am.* **243** (July):40–49, 1980.]

basement membrane under the endothelial cells of the capillary. Depending on the stage of the disease, the deposits can be focal, homogeneous, linear, or, in the most extreme cases, diffuse (Fig. 14.38), and can be demonstrated by immunofluorescent staining with antibodies to immunoglobulins or complement components. The excessive deposit of immune complexes initiates an inflammatory reaction in the glomeruli that can cause varying degrees of damage to the kidney. This inflammation, referred to as *glomerulonephritis* (glomerulus + Gr. *nephros*, kidney, *-itis*, inflammation), is one of the most constant companions of SLE. However, glomerulonephritis also occurs in many other diseases, some associated with immune complex deposit, others not. The condition displays all the complexities of inflammation described in Section 14.2 and in the preceding section dealing with rheumatoid arthritis. It is accompanied by cellular infiltration, destruction of normal kidney architecture, and abnormal proliferation of certain cellular elements. The damaged glomeruli are unable to function properly and fail to remove all the toxic material from the blood; in extreme cases, the kidney fails altogether. The sign of glomeruli malfunction is the appearance of abnormal levels of protein in the urine (*proteinurea*) and sometimes also of blood (*hematurea*). The disease may assume many specific forms, determined by a variety of

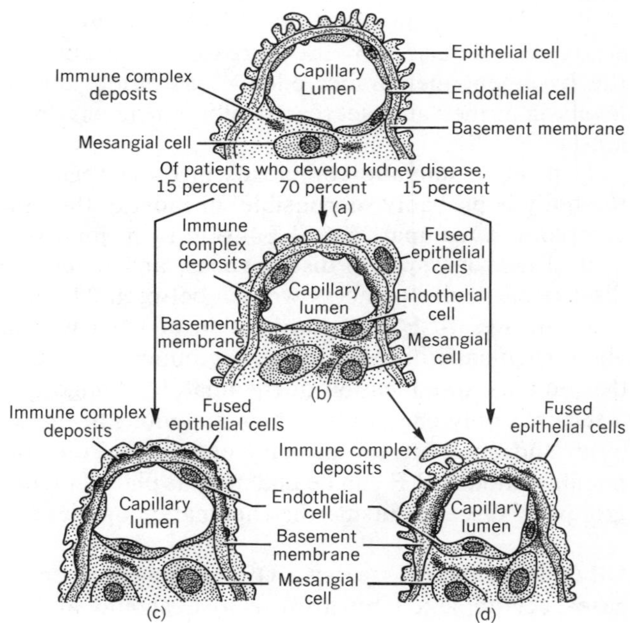

Figure 14.38. Immune complex deposit in the kidney at the different stages of systemic lupus erythematosus. (*a*) Deposit of complexes in the glomerulus of a healthy individual. (*b*) Complex deposit in a patient with a focal proliferative glomerulonephritis. (*c*) Complex deposit in a patient with membranous glomerulonephritis. (*d*) Complex deposit in a patient with diffuse proliferative glomerulonephritis. [From D. Koffler: *Sci. Am.* **243** (July):40–49, 1980.]

factors, among which the nature and size of the deposited immune complexes rank first. In *focal proliferative glomerulonephritis* (Fig. 14.38*b*), immune complex deposits can be demonstrated by immunofluorescence or electron microscopy in all glomeruli, but they are confined to the mesangium. Only certain glomeruli appear diseased and within these, only certain capillary loops appear abnormal. The grossly affected areas show abnormal proliferation of mesangial and endothelial cells and infiltration by neutrophils. Although hematurea and mild proteinurea occur, the kidneys still function reasonably well. In *diffuse proliferative glomerulonephritis* (Fig. 14.38*d*), heavy immune complex deposits can be demonstrated by immunofluorescence throughout the mesangium and in the subendothelium in virtually all glomeruli, nearly all of which are also morphologically abnormal. The abnormalities involved are irregular proliferation of both mesangial and endothelial cells, thickening of the basement membrane, and neutrophilic infiltration. If unchecked, this form of the disease often leads to complete kidney failure. In *membranous glomerulonephritis* (Fig. 14.38*c*), the immune complexes, detectable by immunofluorescence throughout the glomeruli, form a diffuse, finely granular pattern. There is a diffuse overgrowth of the glomerular basement membrane and degeneration of mesangial cells. Patients with this form of the disease often show the so-called *nephrotic syndrome*, characterized by the increased permeability of the basement membrane, edema, increased albumin levels in urine, and decreased albumin levels in the blood.

Deposit of immune complexes in other regions of the body is probably responsible for most of the other symptoms accompanying SLE—skin rash, joint pain, central nervous system disturbances, and fever. The disease particularly affects women between 20 and 40 years of age. SLE is an illustration of what we said about rheumatic diseases at the beginning. The pain in the joints is an indication of rheumatoid changes, but arthritis is only one of many manifestations of the disease, and not even the primary one. Based on other manifestations, SLE can be and often is placed in other groups of disease outside the rheumatic complex.

Other Rheumatic Diseases. Of the many other diseases accompanied by arthritis, we should at least mention *ankylosing spondylitis,* an arthritis of the spine (see Chapter 8); *Sjögren's syndrome* (named after the Swedish ophthalmologist Henrik S. C. Sjögren), characterized by dry eyes (keratoconjunctivitis sicca) and dry mouth (xerostomia) and often accompanying rheumatoid arthritis; and *necrotizing angitis*, an inflammation of the blood vessels resulting from fibrinoid necrosis of tissues supplied by the affected vessels. (Necrotizing angitis is a complex of diseases encompassing, for example, *polyarteritis nodosa*—an inflammation of the medium-sized and small arteries in the kidney muscles, gastrointestinal tract, and heart, and *Henoch-Schönlein purpura*, characterized by bleeding into the skin and accompanied by joint pains and swelling.)

Immune Complex Disease of New Zealand Mice

An animal model that comes closest to human SLE is the disease occurring in the strains of New Zealand (NZ) mice developed in New Zealand by M. and F. Bielschowsky and coming in two coat colors, black (the NZB strain) and white (the NZW strain). Although not bred for manifesting an autoimmune disease, they—like the OS chickens—apparently happened to fix several genes that strongly predispose them to autoimmunity. The NZB mice express several abnormalities that cause their premature death; the NZW mice usually do not show any clinical signs of the disease, but when crossed to NZB mice, they produce hybrids that are affected even more severely than the NZB parent. The NZW mice must therefore carry some genes that intensify the disease when combined with the genes of the NZB mice.

Genetic segregation analysis indicates an influence of at least three genes—one contributed by the NZB parent and two by the NZW parent. One of these three genes appears to belong to the *H*-2 complex, another is linked to *H*-2, and the third segregates independently of *H*-2. The nature of these genes and the mechanism of their influence have not been established.

The NZB mice manifest the following abnormalities.

Autoimmune Hemolytic Anemia. At three months of age, some of the NZB mice give positive Coombs tests, indicating that their erythrocytes are coated with antibodies. By the time they are 12 months old, virtually all the mice are Coombs test-positive. In the serum, autoantibodies can first be demonstrated two or three months after they have become detectable on erythrocytes, and several months after the appearance of serum autoantibodies, the mice develop autoimmune hemolytic anemia, characterized by an increased number of circulating reticulocytes and by the presence of spherocytes in the blood. Anemia is one of the main reasons that NZB mice die prematurely (at 15 to 18 months).

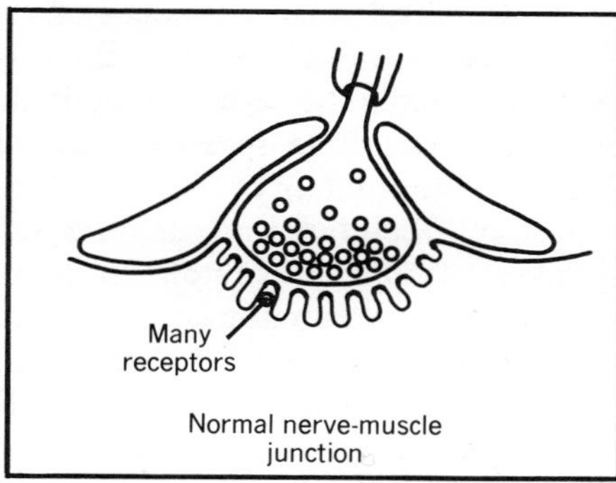

Figure 14.39. Neuromuscular junction—the target of autoantibodies in myasthenia gravis. (From R. Lewin: *Science* **211**:38–41, 1981.)

Immune-Complex Glomerulonephritis. At nine months of age, immunofluorescent staining reveals the presence of immune complex deposits in the kidneys of about 50 percent of the mice. About half of the kidney-bound IgG has specificity for nuclear antigens, and autoantibodies against various forms of DNA are circulating in the serum of these mice. Histological examinations of the affected animals reveal severe membranous glomerulonephritis. An examination of the blood reveals an excess of urea (uremia) and other nitrogenous wastes (azotemia)—an indication of kidney malfunction. However, the kidney disease is much more pronounced in the (NZB × NZW)F_1 hybrids than in the NZB parents. In addition to antinuclear immunoglobulins, one finds other autoantibodies, as well as antibodies to antigens of the Gross leukemia virus, in the immune complexes.

Lymphoproliferation. From the age of three months, there is a pronounced proliferation of lymphoid cells in the spleen, lymph nodes, thymus, lungs, and liver. This widespread proliferation leads to the enlargement of the affected organs—the spleen and lymph nodes, in particular.

Changes in the Thymus. The thymus of the NZB mice has a markedly decreased number of epithelial cells and contains characteristic follicular aggregates of lymphoid cells. Some NZB mice develop true neoplasms, mostly thymomas and lymphomas.

Immunological Dysfunctions. The immune system of the NZB mice displays a number of abnormalities: accelerated maturation of both the humoral and cellular arms of the immune system; enhanced humoral responsiveness throughout the life of the animal; diminishing cellular responsiveness with age; loss of ability to be tolerized; production of natural cytotoxic antibodies to thymocytes; and the disappearance of thymosin-like activity from serum.

Myasthenia Gravis

In this disease, the patient forms autoantibodies against muscle-cell receptors that normally recognize and bind acetylcholine—the neurotransmitter released from nerve endings. The antibodies block the receptors and prevent acetylcholine molecules from transmitting the signal for muscle movement (Fig. 14.39). The result is muscular weakness (hence the designation: Gr. *mys,* muscle, *asthenia,* weakness), with the muscles about the head and the neck most seriously affected. Toward the end of a meal, the jaw muscles may be so tired that further chewing is impossible. Although the ability to move the muscles returns after awhile, they tire again quickly. The patients also have difficulty in swallowing and keeping their eyes open. The condition is serious (hence the adjective *gravis* which means "heavy" in Latin, "dangerous" in medicine), death often resulting from fatigue of the heart or respiratory muscles.

Myasthenia-like conditions can be induced experimentally in animals by injecting them with purified acetylcholine receptors. The complete clinical syndrome can be transferred to a healthy animal with the IgG fraction of a serum obtained from the affected individuals.

In addition to antibodies against the acetylcholine receptors, patients with myasthenia gravis produce autoantibodies directed against striated muscle fibers and thymic tissue, and occasionally, antibodies against nucleoproteins and the thyroid. This broadness of response suggests that there may be some general defect in the immune system of myasthenia gravis patients. The immunity to acetylcholine is not only of the humoral, but also of the cellular type: lymphocytes from myasthenia gravis patients respond by blast transformation when challenged with purified acetylcholine in vitro, whereas lymphocytes from healthy individuals or from patients with other neuromuscular disorders respond only weakly to this antigen, if at all.

The development of myasthenia gravis is somehow connected to a malfunction of the thymus. The involvement of the thymus is indicated by the high incidence of thymic overgrowth and thymic tumors among myasthenia gravis patients and by the observation that thymectomy often decreases the severity of the disease. Cells in the thymus have been demonstrated to carry molecules that crossreact with the acetylcholine receptors. These crossreactive molecules are present on the myoid cells in the thymus, which can transform in culture into skeletal muscle cells, on the thymic epithelial cells, and on thymocytes. However, the crossreactive molecule of the lymphocyte is not an active nicotinic receptor because it does not bind toxins (the lymphocyte receptor appears to be of the muscarinic type). What the primary stimulator of myasthenia gravis is—the acetylcholine receptors on muscle cells or the crossreactive molecule on the thymocytes—is not known.

Myasthenia gravis is a rare disease, affecting about one in every 30,000 people. The disease is significantly associated with HLA-A1 and B8 antigens, indicating that genetic predisposition plays an important role in its development.

14.4.2 How Do Autoimmune Diseases Arise?

Despite their great diversity, the individual autoimmune diseases have certain features in common that may be taken as clues in the consideration of what exactly goes awry when an autoimmune condition arises. The first common feature is that in each disease, a multiplicity of factors must coalesce in a single individual to turn the immune system against the body's own tissue. First among these factors we must place *genetic predisposition*, for which there is evidence in all the diseases we have examined. The pattern of inheritance is always complex, indicating that several genes are involved in each particular case. It is unlikely that the genes are the same for the different diseases, although one gene complex—the major histocompatibility complex—consistently emerges as being implicated in the control. Although the intensity with which this complex has been studied may contribute to the consistency of this finding, the known involvement of the MHC in the control of the immune response suggests that it may, indeed, play a major role in the development of autoimmune disease. What exactly this role is we will not know until we understand just how the MHC controls the immune response in general. We have almost no knowledge of what other genes are involved in the induction of autoimmunity. We should emphasize, however, that genes merely *predispose* a person to the disease; the disease does not develop unless the other factors play along.

The second group of factors stems from the *malfunction of the immune system*. There is plenty of evidence that the immune system in autoimmune conditions does not function normally, but the exact defects cannot yet be pinpointed in one single case. Although the immediate symptoms of the disease are almost always induced by antibodies, the primary defect is probably not in the humoral, but in the cellular arm of immunity. In many of the diseases there appears to be something wrong either with the thymus or with the T cells. Defects in suppressor T-cell function are often suspected, but direct evidence for this presumption is lacking. The possibility that the autoimmune status represents a breakdown in immunoregulation, a disturbance of the homeostatic control, is so far the most appealing. Autoimmune reactions probably occur at a low level all the time but are prevented from taking over the immune system by a complex system of checks and controls. It is only when the regulatory mechanisms fail that the system shifts strongly in a direction unfavorable to the body. Unfortunately, we know too little about normal regulation of the immune system to design testable hypotheses concerning regulatory defects. This second group of factors is undoubtedly linked with the first group in that at least some of the malfunctions are probably caused by faulty genes.

The third group of factors is made up of the various *exogenous agents* that may well be the prime movers of the reaction. Viruses are the most likely candidates for this role and viral etiology is indeed suspected in many of the diseases. However, solid evidence implicating viruses is lacking. In some instances, the factors may not really be exogenous, but rather somewhere between self and nonself, as in the case of the C-type viruses. The case for the involvement of the C-type viruses is strongest in the NZB mice, but here again, fully convincing proof is not available. The exogenous factors may provide for the persistence of the stimulus and so for the chronicity of the disease.

The *self components* themselves make up the fourth group of factors involved in the induction of autoimmunity. They are probably not, as was once thought, the primary inducers of the disease, but they probably are its prime target. There may be a variety of ways in which these molecules become immunogenic to the body's immune system—they may be modified (for example, by drugs), they may be degraded into immunogenic components, or may simply be exposed in their hiding places inside the cell or inside an organ normally inaccessible to lymphocytes.

Finally, the fifth group is made up of the *physiological factors*. Since most autoimmune conditions are diseases of aging individuals, there must be some changes associated with the aging process that provide conditions for malfunction of the immune system. The prevalence of many autoimmune diseases in one sex (females) suggests that one of the contributing factors may be hormones, but the way in which this contribution occurs is totally obscure to us.

The main problem in the study of autoimmunity is how to arrange the individual factors into a causal chain. What comes first and what comes next? What is the cause and what the consequence? Probably there is no single causal chain, but rather a complex network of interactions. To identify the outlines of this network and to draw the lines that connect the dots to produce the whole picture may be one of immunology's most challenging tasks.

REFERENCES

General

Becker, F. F. (Ed.): *Cancer: A Comprehensive Treatise*, Vols. 1–4. Plenum, New York, 1975.

Beveridge, W. I. B.: *Influenza. The Last Great Plague*. Heinemann, London, 1977.

Braun, A. C.: *The Story of Cancer*. Addison-Wesley, London, 1977.

Cairns, J.: *Cancer, Science and Society*. Freeman, San Francisco, 1978.

Cochran, A. J.: *Man, Cancer and Immunity*. Academic, London, 1978.

Currie, G.: *Cancer and the Immune Response*, 2nd ed. Arnold, London, 1980.

Davis, B. D., Dulbecco, R., Eisen, H. N., Ginsberg, H. S., and Wood, W. B.: *Microbiology*, 2nd ed. Harper and Row, Hagerstown, Maryland, 1973.

Fenner, F., McAuslan, B. R., Mims, C. A., Sambrook, J., and White, D. O.: *The Biology of Animal Viruses*, 2nd ed. Academic, New York, 1974.

Gross, L.: *Oncogenic Viruses*, 2nd ed. Pergamon, Oxford, 1966.

Heidelberger, C.: Chemical carcinogenesis. *Annu. Rev. Biochem.* **44**:79–121, 1975.

Herberman, R. B.: Immunogenicity of tumor antigens. *Biochim. Biophys. Acta* **473**:93–119, 1977.

Kilbourne, E. D.: Molecular epidemiology—influenza as archetype. *Harvey Lect.* **73**:225–258, 1978.

Klein, G. (Ed.): *Viral Oncology*. Raven, New York, 1980.

Joklik, W. K. and Willett, H. P. (Eds.): *Zinsser Microbiology*, 16th ed. Appleton-Century-Crofts, New York, 1976.

Lindstrom, J.: Autoimmune response to acetylcholine receptors in myasthenia gravis and its animal models. *Adv. Immunol.* **27**:1–50, 1979.

Maini, R. N.: *Immunology of the Rheumatic Diseases. Aspects of Autoimmunity*. Arnold, London, 1977.

Mims, C. A.: *The Pathogenesis of Infectious Diseases*. Academic, London, 1977.

Mitchel, G. F.: Responses to infection with metazoan and protozoan parasites in mice. *Adv. Immunol.* **28**:451–511, 1979.

Panayi, G. S. and Johnson, P. M. (Eds.): *Immunopathogenesis of Rheumatoid Arthritis*. Reed Books, Chertsey, Surrey, 1979.

Raven, R. W. (Ed.): *Cancer*, Vols. 1–6. Butterworth, London, 1957–1960.

Rose, N. R., Kong, Y.-C. M., and Sundick, R. S.: The genetic lesions of autoimmunity. *Clin. Exp. Immunol.* **39**:545–550, 1980.

Shimkin, M. B.: *Contrary to Nature*. National Institutes of Health, Bethesda, Maryland, 1977.

Stanier, R. Y., Adelberg, E. A., and Ingraham, J. L.: *General Microbiology*, 4th ed. MacMillan, London, 1977.

Theofilopoulos, A. N. and Dixon, F. J.: The biology and detection of immune complexes. *Adv. Immunol.* **28**:89–220, 1979.

Thompson, R. A.: *The Practice of Clinical Immunology*, 2nd ed. Arnold, London, 1978.

Tooze, J.: *The Molecular Biology of Tumor Viruses*. Cold Spring Harbor Laboratory, Cold Spring Harbor, New York, 1973.

Weiss, D. W.: *Tumor Antigenicity and Approaches to Tumor Immunotherapy*. Springer-Verlag, Berlin, 1980.

Weissmann, G., Samuelson, B., and Paoletti, R. (Eds.): *Advances in Inflammation Research*, Vol. 1 onwards. Raven, New York, 1978.

Witz, I. P. and Hanna, M. G. (Eds.): *In Situ Expression of Tumor Immunity. Contemp. Top. Immunobiol.*, Vol. 10. Plenum, New York, 1980.

Original Articles

Abelev, G. I., Perova, S. D., Khramkova, N. I., Postnikova, Z. A., and Irlin, I. S.: Production of embryonal α-globulin by transplantable mouse hepatomas. *Transplantation* **1**:174–180, 1963.

Bittner, J. J.: Some possible effects of nursing on the mammary gland tumor incidence in mice. *Science* **84**:162, 1935.

Ellerman, V. and Bang, O.: Experimentelle Leukämie bei Hühnern. *Centralbl. Bakteriol.* **46**:595–609, 1908.

Foley, E. J.: Antigenic properties of methylcholanthrene-induced tumors in mice of the strain of origin. *Cancer Res.* **13**:835–837, 1953.

Gold, P. and Freedman, S. O.: Specific carcinoembryonic antigen of the human digestive system. *J. Exp. Med.* **122**:467–481, 1965.

Gross, L.: Spontaneous leukemia developing in C_3H mice following inoculation, in infancy, with AK-leukemic extracts, or AK-embryos. *Proc. Soc. Exp. Biol. Med.* **76**:27–32, 1951.

Gross, L.: A filterable agent, recovered from AK leukemic extracts, causing salivary gland carcinomas in C_3H mice. *Proc. Soc. Exp. Biol. Med.* **83**:414–421, 1953.

Huebner, R. J. and Todaro, G. J.: Oncogenes of RNA tumor viruses as determinants of cancer. *Proc. Natl. Acad. Sci. U.S.A.* **64**:1087–1094, 1969.

Isaacs, A. and Lindenmann, J.: Virus interference. I. The interferon. *Proc. R. Soc. Lond.* (*Biol.*) **147**:258–267, 1957.

Klein, G., Sjögren, H. O., Klein, E., and Hellström, K. E.: Demonstration of resistance against methylcholanthrene-induced sarcomas in the primary autochthonous host. *Cancer Res.* **20**:1561–1572, 1960.

Prehn, R. T. and Main, J. M.: Immunity to methylcholanthrene-induced sarcomas. *J. Natl. Cancer Inst.* **18**:769–778, 1957.

Rous, P.: A sarcoma of the fowl transmissible by an agent separable from the tumor cells. *J. Exp. Med.* **13**:397–411, 1911.

Shope, R. E.: Infectious papillomatosis of rabbits. *J. Exp. Med.* **58**:607–624, 1933.

Stewart, S. E., Eddy, B. E., Gochenour, A. M., Borgese, N., and Grubbs, G. E.: The induction of neoplasms with a substance released from mouse tumors by tissue culture. *Virology* **3**: 380–400, 1957.

Sweet, B. H. and Hilleman, M. R.: The vacuolating virus, S.V.40. *Proc. Soc. Exp. Biol. Med.* **105**:420–427, 1960.

Temin, H.: The protovirus hypothesis: speculations on the significance of RNA-directed DNA synthesis for normal development and for cancer. *J. Natl. Cancer Inst.* **46**:iii–vii, 1971.

Thomas, L.: Discussion. *In* H. S. Lawrence (Ed.): *Cellular and Humoral Aspects of the Hypersensitivity States*, pp. 529–532. Cassell, London, 1959.

Yamagiva, K. and Ichikawa, K.: Experimentelle Studie über die Pathogenese der Epithelialgeschwülste. *Mitteil. Med. Fac. Kais. Univ. Tokyo* **15**:295–344, 1915.

CHAPTER 15

THE SPLENDOR AND MISERY OF IMMUNOLOGY

15.1 SARTOR RESARTUS

The Fourth International Congress of Immunology, held in Paris in 1980, attracted some 8000 researchers from a number of countries all over the world. Assuming that about a third stayed home, one can estimate that there are about 12,000 practicing immunologists in the world today.

There are more than 40 journals publishing exclusively immunologically oriented articles (Table 15.1), and at least that number publishing such articles occasionally. The first group of journals publishes somewhere around 50,000 pages yearly. Although fewer pages were printed in the past, still, if one were to collect all immunologically oriented literature into one pile, it would make a small mountain. Pity the poor mountain climber, attempting to conquer this peak (Fig. 15.1)! How can anyone digest so much information? The answer is, of course, that no one can. Fortunately, it does not matter so much because one can do research in immunology even if one does not read 90 percent of what is published today. I used to think this was a sad situation, but with the years I have grown more compassionate. I have come to consider immunology to be one of the sciences engaged in the construction of a hunger wall.

In the fourteenth century, there lived in Bohemia an enlightened king, Charles IV. He did many good things for the country—built beautiful cathedrals, castles, and bridges, and, in general, tried to keep the citizens reasonably happy. So when unemployment in Prague rose to threatening proportions, he thought of an ingenious way to bring it back to normal. He ordered the building of a new wall around the city of Prague. The wall was not an absolute necessity—the city could have lived without it. The ruins scattered all over Europe testify to the fact that walls never did provide much protection. But the construction created new jobs and saved people from dying of hunger. This wall still stands, and the Czechs still call it the hunger wall.

I see such a hunger wall being erected in immunology today. Not a castle, not a cathedral, not even a bridge—but a plain wall, and not a very functional wall, at that. Stone after stone, article after article—they disappear as the wall grows longer and longer. There is always another *Ir* gene to discover, another organism to study, and the supply of T-cell factors seems to be inexhaustible. A gene, a phenotype, an

Table 15.1 Immunological Journals and Review Series

Journal	Number of Printed Pages per Year
Established journals publishing mainly original articles	
Annales d'Immunologie	900
Annals of Allergy	750
Cancer Immunology and Immunotherapy	550
Cellular Immunology	900
Clinical Allergy	700
Clinical and Experimental Immunology	2200
Clinical Immunology and Immunopathology	1500
Developmental and Comparative Immunology	800
European Journal of Immunology	1000
Immunochemistry	1000
Immunogenetics	1200
Immunology	2500
Immunological Communications	600
Infection and Immunity	4000
Inflammation	500
International Archives of Allergy and Applied Immunology	1400
Journal of Allergy and Clinical Immunology	1100
Journal of Clinical and Laboratory Immunology	600
Journal of Immunogenetics	470
Journal of Immunology	5600
Journal of Immunological Methods	2800
Journal of the Reticuloendothelial Society	1500
Scandinavian Journal of Immunology	600
Tissue Antigens	850
Transplantation	950
Transplantation Proceedings	2000
Zeitschrift für Immunitätsforschung (Immunobiology)	900
Journals Initiated Since 1979	
American Journal of Reproductive Immunology	
Comparative Immunology, Microbiology and Infectious Diseases	
Human Immunology	
Immunology Letters	
Immunology Today	
Immunopharmacology	
International Journal of Immunology	
Journal of Clinical Immunology	
Journal of Immunoassay	
Journal of Immunopharmacology	
Journal of Neuroimmunology	
Journal of Reproductive Immunology	
Lymphokine Reports	
Parasite Immunology	
Thymus	
Veterinary Immunology and Immunopathology	
Review Series	
Advances in Immunology	
Clinical Immunobiology	
Clinical Immunology Newsletter	
Contemporary Topics in Immunobiology	
Contemporary Topics in Molecular Immunology	
Current Topics in Microbiology and Immunology	
Immunological Reviews (formerly *Transplantation Reviews*)	
Progress in Allergy	
Springer Seminars in Immunopathology	

organism—a publication. A stone in the wall. And when the stone does not fit, when the results are not reproducible, there is always the difference in experimental conditions to explain away a discrepancy. Whether it fits or not, the stone becomes anonymous within a few years after it has been quarried. The wall keeps many scientists busy, employed, and happy. One has to make a living somehow.

Paraphrasing Honoré de Balzac, one can say that this accumulation of only marginally useful knowledge is the misery of immunology. But in addition to hunger walls, scientists also build cathedrals, castles, and bridges, and in those brilliant and useful constructions lies the splendor of the discipline.

15.2 IMMUNOLOGY AS A BIOLOGICAL DISCIPLINE

Scientific immunology began in the last quarter of the nineteenth century as an insignificant branch of microbiology. As the microbe hunters came to realize that

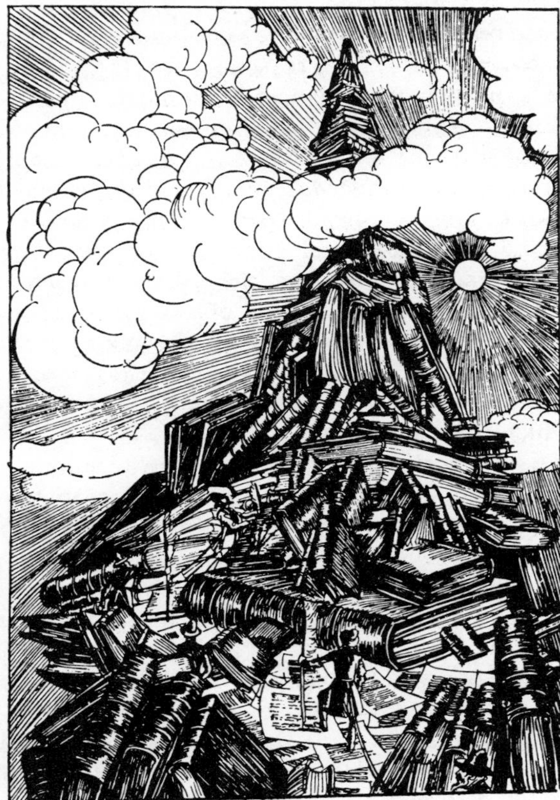

Figure 15.1. Climbing the immunological mountain. E. J. Sullivan's engraving from Thomas Carlyle's *Sartor Resartus*.

immunity played an important role in the body's defense against infectious diseases, some of them made the study of immunity their lifelong occupation. However, progress in elucidating immune mechanisms was slow. The mechanisms proved to be more complex than anyone had imagined, and the immunological phenomena remained elusive. Because of its reputation as an obscure science, immunology did not attract many researchers, and the few who did enter the discipline, despite its reputation, worked in isolation. They fought solitary battles and produced data that were difficult to arrange into a unified concept. Things became even more confusing when researchers realized that allergies, too, had an immunological basis. The notion that antibodies and immune cells could protect and harm at the same time did not seem to make sense.

But then, after World War II, things began to fall into place, and the isolated battles developed into a unified full-scale attack. While one war ended in the world of politics and territories, a new one began in the world of science. In mounting the attack, immunologists were first joined by biochemists, then by cellular biologists, and finally by geneticists. The invasion of these three sciences—biochemistry, cellular biology, and genetics—into immunology eventually led to the development of a unified concept of immunological reactions, and so to the establishment of immunology as a scientific discipline in its own right. Immunology separated from microbiology—but not from medicine. To this day, immunology is considered to be largely a medical discipline, as is evidenced by the fact that it is taught in medical schools but only seldom in natural science departments. Yet immunology is clearly *not* a medical discipline—it is a biological discipline. (Of course, one could argue that so is medicine.) I have tried to reason, throughout this book, that bodily defense is one of the basic characteristics of life, in the same way that inheritance or reproduction is, and that without mechanisms to preserve the body's integrity, life could not exist. Defense reactions are not limited to humans; they are present in all forms of life. In biology textbooks, defense mechanisms should, therefore, be allotted the same amount of space as inheritance and evolution receive; and in biology departments, immunology courses should be firmly incorporated into the curriculum. This is not to say that immunology should not be taught in medical schools. Clinical immunology will remain an important subdiscipline of immunology, just as clinical genetics is of genetics. However, the treatment of patients suffering from immunological diseases is not the sole goal of immunology, which has much broader and more general goals. The association of immunology with medicine is an historical accident that will undoubtedly be rectified by future developments.

15.3 THE FUTURE OF IMMUNOLOGY

In 1967, Niels K. Jerne, one of today's most incisive immunologists, concluded the prestigious XXII Cold Spring Harbor Symposium on Quantitative Biology with these words: "As this younger generation of professionals is pressing rapidly toward the definitive solution of the antibody problem, we older amateurs had perhaps better sit back, waiting for the End." When immunologists met at Cold Spring Harbor again, nine years later, Jerne was forced to observe that the "younger generation of professionals," who had aged somewhat in the meantime, had not only failed to reach the predicted "End" of immunology, but had even failed to provide the "definitive solution of the antibody problem." Unexpectedly to Jerne, in 1976 immunology was flowering as never before, and was entering avenues of research of which no one had dreamed in 1967.

This anecdote only demonstrates how unreliable predictions about the future of science are, especially those that forecast its end. It would be foolish of me to think that I could do better than Niels Jerne and set myself up as a more accurate oracle. Instead, all I would like to do here is to consider what I would do if I were about to begin a career in immunology today. What topics would I choose to study? Actually, it is easier for me to say what topics I would *not* study. There are several of these. First, I would not want to study the molecular genetics of immunoglobulin genes, simply because most of the important questions would be resolved before I could even get my research going. I make this prediction on much firmer ground than Jerne had to stand on in 1967 when the methods for the final solution of the antibody problem had not yet been developed. Today they are, and there are several laboratories exploiting these methods to the hilt. It is now just a matter of how fast one can clone and sequence the DNA of the immunoglobulin genes before all principal facts about these genes and about the generation of antibody diversity will be known.

Second, I would not become involved in the study of the major histocompatibility complex, not because everything important concerning this system will be known within a few years, but because there are already too many immunologists interested in this area of research. The mass generates a pressure that, in the end, leads to the "hunger wall syndrome" and to the acceptance of mediocre research. (As a young investigator, I would, of course, want to do high-quality research.)

Third, for the same reason, I would want to avoid studying the T-cell receptor. Although it is impossible to predict how long it will take for the T-cell receptor problem to be solved, it is increasingly evident that, because of the crowding effect, the research efforts in this area of immunology are becoming counterproductive. If I were to begin such a study, I might be lucky and stumble onto an important clue eventually, but probably I would just dabble, hounded by scientific rumors and constantly seduced by false leads.

And finally, I would probably not enter parasitic immunology either. Although this branch of science is just beginning, it is also producing an enormous bandwagon, which is already creaking with the weight of massed passengers. I simply would not feel right in the crowds that are going to take over this area of research.

If I were biologically oriented, I would probably consider seriously the study of the phylogeny of immune reactions. This rather barren area offers many possibilities to an inventive immunologist. As was pointed out in Chapter 1, little is known about the defense reactions of primitive vertebrates and of invertebrates, and part of the reason for this lack of knowledge is the lack of sophisticated approaches that could lead to the discovery of novel defense systems. Most of those currently working in this area seem simply to be applying the knowledge obtained in the mouse and human to nonmammalian species. This is an insensitive and unphysiological approach that amounts to teaching monkeys to sing Schubert's *Erlkönig*. To elucidate the defense reactions of less advanced vertebrates and invertebrates will require taking into account the entire physiology of a given taxon and designing experiments so as to reflect natural situations in which these forms live.

If I were oriented more toward cellular immunology, I would consider studying the differentiation of lymphocytes and macrophages. While some knowledge has been accumulated concerning the ontogeny of B lymphocytes, almost nothing is known about the ontogeny of T lymphocytes or of macrophages. To define the individual stages of T-cell and macrophage differentiation, one will probably have to develop a whole new methodology, although even the application of the existing methodology to the study of this problem should yield useful information. Such a study would probably also help to sort out the types of mature T cells and macrophages. The three or four presently known types of T cell are probably not the whole story of T-cell ontogeny. More cell types will probably be found when more T-cell markers (membrane or intracellular) become available. Macrophages, which at present seem to be rather uniform, will probably also prove to be quite heterogeneous. Again, markers will have to be found to sort out such a heterogeneity. Macrophages have lately been somewhat neglected by immunologists in general. The original enthusiasm, fueled mainly by Metchnikoff and his colleagues when macrophages seemed to provide all the answers to immunological questions, has evaporated and the level of interest in this cell has moved to the opposite extreme. In contemporary immunology, the macrophage is often regarded as a kind of *Mädchen für alles*, an all-purpose maid that is called upon to perform only housekeeping functions. Immunologists got into the bad habit of invoking the macrophage only when all other explanations had failed. As a consequence, the macrophage has gained the reputation of being something vague and ill-defined. This reputation is enhanced by poor reproducibility of many macrophage experiments, which often discredit the cell's reputation.

I believe, however, that the time will soon come when the macrophage will be rehabilitated and proved to play a much more important role than many immunologists are willing to grant it today. This phylogenetically old cell may still have a few surprises in store for researchers.

Only after the different lymphocyte and macrophage cell types have been characterized would I begin to study their interaction. What we now know about cellular interactions during the immune response is only the proverbial tip of the iceberg; the bulk is still submerged in the dark waters surrounding it.

Naturally, the study of cell interactions will lead to the question of how these interactions are regulated. Immunoregulation is a wide-open area of research in which lie the clues to the most basic problem of immunology—the problem of how an organism distinguishes self from nonself. Furthermore, without understanding the principles of immunoregulation, it may not be possible to explain the mechanisms of such medically important phenomena as tolerance and autoimmunity. To study immunoregulation will not be easy; but those who persist and are lucky may be rewarded by the most fascinating insights into the workings of bodily defense.

If I were a biochemist, I would probably work on complement. Although the classical pathway of complement activation is reasonably well understood and its components will soon be well characterized, the study of the alternative pathway is still in its infancy. No new methodology will be necessary to elucidate this pathway; all one will have to do is apply the knowledge obtained in the study of the classical pathway.

Lastly, if I were medically oriented, I would opt, probably after some hesitation, for the study of tumor immunology and autoimmunity. These fields are far from being underpopulated, but they are so important that they need every bit of help they can get. Although one must have guts to enter these research areas because they are in such a hopelessly confused state, a series of breakthroughs may quickly alter this situation.

Another clinically important area is allergy, in the broadest sense of the word. Although research in allergy is more than 80 years old, it still offers many opportunities for an innovative scientist.

Transplantation biology is currently in a period of stagnation, but again, a few crucial discoveries in cellular immunology may drastically change this situation. As long as prevention of the allograft reaction is virtually the only solution to spare-part surgery, immunologists should, and will, keep trying to find a way to interfere with the rejection process.

I would not exclude the possibility that new forms of immunity will be discovered, particularly in nonmammalian species. But I would not know where to begin the search for them except, of course, with the study of evolution. And I would keep my eyes open for the unexpected.

15.4 "A HEAP OF BROKEN IMAGES"

As for the future of the entire discipline, I am optimistic. If, in a textbook such as this one, the author must repeat, again and again, the phrase "is not known," the discipline cannot be nearing its end. T. S. Eliot's

> *Son of man*
> *You cannot say, or guess, for you know only*
> *A heap of broken images . . .*

may apply here.

Progress in science often resembles the metamorphosis of a butterfly. It starts as an ugly caterpillar, sluggish and earthbound, that seems to have nothing to do with the butterfly it will eventually become. The caterpillar then changes into an imago, which, on the surface, looks lifeless and static, but inside is teeming with activity. Then, one day, the imago bursts and the butterfly emerges—shaking out its crinkled wings and preparing for flight. The impression one receives, if one observes only the spectacular conclusion to this process, is that the butterfly was generated from inactivity.

Many areas of immunology are still in the caterpillar or the imago stage, waiting to be transformed into magnificent butterflies, and, I believe, it will be a long time yet before all the butterflies have flown.

INDEX